D0771389

MATERNAL, FETAL, & NEONATAL PHYSIOLOGY

A Clinical Perspective

SECOND EDITION

MATERNAL, FETAL, & NEONATAL PHYSIOLOGY

A Clinical Perspective

Susan Tucker Blackburn, PhD, RNC, FAAN

Professor, School of Nursing

Department of Family and Child Nursing

University of Washington

Seattle, Washington

with 263 illustrations

SAUNDERS
An Imprint of Elsevier

SAUNDERS
An Imprint of Elsevier

11830 Westline Industrial Drive
St. Louis, MO 63146

MATERNAL, FETAL, & NEONATAL PHYSIOLOGY: A CLINICAL PERSPECTIVE

NOTICE

Pharmacology is an ever-changing field. Standard safety precautions must be followed, but as new research and clinical experience broaden our knowledge, changes in treatment and drug therapy may become necessary or appropriate. Readers are advised to check the most current product information provided by the manufacturer of each drug to be administered to verify the recommended dose, the method and duration of administration, and contraindications. It is the responsibility of the appropriately licensed health care provider, relying on experience and knowledge of the patient, to determine dosages and the best treatment for each individual patient. Neither the publisher nor the editor assumes any liability for any injury and/or damage to persons or property arising from this publication.

First edition copyrighted 1992.

Library of Congress Cataloging-in-Publication Data
Blackburn, Susan Tucker.
  Maternal, fetal & neonatal physiology : a clinical perspective / Susan Tucker
Blackburn.—2nd ed.
    p. ; cm.
  Includes bibliographical references and index.

  ISBN-13: 978-0-7216-8012-5   ISBN-10: 0-7216-8012-7

    1. Pregnancy. 2. Fetus—Physiology. 3. Infants (Newborn)—Physiology. I. Title:
  Maternal, fetal, & neonatal physiology. II. Title.
    [DNLM: 1. Pregnancy— physiology. 2. Fetus—physiology. 3. Infant,
  Newborn—physiology. WQ 205 B628m 2003]
  RG558 .B58 2003
  612.6'3—dc21

Vice President, Publishing Director: Sally Schrefer
Executive Editor: Michael S. Ledbetter
Senior Developmental Editor: Laurie K. Muench
Publishing Services Manager: Catherine Jackson
Project Manager: Clay S. Broeker
Designer: Amy Buxton

TG / MVY
ISBN-13: 978-0-7216-8012-5
ISBN-10: 0-7216-8012-7

Printed in the United States of America.
Last digit is the print number: 9   8   7   6   5

CONTRIBUTOR & REVIEWERS

CONTRIBUTOR

Robin Webb Corbett, PhD, RN, C
Associate Professor, School of Nursing
East Carolina University
Greenville, North Carolina

REVIEWERS

Mary Brucker, CNM, DNSc, FACNM
Certified Nurse-Midwife, Parkland School of
  Nurse-Midwifery
University of Texas Southwestern at Dallas Medical
  Center
Arlington, Texas

Kathrine Peters, BNSc, MN, PhD
Associate Professor
Coordinator, Neonatal Nursing Programmes
University of Alberta
Edmonton, Alberta, Canada

PREFACE

Accurate assessment and clinical care appropriate to the developmental and maturational stage of the mother, fetus, and neonate depend on a thorough understanding of normal physiologic processes and the ability of the caregiver to understand the effect of these processes on pathologic deviations. Information on normal perinatal physiology and its clinical implications can be found in scattered sources, including journal articles, general physiology texts, core nursing texts, and medical references. In teaching students and staff, I found that these sources were either fragmented, too basic in level, too focused on one phase of the perinatal period (and thus lacking integration within the maternal-fetal-neonatal unit), too medically oriented, or lacking in the clinical applications relevant to patient care. Thus they did not adequately meet the needs of nurses in specialty and advanced clinical nursing practice.

Therefore the goal was to create a single text that brought together detailed information on the physiologic changes that occur throughout the perinatal period, with emphasis on the mother, fetus, and neonate and the interrelationships between them. The purpose of this book is not to provide a manual of specific assessment and intervention strategies nor to focus on pathophysiology; it is to provide the practitioner with information on the normal physiologic adaptations and developmental physiology that provide the scientific basis and rationale underlying assessment and management of the low- and high-risk pregnant woman, fetus, and neonate. Because the focus of this book is on physiologic adaptations, psychologic aspects of perinatal nursing are not addressed. These aspects are certainly important, but not within the realm of this text.

This book provides detailed descriptions of the physiologic processes associated with the perinatal patient: the mother, fetus, or neonate. The major focus is on the normal physiologic adaptations of the pregnant women during the antepartum, intrapartum, and postpartum periods; anatomic and functional development of the fetus; transition and adaptation of the infant at birth; and developmental physiology of the neonate (term and preterm), including a summary of the maturation of each body system during infancy and childhood. Clinical implications of these physiologic adaptations as they relate to the pregnant woman, maternal-fetal unit, and neonate are also examined. Each chapter relates the effect of normal physiologic adaptations to clinical assessment and interventions with low- and high-risk women and neonates with selected health problems. Of special interest to those seeking quick access to clinical information are the tabular recommendations for clinical practice, which index relevant content that provides the scientific basis and rationale underlying each recommendation.

Given the growing recognition that advanced practice nursing must be based on a sound physiologic base as well as a sound theoretical base, I hope that this book will be a useful foundation reference for specialty and advanced practice nurses in both primary and acute care settings, as well as for graduate programs in maternal, perinatal, and neonatal nursing and nurse midwifery. As the collaborative perspective on perinatal care gains power, this book may also hold appeal for other health care professionals, including physicians, physical and occupational therapists, respiratory therapists, and nutritionists involved in obstetrics and neonatology.

ACKNOWLEDGMENTS

The help and support of many individuals were critical in making this book a reality. These include former and current students, nursing staff, and faculty colleagues who stimulated me to expand my knowledge of perinatal physiology and examine the scientific basis for nursing interventions with pregnant women and neonates. The women, neonates, and their families for whom I have cared and from whom I have learned a great deal also stimulated development of this book. I want to acknowledge my coauthor for the first edition, Donna Lee Loper, whose vision and contributions were critical to the development of that edition. Also, thank you to Robin Webb Corbett for developing a new chapter for this edition. I am grateful for the efforts of the reviewers, whose constructive comments and suggestions helped in refining the content and in making this book more useful for the intended audience. My appreciation also goes to Laurie Muench and Michael Ledbetter at Elsevier Science for their patience, support, and encouragement. Finally I would like to thank my family for their support, guidance, and encouragement in all of my endeavors.

Susan Tucker Blackburn

CONTENTS

Biologic Basis for Reproduction

The biologic basis for reproduction includes genetic mechanisms and principles, gametogenesis, and embryonic development of the reproductive system. Genetic knowledge has expanded significantly in recent years, increasing our understanding of biologic processes and many disorders. The ability to reproduce is modified throughout the life span and is influenced by deoxyribonucleic acid (DNA) and chromosomal structure and function. Reproduction is also influenced by physiologic processes such as hormonal control mechanisms and the hypothalamic-pituitary-ovarian axis. These processes are described in Chapter 2.

CHROMOSOMES AND GENES

The human genome is the totality of the DNA sequences, containing all of an individual's genetic information. Each human cell, except for the gametes (ovum and sperm), normally contains 46 chromosomes (diploid number) consisting of 22 pairs of autosomes and 1 pair of sex chromosomes. Autosomal genes are located on the autosomes (chromosomes common to both sexes) and are homologous (a pair of chromosomes with identical gene arrangements). Males have a pair of nonhomologous chromosomes, the X and Y sex chromosomes. In the female the sex chromosomes (XX) are homologous. One of each chromosome pair comes from the mother and one from the father. The ovum and sperm have only 23 chromosomes (haploid number). This reduction in the number of chromosomes occurs during meiosis. With fertilization and union of the nuclei of the sperm and ovum, the diploid number of 46 chromosomes is restored in the zygote.

Chromosomes

Chromosomes are classified by structure and banding pattern, which varies depending on the stain used, or by color if spectral analysis is used. Structural characteristics include the location of the centromere (metacentric, submetacentric, or acrocentric) and the length or size of the chromosomes (Figure 1-1). The upper arm of each chromosome is referred to as the p arm; the lower arm is the q arm. Sections of the p and q arm are numbered according to the banding patterns of mitotic chromosomes so specific loci along each chromosome can be identified. Gismo-trypsin banding (G-banding) is the most widely used technique, producing up to 300 to 400 metaphase bands.[38] Each band contains many genes. High-resolution banding during late prophase or early metaphase increases the resolution twofold. Newer spectral methods of karyotyping and fluorescent in situ hybridization (FISH) techniques such as chromosome painting, locus-specific mutations FISH, and interphase FISH allow for even greater resolution and specificity of chromosomes segments and genes.[38] The karyotype is a pictorial display of chromosomes.

Chromosomes are composed of the DNA double helix and several types of proteins that together are known as *chromatin.* In each chromosome the continuous DNA helix is wound around histone (protein) spools that are coiled around each other to form solenoids. The solenoids are coiled into chromatin threads (Figure 1-2). The DNA double helix is similar to a flexible ladder, with the sides composed of deoxyribose and phosphate and each rung composed of two nitrogen bases connected by hydrogen bonds (see Figure 1-2). The human genome contains approximately 3 million bases, with 50 to 250 million pairs in each chromosome.[47]

Genes

Genes are DNA sequences. Currently, each human is thought to have approximately 30,000 to 40,000 genes.[47] Genes make up only about 10% of the human genome. The rest of the DNA consists of noncoding sequences whose exact role is unclear. Interspersed between these noncoding sequences are many series of repeated nucleotides whose function is also unclear.[25] Genes are essential in determining and maintaining structural integrity and cell function and in regulating biochemical and immunologic processes.[21] Some genes control the function of other genes, whereas others regulate the

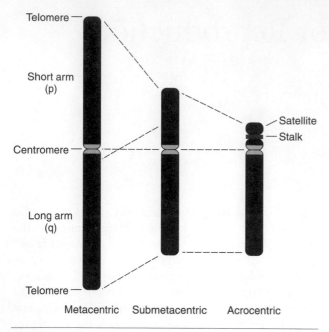

FIGURE **1-1** Schematic diagram of human chromosomes demonstrating metacentric, submetacentric, and acrocentric chromosomes. The location of the centromere, telomere, and short *(p)* and long *(q)* arms are indicated. (From Morton, C.L. & Miron, P. [1999]. Cytogenetics in reproduction. In S.S.C. Yen, R.B. Jaffe & R.L. Barbieri [Eds.]. *Reproductive endocrinology: Physiology, pathophysiology and clinical management* [4th ed.]. Philadelphia: W.B. Saunders.)

process of embryonic and fetal development (Chapter 3). Genes direct protein synthesis and regulate the rate at which proteins are synthesized. The specific proteins synthesized vary depending on the type of cell. For example, a muscle cell synthesizes myosin for muscle contraction; the pancreatic islet cells synthesize insulin; and the liver cells produce gamma globulin. Although the full complement of genes is present in all cells, genes are selectively switched on and off. Therefore, all genes are not active at the same time. This activation process is important during development and is influenced by age, cell type, and function.

Genes are arranged on chromosomes in linear order and in pairs on homologous chromosomes. Each gene has a specific location, called a *locus*, on the chromosome. One copy of a gene normally occupies any given locus. In somatic cells the chromosomes are paired so that there are two copies of each gene (alleles). These corresponding genes at a given locus on homologous chromosomes govern the same trait, but not necessarily in the same way. If gene pairs are identical, they are homozygous; if they are different, the pair is said to be heterozygous. In the het-

erozygous state, one of the alleles may be expressed over the other. This allele is considered dominant, meaning that the trait is expressed if the dominant allele is present on at least one of the pair of chromosomes. Recessive traits can be expressed only when the allele responsible for that trait is present on both chromosomes or when the dominant allele is not present (as with X-linked genes in the XY male). *Genotype* refers to the genetic makeup of an individual or a particular gene pair. The observable expression of a specific trait is referred to as the *phenotype*. A trait may be a biochemical property, an anatomic structure, a cell or organ function, or a mental characteristic. Thus traits are derived from the action of the gene and not from the gene itself.[21,24,46]

DNA Structure and Function

The transmission of hereditary information from one cell to another is a function of DNA. DNA also contains the instructions for the synthesis of proteins that then determine the structure and function of that cell. The nucleus contains DNA; protein assembly occurs within the cytoplasm. The transfer of information from the nucleus to the site of synthesis is the role of messenger ribonucleic acid (mRNA), which is synthesized on the surface of DNA.

Both DNA and RNA are nucleic acids made up of a nitrogenous purine (adenine and guanine) or pyrimidine (cytosine and thymine) base, a sugar (deoxyribose for DNA and ribose for RNA), and a phosphate group (see Figure 1-2). Together these substrates form a structure that is linked in a linear sequence by phosphodiester bonds. DNA is composed of two antiparallel complementary chains of opposite polarity. These strands form a double helix in which the sides are the phosphate and sugar groups and the crossbars are complementary bases joined by hydrogen bonds. Only complementary bases form stable bonds; therefore adenine (A) always pairs with thymine (T), and guanine (G) always pairs with cytosine (C). Thus the sequence of the bases on one strand determines the sequence of bases on the other.

RNA is a single strand rather than a double helix and contains adenine, cytosine, guanine, and uracil (U), which pairs with adenine, because thymine is not present. There are three major types of RNA: (1) mRNA, (2) ribosomal RNA (rRNA), and (3) transfer RNA (tRNA). Messenger RNA receives information from the DNA and serves as the template for protein synthesis. Transfer RNA brings the amino acids to mRNA and positions them correctly during protein synthesis. One of the structural components at the protein assemblage site (ribosome) is rRNA. The passage of information from DNA to RNA is called *transcription;* the assemblage of the proper sequence on amino acids

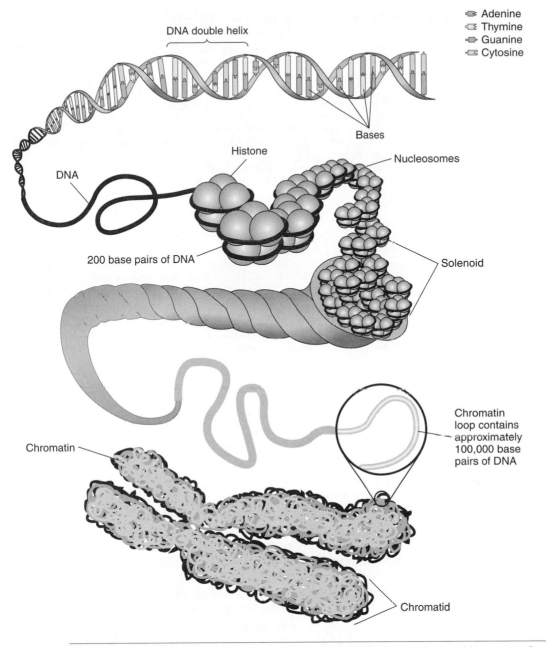

DNA double helix

Adenine
Thymine
Guanine
Cytosine

Bases

Histone

Nucleosomes

DNA

200 base pairs of DNA

Solenoid

Chromatin loop contains approximately 100,000 base pairs of DNA

Chromatin

Chromatid

FIGURE **1-2** Structure of DNA and patterns of DNA coiling. DNA is wound around histones to form nucelosomes. These are organized into solenoids that in turn compose chromatin loops. (From Jorde, L.B., et al. [1999]. *Medical genetics* [2nd ed.]. St. Louis: Mosby.)

Sequence of Events in Transcription and Translation

TRANSCRIPTION

1. The two strands of the DNA double helix separate in the region of the gene to be transcribed. One strand acts as a template.
2. Free nucleotide bases pair with the nucleotide bases in DNA.
3. The nucleotide triphosphates paired with one strand of DNA are linked together by DNA-dependent RNA polymerase to form mRNA containing a sequence of bases complementary to the DNA base sequence.
4. Once the mRNA has formed, the DNA strand rewinds.
5. mRNA is processed before leaving the nucleus. Introns (noncoding areas of DNA) are removed and promoter and terminator structures are added to promoted stability and efficiency of translation.

TRANSLATION

6. The processed mRNA passes from the nucleus to the cytoplasm, where one end of the mRNA binds to a ribosome.

7. The ribosome is formed from rRNA and proteins. The mRNA codons are "read" by the ribosome and translated into amino acids.
8. Free amino acids combine with their corresponding tRNA in the presence of specific aminoacyl-tRNA synthetase enzymes in the cytoplasm.
9. Amino acid-tRNA complexes bind to sites on the ribosome and the three base anticodons in tRNA pair with the corresponding codons in mRNA.
10. Each amino acid is then transferred from its tRNA to the growing peptide chain, which is attached to the adjacent tRNA.
11. The tRNA freed of its amino acid is released from the ribosome.
12. A new amino acid–tRNA complex is attached to the vacated site on the ribosome.
13. mRNA moves one codon step along the ribosome.
14. Steps 9 to 13 are repeated over and over until all the codons have been read.
15. The completed protein chain is released from the ribosome when the termination codon in mRNA is

Adapted from Vander, A., Sherman, J., & Luciano, D. (2000). *Human physiology: The mechanism of body function* (8th ed.). New York: McGraw-Hill.

is *translation*. Protein synthesis is summarized in the box above.

The sequence of bases along the DNA make up the genetic code that specifies the sequence of amino acids in each protein. Each of the 20 amino acids is designated by a specific sequence of three bases (codon). A gene is a single protein, which is a series of amino acids. The four bases (A, T or U, C, and G) can be arranged in 64 triplet combinations, of which 61 are used to specify the 20 amino acids. Most amino acids are represented by several codons. For example, AUG codes for methionine, and CAU and CAC both code for histidine. The other three codes are termination codes, which designate the end of a gene (see the box above).

CELL DIVISION

Genetic material is passed to daughter cells in two ways: via mitosis in somatic cells and meiosis in germ cells. Before onset of either mitosis or meiosis, DNA replication must occur. When a cell divides, the accurate replication of the genetic material stored within the DNA of the parent cell is essential. During DNA replication the strands of the double helix uncoil, relax, and separate. The exposed bases pair with complementary free nucleotides. DNA polymerase links the nucleotides together, resulting in two identical molecules of DNA to pass on to daughter cells. Enzymes

within the cell nucleus "read" the replicated DNA and repair errors. If errors are not repaired, a mutation results. DNA replication is illustrated in Figure 1-3.

Mitosis

Mitosis is the process by which growth of the organism occurs and cells repair and replace themselves. This process maintains the diploid chromosome number of 46, forming two daughter cells that are exact replicas of the parent (unless a mutation occurs). The cell cycle consists of 4 stages: gap 1 (G1), synthesis (S), gap 2 (G2), and mitosis (M). G1, S, and G2 comprise interphase. During G1, the longest stage, proteins needed by the cell are synthesized and substances needed for DNA replication are amassed; DNA replication occurs in S. G2 is a resting stage, during which errors in DNA are corrected and the cell prepares for the final M stage, in which the cell divides.[25] The length of time for a cell to complete the entire cycle varies with the type of cell and may last hours (epithelial tissues) to months (liver cells).[6] The cell cycle is regulated by enzymes such as cell-dependent kinases, which are control switches for the cycle (i.e., switching from G1 to S or from S to G2); maturation promoting factor, which triggers progression through the cell cycle; protein 63, which blocks the cycle if the DNA is damaged to allow time for DNA repair; and protein 27, which can also block the cycle by binding to cy-

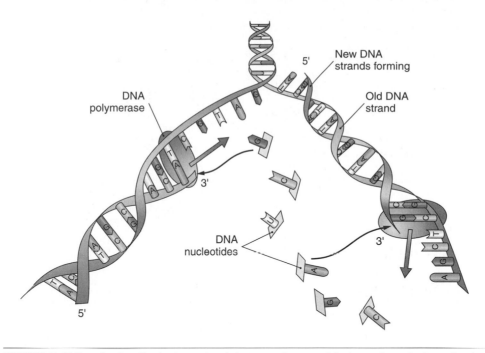

FIGURE **1-3** DNA replication. The hydrogen bonds between the two original strands are broken, allowing the bases in each strand to undergo complementary base pairing with free bases. The process forms two new double strands of DNA. (From Jorde, L.B., et al. [1999]. *Medical genetics* [2nd ed.]. St. Louis: Mosby.)

clins and blocking entry into S.[22] Alterations in these substances can lead to production of cancerous cells.[6,22]

Thus, before initiation of mitosis, DNA replication has occurred. At this point each cell still has 46 chromosomes, but each chromosome has twice the usual amount of DNA. Just before cell division, the duplicated DNA threads, known as chromatin, change from a loose, relaxed mass and become condensed and tightly coiled, forming rod-shaped structures called chromosomes. This condensing process facilitates the transfer of DNA to the daughter cells. This change is the first sign of cell division.

As the cell enters prophase, the chromosomes are double, each consisting of two DNA threads (called *sister chromatids*). The two chromatids are joined at a single point called the centromere. Late in prophase the nuclear membrane begins to disintegrate. The centrioles (two small cylindrical bodies) separate and move to opposite sides of the cell. A number of microtubules are observable at this stage. These are spindle fibers that extend from one side of the cell to the other, between the centrioles.

During metaphase the chromatids line up on the metaphase plate in the center of the cell. Other spindle fibers now extend from the centrioles and are attached to the centromere region of the chromosome. In anaphase the chromosomes divide at the centromere into sister chromatids that are pulled to opposite poles. As the chromosomes reach their respective poles, they begin to uncoil and elongate. A ring of protein appears around the center of the cell and the cell begins to constrict along a plane perpendicular to the spindle apparatus, creating a division in the cell membrane and cytoplasm (cytokinesis). This constriction continues, creating two cells. At the end of this phase (telophase), the nucleus and nuclear membrane re-form and the spindle fibers disappear. Division is complete, and the two daughter cells move into interphase.

Meiosis

Meiosis is the process of germ cell division that is designed to reduce the number of chromosomes from the diploid

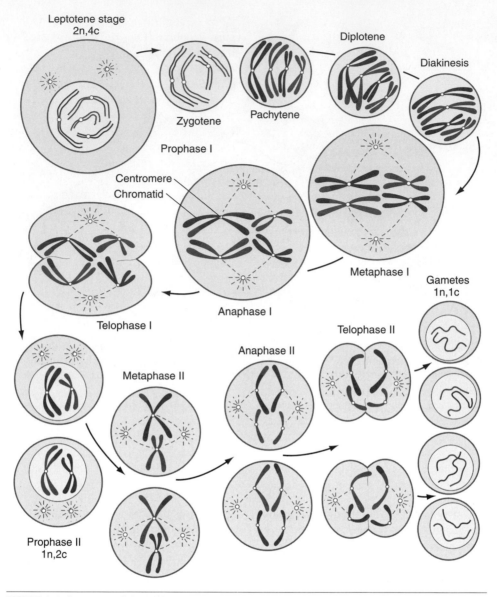

FIGURE 1-4 Summary of the major stages in meiosis in a generalized germ cell. (From Carlson, B.M. [1999]. *Human embryology and developmental biology* [2nd ed.]. St Louis: Mosby.)

(2n, or 46) to haploid (n, or 23) number. In this process there are two sequential divisions. The first meiotic division is a reduction division; the second is an equational one (Figure 1-4). Meiosis results in daughter cells that have 23 chromosomes: one chromosome from each pair of autosomes and one sex chromosome. Fusion of sperm and ovum through fertilization restores the cell to the diploid number of chromosomes. Oogonia and spermatogonia arise from the primordial germ cells (see Embryonic and Fetal Development of the Reproductive System). Before

initiation of meiosis, the primary oocyte or spermatocyte forms as DNA replicates, so each chromosome consists of 2 chromatids joined at the centromere.

The first meiotic division consists of four phases (prophase, metaphase, anaphase, and telophase). Prophase is the longest and most complex and is divided into five stages (see Figure 1-4). In the first stage (leptotene) the chromosomes are threadlike but already duplicated. Although consisting of two chromatids, the chromosome appears as a single strand. The nuclear membrane is intact.

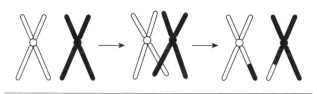

FIGURE 1-5 Illustration of chiasma formation and crossing over during meiosis. Genetic material is exchanged between homologous chromosomes. (From Levine, F. [1998]. Genetics. In R.A. Polin & W.W. Fox (Eds.). *Fetal and neonatal physiology* [2nd ed.]. Philadelphia: W.B. Saunders.)

As the cell moves into the zygotene stage, homologous chromosomes pair up (synapse).

The chromosomes shorten and condense during the pachytene stage. The two chromatids in each chromosome are distinct and can now be seen clearly. Crossover and exchange of segments of genetic material (recombination) occurs at this time between the maternally derived chromatids of one of the chromosome pairs and the paternally derived chromatids of the other homologous chromosomes (Figure 1-5). The sites of exchange are called *chiasmata*. Crossing over allows an individual to inherit a mixture of genetic material from maternal and paternal sides, increasing genetic diversity. The pairs of chromatids separate from each other during the diplotene stage. Once this separation is completed, the nuclear membrane dissolves (diakinesis stage). The chromosomes are maximally condensed, chiasmata are terminated, and normal disjunction (separation of chromosomes) occurs.[6,46]

Between diakinesis and metaphase I, the nucleus disappears and spindle fibers form. In metaphase the chromosomes line up on the metaphase plate. Homologous chromosomes are paired and attached to spindle fibers at the centromere. The centrioles are at opposite poles. In anaphase I, the centromeres are not divided and the chromatids are not pulled to opposite poles as occurs with mitosis. Instead, each pair of chromosomes separates, with one of each chromosome pair going to each pole (see Figure 1-4). In telophase I, the nuclear membranes re-form and the cell divides to form a secondary oocyte or spermatocyte.[6,46] Each has 23 chromosomes, one member of each original chromosome pair; each chromosome has 2 chromatids attached at the centromere (i.e., each chromosome has twice the usual amount of DNA). In the female, cell division is unequal, with one daughter cell receiving 23 chromosomes and most of the cytoplasm; the other cell receives 23 chromosomes and minimal cytoplasm (Figure 1-6). This cell is called the *first polar body* and eventually disintegrates.

In the second meiotic division, no DNA replication occurs. Prophase II is similar to mitosis. During metaphase the chromosomes (only 1 of each pair is present, each with twice the usual DNA) align along the equator of the cell. Centrioles again appear at the cell poles, and spindle fibers form. As the cell moves from metaphase II to anaphase II, the centromeres divide and the two chromatids from each chromosome separate and move to opposite poles. In telophase II, the nuclear membrane re-forms and cell division occurs, forming the spermatid or ovum.[6,46] The end result is haploid (23 chromosome) cells, with one of each chromosome pair in each cell (see Figure 1-4); each chromosome now has the normal amount of DNA. Again cell division in the females is unequal, resulting in formation of one ovum and the second polar body (see Oogenesis).

GAMETOGENESIS

Gametogenesis is the process by which the primordial germ cell develops into mature gametes. These processes are known as *oogenesis* (female) and *spermatogenesis* (male). Oogenesis and spermatogenesis are illustrated in Figure 1-6.

Oogenesis

Oogenesis is the process of ovum development, which, unlike spermatogenesis, begins in fetal life. The primordial germ cells arrive in the ovary from the yolk sac during the fifth week of embryonic life and begin to differentiate into oogonia. During early fetal life, proliferation of the oogonia is rapid. The oogonia continue to enlarge, their DNA replicates, and they become primary oocytes. The primary oocytes enter meiosis I, then arrest in the diplotene stage of prophase I (see Figure 1-4) and remain dormant until puberty. The mechanism for this arrest is unknown but is probably due to a meiosis-inhibiting factor from the surrounding granulosa cells. All primary oocytes are formed by the fifth month of gestation. By birth a layer of follicular cells surrounds the primary oocytes. These structures are the primordial follicles. By 20 weeks' gestation there are between 5 million and 7 million oocytes (Figure 1-7).[6] This peak is followed by a gradual decrease in ova. By puberty less than 300,000 follicles remain; only about 400 of these oogonia will become secondary follicles.[6]

During each ovarian cycle after puberty, a small number of primary oocytes (10 to 43) develop further.[6] Follicle-stimulating hormone (FSH) and luteinizing hormone (LH) from the pituitary gland cause an increase in the size of the oocyte as well as formation of the zona pellucida (see Chapter 2). Before ovulation the first meiotic division is completed, with an unequal division of the cytoplasm, yielding one secondary oocyte and the first polar

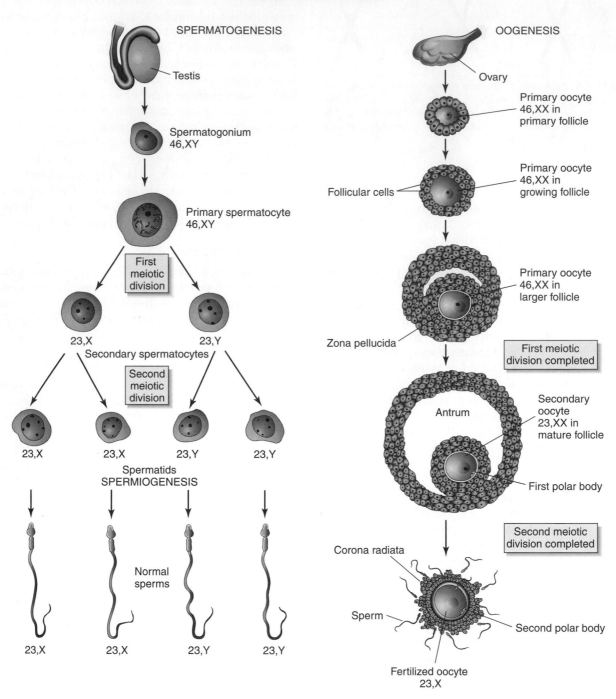

NORMAL GAMETOGENESIS

SPERMATOGENESIS

Testis

Spermatogonium
46,XY

Primary spermatocyte
46,XY

First meiotic division

23,X   23,Y
Secondary spermatocytes

Second meiotic division

23,X   23,X   23,Y   23,Y
Spermatids
SPERMIOGENESIS

Normal sperms

23,X   23,X   23,Y   23,Y

OOGENESIS

Ovary

Primary oocyte
46,XX in
primary follicle

Follicular cells

Primary oocyte
46,XX in
growing follicle

Primary oocyte
46,XX in
larger follicle

Zona pellucida

First meiotic division completed

Antrum

Secondary oocyte
23,XX in
mature follicle

First polar body

Second meiotic division completed

Corona radiata

Sperm

Second polar body

Fertilized oocyte
23,X

FIGURE 1-6 Comparison of spermatogenesis and oogenesis. Oogonia are not shown because they differentiate primarily into oocytes before birth. The chromosome complement of the germ cells is shown at each stage. The number designates the total number of chromosomes, including the sex chromosome(s) shown after the number. Note that: (1) following the two meiotic divisions, the diploid number of chromosomes (46) is reduced to the haploid number (23); (2) four sperms form from one primary spermatocyte, whereas only one mature oocyte results from the maturation of a primary oocyte; and (3) the cytoplasm is conserved during oogenesis to form one large cell, the mature oocyte or ovum. The polar bodies are small, nonfunctional cells that eventually disintegrate. (From Moore, K.L. & Persaud, T.V.N. [1998]. *The developing human: Clinically oriented embryology* [6th ed.]. Philadelphia: W.B. Saunders.)

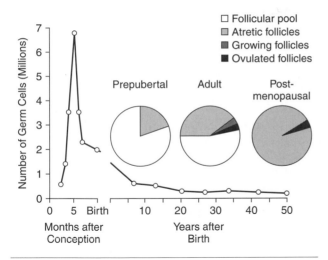

FIGURE **1-7** Changes in the number of germ cells and proportions of follicle types in the human ovary with increasing age. (Based on studies by Baker, T.G. [1970]. In C.R. Austin & R.V. Short [Eds.]. *Germ cells and fertilization [reproduction in mammals]* [vol. 1]. Cambridge, England; and Goodman, A.L. & Hodgen, C.D. [1983] *Recent Prog Hormone Res, 39,* 1-73.)

body, which degenerates. Although the polar body is non-functional, it may divide during the second meiotic division.[6] Once the first meiotic division is completed, the secondary oocyte begins the second meiotic division. Ovulation occurs when the secondary oocyte enters metaphase II, where it again arrests. Meiosis II is completed only if the sperm penetrates the ovum. This division is also characterized by unequal division of the cytoplasm in the female, resulting in formation of a mature oocyte and the second polar body, which disintegrates. The remaining primary oocytes remain arrested in meiosis I. Reproductive endocrinology and follicle maturation are discussed in Chapter 2. Ovulation and fertilization are described in Chapter 3.

Spermatogenesis

Sperm development in the seminiferous tubules involves three stages: (1) mitosis (spermatogonial multiplication), (2) meiosis (production of haploid cells), and (3) spermiogenesis (maturation of spermatids to mature spermatozoa). The androgens and proteins produced locally modulate the stage of spermatogenesis seen within the tubule.[5] The primordial germ cells arrive in the testes during the fifth week of embryonic life and remain dormant until puberty.

Spermatogenesis begins at puberty with the release of androgen. Once begun, the process is continuous. The spermatogonia are located inside the seminiferous tubules. The seminiferous tubule is divided into two zones: the basal compartment, or outer layer (zone 1), of the tubule, and the luminal compartment, or inner layer. The basal compartment is composed of type A spermatogonia that are renewed through mitosis. Some of these continue to proliferate and serve as stem cells, whereas others separate from the basal membrane and begin to migrate toward the lumen. These cells are known as *preleptotene spermatocytes* (type B spermatogonia). As migration progresses, the cells undergo further morphologic changes, becoming primary spermatocytes. The first and second meiotic divisions occur with further differentiation in the luminal zone, resulting in formation of secondary spermatocytes and spermatids.

During the first meiotic division, the primary spermatocytes reduce their chromosome count to half (haploid)—each chromosome having 2 chromatids joined at the centromere—and become two secondary spermatocytes. The second meiotic division involves separation of the two chromatids of each chromosome (with one going to each daughter cell), forming four spermatids, each with 23 chromosomes (see Figure 1-6). The luminal spermatids undergo spermiogenesis, which is the transformation process from ordinary cell structure to sperm cell with head, acrosome, neck, body, and tail (Figure 1-8). From the initial growth phase of the spermatogonia to the final product, the process takes approximately 64 to 74 days. Once completed, the sperm are set free in the seminiferous tubules and transported via the fluid to the epididymis and ductus deferens, where they are stored until ejaculation (see Chapter 3). At the time of their release into the tubules, the spermatozoa are still morphologically immature and lack motility. While traversing the epididymis (which takes 14 to 21 days), they continue to differentiate. Forward motility is achieved in the proximal epididymis.[5]

Abnormal Gamete Development

Abnormal gamete development is the result of either chromosomal or morphologic abnormalities. The impact of maternal or paternal age at the time of conception can be seen in fresh gene mutations. The older the parents are, the greater the likelihood that they will generate germ cells that contain gene mutations that can be passed on to the embryo. The likelihood of chromosomal abnormalities increases after the age of 35, particularly in females, and this may be because of nondisjunction from prolongation of meiosis over many years. DNA damage and replication error are more likely to occur in males because spermatogenesis involves continual cell division and DNA replication, whereas nondisjunction is more common in the females.[30,31]

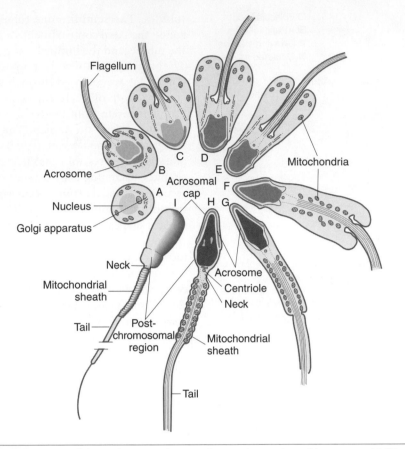

Flagellum

Acrosome

Nucleus

Golgi apparatus

Mitochondria

Acrosomal cap

Neck

Mitochondrial sheath

Tail

Post-chromosomal region

Acrosome

Centriole

Neck

Mitochondrial sheath

Tail

FIGURE **1-8** Summary of the major stages in spermiogenesis, starting with a spermatid *(A)* and ending with a mature spermatozoon *(I)*. (From Carlson, B.M. [1999]. *Human embryology and developmental biology* [2nd ed.]. St Louis: Mosby.)

Nondisjunction during meiosis is an error in meiotic division in which homologous chromosomes fail to separate and move to opposite poles of the cell. For example, in the case of formation of gametes with a trisomy or monosomy, one gamete will have 24 chromosomes and the other will have only 22 (Figure 1-9). Once fertilization occurs, the gamete with 24 chromosomes forms a zygote with 47 chromosomes (trisomy with an extra copy of one chromosome, such as an extra 21 in trisomy 21). About 95% of Down syndrome cases are due to trisomy 21. In the alternative situation, a 45-chromosome zygote (monosomy for a specific chromosome) is formed from the joining of a 22- and a 23-chromosome gamete, with one chromosome missing. Most autosomal trisomies and all autosomal monosomies are nonviable.

Nondisjunction in the autosomes during meiosis, and usually in the first meiotic division, occurs more frequently in the female. For example, maternal nondisjunction accounts for approximately 88% of trisomy 13, 92% of trisomy 18, and 91% of trisomy 21.[31,34] On the other hand, paternal nondisjunction accounts for 80% of Turner syndrome (XO females), while the nondisjunction leading to Klinefelter syndrome (XXY male) occurs equally in the mother and father.[31] Chromosomal abnormalities are described further in the next section.

Nondisjunction can also occur during mitosis after formation of the zygote. If nondisjunction occurs in the first cell division after fertilization, one daughter cell receives 45 chromosomes and one 47 chromosomes. The cell with 45 chromosomes usually does not survive; the zygote continues to develop from the 47 chromosome cell and is a trisomy. If mitotic nondisjunction occurs later in development, some cell lines have the normal number of cells and some have an abnormal number. This is called *mosaicism.* Approximately 1% to 2% of individuals with Down syndrome are mosaics; that is, they have some cells with the normal 46 chromosomes and some cells with 47 chromosomes as a result of an extra chromosome 21.

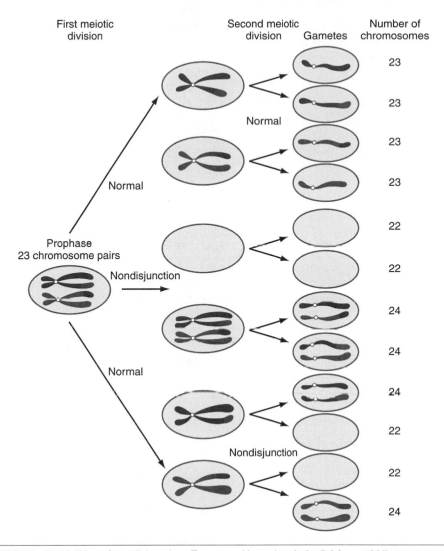

FIGURE **1-9** Possibilities of nondisjunction. *Top arrow,* Normal meiotic division; *middle arrow,* nondisjunction during the first meiotic divisions; *bottom arrow,* nondisjunction during the second meiotic division. (From Carlson, B.M. [1999]. *Human embryology and developmental biology* [2nd ed.]. St Louis: Mosby.)

Gametes may also experience alterations in morphology. This is much less common in oocytes than in sperm. Although some oocytes may have two or more nuclei, they probably never mature. In each ejaculate up to 20% of the sperm are grossly abnormal, having either two heads or two tails. Their ability to fertilize the ovum is probably limited because of decreased or abnormal motility and inability to pass through the cervical mucus, thereby terminating their access to the ovum. An increase in the percentage of abnormal sperm can reduce fertility.[30]

GENETIC AND CHROMOSOMAL DISORDERS

Genetic diseases are the result of detrimental changes in the structure of individual genes (gene disorders) or in the entire chromosome (cytogenetic or chromosomal disorders). These disorders can be inherited (see Modes of Inheritance) or arise as new mutations or from alterations in chromosomal number or structure during cell division. Mutations are not always deleterious, but rather may introduce genetic variation into the species.[41] Cytogenetic or chromosomal disorders result when a large number of genes are damaged.[25] Individuals born with chromosomal defects often demonstrate both physical and mental handicaps.[24] Most gene disorders are mutations in a single or small number of genes, whereas major chromosome errors involve a change in chromosome number or structure. Chromosomal alterations are seen in 60% of spontaneous abortions, 6% to 7% of stillborn infants, and 0.7% of live born infants.[22,31] Chromosomal abnormalities can also be a cause of infertility. Most chromosomal abnormalities arise during gametogenesis, although errors can also occur during fertilization or postfertilizaiton.[31]

Alterations in Chromosome Number

Deviations from euploidy (the correct number of chromosomes) are of two types. *Polyploidy* refers to an exact multiple of the haploid (23) set of chromosomes. For example, *triploidy* refers to a zygote with 69 chromosomes (3 of each). Triploidy may arise from fertilization of an ovum (23 chromosomes) with 2 sperm (each carrying 23 chromosomes) or from fusion of the ovum (23 chromosomes) and polar body (23 chromosomes), which is then fertilized by a sperm (23 chromosomes). *Aneuploidy* is the term used for cases in which there is not an exact multiple. Monosomy is a subset of the latter, in which one member of a pair of chromosomes is missing. Monosomies are rarely viable. The most common monosomy seen in live born infants is a female with Turner syndrome who has only one X chromosome. Trisomy refers to the presence of an extra chromosome. The most common trisomies seen in live born infants are trisomies 21 (Down syndrome), 13 (Patau syndrome), and 18 (Edward syndrome). Individuals with Klinefelter syndrome—another example of an alteration in numbers of sex chromosomes—are XXY males.

Alterations in Chromosome Structure

Variations in chromosomes are more common than alterations in chromosomal number. Some have very little effect, while others are devastating. Alterations in chromosome structure include the following: (1) deletions, (2) duplications, (3) inversions, (4) isochromosomes, (5) instability syndromes, (6) unstable triplet nucleotide repeats, and (5) translocations (Figure 1-10).

Deletions, the loss of part of a chromosome, can occur anywhere on the chromosome. Terminal deletions (see Figure 1-10, *B*) are those occurring on the ends. For example, persons with cri du chat syndrome have a terminal deletion of part of the short (p) arm of chromosome 5. Interstitial deletions occur along the body of the chromosome, with the ends reattaching. If the broken piece is without a centromere, the piece will be lost during cell division. Occasionally, broken fragments may be incorporated into another chromosome. Other examples of deletion syndromes are Wilms tumor (deletion of part of the short arm of chromosome 11), retinoblastoma (deletion of part of the long arm of chromosomes 13), Prader-Willi syndrome (deletion of part of the long arm of the paternally derived chromosome 15), Angelman syndrome (deletion of part of the long arm of the maternally derived chromosome 15), Duchenne muscular dystrophy (deletion of part of the short arm of the X chromosome), and DiGeorge syndrome (deletion of part of the long arm of chromosome 22).[21,22] A variation of deletion defects are ring chromosomes (see Figure 1-10, *C*), in which part of each end of the chromosomes are broken off and the ends attach to each other.

Duplications (see Figure 1-10, *D*) occur when extra copies of genes are created or obtained during crossing-over. The results of this duplication may or may not be visible. Inversions (such as a paracentric inversion) (see Figure 1-10, *E*) result from two breaks and the subsequent 180-degree rotation of the broken segment. This results in a sequence change and rearrangement of genes in reverse order. Chromosome pairing cannot occur normally during meiosis, resulting in an increased incidence of spontaneous abortions. This may explain some cases of infertility. Isochromosomes occur when the chromosome, with its replicated DNA, divides across the centromere (instead of dividing into two sister chromatids), resulting in one chromosome with just upper arms and one with just the lower arms (see Figure 1-10, *F*). Instability syndromes such as Fanconi anemia and xeroderma pigmentosum involve alterations in DNA repair.[22]

Unstable nucleotide repeats are multiple repetitions of a series of three bases at a certain point along the chromosomes. Examples of disorders in which this defect is seen are Huntington's disease (chromosome 4) and fragile X syndrome (X chromosome). For example, in fragile X syndrome the unstable CGG nucleotide repeat occurs at the end of the X chromosome. Instead of the usual number of CGG repeats (less than 50), there are many more, with severity of the disorder associated with the number of repeats. Expansion of the number of repeats occurs during meiosis in females. Fragile X syndrome is the most common cause of inherited developmental delay and mental retardation and is more common in males than females. In Huntington's disease the expansion on chromosome 4 occurs primarily in sperm cells; thus the disorder is more likely to occur when passed through males. Age of onset is usually between 40 and 60 years of age. Increased numbers of repeats are associated with a younger age of onset.[22]

Translocations occur after breaks have happened. Genetic material is transferred to another chromosome. In reciprocal translocation no genetic material is lost, because two chromosomes exchange pieces (balanced transloca-

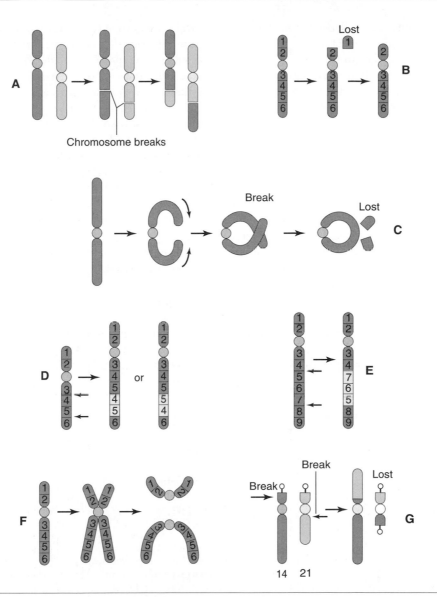

FIGURE **1-10** Diagrams illustrating various structural abnormalities of chromosomes. **A,** Reciprocal translocation. **B,** Terminal deletion. **C,** Ring chromosomes. **D,** Duplication. **E,** Paracentric inversion. **F,** Isochromosome. **G,** Robertsonian translocation. (From Moore, K.L. & Persaud, T.V.N. (1998). *The developing human: Clinically oriented embryology* [6th ed.]. Philadelphia: W.B. Saunders.)

tion). If material is gained or lost, that is considered an unbalanced translocation. Children with balanced translocations appear normal; those with unbalanced translocations may have multiple anomalies. Reciprocal translocations (see Figure 1-10, *A*) involve breaks in two chromosomes, with exchange of genetic material. Translocations are also seen with some forms of leukemia and solid tumors.[22]

Robertsonian translocations (see Figure 1-10, *G*) involve chromosomes 13 through 15 and 21 and 22; these

occur when the short arms of 2 chromosomes break off and are lost, and the long arms fuse together at the centromere to form a single chromosome. For example, an individual with normal 14 and 21 chromosomes and a 14/21 translocation has an abnormal karyotype and number of chromosomes (i.e., only 45 chromosomes) but a normal phenotype (normal amount of genetic material). However, depending of which combination of 21 and 14 chromosomes are transferred to the gametes, this individual can produce normal, carrier, monosomic (for 21 or 14), or trisomic (for 21 or 14) offspring. Approximately 3% to 4% of Down syndrome are due to translocations, most commonly between chromosomes 14 and 21. These individual have 46 chromosomes, because the abnormal dose of chromosome 21 is attached to a chromosome 14.

Gene Disorders

Mutations are permanent changes in DNA. Mutations can involve changes in the sequence of bases, involving large amounts of DNA, as occurs with chromosomal abnormalities, or alterations in one or a few bases that result in production of deficient or defective protein that can be spontaneous or inherited. If the mutation occurs in a somatic cell, it is transmitted only within that cell line; all other cell lines are free of that mutation. However, if a mutation occurs in a germ cell or gamete, it is transmitted to all somatic and germ cells of the offspring.

Gene mutations result in inherited biochemical or structural disorders characterized by defective or deficient cellular functioning or altered production of structural components (e.g., skin, muscles, hemoglobin, connective tissue). The consequences of these alterations depend on the type of molecule affected, defect, metabolic reaction, site of action, remaining residual activity, gene interactions, environment, and degree of adaptation.[24] General categories of gene disorders include hemoglobinopathies, disorders of metabolism (carbohydrate, lipid, amino acid, or degradative pathways), deficient or abnormal circulating proteins, alterations in membrane receptors or transport molecules, immunologic disorders, and cancer genetics. There are hundreds of known gene disorders. Table 1-1 lists examples of each major category; several examples are described further in this section.

Hemoglobinopathies may arise from qualitative or quantitative changes in hemoglobin. For example, both sickle cell anemia and beta thalassemia involve mutations in the gene on chromosome 11 for production of beta chains. Sickle cell anemia involves a single point mutation (change in just one amino acid, with a valine instead of a glutamic acid inserted into the 146 amino acid sequence that makes up beta chains). This mutation results in formation of qual-

TABLE **1-1** Examples of Gene Disorders

TYPE OF DISORDER	EXAMPLES
Hemoglobin disorders	Sickle cell anemia
	β-Thalassemia
	α-Thalassemia
Disorders of metabolism: amino acid metabolism	Enzyme defects (phenylketonuria, congenital adrenal hyperplasia)
	Deficient reabsorption in intestines or kidneys (Hartnup's disease)
Disorders of metabolism: carbohydrate metabolism	Enzyme defects (galactosemia)
	Excess glycogen accumulation (glycogen storage disorders)
Disorders of metabolism: lipid metabolism	Altered transport (hyperlipidemia)
	Enzyme defects (medium chain Acyl-CoA dehydrogenase deficiency)
Disorders of metabolism: altered degradation pathways	Lysosomal storage disorders
	Uric acid cycle disorders
Deficient or abnormal circulating proteins	Globulins (immunologic defects)
	Clotting factors (hemophilia)
Alterations in membrane receptors or regulators	Hypercholesterolemia
	Cystic fibrosis
Immunologic disorders	Major histocompatibility antigen disease associations (type 1 diabetes, celiac disease, Graves' disease)
	Immunodeficiency disorders
Cancers	Familial breast and ovarian cancers (BRCA1, BRCA2)
	Hereditary nonpolyposis colorectal cancer
	Wilms' tumor
	Retinoblastoma

Compiled from Jorde, L.B., et al. (1999). *Medical genetics* (2nd ed.). St. Louis: Mosby; and Lashley, F.R. (1998). *Clinical genetics in nursing practice* (2nd ed.). New York: Springer.

itatively different beta globulin chains (HbS). With beta thalassemia, fewer beta chains of normal length are produced. The alpha chains have fewer beta chains to pair with and accumulate and precipitate. Over 70 different mutations in the beta chain gene have been identified in individuals with various forms of beta thalassemia. Two pairs of genes (or a total of 4 alleles) control synthesis of alpha chains for hemoglobin on chromosome 16. The clinical status of individuals depends on the number of genes in the two gene pairs that are absent or abnormal. If just one of the four alleles is absent, the individual is a "silent" carrier. If two alleles are absent, the individual will have minimal anemia; three absent alleles leads to mild to moderate anemia. Two absent and one abnormal allele lead to moderate to severe anemia. If all four alleles are absent, these infants are stillborn or die soon after birth.[22]

Metabolic defects result in blocked metabolic pathways, accumulation of toxic precursors, lack of end-product production, and loss of feedback inhibition. For example, phenylalanine is a precursor for tyrosine formation. Tyrosine is then broken down (mediated by tyrosinase), to produce substances such as melanin and byproducts used in synthesis of neurotransmitters. Phenylalanine catabolism is mediated by the enzyme *phenylalanine hydrolase.* Individuals with phenylketonuria (PKU) have a mutation of the gene required for production of this enzyme. As a result, these individuals have altered enzyme production and cannot convert any or some (depending on the specific mutation) phenylalanine to tyrosine. As a result, phenylalanine and byproducts of alternative metabolic pathways accumulate with a deficiency of tyrosine. The accumulated phenylalanine and alternative pathway byproducts are excreted in the urine (leading to a musky odor), interfere with tyrosinase function, and are toxic to the central nervous system. The decreased tyrosine results in lack of melanin (leading to the light skin and eye color observed in these cases), altered neurotransmitters, and neurologic abnormalities.

MODES OF INHERITANCE

The way in which a particular trait is transmitted to offspring is referred to as the *mode of inheritance.* The major modes of inheritance are those that follow traditional Mendelian patterns (autosomal and sex-linked inheritance), multifactorial inheritance, and nontraditional patterns. Mendelian patterns follow the principles identified by Mendel (Table 1-2) and influence inheritance of both normal traits and mutated genes. Autosomal dominant traits are the result of a dominant allele at a particular locus on an autosome. When a characteristic is the result of a recessive allele, the mode of inheritance is known as autoso-

mal recessive. Genetic diseases resulting from the mutation of a single allele are called *dominant;* those that result from mutation of both alleles are called *recessive.* The traits or disorders expressed by autosomal genes usually occur with the same frequency in males as in females. The latter is not true of sex-linked traits and disorders, which occur with higher frequency in males than in females. This is because the genes located on the X chromosome are present in only one copy in males. Therefore the genes that are on that chromosome are expressed and are considered hemizygous.[24] Polygenic traits are governed by the additive effect of two or more alleles at different loci.[24]

There are several types of dominance (simple, or complete; partial, or incomplete) and codominance that affect the phenotype.[22,24] In simple, or complete, dominance, the heterozygous genotype (dominant allele present on one of the chromosome pair) produces a phenotype similar to that produced by the homozygous genotype (dominant allele present on both of the chromosome pair) for dominant traits. With partial, or incomplete, dominance, the heterozygous genotype (one copy of the recessive gene and one copy of the dominant gene) produces a phenotype that is intermediate between the recessive homozygous (i.e., two copies of a recessive gene) and dominant homozygous (i.e., two copies of a dominant gene) phenotypes. For example, an individual who is a heterozygote (carrier) for PKU may have elevated levels of phenylalanine, though these levels are not high enough to produce PKU.[22,24]

TABLE 1-2   Mendelian Principles of Inheritance

PRINCIPLE	DESCRIPTION
Dominance	In the competition of two genes at the same locus on paired chromosomes, one gene may mask or conceal the other. The individual manifests the dominant gene's characteristic. The concealed trait is termed *recessive.*
Segregation	During meiosis, paired chromosomes are separated to form two gametes. Therefore the genes remain unchanged and are transferred from one generation to the next.
Independent Assortment	When displayed traits have alleles at two or more loci, each is distributed within the gametes randomly, independent of each other.

Codominance occurs when both alleles are expressed, so that in the heterozygous state, both the dominant and recessive gene products are produced. The gene producing normal beta chains for adult hemoglobin (HbA) and the gene producing abnormal beta chains (HbS) seen with sickle cell anemia are examples of codominance. If both chromosomes in the pair have the normal beta chain gene, HbA is produced; if both chromosomes have the abnormal genes, HbS is produced and the individual has sickle cell anemia. However, if one of the chromosomes has the normal gene and one has the abnormal gene (heterozygote), both HbA and HbS are produced. This individual has the sickle cell trait.

For some traits, such as the ABO blood type, multiple alleles are present. Although any given individual has only two genes for blood type (one on each chromosome in the pair), there are more than two forms of the gene present in the population. For example, although there are genes for types A, B, and O present in humans, any one person has only two alleles. That person may have two identical alleles (AA, BB, or OO), or may have two different alleles (AO, BO, and AB). In the ABO system, A and B are codominant and O is recessive to both A and B. Thus someone who has the AO genotype has the A blood type phenotype. Similarly, a BO individual has the B phenotype. However someone with the AB genotype has AB blood, because A and B are codominant and thus are both expressed.[22,24]

Other factors that influence whether or not an individual with a certain genotype actually manifests the trait are penetrance and variable expression. With differences in penetrance, not everyone with the abnormal gene(s) actually manifest the trait or disorder. This is an "all-or-nothing" type of phenomenon. Reduced penetrance is often seen with autosomal dominant conditions such as retinoblastoma. *Variable expression* refers to the different manifestations of the phenotype that can be observed in individuals with the same genotype. This leads to wide variations in the clinical severity of individuals with some disorders. Examples of disorders with variable expression include neurofibromatosis and osteogenesis imperfecta.[22]

Autosomal Inheritance

The inheritance of these traits is dependent upon the differences between alleles of a particular locus on an autosomal pair. In this type of inheritance, it makes no difference which parent carries the genotype, because the autosomes are the same in both sexes.

Autosomal Recessive Inheritance

A trait governed by a recessive allele is expressed only when the homozygous condition exists.[24] In order for an individual to demonstrate the trait or disorder, both parents must carry the recessive allele. If an affected person reproduces with a homozygous unaffected person, their children will be heterozygous for the trait and will not manifest the disease, but they will be carriers. If two carriers reproduce, then the probability (for each pregnancy) is about 25% that the child will manifest the disease, 50% that the child will be a carrier, and 25% that the child will neither have the disease nor be a carrier. When an affected person reproduces with a carrier, the probability is about 50% that a child will have the disease and 50% that the child will be a carrier. Usually an affected child is the offspring of two heterozygotes who are themselves normal.

Disorders transmitted by recessive inheritance often involved altered enzymes, since normally only 50% of the normal amount of these enzymes is sufficient for normal function.[25] Examples of autosomal recessive disorders include cystic fibrosis, PKU, hypothyroidism, Tay-Sachs disease, congenital adrenal hyperplasia, and galactosemia. Hemoglobinopathies such as sickle cell disease are also transmitted by autosomal recessive inheritance. Characteristics of disorders inherited by autosomal recessive inheritance are listed in Table 1-3.

Autosomal Dominant Inheritance

In autosomal dominant inheritance, traits and disorders are expressed in the heterozygote state and the probability of transmission to the offspring is 50% with each pregnancy. Autosomal dominant disorders often involve mutations in genes that regulate complex metabolic pathways or produce structural proteins. Examples of autosomal dominant disorders include Huntington's disease (triplet nucleotide repeats), osteogenesis imperfecta (mutations in collagen gene), and familiar hypercholesterolemia (mutations in receptor for very-low-density lipoproteins).[25] Whenever the gene is present, it is expressed in the phenotype and can be traced through a number of generations. Expression of these genes rarely skips a generation, and a person not affected will not transmit the gene. Therefore the affected individual will have an affected parent, unless the condition is the result of fresh mutation, which is a common finding in most autosomal dominant conditions. An exception to this is Huntington's disease, in which new mutations are extremely rare.[22]

Some autosomal dominant disorders (e.g., achondroplasia) are apparent at birth, whereas others (e.g., Huntington's disease, adult-onset polycystic kidney disease) have a variable and usually adult onset. Other characteristics of autosomal dominant inheritance include a wide variation in expression in those individuals affected.

TABLE **1-3**   Major Characteristics of Autosomal Recessive and Dominant Inheritance and Disorders

AUTOSOMAL RECESSIVE INHERITANCE	AUTOSOMAL DOMINANT INHERITANCE
The mutant gene is located on an autosome.	The mutant gene is on an autosome.
Two copies of the mutant gene are needed for phenotypic manifestations.	Only one copy of the mutant gene is needed for effects to be evident.
Males and females are affected in equal numbers, on average.	Males and females are affected in equal numbers on average.
There is usually no sex difference in clinical manifestations.	There is no sex difference in clinical manifestations.
Affected individual receives one mutant gene from each parent.	Vertical family history through several generations may be seen.
Family history is usually negative, especially for vertical transmission (in more than one generation).	There is wide variability of expression.
Other affected individuals in family in same generation (horizontal transmission) may be seen.	Penetrance may be incomplete, so the gene may appear to "skip" a generation.
Consanguinity is present more often than in other modes of inheritance.	There is an increased paternal age effect.
Fresh gene mutation is rare.	Fresh gene mutation is frequent.
Age of disease onset is early newborn, infancy, and early childhood.	Later age of onset is frequent.
Often involves enzyme defect or deficiency.	Male-to-male transmission is possible.
Disease course is usually severe.	Normal offspring of an affected person have normal children.
	Structural protein defect is often involved.

Adapted from Lashley, F.R. (1998). *Clinical genetics in nursing practice* (2nd ed.). New York: Springer.

Penetrance may also not be complete. *Penetrance* refers to whether or not there is phenotypic recognition of the mutant gene. If a gene is fully penetrant, the trait it controls is always manifested in the individual. If it is not fully penetrant, the disease may appear to skip a generation; that is, a particular genotype produces a particular trait in some individuals but not in others. A parent may be diagnosed with a particular disorder only after having several affected offspring.[25] A paternal age effect is seen with some autosomal dominant disorders.[24] Table 1-3 summarizes characteristics of autosomal dominant inheritance.

Sex-Linked Inheritance

Genes on the X chromosome are identified as X-linked, whereas those on the Y chromosome are Y-linked. There are many such X-linked genes; however, there is limited evidence for Y-linked genes except for some associated with the male phenotype. Males can transmit X-linked genes to their daughters but not to their sons, and sons can receive X-linked genes only from their mothers. Female offspring can be either homozygous or heterozygous for X-linked genes because of their dual X chromosomes. Males, on the other hand, are hemizygous for X-linked genes, because they have only one X chromosome.

X-linked inheritance in females is influenced by X-chromosome inactivation. In all of a woman's somatic cells (but not in her germ cells), one of the two X chromosomes is inactivated (lyonization) and remains condensed. However, recent evidence suggests that some genes on the inactive X

remain active.[27,31] The inactive X is seen in interphase as the Barr body. The inactive X is reactivated in the oogonium, so that with gametogenesis the woman produces only ova with active X chromosomes. In the female zygote, inactivation begins in the morula stage at about 3 days after fertilization and is complete by the blastocyst stage (5 to 6 days). The inactivated X is random in each cell—it could be the X the zygote received from its mother or the one it received from its father—and the same X is inactive in all descendants of that cell. Exceptions to the random inactivation are seen in some single gene disorders such as Duchenne muscular dystrophy, in which the normal X tends to be the active one.[27,31] Inactivation is thought to occur via methylation of critical segments of DNA and to be initiated by the XIST gene on the long arm (q13) of the X chromosomes.[31]

X-Linked Recessive Inheritance

In males, an X-linked recessive gene is always expressed, because there is no corresponding gene on the Y chromosome to be dominant. In females, recessive genes of this nature are usually expressed only when the recessive allele is present in the homozygous form (i.e., on both of the woman's X chromosomes). Occasionally a female may demonstrate the trait secondary to the random inactivation of one of the X chromosomes in each cell. The degree to which this individual expresses the trait depends on the proportion of cells in which the dominant gene has been inactivated. The larger the proportion is, the greater the likelihood that the

X-linked trait will be visible (Table 1-4). Examples of X-linked recessive inheritance include hemophilia, color blindness, and Duchenne muscular dystrophy.

X-Linked Dominant Inheritance

In this type of inheritance, the trait will be demonstrated in both males and females. Who will be affected and to what degree depend on the genotype of the parents. All the daughters of an affected father will receive the X chromosome with the dominant gene and will express the disease. However, none of the sons of this father will be affected. When the mother is heterozygous, half the offspring will likely be affected. If the mother is homozygous, all the children will be affected, regardless of the father's status. If the father is also affected, the daughters will be homozygous for the disease. In situations in which the father does not exhibit the trait and the mother is heterozygous, the risk of affected offspring is 100% for their daughters and 50% for their sons (see Table 1-4). X-linked dominant disorders are rare; an example is X-linked hypophosphatemia, or vitamin D–resistant rickets.

Y-Linked Inheritance

Since only males have Y chromosomes and there is no corresponding allele on the X chromosome, these traits occur only in males. If a Y-linked trait is present, it will be expressed. There is no dominance or recessiveness. When a father with a Y-linked chromosome transfers genetic material, all the sons will be affected and none of the daughters will. The Y chromosome also contains the testes-determining gene (see Development of the Gonads).

Multifactorial Inheritance

Multifactorial inheritance does not follow Mendelian patterns but is due to the interaction of genetic and environmental factors. Multifactorial disorders include birth defects (e.g., neural tube defects, some congenital heart defects, congenital dislocated hips, cleft lip and palate, pyloric stenosis, Hirschsprung's disease) and adult-onset disorders (e.g., some forms of breast and other cancers, bipolar affective disorders, coronary heart disease, types 1 and 2 diabetes). These disorders can also arise from purely environmental causes as well as via multifactorial inheritance. For example, although some congenital heart defects have a multifactorial inheritance, others arise as the result of teratogen exposure. Multifactorial disorders are thought to be polygenic and additive. The risk increases with the number of individuals in the family that are affected, closeness of the relationship (highest in first-degree relatives, i.e., parents, siblings, offspring), and severity of the disorder. For example, the greater the severity of a birth defect is, the greater the risk of recurrence in first-degree relatives.[22,24]

Nontraditional Inheritance

Nontraditional inheritance involves patterns that do not follow traditional Mendelian principles. Examples of these patterns include genomic imprinting, uniparental disomy, gonadal (germline) mosaicism, and mitochondrial inheritance.

Genomic imprinting is a "phenomenon that sets a parental signature on a specific DNA segment during gametogenesis or before fertilization so that it is modified and functions differently depending on the parental origin of the DNA segment."[23] Thus, with genomic imprinting, gene

TABLE **1-4**   **Major Characteristics of X-Linked Recessive and Dominant Inheritance and Disorders**

X-Linked Recessive Inheritance	X-Linked Dominant Inheritance
The mutant gene is on the X chromosome.	The mutant gene is located on the X chromosome.
One copy of the mutant gene is needed for phenotypic effect in males.	One copy of the mutant gene is needed for phenotypic manifestation.
Two copies of the mutant gene are usually needed for phenotypic effect in females.	X inactivation modifies the gene effect in females.
Males are more frequently affected than females.	Often lethal in males and so may see transmission only in female line.
Unequal X inactivation can lead to manifesting heterozygote female carriers.	Affected families show excess of female offspring.
Transmission is often through heterozygous (carrier) females.	Affected male transmits gene to all his daughters and none of his sons.
All daughters of affected males are carriers.	Affected males have affected mothers (unless it is a new mutation).
All sons of affected males are normal.	There is no male-to-male transmission.
There is no male-to-male transmission.	There is no carrier state.
There may be fresh gene mutations.	Disorders are relatively uncommon.

Adapted from Lashley, F.R. (1998). *Clinical genetics in nursing practice* (2nd ed.). New York: Springer.

expression differs depending on the parent from which the chromosome originated. This process is not completely understood but involves methylation and thus inactivation of certain sites on the chromosome. For example, with triploidy (severe growth failure and mental retardation, with most spontaneously aborted), if the extra set of chromosomes comes from the father (i.e., the zygote has 46 paternal chromosomes and 23 maternal), there is marked growth failure in the embryo, with overgrowth of placental tissue. Conversely, if there are two sets of maternal and one set of paternal chromosomes, early embryo growth is normal, with poor placental and chorion development. Complete hydatidiform moles (see Chapter 3) have two sets of paternal chromosomes and none of maternal origin.[31] Loss of imprinting of growth factors may play a role in childhood cancers such as Wilms' tumor. [50]

Another example of genomic imprinting is seen with deletions on the long arm of chromosome 15(q11-13). If the deletion comes from the father, the offspring has Prader-Willi syndrome; if the deletion is on the maternal chromosomes, the offspring has Angelman syndrome. These syndromes have completely different phenotypes. Angelman syndrome is characterized by mental retardation, seizures, absence of speech, frequent smiling, and paroxysmal laughing; Prader-Willi syndrome is characterized by overeating and obesity, behavior problems, and mild to moderate mental retardation. These syndromes can also arise with uniparental disomy, in which the offspring gets both copies of a chromosome from the same parent (e.g., both chromosome 15s from either the mother or father). Other disorders associated with uniparental disomy are Beckwith-Wiedemann syndrome (two paternal chromosome 11s), Silver-Russell syndrome (two maternal chromosome 7s) and transient neonatal diabetes mellitus (two paternal chromosome 6s).[23]

Gonadal (or *germline*) *mosaicism* refers to mutations that occur in some germ cells. The germ cells (oogonia or spermatogonia) initially undergo mitosis before meiosis and gametogenesis begin. If the mutation occurs at some point during these cell divisions, some cell lines entering meiosis and forming gametes will have the mutation, whereas others will not. This can produce pedigrees that are inconsistent with either dominant or recessive inheritance. For example, a dominant disorder may appear in two offspring of normal parents, or an unaffected parent may have affected children by two different partners. Examples of disorders that have been transmitted by this mechanism are achondroplasia and some forms of osteogenesis imperfecta.[22]

The mitochondria, which are cytoplasmic organelles involved in cellular respiration and production of energy, have their own unique circular DNA (mtDNA) and genes.

Mitochondrial genes code for different amino acids than do nuclear DNA. Mitochondria are present in the cytoplasm of the ovum; the sperm does not have any cytoplasm to pass on to the offspring. Thus each person, whether male or female, inherits mitochondrial DNA only from the mother. Mitochondrial disorders are rare and generally involve disorders of the central nervous system, skeletal muscles, eyes, or heart. When they occur, all of the mother's offspring are affected.[22,50]

EMBRYONIC AND FETAL DEVELOPMENT OF THE REPRODUCTIVE SYSTEM

Embryonic and fetal development of the reproductive system involves the formation of the gonads, genital ducts, and external genitalia from undifferentiated primordial structures (indifferent stage) within the embryo that are adapted to meet the functional need of the two sexes (Figure 1-11). For the male, the gonads differentiate into the testes, and the duct system becomes the efferent ductules of the testes, the duct of the epididymis, the ductus deferens, the seminal vesicles, and most of the urethra. The external genitalia become specialized to form the penis and scrotum. For the female, the gonads differentiate into the ovaries, and the duct system becomes the uterine (fallopian) tubes, uterus, and vagina. The vulva constitutes the external genitalia.

This developmental process begins at fertilization with the determination of genetic sex, passing through three other stages before birth. These include differentiation of gonadal sex, somatic sex, and neuroendocrine sex. After birth, sexual differentiation continues with the development of social sex, psychologic sex, and secondary sex characteristics.[37] These stages determine the final sexual characteristics and behavior of the individual.[29]

Genetic sex is determined at the time of fertilization by the genes. Chromosomal sex is defined by the sex chromosome complement. Gonadal sex is defined by the structure and function of the gonads; somatic sex involves all other genital organs; and neuroendocrine sex is established by the cyclic or continuous production of gonadotropin-releasing hormones (GnRHs).[37]

Prenatally the reproductive system develops from analogous undifferentiated structures in both sexes. Table 1-5 illustrates the indifferent structures and their male and females derivatives. The basic pattern is the female phenotype; the male system develops only when the Y chromosome, testosterone, and other organizing substances are present. This is true of the external genitalia as well. Prenatal reproductive system development involves three areas: the gonads, the genital ducts, and the external genitalia.

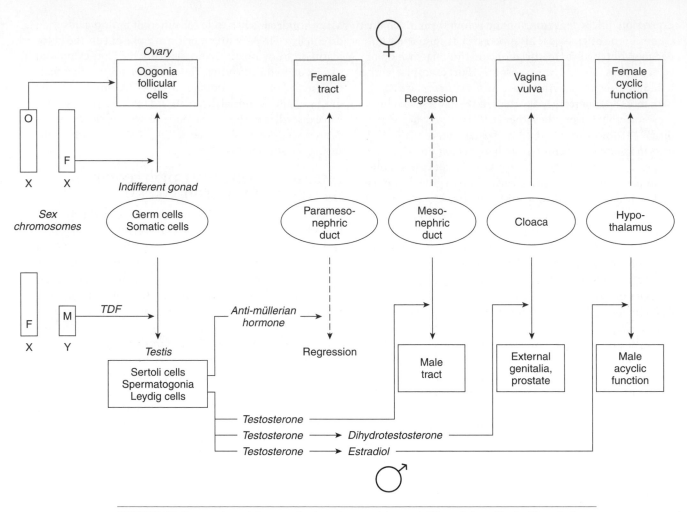

FIGURE 1-11 Proposed regulatory mechanisms in prenatal sexual differentiation. The indifferent stages are in the middle oval blocks. Female structures differentiate upward and male structures downward (solid vertical arrows). Regulatory factors and their source and target are indicated by solid horizontal arrows. Regression is indicated by dashed arrows. *F,* Gene for ovarian differentiation; *M,* gene for testicular differentiation; *O,* gene for further ovarian development; *TDF,* testis-determining gene. (From Pelliniemi, L. & Dym, M. [1994]. The fetal gonad and sexual differentiation. In D. Tulchinsky & A.B. Little [Eds.]. *Maternal-fetal endocrinology* [2nd ed.]. Philadelphia: W.B. Saunders.)

Development of the Gonads

The gonads in the human consist of the ovaries in the female and the testes in the male. These structures are derived from three cellular sources: (1) primordial germ cells, (2) underlying mesenchyme, and (3) coelomic epithelium. The primordial germ cells originate in the endodermal cells of the wall of the yolk sac, near the origin of the allantois, and migrate by ameboid movements along the dorsal mesentery of the hindgut to the gonadal ridge. Mitotic cell proliferation, stimulated by mitogenic factors, continues during this migration. By the end of the fifth week, approximately 1000 to 2000 germ cells arrive in the gonadal ridge, where they are incorporated into the mesenchyme of the gonadal ridge. The exact mechanism

of attraction between the gonadal tissue and the primordial germ cells is unknown, although this migration may be influenced by chemotactic factors excreted by the primitive gonad.[6] Testicular development of the indifferent gonad occurs regardless of whether viable germ cells are present; however, the germ cells must be present for the ovaries to differentiate.[6]

Indifferent Stage

During the fifth week of gestation, a thickening of the coelomic epithelium on the medial side of the mesonephros can be seen; this becomes the gonadal ridge.[30] The surface cells proliferate to form a solid cord of cells that grow downward with fingerlike projections into the mesenchyme,

TABLE **1-5**　Comparison of Male and Female Derivatives of Indifferent Structures in Reproductive System Development

INDIFFERENT STRUCTURE	MALE DERIVATIVE	FEMALE DERIVATIVE
Genital ridge	Testes	Ovary
Primordial germ cells	Spermatozoa	Ova
Sex cords	Seminiferous tubules (Sertoli cells)	Follicular cells
Mesonephric tubules	Efferent ductules	Epoöphoron
	Paradidymis	Paroöphoron
Mesonephric (wolffian) ducts	Appendix of epididymis	Appendix of ovary
	Epididymal duct	Gartner duct
	Ductus deferens	
	Ejaculatory duct	
Paramesonephric (müllerian) ducts	Appendix of testes	Uterine (fallopian) tubes
	Prostate utricle	Uterus
		Upper vagina
Definitive urogenital sinus (lower part)	Penile urethra	Lower vagina
		Vaginal vestibule
Early urogenital sinus (upper part)	Urinary bladder	Urinary bladder
	Prostatic urethra	Urethra
Genital tubercle	Penis	Clitoris
Genital folds	Floor of penile urethra	Labia minora
Genital swellings	Scrotum	Labia majora

From Carlson, B.M. (1999). *Human embryology & developmental biology* (2nd ed.). St. Louis: Mosby.

forming the primary sex cords.[30] At the end of 6 weeks, the gonads remain sexually indistinguishable. Two layers can be identified within the gonads: the cortex (coelomic epithelium) and the medulla (mesenchyme). In the XX embryo, the cortex differentiates into the ovary and the medulla essentially regresses. In the XY embryo, however, the medulla differentiates into the testes and the cortex regresses.

Development of the Testes

The Y chromosome has a strong testis-determining effect on the medulla of the indifferent gonad.[30] The primary sex cords condense and extend even farther into the medulla. Here they branch, canalize, and anastomose to form a network of tubules, the rete testis. These cords are separated from the surface epithelium by a dense layer of connective tissue, the tunica albuginea. Septa grow from the tunica into the medulla to divide the testis into wedge-shaped lobules. Each lobule contains approximately one to three seminiferous tubules, interstitial cells, and supporting cells.

Canalization of the seminiferous cords results in formation of the walls of the tubules by Sertoli (supporting) cells and spermatogenic (germinal) epithelium, which is derived from the primary germ cells.[30] The Sertoli cells multiply during growth of the cords until they constitute the majority of the epithelium during fetal life and provide nutrients for the maturing spermatids in adult life.[30,37] The Sertoli cells produce müllerian inhibiting substance, which

stimulates involution of the paramesonephric ducts.[32] These cells may also secrete a meiosis-inhibiting factor to inhibit spermatogonia meiosis until puberty.[6]

The process of cellular reorganization is the first step in male differentiation and is most likely controlled by the sex-determining genes associated with the Y chromosome. Several candidates for these genes have been identified: the H-Y (histocompatibility-Y) antigen gene on the long arm of the Y chromosomes; the ZFY gene on the short arm of the Y chromosomes; and, most recently, the SRY gene, also on the short arm of the Y chromosome, which appears most promising as the site of the testes-organizing gene.[6,20,31] The products of this gene result in development of the testicular cords and interstitium from the blastema.[37]

The mesenchyme contributes masses of interstitial cells (Leydig cells), which proliferate between the tubules. These cells produce testosterone and are functional almost immediately. The Leydig cells are highly active in the third through fifth gestational months. The rise in testosterone parallels the increase in Leydig cells; after 18 weeks, the number of Leydig cells and testosterone levels decrease. Testosterone and other androgens induce formation of the male genital ducts and masculinization of the external genitalia. In addition, the Leydig cells suppress the development of the paramesonephric ducts.[30] The testicles start to descend into the inguinal canal during the sixth month, entering the scrotal swellings shortly before birth.[37]

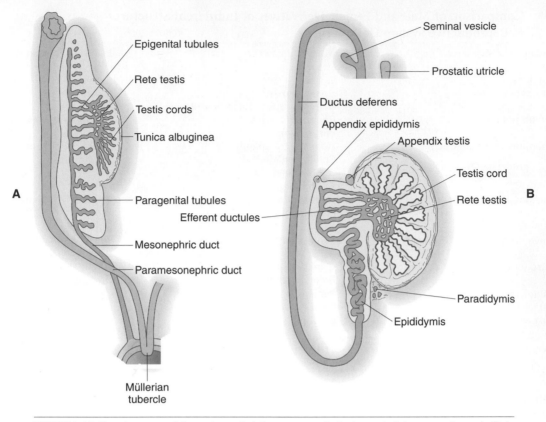

Epigenital tubules

Rete testis

Testis cords

Tunica albuginea

Paragenital tubules

Efferent ductules

Mesonephric duct

Paramesonephric duct

Müllerian
tubercle

A

Seminal vesicle

Prostatic utricle

Ductus deferens

Appendix epididymis

Appendix testis

Testis cord

Rete testis

B

Paradidymis

Epididymis

FIGURE **1-12** Development of the male genital duct system. **A,** At the end of the second month. **B,** In the late fetus. (Modified from Sadler, T. [1990]. *Langman's medical embryology* [6th ed.]. Baltimore: Williams & Wilkins.)

Development of the Ovaries

In XX embryos, gonadal development occurs more slowly; the ovary is not clearly identifiable until 9 to 10 weeks.[30] The primary sex cords do develop and extend into the medulla of the developing ovary but are not prominent and later degenerate. By the twelfth week, the medulla is mainly connective tissue, with scattered groups of cells that represent the prospective rete ovarii.[37] The rete ovarii appears to be derived from migrating mesonephric cells, which may later give rise to the follicular cells.

During the fourth month, secondary sex cords (cortical cords) are thought to grow into the gonad from the germinal epithelium (surface epithelium).[30] As the cortical cords enlarge, the primordial germ cells are incorporated into them. At around 16 weeks the cords begin to break up into clusters, surrounding the primitive ova (oogonia) with a single layer of flattened follicular cells derived from the cortical cords.[30] This complex is the primordial follicle and later develops into the primary follicle once the oocyte is formed (see Chapter 1).[30] The surface epithelium becomes separated from the follicles, which lie in the cortex, by a thin fi-

brous capsule, the tunica albuginea. The ovary, like the testis, separates from the regressing mesonephros, becoming suspended by its own mesentery (mesovarium).[30]

Female gonadal differentiation occurs in the absence of the testes-inducing or -organizing gene on the Y chromosome. There may be an ovarian inducing or organizing gene on the X chromosomes that acts only if the testes-organizing gene on the Y chromosome is not active.[37] For primary ovarian differentiation, only one X chromosome need be present; however, in most 45,X individuals (Turner syndrome) the ovary degenerates before birth.[30,37] Androgen conversion into estrogen has been demonstrated from the fetal age of 8 weeks, although serum increases are not encountered. This may indicate that estrogens act locally, stimulating follicle development.[37] The ovary, probably the rete tissue, secretes a meiosis-inducing substance that inhibits meiosis of the oogonia.[37]

Development of the Genital Ducts

Both male and female embryos have two pairs of genital ducts, the mesonephric (wolffian) duct and the paramesonephric (müllerian) duct (Figures 1-12 and 1-13).

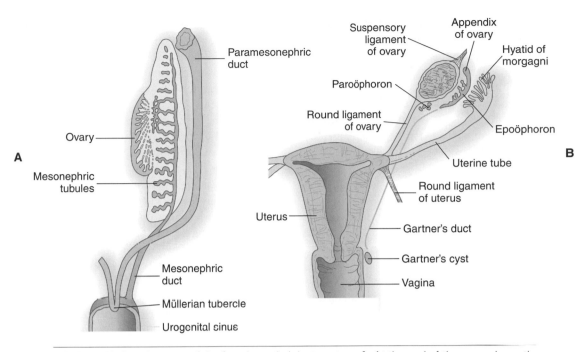

FIGURE **1-13** Development of the female genital duct system. **A,** At the end of the second month. **B,** Mature system. (Modified from Sadler, T. [1990]. *Langman's medical embryology* [6th ed.]. Baltimore: Williams & Wilkins.)

The mesonephric duct originates as part of the urinary system and is incorporated into the developing gonad during the sixth week of gestation. The paramesonephric ducts initially develop alongside the mesonephric ducts in both sexes but reach complete development only in females. The female ducts differentiate autonomously without external regulatory factors, whereas the male system is regulated by testicular androgens and müllerian inhibiting substance.[37]

Indifferent Stage

The mesonephric (wolffian) ducts drain the mesonephric kidneys and develop into the ductus deferens, the epididymis, and the ejaculatory ducts in the male when the second kidney tubules degenerate. In the female the mesonephric ducts almost completely degenerate. The paramesonephric (müllerian) ducts develop bilaterally alongside the mesonephric ducts. The paramesonephric ducts run caudally parallel to the mesonephric ducts, then cross in front of them, fusing to form a Y-shaped canal.[30]

Development of the Male Genital Ducts

Müllerian inhibiting substance stimulates involution of the paramesonephric ducts in the male.[37] Under the influence of testosterone and other androgens, the mesonephric ducts are retained and incorporated into the genital system (see Figure 1-12). The majority of the mesonephric tubules disappear, except those that are in the region of the testes. These 5 to 12 mesonephric tubules lose their glomeruli and join with the rete testis. This creates a communication between the gonads and the mesonephric duct. At this point the tubules are called the efferent ductules; these greatly elongate and become convoluted, making up the majority of the caput epididymis. The mesonephric duct becomes the ductus epididymis in this region. Below this area, the mesonephric duct incorporates muscle tissue and becomes the ductus deferens (vas deferens). The urethra makes up the remainder of the male genital duct system (see Figure 1-12).[22,30]

Development of the Female Genital Ducts

In the female embryo, the mesonephric ducts regress due to lack of testosterone and other androgens, whereas the paramesonephric ducts are retained due to lack of müllerian inhibiting substance (see Figure 1-13). Female sexual development is not dependent upon the presence of ovaries.[30] The paramesonephric ducts become the fallopian tubes, uterus, and proximal vagina in the female. The cranial unfused portions of the paramesonephric ducts develop into the fallopian tubes; the caudal portion fuses to form the uterovaginal primordium. The latter gives rise to the epithelium and glands of the uterus and to the vaginal wall. The endometrial lining and the myometrium are derived from the surrounding mesenchymal tissue. The vaginal epithelium is derived from the endoderm of the urogenital sinus, and the fibromuscular wall of the vagina develops from the uterovaginal primordium. Initially the vagina is a solid cord (the vaginal plate); the vaginal lumen is formed as the central cells of the plate break down.

The broad ligaments are formed from the peritoneal folds that occur during fusion of the paramesonephric ducts. The broad, winglike folds extend from the lateral portions of the uterus to the pelvic wall. The folds of the broad ligaments are continuous with the peritoneum and divide the pelvis into anterior and posterior portions. Between the layers of the broad ligament, the mesenchyme proliferates to form loose connective tissue and smooth muscle. This complex of tissue provides support and attachment for the uterus, fallopian tubes, and ovaries.

Development of the External Genitalia

The early development of the external genitalia is similar in male and female embryos. Distinguishing characteristics can be seen during the ninth week of gestation, with definitive characteristics being fully formed by the twelfth week.[30]

Indifferent Stage

The external genitalia initially appear similar. Early in the fourth week, a swelling can be identified at the cranial end of the cloacal membrane; this is the genital tubercle. Labioscrotal swellings and urogenital folds soon develop alongside the cloacal membrane. The genital tubercle elongates at this time and is the same length in both sexes. The urorectal septum fuses with the cloacal membrane, dividing the membrane into a dorsal anal membrane and a ventral urogenital membrane. These membranes rupture around the eighth week, forming the anus and urogenital orifice. The urethral groove, which is continuous with the urogenital orifice, forms on the ventral surface of the genital tubercle at this time (Figures 1-14 and 1-15).[30]

Development of the Male External Genitalia

The androgens produced by the fetal testes induce the masculinization of the external genitalia of the male embryo. The genital tubercle continues to elongate, forming the penis and pulling the urogenital folds forward. This results in the development of the lateral walls of the urethral groove

by the urogenital folds (see Figure 1-14). The posterior-to-anterior fusion of the urogenital folds as they come in contact results in the development of the spongy urethra and the progressive movement of the urethral orifice toward the glans of the penis. The opening, however, remains on the undersurface of the phallus.[30] Backward growth of a plate of ectodermal tissue from the tip of the phallus to the urethra forms the terminal part of the urethra. Once canalized, the urinary and reproductive systems will have achieved an open system. This, along with the descent of the testes into the genital swellings (scrotum), completes the development of the external genitalia (see Figure 1-14).

After the penile urethra has formed, the connective tissue surrounding the urethra becomes condensed to form the corpus cavernosum urethrae, in which numerous wide and convoluted blood vessels having many arteriovenous anastomoses develop. The labioscrotal swellings also grow toward each other and fuse to form the scrotum. Tissue swelling occurs in order to dilate the inguinal canal and scrotum in preparation for the descent of the testes in the seventh or eighth month of gestation.

Descent of the testes is moderated by many forces, including the enlargement of the pelvis, trunk growth, and the testes' remaining relatively stationary, as well as the influence of gonadotropins and androgens.[30] At about 32 weeks, the testes actually enter the scrotum. Once passage is complete, the inguinal canal contracts around the spermatic cord. The spermatic cord consists of the vas deferens, blood vessels, and nerves. In most situations (97% of cases), the testes have descended bilaterally before delivery. During the first 3 months following delivery, the majority of undescended testes will descend without intervention.[30]

Development of the Female External Genitalia

Without androgens, feminization of the neutral external genitalia occurs. Initially the genital tubercle grows rapidly; however, it gradually slows, becoming the relatively small clitoris. The clitoris develops like the penis, except that the urogenital folds do not fuse. Both the urethra and the vagina open into the common vestibule, which is widely open after the disappearance of the urogenital membrane. The opening is flanked by the urethral folds and the genital swellings, which become the labia minora and majora, respectively (see Figure 1-15).

CLINICAL IMPLICATIONS
Common Anomalies of the Genital Tract

Anomalies encountered in the reproductive systems may be secondary to any of three major factors: (1) genetic makeup, (2) endocrine and hormonal environment, and

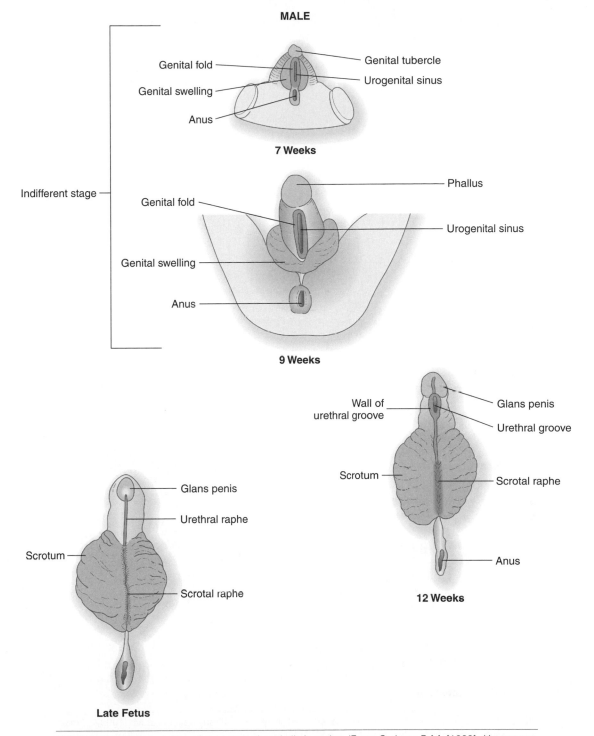

FIGURE **1-14** Differentiation of the external genitalia in males. (From Carlson, B.M. [1999]. *Human embryology* & *developmental biology* [2nd ed.]. St Louis: Mosby.)

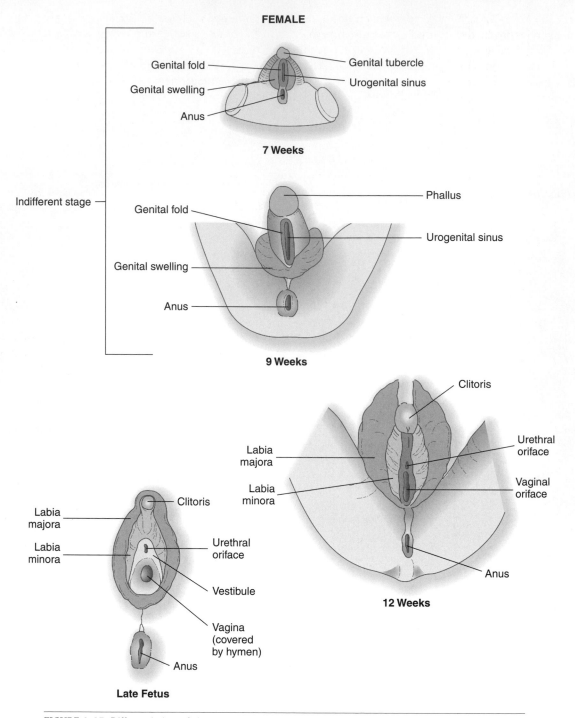

FIGURE **1-15** Differentiation of the external genitalia in females. (From Carlson, B.M. [1999]. *Human embryology & developmental biology* [2nd ed.]. St Louis: Mosby.)

(3) mechanical events. Each may lead to alterations in development and reproductive ability. Because the embryo is bipotential, when genetic or hormonal factors alter development, the embryo may develop various degrees of intermediate sex (intersexuality or hermaphroditism). True hermaphrodites have both ovarian and testicular tissue, whereas pseudohermaphrodites have either one or the other but have incongruence between chromosomal sex and gonadal sex. True hermaphroditism is extremely rare, and pseudohermaphroditism occurs only once in 25,000 births.[29,30] Table 1-6 provides a classification of intersexuality. Mechanical congenital anomalies are somewhat more common and are related to developmental arrests, interference, or failures that result in changes in normal morphologic patterns.

Disorders of Gonadal Development

Gonadal agenesis. Absence of one or both gonads is a rare disorder. If gonadal agenesis is unilateral, absence of the renal system on the affected side is common.[37] Failure or defective development of nephrogenic mesenchyme is probably the cause, although the etiology of such failure is not known.

Gonadal dysgenesis (Turner syndrome). One of the most common sex chromosome abnormalities is Turner syndrome. This syndrome is seen in an estimated 0.8% to 1% of spontaneously aborted fetuses and once in every 4000 to 5000 live births. The absence or deletion of an X chromosome usually results in an individual with a 45, XO karyotype, with 80% due to paternal nondisjunction.[20,31] Mosaics (46,XX/45, XO) often have functioning ovaries. In most other cases, however, there is ovarian dysgenesis associated with other somatic abnormalities.[20]

Hermaphroditism. Hermaphrodites are extremely rare; chromosomal constitution may be either 46,XX; 46,XY; or mosaic XX/XY. These individuals have both ovaries and testes, either as separate organs or as a single ovotestis. Usually the gonadal tissue is not functional, but in some individuals oogenesis and spermiogenesis may occur simultaneously. The external genitalia are ambiguous, but the rest of the physical appearance may be either male or female. This abnormality seems to be the result of an error in sexual determination and lack of dominance of the cortex or medulla of the genital ridge.[29,30] Possible causes include translocation of testicular differentiation genes to the X chromosome, a mutant gene, or undetected XY cells in

---

TABLE **1-6** Classification of Intersexuality

DISORDERS OF GONADAL DEVELOPMENT	Male pseudohermaphroditism, with partial failure of virilization
Kleinfelter syndrome	Abnormalities of müllerian inhibiting factor synthesis
Gonadal dysgenesis	or action
Turner syndrome	Defects in testosterone action
Mosaicism	Complete androgen-binding protein deficiency
Structural abnormality of the second X chromosome	(complete testicular feminization)
Normal karyotype (pure gonadal dysgenesis)	Partial defects of androgen cytosol receptors
True hermaphroditism	(incomplete testicular feminization; familial
Male pseudohermaphroditism	incomplete male pseudohermaphroditism type I)
Primary gonadal defect	5α-Reductase deficiency (familial incomplete male
Y chromosomal defect	pseudohermaphroditism type II)
DISORDERS OF FETAL ENDOCRINOLOGY	Testosterone biosynthesis defect
Female pseudohermaphroditism with partial virilization	Pregnenolone synthesis defect (lipid adrenal
Congenital adrenal hyperplasia	hyperplasia)
21-Hydroxylase deficiency without salt wasting	3β-Hydroxysteroid dehydrogenase deficiency
21-Hydroxylase deficiency with salt wasting	17α-Hydroxylase deficiency
11β-Hydroxylase deficiency (hypertensive)	17,20-Desmolase deficiency
3β-ol Dehydrogenase deficiency	17β-Hydroxysteroid dehydrogenase deficiency
Nonadrenal female pseudohermaphroditism	
Maternal androgenization	
Exogenous androgen	
Virilizing tumors	
Idiopathic	

From Mishell, D.R. & Goebelsmann, U. (1991). Disorders of sexual differentiation. In D.R. Mishell, V. Davajan, & R.A. Lobo (Eds.). *Infertility, contraception & reproductive endocrinology* (3rd ed.). Boston: Blackwell Scientific Publishers.

the gonad. The presence of uterus and fallopian tubes indicates defective functioning of müllerian inhibiting substance. In those individuals who are mosaic 46,XX/XY, the etiology involves the union of two zygotes of different genetic sex. The two cell lines develop normally, limits being set by their topographic distribution during ontogeny.[37]

Disorders of Fetal Endocrinology

Male pseudohermaphroditism. These male infants have more or less dysgenetic testes with an XY constitution. There is incomplete differentiation of the external genitalia secondary to testicular dysgenesis and insufficient testosterone production.[20] This abnormality may be associated with ambisexual internal genitalia due to inadequate production of müllerian substance.[20] Causes may include a deficiency in the 5α-reductase enzyme necessary to convert testosterone to dihydrotestosterone so that external virilization can occur. In testicular feminization syndrome, there is an inability to bind androgens in target tissues; in other situations, transmission of androgens from the receptor to the nucleus is blocked.[20,30]

Externally the genitalia may be either ambiguous or feminine. Internal structures may also vary. These male infants have varying degrees of phallic and paramesonephric duct development, even though their karyotype is 46,XY. When differentiation occurs, males with 5α-reductase deficiencies have testosterone and its derivatives in the external genitalia tissue but not in the developing mesonephric duct. It would seem that testosterone appears in the mesonephric ducts after the period of tissue sensitivity has passed.[20,30]

Males with the X-linked gene for testicular feminization (46,XY) have normally differentiated testes; however, these children look like normal females. The vagina ends in a blind pouch, and the uterus and fallopian tubes are nonexistent or rudimentary.[30] The testes are usually intraabdominal or inguinal, or they may descend into the labia majora. There are high levels of circulating testosterone with elevated levels of gonadotropins. Unfortunately, testosterone receptor sites will not bind or incorporate testosterone into the cells at the labioscrotal and urogenital folds.[30] These individuals may represent an extreme form of male pseudohermaphroditism.[30] They have female genitalia, and at puberty there is development of female secondary sex characteristics; however, menstruation does not occur. The psychosexual orientation of these children is female.[20,30]

Female pseudohermaphroditism. The chromosome composition of these female infants is 46,XX, but there is congenital virilization of the external genitalia. This is usually termed *adrenogenital syndrome* or *congenital adrenal hyperplasia* (CAH), meaning hyperfunction of the adrenal cortices associated with ambiguous genitalia. The most common cause is an excessive production of androgens, which may be due to maternal disease (e.g., adrenal tumor) but is more likely to be of fetal origin. Lack of 21-hydroxylase (an enzyme involved in steroid metabolism) is usually the cause of CAH.

Most often these cases involve clitoral hypertrophy, partial fusion of the labia majora, and a persistent urogenital sinus. The infants who are afflicted with this syndrome do have functioning ovaries, fallopian tubes, uterus, and cervix. The mesonephric duct does not develop. Often there are other metabolic disorders that require complex care.[20] (CAH is described in more detail in Chapter 18.)

Hypospadias and Epispadias

Hypospadias (urethral orifice on the ventral surface of the penis) may be an isolated abnormality or a variety of pseudohermaphroditism, especially if the penis is very abnormal. The more severe the degree of hypospadias is, the higher the possibility of testicular dysgenesis and of cryptorchidism. This defect occurs once in every 300 live births and is probably due to inadequate androgen production, resulting in failure of urogenital fold fusion and incomplete spongy urethra formation.[30] There are four types of hypospadias, with 80% being either glandular or penile. The other 20% are penoscrotal or perineal. Variations in this defect are due to the timing and degree of hormonal failure.[6,30]

Epispadias is a relatively rare congenital anomaly, occurring once in every 30,000 live births. The dorsal surface urethral opening is often associated with exstrophy of the bladder. Epispadias may be glandular or penile and is probably due to caudal development of the genital tubercle, resulting in the urogenital sinus's being on the dorsal surface once the membrane has ruptured.[6,30]

Uterovaginal Malformation

Fusion defects of the paramesonephric ducts result in varying degrees of structural duplication. Complete fusion failure leads to the development of two complete genital tracts, in which the vagina is divided in two by a septum, with a separate cervix and uterine body associated with each half (didelphia). If one of the paramesonephric ducts fails to develop entirely, the result will be uterus unicornis. Various other anomalies may also result, including a single vagina with double cervices, a single vagina and cervix associated with a uterus subdivided into halves, or a single uterus that is incompletely separated by a septum (bicornate, unicornous, vagina simplex). Any of these anomalies may result in infertility.[30]

Prenatal Screening and Diagnosis

Genetic screening and use of diagnostic techniques such as amniocentesis and chorionic villus sampling (CVS) allow for prenatal identification of increasing numbers of chromosomal, genetic, and other congenital anomalies. These techniques, along with ultrasound and percutaneous umbilical cord blood sampling, are discussed in this section. Timing of these techniques is illustrated in Figure 1-16. Recent documentation of fetal DNA in maternal plasma may lead to new techniques in the future.[26] All of these techniques are associated with increased parental anxiety and concern.[13,45]

Prenatal Screening

Several techniques are available for prenatal screening: history, first trimester screening, second trimester screening, and routine ultrasound. A genetic history should be a routine part of prenatal care to identify women with an increased risk of genetic disorders and birth defects.

Components of genetic history include family and obstetric history (including a history of pregnancy loss or early infant death, mental retardation or learning disabilities, known genetic disorders, or having infants with anomalies in either of the parents or their families), ethnic background (some recessive disorders occur with markedly increased frequency in specific ethnic groups), maternal and paternal age, and potential teratogen exposures.[15,40,41] Routine ultrasounds provide an opportunity to observe for major anomalies in the fetus. Ultrasound markers that may allow noninvasive diagnosis have also been identified for infants with Down syndrome.[2,48,49]

First trimester screening. First trimester screening is a recently developed technique that is being used in some areas, although additional research is ongoing. Methods include maternal serum screening and ultrasound for increased nuchal translucency (due to accumulation of fluid behind the fetal neck).[2,43,48,49] Maternal serum is screened for the free beta subunit of human chorionic gonadotropin

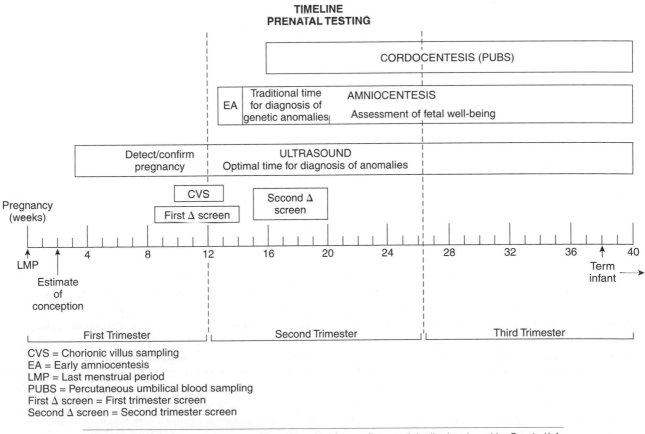

FIGURE **1-16** Timeline for prenatal testing. (Modified from a figure originally developed by Brock, K.A. [1990]. Seattle: University of Washington.)

(hCG) and pregnancy-associated plasma protein P (PAPP-P) from 8½ to 13 weeks. Altered levels may indicate Down syndrome or trisomy 18, with reported detection rates of 68% to 70% for Down syndrome and 90% for trisomy 18. Addition of nuchal translucency reportedly increases the detection rate to 88% to 91% for Down syndrome and as high as 97% for trisomy 18.[8,15,17,42] Nuchal translucency may also be useful in early diagnosis of some congenital heart defects.[10] First trimester screening does not screen for neural tube or ventral wall defects.

Second trimester screening. Second trimester screening has become a standard of prenatal care.[36] Second trimester screening is called maternal serum multiple marker screening (MMS), enhanced or expanded maternal serum α-fetoprotein screening, triple screen, or quad screen (depending on the components used).[18] Screening is done on maternal serum at 15 to 20 weeks (optimum is 16 to 18½ weeks). Different combinations (2, 3, or 4) of components are used. The most common screen involves three components: α-fetoprotein (AFP), unconjugated estriol (uE3), and the free beta subunit of hCG. Recently, inhibin A has been added (i.e., in quad screen) in some settings, which reportedly may lower false positive rates or increased detection of fetuses with Down syndrome.[1,7] Maternal serum MMS is used to screen for Down syndrome, trisomy 18, and neural tube defect (spina bifida and anencephaly). Some infants with Turner syndrome may also be identified.[39] AFP and hCG are most useful in screening for Down syndrome, whereas AFP is most useful for screening for neural tube defects (see Chapter 14).[54] AFP may also be elevated in infants with ventral wall defects such as omphalocele and gastroschisis, esophageal atresia, and renal nephrosis. Each laboratory has its own cut-off for positive screen, so results are usually reported in multiples of the median (MoM). Abnormal values are generally greater than 0.5 and less than 2.5 MoM.[51,54] About 100 in 1000 women will have a positive screen; of these women, only 2 or 3 will have a fetus with a defect.[19] Factors that can influence screen results include maternal age, race and weight, gestational age, and maternal diabetes. If a woman has a positive screen, follow-up ultrasound and/or amniocentesis is indicated.[45,58] Reported detection rates with second trimester screening are 50% to 60% of trisomy 18, 60% of Down syndrome, 80% of spina bifida, and 90% of anencephaly.[3,15,16] Addition of inhibin A is reported to increase detection rates for Down syndrome by 7%.[8] Increased levels of AFP and hCG in women with normal fetuses have been associated with an increased risk of stillbirth, abruption, preterm labor, pregnancy-induced hypertension, miscarriage, and low birthweight.[54] Similarly, decreased uE3 has been associated with increased risk of pregnancy-induced hypertension, intrauterine growth restriction, miscarriage, and intrauterine fetal death.[54]

Prenatal Diagnosis

The goal of prenatal diagnosis is to provide parents the assurance that they will have a child who is unaffected by the specific disorders being evaluated. Most women participate in prenatal testing for reassurance; 90% to 95% will have a normal fetus. If an abnormality is identified, prenatal diagnosis provides parents with an opportunity to prepare for the birth of an affected infant; plan for delivery, care, and management of the infant; or elect to terminate the pregnancy. In some cases, early diagnosis provides options for fetal therapy, such as surgical intervention for urinary tract obstructions to reduce prenatal renal damage, transfusions for hematologic conditions, or pharmacologic interventions (see Chapter 6).[14] Indications for prenatal diagnosis include maternal age greater than 35; paternal age greater than 50 or 55; history of two or more miscarriages; previous pregnancy or family history of genetic or chromosomal disorder; parents who are known or suspected carriers of a specific genetic disorder; previous child or family history of a neural tube or other birth defect, especially defects known to have a multifactorial inheritance pattern; exposure to known teratogens; and women with positive first or second trimester screening results.[28,35,40,53]

Amniotic fluid analysis and amniocentesis. Cellular and biochemical components of amniotic fluid change with gestational age and are useful indicators of fetal maturity and well-being. Amniotic fluid samples are removed via amniocentesis, and the constituents are examined. Amniotic fluid contains cells from the amnion, fetal skin, buccal and bladder mucosa, and tracheal lining. Amniotic fluid cells can be examined early in pregnancy to determine fetal sex (important with sex-linked disorders) and to diagnose genetic and chromosomal disorders. Later, cellular and biochemical components of amniotic fluid can be used to evaluate fetal health and maturity, including fetal lung maturity (Chapter 9).

Genetic amniocentesis has traditionally been performed in most centers at 15 to 16 weeks (range, 14 to 20 weeks) (see Figure 1-16), because at this time amniotic fluid volume has reached 150 to 250 ml (so approximately 20 ml can easily and safely be removed), the uterus has reached the pelvic brim (so a transabdominal approach can be used), adequate fetal cells are available, diagnostic studies can be completed in time for a second trimester abortion (if that option is chosen by the parents), and the incidence of maternal and fetal complication (spotting, fluid leak, bleeding, infection, spontaneous abortion) is relatively low.[52] Rapid detection of trisomies 21, 13, and 18 and alterations in sex chromosome numbers can be obtained within 24 hours using fluorescent in situ hybridization (FISH) techniques with uncultured cells.[38,52] Amniotic fluid can be cultured for karyotype (to identify chromosomal abnormalities) or for biochemical assay (to identify specific inherited metabolic disorders), analyzed using DNA hybridization and restriction enzyme techniques (for detecting gene deletions that occur with disorders such as hemoglobinopathies), and analyzed for quantification of (α-fetoprotein (screening for neural tube defects and other anomalies).[44] Early amniocentesis before 14 to 15 weeks is also used in some centers.[11,12] An increased risk of fetal loss, amniotic fluid leakage, and talipes equinovarus has been reported with early amniocentesis performed before the thirteenth week.[52]

Chorionic villus sampling. CVS is an alternative to genetic amniocentesis. CVS is generally performed 10 to 13 weeks after the last menstrual period (see Figure 1-16). Earlier, chorionic villi may not be sufficiently developed for adequate tissue sampling and risk of limb anomalies is increased; later the chorion laeve is disappearing and the chorion frondosum is forming the definitive placenta (see Chapter 3).[4,9,32] A transcervical approach is used (because the uterus is still in the pelvis) after the gestational sac and implantation site are located by ultrasound. Transabdominal approaches have also been used.

Living trophoblast tissue is aspirated from several sites on the chorion. This tissue can be analyzed for chromosome anomalies or with enzyme assay (for inborn errors of metabolism) or DNA analysis (hemoglobinopathies).[32,40] Advantages of CVS include early diagnosis before the pregnancy is obvious to others and, for some assays, a decreased waiting period for results. Disadvantages include a risk of spontaneous abortion, infection, bleeding, and amniotic fluid leakage; uncertainty about long-term effects on the infant; and inability to do α-fetoprotein assays for diagnosis of neural tube defects at this stage of gestation.[40,45,52] In addition, CVS before 10 weeks' gestation has been associated with an increased risk of limb defects and is not recommended.[52] Wilson concludes that, although not without risk, CVS between 10 and 13 weeks appears to be a safer alternative for first-trimester prenatal diagnosis than early amiocentesis.[52]

Umbilical blood sampling. *Cordocentesis,* or percutaneous umbilical blood sampling (PUBS), involves use of the umbilical cord to obtain fetal blood samples. Umbilical blood sampling has been used in the prenatal diagnosis of inherited blood disorders (hemoglobinopathies and coagulopathies), in detection of congenital infection, to assess fetal anemia (in Rh isoimmunization and in thrombocytopenia), and in fetal therapy such as blood transfusions.[9,33] This technique is performed using real-time ultrasound as early as 16 weeks after the last menstrual period (Figure 1-16).[9] Complications include infection, preterm labor, bleeding, thrombosis, and transient fetal arrhythmia.

SUMMARY

The biologic basis for reproduction includes an understanding of basic genetic mechanisms and principles, including cell division, gametogenesis, chromosomal and genetic alterations, and modes of inheritance. Our knowledge in these areas remains limited but is increasing rapidly. The current revolution in genetic knowledge has markedly altered and challenged our understanding of health and disease and provision of health care, and it will continue to do so. The more nurses and other health care providers understand about the areas and the reproductive processes described in Chapter 2, the more they can work toward ways to improve perinatal outcome. (Clinical implications for mothers and neonates can be found in Table 1-7.)

TABLE **1-7**   Chromosomes and Reproductive Biology: Clinical Implications for the Care of Mothers and Neonates

Understand the biologic basis for genetic and chromosomal disorders (pp. 9-15).
Understand modes of inheritance (pp. 15-19; see also Tables 1-3 and 1-4).
Provide counseling and health teaching to parents regarding genetic disorders and modes of inheritance (pp. 15-19 and Table 1-1).
Perform a genetic history as part of routine care (p. 29).
Counsel parents about prenatal screening and assist them in interpreting results (pp. 29-30).
Provide support to families undergoing prenatal diagnosis (pp. 29-31).
Understand the bases and risks of prenatal diagnostic tests (pp. 29-31).
Teach parents with a familial history of chromosomal or genetic abnormalities about the basis for the disorder (pp. 15-19).
Refer parents with a familial history of chromosomal or genetic abnormalities for genetic counseling (pp. 15-19).
Refer neonates born with abnormal genitalia for complete endocrine evaluation, ultrasonography of internal structures, and chromosomal assessment (pp. 24-29).

REFERENCES

1. Aitken, D.A., et al. (1996). Dimeric Inhibin A as a marker for Down's syndrome in early pregnancy. *N Engl J Med, 334,* 1231.
2. Bahado-Singh, R., et al. (1998). An alternative for women initially declining genetic amniocentesis: Individual Down syndrome odds on the basis of maternal age and multiple ultrasonographic markers. *Am J Obstet Gynecol, 179,* 514.
3. Benn, P.A., et al. (1999). Maternal serum screening for fetal trisomy 18: A comparison of fixed cutoff and patient specific risk protocol. *Obstet Gynecol, 93,* 707.
4. Blackmore, K.J. (1988). Prenatal diagnosis by CVS. *Obstet Gynecol Clin North Am, 15,* 179.
5. Buster, J.E. & Saurer, M.V. (1989). Endocrinology of conception. In S.A. Brody & K. Ueland (Eds.). *Endocrine disorders in pregnancy.* Norwalk, CT: Appleton & Lange.
6. Carlson, B.M. (1999). *Human embryology & developmental biology* (2nd ed.), St. Louis: Mosby.
7. Cuckle, H.S., et al. (1996). Combining Inhibin A with existing second-trimester markers in maternal serum screening for Down's syndrome. *Prenatal Diag, 16,* 1095-1100.
8. Cuckle, H. (2000). Biochemical screening for Down syndrome. *Eur J Obstet Gynecol Reprod Biol, 92,* 97.
9. Daffos, F. (1989). Access to the other patient. *Semin Perinatol, 13,* 252.
10. Devine, P.C. & Simpson, L.L. (2000). Nuchal translucency and its relation to congenital heart disease. *Semin Perinatol, 24,* 343.
11. Evans, M.I., Johnson, M.P., & Drugan, A. (1990). Amniocentesis. In R.D. Eden & F.H. Boehm (Eds.). *Assessment and care of the fetus.* Norwalk, CT: Appleton & Lange.
12. Evans, M.I., et al. (1988). Early genetic amniocentesis and chorionic villus sampling. *J Reprod Med, 33,* 450.
13. Filly, R.A. (2000). Obstetrical sonography: The best way to terrify a pregnant woman. *J Ultrasound Med, 19,* 1.
14. Flake, A.W. (1999). Fetal therapy: medical and surgical approaches. In R.K. Creasy & R. Resnik (Eds.). *Maternal-fetal medicine: Principles and practice* (4th ed.). Philadelphia: W.B. Saunders.
15. Grant, S. (2000, September 30). Prenatal genetic screening. *Online J Issues Nurs, 5*(3), 3. Available online at www.nursingworld.org/ojin/topic13/tpc13_3.htm.
16. Haddow, J.E., et al. (1992). Prenatal screening for Down syndrome with the use of maternal serum markers. *N Engl J Med, 327,* 588.
17. Haddow, J.E., et al. (1998). Screening of maternal serum for fetal Down's syndrome in the first trimester. *N Engl J Med, 338,* 955.
18. Haddow, J.E. & Palomaki, G.E. (1999). Biochemical screening for neural tube defects and Down syndrome. In C.H. Rodeck & M.J. Whittle (Eds.). *Fetal medicine: Basic science and clinical practice.* London: Churchill-Livingstone.
19. Hall, S., et al. (2000). Psychological consequences for parents of false negative results on prenatal screening for Down's syndrome: Retrospective interview study. *BMJ, 320,* 407.
20. Jaffe, R.B. (1999). Disorders of sexual development. In S.S.C. Yen, R.B. Jaffe, & R.L. Barbieri (Eds.). *Reproductive endocrinology: Physiology, pathophysiology and clinical management* (4th ed.). Philadelphia: W.B. Saunders.
21. Jones, O.W. & Cahill, T.C. (1999). Basic genetics and patterns of inheritance. In R.K. Creasy & R. Resnik (Eds.). *Maternal-fetal medicine: Principles and practice* (4th ed.). Philadelphia: W.B. Saunders.
22. Jorde. L.B., et al. (1999) *Medical genetics* (2nd ed.). St. Louis: Mosby.
23. Kalousek, D.K. & Vekemons, M. (2000). Confirmed placental mosaicism and genomic imprinting. *Baillieres Best Pract Res Clin Obstet Gynecol, 14,* 723.
24. Lashley, F.R. (1998). *Clinical genetics in nursing practice* (2nd ed.). New York: Springer.
25. Levine, F. (1998). Genetics. In R.A. Polin & W.W. Fox (Eds.). *Fetal and neonatal physiology* (2nd ed.). Philadelphia: W.B. Saunders.
26. Lo, Y.M.D. (2000). Fetal DNA in maternal plasma: Biology and diagnostic applications. *Clin Chem, 46,* 1903.
27. Lyon, M.K. (1999). X-chromosome inactivation. *Curr Biol, 9,* R235.
28. Mahoney, M. (1999). Genetic and post-pregnancy counseling. In C.H. Rodeck & M.J. Whittle (Eds.). *Fetal medicine: Basic science and clinical practice.* London: Churchill-Livingstone.
29. Mishell, D.R. & Goebelsmann, U. (1986). Disorders of sexual differentiation. In D.R. Mishell & V. Davajan (Eds.). *Infertility, contraception & reproductive endocrinology* (2nd ed.). Oradell, NJ: Medical Economics Books.
30. Moore, K.L. & Persaud, T.V.N. (1998). *The developing human: Clinically oriented embryology* (6th ed.). Philadelphia: W.B. Saunders.
31. Morton, C.L. & Miron, P. (1999). Cytogenetics in reproduction. In S.S.C. Yen, R.B. Jaffe, & R.L. Barbieri (Eds.). *Reproductive endocrinology: Physiology, pathophysiology and clinical management* (4th ed.). Philadelphia: W.B. Saunders.
32. Newton, E.R. (1989). The fetus as patient. *Med Clin North Am, 73,* 517.
33. Nicolaides, K.H., Thorpe, J.G. & Noble, P. (1990). Cordocentesis. In R.D. Eden & F.H. Boehm (Eds.). *Assessment and care of the fetus.* Norwalk, CT: Appleton & Lange.
34. Nicolaidis, P. & Peterson, M.B. (1998). Origin and mechanisms of non-disjunction in human autosomal trisomies. *Hum Reprod, 13,* 313.
35. O'Connor, M.A. (1997). Fetal maternal case management. *Nursing Case Management, 2,* 55-67.
36. Palomaki, G.E., et.al. (1997). Maternal serum screening for Down syndrome in the United States: A 1995 survey. *Am J Obstet Gynecol, 176,* 1046.
37. Pelliniemi, L. & Dym, M. (1994). The fetal gonad and sexual differentiation. In D. Tulchinsky & A.B. Little (Eds.). *Maternal-fetal endocrinology* (2nd ed.). Philadelphia: W.B. Saunders.
38. Pergament, E. (2000). New molecular techniques for chromosome analysis. *Baillieres Best Pract Res Clin Obstet Gynaecol, 14*(4), 677.
39. Ruiz, C., et al. (1999). Turner syndrome and multiple-marker screening. *Clin Chem, 45,* 2259.
40. Scioscia, A.L. (1999). Prenatal genetic diagnosis. In R.K. Creasy & R. Resnik (Eds.). *Maternal-fetal medicine: Principles and practice* (4th ed.). Philadelphia: W.B. Saunders.
41. Seashore, M.R. (1999). Clinical genetics. In G.N. Burrow & T.F. Ferris (Eds.). *Medical complications during pregnancy* (5th ed.). Philadelphia: W.B. Saunders.
42. Spencer, K., et al. (1999). A screening program for trisomy 21 at 10-14 weeks using fetal nuchal translucency, maternal serum free beta-human chorionic gonadotropin and pregnancy-associated plasma protein A. *Ultrasound Obstet Gynecol, 13,* 231.
43. Stewart, T.L. & Malone, F.D. (1999). First trimester screening for aneuploidy: nuchal translucency sonography. *Semin Perinatol, 23,* 369.
44. Thomas, R.L. & Blakemore, K.J. (1990). Evaluation of elevations in maternal serum alpha-fetoprotein: A review. *Obstet Gynecol Surv, 45,* 269.
45. Tymstra, T. (1991). Prenatal diagnosis, prenatal screening and the rise of the tentative pregnancy. *Int J Technol Assess Health Care, 7*(4), 509.
46. Vander, A., Sherman, J. & Luciano, D. (2000). *Human physiology: The mechanism of body function* (8th ed.). New York: McGraw-Hill.
47. Venter, J.C., et al. (2001). The sequence of the human genome. *Science, 291,* 1304.

48. Vintzileos, A.M., et al. (1997). Choice of second-trimester genetic sonogram for detection of trisomy 21. *Obstet Gynecol, 90,* 187.

49. Vintzileos, A.M., et al. (1999). Indication-specific accuracy of second trimester genetic ultrasonography for the detection of trisomy 21. *Am J Obstet Gynecol, 181,* 1045.

50. Wagstaff, J. (2000). Genetics beyond Mendel. Understanding nontraditional inheritance patterns. *Postgrad Med, 108,* 131.

51. Wald, N.J., et al. (2000). Assay precision of serum alpha fetoprotein in antenatal screening for neural tube defects and Down's syndrome. *J Med Screen, 7,* 74.

52. Wilson, R.D. (2000). Amniocentesis and chorionic villus sampling. *Curr Opin Obstet Gynecol, 12,* 81.

53. Wright, L. (1994). Prenatal diagnosis in the 1990s. J *Obstet Gynecol Neonatal Nurs, 23,* 506.

54. Yaran, Y., et al. (1999). Second-trimester maternal serum marker screening: maternal serum alpha-fetoprotein, beta-human chorionic gonadotropin, estriol and their various combinations as predictors of pregnancy outcome. *Am J Obstet Gynecol, 181,*968.

Physiologic Basis for Reproduction

HYPOTHALAMIC-PITUITARY-OVARIAN AXIS

During reproductive life, ovarian function is regulated by cyclic reproductive neuroendocrinology, which is dependent upon the complex interplay of a feedback system involving the ovary, hypothalamus, and anterior pituitary. Expression of hypothalamic-pituitary hormones stimulates ovarian steroid secretion and subsequent folliculogenesis (Figure 2-1). These gonadotropins (follicle-stimulating hormone [FSH] and luteinizing hormone [LH]) and gonadal steroids (estrogen and progesterone) evoke follicular maturation, ovulation, and pregnancy. Thus a woman's reproductive status is entrained to her cyclic neuroendocrine environment.

Hormones

A hormone is a chemical substance secreted into body fluids by a cell or a group of cells that exerts a physiologic effect on other cells of the body, its target cells. Hormones are released into the bloodstream by endocrine glands. The blood carries the hormones to specific cells or organs, hormonal target sites. Thus far, over 50 hormones have been identified. Hormones regulate differentiation of the reproductive and central nervous system in the developing fetus; stimulation of sequential growth and development during childhood and adolescence; and coordination of male and female reproductive systems. Hormones facilitate sexual reproduction; maintenance of an optimal internal environment; and initiation of corrective and adaptive responses with emergencies.[73] These important physiologic processes are regulated by two major systems: the nervous system and the hormonal system (Figure 2-2). Hormonal regulation of reproductive processes is via the hypothalamic-pituitary-ovarian system in the female and the hypothalamic-pituitary-testes system in the male.

Hypothalamic and Pituitary Glands

The pituitary gland, also known as the hypophysis, is composed of two segments: the anterior and posterior lobes (Figure 2-3). The hypophysis is pea sized and approximately 15 mm long, sitting in a protected saddle-shaped sphenoid bone cavity (the sella turcica) at the base of the brain, directly behind the nasal base. The pituitary gland is slightly heavier in women and may double in size during pregnancy. The pars tuberalis, pars distalis, and the intermediate lobe comprise the anterior lobe, the adenohypophysis.[22] The neurohypophysis (i.e., posterior lobe) is composed of the median eminence, infundibular stem, and neural lobe.[22]

Most hormones are secreted by the anterior pituitary, including growth hormone, adrenocorticotropin, thyroid-stimulating hormone, FSH, LH, and prolactin. Specific to reproductive physiology, anterior pituitary gland cells known as *gonadotrophs* secrete FSH and LH. About 60% of gonadotrophs (5% to 10% of pituitary cells) are multihormonal, secreting both FSH and LH.[62] Only two hormones are secreted by the posterior hormone: antidiuretic hormone and oxytocin.

To regulate physiologic processes, communication must occur between the pituitary gland, the hypothalamus, and the target glands and cells. The pituitary gland connects to the hypothalamus directly above the pituitary stalk. The anterior pituitary gland is linked to the hypothalamus via blood vessels known as the hypothalamic-hypophyseal portal system (Figure 2-3). The pituitary receives blood from the paired superior hypophyseal arteries, which arise from the internal carotid arteries and merge at the upper pituitary stalk.[74] The inferior hypophysial arteries supply the neural lobe.[74] The anterior pituitary sinusoids receive blood from the hypophyseal portal vessels that arise in the median hypothalamic eminence.

Hypothalamic hormones are either releasing hormones (RHs) or inhibiting hormones (IHs), which control expression of the anterior pituitary hormones. RHs and IHs are discharged into the blood vessels of the hypothalamic-hypophyseal portal system. The vascular system permits transport of gonadotropin-releasing hormones (GnRHs) from the hypothalamus down the pituitary stalk to the anterior pituitary lobe, where they trigger

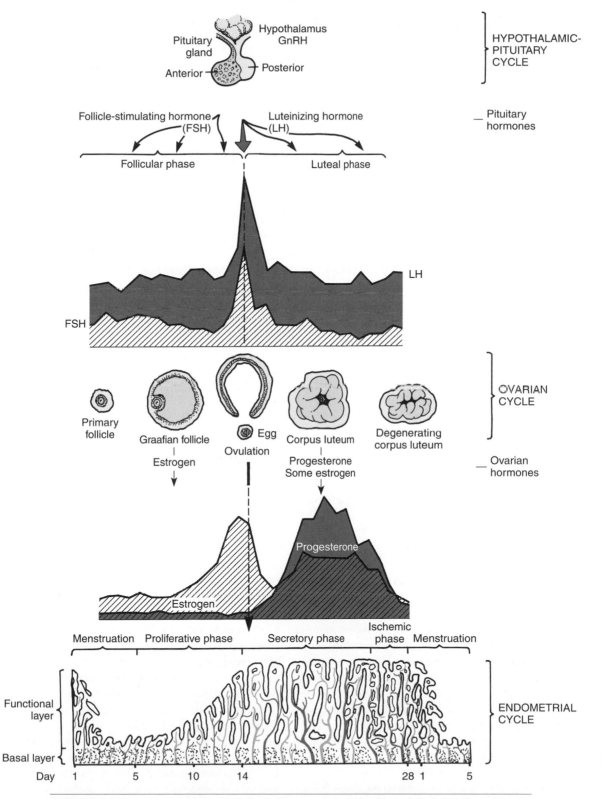

FIGURE **2-1** Menstrual cycle: hypothalamic-pituitary, ovarian, and endometrial. *GnRH,* Gonadotropin-releasing hormone. (From Lowdermilk, D.L., Perry, S.E. & Bobak, I.M. [2000]. *Maternity and women's health care* [7th ed.]. St. Louis: Mosby.)

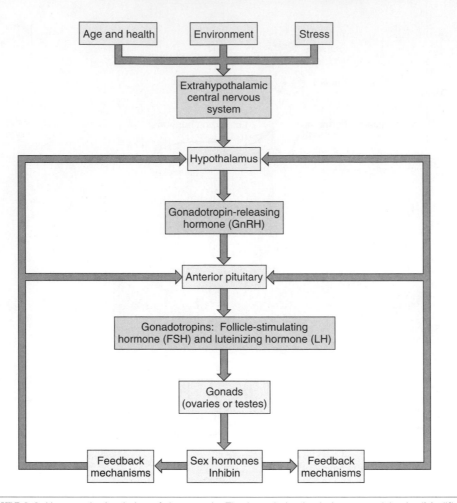

FIGURE **2-2** Hormonal stimulation of the gonads: The hypothalamic-pituitary-gonadal axis. (Modified from McCance, K.L. & Huether, S.E. [2002]. *Pathophysiology: The biologic basis for disease in adults and children* [4th ed.]. St. Louis: Mosby.)

the release of anterior pituitary gonadotropins (FSH and LH). Blood vessels end in capillaries at both ends, allowing movement of RHs from the hypothalamus that moderate pituitary secretion (see Figure 2-3). When hypothalamic neurons are stimulated and neurosecretory cells respond by RHs, neurosecretory products are released into the portal circulation and travel to the anterior pituitary. Hypothalamic regulating hormones travel via nerve fibers to the infundibulum of the neurohypophysis and enter the peripheral circulation by the perigomitolar capillary network.[22] Long and short portal vessels travel parallel to the pituitary stalk and terminate in the anterior pituitary capillaries.

The posterior pituitary lobe receives nerve fibers from the supraoptic and paraventricular nuclei of the anterior hypothalamus through the pituitary stalk, known as the neurohypophysis. The posterior pituitary, an extension of the hypothalamus, is composed of glial-like cells (i.e., pituicytes), the supporting structure for terminal nerve fibers and terminal nerve endings. Magnocellular neurons of the hypothalamus—specifically the paraventricular nuclei and supraoptic nuclei—secrete the hormones expressed by the posterior pituitary (see Figure 2-3).[22] Posterior pituitary hormones travel from the hypothalamus to the neurohypophysis via nerve fibers.[26] Neurohypophyseal hormones travel to the neurohypophyseal tract through the pituitary stalk for storage in the posterior pituitary capillary nerve endings via neurophysins (protein binders).[26] Nerve endings, which are shaped like bulbous knobs, lie on the surfaces of the capillaries, onto which are secreted the hormones, vasopressin, and oxytocin.

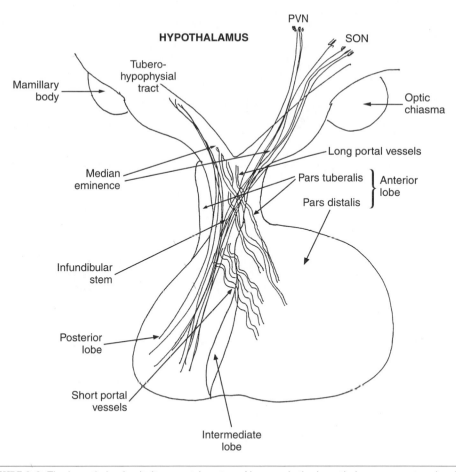

FIGURE **2-3** The hypothalamic-pituitary portal system. Neurons in the hypothalamus secrete releasing hormones into veins that carry these hormones directly to the pituitary, thus bypassing the normal circulatory route. *PVN,* Paraventricular nucleus; *SON,* supraoptic nuclei. (From Gordon, K. & Oehninger, S. [2000]. Reproductive physiology. In L.J. Copeland [Ed.]. *Textbook of gynecology* [2nd ed.]. Philadelphia: W.B. Saunders.)

Hormone Activators, Receptors, and Messenger Systems

Hormones are chemical messengers that have specific rates and patterns of secretion (e.g., diurnal patterns). These patterns—which are pulsatile and have circadian or ultradian rhythmicity—depend on the levels of circulating substrates, calcium, sodium, or the hormones.[74] Various factors affect the circulating level of hormones. Receptor affinity and concentration are regulated by the intracellular and extracellular environment as body temperature, calcium and sodium concentrations, and serum pH. Other physiochemical factors affecting hormone release include urea concentration and the lipid matrix of the plasma membrane. Lastly, circulating hormone levels are regulated by growth and development, diet, drugs, and exercise. Hormones are constantly excreted by kidneys or deacti-

vated by the liver. Hormones are classified by structure, target gland or origin, effects, or chemical classes. Structural categories of hormones include proteins (prolactin), glycoproteins (FSH and LH), polypeptides (oxytocin), steroids (estrogens, progestins, and testosterone), and fatty acids (prostaglandins and thromboxanes).

For each hormone there is a specific cellular receptor, located on the cell surface or within the cell. The majority of hormonal receptors are very large proteins. Hormones bind with cells with appropriate receptors, forming a hormone receptor complex, and then act on these cells to initiate specific cell functions or activities. Each cell has approximately 2,000 to 10,000 receptors.[26] Receptor locations vary with the types of hormones. For example, protein or peptide hormone receptors are located in or on the cell membrane, while steroid hormones such as estrogen

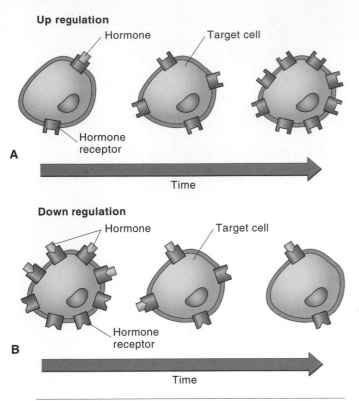

Up regulation

Hormone — Target cell

Hormone receptor

A

Time

Down regulation

Hormone — Target cell

Hormone receptor

B

Time

FIGURE **2-4** Regulation of target cell sensitivity. If synthesis of new receptors occurs faster than degradation of old receptors, the target cell will have more receptors and thus be more sensitive to hormone. This phenomenon **(A)** is called *upregulation* because the number of receptors goes up. If the rate of receptor degradation exceeds the rate of receptor synthesis, the target cell's number of receptors will decrease **(B)**. Because the number of receptors and thus the sensitivity of the target cells goes down, this phenomenon is called *downregulation*. Shading represents hormone concentration. (From Thibodeau, G.A. & Patton, K.T. [1999]. *Anatomy and physiology* [4th ed.]. St. Louis: Mosby.)

TABLE **2-1** Second Messengers Identified for Specific Hormones

Second Messenger	Associated Hormones
Cyclic AMP	Adrenocorticotrophic hormone (ACTH)
	Luteinizing hormone (LH)
	Human chorionic gonadotrophin (hCG)
	Follicle-stimulating hormone (FSH)
	Thyroid-stimulating hormone (TSH)
	Antidiuretic hormone (ADH)
	Thyrotropin-releasing hormone (TRH)
	Parathyroid hormone (PTH)
	Glucagon
Cyclic GMP	Atrial natriuretic hormone
Calcium	Angiotensin II
	Gonadotropin–releasing hormone (GnRH)
	Antidiuretic hormone (ADH)
IP$_3$ and DAG	Angiotensin II
	Luteinizing hormone–releasing hormone (LHRH)

From McCance, K.L. & Huether, S.E. (2002). *Pathophysiology: The biologic basis for disease in adults and children* (4th ed.). St. Louis: Mosby. *AMP*, Adenosine monophosphate; *DAG*, diacylglycerol; *GMF*, guanosine monophosphate; *IP$_3$*, inositol triphosphate.

diffuse freely across the plasma membrane and have their receptors in the cell cytoplasm. Thyroid hormone receptors are located in the nucleus. Hormone binding with the target cell receptor will cause the number of receptors to decrease, a process known as downregulation (Figure 2-4). In contrast, with upregulation, low concentrations of hormones will increase the number of receptors per cell. As the receptors decrease with downregulation, there is decreased responsiveness of the target tissue. In the unbound state, receptors are inert.

Receptor activation on the target cell may be initiated by a variety of mechanisms such as a first messenger system, a second messenger system, and genetic sequencing. In the first messenger system, the hormone recognizes and binds with its specific receptor. With formation of the

hormone receptor complex, enzymes are activated within the cell subsequent to phosphorylation. The second messenger system may act synergistically or antagonistically to regulate cell activities. Second messengers (which are small molecules) include cyclic adenosine monophosphate (cAMP), inositol triphosphate, calcium ions, phospholipids, and the calcium-calmodulin complex. Cellular responses are initiated by transmission of an intracellular signal via a second messenger (Table 2-1) that signals the effect of the hormone on the target cell as membrane transport. Hormone receptor binding increases the intracellular level of the second messengers as cAMP (Table 2-2). The cAMP second messenger system binds with a G protein and converts ATP into cAMP, which then activates a protein kinase, leading to phosphorylation and enzyme activation (Figure 2-5). FSH, LH, and human chorionic gonadotropin (hCG) are hormones responding to the cAMP second messenger system.[26,60] FSH and LH act on the ovary via the cAMP intracellular signaling pathway.[76] Cyclic adenosine monophosphate is a common intracellular messenger during both follicular and luteal phases.[76]

GnRH is activated via the phospholipase C second messenger system (Table 2-3). Hormones bind with the receptor at the cell membrane, catabolizing the phosphatidylinositol biphosphate into inositol triphosphate and

TABLE **2-2**   Hormones That Use the Adenyl Cyclase-
cAMP Second Messenger System

Adrenocorticotrophic hormones (ACTH)	Glucagon
Angiotensin II (epithelial cells)	Human chorionic gonadotropin (hCG)
Calcitonin	Luteinizing hormone (LH)
Catecholamines (β-receptors)	Parathyroid hormone (PTH)
Corticotropin-releasing hormones (CRH)	Secretin
Follicle-stimulating hormone (FSH)	Thyroid-stimulating hormone (TSH)
	Vasopressin (V₂ receptor, epithelial cells)

From Guyton, A.C. & Hall, J.E. (2000). *Textbook of medical physiology* (10th ed.). Philadelphia: W.B. Saunders.

TABLE **2-3**   Hormones That Use the Phospholipase
C Second Messenger System

Angiotensin II (vascular smooth muscle)	Oxytocin
Catecholamines (α-receptors)	Thyroid-releasing hormone (TRH)
Gonadotropin-releasing hormone (GnRH)	Vasopressin (V₁ receptor, vascular smooth muscle)
Growth hormone–releasing factor (GHRF)	

From Guyton, A.C. & Hall, J.E.(2000). *Textbook of medical physiology* (10th ed.). Philadelphia: W.B. Saunders.

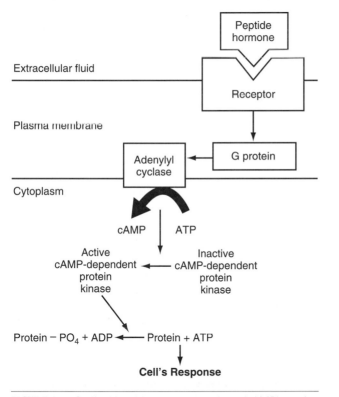

FIGURE **2-5** Cyclic adenosine monophosphate (cAMP) mechanism, by which many hormones exert their control of cell function. *ADP,* Adenosine diphosphate; *ATP,* adenosine triphosphate. (From Guyton, A.C. & Hall, J.E. [2000]. *Textbook of medical physiology* [10th ed.]. Philadelphia: W.B. Saunders.)

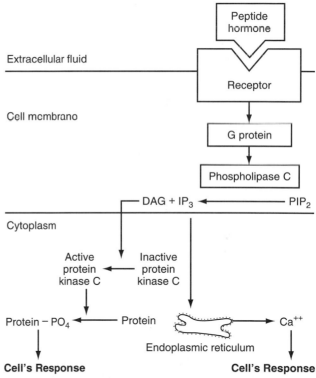

FIGURE **2-6** The cell membrane phospholipid second-messenger system, by which some hormones exert their control of cell function. *DAG,* Diacylglycerol; *IP₃, inositol triphosphate; PIP₂,* phosphatidyl-inositol biphosphate. (From Guyton, A.C. & Hall, J.E. [2000]. *Textbook of medical physiology* [10th ed.]. Philadelphia: W.B. Saunders.)

diacylglycerol. Similar to cAMP, the second messenger diacylglycerol activates a protein kinase, phosphorylates, and initiates the cellular response (Figure 2-6). Diacylglycerol activity may result in the synthesis of prostaglandins or combine with calcium, activating cellular metabolic ac-

tion. Calcium is accessed from the intracellular endoplasmic reticulum and mitochondria by inositol triphosphate that activates the cell functions. Calcium is also mobilized in the calcium-calmodulin second messenger system by binding with calmodulin intracellularly. This binding mediates the use of calcium in the activation, inhibition, or phosphorylation of protein kinases, with subsequent cellular response.[26] Lastly, after binding with specific receptors, steroid hormones synthesize proteins, which in the nucleus bind with chromosomal deoxyribonucleic acid (DNA) to facilitate the formation of messenger ribonucleic acid (mRNA) and subsequent proteins via genetic instructions.[26]

Hormone Storage

There is no single way in which endocrine glands store and secrete hormones. The amount of hormone stored in the glandular cells is minuscule, but the large amounts of precursor molecules, such as cholesterol and its intermediaries, are present intracellularly. With specific stimulation, enzymes initiate conversion to the final hormone followed by hormone expression. For example, the protein hormone prolactin is initially formed by the endoplasmic reticulum. Known as a *preprohormone,* this protein is larger than the active hormone and is cleaved while still in the endoplasmic reticulum, yielding a smaller protein molecule— prohormone. The prohormone is transported in vesicles to the Golgi apparatus, where the protein is further processed to form the final active protein hormone. The Golgi apparatus compacts the hormone molecules into small membrane-encapsulated vesicles known as *secretory vesicles.* There the final hormone is stored in the cytoplasmic compartment of the endocrine cell, awaiting its specific signal (nerve, hormonal, or chemical) for hormone secretion.

Reproductive Hormones

The hypothalamic-pituitary-ovarian axis is regulated by hormones synthesized and expressed by the hypothalamus, pituitary, ovaries, and adrenals (Figure 2-7). Some of these hormones and their physiology are well known. These hormones include FSH, LH, estrogens, progesterone, dehydroepiandrosterone sulfate (DHEAS), dehydroepiandrosterone (DHEA), androsterone, testosterone, activin, and inhibin (Table 2-4). Other hormones are less well known. These include oocyte maturation inhibitor, luteinization inhibitor, and gonadotropin surge–inhibiting factor. Hormonal innervation is independent but also interdependent with other hormones, specifically dose response and receptor proliferation and sensitivity.

Hormones synthesized by the hypothalamus include GnRHs, which mediate anterior pituitary hormone secretion. In response to stimulation by GnRH the anterior pituitary expresses the hormones known collectively as *gonadotropins* (i.e., FSH, LH) that enhance follicular proliferation and maturation and subsequent ovulation.

The ovaries and adrenal cortices synthesize DHEA, the precursor hormone for the steroidal hormones estrogen, progesterone, and testosterone. Steroidal hormones and gonadotropins enhance follicular proliferation and maturation of the dominant follicle in preparation for the midcycle LH surge and ovulation.

Follicle-Stimulating Hormone

FSH is a glycoprotein secreted by the anterior pituitary. FSH, a gonadotropin, promotes follicular growth and differentiation, FSH and LH receptors, inhibin and activin activities, and estrogen synthesis. Receptors for FSH are located on the granulosa cells. FSH is instrumental in estrogen formation, pubertal development, and follicular maturation.[37] Although not mandatory for early follicular development, FSH is necessary for follicular development beyond the small antral follicle size.[37] Antral formation is enhanced in response to FSH expression.[52] In concert with estradiol, FSH increases FSH receptors and LH receptors located on the granulosa.[72]

Luteinizing Hormone

LH is also a glycoprotein that is secreted by the anterior pituitary. LH is the primary hormone involved in ovulation. This hormone promotes theca interstitial cell androgen biosynthesis with the eventual conversion to estradiol in the presence of FSH.[22] Small but sustained increments of LH enhance the development and growth of small antral follicles to preovulatory stage.

Under the influence of FSH and LH, granulosa cells acquire LH receptors in mid to late follicular phase. These gonadotropins synergistically promote follicular development, increase granulosa cells, and produce inhibin.[40] In the preovulatory phase, LH levels rise dramatically, a process known as the LH surge. Within 10 to 12 hours of the LH peak levels (or 28 to 32 hours of the onset of the LH surge), ovulation occurs.

Steroid Hormones

The steroidal hormones—androgens, estrogens, and progestogens—are primarily produced by the gonads and adrenals (see Table 2-3).[30] Cholesterol is the precursor for steroid hormones (Figure 2-8). Steroidogenic cells express low-density lipoprotein (LDL) receptors in particular and HDL receptors to uptake cholesterol. Steroidogenesis commences with LH stimulating the conversion of cholesterol to pregnenolone within the mitochondria of the cells of the theca interna cells.[51] (Figure 2-9). Transfer of the cholesterol within the mitochondria is enhanced by a steroidogenic acute regulatory protein (StAR).[51] Steroid synthesis

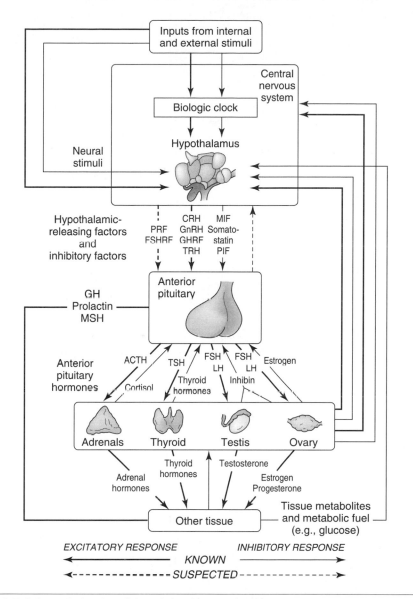

FIGURE 2-7 Schematic drawing of the relationships and feedback mechanisms of the hypothalamus and pituitary glands. Hypothalamic releasing and inhibitory factors include the following: corticotropin-releasing hormone (CRH), gonadotropin-releasing hormone (GnRH), growth hormone–releasing factor (GHRF), thyrotropin-releasing hormone (TRH), dopamine, somatostatin, prolactin-inhibiting factor (PIF), and prolactin-releasing factor (PRF). Anterior pituitary hormones include the following: growth hormone (GH); prolactin; adrenocorticotropin (ACTH); thyrotropin, or thyroid-stimulating hormone (TSH); follicle-stimulating hormone (FSH); and luteinizing hormone (LH). Posterior pituitary hormones include arginine vasopressin and oxytocin. *FSHRF*, Follicle-stimulating hormone–releasing factor; *MIF*, melanocyte-stimulating hormone–inhibiting factor; *MSH*, melanocyte-stimulating hormone. (From Frohman, L.A. [1980]. In D.T. Krieger and J.C. Hughes [Eds.]. *Neuroendocrinology*. A Hospital Practice book. Sunderland, MA: Sinauer Associates. Illustration by Nancy Lou Gahan and Albert Miller. Copyright by The McGraw-Hill Companies, Inc.)

TABLE 2-4 Reference Ranges for Selected Reproductive Steroids in Adult Human Serum

STEROID	SUBJECTS	REFERENCE VALUES
Adrostenedione	Men	2.8-7.3 nmol/L
	Women	3.1-12.2 nmol/L
Testosterone	Men	6.9-34.7 nmol/L
	Women	0.7-2.8 nmol/L
Dihydroestosterone	Men	1.03-3.10 nmol/L
	Women	0.07-0.86 nmol/L
Dehydroepiandrosterone	Men and women	5.5-24.3 nmol/L
Dehydroepiandrosterone sulfate	Men and women	2.5-10.4 µmol/L
Progesterone	Men	<0.3-1.3 nmol/L
	Women	
	Follicular	0.3-3.0 nmol/L
	Luteal	19.0-45.0 nmol/L
Estradiol	Men	<37-210 pmol/L
	Women	
	Follicular	<37-360 pmol/L
	Midcycle	625-2830 pmol/L
	Luteal	699-1250 pmol/L
	Postmenopausal	<37-140 pmol/L
Estrone	Men	37-250 pmol/L
	Women	
	Follicular	110-400 pmol/L
	Luteal	310-660 pmol/L
	Postmenopausal	22-230 pmol/L
Estrone sulfate	Men	600-2500 pmol/L
	Women	
	Follicular	700-3600 pmol/L
	Luteal	1100-7300 pmol/L
	Postmenopausal	130-1200 pmol/L

From O'Malley, B.W. & Strott, C.A. (1999). Steroid hormones: Metabolism and mechanism of action. In S.C. Yen, R.B. Jaffe, & R.L. Barbieri (Eds.). *Reproductive endocrinology: Physiology, pathophysiology, and clinical management* (4th ed.). Philadelphia: W.B. Saunders.

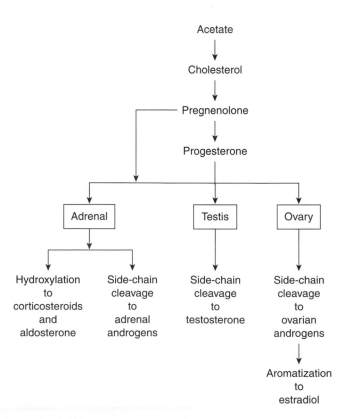

FIGURE 2-8 The unified concept of steroid hormone synthesis. Characteristic steroid secretory functions of the ovary, testes, and adrenal gland are shown. The pathway from acetate to progesterone is common to all. (From Ryan K.J. [1972]. Steroid hormones and prostaglandins. In D.E. Reid, K.J. Ryan, & K. Benirschke [Eds]. *Principles and management of human reproduction.* Philadelphia: W.B. Saunders.)

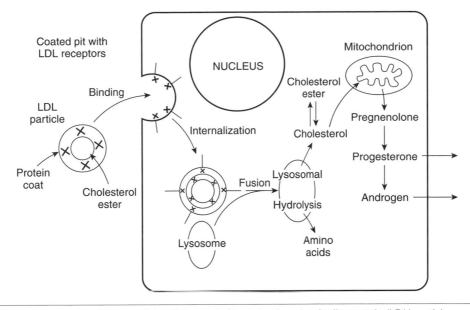

FIGURE **2-9** Source of ovary cellular cholesterol. Circulating low-density lipoprotein (LDL) particles, containing a cholesterol ester core surrounded by a protein coat, bind to specific cell membrane receptors. The LDL receptor complex is internalized and fuses to lysosomes. The cholesterol ester is hydrolyzed to cholesterol and the protein coat to amino acids. The free cholesterol is either stored as re-esterified cholesterol or transferred to mitochondria, where the side chain cleavage enzymes convert it to pregnenolone. (From Adashi, E.Y. (1999). The ovarian life cycle. In S.C. Yen & R.B. Jaffe [Eds.], *Reproductive endocrinology: Physiology, pathophysiology, and clinical management* [4th ed.]. Philadelphia: W.B. Saunders.)

employs a number of enzymes. These enzymes include five different hydroxylases, two dehydrogenases, one reductase, and an aromatase (Table 2-5).[51] The hydroxylases and aromatase descend from the P450 family and act as a catalyst to steroidogenesis.[30,51] Aromatase transcription for hormonal synthesis is evoked with follicular development at the 7-mm stage.[58]

The gonads (i.e., ovaries, testis) produce the majority of the steroidal hormones; the adrenal cortex produces minimal amounts of estrogens and dihydrotestosterone.[51] Progesterone and pregnenolone are also synthesized by the placenta from cholesterol precursors. Synthesis of steroidal hormones may follow one of two pathways: the pregnenolone pathway and the progesterone pathway (Figure 2-10).[51] From the pregnenolone pathway the hormones dehydroepiandrosterone and androstenediol are produced. Dehydroepiandrosterone and androstenediol, hormones derived from the pregnenolone pathway, may enter the progesterone pathway in the synthesis of the hormones androstenedione and testosterone, respectively. The progesterone pathway synthesizes the prohormones androstenedione and testosterone, with final conversion to the hormone dihydrotestosterone. Also from this path-

TABLE 2-5 Enzymes Used in Steroidogenesis

ENZYME	DESIGNATION
Cholesterol side chain cleavage	CYP11A
17α-Hydroxylase	CYP17
17,21-Lyase	CYP17
21-Hydroxylase	CYP21
11β-Hydroxylase	CYP11B1
Aldosterone synthetase	CYP11B2
Aromatase	CYP19
3β-Hydroxysteroid dehydrogenase	3βHSD
17β-Hydroxysteroid dehydrogenase	17βHSD
5α-Reductase	5αRed

From O'Malley, B.W. & Strott, C.A. (1999). Steroid hormones: Metabolism and mechanism of action. In S.C. Yen, R.B. Jaffe, & R.L. Barbieri (Eds.). *Reproductive endocrinology: Physiology, pathophysiology, and clinical management* (4th ed.). Philadelphia: W.B. Saunders.

way, androstenedione is converted to estrone (E1) and testosterone is converted to estradiol.[51] In women, approximately 60% of circulating testosterone is derived from the peripheral conversion of androstenedione in women.[51] Steroidal hormonal levels vary in the

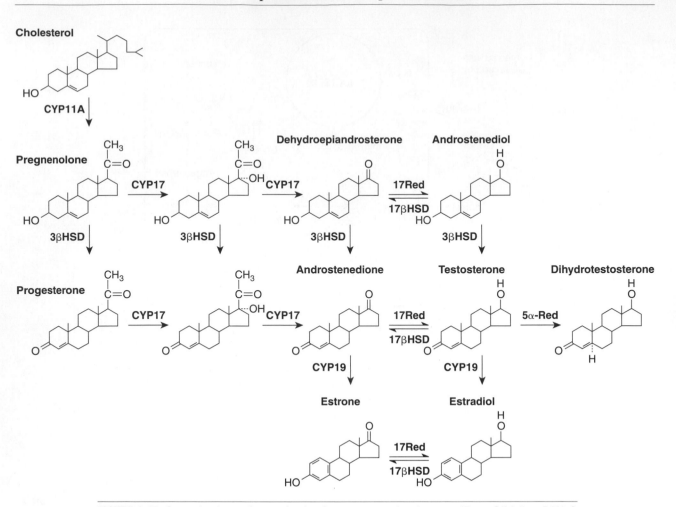

FIGURE **2-10** General scheme for synthesis of estrogens and androgens. (From O'Malley, B.W. & Strott, C.A. [1999]. Steroid hormones: Metabolism and mechanism of action. In S.C. Yen, R.B. Jaffe & R.L. Barbieri [Eds.]. *Reproductive endocrinology: Physiology, pathophysiology, and clinical management* [4th Ed.]. Philadelphia: W.B. Saunders.)

reproductive cycle and in the reproductive life of the woman (see Table 2-5).[51]

Dehydroepiandrosterone sulfate, dehydroepiandrosterone, and androstenedione. Major androgen precursors are DHEAS, DHEA, and androstenedione. These androgen precursors precede steroidal synthesis. Secreted by the ovaries and adrenals, the androgen precursors begin to increase in early adolescence and decline in the fifth and sixth decades. Follicular maturation, increased estradiol levels, and LH stimulation are necessary for ovarian androgen synthesis. Androgens are the precursors of estrogen and progesterone synthesis.

During the menstrual cycle, particularly the follicular phase, two thirds of testosterone is derived from peripheral conversion of androstenedione.[30] During pregnancy the fetal adrenal produces DHEA, the precursor of placental estrogen synthesis.[42]

DHEA is a hormone produced primarily by the adrenals and less so by the ovaries. The physiologic role of dehydroepiandrosterone is unknown.[14] Age is the most important determinant in DHEA hormonal variance, although the cause of the decreased levels with aging is unknown.[67] Hormonal concentrations of DHEA decline with age more than so than estrogen, progesterone, or testosterone.[67]

Estrogens. Estrogens include estrone (E_1), estradiol, and estriol (E_3) (Figure 2-11). In nonpregnant women, the ovaries are the primary source of estrogens; the adrenal

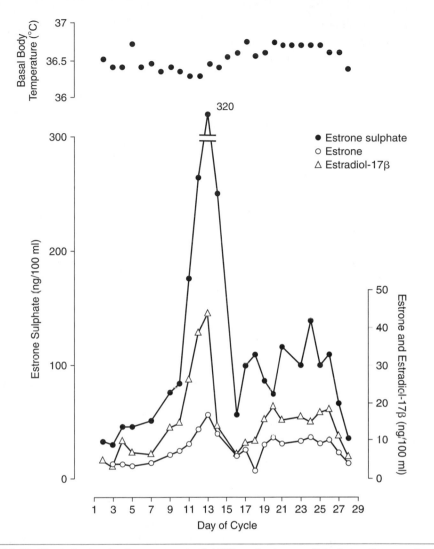

FIGURE **2-11** Circulating levels of estrone, estradiol-17β, and estrone sulfate during the menstrual cycle. (From Fraser, I.S., et al. [1998]. *Estrogens and progestogens in clinical practice.* Philadelphia: Churchill Livingstone.)

cortices also produce small amounts. Before ovulation, the follicles secrete estradiol, which is dependent upon the thecal cell androgen production. During pregnancy the placenta produces significant quantities of estrogens. The principal estrogen of the reproductive years is estradiol that is produced by the ovaries. Estriol, a weak estrogen, is derived from the conversion of either estradiol or estrone.[65] Estrone is derived from androgens of the adrenals and ovaries. Estradiol has 12 times the estrogenic potency of estrone and 80 times that of estriol.[26,65] During the reproductive years, estrone concentrations are greater than those of estradiol, with levels ranging from 1000 pg/ml in the fol-

licular phase to luteal levels of 1800 pg/ml.[65] The greater biologic potency of estradiol establishes it as the dominant estrogen at this time. Conversely, estradiol levels dramatically decrease with menopause and there is a higher estrone/estradiol ratio, with estrone becoming the dominant estrogen of the menopausal period.

The "two-cell, two gonadotropin" theory proposes that two cells (i.e., thecal, granulosa cells) and the two gonadotropins (i.e., FSH, LH) stimulate estrogen synthesis.[22,43] Androgen formation from cholesterol occurs in the theca interna with LH stimulation. Androgen is then converted to estrogens. In addition, antral follicles produce estradiol and these follicles ovulate in response to gonadotropin stimulation (Figure 2-12).[16,55] Stress is known to negatively affect hormonal stimulation. Estradiol blood levels are significantly lower in women diagnosed with depression.[75]

Estradiol stimulates follicular maturation, and increased levels of estrogen by day 5 in the ovarian cycle act to inhibit FSH and LH release. Estrogen priming facilitates FSH development of granulosa LH receptors. Increasing estrogen levels stimulate LH secretion. During the follicular phase, estrogen facilitates the endometrial changes of the proliferative phase. Endometrial tissue depth increases from 1 to 2 mm to 3.5 to 5 mm, with tortuous gland development, increased mitotic activity, and expansion of the spiral arteries. In response to estrogen, the cervical mucus becomes more watery and clear, with increased stretchability prior to ovulation (spinnbarkeit).[47] During the follicular phase the cervical os opens, closing during the luteal phase.[47] Uterine and fallopian tube changes in response to rising estrogen levels include rhythmic contractions to facilitate sperm motility and ovum retention, respectively.

Increased breast sensitivity during the luteal phase is thought to be related to estrogen levels.[47] Following ovulation, the corpus luteum produces estrogen and progesterone. Increased levels of estrogen, in concert with progesterone, inhibit FSH and LH secretion. As the corpus luteum degenerates, estrogen levels decrease. GnRH levels rise in response, with a subsequent increase in FSH and LH to initiate folliculogenesis.[47]

Progestogens. Progesterone is the only naturally occurring steroidal progestogen.[65] The ovaries produce progesterone primarily early in the follicular phase, but large amounts of progesterone are converted by the granulosa cells to estrogens. With the LH surge there is a subsequent increase in progesterone. In concert with estrogen, progesterone stimulates significant FSH secretion and a subsequent increase in granulosa LH receptors (Figure 2-13).[7] Follicular wall elasticity is secondary to increased progesterone levels.

Progesterone production in the follicular phase is 2.5 mg/day, while luteal phase production is 25 mg/day.[41] For the first 6 to 10 weeks following conception, the primary site of progesterone production is the corpus luteum.[41] Progesterone levels rise significantly, peaking at approximately day 8 of the luteal phase. Increased levels of progesterone—along with estrogen via negative feedback—limit the expression of FSH and LH. With involution of the corpus luteum, progesterone levels drop dramatically. In contrast with fertilization of the oocyte, the placenta becomes the primary producer of progesterone after approximately 10 gestational weeks.

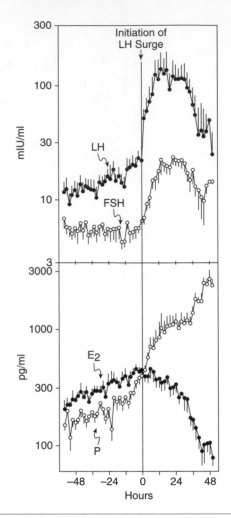

FIGURE **2-12** Mean (±SE) luteinizing hormone (LH), follicle-stimulating hormone (FSH), estradiol (E₂), and progesterone (O) levels measures every 2 hours for 5 days at midcycle in seven studies. Data were centered at the initiation of the gonadotrophin surge. Note that the data were plotted on a logarithmic scale. (From Hoff, J.D., Quigley, M.E., & Yen, S.S.C. [1983]. Hormonal dynamics at midcycle: A reevaluation. *Endocrinol Metab, 57,* 792.)

Progesterone modulates the effects on the reproductive organs, including the "quieting" of the fallopian tubes during the luteal phase to assist the fertilized ovum in its transport to the uterus. This quieting also extends to the uterus to facilitate trophoblast implantation. Progesterone levels are negatively correlated with body mass index.[67] Ethnicity also contributes significantly to variances in progesterone levels.[67]

Testosterone. Testosterone is an androgen derived from the androgenal precursors DHEA and DHEAS.[54] From 30% to 50% of androgens originate in the adrenals and

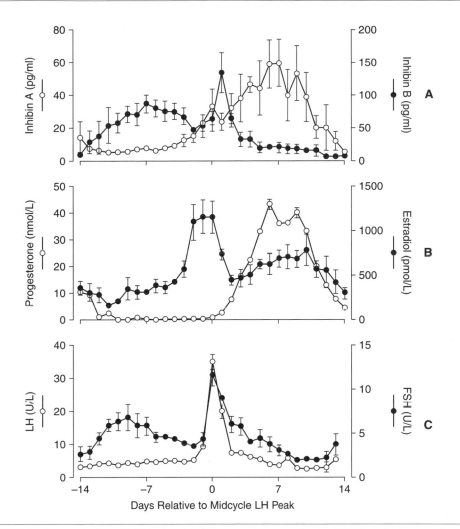

FIGURE **2-13** Concentration of inhibin A and B **(A)**, progesterone and estradiol **(B)**, and luteinizing hormone (LH) and follicle-stimulating hormone (FSH) **(C)** throughout the menstrual cycle. (From Groome N.P., et al. [1996]. Measurement of dimeric inhibin B throughout the human menstrual cycle. *J Clin Endocrinol Metab, 81,* 1401-1405.)

ovaries, with the remainder deriving from peripheral tissue conversion as liver and adipose tissue.[54] Secretion of androgens commences at approximately 6 to 8 years of age as influenced primarily by elevated DHEAS and less so by androstenedione levels.[54] Levels begin to reach adult levels during adolescence and begin to decline after the age of 50. Premenopausally, mean testosterone production rates decrease from 200 μg/day to 150 μg/day perimenopausally.[49]

Synthesis of testosterone occurs early in the follicular cycle by the ovaries. The majority of testosterone is converted into estrogens by the granulosa cells. Testosterone levels decline with age.[67] Body mass index is the most important predictor of testosterone levels.[67]

Activin

Activin is a glycoprotein that activates the release of FSH.[71] Composed of dimers of the β-inhibin subunits, activin A is synthesized in gonadal tissue but may also be synthesized in nongonadal organs, such as bone marrow.[9,72] Higher activin concentrations overcome the effect of inhibin, with a resulting increase in FSH expression. Activin levels are independent of FSH stimulation.[9] Activin levels are highest midcycle and in the late luteal–early follicular phase. Levels are even higher in pregnancy. Activin of the granulosa promotes FSH-induced growth of LH receptors on granulosa cells and inhibits synthesis of thecal cell LH, progesterone, and estrogen.[72] Activin A concentrations during the menstrual cycle range from 100 to 200 pg/ml, whereas postmenopausal levels may be five times higher than those levels.[33]

Inhibin

Inhibin, another glycoprotein, suppresses FSH secretion from the hypophysis.[71] Inhibin is synthesized primarily by the granulosa cells and is secreted into the follicular fluid.[22] Synthesis of inhibin is regulated in response to gonadotropins or factors that increase intracellular cAMP. There are two different forms of inhibin: inhibin A and inhibin B. Inhibin A and B have similar biologic characteristics; the primary difference is that hormonal synthesis is regulated differently during the follicular and luteal phases (see Figure 2-13). FSH regulates inhibin production by the ovarian granulosa cells. LH augments inhibin production in the granulosa cells with the acquisition of its LH receptors. In addition, ovarian insulin growth factor 1 (IGF-I) and vasoactive intestinal peptide stimulate inhibin synthesis.[73] Levels of inhibin vary in the menstrual cycle from 100 IU/L to 1500 IU/L.[39] In the follicular phase, inhibin concentrations are low, with increased levels in the luteal phase.[13] In response to rising FSH levels in the luteal-follicular phase, inhibin levels drop dramatically.[13] With menopause, inhibin concentrations are reduced.[12]

Inhibin A is produced and expressed by the dominant follicle or corpus luteum.[29] Inhibin A slowly increases during the late follicular phase, stimulated by incremental LH expression, and is present in high levels during midluteal phases.[25] An initial reduction in inhibin A is followed by a decreased but consistent level. During the second half of the menstrual cycle, concentrations of inhibin A increase markedly parallel to increasing concentrations of estradiol.

Inhibin B decreases FSH synthesis and obscures the effects of low activin levels. In the early follicular phase there are increased levels of FSH and estradiol.[70] These hormones stimulate inhibin B expression from the luteinized granulosa cells.[69] Thus inhibin B levels increase during the early follicular phase and reach their highest point at the early to midfollicular phase of menstrual cycle. Levels are highest in the granulosa cells of luteal antral follicles. Then inhibin B levels continuously decrease, becoming undetectable following the LH surge.[9,33]

Follistatin

Follistatin is derived from the granulosa cells of the small antral and preovulatory follicles. It is a polypeptide that, like inhibin, also suppresses FSH expression.[72] However, follistatin is only about one third as active as inhibin.[28] Other physiologic roles of follistatin include the protein binding of activin (which restricts the bioavailability of activin) and the synthesis of progesterone.[63,72] Concentrations of follistatin remain relatively constant throughout the menstrual cycle.[28]

Oocyte Maturation Inhibitor

The factor leading to oocyte meiotic arrest in the prophase stage is thought to be oocyte maturation inhibitor.[26,43] It is postulated that meiosis resumes with the complex interplay of oocyte maturation inhibitor and granulosa cumulus cells.[72]

Luteinization Inhibitor

The existence of another chemical factor, luteinization inhibitor, is suggested by the ability of granulosa cells from large preovulatory follicles to initiate spontaneous luteinization.[72]

Gonadotropin Surge–Inhibiting Factor

Gonadotropin surge–inhibiting factor is a nonsteroidal substance that inhibits the LH surge and FSH expression as normally occurs by either estradiol or GnRH.[72] In contrast to inhibin, which inhibits only FSH expression, gonadotropin surge–inhibiting factor suppresses both FSH and LH. The ovaries are the source of this short-acting factor.[72]

Feedback Systems

Hormone secretion is regulated by feedback systems, which can be negative or positive (Figure 2-14). The negative feedback system is the most common. As the level of a hormone rises, it inhibits the initiation of further release of that hormone. Secretion of the pituitary hormone to a level above the set point causes a decrease in secretion of that same pituitary hormone into the blood. For example, the administration of moderate amounts of estrogen will lower the secretion of FSH and LH into the blood. In the normal menstrual cycle, high levels of progesterone and moderate levels of estrogen during the luteal phase will lower gonadotropin secretion by a long-loop negative feedback. With positive feedback, a rising hormone level will increase secretion of the same hormone. High levels of estrogen in blood increase the secretion of LH and FSH from the adenohypophysis, resulting in a surge of gonadotropins (FSH and LH).

Physiologic effects are produced by peripheral target tissues (gonads) and travel via the bloodstream to the brain and pituitary gland. In addition to the negative and positive feedback loops, there are long, short, and ultrashort loops. In the long-loop feedback, the gonadotropins (FSH and LH) increase the gonadal secretion of steroidal hormones. These steroidal hormones (i.e., estrogen, progesterone) influence the secretion of LH and FSH by their feedback effects on the

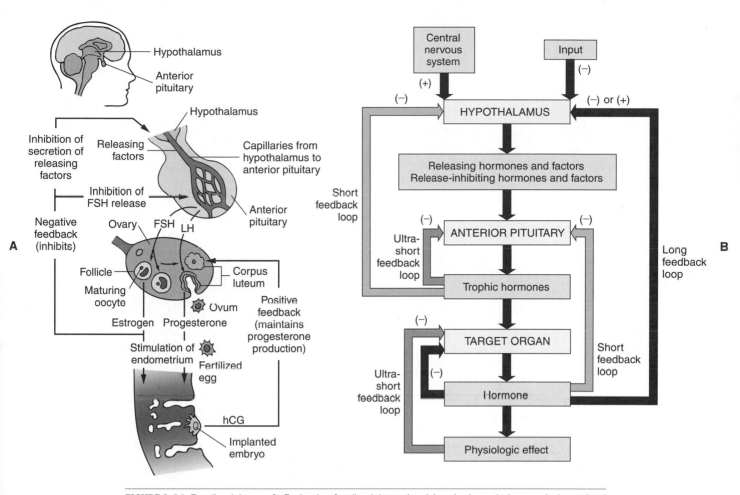

FIGURE 2-14 Feedback loops. **A,** Endocrine feedback loops involving the hypothalamus-pituitary gland and end organs (endocrine regulation). **B,** General model for control and negative feedback regulation is possible at three levels: target organ (ultrashort feedback), anterior pituitary (short feedback), and hypothalamus (long feedback). (From McCance, K.L. & Huether, S.E. [2002]. *Pathophysiology: The biologic basis for disease in adults and children* [4th ed.]. St. Louis: Mosby.)

systems controlling gonadotropin secretion. In the short-loop feedback system, LH or FSH circulates in the vascular system, returns to the median eminence of the hypothalamus, and subsequently decreases the secretion of GnRH from the neurosecretory axons.[26] This is a more direct negative feedback system that does not involve gonadal steroid hormones. In the ultrashort-loop feedback, the GnRH may directly stop GnRH secretion from the neurosecretory axons in the median eminence. At present, only the short and ultrashort feedback loops have been demonstrated to be negative. On the other hand, the long-loop feedback system may be either positive or negative. High serum levels of estrogen increase the secretion of LH and FSH from the adenohypophysis, resulting in an LH surge with ovarian release of the ovum.

Gonadotropin-Releasing Hormone

Gonadotropin-releasing neurons are located in the arcuate nucleus of the medial basal hypothalamus and in the preoptic area of the anterior hypothalamus.[22,74] The GnRH pulse generator exhibits pulsatile secretion, at 60- to 90-minute intervals, from the medial basal hypothalamus with ultradian rhythm.[74] Pulsation frequency and amplitude vary depending on hormonal stimulation or inhibition, substrates, and other hormones.[34] Continuous exposure to GnRH decreases the responsiveness of the receptors, leading to increased downregulation.[5] For example, during the luteal phase, there is a significant decrease in the GnRH pulse generator.[22]

In response to GnRH, the anterior pituitary gland secretes FSH and LH. GnRH pulse frequency during the luteal follicular phase modulates FSH secretion to initiate

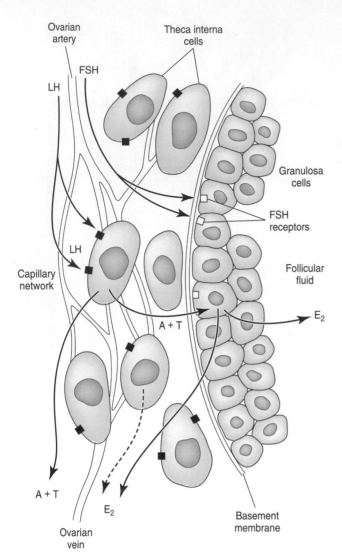

FIGURE **2-15** Diagram of action of gonadotropins on the follicle and the synthesis of estrogens. Luteinizing hormone (LH) interacts with receptors on the theca cells to stimulate production of androgens and small amounts of estradiol (E_2). Follicle-stimulating hormone (FSH) activates the aromatase enzyme system in the granulosa cells by interacting with receptors. *A*, Androstenedione; *T*, testosterone. (From Band, D.T. [1984]. The ovary. In C.R. Austin & R.V. Short [Eds.]. *Hormonal control of reproduction* [vol. 3]. Cambridge: Cambridge University Press.)

folliculogenesis.[70] Both hormones are small glycoproteins that stimulate the ovary by combining with specific FSH and LH receptor cells located in the cell membranes (Figure 2-15). Cyclic AMP, the second messenger system in the cell cytoplasm, promotes mobilization and expression of FSH and LH from storage granules in the gonadotropes.[22]

REPRODUCTIVE PROCESSES IN THE FEMALE
Oogenesis

In utero, the ovaries function in response to placental secretion of chorionic gonadotropin. In utero oogenesis commences between weeks 6 and 16 of gestation.[43,72] Fetal pituitary FSH secretion has been detected at times as early as 12 to 14 gestational weeks.[5] Serum FSH levels at 20 to 28 gestational weeks are comparable to levels postmenopausally.[72] Whereas the adult pulse generator frequency is from 60 to 120 minutes, the fetal GnRH frequency pulsates every 60 minutes.[73] At approximately 20 gestational weeks, the maximal number of primordial follicles are present; this number decreases throughout the reproductive life of the woman, until depletion at the climacteric.[72,43] Oogenesis ceases at approximately 28 gestational weeks, with no further ova production.[5] At birth the newborn ovaries contain approximately 200,000 to 400,000 follicles arrested in the prophase stage phase of meiosis.[43] (Oogenesis is described further in Chapter 1.)

Puberty

Following birth, the ovaries are dormant until puberty. At puberty, 40,000 follicles[46] to 300,000 follicles[72] exist and await activation; however, only approximately 400 oogonia mature as secondary follicles for ovulation.[46] Oocytes are arrested in the prophase stage of the first meiotic division, converting oogonia to primary oocytes until ovulation.[72] With ovulation, meiosis commences and the first polar body is formed.[72] Atresia of the remaining ovarian follicles occurs in response to apoptosis. Apoptosis is the programmed cell self-destruction without an accompanying inflammatory response. (Meiosis is discussed further in Chapter 1.)

GnRH episodic pulses increase in frequency at about 10 years of age[64] (Figure 2-16), beginning at night during sleep (Figure 2-17).[2] With puberty, estradiol stimulus via positive feedback initiates the hypothalamic pulse generator (Figure 2-18).[43] This hormonal stimulus is dependent upon an adequate LH pool for the LH surge, ovarian follicles responsive to FSH, and a pituitary gland responsive to GnRH. LH pulses have been detected as early as mid-childhood. With the onset of puberty, there is a greater increase in LH pulse amplitude in comparison to pulse frequency.[2] There is a progressive increase in FSH and LH daytime pulsatility, with a subsequent decrease in sleep-entrained pulse amplification (Figure 2-19).[2] Prepubertal girls have high FSH concentrations.[2] FSH is necessary for pubertal development, and rising FSH levels accompany follicular development.[37,49] Ovary activation occurs in response to increasing LH pulses.[64]

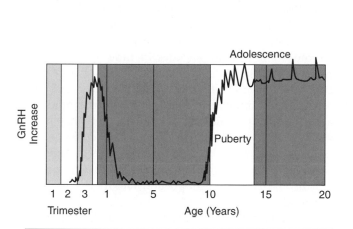

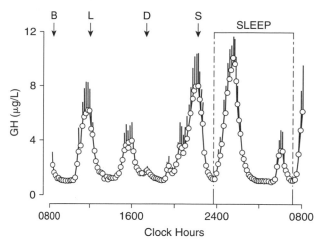

FIGURE **2-16** Diagrammatic representation of the ontogeny of gonadotropin-releasing hormone (GnRH) secretion from fetal life to adolescence. Note the prepubertal nadir and upswing of GnRH secretory activity at the onset of puberty. This is followed by irregular luteinizing hormone surges during adolescence. (From Yen, S.S.C. (1987). Reproductive strategy in women: Neuroendocrine basis of endogenous contraception. In R. Rolland [Ed.]. *Neuroendocrinology of reproduction.* Amsterdam: Excerpta Medica.)

FIGURE **2-17** Mean (±SE) growth hormone (GH) pulsitile secretory pattern during the 24-hour sleep-wake cycle in healthy women. Arrows denote mealtimes. Note large episode of release at sleep onset and the uniformity of the pattern of GH pulses when the timing, content, and duration of meals, as well as sleep time, are controlled. (From Laughin, G.A., et al. [1998]. Nutritional and endocrine-metabolic aberrations in women with functional hypothalamic amenorrhea. *J Clin Endocrinol Metab, 83,* 25.)

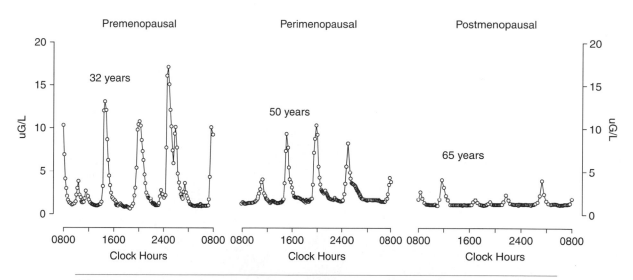

FIGURE **2-18** Age-related decline in growth hormone 9GH pulse amplitude but not frequency, independent of menstrual status. (From Yen, S.C., Jaffe, R.B., & Barbieri, R.L. [1999]. *Reproductive endocrinology: Physiology, pathophysiology, and clinical management* [4th ed.]. Philadelphia: W.B. Saunders.)

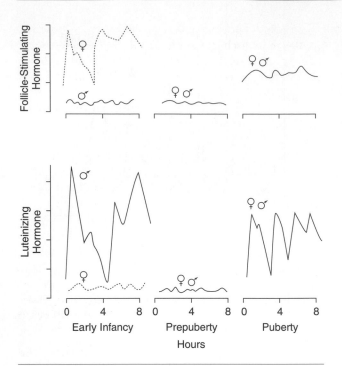

FIGURE **2-19** Changes in the patterns of follicle-stimulating hormone and luteinizing hormone secretion at puberty. (From Klein, K., et al. [1996]. In S.G. Hillier, H.C. Kitchener, & J.P. Neilson [Eds.]. *Scientific essentials of reproductive medicine.* Philadelphia: W.B. Saunders.)

There is increased gonadotropin sensitivity to GnRH with the cessation of the gonadostat.[20] Control of GnRH release is mediated via a neuroendocrine cascade composed of neuropeptides, neurotransmitters, and neurosteroids. These neuropeptides include opioids, neuropeptide Y, galanin, and corticotropin-releasing factor (CRF). Neurotransmitters include dopamine, melatonin, serotonin, γ-aminobutyric acid (GABA), and noradrenaline. The neurotransmitters dopamine, norepinephrine, and epinephrine stimulate GnRH secretion. Serotonin is norepinephrine mediated. DHEA (an antagonistic neurosteroid) and allopregnalnolone (an agonistic neurosteroid) are also important factors in initiating puberty.[20]

After puberty, with increased FSH and LH expression, the ovaries and follicles are stimulated. Oocytes are surrounded by a single layer of granulosa cells that are believed to nourish the ovum and secrete oocyte maturation inhibiting factor. Oocyte maturation inhibiting hormone maintains the ova as primordial follicles in the first stage of meiotic division as in fetal development.[43,72]

Ovarian Cycle

The ovarian cycle consists of the follicular phase and the luteal phase (Figure 2-20). During the follicular phase there is ovarian follicular maturation and ovulation. The

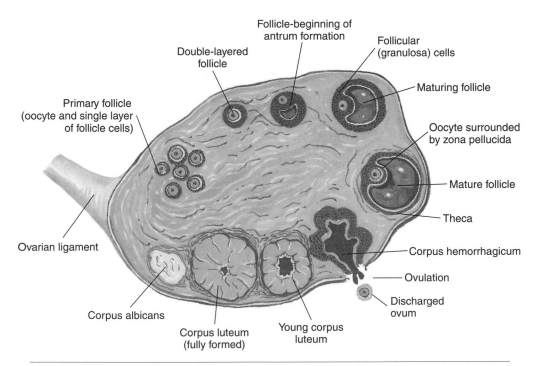

FIGURE **2-20** Cross-section of the ovary during reproductive years. (From Thibodeau, G.A. & Patton, K.T. [1999]. *Anatomy and physiology* [4th ed.]. St. Louis: Mosby.)

luteal phase includes the development of the corpus luteum from luteinization of the granulosa and theca interna cells. With involution of the corpus luteum, a new ovarian cycle begins.

The follicular phase commences with follicular growth in response to gonadotropin stimulation. A primordial follicle contains an oocyte with a single layer of granulosa cells. Developing into preantral follicles or primary follicles, the oocyte is covered with multiple layers of granulosa cells. FSH expression by the granulosa cells parallels formation of the antral cavity. Follicles mature from primordial to preantral follicles even without LH and FSH stimulation, but subsequent maturation does not occur without FSH stimulation.[37]

Follicular maturation to the antral stage is thought to require a 3-month trajectory.[22,23,43] The "trajectory of follicle growth"—from follicle recruitment to follicle selection to dominant follicle—is interdependent upon gonadotropins (Figure 2-21).[21,22] Gonadal steroids act to "guide" the process from primordial follicle to the secondary follicular stage.[21,22]

The GnRH pulse generator has a frequency of approximately one discharge per hour (60 to 120 minutes), resulting in a GnRH pituitary portal circulation bolus. Research suggests that there is a corresponding LH pulse for each GnRH pulsation.[22] Hormone priming (i.e., small doses over a period of time) induces an increased LH pulse amplitude, which over 4 hours enhances GnRH receptors.[73] Activation of the system initiates a sequence of reproductive endocrinology events (Figure 2-22). Specialized neurons in the hypothalamus synthesize and secrete GnRH in response to hormonal and neural stimuli. The GnRH pulse generator varies dependent upon cycle timing. In the early follicular phase the GnRH generator pulses approximately every 94 minutes (compared to late follicular phase pulsations every 71 minutes and late luteal phase pulsations every 216 minutes).[17] Both ovaries have an equal opportunity for stimulation and alternate ovulation.[49]

The neurosecretory cells integrate neuronal input from the feedback signals of the developing ovarian follicle. GnRH is secreted into the capillary venous network, bathing the anterior pituitary gland through the portal circulation. GnRH binds to membrane receptors located in the pituitary gonadotropes via cAMP and calcium mobilization, stimulating gonadotropin release.[76] Then pituitary gonadotropes secrete LH and FSH in pulses into the peripheral circulation. During the follicular phase of the ovarian cycle, the GnRH pulse generator operates at the

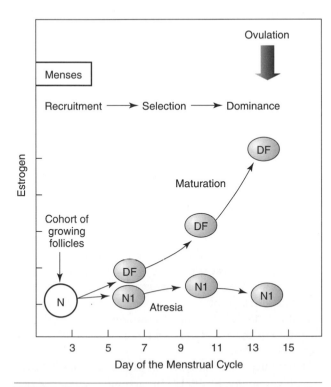

FIGURE **2-21** Time course for recruitment, selection, and ovulation of the dominant ovarian follicle (DF) with onset of atresia among other follicles of the cohort. (From Hidgen, G.D. [1986]. Physiology of follicular maturation. In H.W. Jones, Jr., G.S. Jones, G.D. Hodgen, & Z. Rosenwaks [Eds.]. *In vitro fertilization.* Baltimore: Williams &

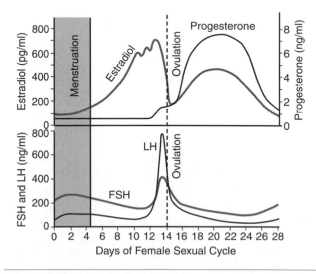

FIGURE **2-22** Approximate plasma concentrations of the gonadotropins and ovarian hormones during the normal female sexual cycle. *FSH,* Follicle-stimulating hormone; *LH,* luteinizing hormone. (From Guyton, A.C. & Hall, J.E. [2000]. *Textbook of medical physiology* [10th ed.]. Philadelphia: W.B. Saunders.)

same frequency as in its unmodulated state (i.e., independent of hypothalamic-pituitary-ovarian stimulation), releasing GnRH from secretory packets. Differentiation of follicles is believed to be multifactorial. Endocrine, paracrine, and autocrine factors modulate the effect of FSH on the growing follicles.[57]

Rising FSH levels are noted in the early follicular phase, stimulating increased inhibin B secretion (Figure 2-23).[49,69,70] FSH and LH secretion increases significantly. The increase in FSH precedes that of LH by several days. With FSH stimulation, follicular development progresses. Follicular recruitment consists of follicular maturation from a primordial follicle to a secondary follicle. A primordial follicle (30 to 60 μm in diameter) is a primary oocyte in the late diplotene phase that is surrounded by a single layer of approximately 15 pregranulosa cells.[72] Primordial follicles have been detected as early as 16 gestational weeks, with formation ceasing by 6 months postpartum.[72] Follicular growth is accelerated when the germinal vesicle reaches approximately 20 μm in diameter.

Primary follicles (greater than 60 μm in diameter) are primary oocytes surrounded by a single layer of granulosa cells.[72] Spindle cells of the ovarian stroma develop into granulosa cells, which rapidly proliferate. Granulosa cells give rise to the theca follicular cells, which are composed of two sublayers: the theca interna and theca externa (see Figure 2-20). The theca interna (the inner sublayer) develops the follicular blood supply and secretes steroidal hormones. The theca externa (the external layer) becomes the capsule of the maturing follicle as it comes in contact with the surrounding stroma. The theca externa is thought to produce an angiogenic factor. Differentiation of the thecal cells concludes the primary follicle stage. Development of the zona pellucida is characteristic of a preantral primary follicle.[72] Mucopolysaccharides secreted by the granulosa cells comprise the zona pellucida.[10]

Secondary follicles (less than 120 μm) are primary oocytes surrounded by approximately 600 granulosa cells, arranged in several layers.[72] Follicular enlargement is secondary to oocyte growth, proliferation of granulosa cells, and thecal cell differentiation. Accompanying the proliferation of granulosa cells and secondary follicles is the development of FSH, estrogen, and androgen receptors.[72]

Ovarian activin promotes FSH expression. Rising FSH levels in turn promote accelerated growth of 6 to 12 primordial follicles each cycle.[26] Follicular recruitment of secondary follicles follows FSH and LH expression and occurs in the first 4 to 5 days of the cycle, leading to a selected follicle cohort from days 5 to 7. Until day 7 of the early follic-

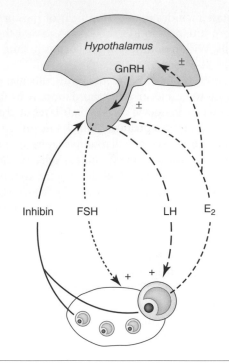

FIGURE **2-23** Diagrammatic representation of the hypothalamic-pituitary-ovarian axis in women during the follicular phase. Estradiol (E₂) feeds back at both the hypothalamus and anterior pituitary to inhibit the secretion of follicle-stimulating hormone (FSH) and luteinizing hormone (LH) (negative feedback). Under certain conditions, it can provoke the discharge of LH (positive feedback). Inhibin arising from both dominant and small antral follicles suppresses the synthesis and release of FSH by the anterior pituitary. *GnRH,* Gonadotropin-releasing hormone. (From Hillier, S.G. [1998]. Biosynthesis and secretion of ovarian and adrenal steroids. In I.S. Fraser, et al. [Eds.]. *Estrogens and progestogens in clinical practice.* Philadelphia: Churchill Livingstone.)

ular phase, all maturing follicles possess gametogonic potential or follicular selection.[22]

As follicles develop (ranging from 200 to 400 μm in diameter), antral formation follows. Follicular fluid that is high in estrogen is expressed by the granulosa cells (see Figure 2-20). Antral development heralds follicle maturation as a vesicular follicle and graafian follicle. With antral formation, the follicle is called a *vesicular follicle;* rapid proliferation of the granulosa and theca cells continues with estradiol expression.[55]

Continued follicular maturation as a vesicular follicle is dependent upon activation of the granulosa and thecal cells by increased FSH and follicular estrogen. In response to the rising follicular estrogen levels, the granulosa cells develop increased FSH receptors and sensitivity.[22] Receptors for

FSH and LH are present on the follicular granulosa cells and thecal cells (antral follicles), respectively.[5] Vesicular follicular enlargement results.

The follicle dominance attained during the midfollicular and late follicular phases is determined by rising serum FSH levels and by specific follicular sensitivity to FSH.[57,72] Initially, there is an intercycle rise in FSH that promotes follicular development. Dominant follicles have a greater sensitivity to FSH than the remaining growing follicles. Granulosa cells secrete inhibin and follistatin, both peptides that suppress FSH secretion during the midfollicular phase. Also, with increasing ovarian levels of follistatin and inhibin B in the middle to late follicular phase (the time of follicle selection), there is a corresponding decrease in FSH secretion.[49,73] During the mid and late follicular phases, the number of developing dominant follicles decrease in response to lower serum FSH levels and sensitivity.[57] With follicle selection, secondary to gonadotropic stimulus, one single follicle matures and is dominant (days 8 to 12). Follicle dominance is determined by the late follicular phase (approximately 7 days before ovulation) and is established when the follicle is 8 to 10 mm.[58,72] When follicular cells are 10 mm, LH receptors are located on the granulosa cells.[5] In contrast to follicular recruitment that transcends ovarian cycles, the follicular selection and dominant phase is completed within one cycle.

Factors contributing to follicle dominance include the ability of the follicle to aromatize androgens from the midfollicular phase on, specifically estradiol and a high granulosa cell mitotic index.[72] As the dominant follicle matures, it expresses increased estradiol, with a subsequent rise in serum estradiol levels.[22,52,73] About 90% of circulating estradiol is secreted by the dominant follicle.[5,22] In addition, the dominant follicle contains FSH and estrogen intrafollicularly.[72] Late follicular phase estradiol levels are at their highest levels within the follicle and blood.[72] During follicular maturation when plasma estradiol levels exceed a threshold level of approximately 250 pg/ml for 36 hours, the negative feedback system is overridden by a positive feedback result.[73] Estrogen's positive system feedback relationship with the hypothalamus stimulates increased secretion of GnRH and follows the "priming" of the adenohypophysis by high-frequency GnRH.[5,73] Estrogen modulates the release of FSH and LH by the gonadotropin pulse generator when "read" by the pituitary gland.[73]

Higher levels of interleukin-8 (IL-8) and interleukin-11 (IL-11), both chemotaxic cytokines, are found in more dominant follicles.[8,56] IL-8 activates neutrophils and promotes cell proliferation and angiogenesis.[56]

Follicular growth may also be categorized by class or phase (Figure 2-24).[72] The tonic growth phase involves the conversion of a preantral follicle (class 1) to an antral follicle up to 2 mm in diameter (class 4). Follicular development during the tonic growth phase is gonadotropin dependent.[72] With development of the theca interna, class 1 follicles are activated by gonadotropin stimulation.[72] Tonic follicular growth occurs over three menstrual cycles.[72] During the first menstrual cycle, secondary follicles mature as class 1 follicles in the early luteal phase (days 15 to 19).[72] In the following menstrual cycle, which is designated the second cycle, class 1 follicles are converted into class 2 follicles (days 11 to 15 of the second cycle). Early antral development is noted in class 2 follicles. Also during the second cycle, approximately 20 days later, class 2 follicles mature to class 3 follicles (end of luteal phase).[72] In the late follicular phase of the third menstrual cycle, class 3 follicles become class 4 follicles.

Conversion of class 4 follicles to class 5 is gonadotropin dependent and occurs in the late luteal phase of cycle 3. All follicular maturation beyond class 4 is strongly dependent upon FSH and LH.[72]

Follicular recruitment during the late luteal phase for the succeeding cycle will occur from class 5 follicles. During this phase, which is even more gonadotropin dependent, follicles mature from class 5 to class 8 prior to ovulation, averaging 5 days per class.[72] Follicular selection and dominance occurs during this gonadotropin growth phase. Maturation of the follicle is accompanied by follicular growth, with an increase from 5 to 20 mm in diameter.[72]

Via negative feedback, the hypothalamus responds to the moderately increased estrogen levels by inhibiting the secretion of gonadotropins. Decreasing FSH concentration and FSH sensitivity initiate follicle atresia of the nondominant follicles.[22,72] Higher follicular fluid levels of IL-11 have been noted in atretic follicles.[8]

Over 2 to 3 days, the rising ovarian estradiol levels sensitize the LH pulse generator in the anterior pituitary gland to secrete LH but suppress FSH expression.[73] In the mid-late follicular phase, rising estrogen and inhibin B levels result in reduced FSH but increased LH secretion.[69,73] The pituitary gland gonadotropes respond with a preovulatory surge of gonadotropins (specifically LH) into the peripheral circulation.[22] Thus estrogen levels signal the hypothalamus, which regulates the pulsatile expression of gonadotropins. Follicles greater than 18 mm in diameter are the source of the increased estradiol secretion, which subsequently signals the LH surge.[5,9] The LH surge of ovulation is accompanied by decreases in intrafollicular estradiol and androstenedione.[72] In contrast, increases in progesterone and

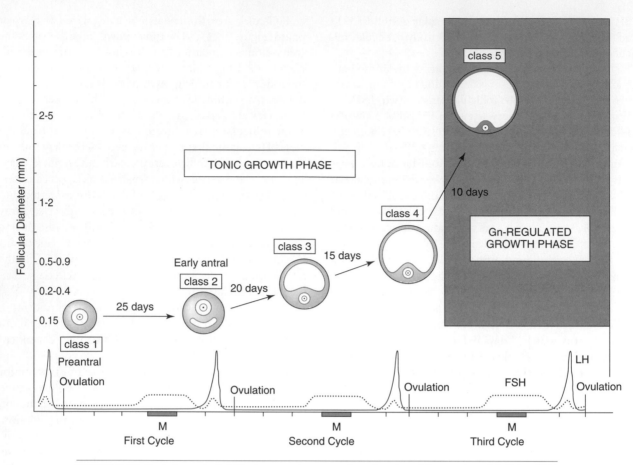

FIGURE **2-24** Tonic (preantral) follicular growth: conversion of a class 1 into a class 5 follicle. *FSH,*
Follicle-stimulating hormone; *Gn,* gonadotrophin; *LH,* luteinizing hormone; *M,* menses. (Courtesy A,
Gougeon; from Yen, S.C., Jaffe, R.B., & Barbieri, R.L. (1999). *Reproductive endocrinology: Physiology,*
pathophysiology, and clinical management [4th ed.]. Philadelphia: W.B. Saunders.)

17α-hydroxyprogesterone are noted intrafollicularly.[72]
Inhibin A levels increase concurrently with rising estradiol
levels and follicular maturation. Thecal vascularity of the
dominant follicle is more than twice that of the nondominant follicles by day 9.[72] This increased vascularity contributes to the elevated LH secretion on day 12 in the ovarian cycle, approximately 2 days before ovulation.

Ovulation

LH secretion increases significantly (i.e., six- to tenfold),
peaking approximately 12 to 24 hours before ovulation.[46]
Known as the LH surge, this dramatic increase in LH precedes ovulation by up to 36 hours (see Figure 2-1).[72] In addition, the LH surge stimulates resumption of the first meiotic division, so the mature follicle contains secondary
oocytes.[22] FSH also increases, but to a lesser degree (approximately twofold).

The ovum surrounded by loosely packed follicular cells is
known as the cumulus oophorus and is located to one side
of the follicle. Follicular swelling results from the synergistic
effect of the increased FSH and LH levels before ovulation.
Follicular hyperemia and prostaglandins secreted in the follicular tissues contribute to plasma transudation and subsequent follicular swelling. LH's acting on the granulosa cells
2 to 3 days before ovulation causes decreased estrogen secretion but, conversely, increased inhibin and progesterone levels.[5,73] Therefore, 1 day before ovulation, estrogen levels are
decreasing with increasing incremental levels of progesterone.

The LH surge lasts, on average, 48 hours, with a rapid
ascension for approximately 14 hours and with a descending limb of approximately 20 hours.[73] In response to the
ovulation-inducing LH surge, the dominant follicle ruptures (days 13 to 15), with subsequent formation of the
corpus luteum.[30,73] While accompanied by drastic de-

creases in estradiol and inhibin B, there are rising levels of inhibin A and the second increase in progesterone at approximately 36 hours after initiation of the LH surge.[73] Ovulation occurs approximately 35 to 44 hours after the LH surge.[73,74]

As the follicle enlarges, a small cystlike protrusion (i.e., the stigma) develops in the outer follicular wall. Proteolytic enzymes' digestion of the mature follicle capsule's wall, prostaglandins' contraction of the thecal externa smooth muscle, and increased intrafollicular pressure together promote stigma rupture. Initially, fluid oozes from the follicle. Then the oocyte, surrounded by the zona pellucida, extrudes and is carried out by the viscous follicular fluid (see Figure 3-2).

Luteal Phase

Progesterone dominates during the luteal phase of the ovarian cycle. The remaining granulosa cells of the ruptured follicle are changed into lutein cells via stimulation by LH remaining from the LH surge.[22] With luteinization, granulosa cells fill with lipids and become yellowish. Thecal cells of the corpus luteum produce androgens. Androgens are progressively converted to androgenic steroids and then to estrogens and progesterone. The luteinization process is enhanced by rising LH levels accompanying the LH surge and is dependent on the degree of exposure. The process continues with only the initial LH surge, though with decreased secretions of androgens and a shortened corpus luteum life span. The corpus luteum, along with lutein cells, secretes increasing amounts of estrogen and progesterone, particularly progesterone (Figure 2-25). In the midluteal phase, as much as 40 mg/day of progesterone may be secreted by the corpus luteum.[22]

During the luteal phase of the ovarian cycle, FSH and LH levels drop drastically in response to high levels of estrogen and, to a lesser extent, progesterone as secreted by the corpus luteum. Gonadotropin concentrations, especially that of FSH, further decrease secondary to the increased hormone concentration of inhibin A secreted by the luteal cells as signaled by the anterior pituitary gland.[5] Secretion of the hypothalamic pulsatile GnRHs declines, leading in turn to decreased LH pulses in response to increased progesterone levels and hypothalamic signaling.[5] In contrast to the early follicular phase, secretion of the LH pulse generator declines from pulses every 60 to 90 minutes to one pulse every 7 to 8 hours with an increase in the pulse amplitude.[15]

Luteal cells of the corpus luteum constitute the principal source of progesterone (the hormone of pregnancy) and, to a lesser degree, estrogen.[30] Progesterone levels during the

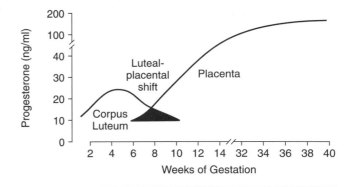

FIGURE **2-25** Diagrammatic representation of the shift in progesterone production from the corpus luteum to the placenta between the seventh and ninth weeks of gestation. (From Liu, J.H. & Rebar, R.W. [1999]. Endocrinology of pregnancy. In R.K. Creasy & R. Resnik [Eds.]. *Maternal-fetal medicine* [4th ed.]. Philadelphia: W.B. Saunders.)

luteal phase suppress FSH levels. Decreased FSH levels (lowest of the cycle) prevent folliculogenesis.[73] LH levels after ovulation differ little from those of the follicular phase secondary to the increased amplitude of the LH pulse generator.[22] LH provision is necessary to maintain the corpus luteum.

Midluteally, peak levels of progesterone and estrogen are noted.[73] These peak ovarian steroid levels are coupled with an endometrium favorable to trophoblastic implantation.[73] During the luteal phase, uterine contractility decreases, becoming nearly quiescent at the time of blastocyst implantation.[16]

The placental hormone hCG (see Chapter 3) also enhances corpus luteum development and continuation during its first 3 to 4 months.[22] Luteinization-inhibiting hormone prevents corpus luteum formation and the subsequent luteinization process until ovulation has occurred.

Corpus Luteum Demise

The corpus luteum involutes in approximately 14 days (give or take 2 days) unless the oocyte is fertilized.[72] FSH levels rise, paralleling the demise of the CL.[22] Decreased FSH and LH levels signal the corpus luteum (approximately 1.5 cm) to begin the involution process at day 21. Declining progesterone, estrogen, and inhibin A levels characterize the remaining 4 to 5 days of the corpus luteum. By day 26 the corpus luteum has progressively involuted to become the corpus albicans, which over the following weeks is replaced by connective tissue. As the corpus luteum involutes, estrogen, progesterone, and inhibin levels fall, removing the feedback inhibition of the anterior pituitary gland. As a result the anterior pituitary begins to secrete progressively more FSH and, in a few days, LH.

With involution, progesterone continues to decrease to a level similar to that of the follicular phase. Declining inhibin A levels 48 hours before menstruation (in concert with rising FSH levels) contribute to follicular recruitment.[73] One day before menstruation, the LH pulse generator frequency increases and amplitude decreases, with a subsequent increase in inhibin B and follicular development.[73] Increased GnRHs are secreted in response to the lower progesterone and estrogen levels, initiating a new ovarian cycle. Menstruation begins. The new ovarian cycle commences with follicular recruitment, selection, and dominance.

Menstruation

Menarche is the first menstrual cycle; the mean age of menarche is 12.7 years of age in the United States.[45] Declines in age of menarche are thought to be associated with improved nutrition. According to Tanner's staging, menarche commonly occurs at stage 4.[45]

With early menstrual cycles the developing follicles secrete only estrogens. Estrogen secretion is variable and is unopposed by progesterone.[64] As a result, early cycles are anovulatory and irregular for 1 to 2 years, with variable menstrual flow.[2,64] Generally within 1 to 2 years, menstrual frequency stabilizes at 28 days, ranging from 26 to 34 days, with pattern variations noted at the extremes of reproductive ages.[22,49] The interval between menstrual cycles averages 28.1 days for women reporting cycle lengths ranging from 15 to 45 days.[11] Cycle length variations primarily occur in the follicular-proliferative phase.[22,49] Lasting 4 days (give or take a day), most menstrual discharge occurs within the first 24 hours,[6,22] with the maximal flow occurring on day 2.[6,49]

Over 3 to 8 days, uterine blood loss averages approximately 35 ml (ranging from 25 to 80 ml), with an equal amount of serous fluid loss per menstrual cycle.[6,11,73] Intersubject menstrual blood loss variations are also noted.[6,27] Iron loss accompanying menstruation is believed to be approximately 0.4 to 1 mg/day of the cycle up to 12 mg/cycle.[6,11,59] Menstrual discharge has a distinctive fleshy, musky odor secondary to tissue necrosis and endometrial ischemia and anoxia.

Endometrial Cycle

The endometrial cycle is composed of proliferative and secretory phases. Whereas the ovary is sensitive to FSH and LH, the uterus is more sensitive to estrogen and progesterone (Figure 2-26). The uterine endometrium is comprised of three layers: the functionalis, containing the stroma (mesenchymal connective tissue); the spongy zone; and the germinal basalis layer, which is adjacent to the myo-

metrium (Figure 2-27).[22] Whereas the functionalis layer is denuded each menstrual cycle, the germinal basalis remains constant throughout.[22] With fertilization, the endometrial tissue changes from secretory tissue to decidual tissue in preparation for implantation.[11] Under the influence of progesterone, the endometrial stroma is transformed to decidual cells.[11] The decidual tissue contains bone marrow cells and immunologic properties to facilitate "acceptance" of the implanting trophoblast: cytokines, relaxin, inhibin, growth factors, and prorenin.[11] Uterine blood is supplied by the uterine and ovarian arteries, which branch to form the arcuate arteries. These arcuate arteries further branch to form the spiral (coiled) arteries and the basal (straight) arteries (Figure 2-27). Spiral arteries supply primarily the endometrial basal layer and are responsive to vasoconstrictive factors; basal vessels are not responsive to vasoconstrictive factors.[11] Spiral arteries underlying the placenta undergo marked changes with pregnancy (see Chapter 3).

Menstrual Phase

Menstrual bleeding is initiated with arterial vasoconstriction, subsequent hematoma formation, and relaxation of the endometrial arteries, followed by bleeding, with resultant anoxia.[11,66] Apoptotical changes occur in the endometrial tissue throughout the endometrial cycle.[61] Fissures form in the functionalis layer, and necrotic outer endometrial fragments of the functionalis detach at the hemorrhagic sites for approximately 48 hours following the initiation of menstruation.[66] This results in desquamation of the superficial endometrial layers down to the basalis layer within 48 to 72 hours, leaving a thin endometrium that cyclically regenerates from the spongy layer.[49] Endometrial tissue and seeping blood evoke uterine contractions.

Menstrual blood clotting and fibrinolysis are orchestrated by hormonal endometrial stimulation.[11] Progesterone facilitates production of tissue factor and plasminogen activator inhibitor–1 for blood coagulation. In contrast, plasminogen activator is released with the necrotic endometrium and enhances the nonclotting properties of the menstrual fluid.[11] In addition, leukocytes and prostaglandins are released with the desquamated tissue and blood.[11] Uterine leukocytes are thought to protect the uterus from infection, though the endometrium is completely desquamated.

Proliferative Phase

The proliferative phase (the first 11 days of the cycle) is also known as the estrogen phase, corresponding to the follicular phase of the ovarian cycle. Proliferative phase variations account for most of the menstrual cycle irregularities.[22]

Approximate Relationship of Useful Morphologic Factors

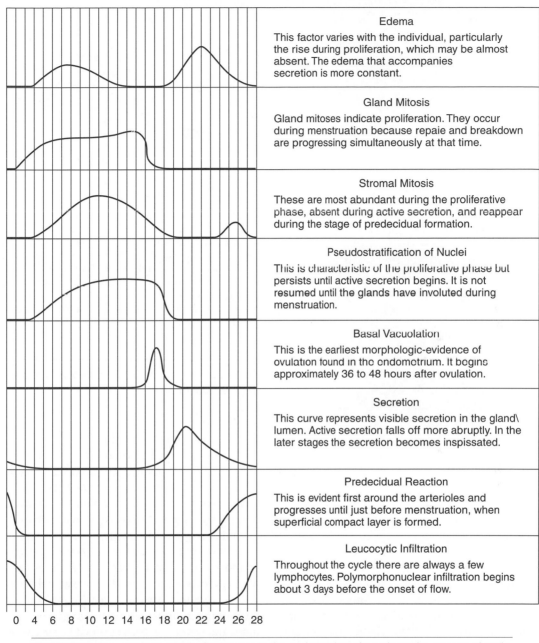

FIGURE **2-26** Characteristic histologic changes in the endometrium throughout the menstrual cycle. (From Noyes, R.W., Hertig, A.T., & Rock, J. [1950]. Dating of the endometrium biopsy. *Fertil Steril, 1,* 3.)

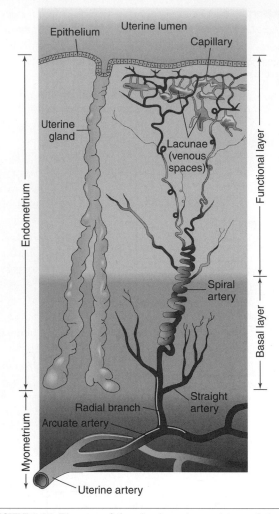

FIGURE **2-27** Diagram of the glands and vasculature of the endometrium. (From Moore, K.L. & Persaud, T.V.N. [1998]. *The developing human: Clinically oriented embryology* [6th ed.]. Philadelphia: W.B. Saunders.)

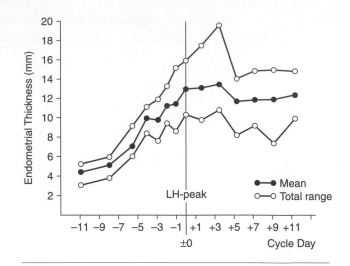

FIGURE **2-28** The endometrial thickness (in mm) measured by transvaginal ultrasound, presented as mean and total range, in 16 women during an ovulatory cycle. Each point on the curve represents a minimum of six observations. (From Bakos, O., Lundkvist, O., & Bergh, T. [1993]. Transvaginal sonographic evaluation of endometrial growth and texture in spontaneous ovulatory cycles: A descriptive study. *Human Reproduction, 8*[6], 799-806.)

the endometrial tissue ranges from 0.5 mm to 5 mm (Figure 2-28).[11,22]

Secretory Phase

The secretory phase, or the following 12 days, corresponds to the luteal phase of the ovarian cycle, with increased secretion of estrogen and progesterone. At ovulation, the endometrium is 3 to 4 mm thick and the endometrial glands secrete a thin, stringy mucus. These mucus strings line the cervical canal, providing channels to guide the sperm. There are increased endometrial lipid and glycogen deposits, along with stromal cytoplasm and tortuosity of blood vessels.[22,49,66] In response to progesterone, vacuoles are formed approximately 36 to 48 hours after ovulation.[11] Stromal edema contributes to enlargement of the endometrium.[66] Increased endoplasmic reticulum and mitochondria are noted in the endometrial epithelial cells.[66]

Midsecretory and Late Secretory Phases

Spotting or breakthrough bleeding may result from decreased estradiol levels at ovulation. Midcycle pain, also referred to as *mittelschmerz,* occurs on the side of the dominant follicle.[49] Accompanying the LH surge is a basal temperature nadir.[24] The basal temperature increases 0.5° to 1° F (0.3° to 0.6° C) on day 16 of the cycle (following the LH surge) and remains elevated for approximately 11 to

Following menstruation, a thin layer of endometrial stroma is left, with few epithelial cells in the endometrial glands and crypts. In the early proliferative phase the endometrial glands are simple and straight.[22,49] With increasing ovarian estrogen the endometrium spongy layer, stromal and epithelial cells, and glandular and stromal mitoses proliferate.[11,49,61] Neutrophils adherent to the endometrium may be the source of vascular endothelial growth factor, promoting endometrial angiogenesis.[19] During the late proliferative phase there is continued growth of the stroma and glands, with corkscrew convolutions, edema, lymphocytes, and macrophages. Cervical mucus significantly increases.[49] From days 12 to 14 of the cycle, there is maximized endometrial growth and proliferation. Growth of

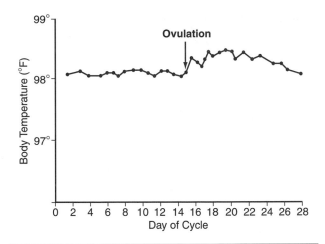

FIGURE **2-29** Elevation of body temperature shortly after ovulation. (From Guyton, A.C. & Hall, J.E. [2000]. *Textbook of medical physiology* [10th ed.]. Philadelphia: W.B. Saunders.)

14 days (Figure 2-29).[24,49] The endometrium responds to the increased progesterone with edema and further secretory development. Endometrial venules and sinusoidal spaces fill with blood and stromal cells accumulate cytoplasm, forming the predecidual endometrial layer. Decidualization is facilitated by transforming growth factor–β and progesterone.[11] Endometrial spiral arteries coil and lengthen,[49,66] and the endometrial glands become increasingly tortuous.[49,66] Endometrial secretory activity is greatest 6 days after ovulation.[22] Increased estradiol and progesterone contribute to maximal stroma edema on day 22.[22] The highly vascularized endometrium is now 5 to 6 mm thick and secreting tissue factors, coagulation factor, plasminogen activator inhibitor–1, and other factors.[11,66] Coiled arteries lengthen rapidly in the thickening endometrium.[49,73] Endometrial secretions increase, preparing for implantation of the fertilized ovum.

If fertilization of the oocyte does not occur, the corpus luteum degenerates secondary to decreased estrogen and progesterone levels. Blood vessels of the secretory endometrium undergo vasoconstriction, arterial relaxation, bleeding, ischemia, and endometrial tissue necrosis. Menstruation occurs.

With fertilization, the secretory endometrium is further transformed to decidual tissue (see Chapter 3). In response to increased estrogen and progesterone, the endometrial stromal cells become decidual cells surrounded by a membrane.[11] Growth of the decidua ranges from 5 to 10 mm in depth in preparation for implantation.[11] Embryonic expression of the heparin-binding epidermal growth factor promotes implantation and tro-

phoblast invasion through paracrine and autocrine signaling.[38] This process helps cells penetrate the stroma and displace the arteriole endothelium. hCG produced by the syncytiotrophoblast (outer layer of the trophoblast) rescues the corpus luteum, thereby increasing estrogen and progesterone levels.[1] The blastocyst implants and pregnancy occurs. (Implantation is discussed further in Chapter 3.)

Premenstrual/Ischemic Phase

The uterus responds to the declining gonadal steroids by stimulating the uterine endometrial cells followed by involution on days 26 to 28. Without support from the corpus luteum, vasospasm occurs in the arterioles and coiled arteries and blood vessels in the endometrial mucosa from 4 to 24 hours before menstruation.[11,26] Endothelin 1 of the endometrium epithelium or stroma promotes vasospasm and vasoconstriction of the endometrial arteries.[66] With vasospasm and decreased estrogen and progesterone, necrosis of the basal layer of the endometrium and stratum vascular blood vessels results and blood pools beneath the endometrium.[22] About 1 to 2 days before menstruation, stroma and epithelial cells of the endometrium produce IL-8 and monocyte chemotactic protein–1, which are chemotactic factors for neutrophils and monocytes.[3,11] As the corpus luteum ceases to function, there is resorption of the endometrial edema, with subsequent endometrial shrinking.[49]

Gestational Follicular Development

During pregnancy, limited follicular maturation continues in response to gonadotropin stimulation. Although follicular growth may continue until delivery, atresia soon follows. Atresia of the follicles occurs before the follicles can grow to ovulatory size.[48]

Climacteric

Menopause and the climacteric are both terms referring to a woman's transition from a reproductive to a nonfertile state. This transition encompasses a myriad of physiologic and psychosocial changes. Although they are sometimes used interchangeably, the terms *climacteric* and *menopause* have different meanings. *Climacteric* is the transitional period encompassing the perimenopausal, menopausal, and postmenopausal years.[31] From 35 years of age onward, there is increased follicular atresia and the ovaries are less responsive, resulting in decreased female fertility.[12] Decreased female fertility precedes menopause.[43] The climacteric continues for approximately 2 to 5 years after menopause and includes the physiologic and psychosocial changes accompanying estrogen deprivation.

TABLE **2-6**   Reproductive Hormone Levels in Postmenopausal Versus Premenopausal Women

HORMONE	PREMENOPAUSAL		POSTMENOPAUSAL		
	PLASMA LEVEL	DAILY PRODUCTION RATE	PLASMA LEVEL	DAILY PRODUCTION RATE	TIGHTLY BOUND (%)
Androstenedione	150 ng/dl	2.7 mg	90 ng/dl	16 mg	0
Testosterone	35 ng/dl	200 μg	25 ng/dl	150 μg	>90
Dehydroepiandrosterone	4-5 ng/dl		1.8 ng/ml		0
Dehydroepiandrosterone sulfate	1500 ng/ml		300 ng/ml		
Estrone	40-200 pg/ml	80-4000 μg	35 pg/ml	55 μg	0
Estradiol	40-350 pg/ml	50-500 μg	13 pg/ml	12 μg	50
Luteinizing hormone	10-40 mIU/ml		70 mIU/ml		
Follicle-stimulating hormone	10-40 mIU/ml		80 mIU/ml		
Prolactin	10 ng/ml		8 ng/ml		

From Korenman, S.G. (1982). Menopausal endocrinology and management. *Arch Int Med, 142,* 1131.

The term *menopause* (from the Greek word for "to stop") means cessation of menses and is confirmed by amenorrhea for 12 months. The mean age of menopause is 51.4 years of age, with a range of 48 to 55 years.[12,72] The 2 years preceding and following menopause are referred to as *perimenopause.*[12]

With reproductive aging, the primary changes occur in the ovary and follicles (particularly the oocytes).[32] Oocytes in women of advanced reproductive age (40 to 45 years) have been found to have abnormal chromosomal alignment at metaphase.[7] Although ovarian follicles may form more rapidly, they are the same size as in earlier years. At menopause, the ovaries are atrophic and weigh less than 10 g. The ovarian medulla is large and contains sclerosed blood vessels. With aging, there is a decrease in the total follicular population and in each type of follicle, though no difference has been noted in the total number of follicles of the right and left ovaries.[23] The ovaries secrete primarily androstenedione at levels 4 times the premenopausal levels, and this contributes to increased ovarian vein testosterone levels (15 times higher).[72] During perimenopause, minimal follicles are present at various stages (i.e., primordial to atretic) of development. It is thought that in the decade before menopause there is a significant increase in follicular atresia, which accounts for the minimal ovarian follicles.[72] For 1 to 5 years perimenopausally, menstrual cycles lengthen, and ovulation frequency and reproductive hormone levels vary (Table 2-6).[50] In a woman's midthirties and early forties, the hormone inhibin begins to progressively decline.[44] Subsequently, FSH levels increase as a compensatory mechanism.[18,68] Initially, LH levels stabilize at approximately premenopausal levels, though they begin to rise following amenorrhea of 12 months and then plateau.[36] Changes in inhibin and FSH concentration may precede decreased levels of estrogen and progesterone.

During menopause, estrone becomes the major estrogen; it is derived primarily from peripheral aromatization of adrenal androstenedione, mainly adipose tissue.[49] Thus the daily production of estrone is significantly related to the woman's body mass index.[72]

With ovarian aging, there is a decrease in estradiol synthesis. Only about 10% of the ovaries secrete estradiol.[42] With aging, androstenedione decreases, with a subsequent decrease in estradiol production. After menopause, androstenedione expression decreases by approximately 50%. Postmenopausally, estradiol concentrations decline, ranging from 20 to 25 pg/ml.[12] The hypothalamic-pituitary-estrogen positive-feedback mechanism no longer initiates LH secretion.[68] As ovulation frequency decreases, anovulatory cycles increase, with a subsequent decrease in progesterone.

Reproductive hormone levels change with menopause. Hormonal confirmation of menopause includes a 10% to 20% increase in FSH levels and LH levels 3 to 5 times greater than those in earlier menstrual cycles. FSH levels increase gradually but do so significantly. LH levels greater than 40 IU/L and early follicular FSH levels greater than 30 IU/L are frequently clinical markers for ovarian reserve.[43,44] FSH levels maximize approximately 1 to 3 years after menopause.[31] Postmenopausally, testosterone levels decrease from 200 μg/day to 150 μg/day.[49] Therefore an androgen excess state exists.[12]

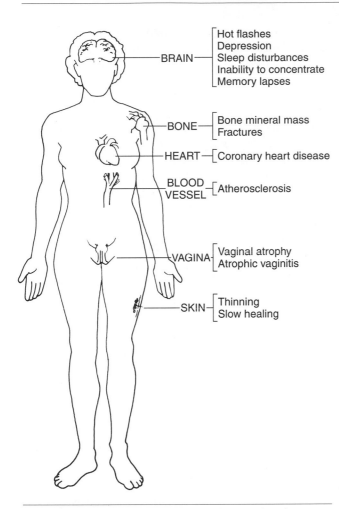

BRAIN — Hot flashes
Depression
Sleep disturbances
Inability to concentrate
Memory lapses

BONE — Bone mineral mass
Fractures

HEART — Coronary heart disease

BLOOD VESSEL — Atherosclerosis

VAGINA — Vaginal atrophy
Atrophic vaginitis

SKIN — Thinning
Slow healing

FIGURE **2-30** Effect of estrogen deprivation or reduced estrogen on different organ and tissue systems at or after menopause. (From Dawood, M. Y. [2000]. Menopause. In L.J. Copeland [Ed.]. *Textbook of gynecology* [2nd ed.]. Philadelphia: W.B. Saunders.)

Menopausal declines in estradiol have numerous physiologic and psychologic effects (Figure 2-30), including vasomotor instability, breast tissue reduction, sleep difficulties, depression, atrophy of urogenital epithelium, atrophy of vaginal tissue and dermis, osteoporosis, coronary heart disease, lethargy, headaches, and concentration difficulties.[12,49]

REPRODUCTIVE PROCESSES IN THE MALE
Endocrinology

The hormones of the male reproductive system are released by the hypothalamus, anterior pituitary, and testes. Release is both systemic and local, being continuous or acyclic after puberty. Slight diurnal changes in plasma testosterone levels

occur. The release of male reproductive hormones is controlled by a negative feedback loop along the hypothalamic-pituitary-testicular axis (see Figure 2-7).

Testosterone is an androgen produced by the Leydig cells of the testes. Initial production of testosterone early in embryonic development is responsible for development of the male reproductive organs and external genitalia. Production becomes active again at puberty. Testosterone is necessary for spermatogenesis, development of male secondary sex characteristics, bone growth, growth and development of male reproductive organs, sexual drive, and potency. The testes also produce small amounts of other androgens.

The hypothalamus regulates the testicular environment by secreting GnRH, which is moderated further by norepinephrine, serotonin, endorphin, melatonin, and dopamine. GnRH secretion occurs once every 70 to 90 minutes. The pulsatile pattern is required for the production and release of LH and FSH by the anterior pituitary.

Both LH and FSH act directly on the testes, stimulating spermatogenesis and testosterone production. Both hormones have a high affinity for their respective receptors. Once bound, they activate the protein kinase cascade via cAMP. LH stimulates the Leydig cells to initiate steroidogenesis by synthesizing androgens from cholesterol precursors. Along with androgen production, LH is responsible for triggering spermatogenesis.

The effects of FSH complement those of LH. FSH binds to receptor sites in the Sertoli cells, stimulating the production of proteins that in turn affect spermatogenesis. FSH is also responsible for facilitating mitosis in the spermatogonia and initiating meiosis in the spermatocyte. Lastly, FSH seems to be necessary for the maturation of the spermatid. Normal levels of FSH are necessary to maintain normal sperm quality.

Testicular testosterone is thought to act directly on the germ cells and Sertoli cells. Through diffusion and active transport, testosterone supports the germinal epithelium and regulates spermatogenesis.

Puberty

Reproductive capability in men begins with spermarche. Unlike menarche, which occurs toward the end of puberty, spermarche begins early in puberty, preceding the peak growth spurt and beginning at an average at 13½ years of age. Puberty generally takes about 4 years to complete, beginning somewhere between 11 and 16 years of age. During this time there are growth and development of the reproductive organs, rapid physical growth, and development of secondary sex characteristics.

The specific stimulus or mechanism for initiating puberty is unclear. There is an increase in the release of pituitary gonadotropins, which stimulates the production of androgens, particularly testosterone. Synthesis of testosterone and other androgens that results in the changes in the reproductive system and somatic tissue.

The major changes include the enlargement of the testes and penis; development of pubic, axillary, facial, and body hair; rapid skeletal growth; hypertrophy of the larynx, with subsequent deepening of the voice; increased activity of the sweat and sebaceous glands; and muscular hypertrophy. Along with these changes, the seminiferous tubules begin sperm production. Before this point, a meiosis-inhibiting factor may be secreted by the Sertoli cells to inhibit spermatogonia meiosis. The earliest observable changes are the enlargement of the testes and scrotum resulting from growth of the seminiferous tubules. Ejaculation generally can occur about a year after the growth of the penis.

Sperm Production

Sperm production takes place within the complex endocrine environment described earlier. The development of mature germ cells in the seminiferous tubules involves three stages: (1) *mitosis,* spermatogonial multiplication; (2) *meiosis,* production of haploid cells; and (3) *spermiogenesis,* maturation of spermatids to mature spermatozoa. The androgens and proteins produced locally modulate spermatogenesis seen within the seminiferous tubule. (See Chapter 1.)

The seminiferous tubule is divided into basal and luminal compartments. The basal compartment is the outer layer (zone 1) of the tubule, while the luminal compartment is the inner layer. The basal compartment is composed of stem cells (type A spermatogonia) that are renewed through mitosis. Some of these continue to proliferate and serve as stem cells, whereas others (preleptotene spermatocytes or type B spermatogonia) separate from the basal membrane and begin to migrate toward the lumen. As migration progresses, the cells undergo further morphologic changes, becoming primary spermatocytes. The first and second meiotic divisions occur with further differentiation in the adluminal zone, resulting in the formation of secondary spermatocytes and spermatids. The luminal spermatids undergo a complex sequence of changes within the cell organelles (spermiogenesis). (Spermatogenesis and spermiogenesis are discussed further in Chapter 1.)

The sperm move down the tubules by contraction and fluid secretion by the Sertoli cells. The evolution process takes approximately 64 to 74 days. At the time of their release into the seminiferous tubules, the spermatozoa are still morphologically immature and lack motility. While traversing the epididymis (which takes 14 to 21 days), they continue to differentiate. Forward motility is achieved in the proximal epididymis. (Ejaculation, sperm transport, and fertilization are described in Chapter 3.)

Climacteric

Males do not experience a cessation in reproductive ability in the same manner that females experience menopause. There is a gradual decline in testosterone production and in spermatogenesis in the thirties and forties. Reproductive ability is usually not compromised, however. In later life, atrophy of the external genitalia occurs. Concomitantly there are involution of the testes and degenerative changes in the Leydig cells, thereby diminishing the production of testosterone. The age at which these events occur is variable among individual men, and some do not experience them at all.

SUMMARY

Reproductive endocrinology is an orchestrated cascade of events initiated in utero and mediated by hormonal control. Episodic pulses of gonadotropin-releasing factors and hormones modulate the secretion of gonadal steroids, estrogen, and progesterone. Cyclical follicular development and maturation, in concert with endometrial changes, prepare for the fertilized oocyte. Knowledge of the hypothalamic-pituitary-ovarian axis undergirds obstetrical, infertility, and gynecologic nursing.

REFERENCES

1. Al-Sebai, M.A.H., et al. (1995). The role of a single progesterone measurement in the diagnosis of early pregnancy failure and the prognosis of fetal viability. *Obstet Gynaecol, 102,* 364.
2. Apter, D. (1997). Development of the hypothalamic-pituitary-ovarian axis. *Ann NY Acad Sci, 816,* 9.
3. Arici, A., et al. (1996). Modulation of the levels of interleukin-8 messenger ribonucleic acid and interleukin-8 protein synthesis in human endometrial stromal cells by transforming growth factor-β1. *J Clin Endocrinol Metab, 81,* 3004.
4. Asselin, E., et al. (2000). Mammalian follicular development and atresia: role of apoptosis. *Biolog Signals & Receptors, 9,* 87.
5. Baird, D.T. (1998). Feedback mechanisms. In I.S. Fraser, et al. (Eds.). *Estrogens and progestogens in clinical practice.* Philadelphia: Churchill Livingstone.
6. Baldwin, R.M., et al. (1961). Measurements of menstrual blood loss. *Am J Obstet Gynecol, 81,* 739.
7. Battaglia, D.E. & Soules, M.R. (1994). Maternal aging and regulation of meiosis in the human oocyte. *Proc Annual Meeting Soc Gynecol Invest,* abstract 0163.
8. Branisteaun, I., et al. (1997). Detection of immunoreactive interleukin-11 in human follicular fluid: correlations with ovarian steroid, insulin-like growth factor 1 levels, and follicular maturity. *Fertil Steril, 67,* 1054.
9. Casper, F.W., et al. (2001). Concentrations of inhibins and activin in women undergoing stimulation with recombinant follicle-stimulating hormone for in vitro fertilization treatment. *Fertil Steril, 75,* 32.

10. Chiquoine, H.D. (1960). The development of the zona pellucida of the mammalian ovum. *Am J Anat., 106,* 149.

11. Cunningham, F.G., et al. (2001). *Williams obstetrics* (21st ed.). New York: McGraw-Hill.

12. Dawood, M.Y. (2000). Menopause. In L.J. Copeland (Ed.). *Textbook of gynecology* (2nd ed.). Philadelphia: W.B. Saunders.

13. Demura, R., et al. (1993). Human plasma free activin and inhibin levels during the menstrual cycle. *J Clin Endocrinol Metab, 76,* 1080.

14. Ebeling, P. & Koivisto, V.A. (1994). Physiological importance of dehydroepiandrosterone. *Lancet, 343,* 1479.

15. Ellinwood, E.H., et al. (1989). Dynamics of steroid biosynthesis during the luteal-placental shift in rhesus monkeys. *J Clin Endocrinol Metab, 69,* 348.

16. Fanchin, R., et al. (2001). Uterine contractility decreases at the time of blastocyst transfers. *Hum Reprod, 16,* 1115.

17. Filicori, M., et al. (1986). Characterization of the physiologic pattern of episodic gonadotropin secretion through out the human menstrual cycle. *J Clin Endocrinol Metab, 62,* 1136.

18. Freeman, E.W., et al. (2001). Hot flashes in the late reproductive years: Risk factors for African-American and Caucasian women. *J Women's Health Gender-Based Med,* 10(1), 67.

19. Gargett, C.E., et al. (2001). Focal vascular endothelial growth factor correlates with angiogenesis in human endometrium. Role of intravascular neutrophils. *Hum Reprod, 16,* 1065.

20. Genazzani, A.R., et al. (2000). Neuropeptides, neurotransmitters, neurosteroids, and the onset of puberty. *Ann N Y Acad Sci, 900,* 1.

21. Goodman, A.L. & Hodgen, G.D. (1983). The ovarian triad of the primate menstrual cycle. *Recent Prog Horm Res, 39,* 1.

22. Gordon, K. & Oehninger, S. (2000). Reproductive physiology. In L.J. Copeland (Ed.). *Textbook of gynecology* (2nd ed.). Philadelphia: W.B. Saunders.

23. Gougeon, A. & Chainy, B.B.N. (1987). Morphometric studies of small follicles in ovaries of women at different ages. *J Reprod Fert, 81,* 433.

24. Greene, C.A. & O' Keane, J.A. (2000). Investigation of the infertile couple. In L.J. Copeland (Ed.). *Textbook of gynecology* (2nd ed.). Philadelphia: W.B. Saunders.

25. Groome, N.P., et al. (1996). Measurement of dimeric inhibin-B throughout the human menstrual cycle. *J Clin Endocrinol Metab, 81,* 1401.

26. Guyton, A.C. & Hall, J.E. (2000). *Textbook of medical physiology* (10th ed.). Philadelphia: W.B. Saunders.

27. Hallberg, L., et al. (1966). Menstrual blood loss—A population study. *Acta Obstetricia Gynecologica Scandinavica, 45,* 320.

28. Halvorson, L.M. & Chin, W.W. (1999). Gonadotropic hormones: Biosynthesis, secretion, receptors, and action. In S.C. Yen, R.B. Jaffe, & R.L. Barbieri (Eds.). *Reproductive endocrinology: physiology, pathophysiology, and clinical management* (4th ed.). Philadelphia: W.B. Saunders.

29. Hayes, F.J., et al. (1998). Differential control of gonadotropin secretion in the human: Endocrine role of inhibin. *J Clin Endocrinol Metab, 83,* 1835.

30. Hillier, S.G. (1998). Biosynthesis and secretion of ovarian and adrenal steroids. In I.S. Fraser, et al. (Eds.). *Estrogens and progestogens in clinical practice.* Philadelphia: Churchill Livingstone.

31. Kass-Annese, B. (1999). *Management of perimenopausal & postmenopausal woman: A total wellness program.* Philadelphia: Lippincott.

32. Klein, N.A., et al. (1996). Ovarian follicular development and the follicular fluid hormones and growth factors in normal women of advanced reproductive age. *J Clin Endocrinol Metab, 81,* 1946.

33. Knight, P.G., et al. (1996). Development and application of a two site enzyme immunoassay for the determination of "total" activin-A concentrations in serum and follicular fluid. *J Endocrinol, 148,* 267.

34. Knobil, E. (1989). The electrophysiology of the GnRH Pulse generator in the rhesus monkey. *J Steroid Biochem, 33,* 669.

35. Krsmanovic, L.Z., et al. (1996). Pulsatile gonadotropin releasing hormone release and its regulation. *Trends Endocrinol Metab, 7,* 56.

36. Kwekkeboom, D.J., et al. (1990). Serum gonadotropins and a subunit decline in aging normal postmenopausal women. *J Clin Endocrinol Metab, 70,* 944.

37. Layman, L.C. & McDonough, P.G. (2000). Mutations of follicle stimulating hormone-β and its receptor in human and mouse: Genotype/phenotype. *Molecular Cellular Endocrinol, 161,* 9.

38. Leach, R.E., et al. (1999). Multiple roles for heparin-binding epidermal growth factor-like growth factor are suggested by its cell-specific expression during the human endometrial cycle and early placentation. *J Clin Endocrinol Metab, 84,* 3355.

39. Lenton, E.A., et al. (1991). Inhibin concentrations throughout the menstrual cycles of normal, infertile, and older women compared with those during spontaneous conception cycles. *J Clin Endocrinol Metabol, 73,* 1180.

40. Lévy, D.P., et al. (2000). The role of LH in ovarian stimulation-exogenous LH: Let's design the future. *Hum Reprod, 15,* 2258.

41. Liu, J.H. & Rebar, J.R. (1999). Endocrinology of pregnancy. In R.K. Creasy & R. Resnik (Eds.). *Maternal-fetal medicine* (4th ed.). Philadelphia: W.B. Saunders.

42. Longcope, C. (1998). Metabolism of estrogens and progestogens. In I.S. Fraser, et al. (Eds.). *Estrogens and progestogens in clinical practice.* Philadelphia: Churchill Livingstone.

43. Macklon, N.S. & Fauser, B.C.J.M. (1999). Aspects of ovarian follicle development throughout life. *Horm Res, 52,* 161.

44. Metcalf, M.G. & Livesay, J.H. (1985). Gonadotrophin excretion in fertile women: Effect of age and the onset of the menopausal transition. *J Endocrinol, 105,* 357.

45. Mitan, L.A.P. & Slap, G.B. (2000). Adolescent menstrual disorders. *Adolescent Medicine, 84,* 851.

46. Moore, K.L. & Persaud, T.V.N. (1998). Before we are born: Essentials of embryology and birth defects (5th ed.). Philadelphia: W.B. Saunders.

47. Murphy, P.A. (1990). Anatomy and physiology of the female reproductive system. In R. Litchtman & S. Papera (Eds.). *Gynecology: Well-woman care.* Norwalk, CT: Appleton & Lange.

48. Nelson, W.W. & Greene, RR. (1958). Some observations on the histology of the human ovary during pregnancy. *Am J Obstet Gynecol, 76,* 66.

49. Norman, R.J. & Phillipson, G. (1998). The normal menstrual cycle: changes throughout life. In I.S. Fraser, et al. (Eds.). *Estrogens and progestogens in clinical practice.* Philadelphia: Churchill Livingstone.

50. O'Connor, K.A., et al. (2001). Menstrual cycle variability and the perimenopause. *J Human Biology, 13,* 465.

51. O'Malley, B.W. & Strott, C.A. (1999). Steroid hormones: metabolism and mechanism of action. In S.C. Yen, R.B. Jaffe, & R.L. Barbieri (Eds.). *Reproductive endocrinology: Physiology, pathophysiology, and clinical management* (4th ed.). Philadelphia: W.B. Saunders.

52. Palter, S.F., et al. (2001). Are estrogens of import to primate/human ovarian folliculogenesis? *Endocr Rev, 22,* 389.

53. Persaud, T.V.N. (2000). Embryology of the female genital tract and gonads. In L.J. Copeland (Ed.). *Textbook of gynecology.* Philadelphia: W.B. Saunders.

54. Rittmaster, R.S. (2000). Hyperandrogenism. In L.J. Copeland (Ed.). *Textbook of gynecology* (2nd ed.). Philadelphia: W.B. Saunders.

55. Rogers, R.J., et al. (2001). Dynamics of the membrana granulosa during expansion of the ovarian follicular antrum. *Molecular Cellular Endocrinol, 171,* 41.

56. Runesson, E., et al. (2000). Gonadotropin- and cytokine-regulated expression of the chemokine interleukin 8 in the human preovulatory follicle of the menstrual cycle. *J Clin Endocrinol Metab, 85,* 4387.

57. Scheele, F. & Schoemaker, J. (1996). The role of follicle-stimulating hormone in the selection of follicles in human ovaries: a survey of the literature and a proposed model. *Gynecol Endocrinol, 10,* 55.

58. Schneyer, A.L., et al. (2000). Dynamic changes in the intrafollicular inhibin/activin/follistatin axis during human follicular development: relationship to circulating hormone concentrations. *J Clin Endocrinol Metab, 85,* 3319.

59. Scott, D.E. & Pritchard, J.A. (1967). Iron deficiency in healthy young college women. *JAMA, 199,* 147.

60. Seger, R., et al. (2001). The ERK signaling cascade inhibits gonadotropin-stimulated steroidogenesis. *J Biological Chemistry, 276,* 13957.

61. Shikone, T., et al. (1997). Apoptosis of human ovary and uterine endometrium during the menstrual cycle. *Horm Res, 48,* 27.

62. Shacham, S., et al. (2001). Mechanism of GnRH receptor signaling on gonadotropin release and gene expression in pituitary gonadotrophs. *Vitamins Horm, 63,* 63.

63. Sidis, Y., et al. (2001). Follistatin: Essential role for the N-terminal domain in activin binding and neutralization. *J Biological Chemistry, 276,* 17718.

64. Spence, J.E.H. (1997). Anovulation and monophasic cycles. *Ann N Y Acad Sci, 816,* 173.

65. Stanczyk, F.Z. (1998). Structure-function relationships and metabolism of estrogen and progestogens. In I.S. Fraser, et al. (Eds.). *Estrogens and progestogens in clinical practice.* Philadelphia: Churchill Livingstone.

66. Strauss, J. & Cortifaris, C. (1999). The endometrium and myometrium: regulation and dysfunction. In S.C. Yen, R.B. Jaffe, & R.L. Barbieri (Eds.). *Reproductive endocrinology: Physiology, pathophysiology, and clinical management* (4th ed.). Philadelphia: W.B. Saunders.

67. Ukkola, O., et al. (2001). Age, body mass index, race and other determinants of steroid hormone variability: The HERITAGE Family Study. *Eur J Endocrinol, 145,* 1.

68. Weiss, G. (2001). Menstrual irregularities and the perimenopause. *J Soc Gynecol Investig, 8,* S65.

69. Welt, C.K., et al. (2001). Differential regulation of inhibin A and inhibin B by luteinizing hormone, follicle-stimulating hormone, and stage of follicle development. *J Clin Endocrinol Metab, 86,* 2531.

70. Welt, C.K., et al. (1997). Frequency modulation of follicle-stimulating hormone (FSH) during the luteal-follicular transition: evidence for FSH control of inhibin B in normal women. *J Clin Endocrinol Metab, 82,* 2645.

71. Woodruff, T.K. & Mather, J.P. (1995). Inhibin, activin and the female reproductive axis. *Annu Rev Physiol, 57,* 219.

72. Yeh, J. & Adashi, E.Y. (1999). The ovarian life cycle. In S.C. Yen, R.B. Jaffe, & R.L. Barbieri (Eds.). *Reproductive endocrinology: Physiology, pathophysiology, and clinical management* (4th ed.). Philadelphia: W.B. Saunders.

73. Yen, S.C. (1999). The human menstrual cycle: neuroendocrine regulation. In S.C. Yen, R.B. Jaffe, & R.L. Barbieri (Eds.). *Reproductive endocrinology: Physiology, pathophysiology, and clinical management* (4th ed.). Philadelphia: W.B. Saunders.

74. Yen, S.C. (1999). Neuroendocrinology of reproduction. In S.C. Yen, R.B. Jaffe, & R.L. Barbieri (Eds.), *Reproductive endocrinology: Physiology, pathophysiology, and clinical management* (4th ed.). Philadelphia: W.B. Saunders.

75. Young, E.A., et al. (2000). Alteration in the hypothalamic-pituitary-ovarian axis in depressed women. *Arch Gen Psychiatry, 57,* 1157.

76. Zeleznik, A.J. (2001). Modifications in gonadotropic signaling: A key to understanding cyclic ovarian function. *J Soc for Gynecol Investig, 8,* S24.

Prenatal Period and Placental Physiology

The prenatal period encompasses the period from conception to birth. During this period the pregnant woman experiences major physiologic and psychologic changes that support maternal adaptations and fetal growth and development as well as prepare the mother for the birth process and transition to parenthood. Simultaneously the embryo and fetus are developing from a single cell to a complex organism. Supporting this development are the placenta, fetal membranes (amnion and chorion), and amniotic fluid. These structures protect and nourish the embryo and fetus and are essential for the infant's survival, growth, and development. Alterations in maternal physiology, endocrine function, embryonic and fetal development, or placental function and structure can lead to maternal disorders and fetal death, malformations, poor growth, or preterm birth. Assessment of placental size and function and amniotic fluid volume and composition is useful in evaluating fetal growth and health status during gestation. This chapter describes events that result in conception and provides an overview of pregnancy; related endocrinology; and development of the embryo, fetus, and placenta. Specific clinical implications related to normal and abnormal aspects of the development and functional status are discussed.

PREGNANCY

The duration of pregnancy averages 266 days (38 weeks) after ovulation, or 280 days (40 weeks) after the first day of the last menstrual period (Figure 3-1). This equals 10 lunar months, or just over 9 calendar months. During these months, the almost solid uterus, with a cavity of 10 ml or less, develops into a large, thin-walled organ. The total volume of the contents of the uterus is 5 L or more at term, 500 to 1000 times the original capacity.[35]

Most of the changes encountered during pregnancy are progressive and can be attributed to either hormonal responses or physical alterations secondary to fetal size. The preimplantation endocrine system controls the reproductive cycles in males and females. In the woman, this system is controlled by the cyclic release of pituitary gonadotropins and secretion of estrogen and progesterone by the ovary (see Chapter 2).

The pregnancy-specific or postimplantation endocrine system controls the integrity and duration of gestation. These processes include: (1) prolongation of the corpus luteum by human chorionic gonadotropin (hCG); (2) production of estrogen, progesterone, human placental lactogen (hPL), and other hormones and growth factors by the placenta; and (3) release of oxytocin (by the posterior pituitary), prolactin (by the anterior pituitary), and relaxin (by the ovary, uterus, and placenta). Changes in specific organ systems and metabolic processes during pregnancy and clinical implications are described in detail in Units II and III. This section presents an overview of physiologic changes during each trimester of pregnancy. Concomitant with these adaptations and equally significant are psychologic adaptations; these adaptations are not discussed because the focus of this text is on physiologic changes.

First Trimester

During the first trimester the woman experiences the first signs and symptoms of pregnancy. The first sign of pregnancy is usually cessation of menses. The average cycle length is 28 days (give or take 7 days), with a range of 15 to 45 days. The first missed period is suggestive of pregnancy; by the time the second period is missed, pregnancy becomes probable. Brief or scant bleeding may occur during pregnancy, most commonly in the first trimester around the time of implantation.

Breast tenderness and tingling, especially around the nipple area, often occurs beginning at 4 to 6 weeks. Increased breast size and vascularity are usually evident by the end of the second month and are due to growth of the secretory duct system. Colostrum leakage may occur by 3 months. Enlargement of the sebaceous glands around the nipple (Montgomery's glands) may also be apparent.

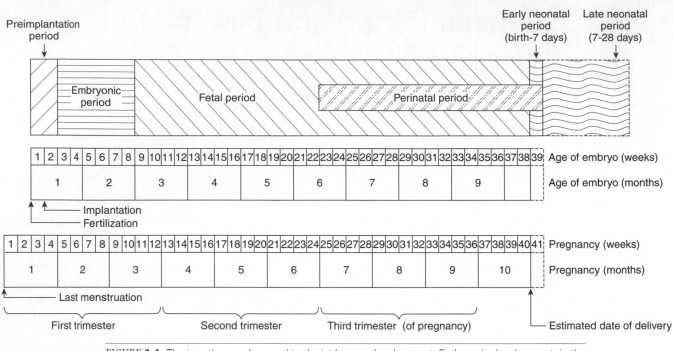

FIGURE **3-1** The two time scales used to depict human development. Embryonic development, in the upper scale, is counted from fertilization (or from ovulation [i.e. postovulatory days]). The clinical estimation of pregnancy is counted from the last menstrual period and is shown on the lower scale. Note that there is a 2-week discrepancy between these scales. The perinatal period is very long because it includes all of the preterm deliveries. (From Williams, P.L. [1995]. *Gray's anatomy: The anatomical basis of medicine and surgery* [38th ed.]. Edinburgh: Churchill-Livingstone.)

Nausea with or without vomiting may occur any time of the day or night. This symptom usually begins about 6 weeks after the onset of the last menstrual period and continues for 6 to 12 weeks or longer in some women. An increase in frequency of urination is seen during the first trimester, subsiding by about 12 weeks. Excessive fatigue is often experienced and may last throughout the first 12 weeks. The cause of this fatigue is unknown, but it may be a response to hormonal shifts. Hormonal changes are also thought to be responsible for the dyspnea experienced during this period.

Physical signs associated with pregnancy include Goodell's sign (softening of the cervix and vagina with increased leukorrheal discharge), Hegar sign (softening and increased compressibility of the lower uterine segment), and Chadwick's sign (bluish-purple discoloration of the vaginal mucosa, cervix, and vulva) by 8 weeks. Although a presumptive sign of pregnancy, Chadwick's sign is only useful in primiparous women.

By 8 to 10 weeks, fetal heart tones can be auscultated by Doppler ultrasonography. Real-time ultrasound can pick up fetal heart movements earlier. Maternal cardiovascular changes are also occurring, with cardiac volume as well as cardiac output already beginning to increase. These changes contribute to increased renal plasma flow and glomerular filtration.[35] Weight gain during the first trimester is usually small.

Second Trimester

This trimester is characterized by marked maternal changes as the fetus's presence becomes more evident. The uterus, which started as a pear-shaped organ, is now ovoid, as length increases over width. With this growth, the uterus moves into the abdominal cavity and begins to displace the intestines. The tension and stretching of the broad ligament may lead to low, sharp, painful sensations. Normally contractions during the second trimester are irregular and usually painless.

The increasing vascularity of the vagina and pelvic viscera may result in increased sensitivity and heightened arousal and sexual interest. Mucorrhea is not uncommon as a result of the hyperactivity of the vaginal glandular tissues. This change may increase the pleasure experienced during sexual intercourse. Spontaneous orgasm and multiple orgasm may occur as a result of the increased congestion.

Leukorrhea often occurs, with thick, white, acidic (pH of 3.5 to 6.0) discharge that may contribute to inhibition of pathogenic colonization of the vagina.[55] Perineal structures also enlarge as a result of the vasocongestion, increased vascularity, hypertrophy of the perineal body, and fat deposition that began during the first trimester.

The breasts become increasingly more nodular. Colostrum can be easily expressed at this stage. The nipples become larger and more deeply pigmented. The areolae have also broadened. Increased skin pigmentation occurs elsewhere as well. The line from the symphysis to the pubis (linea alba) may darken very distinctly and is referred to as the *linea nigra*. Darkening of the skin over the forehead and cheeks (chloasma gravidarum) can also result from the hormonal changes. Deeper pigmentation changes seem to occur in women with darker complexions. Most pigmentation changes resolve following delivery.

Other cutaneous changes include the appearance of spider nevi and capillary hemangiomas. The former usually resolve; the latter may shrink but often do not completely disappear after delivery. The breakdown of underlying connective tissue may result in reddish, irregular stretch marks on the abdomen, buttocks, thighs, or breasts. Although little can be done to prevent the formation of stretch marks, they may fade with time.

Increased estrogen levels may result in hyperemic, soft, swollen gums that bleed easily. Increased salivation also may occur. Good oral and dental care is important. Elevated progesterone levels decrease the motility of the gastrointestinal tract. By the end of the second trimester, esophageal regurgitation may lead to heartburn. Fluid retention and constipation also may occur as pregnancy progresses.

Maternal blood volume rises significantly during these months, and hematocrit and hemoglobin levels fall. Blood pressure decreases slightly, whereas the heart rate increases by 10 to 20 beats per minute. Cardiac output increases slowly from the first trimester. Some women present with a grade II systolic murmur.[224] Glomerular filtration rates increases, especially over the second and third trimesters. Bladder and ureter tone is decreased, and the ureters become more tortuous, increasing the risk of urinary tract infection.

Protein and carbohydrate needs increase markedly, contributing to the weight gain during this phase. The mother first perceives fetal movement (quickening) at 16 to 20 weeks (earlier in successive pregnancies). These movements become perceptible to a hand on the mother's abdomen toward the end of this period. By 20 weeks, the uterus will be at the level of the umbilicus.[55]

Third Trimester

In the third trimester fatigue, dyspnea, and increased urinary frequency are experienced. Fatigue and dyspnea are related to the increased weight and pressure exerted by the greatly enlarged uterus. Thoracic breathing predominates. Increased urinary frequency is due to pressure of the presenting part against the bladder.

The uterine wall is thin (1.5 cm or less). The myometrium softens and is easily indented. The fetus can be easily palpated through the uterine wall, and fetal movements are quite visible. The uterus reaches almost to the liver, and broad ligament pain may become more intense as tension is increased. Uterine contractions become more regular and uncomfortable and are easily detected and palpable at 38 to 40 weeks.

The heart is displaced slightly to the left now as a result of the increased pressure from the enlarged uterus. Blood pressure rises slightly, and cardiac output remains unchanged. Blood volume peaks at 30 to 34 weeks. Dependent edema frequently occurs as blood return from the lower extremities is reduced. Increasing pelvic congestion, relaxation of the smooth muscle in the veins, and the increased pressure of the growing fetus lead to varicosities of the perineum and rectum. Constipation and obesity may lead to development of engorged blood vessels.[35,55]

The growing uterus displaces the intestines and stomach. The upper portion of the stomach may herniate, increasing the hiatus of the diaphragm. This produces heartburn and decreases the stomach's capacity. The bladder is pulled up and out of the true pelvis by the growing uterus. This stretches the urethra and increases the susceptibility to urinary tract infection.

The increased elasticity of connective and collagen tissue leads to relaxation and hypermobility of the pelvic joints. Separation of the symphysis pubis results in instability of the sacroiliac joint. The center of gravity shifts lower with development of a progressive lordosis to compensate for the anterior shift of the uterus. Balance is maintained by an enhanced cervicodorsal curvature, leading to difficulty in walking and the characteristic waddling gait. Stress on the ligaments and muscles of the middle and lower back and spine may lead to discomfort and back pain.[35]

Most women tolerate these changes without difficulty; however, many become tired of pregnancy late in gestation. The process of conception and the changes related to pregnancy are truly remarkable events. The coming together of all factors brings about the appropriate and necessary environment for the nurturance and development of the next generation.

CONCEPTION

For conception to occur, a precise set of sequential events must take place. The probability of a viable conception per menstrual cycle is only 30% at best.[34,42] The process of conception and fetal survival is selective, as evidenced by implantation failures and the approximately 50% anomaly rate encountered in spontaneously aborted fetuses.[121] Gametogenesis is described in Chapter 1. The ovarian and endometrial cycles necessary for conception and early support of the fertilized ovum, as well as follicle maturation, are described in Chapter 2. This section will examine ovulation, sperm transport, fertilization, cleavage, and zygote transport.

The ovary is responsible for two important functions: gametogenesis and steroid hormone synthesis. Integration of ovarian steroid synthesis, follicle maturation, ovulation, and corpus luteum function is essential for fertilization and implantation. Estrogen and progesterone have significant effects on tubal and uterine motility, endometrial proliferation, and the properties of the cervical mucus.[35] The close proximity of the germ cells and steroid-producing cells in the ovary allows the ovary to control follicle maturation; ovulation; and corpus luteum formation, function, and regression. The hypothalamus and anterior pituitary regulate these morphologic changes through secretion of gonadotropin-releasing hormone (GnRH) and gonadotropins. Follicle-stimulating hormone (FSH) and luteinizing hormone (LH) act synergistically (see Chapter 2).

Ovulation

In the fully developed follicle, multiple layers of granulosa cells line the antral side of the basement membrane, and a cumulus of granulosa cells surrounds the oocyte. The oocyte is covered by the zona pellucida (ZP). The theca cells surrounding the follicle are fully vascularized. The follicle produces large amounts of estradiol; the level peaks about 24 hours before ovulation.

LH levels are also rising, which increases production of progesterone by the dominant follicle through interaction of LH with LH receptors on granulosa cells. The rise in progesterone occurs 12 to 24 hours before ovulation and elicits a rapid and marked surge in LH secretion, paralleling the mid-cycle FSH peak (see Chapter 2). This LH peak is essential for ovulation which occurs 28 to 36 hours later.[29,35] The mid-cycle surge of LH initiates ovulation by stimulating prostaglandin (PGE and PGF) synthesis, lead-ing to formation of collagenase and other proteolytic enzymes with disruption of the gap junctions between the oocyte and follicular cells.[29] This disrupts meiotic inhibition and initiates completion of the first meiotic division. The oocyte completes its first meiotic division 10 to 12 hours before ovulation, forming the secondary oocyte (23 chromosomes plus most of the cell cytoplasm) and first polar body (23 chromosomes and minimal cytoplasm). The small polar body is nonfunctional and degenerates (see Chapter 1). The LH surge also causes a decrease in estradiol production.

Ovulation begins with a protrusion or bulge on the ovarian wall. A small avascular spot (stigma) develops, forms a vesicle, and ruptures, extruding the secondary oocyte, follicular fluid, and cells. Rupture is thought to be caused by enzymatic digestion of the follicular wall via the action of proteases (e.g., collagenase, plasmin, and hyaluronic acid), which dissolve connective tissues (Figure 3-2).[58,121] The oocyte is surrounded by the ZP and corona radiata (radially arranged granulosa cells). The second meiotic division begins with ovulation, then arrests and is not completed until fertilization. The oocyte is swept by the fimbriae into the fallopian tube. Muscular contraction of the tube and, primarily, beating of the cilia move the ovum along the tube to the ampulla (the usual site of fertilization). If unfertilized, the ovum usually dies within 24 hours.[121]

Corpus Luteum

After ovulation the follicular walls and theca collapse inward and become vascularized (Figure 3-2). The granulosa cells undergo a luteinizing process to form the corpus luteum, which secretes progesterone with a small amount of estrogen secreted by the theca cells (see Chapter 2). If fertilization has taken place, implantation occurs during the latter part of this week. Around the time of implantation, the trophoblast tissue secretes hCG, a luteotropin that stimulates the corpus luteum to continue to function and may alter the metabolism of the uterus to prevent the release of substances that result in luteal regression. If implantation does not occur, hCG is not produced, the corpus luteum begins to regress, and involution begins. The decline in steroids results in menstruation.

The corpus luteum is not essential for pregnancy maintenance once the placenta has developed the capacity to secrete estrogens and progesterone. The corpus luteum is probably essential for continuation of the pregnancy for the first 6 to 7 weeks. From 6 to 10 weeks, there is a transition period in which both the placenta and corpus luteum are producing hormones; by 7 weeks the pla-

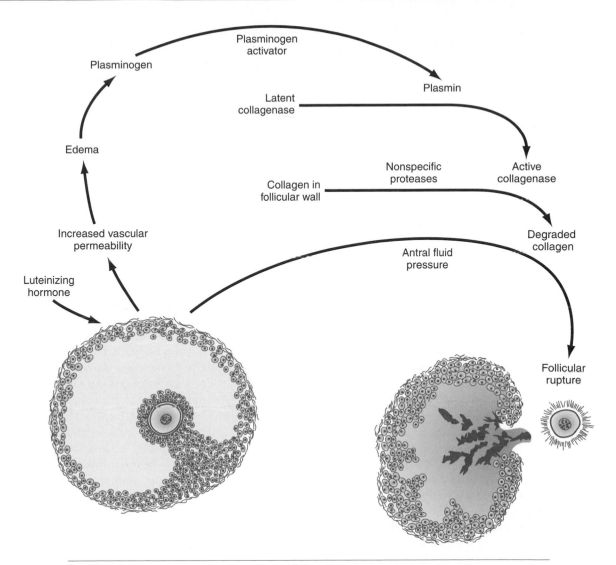

FIGURE **3-2** Factors involved in mammalian ovulation. (From Carlson, B.M. [1999]. *Human embryology & developmental biology* [2nd ed.]. St. Louis: Mosby.)

centa is capable of producing sufficient progesterone to maintain pregnancy.[24] At 6 to 8 weeks, there is a dip in progesterone levels, indicating a decline in corpus luteum functioning. This is followed by a secondary rise in progesterone (presumably as a result of placental takeover) without a rise in the metabolite 17α-hydroxyprogesterone (secreted by corpus luteum). Around 32 weeks there is a more gradual rise in this metabolite, indicating placental utilization of fetal precursors.[24]

Sperm Transport

Spermatozoa have not completely differentiated when they are released into the lumen of the seminiferous tubules (Chapter 1). They are nonmotile and incapable of fertilization. Mature sperm have a condensed and genetically inactive nucleus. Reactivation of the nucleus occurs once the sperm enters the cytoplasm of the ovum.[180] Sperm are moved down the seminiferous tubules and through the epididymis and vas deferens by: (1) the pressure of additional sperm forming behind them, (2) seminal fluid, and (3) peristaltic action. Biochemical and morphologic maturation of the sperm (see Figure 1-8) occurs during their 9- to 14-day passage through the epididymis. Further modifications occur after ejaculation so that the sperm can bind to the ZP of the ovum. Sperm are stored in the vas deferens and epididymis before ejaculation. Ejaculation occurs through the urethra with contraction of the ampulla and the ejaculatory duct upon orgasm.

The volume of ejaculate ranges from 2 to 6 (mean 3.5) ml and usually contains 40 to 250 million sperm per ml.[29] Men with less than 20 million sperm per ml are likely to be sterile.[162] Some spermatozoa are immature, senescent, and abnormal, and generally only the normal and strongest sperm are able to complete the journey within the female reproductive tract to the upper end of the fallopian tube. As sperm move along the epididymis, they begin to gain motility. Sperm become fully motile in the semen after entering the female reproductive tract.[180] Semen provides fructose for energy and an alkaline pH for protection against the acid environment of the vagina and dilutes the sperm to improve motility. Sperm move at 2 to 3 mm per minute. Motility is slower in the acidic vaginal environment, but increases in the alkaline uterine environment.[121] Failure of sperm to achieve motility is a cause of male infertility; for potential fertility at least 40% should be motile by 2 hours after ejaculation.[121]

The neck and midpiece of the spermatozoa contain a pair of centrioles, the base of the tail apparatus, and the mitochondrial sheath. The mitochondria are arranged in a tight helical spiral around the anterior portion of the flagellum (tail). Mitochondria supply the adenosine triphosphate (ATP) required for independent motility. Sperm must reach the ovum within an allotted time or they exhaust their energy supply and die. Sperm survival in the uterus is relatively short because phagocytosis by leukocytes begins within a few hours. Most sperm do not survive for more than 48 hours, although some may survive for up to 80 hours.[29,121]

Once deposited at the external cervical os, some ejaculated sperm cross the cervical mucus facilitated by a decrease in mucus viscosity at mid-cycle, allowing for more rapid migration. Within minutes the sperm enter the uterine cavity, although some get caught in cervical crypts and endometrial glands. The cervical crypts provide a short-term reservoir or storage site from which sperm are gradually released; this may increase the chance of fertilization.[121] Sperm can reach the upper end of the fallopian tube 5 to 20 minutes after ejaculation. Uterine motility, stimulated by prostaglandins in seminal fluid that cause smooth muscle contraction, facilitates initial sperm transport.[60] Other sperm move more slowly or are stored in cervical crypts and may not reach the ampulla for up to 80 hours.[29] Sperm transport in the female reproductive system is illustrated in Figure 3-3.

Sperm chemotaxis (organized movement of the sperm toward the ovum) is stimulated by chemoattractants in follicular fluid, and possibly the cumulus oorphus and ovum.[44] At least one chemoattractant in follicular fluid has been identified. Other components of follicular fluid that may also act as chemoattractants include heparin, progesterone, atrial natriuretic peptide, epinephrine, oxytocin, calcitonin, and acetylcholine.[43] Thus sperm appear to be responsive to chemicals released by the ovum and use these substances to "find" the ovum.

Fertilization

The process of fertilization has been defined in three different ways: (1) the instant of sperm and ovum fusion, (2) time from sperm-ovum fusion to development of the male and female pronuclei, and (3) time from sperm-ovum fusion to the first mitotic division (about 24 hours). Fertilization begins with contact between the sperm and secondary oocyte, arrested in the metaphase of the second meiotic division (see Chapter 1). Fertilization usually occurs in the upper third of the fallopian tube, usually in the ampulla. Before fertilization the sperm must undergo two final maturational changes: capacitation and the acrosome reaction.

Capacitation involves removal of the glycoprotein coat and seminal plasma proteins from the plasma membrane

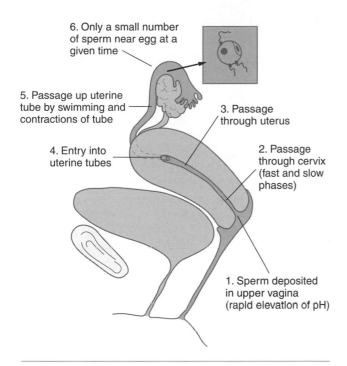

6. Only a small number of sperm near egg at a given time

5. Passage up uterine tube by swimming and contractions of tube

4. Entry into uterine tubes

3. Passage through uterus

2. Passage through cervix (fast and slow phases)

1. Sperm deposited in upper vagina (rapid elevation of pH)

FIGURE **3-3** Sperm transport in the female reproductive system. (From Carlson, B.M. [1999]. *Human embryology & developmental biology* [2nd ed.]. St. Louis: Mosby.)

over the acrosome (head of the sperm), which allows the acrosomal reaction to occur. Capacitation takes about 7 hours and usually occurs in the fallopian tubes but may begin while the sperm is still in the uterus. This process is stimulated by substances in the female genital tract and follicular fluid.[58,121] For example, albumin in genital tract secretions stimulates loss of fatty acids and cholesterol from the sperm plasma membrane. This increases permeability of the sperm plasma membrane and initiates capacitation and the acrosome reaction.[1]

Capacitation is a transient process that, in vitro, lasts 50 to 240 minutes.[44] Capacitated sperm are chemiotaxically active.[43] Approximately 2% to 14% of the sperm are capacitated at any time, with continued replacement of sperm that lose their capacitation with newly capacitated sperm. Each sperm can only become capacitated once in its lifespan.[43] This constant replacement of capacitated sperm extends the time when fertilization is possible by continuous production of "ripe" sperm.[43,44] Thus after ejaculation there are precapacitated, capacitated, and postcapacitated sperm, as well as sperm that have undergone the acrosomal reaction within the female genital tract.[44]

Of the millions of sperm in the ejaculate, only about 200 to 250 (range from 80 to 1400) sperm are found in the fal-

lopian tubes at any given time.[29,178] Similar numbers of sperm appear to enter each fallopian tube, but the ampulla of the ovulatory tube has more sperm than the ampulla of the nonovulatory tube.[178] Although it takes only one sperm to penetrate the ovum, it appears that several hundred are necessary to effect passage of the spermatozoa through the corona radiata to the ovum. The number of spermatozoa that are ejaculated does not appear to influence the number of sperm that enter the fallopian tubes unless very low counts occur.[60]

For successful penetration of the corona radiata and ZP to occur, the acrosome reaction must occur with release of enzymes through small holes in the acrosomal membrane. The acrosome is a saclike structure on the head of the sperm containing many enzymes, including acid glycohydrases, proteases, phosphatases, esterases, and hyaluronidase.[1,121] The capacitated sperm binds to the ZP of the ovum, initiating the acrosome reaction (sperm activation).[1,114] The sperm penetrates the ZP and binds to the outer membrane of the oocyte.

Once a sperm has passed through the ZP, a zonal reaction occurs, with physicochemical alterations in the ZP that make it impenetrable to other sperm. The ZP is an ovum-specific extracellular membrane composed of three glycoproteins (ZP1, ZP2, ZP3) that act as ligands (molecules that bind to receptors) for sperm receptors. The ZP is secreted by the growing oocyte and helps to regulate fertilization.[114] Roles of the ZP include sperm activation (acrosome reaction), preventing fertilization by more than one sperm, protecting the ovum before fertilization, and species specificity.[114]

The sperm head transverses the perivillous space between the plasma membranes and ZP and attaches to the surface of the oocyte, and their plasma membranes fuse. This process is mediated by integrins (adhesion molecules) on the ovum surface along with fertilin and other substances produced by the sperm.[114] The head and tail of the sperm enter the oocyte, leaving the outer plasma membrane of the sperm attached to the outer membrane of the oocyte (Figure 3-4). The ovum has a layer of cortical secretory granules along the inside of its plasma membrane. After sperm entry these granules release proteases and glycosidases into the perivillous space. This modifies the ZP glycoproteins preventing activation and entry of other sperm.[114,142,176]

After entering the cytoplasm of the oocyte, the sperm undergoes rapid morphologic changes. The tail of the sperm degenerates and the head enlarges to form the male pronucleus. Each pronucleus has 23 chromosomes (22 autosomes and 1 sex chromosome). Sex of the offspring is determined by the male and depends on whether

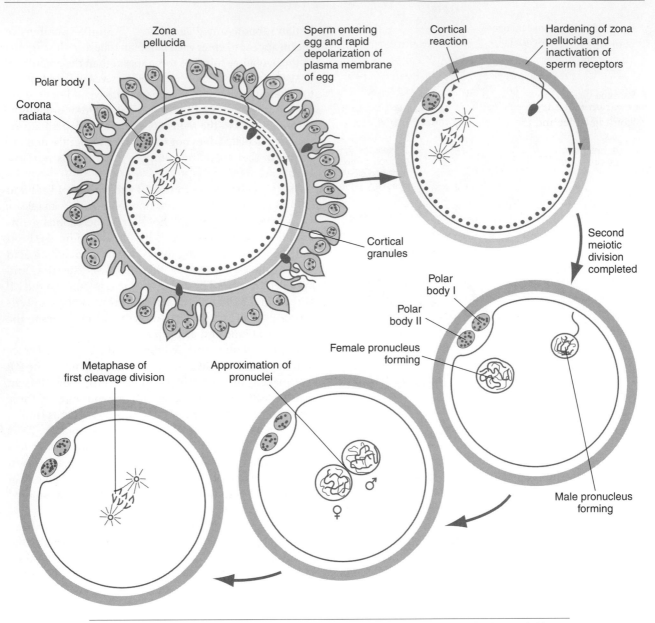

FIGURE **3-4** Summary of the main events involved in fertilization. (From Carlson, B.M. [1999]. *Human embryology & developmental biology* [2nd ed.]. St. Louis: Mosby.)

the sperm that enters the ovum contains an X or Y chromosome. The sperm nucleus becomes reactivated so that it can again synthesize DNA and RNA.[180] This processing involves removal of the nuclear membrane with exposure of the sperm chromatin to the cytoplasm of the ovum. The nuclear protein is remodeled and the nucleus decondenses, becoming larger and more spherical. A new nuclear envelope develops, forming the male pronucleus and activating DNA transcription and replication. The exact mechanisms for this process are unclear but are thought to be mediated by factors in the cytoplasm of the ovum. This process takes about 3 to 4 hours, during which the developing male pronucleus gradually approaches the female pronucleus.[180]

The ovum must also be activated. Entry of the sperm into the ovum triggers two events: (1) the cortical reaction described earlier, which blocks entry of other sperm, and (2) a transient increase in intracellular calcium.[114,142] The increased calcium stimulates the oocyte to complete its second meiotic division with extrusion of the second polar body into the perivitelline space. The nucleus enlarges and is called the *female pronucleus*. The oocyte is now mature and metabolically active.[142,176] Failure of calcium signaling can lead to complete failure (triploidy) or partial failure (abnormalities of chromosomal number of the second meiotic division, cleavage arrest, and alterations in development of the inner cell mass and trophectoderm [trophoblast]). These alterations can result in implantation failure and miscarriage.[169]

The female and male pronuclei approach each other, their membranes disintegrate, and the nuclei fuse (see Figure 3-4). Chromatin strands intermingle, and the diploid number (46) of chromosomes is restored. The zygote (from the Greek, meaning "yoked together") is formed, and mitotic division (cleavage) begins. The zygote measures 0.2 mm in diameter and carries the genetic material necessary to create a unique human being. Fertilization results in species variation, with half of the chromosomes coming from the mother and half from the father, mixing the genes each parent originally received from their parents.[121]

Cleavage and Zygote Transport

Cleavage involves a series of rapid mitotic cell divisions that begins with the first mitotic division of the zygote and ends with formation of the blastocyst. Cleavage is under the control of mitosis-promoting or maturation-promoting factor (MPF).[29] The zygote divides into two daughter cells (blastomeres) about 30 hours after fertilization; each of these cells divides into two smaller cells, which also divide, and so forth (Figure 3-5). The dividing cells are contained by the ZP and become progressively smaller with each sub-

sequent division, with no change in the total mass of the zygote. Cell division occurs every 12 to 24 hours. By 3 to 4 days, the zygote has divided into 8 to 16 blastomeres. Around the 8- to 9-cell stage, the blastomeres realign and form a tight ball of cells mediated by cell surface adhesion glycoproteins. This process, called *compaction*, allows increased interaction between cells needed for formation of the inner cell mass. This occurs via gap and tight junctions.[29]

The zygote remains in the ampulla for the first 24 hours, then is propelled down the fallopian tube by ciliary action over the next few days. At the 12- to 15-cell stage (about 3 days after fertilization), the zygote becomes a solid cluster of cells called the *morula* (from the Greek word for "mulberry," which it resembles).[24,29] The zygote reaches the uterine cavity 3 to 4 days after fertilization (about 90 hours or 5 days after follicle rupture). As fluid from the uterine cavity (which provides nutrients for the organism) enters the morula, the blastocyst is formed. The blastocyst consists of four distinct components: (1) ZP, a thick glycoprotein membrane that is beginning to stretch and thin; (2) trophectoderm (trophoblast), a one-cell-thick outer layer of flattened cells that will form the placenta; (3) inner cell mass (embryoblast), a one- or two-cell-thick, crescent-shaped cluster of cells that will form the embryo; and (4) fluid-filled blastocyst cavity.[33,121] The ZP protects the zygote from adhering to the mucosa of the fallopian tube and from rejection by the maternal immune system (see Chapter 12). Position of individual cells and gene transcription factors influence which cells become trophoblast and which become inner cell mass. If these gene transcription factors are deficient, all or most of the cells in the blastocyst become part of the trophectoderm, resulting in a molar pregnancy (see Gestational Trophoblast Disease).[33] The blastocyst floats free in the uterine cavity from 90 to 150 hours after ovulation, then begins to implant (Figure 3-6).

EMBRYONIC AND FETAL DEVELOPMENT

The infant develops progressively from the single-cell fertilized egg to a highly complex multicellular organism. The genetic constitution of the individual is established at the time of fertilization. During development of the embryo and fetus, genetic information is unfolded to control morphologic development. Alterations in genetic information or morphologic development can modify structure and function of cells and organs and result in congenital defects. This section provides an overview of embryonic and fetal development and includes a discussion of basic principles of morphogenesis and implications for the

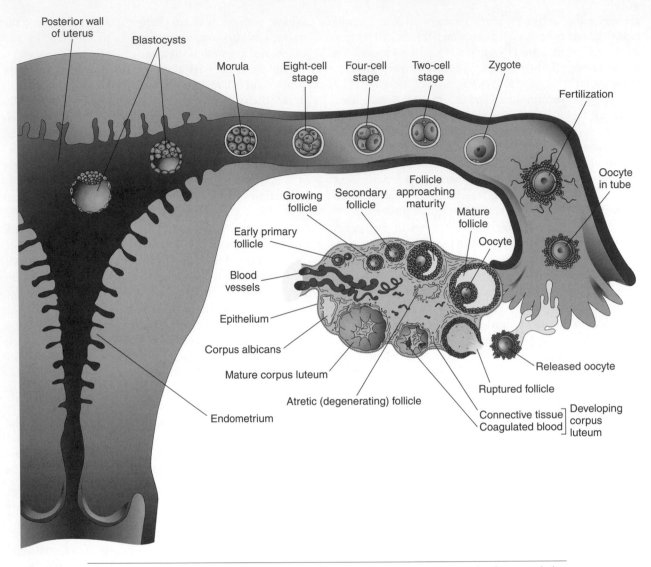

FIGURE **3-5** Diagrammatic summary of the ovarian cycle, fertilization, and human development during the first week. (From Moore, K.L. & Persaud, T.V.N. [1998]. *The developing human: Clinically oriented embryology* [6th ed.]. Philadelphia: W.B. Saunders.)

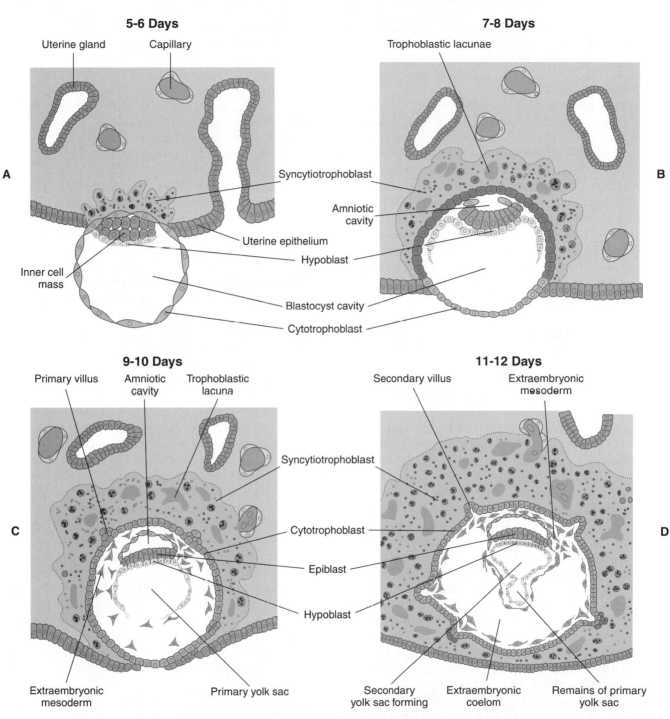

5-6 Days

Uterine gland
Capillary

Syncytiotrophoblast

Uterine epithelium

Hypoblast

Inner cell mass

Blastocyst cavity

Cytotrophoblast

A

7-8 Days

Trophoblastic lacunae

Amniotic cavity

B

9-10 Days

Primary villus   Amniotic cavity   Trophoblastic lacuna

Syncytiotrophoblast

Cytotrophoblast

Epiblast

Hypoblast

Extraembryonic mesoderm   Primary yolk sac

C

11-12 Days

Secondary villus   Extraembryonic mesoderm

Secondary yolk sac forming   Extraembryonic coelom   Remains of primary yolk sac

D

FIGURE **3-6** Implantation and early development of the embryo. **A,** Syncytiotrophoblast invades endometrium. **B,** Most of the embryo is embedded in the endometrium with early formation of trophoblastic lacunae. The amniotic cavity and primary yolk sac are beginning to form. **C,** Implantation is almost complete; primary villi are forming and the embryonic mesoderm is appearing. **D,** Implantation is complete; secondary villi and the secondary yolk sac are forming. (From Carlson, B.M. [1999]. *Human embryology & developmental biology* [2nd ed.]. St. Louis: Mosby.)

pathogenesis of developmental defects. Principles of genetics are discussed in Chapter 1; development of specific body systems is described in Units II and III.

Principles of Morphogenesis

Embryonic development combines growth, differentiation, and organization of cellular components at all levels. As development progresses, differential synthesis is established, resulting in cellular differentiation. Growth is the process of creating more of a substance that is already present through increase in cell size and number. In contrast, differentiation is the creation of new types of substances, cells, tissues, and organs that were not previously present. Organization is the process by which these elements are coordinated into functional integrated units. Morphogenesis is the production of a special form, shape, or structure of a cell or group of cells and occurs by the precise organization of cell populations into distinct organs.[59]

The mechanisms controlling morphogenesis are complex and incompletely understood.[29] Development is controlled by developmental gene families within the embryo.[21,29,32,51,54,57,162] Although the first cell divisions after fertilization are under maternal control, by the 2- to 4-cell stage, the embryonic genome is activated and is producing many intercellular signaling proteins. These proteins regulate cell activities, such as causing a cell to differentiate in a specific way, and are modulated by positive and negative feedback loops.[51] Positive feedback induces further production of regulatory proteins and gene transcription factors that influence that cell or other target cells. Negative feedback results in the production of inhibitors. This process is controlled by interactions of developmental genes with environmental factors that turn the gene on and off at precise intervals. Each gene can produce multiple isotypes, each isotype producing a different product. The different isotypes are produced by splicing and reorganization of the DNA within that gene.[162] Individual developmental genes may have different functions at different stages of development and with development of specific organs.[21,29,32,51] Examples of developmental gene families that control development include the homeobox (HOX) and PAX gene families. For example, the HOX genes are involved with craniocaudal organization; the PAX gene family is involved with development of the urogenital system, central nervous system (CNS), thyroid gland, and eye, among other sites.[29]

Transcription factors remain within the cell and bind to DNA at the promoter or enhancer regions of specific genes or regulate mRNA production. Intercellular signaling molecules (first messengers), many of which are growth factors, influence other cells by binding to receptor molecules (Figure 3-7). Examples of signaling molecules include activin (mesodermal inductor), inhibin (inhibitor of gonadotropin secretion), transforming growth factor–β (TGF-β) (mesoderm inducer, myoblast proliferation) and decapentaplegic (limb development inductor).[21,29,32,51,54,57] Receptor molecules can be intracellular or on the cell surface. Extracellular receptors are binding sites for ligands (hormones, growth factor, or cytokine). Binding to the receptor alters the receptor and stimulates an intercellular response (signal transduction) either directly via a protein kinase or indirectly via a second messenger such as cyclic adenosine monophosphate (cAMP) (see Figure 3-7). Examples of mechanisms for signaling between mesenchymal and epidermal cells are illustrated in Figure 3-8.

The human embryo's progression through stages of development is shared by many other creatures (phylogenetic recapitulation). As a result, animal models can be useful in understanding developmental processes and deviations in humans. Development and maturation generally proceed in a cephalocaudal direction. Morphogenesis is accomplished by a variety of mechanisms.

Cell Differentiation

Initially all cells are similar and unspecialized, but each must eventually become one of 350 different cell types found in the human body.[165] Cells pass through two phases in order to become specialized. In the first phase (determination) the cell becomes restricted in its developmental capabilities and loses the ability to develop in alternative ways (Figure 3-9). Cell determination occurs for the first time in the blastocyst, with formation of the inner cell mass (which forms the embryo) and trophectoderm (which becomes the placenta). In the second phase (differentiation) cells develop distinctive morphologic and functional characteristics. Initially cell position determines the fate of the cell. Specific differentiation is regulated by interactions between cell populations and is controlled by HOX and other gene families that are switched on to produce specific proteins in a sequential manner.[17,126,165]

Induction

Induction is the process by which cells in one part of the embryo influence cells around them to develop in a specific way. Induction requires inductors, or cells that stimulate reactions in surrounding cells via signal transudation and induced tissue, which is made up of cells that have the capacity or competence to respond to the protein signals via cell membrane receptor molecules (see Figure 3-8). At

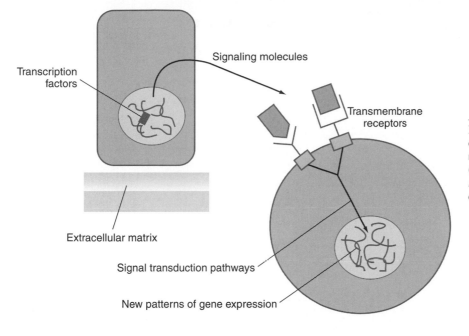

FIGURE **3-7** Schematic representation of types of developmentally important molecules and their sites of action. (From Carlson, B.M. [1999]. *Human embryology & developmental biology* [2nd ed.]. St. Louis: Mosby.)

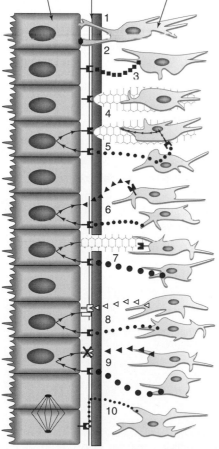

1 Direct cell-cell contact by gap junctions.

2 Cell-cell contact by cell adhesion molecules.

3 A soluble factor (growth factor) reacting with a receptor for that factor on the epithelial cells.

4 Extracellular matrix molecule secreted by the mesenchyme cells interacting with a receptor on the epithelial cell.

5 A soluble factor (growth factor) secreted by a mesenchymal cell having a biphasic action, interacting (1) with a receptor on an epithelial cell, causing it to express a specific extracellular matrix molecule receptor, and (2) with a receptor on a mesenchyme cell, causing it to secrete a specific extracellular matrix molecule that then interacts with the induced epithelial receptor.

6 A soluble factor (growth factor) secreted by a mesenchyme cell interacting with a receptor on an epithelial cell, causing it to express a receptor or secrete a factor, which interacts with another factor synthesized, or receptor expressed, by another mesenchyme cell.

7 A soluble factor secreted by a mesenchyme cell interacting with a receptor on an epithelial cell, causing it to synthesize an extracellular matrix molecule (or a receptor for such a molecule) that then interacts with a specific receptor for that molecule on another mesenchyme cell.

8 A soluble factor secreted from a mesenchyme cell interacting with a receptor on an epithelial cell, causing it to synthesize a molecule that stabilizes or enhances the interaction between a mesenchymal derived factor and its epithelial receptor.

9 A soluble factor secreted by a mesenchyme cell interacting with a receptor on an epithelial cell, causing the inhibition of synthesis or assembly of a factor or receptor.

10 A soluble factor secreted by a mesenchyme cell binding to the extracellular matrix of the basal lamina where it remains active and subsequently interacts with a receptor on an epithelial cell that appears at a later developmental time.

FIGURE **3-8** The many ways by which mesenchyme cells can signal to epithelial cells. Precisely the same mechanisms can operate in reverse for epithelium to mesenchyme. (From Williams, P.L. [1995]. *Gray's anatomy: The anatomical basis of medicine and surgery* [38th ed.]. Edinburgh: Churchill-Livingstone.)

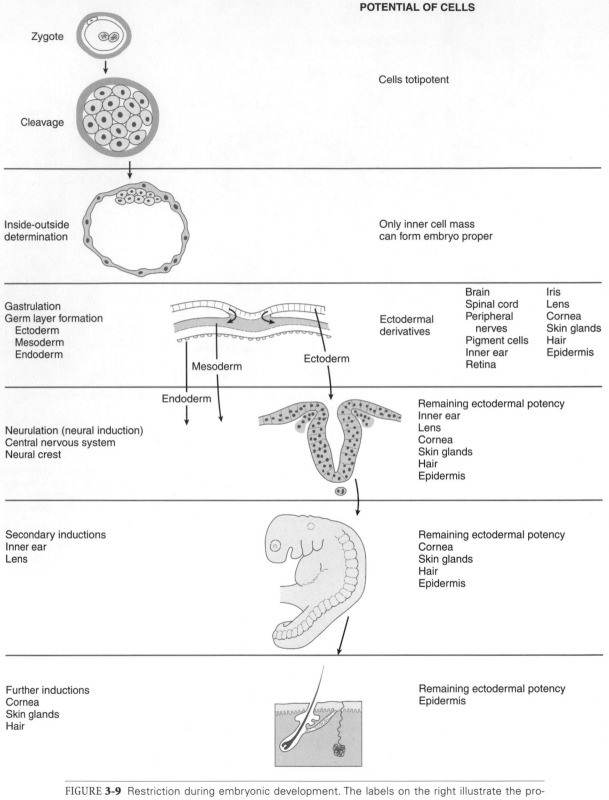

POTENTIAL OF CELLS

Zygote

Cleavage

Cells totipotent

Inside-outside
determination

Only inner cell mass
can form embryo proper

Gastrulation
Germ layer formation
  Ectoderm
  Mesoderm
  Endoderm

Mesoderm

Ectoderm

Endoderm

Ectodermal
derivatives

Brain	Iris
Spinal cord	Lens
Peripheral	Cornea
nerves	Skin glands
Pigment cells	Hair
Inner ear	Epidermis
Retina	

Neurulation (neural induction)
Central nervous system
Neural crest

Remaining ectodermal potency
Inner ear
Lens
Cornea
Skin glands
Hair
Epidermis

Secondary inductions
Inner ear
Lens

Remaining ectodermal potency
Cornea
Skin glands
Hair
Epidermis

Further inductions
Cornea
Skin glands
Hair

Remaining ectodermal potency
Epidermis

FIGURE **3-9** Restriction during embryonic development. The labels on the right illustrate the progressive restriction of the developmental potential of cells that are in a line leading to the formation of the epidermis. On the left are the developmental events that remove groups of cells from the epidermal track. (From Carlson, B.M. [1999]. *Human embryology & developmental biology* [2nd ed.]. St. Louis: Mosby.)

some point, inductors and inducers lose their ability to perform these actions.[32,57,61]

Secondary induction is a chain of developmental events and is a common way many parts of the embryo are formed. For example, in the nervous system the notochord is a primary inductor or organizer for brain development. The forebrain reacts to secondary inductors in the mesoderm to form the optic cup, which then induces adjacent ectoderm to form the eye lens. The eye lens then induces epidermis around it to form the corneal epithelium. If any of these steps is interfered with, the next stage in development may not occur, or may occur abnormally. If these alterations occur early in the developmental sequence, complete organ agenesis may result.[17,61,121] An example of chemical pathway activity during secondary induction is the interaction of activin and TGF-β, which influences branching of epithelial tubes in the kidney, pancreas, and salivary glands.[54]

Differential Cell Proliferation

Differential cell proliferation results from localized differences in rates of cell division. Proliferation is controlled by cell signaling mechanisms and growth factors. These differences may lead to a buildup of cells in certain areas or may result in a phenomenon called invagination, in which cells growing more slowly than surrounding cells appear to be "sinking" into tissues. In fact, one set of cells is overtaking the other cells in growth. This phenomenon can be seen during the development of the neural groove, the oral cavity, and the nostrils. The rate of cell proliferation is modulated by interactions of receptor molecules on the surface of the cells with systemic and local growth factors that stimulate proliferation during organogenesis. A period of rapid cell proliferation often precedes differentiation.[17,61] Proliferation inhibition by teratogenic agents may cause defects. Growth inhibition can also be caused by lack of space (when space runs out, tissues stop proliferating). For example, with a diaphragmatic hernia, the intestinal contents are in the thoracic cavity and inhibit lung development.

Programmed Cell Death

Cell death is a precisely timed event—under genetic control and cell feedback mechanisms—that occurs in many of the embryonic tissues as part of normal development. The process involves the release of lysosomal hydrolytic enzymes that dissolve cells, thereby altering the tissues. This mechanism is responsible for lumen formation in solid tubes (trachea and parts of the gut) and the disappearance of the webbing between the fingers and toes. If enzyme release is inhibited, syndactyly, some forms of bowel atresia, or im-

perforate anus may result. If enzyme activity is increased, micromelia (shortened limbs) may result.[17,165]

Cell Size and Shape Changes

Cell size and shape changes occur with elongation or narrowing and swelling or shrinkage. Elongation or narrowing is accomplished by the coordinated activities of cell microfilaments and microtubules. Microtubules are long cylinders containing tubulin, a substance that alters its length when polymerized (i.e., joined together to form a molecule of higher molecular weight [MW]). Certain chemicals (including some found in microorganisms) inhibit tubulin polymerization and normal microfilament action. Changes in osmotic balance or interference in transport of elements across the membranes results in swelling or shrinkage of cells.[17,61]

Cell Migration

During development some cells move around in a fashion similar to that of an amoeba. This process is dependent on microtubular and microfilament elongation and contraction. Migration involves the elongation of the leading edge of the cell, followed by adhesion of the cell to a new contact point. Contraction of the cell toward the new adhesion site results in movement of the cell. Alterations or interference with the enzyme system may limit cell migration and result in a defect. Hirschsprung's disease (absence of intestinal ganglion cells) results from failure of neural crest cells to migrate. From 3 to 6 months' gestation there is normally migration of millions of neurons and glial cells within the central nervous system from their point of origin in the periventricular area to their eventual loci in the cerebrum and cerebellum. Alterations in this migration can result in defects in CNS organization and function (see Chapter 14).[17,61,121,165]

Cell Recognition and Adhesion

This mechanism involves the adhesion of certain cells, such as the neural folds, which meet and fuse to form the neural tube. The recognition and adhesion process involves interaction of specific substrates (e.g., integrins, glycoproteins, cell surface enzymes) on one cell with complementary substrates, enzymes, or adhesion molecules on the membrane of another cell. A similar mechanism is seen with adhesion during cell migration. Interference with cellular membrane substrates may prevent adhesion. Alterations in this mechanism may be responsible for cleft palate or neural tube defects.[17]

Folding of the Embryo

The embryo begins as a relatively straight line of cells. As new cells form, the embryo is forced to conform to available space. To adapt to the confined space, the embryo folds (curves) in both transverse and longitudinal planes. Folding in the transverse plane causes the embryo to become cylindric in shape; longitudinal folding results in the head and tail folds. Structures within the embryo (e.g., heart, intestines) also undergo folding to conform to the space available to them.

Differential Maturity

Various tissues and organs are at different stages of maturity throughout development. For example, the gut and bladder are essentially structurally complete at birth, whereas the long bones and lung alveoli do not reach maturity for years after birth. Therefore various organs are more or less vulnerable to insults and toxic agents at different stages of development.

Overview of Embryonic Development

Preembryonic development occurs from the time of conception and zygote formation until 2 weeks' gestation. By the time of implantation the inner cell mass consists of 12 to 15 cells. At about 7 days the first of three germ cell layers that give rise to the embryo—the hypoblast, or primitive endoderm—appears.[29] During the second week the bilaminar embryo develops as the inner cell mass differentiates to form the epiblast along the inner part of the amniotic cavity.

The developing organism appears as a flat disk with a connecting stalk that will become the umbilical cord. During this week, cytotrophoblast cells form an exocelomic membrane around the inner wall of the blastocyst cavity to form the primitive yolk sac (see Figure 3-6) and exocelomic cavity, which serves as transfer interface and nutrient resevoir.[78] Connective tissue (extraembryonic mesoderm) fills in the space between the cytotrophoblast cells and the exocelomic membrane. Near the end of the second week, cavities appear in the extraembryonic mesoderm and fuse to form the extraembryonic coelom. A secondary yolk sac (see Figure 3-6) develops from the primary sac (which gradually disintegrates). This yolk sac provides for early nutrition of the embryo and is eventually incorporated into the primitive gut. The fluid in this cavity is an ultrafiltrate of maternal serum with placental and secondary yolk sac products.[78] An endodermal cell thickening (prochordal plate) appears at one end of the disk and is the future site of the mouth and cranial region.

The embryonic period lasts from 2 weeks after fertilization until the end of the eighth week. This period is the time of organogenesis. Table 3-1 and Figure 3-10 summarize the major stages in development of specific organ systems. Development of specific organ systems is described in detail in Units II and III. This section provides on overview of major events during embryogenesis.

The third week coincides with the first missed menstrual period (Figure 3-1). During the third week, growth becomes more rapid, with development of the mesoderm and establishment of the trilaminar embryo; formation of the neural tube (CNS), somites (bones and other supporting structures), and coelom (body cavities); and development of a primitive cardiovascular system.

The primitive streak (thick band of epiblast cells) appears at 15 days in the midline of the dorsal aspect of the embryonic disc.[121] Cells in the primitive streak migrate between the endoderm and ectoderm to form the mesoderm; the epiblast layer becomes the ectoderm, establishing the trilaminar embryo. Cells from the mesoderm later migrate out into the embryonic body to become mesenchyme and form supporting tissues.

The ectoderm layer eventually forms the central and peripheral nervous systems, epidermis, hair, nails, inner ear, epithelium of the sensory organs, nasal cavity and mouth, salivary glands, and mucous membranes. The middle mesoderm layer develops into the dermis; muscle; connective tissue; skeleton (tendon, bones, cartilage); circulatory and lymphatic systems; kidneys; gonads; and the lining of the pericardial, pleural, and peritoneal cavities. The endoderm forms the epithelium of the digestive, respiratory, and urinary tracts as well as the thyroid and parathyroid.[29,121]

Development is in a cranial-to-caudal direction, with the embryo initially being a pear-shaped disk with a broad cephalic end and a narrow caudal end. The primitive streak elongates cranially to form a midline rod of cells, or *notochord*. The notochord extends to the prochordal plate, where the endoderm and ectoderm fuse into the oropharyngeal membrane. Other cells from the primitive streak migrate around the notochord and prochordal plate to form a cardiogenic area where the heart will develop. At the caudal end the endoderm and ectoderm fuse into the cloacal membrane.[29,121]

The ectoderm over the notochord thickens to form the neural plate, which will eventually form the neural tube, which gives rise to the brain and spinal cord. The mesoderm on either side of the notochord thickens to form two long columns that divide into paired cuboidal bodies (somites). Somites give rise to the skeleton and its associated musculature and much of the dermis. Somite development is used to distinguish the stage of development. The foregut and body cavities begin to develop. Mesoderm cells aggregate in the cardiogenic area at 18 to 19 days to form two endocardial tubes, which fuse by 19 to 20 days.[29,121] Primitive blood cells and vessels develop in the yolk sac, chorion, and embryo, and by 21 days' gestation they link with heart tubes to form a primitive cardiovascular system.

TABLE **3-1** Timetable of Human Development

Age (Days)	Size (mm)	General Body Form	Age (Days)	Size (mm)	Respiratory System
1	0.100	Zygote	27	3.3	Lung primordia appear
5	0.125	Blastocyst	35	5.0	Primary and lobar bronchi formed
18	1.5	Neural plate	49	20.0	Segmental bronchi develop
26	3.0	Closure of anterior neuropore Arm buds appear	180	230.0	Alveolar ducts form
28	3.5	Closure of posterior neuropore Leg buds appear			
35	6.0	Tail regression			
38	8.0	Hand plate Umbilical hernia			
56	25.0	Facial clefts closed Eyelids formed			
70	45.0	Intestines return to abdomen Eyelids fused			
196	240.0	Eyelids open			

Age (Days)	Size (mm)	Nervous System	Age (Days)	Size (mm)	Genitourinary System
18	1.5	Neural plate and groove develop	24	2.5	Pronephros primordium
24	3.0	Optic vesicles appear	28	4.0	Differentiation of mesonephros and mesonephric ducts
26	3.0	Anterior neuropore closed	35	6.0	Primordium of kidney pelvis and differentiation of metanephros Bulging of genital ridge
27	3.3	Posterior neuropore closed Ventral horn cells appear	42	13.0	Division of cloaca Separation of bladder and urachus Primordium of gonad present External genitalia indifferent
31	4.3	Anterior and posterior nerve roots appear	49	20.0	Müllerian duct primordium Degeneration of wolffian duct in females Gonadal tissue differentiation

Continued

TABLE **3-1** Timetable of Human Development—cont'd

Age (Days)	Size (mm)	Nervous System	Age (Days)	Size (mm)	Genitourinary System
35	5.0	Five cerebral vesicles Choroid plexuses appear Dorsal root ganglia present	56	26.0	Body of uterus and cervix complete Testis and ovary distinct
42	13.0	Primordium of cerebellum evident	100	125.0	Primary follicles evident in ovaries
56	25.0	Differentiation of cerebral cortex Meninges distinct			
150	225.0	Five fissures in cerebral cortex Spinal cord ends at L_3			
180	230.0	Myelinization increases			

Age (Days)	Size (mm)	Cardiovascular System	Age (Days)	Size (mm)	Sense Organs
18	1.5	Cardiogenic plate present	24	3.0	Optic vesicle present Auditory placode visible
23	3.0	Primitive vascular system Heart tubes fuse First aortic arch appears	28	3.5	Lens primordium evident Otocyst cut off Olfactory placode present
30	4.5	Septum primum develops Aortic arches present	35	5.0	Lens vesicle separated Olfactory pits present
38	8.0	Septum secundum and interentricular septum appear Absorption of bulbus cordis	42	13.0	Hyaloid artery identifiable Retinal pigmentation present Pinnae forming
42	13.0	Ductus venosus visible Division of truncus arteriosus	49	20.0	Lens solid Eyelids appear Semicircular canals present Cochlear duct
49	20.0	Interatrial septum complete Interventricular septum complete Superior vena cava appears Inferior vena cava appears Pulmonary vein absorption	70	45.0	Eyelids fused

TABLE **3-1**   Timetable of Human Development—cont'd

AGE (DAYS)	SIZE (mm)	CARDIOVASCULAR SYSTEM	AGE (DAYS)	SIZE (mm)	SENSE ORGANS
56	25.0	Sinus venosus absorbed Definitive plan of main blood vessels	196	240.0	Eyelids open

AGE (DAYS)	SIZE (mm)	DIGESTIVE SYSTEM	AGE (DAYS)	SIZE (mm)	SKELETAL SYSTEM
22	2.8	Formation of foregut and hindgut	22	2.0	Appearance of somites
25	3.0	Liver bud appears Rupture of buccopharyngeal membrane	28	4.0	Primordia of upper and lower limbs
28	4.0	Primordium of stomach visible Dorsal pancreas evident Cloaca present	35	5.0	Appearance of myotomes in limbs
35	5.0	Atrophy of tailgut Primordium of ventral pancreas and spleen evident	42	13.0	Subdivision of limbs occurs Finger rays in hand plate evident Cartilaginous models appear
38	8.0	Herniation of intestines Division of cloaca	49	20.0	Primary centers of ossification begin to appear
49	20.0	Rectum and bladder separated Anal membrane ruptured Duodenum occluded Lumen in gallbladder	56	26.0	Palatal processes grow medially Digits of upper and lower limbs clearly separated Pancreas fused
56	25.0	Duodenum recanalized	63	35.0	Fusion of palate completed
63	50.0	Intestines return to abdomen			

The fourth week is a time of body building. The embryo becomes cylindrical and begins to assume a C-shape as a result of transverse and longitudinal folding. The neural tube fuses during days 21 to 28. The cranial area enlarges and develops cephalic and cervical flexure, with the head oriented in the characteristic flexed position. The heart is prominent and begins beating at 22 days. Small swellings become visible on the lateral body walls at 26 (arm buds) and 28 (leg buds) days. The branchial arches (from which the face, mandible, and pharynx will develop) become visible; however, facial structures are not distinct and human likeness is not clear yet. The embryo is now 2 to 5 cm long.[29,121]

As the embryonic period moves into the fifth week, the form develops a humanlike appearance.[121] Head growth is rapid as a result of brain development. The embryo further flexes into the characteristic C-shape and the facial area comes into close approximation with the heart prominence. The forelimbs begin to develop, and paddle-shaped hand plates with digital ridges are visible. The heart chambers are forming, and five distinct areas in the brain are visible. The cranial nerves are present. Retinal pigment and the external ear begin to appear.

Limb differentiation continues in the sixth week, short webbed fingers develop, and toe rays form. The face is much more distinct, the jaws are visible, and the nares and upper lip are present. Heart development is almost complete, and circulation is well established. The liver is prominent and

EMBRYONIC DEVELOPMENT

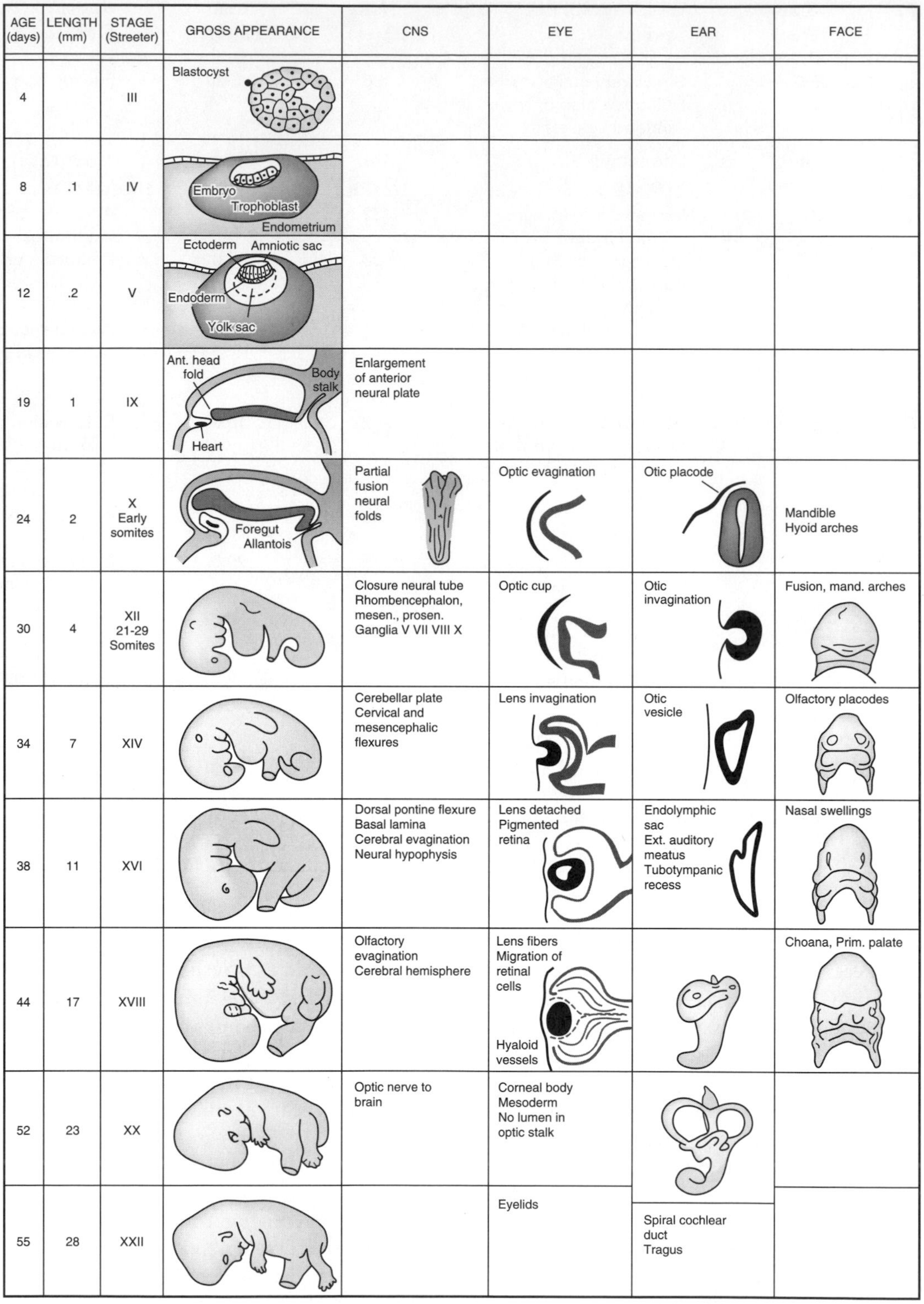

AGE (days)	LENGTH (mm)	STAGE (Streeter)	GROSS APPEARANCE	CNS	EYE	EAR	FACE
4		III	Blastocyst				
8	.1	IV	Embryo / Trophoblast / Endometrium				
12	.2	V	Ectoderm / Amniotic sac / Endoderm / Yolk sac				
19	1	IX	Ant. head fold / Body stalk / Heart	Enlargement of anterior neural plate			
24	2	X Early somites	Foregut / Allantois	Partial fusion neural folds	Optic evagination	Otic placode	Mandible Hyoid arches
30	4	XII 21-29 Somites		Closure neural tube Rhombencephalon, mesen., prosen. Ganglia V VII VIII X	Optic cup	Otic invagination	Fusion, mand. arches
34	7	XIV		Cerebellar plate Cervical and mesencephalic flexures	Lens invagination	Otic vesicle	Olfactory placodes
38	11	XVI		Dorsal pontine flexure Basal lamina Cerebral evagination Neural hypophysis	Lens detached Pigmented retina	Endolymphic sac Ext. auditory meatus Tubotympanic recess	Nasal swellings
44	17	XVIII		Olfactory evagination Cerebral hemisphere	Lens fibers Migration of retinal cells / Hyaloid vessels		Choana, Prim. palate
52	23	XX		Optic nerve to brain	Corneal body Mesoderm No lumen in optic stalk		
55	28	XXII			Eyelids	Spiral cochlear duct Tragus	

FIGURE **3-10** Timetable of human embryonic and fetal development. (From Jones, KL. [1996]. *Smith's recognizable patterns of human malformation* [5th ed.]. Philadelphia: W.B. Saunders.)

The embryonic ages for Streeter's stages XII-XXII have been altered
in accordance with the human data from Iffy, L., et al.: Acta Anat., 66:178, 1967.

EXTREMITIES	HEART	GUT, ABDOMEN	LUNG	UROGENITAL	OTHER
					Early blastocyst with inner cell mass and cavitation (58 cells) lying free within the uterine cavity
					Implantation Trophoblast invasion Embryonic disc with endoblast and ectoblast
		Yolk sac			Early amnion sac Extraembryonic mesoblast, angioblast Chorionic gonadotropin
	Merging mesoblast anterior to prechordal plate	Stomatodeum Cloaca		Allantois	Primitive streak Hensen's node Notochord Prechordal plate Blood cells in yolk sac
	Single heart tube Propulsion	Foregut		Mesonephric ridge	Yolk sac larger than amnion sac
Arm bud	Ventric. outpouching Gelatinous reticulum	Rupture stomato-deum Evagination of thyroid, liver, and dorsal pancreas	Lung bud	Mesonephric duct enters cloaca	Rathke's pouch Migration of myotomes from somites
Leg bud	Auric. outpouching Septum primum	Pharyngeal pouches yield parathyroids, lat. thyroid, thymus Stomach broadens	Bronchi	Ureteral evag. Urorect. sept. Germ cells Gonadal ridge Coelom, Epithelium	
Hand plate, Mesench. condens. Innervation	Fusion mid. A-V canal Muscular vent. sept.	Intestinal loop into yolk stalk Cecum Gallbladder Hepatic ducts Spleen	Main lobes	Paramesonephric duct Gonad ingrowth of coelomic epith.	Adrenal cortex (from coelomic epithelium) invaded by sympathetic cells = medulla Jugular lymph sacs
Finger rays, Elbow	Aorta Pulmonary artery Valves Membrane ventricular septum	Duodenal lumen obliterated Cecum rotates right Appendix	Tracheal cartil.	Fusion urorect. sept. Open urogen. memb., anus Epith. cords in testicle	Early muscle
Clearing, central cartil.	Septum secundum			S-shaped vesicles in nephron blastema connect with collecting tubules from calyces	Superficial vascular plexus low on cranium
Shell, Tubular bone				A few large glomeruli Short secretory tubules Tunica albuginea Testicle, interstitial cells	Superficial vascular plexus at vertex

FIGURE **3-10, cont'd** For legend see opposite page.

Continued

FETAL DEVELOPMENT

AGE (weeks)	LENGTH (cm) C-R	LENGTH (cm) Tot.	WT (g)	GROSS APPEARANCE	CNS	EYE, EAR	FACE, MOUTH	CARDIO-VASCULAR	LUNG
7½	2.8				Cerebral hemisphere Infundibulum, Rathke's	Lens nearing final shape	Palatal swellings Dental lamina, Epithel.	Pulmonary vein into left atrium	
8	3.7				Primitive cereb. cortex Olfactory lobes Dura and pia mater	Eyelid Ear canals	Nares plugged Rathke's pouch detach. Sublingual gland	A-V bundle Sinus venosus absorbed into right auricle	Pleuroperitoneal canals close Bronchioles
10	6.0				Spinal cord histology Cerebellum	Iris Ciliary body Eyelids fuse Lacrimal glands Spiral gland different	Lips, Nasal cartilage Palate		Laryngeal cavity reopened
12	8.8				Cord-cervical and lumbar enlarged, Cauda equina	Retina layered Eye axis forward Scala tympani	Tonsillar crypts Cheeks Dental papilla	Accessory coats, blood vessels	Elastic fibers
16	14				Corpora quadrigemina Cerebellum prominent Myelination begins	Scala vestibuli Cochlear duct	Palate complete Enamel and dentine	Cardiac muscle condensed	Segmentation of bronchi complete
20						Inner ear ossified	Ossification of nose		Decrease in mesenchyme Capillaries penetrate linings of tubules
24		32	800		Typical layers in cerebral cortex Cauda equina at first sacral level		Nares reopen Calcification of tooth primordia		Change from cuboidal to flattened epithelium Alveoli
28		38.5	1100		Cerebral fissures and convolutions	Eyelids reopen Retinal layers complete Perceive light			Vascular components adequate for respiration
32		43.5	1600		Accumulation of fat		Auricular cartilage	Taste sense		Number of alveoli still incomplete
36		47.5	2600						
38		50	3200		Cauda equina, at L-3 Myelination within brain	Lacrimal duct canalized	Rudimentary frontal maxillary sinuses	Closure of: foramen ovale, ductus arteriosus, umbilical vessels, ductus venosus	
First postnatal year +					Continuing organization of axonal networks Cerebrocortical function, motor coordination Myelination continues until 2-3 years	Iris pigmented, 5 months Mastoid air cells Coordinate vision, 3-5 months Maximal vision by 5 years	Salivary gland ducts become canalized Teeth begin to erupt 5-7 months Relatively rapid growth of mandible and nose	Relative hypertrophy left ventricle	Continue adding new alveoli

FIGURE **3-10, cont'd** For legend see page 86.

GUT	UROGENITAL	SKELETAL MUSCLE	SKELETON	SKIN	BLOOD, THYMUS LYMPH	ENDOCRINE
Pancreas, dorsal and ventral fusion	Renal vesicles	Differentiation toward final shape	Cartilaginous models of bones Chondrocranium Tail regression	Mammary gland		Parathyroid associated with thyroid Sympathetic neuroblasts invade adrenal
Liver relatively large Intestinal villi	Mullerian ducts fusing Ovary distinguishable	Muscles well represented Movement	Ossification center Sternum Joints	Basal layer	Bone marrow Thymus halves unite Lymphoblasts around the lymph sacs	Thyroid follicles
Gut withdrawal from cord Pancreatic alveoli Anal canal	Testosterone Renal excretion Bladder sac Müllerian tube into urogenital sinus Vaginal sacs, prostate	Perineal muscles		Hair follicles Melanocytes	Enucleated RBC's Thymus yields reticulum and corpuscles Thoracic duct Lymph nodes; axillary iliac	Adrenalin Noradrenalin
Gut muscle layers Pancreatic islets Bile	Seminal vesicle Regression, genital ducts		Tail degenerated Notochord degenerated	Corium, 3 layers Scalp, body hair Sebaceous glands Nails beginning	Blood principally from bone marrow Thymus—medullary and lymphoid	Testicle— Leydig cells Thyroid— colloid in follicle Anterior pituitary acidophilic granules Ovary—prim. follicles
Omentum fusing with transverse colon Mesoduodenum, asc. and desc. colon attach to body wall Meconium Gastric, intest. glands	Typical kidney Mesonephros involuting Uterus and vagina Primary follicles	In-utero movement can be detected	Distinct bones	Dermal ridges hands Sweat glands Keratinization		Anterior pituitary— basophilic granules
	No further collecting tubules			Vernix caseosa Nail plates Mammary budding	Blood formation decreasing in liver	
						Testes—decrease in Leydig cells
						Testes descend
	Urine osmolarity continues to be relatively low			Eccrine sweat Lanugo hair prominent Nails to fingertips		
			Only a few secondary epiphyseal centers ossified in knee		Hemoglobin 17-18 gm Leukocytosis	
			Ossification of 2nd epiph. centers— hamate, capitate, proximal humerus, femur. New ossif. 2nd epiph. centers till 10-12 yrs. Ossif. of epiphyses till 16-18 yrs.	New hair, gradual loss of lanugo hair	Transient (6 wk) erythroid hypoplasia Hemoglobin 11-12 gm 7S gamma globulin produced by 6 wks. Lymph nodes develop cortex, medulla	Transient estrinization Adrenal— regression of fetal zone. Gonodotropin with feminization of ♀ 9-12 yr. (onset); masc. of ♂ 10-14 yr. (onset)

FIGURE **3-10, cont'd** For legend see page 86.

producing blood cells. The intestines enter the proximal portion of the umbilical cord.

The last 2 weeks of the embryonic period are a time of facial, organ system, and neuromuscular development. The head is rounded and more erect although still disproportionately large. The eyes are open, and the eyelids are developing. The eyelids fuse by the end of the eighth week and do not open again until the twenty-fifth week. The mouth, tongue, and palate are complete. The external ear is distinct, although it is still low on the head. The regions of the limbs are distinct, and elbow and wrist flexion are possible. Fingers are longer and the toes are differentiated. The feet have moved to the midline. The forearms gradually rise above the shoulder level, and the hands often cover the lower face. The abdomen is less protuberant, and the body is covered by thin skin.[29,121]

Neuromuscular development leads to movement, which can be seen on ultrasound although not felt. The gastrointestinal and genitourinary systems have separated, and the kidneys have achieved their basic structure. Although the internal genitalia have differentiated, the external genitalia have not. The rectal passage is complete, and the anal membrane is perforated, resulting in an open digestive system.[29,121]

Overview of Fetal Development

The fetal period extends from the end of the eighth week of gestation until term. All major systems and external features are established or have begun to develop. During the early fetal period (9 to 20 weeks), there is further differentiation of body structures, with a gradual increase in functional ability. By 6 months the fetus has achieved 60% of its eventual length and 20% of its weight.[121] During the late fetal period (20 weeks to term) further maturation of organ and body systems occurs, along with a marked increase in weight. Organization is a prominent feature of this period.

During weeks 9 through 12, the embryo is 5 to 8 cm long and weighs 8 to 14 g. The head is half the body length. The body length doubles during these weeks. Head growth slows down, the neck lengthens, and the chin is lifted off the chest. The face is broad, with widely set eyes, fused lids, and low set ears. Teeth begin forming under the gums, and the palate fuses. Fingernails become apparent, and the arms reach their final relative length.[29,121]

Micturition and swallowing of amniotic fluid begin. The esophageal lumen forms, and the intestines reenter the abdominal cavity and assume their fixed positions. The bone marrow begins blood formation. The external genitalia differentiate, and by 12 weeks sexual determination is possible visually.

From 13 to 16 weeks, rapid growth continues. The length of the embryo almost doubles during these weeks. The embryo weighs 20 g by the end of the sixteenth week.[121] The eyes and ears have achieved more normal positions, giving the face a distinctively human look. Fetal skin is extremely thin, and lanugo is present. There is increased muscle and bone development, which along with establishment of neuromuscular connections results in increased fetal movements. Skeletal ossification continues and can be seen on roentgenogram by 16 weeks. Brown fat deposition and meconium formation begin.[29,121]

Growth slows slightly during the next month (17 to 20 weeks), and the legs reach their final relative positions. During this period, fetal movement is felt by the first-time mother (earlier with successive pregnancies). Fetal heart tones are now audible with a stethoscope. Myelinization of the spinal cord begins. Head hair, eyelashes, and eyebrows can be seen. The sebaceous glands are active, resulting in vernix caseosa deposition. Lung development continues as bronchial branching is completed and terminal air sacs begin to develop. The pulmonary capillary bed is forming in preparation for gas exchange. By 20 weeks the fetus weighs about 300 g and is 25 cm long.[121]

After 20 weeks, weight increases substantially. By 24 to 25 weeks, the fetus weighs 650 to 780 g and is 30 cm long.[121] The body is better proportioned. The skin is translucent, and subcutaneous fat has yet to be laid down. Fingerprint and footprint ridges are formed, and the eye is structurally complete.

During weeks 25 to 28, the gas exchange ability of the lungs improves so that extrauterine life can be sustained. Subcutaneous fat begins to form, and head hair and lanugo are well developed. The eyes open as the lids unfuse. CNS development allows initiation of rhythmic breathing movements and partial temperature control. The testes begin to descend into the scrotum.

From 29 weeks to term, fat and muscle tissue are laid down and skin thickness increases. Although the bones are fully formed, ossification is not complete. Vernix caseosa and lanugo begin to disappear as term gestation is approached and growth slows. The testes descend into the scrotum. The infant fills the uterine cavity, and the extremities are flexed against the body. Myelinization progresses, and sleep-wake cycles are established. By 38 to 40 weeks, fetal size averages 3000 to 3800 g and 45 to 50 cm.[121]

Intrauterine Environment

The uterine environment provides the ideal stimulation for the development and refining of the organ systems so that transition to and interaction with the extrauterine environment are possible. The amniotic fluid provides the space for the developing fetus to grow and protection from the external environment. Amniotic fluid cushions against external pressure, allowing pressure to the uterus to be transmitted from one side to the other with minimal exertion on the fetus. The weightless space allows for the symmetric development of the face and body. Adequate volume facilitates normal lung development and, until late gestation, exercise and neuromuscular development. The amniotic sac and uterine wall give the fetus something to push against during "practice" activities.

The maternal body provides the fetus with a darkened environment, which may become grayer as the uterus grows and stretches. Auditory stimuli are rich and include the sound of blood flow through the placenta. Most of these sounds are patterned and rhythmic. Extrauterine sounds, such as voices and music, are transmitted in a muted form to the fetus. The maternal system maintains a warm thermal environment. Kinesthetic and vestibular stimulation are provided by maternal movement and changes in position. Other, less well-defined patterns of stimulus that have a powerful impact on the activity and responses of the fetus and neonate include maternal biorhythms and diurnal, circadian, and sleep-wake cycles.

Exposure of the fetus to these stimuli and events provides appropriate experiences that enhance neurologic organization and establishment of synaptic connections. These activities are critical for successful transition to extrauterine life and for establishing physiologic and social relationships necessary to ensure survival.

THE PLACENTA AND PLACENTAL PHYSIOLOGY

The human placenta is a hemochorial villous organ that is essential for transfer of nutrients and gases from the mother to the fetus and for removal of fetal waste products. Alterations in placental development and function markedly influence fetal growth and development and the ability of the infant to survive in intrauterine and extrauterine environments.

Placental Development
Implantation

Implantation is mediated by a coordinated sequence of interactions between maternal and embryonic cells.[40,80] Implantation begins at about 150 hours after ovulation and involves three distinct processes: (1) loss of the ZP ("hatching" of the blastocyst) 4 to 5 days after fertilization, followed by rapid proliferation of the trophectoderm to form the trophoblast cell mass; (2) adherence of the blastocyst to the endometrial surface, which occurs in the early luteal phase of the menstrual cycle; and (3) erosion of the ep-

ithelium of the endometrial surface, with burrowing of the blastocyst beneath the surface.[48,88,150] Both implantation and placentation require ongoing communication between the developing blastocyst and maternal endometrium via hormones, cytokines, growth factors, and other immunoregulatory substances.[40,80]

The endometrium must undergo physiologic changes in order for implantation to occur, with a narrow period of maximal uterine receptivity ("window of implantation") for implantation.[40] The endometrium prepares for implantation by the cyclic secretion of 17β-estradiol and progesterone. These hormones regulate the expression of growth factors and cytokines in the uterus, which in turn alter the endometrial surface.[40] Adhesion molecules (integrins) form cell surface receptors that develop from days 20 to 24 of the menstrual cycle. Integrins are glycoproteins with alpha and beta subunits that can be upregulated via interaction with other substances.[77] Specific receptors (for vitronectin) appear on day 20 (opening the implantation window), and other substances (e.g., fibronectin) close the window several days later.[101,102]

Preimplantation, implantation, and placentation signaling by the zygote and blastocyst to maternal tissues involves substances such as: (1) early pregnancy factor (EPF); (2) preimplantation factor (PIF); (3) growth factors such as epidermal growth factor, transforming growth factor–α, platelet-derived growth factor, insulin-like growth factors, tumor necrosis factor–α (TNF-α), and colony stimulating factor–1; (4) immunoregulatory cytokines such as interleukin-1 (IL-1), interleukin-6 (IL-6), and TGF-β; (5) prostaglandin E2; (6) platelet activity factor (PAF); and (7) hCG.[6,9,11,25,40,150,151,159,167] EPF is found a within a few hours after fertilization; PIF is found by 4 days.[40] Immunoregulatory cytokines are present within the first 48 hours after implantation.[40,95,146] hCG can be detected in maternal serum by 20 to 24 days after the last menstrual period, which is about 7 days after fertilization.[16] Growth factors such as TNF-α and CSF-1 are found by the 2- to 8-cell stage; others appear from 8 days onward.[40] The zygote develops receptors for cytokines and growth factors by the 2-cell stage; by the blastocyst stage, these receptors are seen only on trophectoderm tissue.[40] Before implantation the trophoblast is activated. This process occurs on days 5 to 6 and lasts about 24 hours.[91] The initial signaling between the trophoblast and luminal epithelium may be mediated by immunologic mechanisms.[80]

By 5 to 6 days after fertilization (7 to 9 days after follicle rupture), the blastocyst rests on and adheres to the endometrium. Metabolism increases, with localized changes seen at the eventual site of the implantation beginning up to 24 hours before adherence of the blastocyst to the endometrium.[24,62] The place of attachment is usually on the anterior or posterior wall of the upper part of the uterus, but it can occur at various other intrauterine and extrauterine sites.

Initiation of implantation may involve binding of ligands such as oncofetal fibronectin (an extracellular matrix protein on the surface of the trophoblast) with integrins on the endometrium surface epithelium.[102] Ligands (molecules that bind to receptors) such as cytokines, growth factors, and hormones on the trophectoderm of the hatched blastocyst bind to cell surface adhesion molecules on the surface of the luminal endometrium.[9,91] Antiadhesion molecules that inhibit luminal endothelium–blastocyst interaction may be a mechanism for preventing implantation of many abnormal embryos.[9] The blastocyst orients itself so that the embryonic pole containing the embryo-forming inner cell mass contacts the endometrial surface first.

The trophectoderm (trophoblast) attaches to endometrial extracellular matrix proteins and secretes proteases to degrade these proteins. By day 6 or 7, trophoblast cells have begun to invade the endometrium. Fingerlike projections of trophoblast cells protrude between the cells of the endometrial epithelium into the endometrial stroma.[50] The trophoblast cells then migrate between the cells of the endometrial extra cellular matrix until they reach maternal blood vessels.[39] Regulatory substances found on both trophoblast and endometrial tissue enhance invasion and trophoblast proliferation. Trophoblast invasion and proliferation is enhanced by metalloproteinases (e.g., collagenases, gelatinases, stomelysins), plasminogen activation, plasmin regulating factors, cytokines, and growth factors.[25,40] Other factors that limit trophoblast invasion develop as part of the decidual reaction (see Endometrium and Decidua). For example, the decidua (i.e., the altered endometrium during pregnancy) secretes protease inhibitors such as TGF-β and tissue inhibitor of metalloproteinase (TIMP). The trophoblast may also autoregulate its invasion via secretion of TGF-β, TIMP, and hCG.[40] If trophoblast invasion is too extensive, placenta accreta can result; if invasion is too little, the risk of miscarriage or abruptio placentae is increased.[25]

By the seventh day after fertilization, the trophoblast begins to differentiate into two layers: the inner cytotrophoblast and the outer syncytiotrophoblast layer.[50] The mononuclear cytotrophoblast is a mitotically active layer that forms new syncytial cells, the chorionic villi, and the amnion. The syncytiotrophoblast is a thick multinuclear mass, without distinct cell boundaries, that puts out fingerlike projections that invade the endometrial epithelium, engulfing uterine cells (see Figure 3-6).[16] Slight bleeding may occur during this process, which may be mistaken for a scanty, short menstrual period. The trophoblast, primarily the syncytiotrophoblast, produces hCG (which maintains the corpus luteum during early pregnancy) as well as estrogens, progesterone, hPL, and other substances (see Placental Endocrinology). The functions of trophoblast are summarized in Table 3-2.

Two other types of trophoblast derive from cytotrophoblast: junctional trophoblast that attaches the anchoring villi of the placenta to the decidua via trophuteronectin, and an extravillous invasive trophoblast. Invasive trophoblast migrates out from the placenta into the endometrium and spiral arteries. This form of trophoblast has two roles: (1) conversion of the maternal spiral arteries into low-resistance, high-capacity vessels, and (2) formation of plugs at the top of the spiral arteries to limit maternal blood flow into the placenta during the first trimester (see Placental Circulation).[77,96,163]

Many ova that are fertilized never implant. Moore indicates that one third to one half of all zygotes never become blastocysts.[121] Hertig estimates that 70% to 75% of blastocysts implant and 51% of these survive to the second week.[65] Approximately 15% to 19% of this latter group are later spontaneously aborted.[40] Implantation can be selectively inhibited by administration of low-dose estrogen for several days following sexual intercourse ("morning-after" pill). Estrogen preparations such as diethylstilbestrol act by altering the normal balance of estrogen and progesterone during the secretory phase of the endometrial cycle making the endometrial lining unsuitable for implantation.

TABLE **3-2** **Functions of Trophoblast**

Function	Effectors
Erosion of maternal tissue to make space for implantation and growth	Proteases (e.g., plasminogen system, matrix metalloproteinases)
Hormone secretion	hCG, hPL, others
Transport nutrients and waste products	Substrate specific transporters, trophoblast, endothelial plasma membranes
Placental attachment	Adhesion molecules in the extracellular matrix and at the cell surface
Migration and arterial transformation	Adhesion molecules, proteases, extracellular matrix components

From Aplin, J. (2000). Maternal influences on placental development. *Semin Cell Dev Biol, 17,* 116.
hCG, Human chornionic gonadotropin; *hPL,* human placental lactogen.

Estrogen may also accelerate passage of the zygote along the fallopian tube so that it arrives in the uterus before the secretory phase of the endometrial cycle is established.[121]

Implantation is complete by 10 days after fertilization.[50] At 10 days the blastocyst lies beneath the endometrial surface and is covered by a blood clot and cellular debris. By 12 days the endometrial epithelium has regenerated in this area.[88]

Ectopic pregnancy. Extrauterine implantation results in an ectopic pregnancy in 1 in every 80 to 250 pregnancies. The incidence of ectopic pregnancy has tripled since 1970 and accounts for 10% to 11% of maternal mortality in the United States. Ectopic pregnancy is the most common cause of maternal death in the first 20 weeks of pregnancy.[73] The increased incidence in recent years is thought to be a result of the prevalence of sexually transmitted diseases (STDs) and pelvic inflammatory disease (PID).[73] The most common site for an ectopic pregnancy is the fallopian tubes. This probably results from delay in transport of the zygote from the site of fertilization to the uterine cavity. The delay may be due to tubal adhesions or mucosal damage from PID.[121] PID and salpingitis disrupt and damage the tubal mucosa, decreasing the number of cilia, which are essential for timely movement of the zygote along the tube. Alterations in the concentrations of progesterone, estrogen, and prostaglandins may also delay ovum transport.[73] If transport is delayed, the blastocyst emerges from the ZP while in the fallopian tube and adheres to and implants in tubal mucosa.

Endometrium and Decidua

The uterine endometrial lining consists of an epithelial layer that contains ciliated and mucus-secreting cells. These cells penetrate into the endometrial stroma and may enter the underlying myometrium. The endometrium is divided into three functional zones (see Figure 2-27). The deepest basalis layer lies adjacent to the myometrium. This layer responds to progesterone stimulus with secretory activity and provides the base for endometrial regeneration after menstrual sloughing. The two superficial layers of endometrium are the outer compacta and the middle spongiosa, which contains glands and blood vessels.

Early nutrition of the blastocyst is from digestion of substances in endometrial tissue and the capillaries that diffuse into the inner cell mass. Under stimulation of progesterone and estrogen, the epithelium and stromal cells become progressively hypertrophic and develop subnuclear vacuoles rich in glycogen and lipids.[88] These endometrial changes during pregnancy are known as the *decidual reaction,* and the altered endometrial lining is known as the *decidua.* The decidual reaction involves remodeling of the ex-

tracellular matrix with changes in collagen, proteoglycans, and glycoproteins. This process is mediated by substances such as metalloproteinases and the plasminogen system.[10] A poor decidual reaction is associated with placenta accreta and ectopic pregnancy.[40]

Decidualization begins after implantation and is independent of the embryo.[9,96] As decidualization increases, the window of receptivity for implantation is closed.[96] In addition to its role in early nutrition of the embryo, the decidua may protect the endometrium and myometrium from uncontrolled invasion by the trophoblast cell mass.[88] The decidua also acts—as both a physical barrier and via production of cytokines that promote trophoblast attachment, not invasion—to protect the endometrium during the period when trophoblast cells migrate out of the placenta into the maternal spiral arteries (see "Maternal Uteroplacental Circulation").[96] A somewhat hypoxic environment appears to be needed in early pregnancy for trophoblast invasion and differentiation; high oxygen levels may alter morphogenesis.[76,77,96]

The decidua is divided into three sections (Figure 3-11). The decidua capsularis, just above the area of trophoblastic proliferation, initially covers the growing embryo. With development of the chorion, the decidua capsularis gradually disappears. The portion of the decidua on which the blastocyst rests forms a soft, spongy vascular bed known as the *decidua basalis,* site of the future placenta. The remaining portion is known as the *decidua parietalis* (or decidua vera). At the interface between the trophoblast and decidua basalis is a specialized extracellular matrix rich in fibrin and fibronectin that supports trophoblast adhesion and migration.[9,10]

With embryonic growth, the decidua basalis is progressively compressed. The glands and blood vessels become distorted and assume oblique and horizontal courses. The decidua basalis forms the maternal portion of the placenta and the stratum in which separation of the placenta will occur at delivery.[35,121] As the embryo fills the lumen of the uterus, the decidua capsularis disappears. Eventually the chorion laeve and decidua parietalis meet and fuse, obliterating the uterine cavity (see Figure 3-11).[88]

Placentation

As the syncytiotrophoblast proliferates and invades the endometrial stroma, the blastocyst slowly sinks into the endometrium. The syncytiotrophoblast is thought to lack transplantation antigens and therefore is not rejected by the mother.[121] By 9 days, intersyncytial spaces or lacunae are seen in the syncytiotrophoblast (see Figure 3-6). The lacunae fill with a nutritive substance derived from maternal blood containing glandular fluid that diffuses through

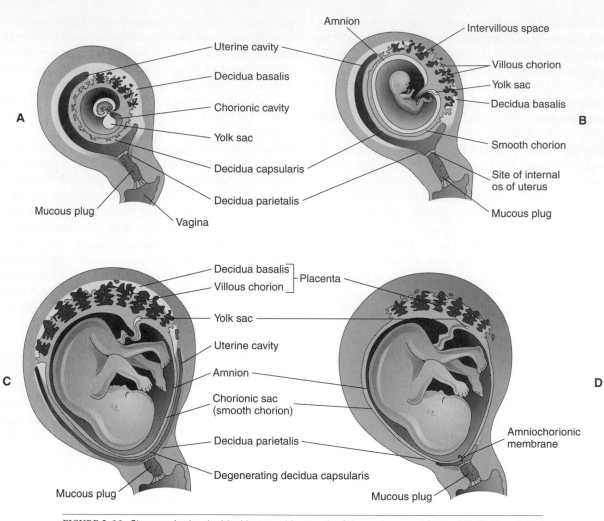

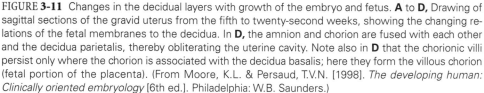

FIGURE **3-11** Changes in the decidual layers with growth of the embryo and fetus. **A** to **D,** Drawing of sagittal sections of the gravid uterus from the fifth to twenty-second weeks, showing the changing relations of the fetal membranes to the decidua. In **D,** the amnion and chorion are fused with each other and the decidua parietalis, thereby obliterating the uterine cavity. Note also in **D** that the chorionic villi persist only where the chorion is associated with the decidua basalis; here they form the villous chorion (fetal portion of the placenta). (From Moore, K.L. & Persaud, T.V.N. [1998]. *The developing human: Clinically oriented embryology* [6th ed.]. Philadelphia: W.B. Saunders.)

the trophoblast to the embryo. Individual lacunae fuse into lacunar networks that will later develop into the intervillous spaces (IVS) and become filled with maternal blood. Endometrial capillaries around the implanted embryo become congested and dilated, forming sinusoids.

For years it was believed that maternal blood seeped into the lacunae early in the first trimester. However, recent data from color ultrasonography demonstrate that blood flow is limited in the first trimester and that the IVS is filled with fluid from the endometrial glands and not blood.[77] The highly oxygenated maternal blood does not fill the IVS until fetal vessels are established in the villi and mechanisms to protect the fetus against oxidative stress are established.[76,77,79,82,96,148] This occurs around 10 to 12 weeks. Before that time, trophoblast plugs fill the tops of the spiral arteries, limiting blood flow into the IVS. Thus initial placental and embryonic development occurs in a relatively hypoxic environment. This environment may stimulate production of vascular endothelia growth factor and stimulate chorionic vascularization.[77] Vascular changes in the uteroplacental vessels are described further in Placental Circulation.

Development of the Amniotic Cavity

The amniotic cavity appears during the second week as the blastocyst is burrowing into the endometrium. Small spaces appear between the inner cell mass and cytotrophoblast. By 8 days these spaces coalesce to form a narrow amniotic cavity that gradually enlarges to completely surround the fetus (Figure 3-12).

The amniotic cavity develops a thin epithelial roof or lining. This lining is the amnion, which arises from amnioblasts (amniogenic cells) from the cytotrophoblast. The floor of the amniotic cavity is formed from the embryonic epiblast germ layer. Initially a small amount of fluid may be secreted by the amniotic epithelial cells, but the major early source of amniotic fluid is probably maternal serum. With advancing gestation, the epithelial cells of the amnion become more cuboidal or columnar and are covered with microvilli.[121]

Development of the Villi

The placenta consists of the outer epithelial layer, derived from trophoblast cells, and an inner vascular network and connective tissue stroma, derived from embryonic mesoderm.[33] Initially the lacunae are separated by trabecular columns of syncytial trophoblast (primary villous stems), which provide the framework for development of the placental chorionic villi. The cytotrophoblast differentiates into vascular cytotrophoblast, which fuses to form chorionic villi and the extravascular invasive trophoblast, which

is involved in remodeling of the spiral arteries (see Placental Circulation).[92] Chorionic villi begin to appear toward the end of the second week as proliferation of the cytotrophoblast layer produces columns of cells or finger-like processes known as *primary chorionic villi* (Figure 3-13).[92] A mesenchymal core grows within these primary villi forming secondary villi. Blood vessels within the villi arise from this mesenchymal core within a few days, forming tertiary villi.[88,92]

As the columns of cytotrophoblast cells proliferate, they extend through the syncytiotrophoblast, expanding laterally to meet and fuse with adjoining cytotrophoblast columns. This forms the cytotrophoblastic shell and divides the syncytiotrophoblast into an inner layer and a peripheral layer. The peripheral layer degenerates and is replaced by fibrinoid material.[50,88] Villous development is stimulated by growth factors such as vascular endothelium growth factor (VEGF) and placental-like growth factor and by the relatively hypoxic environment. VEGF is found in maternal plasma by 6 weeks' gestation and peaks at the end of the first trimester, similar to the pattern seen with hCG. During the third trimester, placental-like growth factor enhances formation of terminal villi.[92] The low-oxygen environment stimulates angiogenesis, trophoblast formation, and increased numbers of highly vascularized terminal villi.[93,94] A recent hypothesis for the nausea and vomiting of pregnancy suggests that decreased energy intake in early pregnancy may result in compensatory placental growth and thus enhanced placental development (see Chapter 11).[49,75]

The cytotrophoblastic shell is the point of contact between the fetal tissue and maternal tissue; it attaches the chorionic sac to the basal plate. The basal plate is formed by the compact and spongy zones of the maternal decidua basalis, remnants of the trophoblast, and fibrinoid material. By the end of the fourth month, the shell has regressed, with replacement of the cytotrophoblast cell columns by fibrinoid material (Rohr layer) and formation of clumps (islands) of cytotrophoblast cells.[50] A layer of fibrinoid material (Nitabuch layer) also develops within the spongy zone of the decidua basalis. This is the level of placental separation at delivery (Figure 3-14).

Villi containing blood vessels arise by 18 to 21 days (see Figure 3-13).[13,92] At 21 to 22 days, a primitive fetoplacental circulation is established between blood in the villi, vessels forming in the embryo, primitive heart, and blood islands in the yolk sac (see Chapters 7 and 8). The villi that arise from the chorionic plate and attach to the maternal decidua basalis are known as *anchoring* (or stem) *villi*. Initially embryonic and fetal blood vessels develop by branching angiogenesis, forming 10 to 16 generations of

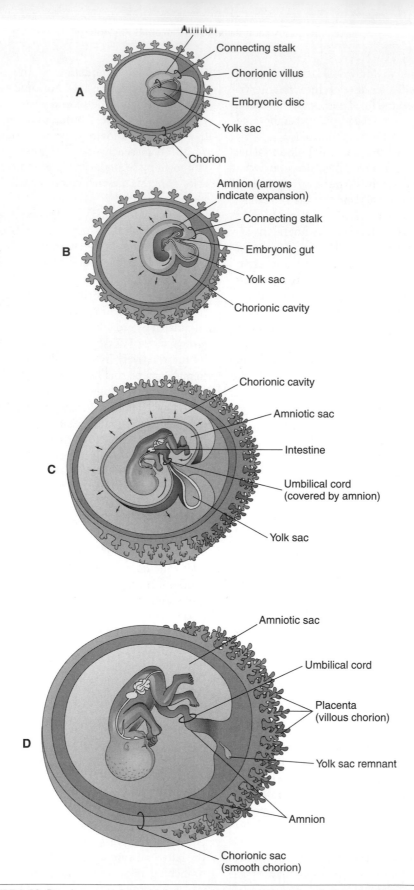

FIGURE 3-12 Development of the amniotic cavity, amnion and chorion. **A,** 3 weeks. **B,** 4 weeks. **C,** 10 weeks. **D,** 20 weeks. (From Moore, K.L. & Persaud, T.V.N. [1998]. *The developing human: Clinically oriented embryology* [6th ed.]. Philadelphia: W.B. Saunders.)

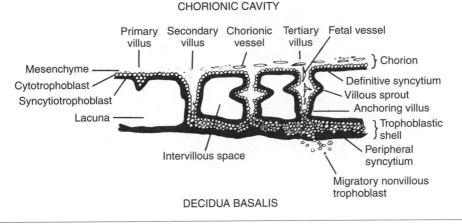

FIGURE **3-13** Early development of the placenta progressing from 9 to 13 days (left side of figure) to 13 to 21 days (right side of figure). (From Lavery, J.P. [1987]. *The human placenta: Clinical perspectives.* Gaithersburg, MD: Aspen.)

stem villi.[92] Stem villi, which contain arteries and veins as well as some arterioles and venules, make up about one third of the villi in the mature placenta.[86] Mature intermediate villi grow from the sides of stem villi and project into the IVS (see Figure 3-13). These intermediate villi, which constitute approximately 25% of the villi in the mature placenta, contain primarily fetal capillaries with a few small arterioles and venules.[50,86] Intermediate villi and their branches (terminal villi), constitute the major area of exchange between maternal and fetal circulations.[50] After fetal viability, terminal villi are formed by nonbranching angiogenesis in mature intermediate villi. Terminal villi (see Figure 3-14) contain multiple dilated capillaries or sinusoids and account for 30% to 40% of the mature villous tree.[86] Terminal villi bulge into the villous cytotrophoblast so that maternal and fetal blood are separated only by a thin syncytiotrophoblast layer.[92]

Initially there are two divisions within the chorionic villi. The chorion laeve forms the chorion; the chorion frondosum forms the fetal portion of the placenta. At first, villi cover the entire surface of the chorionic sac. Beginning around 8 weeks, villi near the decidua capsularis become compressed, blood flow decreases, and the villi degenerate, leaving a bare avascular area (smooth chorion, or chorion laeve). Simultaneously, villi near the decidua basalis (villous chorion, or chorion frondosum) rapidly enlarge, increase in number, and develop a mesenchymal core and blood vessels.

Anchoring villi grow more slowly than other portions of the placenta. As a result, during the third month, folds of the basal plate are pulled up into the IVS (see Figure 3-14). These folds (known as the placental septa) do not extend to the chorionic plate and have no known morphologic or physiologic function.[50,88,177]

By 40 to 50 days after ovulation, the trophoblast has invaded far enough into the endometrium to reach and begin to erode maternal spiral arterioles. Trophoblast plugs fill the tops of the spiral arteries until around 10 to 12 weeks, when the arteries open up and begin to supply blood to the IVS.[10] This is the time when the mature placenta is established. The chorion laeve fuses onto the decidua vera, forming the chorion or outer fetal membrane. The inner membrane, the amnion, is derived from the amniogenic cells (amnioblasts) of the cytotrophoblast. Although the amnion and chorion are often thought of as fusing, they do not actually grow together; rather, the amnion is passively pushed against the chorion.

Placental Growth

By 4 months the placenta has achieved its full thickness, with no new lobules or stem villi added after 10 to 12 weeks.[111] Circumferential placental growth continues with further ramification of stem villi (via growth and extension of new trophoblast sprouts, followed by growth of the mesenchymal core and development of blood vessels), lengthening of existing villi, and increases in the size and number of placental capillaries.[35,121,177] Much of the expansion of villi after 20 weeks is in the terminal villi. Mature intermediate villi elongate in the third trimester, which assists in generation of new terminal villi branches.[112] As a result of the proliferation of terminal villi, the surface area for placental exchange continues to increase until late in gestation. In addition, the thickness of the tissue layers separating maternal and fetal blood thins, thus enhancing

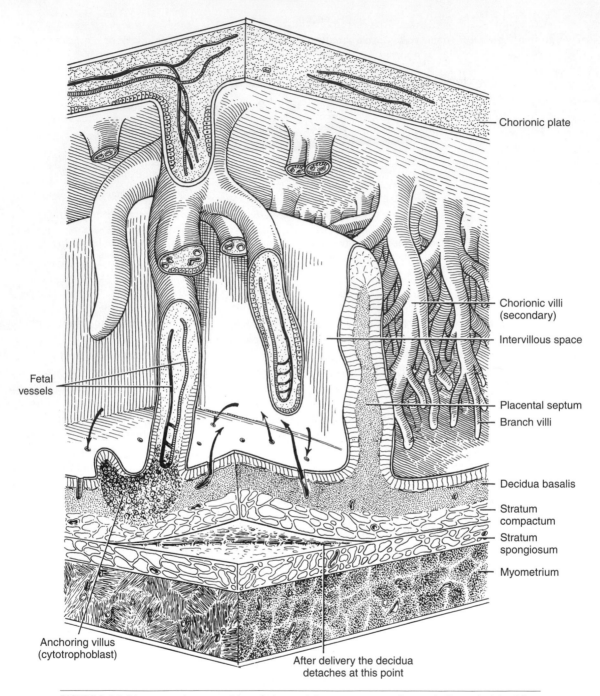

Chorionic plate

Chorionic villi
(secondary)

Intervillous space

Placental septum

Branch villi

Decidua basalis

Stratum
compactum

Stratum
spongiosum

Myometrium

Fetal
vessels

Anchoring villus
(cytotrophoblast)

After delivery the decidua
detaches at this point

FIGURE **3-14** Diagrammatic composition of placental tissues near term. Arrows indicate the blood flow from uteroplacental arteries to the intervillous space and back to the uteroplacental veins. (From Duplessis, G. D. T. and Haegel, P. [1971]. *Embryologie.* New York: Masson. English edition by Springer-Verlag; Chapman and Hall; and Masson, [1972].)

diffusion. Occasionally, trophoblast sprouts not used to form new villi may break off, enter the maternal circulation, and lodge in the mother's lung capillaries.

After 30 weeks' gestation, syncytial knots develop, pulling the syncytium and its nuclei into "piles" several layers thick and leaving a thin, attenuated, anuclear membrane in the intervening areas.[177] These areas (known as the vasculosyncytial membrane) appear to, but do not actually, fuse with dilated fetal capillaries and are thought to be specialized regions that facilitate placental gas exchange.[50,88,177]

The placenta eventually occupies one third of the inner uterine surface. Until 15 to 16 weeks, the placenta is larger than the fetus; the fetus then becomes larger than the placenta, so that by term the fetus is five to six times heavier than the placenta.[111,112,132] The early growth of the placenta establishes a wide area of maternal blood flow (so the placenta is not dependent on relatively few blood vessels for perfusion) and adequate trophoblastic tissue for production of sufficient hCG to maintain the corpus luteum and thus the pregnancy.

Increases in villous surface area and thinning of placental tissue layers increase the functional efficiency of the placenta during pregnancy. During the first 2 months the relatively few villi are greater than 170 μm in diameter, are vascularized by a small central fetal vessel, and are covered by two layers of trophoblast (syncytial outer layer and inner layer of cytotrophoblast) of uniform thickness. At this stage the villous stroma consists of a loose network of primitive mesenchymal tissue and many Hofbauer cells (tissue macrophage).[50,177] From 8 to 30 weeks, the number of villi increase and the average diameter decreases to about 70 μm. The stroma is then thinner and more compact and contains fibroblasts and collagen fibers with fewer Hofbauer cells.[50] By term the placental villi are approximately 35 to 40 μm in diameter. The trophoblastic layer and stroma have thinned considerably, and few cytotrophoblast cells are seen.[132,177]

The area-to-volume ratio of the placenta progressively increases. Surface area increases from 3.4 m^2 (28 weeks) to 12.6 m^2 (term), and the syncytium decreases in thickness from 10 mm^2 to 1.7 mm^2 late in gestation.[130] The actual surface area is closer to 90 m^2 because of the presence of extensive microvilli on the surface of the syncytial trophoblast covering the villi.[35,48] Transfer efficiency of placental tissue increases sixfold. The trophoblast layer and connective tissue thin so that the capillaries lie closer to the syncytial trophoblast, decreasing the distance that nutrients and waste products have to travel.

By term the placenta weighs approximately 480 g (give or take 135 g) with a diameter of 18 to 22 cm and thickness of 2 to 2.5 cm, although considerable variation is seen.[158,182] Although villous growth continues to near term, the placenta also undergoes degenerative changes (increased syncytial knots, intervillous thrombi, fibrin deposits, infarcts, calcification). Abnormal growth of the placenta may also occur. Hypoplasia of the syncytial trophoblast can alter implantation and result in abortion, abruptio placentae, or poor development of terminal villi and increase the risk of stillbirth or preterm delivery. Hyperplasia and reactivation of the syncytial growth layer, possibly due to suboptimal oxygenation, have been observed in women with hypertension and with prolonged pregnancy. Although the amount of cytotrophoblast decreases with gestation, the remaining tissue retains its proliferative capacity so the cytotrophoblast can be reactivated to replace damaged or destroyed syncytiotrophoblast.[50] However, this hyperplasia may be followed by degenerative changes.[35,111]

Separation of the Placenta

Placental separation and expulsion occur during the third stage of labor. The "afterbirth" consists of maternal and fetal tissues (see Figure 3-14). Maternal tissues include the decidua basalis (maternal portion of the placenta), decidua parietalis, and any remaining decidua capsularis. Fetal tissues include the chorion frondosum (fetal portion of the placenta), chorion laeve (chorion), amnion, and umbilical cord. Retained fragments of the placenta and membranes can lead to uterine atony, hemorrhage, or infection.

The sudden emptying of the uterus with delivery of the fetus rapidly reduces the surface area of the placental site to an area approximately 10 cm in diameter. This reduction in the base of support for the placenta leads to compression and shearing of the placenta from the uterine wall.[98] The usual site of placental separation is within the spongy layer of the decidua basalis (see Figure 3-14). This layer has been described as being like the "lines of perforation found between postal stamps."[98] The placenta may separate from the central area to the margins with inversion so that the fetal surface presents first (Schultze mechanism), or from the margins toward the center with initial presentation of the maternal surface (Duncan mechanism). Placentas implanted in the fundus of the uterus are more likely to separate via Schultze mechanism; those implanted lower on the uterine wall usually separate by Duncan mechanism (although these placentas may invert before expulsion).

Placental Structure

Although the mature placenta contains maternal and fetal components, it is primarily a fetal structure composed of extensively branching, closely packed fetal villi containing fetal blood vessels (see Figure 3-14). Three main types of villi can be identified: (1) stem (or anchoring) villi, which consist of multiple branches and function to stabilize the villous tree; (2) mature intermediate villi, located between the stem and terminal villi; and (3) terminal villi, which are the major areas of maternal-fetal exchange.[73,88] On the fetal side the placenta is covered by the chorionic plate, a thin membranous structure continuous with the fetal membranes. On the maternal side the outer layer of trophoblast cells fuse to the decidua basalis.

The fetal portion of the placenta is divided into 50 to 60 lobes, each arising as a primary stem villus supplied by primary branches of the umbilical vessels from the chorionic plate. Each lobe is divided into one to five subunits or lobules.[177] Lobules are globular structures with a central cylindrical space that is relatively empty.[50] This space may arise because of preferential growth of villi in relation to entry of maternal arteries into the IVS.[177] Beneath the chorionic plate the primary stem villi divide into secondary stem villi. These villi run parallel to the chorionic plate, dividing into tertiary stem villi, which project downward through the parenchyma of the placenta around the central space and anchor onto the basal plate (see Figure 3-14).[50,177] Each primary stem villus may give rise to varying numbers of secondary stem villi and lobules.[50] The terminal villi branch off of the tertiary stem villi.

The placental septa divide the maternal surface of the placenta into an average of 15 to 20 lobes, each containing two or more main stem villi and their branches.[35,111] The term *cotyledon* is sometimes used to describe these lobes. Fox suggests that, since the maternal lobes are just areas between placental septa with no physiologic or morphologic significance, *cotyledon* should really be used to describe portions of the villus tree that arise from a single primary stem villus.[50]

Maternal and fetal circulations are separated by several layers of tissue. These tissues are called the *placental membrane* or *placental barrier*. A substance, such as oxygen, moving from the maternal circulation to the fetal circulation must pass from maternal blood through five tissue layers to reach the fetal blood: (1) the microvillous membrane of the trophoblast; (2) the syncytiotrophoblast cells of the villus; (3) the basal membrane of the trophoblast; (4) the connective tissue mesoderm of the villus; and (5) the epithelium of the fetal blood vessel (Figure 3-15). The layers of the placental barrier are modified as the cytotrophoblast ceases to form a continuous layer after about 12 weeks and is replaced by a fibrinoid layer.[111,121,125] The connective tissue mesoderm thins, and the fetal capillaries increase in number and size.

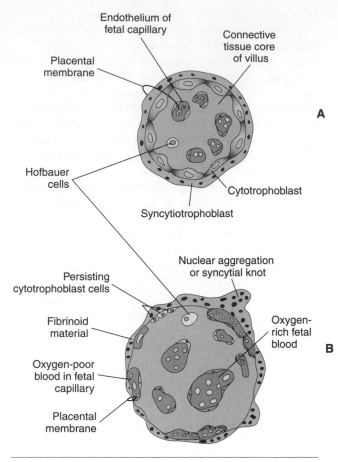

FIGURE **3-15** The placental membrane or barrier. **A** and **B,** Drawings of sections through a chorionic villus at 10 weeks and at full term, respectively. (From Moore, K.L. & Persaud, T.V.N. [1998]. *The developing human: Clinically oriented embryology* [6th ed.]. Philadelphia: W.B. Saunders.)

Placental Circulation

Adequate blood flow to and through the placenta from both fetal and maternal circulations is essential for adequate exchange of nutrients, gases, and waste products. However, nearly half of the combined maternal-fetal blood flow to the placenta is not involved in maternal-fetal transfer due to maternal and fetal shunts within the uteroplacental circulation.[48] The fetal shunt is the portion of umbilical blood flow that does not supply an area of exchange between maternal and fetal blood. Approximately 17% to 25% of the total umbilical blood flow is used to supply the fetal membranes and placental tissue. Maternal shunt is the portion of uterine blood flow that does not supply the IVS. Approximately 20% to 27% of uterine arterial blood supplies the myometrium and cervix. At term the uterus extracts 30 to 35 ml of oxygen per minute from maternal blood.[48]

Fetal-Placental Circulation

Deoxygenated blood from the fetus passes via the two umbilical arteries, which spiral around the umbilical vein, to the placenta. Each artery supplies half of the placenta. Before entering the placenta, the two umbilical arteries are connected by several anastomosed vessels. These arteries tend to fuse close to the surface of the placenta.[60,66] As the cord enters the placenta, the arteries divide and branch radially onto the chorionic plate before entering the villi. The chorionic vessels branch into 20 to 40 villous trunks or lobular arteries, which branch further into multiple smaller villous vessels, forming an extensive arteriovenous system within each villus. The veins converge back into the umbilical vein at the umbilical cord.

The rate of fetal blood flow in the placenta is about 500 ml/minute.[50] Blood flow is dependent on fetal heart activity and regulated by the interaction of blood pressure, fetal right-to-left shunts, and systemic and pulmonary vascular resistance.[4,48] Contraction of smooth muscle fibers in stem villi may help pump blood from the placenta back to the fetus. The placenta is a low-resistance circuit in the fetal circulatory system (see Chapter 8) as a result of minimal umbilical innervation.

Maternal Uteroplacental Circulation

Blood flows to the uterus via the uterine arteries, which are branches of the internal iliac and ovarian arteries from the abdominal aorta. The proportion of the maternal cardiac output supplying the uterus and IVS increases during pregnancy, peaking at 20% to 25% (see Chapter 8). The increased blood flow is mediated by the low-resistance uteroplacental circuit, alterations in maternal cardiac output and systemic and peripheral vascular resistance, and hormonal and chemical influences.[63,175]

Maternal blood enters the IVS via uteroplacental arteries in the endometrium. By term, blood in these spaces is supplied by 100 to 200 maternal uteroplacental arteries and removed by 75 to 175 veins.[88] Blood flow enters the IVS through arterial inlets as a funnel-shaped stream flowing toward the chorionic plate or "roof" of the placenta (see Figure 3-14).[121,141] The blood then flows around the villi, allowing exchange of materials between maternal and fetal circulation. Blood leaves the IVS via wide venous outlets into the uteroplacental veins and subchorial, interlobular, and marginal venous lakes.[48,111,177]

Overall the pressures within this system are low due to anatomic changes in maternal uterine blood vessels. As a result, the maternal arterial blood pressure is not transmitted to the IVS, and pressure gradients from the arterial to venous sides are relatively small (i.e., pressure averages 25 mmHg in the uteroplacental arteries, 15 to 20 mmHg in the IVS, and 5 to 10 mmHg in the uterine veins).[5,50,141] Ramsey and Donner suggest that blood enters the IVS "much as water from an actively flowing brook penetrates a reed-filled marsh."[141]

The IVS in the mature placenta contains about 150 ml of blood, which is completely replenished three to four times a minute.[111] The rate of blood flow within the maternal side of the placenta increases during pregnancy from 50 ml/minute at 10 weeks to 500 to 600 ml/min by term.[35,48] Uterine contractions limit the entry of blood into the IVS but do not squeeze out a significant amount of blood. Thus oxygen transfer to the fetus is decreased during a normal contraction but does not cease, because transfer continues from blood remaining in the IVS.

The arteries of the endometrium (decidua) and myometrium undergo marked physiologic changes during pregnancy that convert the uterine spiral arteries into uteroplacental arteries. These changes are mediated by extravillous invasive trophoblast that invades the spiral arteries in the decidua and upper third of the myometrium, replacing spiral artery endothelium and destroying muscular and elastic elements in the medial tissue.[40,50,82,145] Much of the arterial wall is replaced by a fibrinoid extracellular matrix that arises from maternal fibrin and from proteins secreted by the trophoblast.[150] As a result, the spiral arteries (now called *uteroplacental arteries*) become saclike structures unresponsive to maternal vasoconstrictive agent and able to accommodate the blood needed to supply the IVS.[22,82]

As the trophoblast migrates into the decidua, it acquires an endothelial cell adhesion molecule phenotype, switching from a proliferative function to and invasive function. This switch is controlled by down- and upregulation of specific genes and gene products, including integrins, and mediated by trophoblast and decidual factors, including growth factors, enzymes, and binding proteins.[33,72,124] Proinvasive factors include trophoblast proteases and decidual activators and attractants; antinvasive factors include decidual barrier properties and local inhibitors. If the balance between proinvasive and inhibiting factors is altered, abnormally decreased or increased invasion occurs.[96] The switch from a proliferative to invasive phenotype is abnormal in women with preeclampsia.[184] Lack of invasion is associated with miscarriage, intrauterine growth restriction (IUGR) and preeclampsia.[27] Excessive blood flow to the IVS in the first trimester may result in an oxidative insult to the developing embryo and decreased angiogenesis in the placenta.[77]

The invasive trophoblast not only remodels the spiral arteries but also temporarily plugs the tops of the spiral arteries, preventing maternal blood from entering the IVS

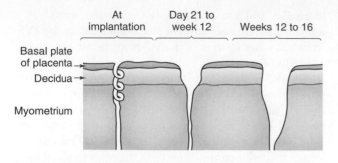

FIGURE **3-16** Diagrammatic representation of the conversion of the spiral arteries in the placental bed into uteroplacental vessels. (From Fox, H. (1997). *Pathology of the placenta* [2nd ed.]. Philadelphia: W.B. Saunders.)

until 10 to 12 weeks.[76,79,82,96] At the same time, as maternal blood begins to flow into the IVS, fetal antioxidant systems increase.[79] Thus first trimester placental circulation is very different from that in the second and third trimesters.[76] During the first trimester, maternal blood is shunted from the spiral arteries to uterine veins via arteriovenous shunts and does not enter the IVS. The IVS is filled with a clear fluid—secretions from the decidual glands rather than blood in the IVS.[76,96] It may be that the low oxygen environment in the first trimester protects the developing embryo, which has not yet developed protective mechanisms against oxidative stress.[76,79,115,148]

The extravillous invasive trophoblast migrates into the maternal tissue in two waves. During the initial wave at 6 to 10 weeks, spiral arteries in the decidua are altered; during the second wave, beginning at 14 to 16 weeks and lasting for 4 to 6 weeks (generally completed by 20 to 22 weeks), spiral arteries in the myometrium—and occasionally distal portions of the radial arteries—are altered (Figure 3-16).[50,72,88,137,145,177]

Changes in the maternal arteries, particularly disruption of the muscular and elastic elements, enhance the capacity of the uteroplacental vessels to accommodate the increased blood volume needed to supply the placenta. These vessels are also functionally denervated due to decreased neurotransmitter sites.[145] As a result of these changes, the arteries underlying the placenta are almost completely dilated and are no longer responsive to systemic circulatory pressor agents or influences of the autonomic nervous system.[155,175,187] Control of the uteroplacental circulation is at the level of the radial arteries and is mediated primarily by local (uteroplacental) influences, including placental production of prostacyclin (PGI$_2$). PGI$_2$, the most potent vasodilator produced by the placenta, is thought to maintain vasodilatation of these vessels, prevent platelet aggregation,

and enhance cell disengagement (needed for disruption of elastic and muscular elements).[145,175]

The importance of these changes for fetal survival and growth can be appreciated by examining situations such as spontaneous abortion, preeclampsia, and IUGR in which invasion of the spiral arteries by invasive cytotrophoblast does not occur or is abnormal (see Figure 3-16).[27,72,77] Recurrent spontaneous abortion in some women may be due to absent or inadequate conversion of spiral arteries to uteroplacental arteries. Absence of changes in decidual arteries has been associated with late first trimester loss, and absence of myometrial artery changes with second trimester loss.[93,136] Failure of the normal cytotrophoblastic invasion of the decidua and myometrium and subsequent arterial changes occurs in some types of IUGR. Underperfusion of the IVS may lead to occlusion of small arterioles within the villi. These changes can markedly alter fetal growth and health status and are similar to changes reported with some growth-restricted fetuses.

Preeclampsia is associated with alterations in the normal invasion of the spiral arteries by the invasive trophoblast (Figure 3-17).[96,152] This defect, which may have a genetic basis, is postulated to be an initial event in the development of preeclampsia.[175] Generally the first invasive trophoblast wave proceeds normally, but there is failure of the second wave.[50,88] Thus decidual spiral arteries undergo the usual physiologic changes, but the myometrial arteries do not. The uninvaded arterial segments may also develop atherosclerosis with necrosis and invasion of the damaged wall by fibrin and other substances. Alterations in the normal changes within the uterine arteries in women with preeclampsia lead to: (1) decreased perfusion of the IVS due to the retained muscular coat and inability of the vessels to dilate sufficiently to accommodate the increased blood flow, and (2) hypertension in the uteroplacental arteries due to continued sensitivity of these vessels to circulatory pressor agents and the influences of the autonomic nervous system.[88,136]

The cause of the defect in preeclampsia is unclear. It may be a primary defect in invasive trophoblast, alterations in endometrial metabolism, altered endometrial immunologic reactions, or an altered environment.[96] Preeclampsia has been associated with abnormal expression of integrin molecules limiting trophoblast invasion to the deciduus, resulting in decreased uteroplacental blood flow.[72] If the spiral arteries are not converted into low-resistance circuits, the placenta secretes vasoactive substances that increase maternal blood pressure.[96] Alterations in production of placental PGI$_2$ and thromboxane (TXA$_2$) occur with preeclampsia. Prostacyclin is produced in many tissues and is a potent vasodilator and inhibitor of platelet aggregation

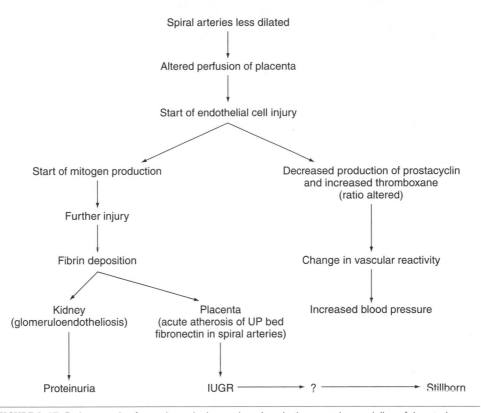

FIGURE **3-17** Pathogenesis of preeclampsia due to alterations in the normal remodeling of the uterine vasculature during pregnancy. *IUGR,* Intrauterine growth restriction; *UP,* uteroplacental. (From Fanaroff, A.A. & Martin, R.J. [1997]. *Neonatal-perinatal medicine: Diseases of the fetus and infant* [6th ed.]. St. Louis: Mosby.)

and uterine contractility, which acts to promote increased uteroplacental blood flow during pregnancy. Conversely, TXA_2 is a potent vasoconstrictor that opposes the action of prostacyclin. Women with preeclampsia have been reported to have an imbalance in levels of these mediators produced by the placenta with elevated TXA_2 and decreased prostacyclin (see Chapter 8), which may alter the usual changes in the uterine blood vessels.[175]

Placental Function

The placenta has four major activities: metabolic, endocrine, immunologic, and transport. The placenta also serves as a "radiator," with 85% of fetal heat production transmitted to the mother via the placenta.[157]

Placental Metabolism

Placental metabolism contributes to the quality and quantity of the fetal nutrient supply.[53] Placental metabolic functions are particularly important early in pregnancy in providing nutrition and energy for the developing fetus and for the placenta itself. The placenta has a high metabolic

rate. Rates of oxygen consumption and glucose utilization by the placenta approximate those of the brain.[92] Glucose use by the placenta equals 50% to 70% of the uterine glucose uptake.[53]

The placenta is an active synthesizer of glycogen, fatty acids, cholesterol, and enzymes. The placenta produces protective and enhancement enzymes such as sulfatase, which enhances the excretion of fetal estrogen precursors, and insulinase, which increases the barrier to the transfer of insulin.[48] Relatively large amounts of ammonia and lactate are produced by the placenta and may be important in stimulating metabolic activity of the fetal liver. The impact of alterations in these metabolic processes on placental function and transport during pathologic states is not clear, but they decrease the capacity of the fetus to tolerate labor and transition to extrauterine life. Placental metabolism is described further in Chapter 15.

Placental Endocrinology

Placental endocrine activities are important in maintaining pregnancy and inducing metabolic adaptations in the mother and fetus. The placenta synthesizes polypeptide hormones (hCG and hPL) and steroid hormones (estrogens and progesterone) as well as mediators such as pregnancy-associated plasma proteins (PAPP), neurohormones and neuropolypeptides, binding proteins, cytokines, and growth factors (Table 3-3). Growth factor receptors appear on the trophoblast early in gestation. Growth factors are short polypeptides that are produced in many different types of tissues. Growth factors act in paracrine and autocrine manner on specific localized target tissues by interacting with receptors on the target cell's membrane. This stimulates, via second messengers, signal transduction within the cell, initiating specific changes within the cell such as glucose uptake, RNA and protein synthesis, amino acid transport, or DNA synthesis and cell replication.[53,104]

The four main hormones synthesized by the placenta are hCG, hPL, progesterone, and estrogens. The placenta also produces pituitary-like and gonad-like peptide hormones (i.e., placental corticotrophin, human chorionic thyrotropin, melanocyte stimulating hormone, β-endorphin, β-lipoprotein), hypothalamus-like releasing hormones (i.e., human chorionic somatostatin, corticotrophin-releasing hormones [CRH]), and gut hormones (i.e., gastrin, vasoactive intestinal peptide).The placenta, membranes, and fetus also synthesize a variety of peptide growth factors including epidermal growth factor (EGF), nerve growth factor (NGF), platelet-derived growth factor (PDGF), skeletal growth factor, and insulin-like growth factor 1 (IGF-1) (somatomedin C) and IGF-2.[6,47,53,63,104]

Placental growth factors regulate cell growth and differentiation, hormone release at the local level, and uterine contractility.[104] For example, IGF-1 and IGF-2 regulate cell proliferation and differentiation to maintain normal fetal growth. IGF works by enhancing amino acid and glucose uptake and preventing protein breakdown.[53] Transforming growth factor–α (TGF-α) and EGF have primarily roles in regulating cell differentiation.[104] TGF-β has both proliferative and antiproliferative actions to stimulate and inhibit cell differentiation. This factor is involved in embryogenesis and neural migration and differentiation.[53] Activin stimulates and inhibin decreases placental hCG and progesterone.[134,140] Follistatin inhibits FSH release.[104,140] Human placental growth hormone (hPGH) regulates IGF-1. Until 15 to 20 weeks, maternal pituitary GH is the major maternal growth hormone; after that time, levels of hPGH increase and maternal pituitary GH is supressed.[47,104] hPGH may alter maternal metabolism by stimulating gluconeogenesis and lipolysis in the second half of pregnancy to increase nutrient availability for the fetus.[6,47] PDGF has insulin-like activity to stimulate growth.[53]

Parathyroid hormone–related protein (PTHrP) mediates placental calcium transport (Chapter 16). PTHrP also has a role in development of the bone and epithelial organs and in the interaction of epithelial and mesenchymal cells.[166,181] Leptin is involved in regulating energy homeostasis, weight, and reproductive processes in pregnancy and may play a role in regulating fetal growth and development and possibly in placental development, angiogenesis, and hematopoiesis.[47,64,71,110] CRH is synthesized by the

TABLE **3-3**   **Examples of Growth Factors, Neuropeptides, and Proteins Identified in Placental Tissues**

Protein and Peptide Hormone	Neurohormone or Neurpeptiodes	Growth Factors	Binding Proteins	Cytokines
Human chorionic gonadotrophin	Gonadotrophin-releasing hormone	Activin	Corticotrophin-releasing-hormone-binding protein (CRH-BP)	Interleukin-I (IL-1)
Human placental lactogen	Thyroid-releasing hormone	Follistatin		IL-2
Growth hormone variant	Growth hormone-releasing hormone	Inhibin	Insulin-like growth factor-binding protein-1 (IGFBP-1)	IL-6
Adrenocorticotrophic hormone	Somatostatin	Transforming growth factor (β and α)		IL-8
	Corticotrophin-releasing hormone	Epidermal growth factor		Interferon-α
	Oxytocin	Insulin-like growth factor 1 (IGF-1)	IGFBP-2	Interferon-β
	Neuropeptide Y	IGF-2	IGFBP-3	Interferon-γ
	β-Endorphin met-enkephalin dynorphia	Fibroblastic growth factor	IGFBP-4	Tumor necrosis factor-α
		Platelet-derived growth factor	IGFBP-5	
			IGFBP-6	

From Liu, J.H. & Rebar, R.W. (1999). Endocrinology of pregnancy. In R.K. Creasy & R. Resnik (Eds.). *Maternal-fetal medicine* (4th ed.). Philadelphia: W.B. Saunders.

placenta, amnion, chorion, and decidua and stimulates release of prostaglandins. CRH has a major role in initiation of myometrial contractility and labor onset (see Chapter 4).

The placenta also produces cytokines (see Table 3-3). Cytokines are regulatory peptides or glycoproteins produced by most nucleated cells that regulate cell function via paracrine (intercellular) or autocrine (intracellular) signals.[150,151] For example, interleukins induce syncytiotrophoblast release of hCG that in turn stimulates release of progesterone from the corpus luteum. Other cytokines and peptides produced by the placenta are involved in immunoregulation (see Chapter 12).[26]

Human chorionic gonadotrophin. hCG is a glycoprotein with alpha and beta subunits that is biologically similar to luteinizing hormone. The major function of hCG is to maintain the corpus luteum during early pregnancy in order to ensure progesterone secretion until placental production is adequate.[53] In addition, hCG may stimulate the fetal testes and adrenal gland to enhance testosterone and corticosteroid secretion, stimulate production of placental progesterone, and suppress maternal lymphocyte responses thereby preventing rejection of the placenta by the mother.[53,63,131,132] Release of hCG is enhanced by GnRH, IL-1, IL-2, IGF, EGF, and activin and inhibited by inhibin, opioids, and TGF-β.[135] hCG is produced primarily by syncytiotrophoblast cells in the placenta, although small amounts may be produced by other types of trophoblast tissue.[50]

hCG can be detected in maternal circulation around the time of implantation and has been found in the preimplantation blastocyst.[53] Significant serum concentrations of hCG can be detected about 12 days after follicle rupture in normal pregnancies. Concentrations of hCG in maternal serum double every 2 to 3 days until peak values are reached 60 to 90 days after conception (Figure 3-18).[53,73,131] Concentrations of hCG decrease after 10 to 11 weeks and reach a plateau at low levels by 100 to 130 days. By 2 weeks after delivery, hCG disappears. Persistently low levels may indicate an abnormal placenta or ectopic pregnancy; levels remain elevated in women with hydatidiform moles.[35] Urine hCG can be detected 26 to 28 days after conception and is identified by isoimmunologic analysis. Home pregnancy tests of maternal urine are now usually positive as early as 1 day after the first missed period. These tests have a sensitivity of 80% to 90% and a specificity of 95%.[127]

Human placental lactogen. hPL, also called *human chorionic somatomammotropin* (hCS) or *chorionic growth hormone,* consists of a single polypeptide chain similar in structure to that of human growth hormone. hPL promotes fetal growth by altering maternal protein, carbohydrate, and fat metabolism (see Chapter 15). The primary role of hPL is regulating glucose availability for the fetus, and it is an insulin antagonist that increases maternal metabolism and use of fat as an energy substrate and reduces glucose uptake and use by maternal cells. As a result, more glucose is available for transport to the fetus.[50,63] Thus hPL

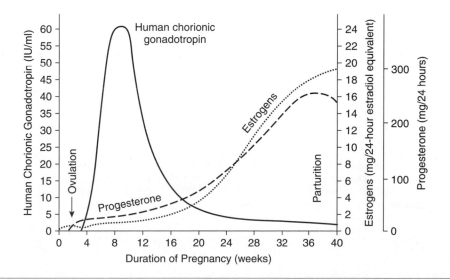

FIGURE **3-18** Patterns of excretion of human chorionic gonadotropin, progesterone, and estrogen during pregnancy. (From Guyton, A.C. [1987]. *Human physiology and mechanisms of disease* [4th ed.]. Philadelphia: W.B. Saunders.)

acts as a growth-promoting hormone, promoting fetal growth by altering maternal metabolism.[53]

Production of hPL by the syncytiotrophoblast begins 12 to 18 days after conception (5 to 10 days after implantation), rises during pregnancy, and peaks near term.[53] Secretion of hPL is regulated by glucose; decreased serum glucose leads to increased hPL secretion and increased maternal lipolysis.[63] As early as 4 weeks after conception, hPL can be detected in maternal serum; little is found in maternal urine. It has a short half-life, so maternal serum levels reflect the rate of production.

Steroidogenesis. Progesterone and the estrogens are steroid hormones whose synthesis increases rapidly during pregnancy (see Figure 3-18). Early in gestation, the corpus luteum is the main synthesis site, but by 7 weeks the placental syncytiotrophoblast has taken over as the major producer.[53] Steroidogenesis during pregnancy is based on a complex set of interactions by separate organ systems. Each system lacks essential enzymes necessary for creation of the final hormone. Placental production of progesterone and estrogens is an example of a function that requires cooperative efforts of the mother, placenta, and fetus. The placenta lacks certain enzymes needed for production of estriol; these enzymes are present in the fetal adrenal. The fetus is the major source of precursors for the estrogens, and the mother is the major source of precursors for the progesterone (Figure 3-19). Placental progesterone also serves as a precursor for fetal synthesis of corticosteroids, testosterone, and androgens.[35,63,81]

Progesterone. Progesterone is produced by the corpus luteum (under the influence of hCG) during the first 6 to 8 weeks after fertilization. After that period, progesterone is synthesized using maternal cholesterol and low-density lipoproteins (see Figure 3-19). A fetus is not essential for placental progesterone production, which continues even after fetal death.[132] Progesterone production in late pregnancy is about 250 to 300 mg/day; 90% is secreted into maternal circualtion.[50,53,63] The active progesterone metabo-

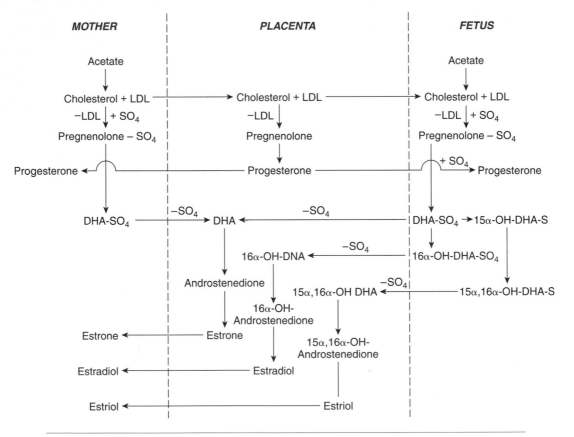

FIGURE **3-19** Steroidogenic pathways in the maternal-placental-fetal unit. *DHA-SO₄,* Dihydro-epiandrosterone sulfate; *LDL,* low-density lipoprotein; *OH,* hydroxy. (From Siler-Khodr, T. M. [1998]. Endocrine and paracrine functions of the human placenta. In R.A. Polin & W.W. Fox [Eds.]. *Fetal and neonatal physiology* [2nd ed.]. Philadelphia: W.B. Saunders.)

lites are 5α-reduced metabolite; 5α-pregnane-3,20-dione; and deoxycorticosterone (DOC). The first two contribute to the altered response to the pressor action of angiotensin II during pregnancy (Chapter 10).[24]

During pregnancy progesterone acts to decrease myometrial activity and irritability; constrict myometrial vessels; decrease sensitivity of the maternal respiratory center to carbon dioxide; inhibit prolactin secretion; help suppress maternal immunologic responses to fetal antigens, thereby preventing rejection of the fetus; relax smooth muscle in the gastrointestinal and urinary systems; increase basal body temperature; and increase sodium and chloride excretion.[35,53]

The most important role of progesterone in the fetus is to serve as the substrate pool for fetal adrenal gland production of glucocorticoids and mineralocorticoids. The fetal adrenal gland lacks enzymes in the 3β-hydroxysteroid dehydrogenase, δ4-5 isomerase system necessary for synthesis of some important corticosteroids. Therefore the fetus must utilize progesterone substrate from the placenta to accomplish this.[24]

Estrogens. The three major estrogens are estrone, estradiol, and estriol. During pregnancy production of estrogens, particularly that of estriol, increases markedly. Estrone and estradiol production increases about 100 times; estriol production increases about 1000 times.[63] During pregnancy estrogens act to enhance myometrial activity, promote myometrial vasodilatation, increase sensitivity of the maternal respiratory center to carbon dioxide, soften fibers in the cervical collagen tissue, increase pituitary secretion of prolactin, increase serum binding proteins and fibrinogen, decrease plasma proteins, and increase the sensitivity of the uterus to progesterone in late pregnancy.[35,53]

Early in pregnancy, estriol is derived from estrone and estradiol. Production of estrogens, and particularly estriol, is dependent on interaction of the maternal-fetal-placental unit. Approximately 90% of the precursors for estriol are derived from the fetus; 40% of the precursors for estrone and estradiol come from the mother and 60% from the fetus.[35] The primary source of estriol precursors (dehydroepiandrosterone sulfate [DHEAS]) is the fetal adrenal gland under stimulation by fetal adrenocorticotropic hormone (ACTH). DHEAS is hydroxylated in the fetal liver and further metabolized by the placenta to form estriol. Estriol is secreted by the placenta into maternal circulation and eventually excreted in maternal urine (see Figure 3-19). Maternal serum and urinary estriol levels rise rapidly during early pregnancy, more slowly between 24 and 32 weeks, and then increase rapidly again in the last 6 weeks. Although seldom used currently, estriol assays were one of the earlier methods of assessing fetal well-being and placental function for management of complicated pregnancies.[35,87]

Placental Immunologic Function

The immunologic functions of the placenta include protection of the fetus from pathogens and prevention from rejection by the mother. The fetus differs in genetic makeup from the mother, yet it is not rejected. Possible explanations for this phenomenon are discussed in Chapter 12. The placenta also protects the fetus from pathogens. Many bacteria are too large to cross placenta, although most viruses and some bacteria are able to cross. The placenta also allows passage of maternal antibodies of the immunoglobulin G (IgG) class primarily via pinocytosis, although some may cross by diffusion. This may also be a disadvantage, because both protective and potentially deleterious antibodies cross the placenta (see Chapter 12).

Placental Transport

Placental transfer or transport involves bidirectional movement of gases, nutrients, waste materials, drugs, and other substances across the placenta from maternal-to-fetal circulation or from fetal to maternal circulation (Figures 3-20 and 3-21). Transport across the placenta increases during the course of gestation due to changes in placental structure (decreased distance between maternal and fetal blood), increased fetal and maternal blood flow, and greater fetal demands. Transfer can be modified by maternal nutritional status; exercise; and disease, such as diabetes mellitus (glucose transport increases due to maternal

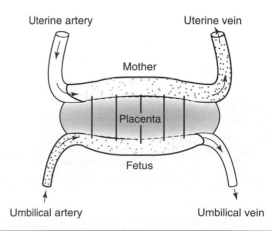

FIGURE **3-20** Schematic representation of the conversion of the placenta as an exchange organ. (From Fox, H. (1997). *Pathology of the placenta* [2nd ed.]. Philadelphia: W.B. Saunders.)

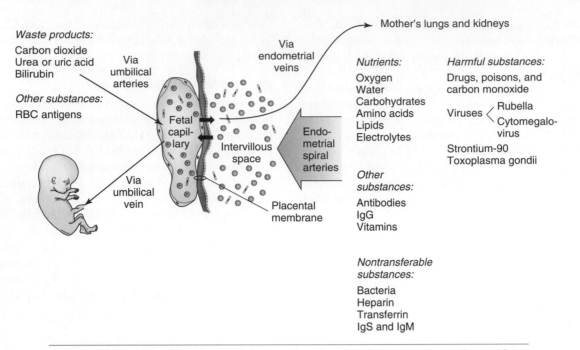

FIGURE **3-21** Summary of transfer of substances across the placenta between the mother and fetus. (From Moore, K.L. [1998]. *The developing human* [6th ed.]. Philadelphia: W.B. Saunders.)

TABLE **3-4**   **Mechanisms by Which Selected Substances are Transported Across the Placenta**

MECHANISM	SUBSTANCE
Simple (passive) diffusion	Water, electrolytes, oxygen, carbon dioxide, urea, simple amines, creatinine, fatty acids, steroids, fat-soluble vitamins, narcotics, antibiotics, barbiturates, and anesthetics
Facilitated diffusion	Glucose, oxygen
Active transport	Amino acids, water-soluble vitamins, calcium, iron, iodine
Pinocytosis and endocytosis	Globulins, phospholipids, lipoproteins, antibodies, viruses
Bulk flow/solid drag	Water, electrolytes
Accidental capillary breaks	Intact blood cells
Independent movement	Maternal leukocytes, organisms such as *Treponema pallidum*

hyperglycemia), hypertension (decreased nutrient transfer as a result of reduced uteroplacental blood flow), and alcoholism (ethanol impairs placental uptake of amino acids and glucose).[125,160] Transfer of specific substances across the placenta is summarized in Table 3-4, while relative con-

centrations of selected materials in fetal and maternal plasma are listed in Table 3-5.

The mechanisms by which substances are transferred across the placenta include simple (passive) diffusion, facilitated diffusion, active transport, pinocytosis, endocytosis, bulk flow, solvent drag, accidental capillary breaks, and independent movement. Facilitated diffusion and active transport are mediated by protein carriers and other transporters. Transporters are located on both the maternal-facing brush border syncytiotrophoblast (facing the IVS) and the fetal-facing basal membrane (facing the fetal villous stroma).[52]

Simple (passive) diffusion. Diffusion is movement of a substance from higher to lower concentration or electrochemical gradients (Figure 3-22, *A*). The quantity of a substance transferred is illustrated by the Fick diffusion equation:

$$Q/t = \frac{K\,A\,(C1 - C2)}{L}$$

Q/t is the quantity transferred/unit of time, K is the diffusion constant, A is the fetal surface area available for exchange, C1−C2 is the concentration gradient across the placenta, and L is the thickness of the membrane across which the substance is to move.

Diffusion is the major mechanism of placental transfer. Simple diffusion is generally limited to smaller molecules

TABLE **3-5**   **Relative Concentrations of Nutrients and Other Substances in Maternal Versus Fetal Circulation**

HIGHER IN FETUS	SIMILAR IN FETUS AND MOTHER	HIGHER IN MOTHER
Amino acids	Sodium	Total proteins
Total phosphorus	Chloride	Globulins
Lactate	Urea	Fibrinogen
Serum iron	Magnesium	Total lipids
Calcium		Phospholipids
Riboflavin		Fatty acids
Ascorbic acid		Glucose
		Cholesterol
		Vitamin A
		Vitamin E

Compiled from Longo, L. (1981). Nutrient transfer in the placenta. In *Placental transport.* Mead Johnson Symposium on Perinatal and Developmental Medicine (No. 18). Evansville, IN: Mead Johnson.

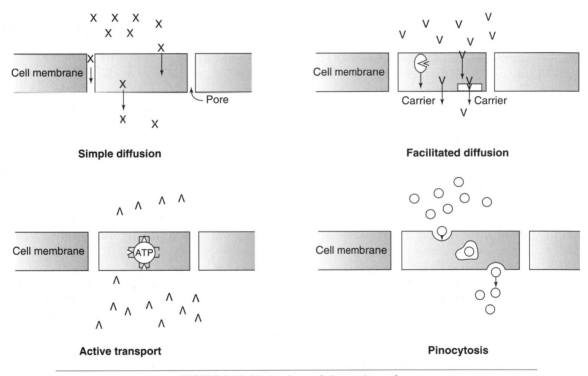

FIGURE **3-22** Mechanisms of placental transfer.

that can pass through pores in the cell wall. Because the cell walls have a high lipid content, some lipid-soluble substances may cross directly through these lipid regions.[19,35,111,144] Water-soluble substances cross easily if less than 100 MW; lipid-soluble molecules less than 600 MW cross unimpeded. The cell walls can act as a barrier to some large non-lipid-soluble substances such as muscle relaxants used with anesthesia. Table 3-4 lists substances that cross the placenta via simple diffusion.[48,111,125] Fat-

soluble vitamins and cholesterol diffuse as lipoprotein complexes.[5] Compounds such as histamine, serotonin, angiotensin, and epinephrine diffuse readily, but significant concentrations may never reach the fetus due to enzymatic deamination within the placenta.[35] Free water crosses at a rate of 180 ml/second, faster than any other known substance.[48]

Carbon dioxide is highly soluble in the placental membrane and diffuses readily. Oxygen diffuses with greater difficulty and therefore requires a considerable gradient of oxygen pressure on either side of the membrane. The average gradient is about 20 mmHg for oxygen and 5 mmHg for carbon dioxide. The oxygen gradient is higher because the placenta and myometrium also extract oxygen.[48] The rate of gas exchange across the placenta is limited by maternal blood flow supplying oxygen to the placenta. The placenta consumes about 10% to 30% of the oxygen delivered to it.[5]

Although the placenta is similar to the lungs in relation to the efficiency of gas exchange, the PO_2 levels of maternal and fetal blood leaving the placenta differ. These differences are due to the previously described vascular shunts in maternal and fetal circulations, nonuniform distribution of maternal and fetal blood flow, and differences in the positions of the maternal and fetal oxygen hemoglobin dissociation curves (see Chapter 9). When maternal blood flow exceeds fetal flow, the exchange of oxygen with fetal blood results in only minimal changes in maternal PO_2. Blood from these compartments contributes heavily to the PO_2 of mixed venous blood leaving the uterus. Conversely, oxygen exchange in areas in which fetal blood flow exceeds maternal flow depletes maternal reserves and equilibrates at a level similar to the fetal PO_2.[121] Placental gas exchange is discussed further in Chapter 9.

Facilitated diffusion. Facilitated diffusion involves transport via protein carriers and other transporters to move substances across the placental membrane (see Figure 3-22, *B*). Movement is from higher to lower concentration or electrochemical gradients. Glucose (fetal levels are 70% to 80% of maternal values) and possibly some oxygen are transported from maternal-to-fetal circulation via facilitated diffusion. Placental glucose metabolism may partially account for differences in maternal and fetal glucose concentrations. Glucose transport systems may become saturated at high concentrations (See Chapter 15).[14,143] Waste products such as lactate are transported from fetus to mother via facilitated diffusion.[144]

Active transport. Active transport utilizes energy-dependent carrier systems and other transporters to move substances against concentration or electrochemical gradient (see Figure 3-22, *C*). Amino acids, potassium, water-soluble vitamins, calcium, phosphate, iron, and iodine cross the placenta via active transport (see Table 3-4).[48,135,141,161] Active transport systems become saturated at high concentrations. Similar molecules may compete, reducing the movement of some substances across the placenta.

Amino acids such as alanine, glutamine, threonine, and serine that are transported by multiple carrier systems are found in high concentrations in placental tissue.[125] The net movement of many amino acids is greater than that estimated for fetal growth needs, suggesting that the fetus also uses these substances for energy or the synthesis of other amino acids.[125,161] The amount of amino acids transported across the placenta increases markedly late in pregnancy due to increased numbers of carriers. Most polypeptides and larger proteins that cross the placenta do so via pinocytosis or accidental capillary breaks. The only proteins transported in significant quantities are IgG (see Chapter 12) and retinol-binding protein.

Pinocytosis and endocytosis. These mechanisms involve the engulfing of microdroplets of maternal plasma (pinocytosis) (see Figure 3-22, *D*) or solid substances (endocytosis) by trophoblast cells. Substances in maternal plasma such as globulins, phospholipids, lipoproteins, and antibodies are transferred to the fetus or metabolized by the placenta. These mechanisms are necessary to transfer molecules too large for diffusion or for which no carrier transport exists and allow molecules of up to 150,000 MW to cross the placenta.[19]

Maternal antibodies of the IgG class readily cross the placenta during the third trimester. Maternal immunoglobulin A (IgA) antibodies do not cross in significant amounts; immunoglobulin M (IgM) antibodies are not transferred. IgG antibodies from the mother can be protective (e.g., antibodies against diphtheria, measles, mumps, herpes simplex virus) or potentially damaging (as occurs in Rh incompatibility or with maternal Graves' disease or myasthenia gravis) to the fetus (see Chapter 12).

Bulk flow and solvent drag. Water crosses the placenta very rapidly. Bulk movement may occur with changes in hydrostatic or osmotic forces. Ions cross either by simple diffusion or by solvent drag as dissolved electrolytes are pulled across the placenta by the movement of water. This mechanism is useful in maintaining water and osmotic balances between maternal and fetal circulations.[48,111,125] This mechanism may involve (hypothetical) aqueous pores and thus is most effective for molecules with low MW.[144] Water movement varies within the placenta depending on the concentrations of various osmotically active substances and the hydrostatic pressure.[161]

Accidental capillary breaks. Accidental capillary breaks and breaks in the villous covering permit passage of intact blood cells between maternal and fetal circulations. Small amounts (0.1 to 0.2 ml) of fetal cells can be found in maternal circulation intermittently during pregnancy. More extensive (>1 to 2 ml) fetomaternal hemorrhage may occur with placental separation and affect development of isoimmunization (see Chapter 12).[48,111]

Independent movement. Maternal leukocytes or organisms such as *Treponema pallidum* may cross the placenta under their own power. Although many viruses can infect the fetus, the specific mechanisms through which they cross the placenta are unclear. Some viruses may be carried across via pinocytosis.[214]

UMBILICAL CORD

The umbilical cord normally contains two arteries and one vein surrounded by Wharton jelly, a substance containing collagen, muscle, and mucopolysaccharide. The cord epithelium is formed by amnion. No other blood vessels are found in the cord; neural tissue is also absent. The umbilical vessels are longer than the cord and tend to twist and spiral within the cord. The umbilical arteries contain four muscle layers: an inner circular layer, a longitudinal layer, and two helical layers. The helical layers function independently to coil both the arteries and the umbilical cord.[66] The twist or spiral of the cord is established by 9 weeks' gestational age. A left (counterclockwise) twist is more common than a right (clockwise) twist; however, bidirectional twisting is sometimes seen. The direction of the twist is not significant.[82,158] Vasoresponsiveness of the cord to stimuli or drugs is thought to be myogenic.[99]

The cord is usually inserted into the center of the placenta but may be attached at any point. Centric and eccentric insertion of the cord have no significance and reflect differences in the plane of implantation and placental growth.[84] However, velamentous and marginal insertion of the cord are abnormal. The cord arises from fusion of the connecting stalk with the yolk sac stalk and allantois at the end of the fourth week of gestation.[121] The umbilical vessels arise from the allantois and initially consist of four vessels. One of the two original umbilical veins invariably atrophies by 6 weeks after fertilization, followed by dilation of the remaining (left) vessel.[66] Occasionally the right umbilical artery also regresses or does not form, resulting in a two-vessel cord, which may be associated with other anomalies (see Abnormalities of the Cord and Placenta). The cord reaches its maximal length by 30 weeks and averages 55 to 60 cm (range, 40 to 70 cm) with a width of 2 to 2.5 cm.[84,158,187] Cord length is determined both genetically and by intrauterine space and fetal activity, which places tension on the cord.[187] The minimum cord length for vaginal delivery is 32 cm.[84,158] Occasionally the arteries may fuse near the placenta, so observation of the number of placental vessels should occur at least 3 cm from the placenta.[84,158]

The umbilical vessels constrict soon after delivery. Constriction of the umbilical arteries begins within 5 seconds of birth and is complete by 45 seconds; the umbilical vein begins to constrict within 15 seconds of delivery and is functionally closed by 3 to 4 minutes.[99] Placental transfu-sion and issues regarding timing of cord clamping are discussed in Chapter 7.

AMNION AND CHORION

The amnion and chorion begin to develop soon after fertilization and continue to grow until about 28 weeks' gestation. After this point, further mitotic activity is rare, and enlargement takes place by stretching of the existing membranes.[99] Development of the amnion and chorion is described in The Placenta and Placental Physiology.

The chorion or outer membrane contains blood vessels that atrophy as pregnancy advances, but no nerves. The blood vessels carry nutrients for the chorion that cross via diffusion to supply the amnion. The chorion is composed of 2 to 10 layers of polygonal cells and is up to 0.4 mm.[138] The amnion is a single-layer-thick (0.08 to 0.12 mm), avascular, and nerveless membrane with cuboidal and columnar cells. Its surface is strengthened by surface desmosomes and microvillar interdigitations that lie over a basement membrane with a collagenous extracellular matrix.[138]

The amnion and chorion are not fused and up to 200 ml of amniotic fluid may accumulate in the intermembrane space. The chorion is relatively fixed. The amnion is passively pushed against and moves over the chorion aided by mucus from the spongy layer. As a result, the amnion can rupture, forming shreds of tissue (amniotic bands), while chorion remains intact. The amniotic bands may wrap around, constrict, or amputate fetal parts. The reason for rupture of the amnion is unknown but may be related to trauma.[83]

The fetal membranes are metabolically active and are involved in amniotic fluid turnover and initiation of labor (see Chapter 4). The amnion is a reservoir for storage of arachidonic acid, an essential prostaglandin precursor, and the chorion is a reservoir for progesterone.[99] The membranes and decidua are rich sources of enzymes (e.g., phospholipase A_2) needed for formation of prostaglandins.[69] Cells of the amnion are involved in protein synthesis; protein and lipid secretion; and exchange of water, electrolytes, and other solutes. The amnion has a metabolic rate similar to that of the liver. The chorion synthesizes substances such as renin and prostaglandins.

The ability of the membranes to stretch and resist rupture from increasing fetal size and amniotic fluid volume until the end of pregnancy is thought to be related to the collagen-rich tissue of the amnion, which has great tensile strength that is maintained throughout gestation.[183] Rupture of the membranes during labor or with delivery is primarily due to hyperdistention with pressure of the presenting part along with increased hydrophobicity. This involves loss of phospholipids that normally lubricate the chorion-amnion interface, leading to increased shear force with cellular fracturing and rupture.[138] Premature rupture of the membranes (PROM), or rupture before onset of uterine contractions, may be due to factors such as mechanical stress (polyhydramnios, multiple gestation), alterations in membranous collagen, or chorioamnionitis. In chorioamnionitis a variety of vaginal and cervical microorganisms have been demonstrated to produce proteases that alter membrane integrity and reduce the pressure needed for rupture.[56] PROM may be mediated by collagenetic enzymes from the placenta and amniotic fluid that increase in activity with increasing gestational age.[138]

AMNIOTIC FLUID

Amniotic fluid provides space for symmetric fetal growth, maintains constant temperature and pressure, protects and cushions the fetus, allows free movement of the fetus, and distributes pressure from uterine contractions evenly over the fetus.[35,121] Amniotic fluid antibacterial factors, such as transferrin (which binds iron needed by some bacteria and fungi for growth), fatty acids (which have a detergent effect on bacterial membrane), immunoglobulins (e.g., IgG, IgA), and lysozyme (which is bactericidal for gram-positive bacteria), help protect the fetus from infection (see Chapter 12).[155]

Amniotic Fluid Volume and Turnover

The exact mechanisms for regulation of amniotic fluid volume are unclear, although the primary components of flow (fetal swallowing, urination, and lung fluid) are highly regulated.[23] Amniotic fluid first appears as a droplet dorsal to the embryonic pole at about 3 weeks.[20,121] There are approximately 7 ml of amniotic fluid by 8 weeks, 10 to 20 ml by 10 weeks, and 200 ml by 16 weeks.[23] Volume increases by about 50 ml/week to around 32 weeks, then remains stable at 700 to 800 ml until term, decreasing to about 400 ml by 42 weeks.[122] Amounts of amniotic fluid vary widely in the third trimester (Figure 3-23).[23,108] The net volume turnover of amniotic fluid is about 1000 ml/day.[23] Turnover rate is independent of volume.

Amniotic Fluid Production and Disposition

The cells of the amnion are separated by intracellular channels leading directly into the amniotic cavity that allow bulk flow of water and solutes. Transfer of water and most solutes across the amnion and chorion is governed by hydraulic, osmotic, and electrochemical forces. Water movement occurs as a result of a net imbalance between transmembrane hydrostatic pressure and effective osmotic pressure.[121] Some of the free water in amniotic fluid is thought to come from this transmembrane pathway. In the

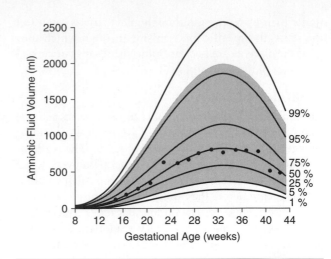

FIGURE **3-23** Amniotic fluid volumes as a function of gestational age in pregnancies with a normal fetus. Shaded area represents the 95% confidence interval. (From Brace, R.A. & Wolf, E.J. [1989]. Normal amniotic fluid volume changes throughout pregnancy. *Am J Obstet Gynecol, 161*, 382.)

last half of pregnancy, fetal urine output is the major source of amniotic fluid; the primary removal pathways are fetal swallowing and transmembranous movement. Major sources for amniotic fluid production and exchange include the following:

1. *Placenta, fetal membranes, and umbilical cord.* The fetal membranes are thought to be the second most important route of amniotic fluid clearance (after fetal swallowing) during the second half of gestation and account for an estimated 200 to 500 ml/day of amniotic fluid removal.[23,122] Water crosses the membranes by either nondiffusional fast bulk flow or slower diffusional flow. The net transfer of water is probably small except at the site of the placenta, where the chorioamniotic membrane is relatively close to maternal blood.[105] The umbilical cord arises from the same cell type as the amnion and is involved in fluid exchange after 4 weeks, with development of intracellular channels in cord membranes.

2. *Uterine wall via sinusoidal vessels of the decidua.* This is probably a minor pathway, with only small amounts (~10 ml/day) of fluid removed via this pathway near term.[23]

3. *Fetal skin.* Before complete keratinization of the fetal skin at 24 to 25 weeks (see Chapter 13), the skin is a site for transfer of water and solutes.

4. *Fetal gastrointestinal tract.* Fetal swallowing is a major route for disposal of amniotic fluid. The fetus swallows approximately 500 to 1000 ml/day late in pregnancy,

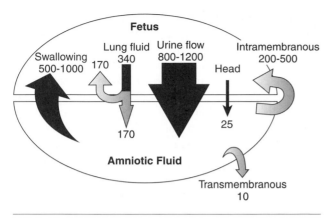

FIGURE **3-24** Summary of volume flows in and out of the amniotic space in late gestation. Arrow size is proportional to flow rate. (From Brace, R.A. [1997]. Physiology of amniotic fluid volume regulation. *Clin Obstet Gynecol, 40,* 286. Modified from original from Gilbert, W.M. & Brace, R.A. [1993]. Amniotic fluid volume and normal flows to and from the amniotic cavity. *Semin Perinatol, 17,* 150-157.)

or an amount equivalent to 20% to 25% of the fetal weight.[23,149]

5. *Fetal respiratory tract.* The fetal lung secretes 300 to 400 ml of fluid/day or an amount equivalent to 5% to 10% of the fetal weight.[23,105,122] Oral and nasal secretions may also contribute to amniotic fluid in a small way.[23]

6. *Fetal renal/urinary tract.* Hypotonic urine is present in the bladder by 11 weeks. The fetus produces 800 to 1200 ml/day or an amount equivalent to 30% of its weight in the third trimester.[23] After 40 weeks, fetal urine production declines.

These pathways are summarized in Figure 3-24. Amniotic fluid volume may also be influenced by other factors, including changes in tonicity of maternal serum and amniotic fluid prolactin, which seems to influence permeability of the amnion and chorion membranes.[122]

Composition of Amniotic Fluid

Amniotic fluid is 98% to 99% water, with the remainder consisting of electrolytes, creatinine, urea, bile pigments, renin, glucose, hormones, fetal cells, lanugo, and vernix caseosa. The composition of amniotic fluid changes with gestation. In early pregnancy, amniotic fluid is similar to maternal and fetal serum with little particulate matter. During the second half of gestation, amniotic fluid osmolality decreases to 92% of maternal serum values at term and is similar to dilute fetal urine with added phospholipids and other substances from the fetal lungs.[153] Urea, creatinine, and uric acid concentrations increase as preg-

nancy progresses; whereas sodium and chloride levels decrease as fetal renal function matures.[105,173,174]

CLINICAL IMPLICATIONS
Assisted Reproductive Technology

Issues surrounding conception relate to the ability of couples to conceive and maintain pregnancies until the fetus can survive outside the uterus. Infertility is the principal symptom of conception failure. Failure to conceive can result from disorders of ovulation, spermatogenesis, and gamete transport. Recent years have brought increased knowledge of these factors, with development of assisted reproductive technologies (ART) such as artificial insemination, therapeutic donor insemination, ovulation induction, microsurgery, laser surgery, in vitro fertilization (IVF), gamete intrafallopian transfer (GIFT), zygote intrafallopian transfer (ZIFT), intracytoplasmic sperm injection (ICSI), cryopreservation, frozen embryo transfer (FET), donation of eggs or preembryos, and surrogate mothering for couples having difficulty achieving conception.[171] Emotional, physical, and financial stress is high for these families.

The most common ART procedure used in the United States in 1998 was IVF (73.3%); GIFT (1.8%) and ZIFT (1.4%) were used significantly less frequently. The success rates for using fresh nondonor eggs or embryos was 30.5% (18.5% single fetus and 11.9% multiple fetus), with no pregnancy in 69.5%; the success rate for frozen embryos was 17% to 19%. The major reasons for ART in 1998 were tubal factors (26%), male factor infertility (27%), endometriosis (14.7%), and ovulatory dysfunction (12.4%).[30]

Artificial insemination with donor sperm has been used to treat infertility since the nineteenth century.[46] This therapy may be employed when azoospermia, oligospermia, decreased sperm motility, or other sperm abnormalities are present. When vasectomy is nonreversible or genetic disorders are possible, artificial insemination may be an option. Single women who desire a child may also opt to use this method in order to conceive. Candidates for insemination must ovulate regularly or respond to ovulation-inducing drug therapy. The techniques used include deposition of sperm into the upper vagina at the cervical os, or inside the cervical canal, or directly into the uterus. Reported success rates are 5% to 20% per month with 70% to 90% of couples conceiving within 6 months. Fresh semen is rarely used, because of concern over sexually transmitted diseases and HIV infection.

In vitro fertilization means fertilization that takes place outside the body in test tubes or in a Petri dish. The first infant conceived in this manner was born in 1978. Since that time, thousands of infants have been born utilizing this technique.[24] Originally, IVF was developed for women with blocked or absent fallopian tubes. This continues to be the main reason for use of IVF, but other indications include endometriosis unresponsive to conventional therapy, low sperm counts, immunologic disorders unresponsive to therapy, hostile cervical mucus or sperm antibodies, control of sex-linked disorders, and idiopathic infertility.

The procedure is done in four stages: ovulation induction and monitoring, follicular aspiration, fertilization, and embryo transfer. The goal of ovulation induction is recruitment of a large number of follicles to increase the number of embryos that can be transferred and thus the percentage of successful pregnancies per IVF cycle. Drugs given on day 2 or 3 of the menstrual cycle induce maturation of more than one follicle. The maturing ova are monitored and, once adequate follicular size is achieved or preovulatory estradiol levels are appropriate, follicular aspiration can occur.[29,121]

The woman is given hCG to enhance the final stages of follicular maturation and to control timing of ovulation. After follicle aspiration and processing of the semen sample from the father, the ova are identified, placed in a special nutrient culture medium and incubated at body temperature. Capacitated sperm are then mixed with the ova, and the mixture is incubated again for 48 to 72 hours to allow for fertilization and adequate early cell division.[24] Approximately 50,000 to 200,000 sperm are needed, and at least 100,000 sperm per oocyte are preferred.

Embryo transfer generally occurs when the zygote has reached a 2- to 8-cell stage (after 35 to 60 hours), with timing varying between different centers. The zygotes are injected via a catheter into the cervix. Up to four zygotes are usually transferred to increase the likelihood of pregnancy. Progesterone by injection is begun on the day of transfer and is continued for 2 weeks to support the corpus luteum. A serum β-hCG assay is done at 2 weeks to determine if implantation has occurred. Progesterone supplements are continued for up to 10 weeks if implantation has taken place. Unused zygotes may be frozen and stored.[24]

GIFT is the process of transferring eggs and sperm directly into the fallopian tube via a fine catheter. This therapy was developed for use in infertile couples when there was doubt that the gametes would be able to reach the fallopian tubes or when male factor or idiopathic infertility existed.[24,121] Women must have at least one healthy patent fallopian tube in order to qualify for this treatment modality. The three stages of GIFT are induction, oocyte retrieval, and gamete transfer to fallopian tubes. Ovarian induction is the same as in IVF. Oocyte retrieval is by laparotomy or transvaginal using ultrasonographic techniques. The ova are mixed with capacitated sperm, and the mixture is trans-

ferred to the fallopian tubes. Fertilization takes place within the natural environment and successive events progress normally.

The process for ZIFT is similar to IVF, but after fertilization the zygote is returned to the fallopian tube without further incubation. As with GIFT, women must have one patent fallopian tube. Procedures used in conjunction with other ARTs include use of donor oocytes, assisted hatching (creation of an opening in the ZP to assist with implantation) and ICSI.[37,171] ICSI is used with about one third of IVF and ZIFT and involves injecting the sperm into the ova.[30] ICSI can be used for males who have had vasectomies, who have severe sperm abnormalities, or who are unable to ejaculate.

Critical Periods of Development and Birth Defects

Growth and development in the uterus is usually a peaceful yet richly stimulating experience. Early on, the infant develops morphologic characteristics upon which functional and neurobehavioral characteristics develop later in gestation and after birth. Embryonic and fetal development can be altered by a variety of internal and external events and teratogens, which result in structural and functional defects. Fetal defects can result from malformation, deformation, or disruption. A malformation is an embryonic alteration in morphogenesis due to an intrinsically abnormal developmental process such as may occur with a chromosome or multifactorial disorder (Chapter 1).[81] Deformation defects are the abnormal form, shape, or position of a body part arising from extrinsic mechanical forces (e.g., clubfoot due to fetal restraint or lung hypoplasia due to congenital diaphragmatic hernia); a disruption is caused by an external force that alters a previously normal tissue (e.g., teratogenic effects or amputation of a fetal part by an amniotic band).[81] Teratogenesis is discussed in Chapter 6. Birth defects may be major or minor abnormalities. Minor abnormalities may be normal variations, family traits, or isolated defects or may provide clues to the presence of internal malformations, genetic disorders, or chromosomal problems. Three or more minor abnormalities are associated with an increased risk for a major birth defect.[18,81,100] Causes of birth defects are listed in Table 3-6.

The most likely period for structural defects to occur is during organogenesis, since exposure of the embryo to a teratogenic agent either during or before a critical stage in development of that organ can lead to anomalies.[29,121] The time of greatest susceptibility during development is defined as the time when the highest incidence of defects occurs (usually gross anatomic defects). Other defects, especially functional defects, have peaks in sensitivity at different times during development. These periods of sen-

TABLE **3-6** **Causes of Congenital Anomalies**

Cause	Percentage
Chromosomal abnormalities	6-7
Gene abnormalities	7-8
Environmental agents	7-10
Multifactorial inheritance	20-25
Unknown etiology	50-60

Data from Moore, K.L. & Persaud, T.V.N. (1998). *The developing human: Clinically oriented embryology* (6th ed.). Philadelphia: W.B. Saunders.

sitivity vary depending on the timing and duration of the period of cell proliferation (e.g., brain growth and development extend into early childhood and thus are vulnerable for a longer period of time).[121,179]

Before conception, damage can occur to the chromosomes of one or both parents, or they may have inherited defective genes from their parents. Alterations in spermatogenesis; in seminal fluid or sperm transport in the male; or in oogenesis or the environment of the vagina, cervix, or uterus of the female may also alter development.

The preembryonic stage (up to 14 days) is a time of little morphologic differentiation. During the first part of this period, the zygote is protected by the ZP. Exposure to teratogens during this period usually has an all-or-nothing effect; that is, either the damage is so severe that the zygote is aborted or there are no apparent effects. However, this may also be the time that syndromes affecting multiple organ systems arise. Teratogens or environmental disturbances may interfere with implantation of the blastocyst or cause death and early abortion. However, most congenital anomalies probably do not arise during this period, probably due to the lack of differentiation, at least in the early part of this period. Many cells within the inner cell mass are not yet programmed to become specific structures. Thus damage to a few cells does not alter development if the preembryo is able to produce sufficient cells to restore the volume.[179] If a teratogen is potent or the dosage is high, the effect is death or possibly mitotic disjunction during cleavage, with chromosomal alterations that subsequently cause malformation syndromes rather than local defects.[81] If only a few cells are damaged, development continues, although the schedule programmed by genetic material may be delayed.[179]

The period of organogenesis (15 to 60 days after conception) is a period of extreme sensitivity to teratogens and the period when most congenital malformations de-

velop. Insults early in this period (15 to 30 days) are likely to result in death if the embryo is damaged. Early events in organ formation are generally most sensitive to extraneous forces, although, in some systems (e.g., sensory organs), critical periods occur during relatively late stages. The more specialized the metabolic requirements of a group of cells, the more sensitive they are to deprivation and damage; therefore, they are more likely to experience malformation.[121,179]

From 11 weeks to term, the fetus becomes increasingly resistant to damage from toxic agents. The ability to produce major structural deviations is reduced as organ systems become organized. Once the definitive form and relationships within a system are established, gross anatomic defects are no longer possible. However, the functional role of the organ system can still be altered.[121,179] Histogenesis of most systems continues postnatally until complete maturation of that system is achieved. Therefore defects can occur at the microscopic level, or functional abilities can be altered, resulting in physiologic defects and delayed growth. Insults during late fetal life and early infancy can lead to dysfunction such as brain damage or deafness, prematurity, growth restriction, stillbirth, infant death, or malignancy.

Transfer of Substances across the Placenta

Dancis offers the following guidelines for thinking of placental transfer: "Ask not whether a maternal nutrient crosses the placenta. Ask rather, how, how much, and how fast. Ask also as to fetal need."[36] There are few compounds—endogenous or exogenous—that are unable to cross the placenta in detectable amounts given sufficient time and sensitivity of detection.[36] Placental transfer is influenced by the area of the placenta, physicochemical characteristics of the diffusing substance, concentration gradients, electrical potential differences, diffusing distance, degree of binding of a substance to hemoglobin or other blood proteins, permeability of the placental barrier, and the rates of maternal and fetal blood flow through the intervillous space and villi (see Table 6-5).[48,111,125]

Diffusion of a substance across the placenta can be expressed as follows:

$$\text{Diffusion} = \frac{\text{Substance characteristics} \times \text{Surface area} \times \text{Concentration gradient}}{\text{Distance}}$$

Increased surface area for exchange (as occurs with growth of the placenta along with the fetus), increased concentration gradient, and decreased diffusing distance enhance transfer across the placenta. As the placenta matures, the distance between maternal and fetal blood decreases due to thinning of the syncytial trophoblast and connective tissue as well as increases in the size and number of capillaries in the villi. Transfer may be reduced with decreased surface area (e.g., small placenta, placental infarcts) or increased diffusing distance (e.g., placental edema, infection).

Physicochemical characteristics that influence movement across the placenta include lipid solubility, MW, degree of ionization, and protein binding. These characteristics can increase, decrease, or prohibit movement of potentially harmful drugs and other substances from maternal-to-fetal circulation (see Chapter 6).[35,48,111] Placental transfer may be increased or enhanced if a substance is lipid soluble (e.g., lipoproteins) or nonionized (e.g., phenobarbital), has an MW less than 600 (e.g., propylthiouracil), or lacks significant binding to albumin (e.g., ampicillin). Increased maternal-to-fetal concentration or electrochemical gradients also increase transfer. A substance may be prevented from crossing the placenta because it has a certain charge or molecular configuration (e.g., heparin) or certain size (e.g., bacteria, IgM), is altered or bound by enzymes within the placenta (e.g., amines, insulin), or is firmly bound to the maternal red blood cell or plasma protein (e.g., carbon monoxide).[48,50,111,125]

The rate of maternal blood flow to and through the IVS and fetal blood flow to and through the villi influence placental transfer. Blood flow is the limiting factor in gas exchange across the placenta but also affects transfer of nutrients and waste products. During uterine contractions the entry of blood into the IVS is limited. Transfer of oxygen and other nutrients to the fetus may decrease but does not cease during contractions.[48,50,125] The decrease in afferent blood flow during a contraction may be due to: (1) compression and obliteration of the uteroplacental veins with increased IVS pressure, (2) occlusion of the uteroplacental arteries, or (3) increased intraluminal pressure within the uterus with alteration in the arteriovenous pressure gradients within the IVS.[3]

The fetus may become hypoxic and acidotic if contractions are hypertonic or if resting time between contractions is insufficient. If placental transfer is compromised by small placental size, infarcts, or edema, fetal distress may arise at lower levels of uterine activity. Because the quantity of oxygen reaching the fetus is primarily flow limited, reduction of uteroplacental blood flow increases the risk of fetal hypoxia.

In addition to uterine contractions, factors that may alter uteroplacental blood flow include maternal position; anesthesia; nicotine and other drugs; emotional or physical stress; and degenerative changes within the placenta that are seen with hypertension, prolonged pregnancy, diabetes,

or renal disease.[111,125] Maternal blood flow to and through the IVS can be altered by: (1) changes in the systemic circulation (cardiac disease, small uterine artery); (2) changes in the number or size of the uteroplacental blood vessels (infection, degeneration); (3) compression of the uteroplacental blood vessels (tetanic or other abnormal contractions, polyhydramnios, multiple pregnancy); and (4) degenerative changes in the IVS associated with high-risk conditions such as maternal hypertension.[48]

Assessment of Fetal Status and Placental Function

Assessment of placental function and analysis of the constituents of amniotic fluid are useful in evaluating the growth and health of the fetus and the ability of the fetus to withstand the stresses of labor and delivery. New techniques have improved monitoring of fetal and placental status with high-risk pregnancies. Techniques for evaluation of placental function consist of biochemical monitoring of the fetoplacental unit, antepartum fetal heart rate surveillance, fetal blood gas monitoring, and the biophysical profile (see Chapter 9). Amniocentesis and chorionic villus sampling allow for prenatal diagnosis of increasing numbers of chromosomal, genetic, and other congenital anomalies. These techniques and percutaneous umbilical blood sampling, which can be used for both prenatal diagnosis and therapy, are discussed (along with ultrasound) in Chapter 1. Ultrasound can be used to detect birth defects and to monitor fetal growth and well-being.

Cellular and biochemical components of amniotic fluid change with gestational age and are useful indicators of fetal maturity and well-being. Amniotic fluid samples are removed via amniocentesis, and the constituents are examined. Amniotic fluid contains cells from the amnion, fetal skin, buccal and bladder mucosa, and tracheal lining. Amniotic fluid cells can be examined early in pregnancy to determine fetal sex (important with sex-linked disorders) and to diagnose genetic and chromosomal disorders. Later, cellular and biochemical components of amniotic fluid can be used to evaluate fetal health and maturity. The most common parameter assessed is fetal lung maturity (see Chapter 9) in women with preterm labor.

Alterations in Placenta, Umbilical Cord, and Amniotic Fluid

An intact and adequately functioning placenta and amniotic fluid are critical for fetal survival and well-being. Without the placenta the fetus could not survive, because it would have no alternatives for essential processes such as respiratory gas exchange and nutrition. This section discusses the roles of the placenta and amniotic fluid in low-

and high-risk pregnancies, the implications for the fetus and neonate from placental dysfunction and alterations in amniotic fluid volume, and the bases for common cord and placental abnormalities.

Alterations in the Appearance of the Placenta and Membranes

The appearance of the placenta (color, size, consistency) often provides clues to maternal or placental dysfunction or pathologic processes in the fetus. The color of the placenta is determined by fetal hemoglobin. The placenta is paler in immature infants and congested in infants of diabetic mothers. Pale placentas suggest fetal anemia. Edematous, pale, and bulky placentas are seen with immune and nonimmune hydrops fetalis, twin-to-twin transfusion syndrome (donor twin), fetal congestive heart failure, and infection.[133,143,177,181] These placentas may also contain more Hofbauer cells, an immature trophoblast layer, and other changes similar to those seen with hypoxia. Placentas less than 2 to 2.5 cm thick are often seen with IUGR; those more than 4 cm thick are seen with diabetes mellitus and fetal hydrops.[182]

The placenta responds to hypoxia and ischemia with formation of excessive syncytial knots, proliferation of villous cytotrophoblast (Langhans) cells, nucleated erythrocytes, fibrinoid necrosis of the villi, increased perivillous fibrin, and thickening of the trophoblast basement membrane.[7,8,50,84,143,177] The placentas from women with preeclampsia often have infarcts, hematomas, and characteristic histologic changes such as excessive proliferation of cytotrophoblast tissue within the villi and fibrin deposits.[83,112,177] Infarctions are seen in placentas of infants with IUGR whose placentas are also small and in placentas from women with elevated (more than 13 g/dl) hematocrits in the second half of pregnancy.[129] In this latter group the infarctions may be due to increased blood viscosity and thrombosis. Placentas of women who smoke demonstrate characteristic changes, including increased thickness of the villous membrane that may reduce efficiency of diffusion.[112]

Thrombi in the veins along the chorionic plate appear as yellow streaks on the surface of the placenta. These thrombi may embolize and are associated with velamentous insertion of the cord. Infarctions are often seen near the margins of the placenta; central infarctions are less common and more serious, since they may disrupt IVS circulation. Infarctions are areas of ischemic necrosis of primary villi resulting from obstruction of IVS blood flow due to thrombi or marked impairment of blood flow in the spiral arteries.[50,177] Initially these infarcted areas are red, later turning brown, gray, and then white with fibrin deposition;

they may be covered with necrotic decidua. Hematomas and thrombi may be seen in the IVS.[84,177] Infarctions may be a way the fetus responds to villi that have inadequate maternal perfusion; that is, the flow of blood to the affected villus is reduced so blood normally flowing to that villus can be redistributed to areas where maternal circulation is adequate.[177]

Multiple plaques or nodules on the fetal surface of the placenta are found with amnion nodosum (associated with oligohydramnios and renal agenesis), squamous metaplasia (benign disorder), and infection.[10,84,177] With chorioamnionitis the placenta often has an opaque surface and may be foul smelling. Infection with *Candida albicans* is associated with white or yellow nodules on the placental surface.[177]

Meconium staining of the membranes occurs in 0.5% to 29% of pregnancies.[3] Because meconium is not discharged until after fetal gastrointestinal peptides (e.g., motilin) have reached critical levels, meconium passage is infrequent in preterm infants and common in postmature infants. Green membranes are not necessarily due to meconium, since accumulations of hemosiderin (as may occur with hemolysis and circumvallation) also stain the membranes green.[143] Green pigment can be found in amniotic macrophages an hour after meconium is discharged and in chorionic macrophage by 2 to 3 hours.[7,8] With extended exposure to meconium, extraplacental membranes become edematous and the membranes and placenta become tan-green or brown.[7]

Alterations in Amniotic Fluid Volume

An understanding of the processes involved in the production of amniotic fluid and the pattern of fluid accumulation during pregnancy is necessary for assessing uterine growth and identifying women who need further evaluation. Alterations in production and removal of amniotic fluid can lead to polyhydramnios (hydramnios) or oligohydramnios.

Polyhydramnios. Polyhydramnios (also called hydramnios), has traditionally been defined as accumulation of more than 2 L of fluid in a single amniotic sac. More recently the amniotic fluid index (AFI) based on the largest amniotic fluid pocket seen on ultrasound has been used.[67,108] Polyhydramnios has an overall incidence of 0.93%.[67] It can occur gradually during pregnancy or rapidly over a few days or weeks. Polyhydramnios is idiopathic in 60% of women but is also associated with maternal disease; multiple gestation; immune and nonimmune hydrops fetalis; Down syndrome and other chromosomal anomalies; and fetal gastrointestinal, cardiac, and neural tube anomalies.[20,28,120] However, women with any of these complications can also have normal amniotic fluid volume.[149] Idiopathic or essential polyhydramnios (i.e., due to no known cause) is thought to arise from an unexplained imbalance in water exchange between the fetus, mother, and amniotic fluid.[174]

Although multiple pregnancy frequently results in increased accumulation of amniotic fluid, in most cases this is not true polyhydramnios, since the fluid is distributed among several sacs, each sac containing usual amounts of fluid. An increased incidence of polyhydramnios has been reported in monozygotic (MZ) monochorionic twins with arteriovenous anastomoses within their shared placenta and twin-to-twin transfusion syndrome. Development of polyhydramnios in these pregnancies may be the result of excessive urination, polycythemia, and transudation of fluids.[13,174] The elevated venous pressure and altered fluid dynamics seen with hydrops fetalis and some cardiovascular disorders may lead to excessive accumulation of amniotic fluid. Polyhydramnios is more frequent in diabetic women, perhaps because of fetal polyuria caused by fetal hyperglycemia or because of alterations in osmotic gradients as a result of increased amniotic fluid glucose.[28]

Congenital anomalies are reported in 12% to 19% of pregnancies complicated by polyhydramnios.[120] Neural tube defects, particularly anencephaly, may result in polyhydramnios as a result of decreased fetal swallowing or transudation of fluid from the exposed meninges.[120] Polyhydramnios associated with chromosomal anomalies may be related to reduced fetal swallowing and, in some infants with Down syndrome, duodenal atresia. Although polyhydramnios is seen in many infants with esophageal or duodenal atresia (presumably due to decreased fetal swallowing and decreased gut absorption), these pregnancies may also have normal amniotic fluid volumes.[149] The basis for this finding is unclear but suggests that amniotic fluid homeostasis is a very complex mechanism involving the interaction of many variables.

Treatment options include fetal therapy (e.g., if the cause is due to fetal hydrops or arrhythmias); serial amniocenteses; and administration of prostaglandin synthetase inhibitors such as indomethacin. Indomethacin is thought to work by increasing fluid reabsorption by the fetal lungs, decreasing fetal urine production, and increasing fluid movement across the membranes to the mother.[120] Indomethacin has potential maternal and fetal side effects.

Oligohydramnios. Oligohydramnios (less than 500 ml at term or less than 50% of the usual accumulation of amniotic fluid at any stage of development) can occur at any time during gestation. Oligohydramnios is rarer than polyhydramnios and is associated with amnion abnormalities, placental insufficiency, and fetal urinary anomalies.[25,122,165]

Oligohydramnios may lead to umbilical cord compression in labor and fetal distress.

Inadequate amniotic fluid during labor can be due to premature rupture of the membranes, oligohydramnios, or early amniotomy.[89] A lack of adequate fluid removes the natural protective cushioning effect of this fluid and increases the risk of cord compression and variable fetal heart rate decelerations during contractions. These decelerations can sometimes be relieved by maternal position, intravenous hydration change and oxygen administration, or by increasing amniotic fluid volume through intrauterine infusion of a saline solution (amnioinfusion).[89,90,170]

Severe fetal renal anomalies (agenesis, dysplasia, or obstructive disorders) may lead to oligohydramnios because of decreased or no urine output. Bilateral renal agenesis in conjunction with pulmonary hypoplasia, musculoskeletal abnormalities, and a characteristic facies is known as Potter syndrome and is associated with oligohydramnios. Several of the findings in Potter syndrome may be deformation defects arising from lack of amniotic fluid.[81]

Movement produced by fetal muscular activity is an integral component of normal morphologic development. Mechanical forces can lead to defects either from intrinsic forces (such as fetal myoneuropathy, development of an organ in an abnormal and excessively small site, or alterations in the normal flow or volume of body fluids) or from external forces (such as a bicornate uterus, fibromas, or oligohydramnios) that interfere with fetal mobility.[118]

The constraints on fetal movement imposed by oligohydramnios can result in a cascade of developmental events resulting in fetal anomalies. These anomalies include congenital contracture (due to relative or complete immobilization of the joints in a confined space); lung hypoplasia (lack of room for development of the thorax and for the subsequent stretch or distention of lung tissue required for normal lung growth); shortened umbilical cord (length is related to fetal activity); dysmorphic facies including micrognathia, low-set ears, small alae nasi, and hypertelorism (molding of the face by compressive forces); growth restriction (fetal motor activity seems important for normal development of muscle mass and weight gain); perhaps microgastria (lack of stretching and distention because the volume of amniotic fluid available for swallowing is reduced); and "loose" skin (stretched by the constrained fetus's attempts to move).[117,119] This sequence has been termed the *fetal akinesia/hypokinesia deformation sequence* (Figure 3-25).[118]

Oligohydramnios is often associated with amnion nodosum. In this disorder, yellow-gray nodules or plaques consisting of desquamated fetal epidermal cells, hair, and vernix

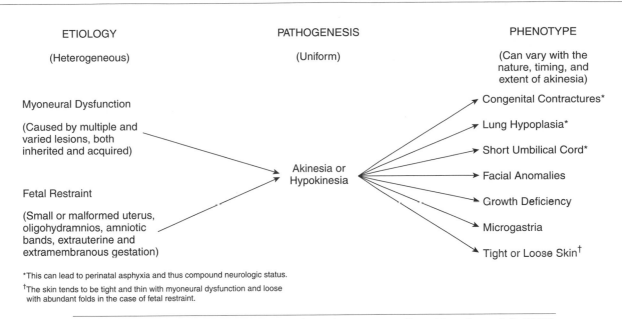

FIGURE **3-25** The fetal akinesia/hypokinesia deformation sequence. (From Moessinger, A.C. [1989]. Morphological consequences of depressed or impaired fetal activity. In W.P. Smotherman & S.R. Robinson [Eds.]. *Behavior of the fetus*. Caldwell, NJ: Telford Press.)

are found in and on the amnion and on the placental surface (fetal side). This debris is probably pressed into the amnion by close approximation of the fetal skin and amnion in the presence of oligohydramnios.[174] Oligohydramnios may also occur with IUGR (as a result of decreased urine flow rates) or with prolonged pregnancy.

Abnormalities of the Cord and Placenta

Abnormalities of the cord and placenta arise from alterations in implantation and placentation or from disorders of the trophoblast. Occasionally these abnormalities may have minimal effect on the fetus and the outcome of the pregnancy; more often, serious and sometimes fatal conditions develop so that the pregnancy cannot be maintained and is terminated early or fetal development and survival are threatened. At times, maternal survival and reproductive function may also be compromised.

Abnormalities of implantation and separation. The major abnormalities of implantation and separation of the placenta are placenta previa, abruptio placentae, and placenta accreta. Placenta previa is implantation of the placenta over or near the internal cervical os so that it encroaches on a portion of the dilated cervix. Placenta previa may be classified as total, partial, or marginal; low-lying placentas are sometimes included in this classification. Various theories have been proposed to explain the pathogenesis of placenta previa, including defective vascularization of the endometrium, alteration of the normal ovum

transport mechanism, and development of the placenta in the decidua capsularis.[35,50]

If the blastocyst implants in endometrium that is poorly vascularized due to atrophic or inflammatory changes, the placenta may develop a larger decidual surface area to compensate for an inadequate blood supply and grow downward into the lower uterine segment.[35] If vascularization of the endometrium in the upper uterine segment is poor, the blastocyst may continue to descend, implanting by chance in healthier endometrium in the lower uterine segment. Altered transport of the blastocyst due to abnormal uterine motility, deviations in the size or shape of the uterine cavity, or fluid in the cavity can also result in displacement of the blastocyst to the lower uterus.[35] A scar from a previous cesarean section also predisposes to later placental previa.[128]

Normally the chorionic villi initially surround the entire embryo but later degenerate beneath the decidua capsularis, forming the chorion laeve. By 4 months, the growing fetus fills the uterine cavity and the decidua capsularis fuses with the decidua vera (see Figure 3-11). If chorionic villi near the lower uterus fail to degenerate as the decidua capsularis fuses with the decidua vera, these villi can become incorporated into the placenta and impinge on the lower uterine segment.[35,50]

Abruptio placentae is separation of a normally implanted placenta before the delivery of the fetus. Abruptio placentae is initiated by hemorrhage into the decidua basalis with formation of a hematoma that leads to separation and compression of the adjacent portion of the placenta. Hemorrhage may develop secondary to degenerative changes in the arteries supplying the intervillous space and with thrombosis, degeneration of the decidua, and vessel rupture with formation of a retroplacental hemorrhage.[50] Possible causes include maternal hypertension (secondary to essential hypertension, preeclampsia, chronic renal disease, or cocaine use), compression or occlusion of the inferior vena cava, circumvallate placenta, or trauma.[35,50] The incidence of abruptio placentae is markedly increased with maternal cocaine and crack use. These drugs induce vasoconstriction of placental blood vessels and a sudden elevation in maternal blood pressure.

Placenta accreta is a general term used to describe any placental implantation in which there is abnormally firm adherence of the placenta to the uterine wall. As a result, there is partial or total absence of the decidua basalis and attachment of the placental villi to the fibrinoid (Nitabuch) layer or to the myometrium. Occasionally the villi invade the myometrium (placenta increta) or penetrate through the myometrial wall (placenta percreta). Placenta accreta usually occurs when decidual formation is defective, such as with implantation over uterine scars or in the lower uterine segment. Placenta accreta is often associated with placenta previa and with significant morbidity including severe hemorrhage, uterine perforation, infection, and hysterectomy.[35,50]

Abnormalities of placentation. The size and configuration of the placenta are influenced by the degree of vascularization of the decidua and the number and arrangement of the primitive villi that later comprise the fetal portion of the placenta.[35] The major clinically significant abnormalities of placental configuration result in circumvallate, marginate, or succenturiate placentas.

With circumvallate placenta, the area of the chorionic plate is reduced. As chorionic villi invade the decidua, the fetal membranes fold back upon themselves, creating a dense, grayish-white raised ring encircling the central portion of the fetal surface (Figure 3-26). The fetal vessels forming the cord stop at this ring rather than covering the entire fetal surface of the placenta. The risk of abruptio placenta is increased with circumvallate placentas. Marginate (or circummarginate) placenta also arises from a chorionic plate that is smaller than the basal plate. In these placentas the white ring composed of the fetal membranes coincides with the margin of the placenta, without the folding back of the membranes seen in circumvallate placentas.[50]

The etiology of circumvallate and marginate placentas is uncertain, although partial or complete forms are seen in up to 25% of gestations.[84,177] Possible causes include sub-

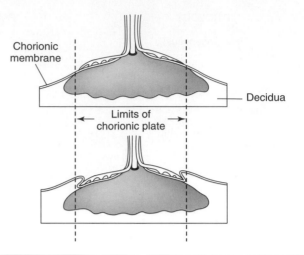

FIGURE **3-26** Diagrammatic representation of a circummarginate placenta *(top)* and a circumvallate placenta *(bottom)* (From Fox, H. (1997). *Pathology of the placenta* [2nd ed.]. Philadelphia: W.B. Saunders.)

chorial infarcts, formation of insufficient chorion frondosum, and an abnormally deep implantation of the blastocyst causing part of the fetal surface to be covered by the decidua vera. These placentas are often asymptomatic, but circumvallate placentas have been linked to threatened abortion, preterm labor, painless vaginal bleeding after 20 weeks, placental insufficiency, and intrapartum and postpartum hemorrhage.[7,35,50,84,177,182]

Succenturiate placenta involves development of one or more smaller accessory lobes in the membranes that are attached to the main placenta by fetal vessels. This abnormality arises when a group of villi distant to the main placenta fail to degenerate, implantation is superficial, or implantation occurs in a confined site (e.g., a bicornate uterus) so that attachment of the trophoblast also occurs on the opposing wall.[35,50,182] The accessory lobes may be retained, leading to postpartum hemorrhage or infection.[84,182] These placentas are often associated with malrotation of the implanting blastocyst with velamentous insertion of the cord.[35]

Abnormalities of the umbilical cord. The umbilical cord may develop knots, loops, torsion, or strictures. These alterations are associated with increased fetal mortality and morbidity.[50,99] Excessively long cords (more than 75 to 100 cm) are more likely to develop knots, torsion, or prolapse. Excessively long cords are associated with increased fetal activity.[182] Abnormally short cords (less than 30 to 32 cm) are associated with asphyxia at birth as a result of traction on the cord with fetal descent.[35,158] Abnormally short cords are also associated with decreased fetal activity because tension on the cord promotes growth. Decreased fetal activity is seen with Down syndrome, neuromuscular disorders, and fetal malformations.[182] A single umbilical artery occurs in 1% of newborns and probably arises from agenesis or degeneration of the missing vessel early in gestation. This anomaly is associated with an increased incidence (up to 50%) of fetal cardiovascular, gastrointestinal, or genitourinary anomalies.[103,158]

Battledore placenta, or insertion of the cord at or within 1.5 cm of the margin of the placenta (seen in 7% of placentas), may be clinically benign but has been linked to preterm labor, fetal distress, and bleeding in labor due to cord compression or vessel rupture.[158] With velamentous insertion (1% of placentas), the cord inserts into the membranes so that the vessels run between the amnion and chorion before entering into the placenta. These variations in insertion of the cord probably arise at the time of implantation.

Normally the blastocyst implants with the inner cell mass adjacent to the endometrium and the trophoblast that will form the placenta. The body stalk, which will become the cord, aligns with the center of the placenta. Rotation of the inner cell mass (and body stalk) gives rise to eccentric insertions of the cord. The degree of rotation will influence how far the umbilical cord will be from the center of the placenta (i.e., eccentric, marginal, velamentous). Velamentous insertion may lead to rupture and fetal hemorrhage associated with a high fetal mortality, particularly with vasa praevia (when the fetal vessels are located along the lower uterine segment, crossing the internal cervical os, and presenting ahead of the fetus).[35,177]

Gestational Trophoblastic Disease

Gestational trophoblastic disease includes hydatidiform mole and gestational trophoblastic tumors (derived from neoplastic hyperplastic changes).[116] Both forms of trophoblastic disease are associated with markedly elevated levels of hCG.[68] Hydatidiform moles result from deterioration of the chorionic villi into a mass of clear vesicles. Histologically, hydatidiform mole is characterized by hyperplasia of the syncytiotrophoblast and the cytotrophoblast, edema of the avascular villous stroma, and cystic cavitations within the villous stroma. The villi become converted into molar cysts connected to each other by fibrous strands.[35] There may be no fetus (complete mole) or the remains of a degenerating fetus or amniotic sac (partial or incomplete mole). Rarely the fetus in an incomplete molar pregnancy survives to delivery.[116]

The karyotype of a complete mole is 46,XX and is thought to be derived from duplication of a haploid X-carrying (23,X) sperm (85% of cases) or from fertiliza-tion of the ovum by two sperm X-carrying with failure of the maternal genome to participate in development (1% of cases).[29,50,156] Thus the mole is androgenic in origin; that is, the ovum develops under the influence of a spermatozoon nucleus. The nucleus of the ovum is inactivated or lost before fertilization. A complete mole is associated with increased risk of choriocarcinoma.

In an incomplete mole the hydatidiform changes are focal; that is, there is slowly progressive swelling of some villi (which are usually avascular), whereas other vascular villi develop with a functioning fetoplacental circulation.[35] The karyotype of this type of mole is usually triploid (69,XXX; 69,XXY; or 69,XYY). An incomplete mole results from fertilization of a normal haploid ovum (23,X) by two haploid sperm (dispermy) or a single diploid sperm.[50,116] A third type involves heterozygous diploid fertilization of an empty ovum with two haploid sperm (46,XX or 46,XY). This form of mole is associated with an increased risk of gestational trophoblastic tumors.[116]

Multiple Pregnancy

The incidence of twins in the United States is 10 in 1000 deliveries, with other forms of multiple births seen less frequently.[70] The arrangement of membranes and placentas in twin and other multiple pregnancies is determined by the type of twin and the stage of gestation at which twinning occurs. The incidence of twin conceptions is greater than that of twin births. Ultrasound studies indicate that 12% of pregnancies begin as twins, with up to 70% converted to singleton pregnancies by the asymptomatic loss of one embryo.[50]

There are basically two types of twins: MZ (arising from division of a single ovum after fertilization) and dizygotic (DZ) (simultaneous fertilization of two ova enclosed within a single follicle or theca, or ovulation of two ova from one or both ovaries that are then fertilized independently). Most (70%) twins are DZ. A third type of twinning, which has been identified by DNA analysis, arises due to simultaneous fertilization of an ovum and the first polar body by two sperm. Its frequency is unknown, but it is thought to be rare.[12,107] This section focuses on twins, because higher-order multiple pregnancies (triplets, quadruplets, etc.) can be MZ, DZ, or multizygotic, with attributes that are variations of findings characteristic of twins.

Twin zygosity cannot be determined solely on the number of placentas. Two types of placentas are seen: monochorionic, which occurs with MZ twins, and dichorionic, which may occur with either MZ or DZ twins. Dichorionic placentas may be separate or fused. Examinations to determine zygosity often require morphologic examination of the chorion, amnion, and yolk sac as well as DNA analysis.

Placentas and membranes of twins and other multiple births should always be saved and sent to pathologic examination for accurate morphologic analysis and placental DNA for restriction fragment length polymorphism (RFLP) analysis.[15]

MZ twins may have one or two placentas (which may be separate or fused). The placentas and membranes of MZ twins may be monochorionic-monoamniotic, monochorionic-diamniotic, or dichorionic-diamniotic (fused or separate). About 70% of MZ twins are monochorionic and 30% are dichorionic.[37] With higher-order multiple births, placentas and membranes may also be multichorionic-multiamniotic. Although DZ twins always have two dichorionic-diamniotic placentas, the placentas may be fused and appear to be single. Fused placentas increase the risk of growth restriction in one or both infants as a result of competition for space and abnormal cord insertions.[14] About 80% of twins can be differentiated according to zygosity (i.e., as MZ or DZ) at or shortly after birth as follows (percentages are approximate): (1) 23% are monochorionic, and therefore the infants are MZ; (2) 30% are dichorionic with a male and female twin who must therefore be DZ; and (3) 27% are same-sex twins but with different blood types and thus DZ.[139] The remaining 20% are same-sex twins with similar blood types who are either MZ twins with dichorionic placentas (either separate or fused) or DZ twins of the same sex (with separate or fused placentas). Determination of the zygosity of these twins requires more intensive investigation such as tissue typing, enzymatic studies, dermatoglyphics, or DNA mapping.

Perinatal mortality is 3 to 11 times higher in twins than in singletons.[70] This risk is affected by zygosity and placental and membrane characteristics.[113] For example, mortality is two to three times higher in monochorionic twins than in dichorionic (either DZ or MZ) twins.[54,113] Monochorionic twins tend to weigh less and are more frequently growth restricted in utero than are dichorionic twins.[45] The incidence of congenital anomalies is higher in MZ twins than in DZ twins.[38,168] Structural defects in MZ twins may arise from deformations due to limited intrauterine space, disruption of blood flow due to placental vascular anastomoses, or localized defects in early morphogenesis.[113,154]

Monozygotic Twins

MZ twins occur in 3.5 to 4 in 1000 births.[48] The rate of MZ twinning is relatively constant worldwide and probably represents an accident in embryonic development. The etiology of this form of twins is unknown, although it has been proposed that MZ embryos arise from a delay in implantation secondary to adverse environmental conditions such as inadequate nutrition or oxygen deprivation or to formation of two cell lines from early mosaicism (see Chapter 1) that trigger separation.[106,107] MZ twins are not completely "identical" but often have minor to major differences in birthweight or congenital defects due to unequal allocation of blastomeres.[107] Postzygotic genetic events that can lead to MZ pair differences include chromosomal mosaicism, altered X-chromosome inactivation in female MZ twins, or late gene mutations. Separation may interrupt left-right axial orientation resulting in "mirror-image" twins.[107] MZ twinning can occur at three different stages of development: (1) during the early blastomere stage, (2) during formation of the inner cell mass, and (3) with development of the embryonic disk (Figure 3-27). The stage of development determines the number of placentas and arrangement of membranes.

Separation of the ovum during the early blastomere stage usually occurs about 2 days after fertilization while the blastomere is in the 2- to 4-cell stage (see Figure 3-27). Since this is before differentiation of any cells, the two blastomeres will develop independently into morulae, blastocysts, and embryos, each with separate placentas, chorions, and amnions (dichorionic-diamniotic). These blastocysts will implant at separate sites. If these sites are close together, the placentas may fuse. Membranes separating the embryos will contain the amnion-chorion of infant 1 and the chorion-amnion of infant 2 separated by their fused placentas.[13] This arrangement of infants, placentas, and membranes, which is identical to that of same-sex DZ twins, requires blood typing, tissue typing, and other analyses to determine zygosity.

Separation and duplication of the inner cell mass during development of the blastocyst 4 to 7 days after fertilization give rise to the most common form of MZ twins (see Figure 3-27). The trophoblast layer that will become the placenta and chorion has already formed in the blastocyst prior to separation of the inner cell mass. The amnion and amniotic cavity, however, have not yet begun to form and will develop independently in each embryo. Thus this form of twinning is monochorionic-diamniotic with a single placenta. The membranes separating the embryos consist of two layers of amnion and one chorion. The placenta of these infants is larger than the placenta found with a single infant but smaller than two single placentas. These placentas have an increased frequency of abnormal configurations and cord attachments.[13]

Less frequently, twinning occurs as a result of separation and duplication of the rudimentary embryonic disk, with appearance of two embryonic nodes instead of one at 7 to 15 (possibly up to 17) days after fertilization. Because the placenta, chorion, and amnion have all formed at this

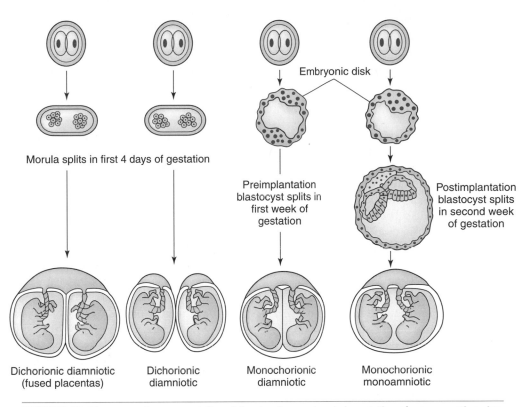

Morula splits in first 4 days of gestation

Embryonic disk

Preimplantation blastocyst splits in first week of gestation

Postimplantation blastocyst splits in second week of gestation

Dichorionic diamniotic (fused placentas)

Dichorionic diamniotic

Monochorionic diamniotic

Monochorionic monoamniotic

FIGURE **3-27** Diagrammatic representation of the development and placentation of monozygotic twins. (From Fox, H. [1997]. *Pathology of the placenta* [2nd ed.]. Philadelphia: W.B. Saunders.)

time, these twins are monochorionic-monoamniotic (see Figure 3-27). Monochorionic-monoamniotic infants account for only 1% to 2% of all MZ twins.[13] Perinatal mortality rate for this type of twins is 30% to 50% because of twisting, knotting, and entanglement of the two umbilical cords within the single amniotic sac.[15,50] If this form of twinning occurs at 7 to 13 ½ days, two separate embryos are formed (see Figure 3-27).

Separation after 13 days is usually incomplete; that is, the embryonic disk divides but remains united at one or more points (fission theory), resulting in the formation of conjoined twins. Incidence of conjoined twins has also been explained as arising after normal division of the embryonic disk into two cell masses that subsequently abut and join together (collision theory). Conjoined twins occur in 1.3 of 100,000 live births.[168] The most common areas of fusion (either singularly or in combination) are the thorax, abdomen, and umbilical cord.

Dizygotic Twins

The incidence of DZ twins varies markedly among different racial groups, ranging from 1 in 20 to 25 births in certain Nigerian tribal groups to 1 in 80 in U.S. Caucasians, 1:70 in African-American populations, and 1 in 150 in Japanese women.[168] The incidence of DZ twinning is also influenced by a variety of endocrine, endogenous, exogenous, and iatrogenic (administration of gonadotropins for treatment of infertility) factors. With ART, multiple birth rates are increased. DZ twinning has a strong maternal familial tendency. For example, the incidence of twins in female relatives of mothers of twins is 19% versus 10.7% among female relatives of fathers of twins.[13] Endocrine factors suggested in the etiology of DZ twins usually relate to increased levels of follicle-stimulating hormone (FSH) with overstimulation of the ovaries, leading to release of more than one ovum.[15,154] Endogenous factors associated with an increased incidence of DZ twinning include increased parity, maternal age (peaking at 37 years), maternal height and weight (perhaps related to nutrition), and increased frequency of intercourse.[15,54,70,106] Because DZ twins arise from separate ova, they have separate placentas, chorions and amnions (dichorionic-diamniotic), although their placentas may fuse if implanted close to each other.

Placental Abnormalities in Multiple Gestations

Bardawil and colleagues categorize pathologic placental lesions associated with multiple gestation into four groups: (1) specific pathology directly due to the twinning process (conjoined twins, acardiac or amorphous fetuses, and vascular anastomoses); (2) pathologic lesions or conditions that arise as a consequence of group 1 lesions (entanglement of umbilical cords in monoamniotic twins, twin-to-twin transfusion, polyhydramnios, amnion nodosum, chimera in DZ twins); (3) lesions related to physical problems of accommodation due to decreased intrauterine space (circumvallate changes, velamentous or marginal cord insertion, vasa praevia); and (4) incidental lesions that can occur in any placenta and are not related to twinning specifically.[13] Vascular lesions are described in the following paragraphs; other lesions have been discussed earlier in this chapter.

Vascular connections or anastomoses occur in nearly all of the common monochorionic placentas shared by MZ twins.[15,39] Thus twin-to-twin transfusion is a normal event in monochorionic pregnancies, but are not significant since blood flow is balanced.[41] Placental vascular anastomoses can be arterial-arterial, venous-arterial, arterial-venous, or venous-venous. The most common anastomoses, artery-to-artery, are thought to be inconsequential.[13] Significant problems can arise with deep arterial-venous anastomoses, especially without compensatory superficial anastomoses.[41] This type of anastomosis can lead to an imbalance in blood flow and development of fetal acardia and other anomalies or twin-to-twin transfusion. Arterial-venous anastomoses usually occur in a shared lobe supplied by an umbilical artery of one twin and drained by the umbilical vein of the other (Figure 3-28).[15,177] Thus a portion of the blood reentering the placenta from one fetus drains into the placental venous system of the second fetus (sometimes called the "third circulation"). The vascular flow is unidirectional and, unless compensated for by anastomoses in the opposite direction or other artery-to-artery anastomoses, will result in a hydrodynamic imbalance.[13,14,15]

Twin-to-twin transfusion syndrome (TTTS), also called fetal-to-fetal transfusion syndrome (FFTS) is seen in about 10% to 15% of MZ twins.[41] TTTS usually results from arterial-venous anastomoses. The donor twin is smaller, hypovolemic, and anemic and may develop congestive heart failure. The infant has decreased urine volume, and oligohydramnios may be present. The larger, recipient twin is hypervolemic and hypertensive with excessive urination often leading to polyhydramnios. This infant may develop hydrops and cardiomegaly.[15] TTTS may occur with significant differences in volume without significant differences in hemoglobin levels.[38] Although vascular anastomoses are frequent and extensive in monochorionic-monoamniotic twins, especially in those with closely implanted umbilical cords, twin-to-twin transfusion syndrome is rare in this type of MZ twin. This finding may be because the anastomoses are so extensive that there is no net hydrodynamic imbalance.[13]

Placental vascular anastomoses can also be present between a living and a dead twin, with subsequent passage of thromboplastic substances to the living twin. These substances can initiate intravascular coagulation, thrombosis, infarction, necrosis, alterations in organ function, and death.[113] Vascular abnormalities have been suggested as a cause for development of acardia or amorphous fetuses (shapeless mass of necrotic tissue and fibrin).[14,23,38,154,168] This anomaly, called twin reversed arterial perfusion syndrome (TRAP), occurs in 1% of MZ twins. TRAP likely arises in association with large artery-to-artery and vein-to-vein anastomoses. If pressure in the umbilical artery of the normal twin exceeds that in the artery of the other twin, circulation in the recipient twin may be reversed (i.e., blood flows to the twin via the um-

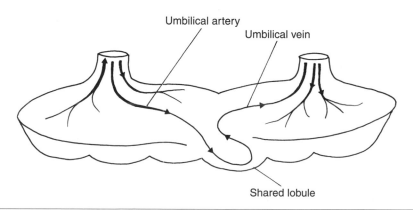

FIGURE **3-28** Vascular anastomoses in shared placental lobules with twin-to-twin transfusion. (From Wigglesworth, J.S. [1996]. *Perinatal pathology*. Philadelphia: W.B. Saunders.)

TABLE 3-7   Summary of Recommendations for Clinical Practice Related to the Prenatal Period and Placental Physiology

Counsel women regarding physical and physiologic changes during pregnancy and postpartum (pp. 67-70 and Chapters 5 to 19).

Understand the basic processes involved in embryonic and fetal development (pp. 75-82, Table 3-1, and Figure 3-10).

Provide teaching to families regarding embryonic and fetal development at each stage of gestation (pp. 82-90).

Recognize critical periods of development (pp. 114-115 and Figure 3-10).

Recognize risks associated with fetal exposure to drugs and other environmental agents during pregnancy (pp. 114-115 and Chapter 6).

Provide appropriate counseling and health teaching to promote optimal fetal development and health (pp. 82-90, 114-115).

Counsel women regarding the use of drugs or exposure to other environmental agents during pregnancy (pp. 114-115 and Chapter 6).

Recognize and monitor women at risk for ectopic pregnancy (p. 93).

Understand the usual patterns of human chorionic gonadotropin production and counsel women regarding home pregnancy testing (p. 105 and Figure 3-18).

Provide health teaching regarding placental development and growth during gestation (pp. 91-99).

Recognize and monitor for factors that can alter placental growth and development or lead to pregnancy loss (pp. 116-117).

Understand the dynamics of placental function throughout gestation and the factors influencing transfer (pp. 103-111, 115-116).

Recognize and monitor for factors that can alter maternal-fetal-placental circulation (pp. 100-103).

Recognize the potential effects of maternal disorders on placental function and fetal development (pp. 102-103, 115-116).

Monitor fetal growth and development (pp. 114-116).

Identify fetal risk situations during the antepartum and intrapartum periods related to alterations in placental function (pp. 102-103, 116-122).

Understand endocrine functions of the placenta and interaction of the maternal-fetal-placental unit (pp. 103-107 and Figure 3-19).

Counsel women regarding the effects of estrogen and progesterone on body function and structure during pregnancy (pp. 106-107).

Recognize factors that may alter the composition, production, and removal of amniotic fluid (pp. 112-113).

Monitor infants with a history of maternal polyhydramnios for congenital defects (p. 117-118).

Monitor infants with a history of maternal oligohydramnios for congenital anomalies and growth retardation (pp. 118-119).

Inspect the placenta, membranes, and umbilical cord after delivery (pp. 117, 119-121).

Know the implications of placental, umbilical cord, and trophoblastic disorders, and monitor at-risk women and their infants (pp. 119-121).

Teach women who have experienced a multiple birth the basis for development of monozygotic and dizygotic twins (or triplets, or quadruplets, and so on) and implications of the arrangements of placentas and membranes (pp. 121-124).

Recognize and monitor for fetal and neonatal effects of placental abnormalities with monozygotic twins (pp. 124-125).

bilical arteries and returns to a large placental vein-to-vein anastomosis via the umbilical artery). The resultant low perfusion pressure, poor oxygenation, and circulatory reversal lead to development of multiple severe structural defects.[113] The abnormal twin continues to develop only if there is perfusion by the normal twin, who may subsequently develop cardiac hypertrophy, congestive heart failure, and hydrops fetalis.[113]

Anastomoses in dichorionic fused placentas are rare (1 in 1000) but may account for chimerism in DZ twins. Chimerism is uncommon but may complicate the determination of zygosity. The chimeric twin carries within its system genetically dissimilar blood or tissue from its fraternal twin. Movement of material from one twin to the other is thought to involve transfer of precursor blood cells or other immature cells through vascular communication during early stages of gestation when the fetal immune system is poorly developed. In chimerism the recipient twin becomes tolerant of the foreign blood cells or tissue.[13,97,132]

SUMMARY

The respiratory, nutritive, and endocrinologic functions of the placenta are critical for fetal growth and development and pregnancy outcome. A major component of nursing care for women with normal, at risk, and complicated pregnancies is providing appropriate counseling and health teaching to promote optimal fetal development and health and to prevent exposure of the fetus to adverse environmental influences. To accomplish this goal and to assess maternal and fetal responses to compromised placental function and identify fetal risk situations during the antepartum and intrapartum periods, the nurse must understand the factors influencing transfer of substances across the placenta. An understanding of endocrine functions and interactions of the maternal-fetal-placental unit provides a basis for assessing, monitoring, and teaching pregnant women undergoing various tests for clinical assessment of placental function and fetal well-being. Recommendations for clinical practice are summarized in Table 3-7.

REFERENCES

1. Abou-Haila, A. & Tulsiani, D.R. (2000). Mammalian sperm acrosome: formation, contents, and function. *Arch Biochem Biophys, 379,* 173.
2. Adamson, E.G. (1983). Growth factors in development. In J.B. Warshaw (Ed.). *The biological basis of reproductive and developmental medicine.* New York: Elsevier Biomedical.
3. Adamsons, K. & Myres, R.E. (1975). Circulation in the intervillous space: Obstetrical considerations in fetal deprivation. In P. Gruenwald (Ed.). *The placenta and its maternal supply line.* Lancaster, England: Medical and Technical Publications.
4. Ahmed, A.G. & Klopper, A. (1985). Early fetal signals: Schwangerschaftsprotein 1 and human chorionic gonadotropin. In C.T. Jones & P.W. Nathanielsz (Eds.). *The physiological development of the fetus and newborn.* Orlando, FL: Academic Press.
5. Ahokas, R.A. & Anderson, G.D. (1987). The placenta as an organ of nutrition. In J.P. Lavery (Ed.). *The human placenta: Clinical perspectives.* Rockville, MD: Aspen.
6. Alsat, E., et al. (1998). Physiological role of human placental growth hormone. *Mol Cell Endocrinol, 25,* 121.
7. Altshuler, G. & Hyde, S.R. (1996). Clinicopathologic implication of placental pathology. *Clin Obstet Gyneol, 39,* 549.
8. Altshuler, G. (1996). Role of the placenta in perinatal pathology (revisited). *Pediatr Pathol Lab Med, 16,* 207.
9. Aplin, J. (1996). The cell biology of human implantation. *Placenta, 17,* 269.
10. Aplin, J. (1999). Maternal influences on placental development. *Semin Cell Dev Biol, 11,* 115.
11. Arck, P. (1999). From the decidual cell internet: Trophoblast-recognizing T cells. *Biol Reprod, 60,* 227.
12. Baldwin, V.J. (1994). *Pathology of multiple pregnancy.* New York: Springer-Verlag.
13. Bardawil, W.A., Reddy, R.L., & Bardawil, L.W. (1988). Placental considerations in multiple pregnancy. *Clin Perinatol, 15,* 130.
14. Benirschke, K. (1990). The placenta in twin gestation. *Clin Obstet Gynecol, 33,* 18.
15. Benirschke, K. (1995). The biology of the twinning process: how placentation influences outcome. *Semin Perinatol, 19,* 342.
16. Bergh, P.A. & Navot, D. (1992). The impact of embryonic development and endometrial maturity on the timing of implantation. *Fertil Steril, 58,* 537.
17. Bernfield, M. (1983). Mechanisms of congenital malformations. In J.B. Warshaw (Ed.). *The biological basis of reproductive and developmental medicine.* New York: Elsevier Biomedical.
18. Bodurtha, J. (1999). Assessment of the newborn with dysmorphic features. *Neonatal Network, 18*(2), 27-30.
19. Bourget, P., Roulot, C., & Fernandez, H. (1995). Models for placental transfer studies of drugs. *Clin Pharmacokinet, 28,* 161.
20. Boylan, P. & Parisi, V (1986). An overview of hydramnios. *Semin Perinatol, 10,* 136.
21. Burdine, R.D. & Schier, A.F. (2000). Conserved and divergent mechanisms in left-right axis formation. *Genes Dev, 14,* 763.
22. Burrows, T.D., King, A., & Loke, Y.W. (1996). Trophoblast migration during human placental implantation. *Hum Reprod Update, 2,* 307.
23. Brace, R.A. (1997). Physiology of amniotic fluid volume regulation. *Clin Obstet Gynecol, 40,* 280.
24. Buster, J.E. & Sauer, M.V. (1989). Endocrinology of conception. In S.A. Brody & K. Ueland (Eds.). *Endocrine disorders in pregnancy.* Norwalk, CT: Appleton & Lange.
25. Cameron, I.T. (1998). Matrix metalloproteinases, prostaglandins and endothelins: Paracrine regulators of implantation. *Gynecol Endocrinol, 12,* 44.
26. Carbillon, L. (2000). Fetal-placental and decidual-placental units: Role of endocrine and paracrine regulations in parturition. *Fetal Diagn Ther, 15,* 308.
27. Carbillon, L., Uzan, M., & Uzan, S. (2000). Pregnancy, vascular tone, and maternal hemodynamics: A crucial adaptation. *Obstet Gynecol Surv, 55,* 574.
28. Cardwell, M.S. (1987). Polyhydramnios: A review. *Obstet Gynecol Surv, 42,* 612.
29. Carlson, B.M. (1999). *Human embryology & developmental biology* (2nd ed.). St Louis: Mosby.
30. Centers for Disease Control Reproductive Health Information Source. (1998). *Assisted reproductive technology success rates: National summary and fertility clinic reports.* Available online at www.cdc.gov/nccdphp/drh/art98/index.htm.
31. Collins. P. (1999). Staging embryos in development. In C.R. Rodeck & M.J. Whittle (Eds.). *Fetal medicine: basic science and clinical practice.* London: Churchill-Livingstone.
32. Collins. P. (1999). Cellular mechanisms in development In C.R. Rodeck & M.J. Whittle (Eds.). *Fetal medicine: basic science and clinical practice.* London: Churchill-Livingstone.
33. Cross, J.C. (2000). Genetic insights into trophoblast differentiation and placental morphogenesis. *Semin Cell Dev Biol, 11,* 105.
34. Croxatto, H.B., et al. (1978). Studies on the duration of egg transport by the human oviduct II. Ovum location at various times following luteinizing hormone peak. *Am J Obstet Gynecol, 132,* 629.
35. Cunningham, F.G. & Whitridge, W.J. (1997). *Williams obstetrics* (20th ed.). Stamford, CT: Appleton & Lange.
36. Dancis, J. (1981). Placental transport of amino acids, fats and minerals. In *Placental transport.* Mead Johnson Symposium on Perinatal and Developmental Medicine (No. 18). Evansville, IN: Mead Johnson.
37. De Vos, A. & Van Steirteghem, A. (2000). Zona hardening, zona drilling and assisted hatching: new achievements in assisted reproduction. *Cells Tissues Organs, 166,* 220.
38. Denbow, M.L. & Fisk, N.M. (1998). The consequences of monochorionic placentation. *Baillieres Clin Haematol, 12,* 37.
39. Dockery, P., Bermingham, J. & Jenkins, D. (2000). Structure-function relations in the human placenta. *Biochem Soc Trans, 28,* 202.
40. Duc-Goiran, P. et al. (1999). Embryo-maternal interactions at the implantation site: a delicate equilibrium. *Eur J Obstet Gynecol Reprod Biol, 83,* 85.
41. Duncan, K.R., Denbow, M.L., & Fisk, N.M. (1997). The etiology and management of twin-twin transfusion syndrome. *Prenat Diagn, 17,* 1227.
42. Edwards, R.G. (1986). Causes of early embryonic loss in human pregnancy. *Hum Reprod, 1,* 185.
43. Eisenbach, M. & Tur-Kaspa, I. (1999). Do human eggs attract spermatozoa? *Bioessays, 21,* 203.
44. Eisenbach, M. (1999). Mammalian sperm chemotaxis and its association with capacitation. *Dev Genet, 25,* 87.
45. Erkkola, R., et al. (1985). Growth discordancy in twin pregnancies: A risk factor not detected by measurements of biparietal diameter. *Obstet Gynecol, 66,* 203.
46. Ethics Committee of the American Fertility Society. (1986). Artificial insemination-donor. *Fertil Steril, 46,* 36s.
47. Evain-Brion, D. (1999). Maternal endocrine adaptation to placental hormones in humans. *Acta Paediatr Suppl, 428,* 12.
48. Faber, J.J. & Thornburg, K.L. (1983). *Placental physiology.* New York: Raven Press.
49. Flaxman, S.M. & Sherman, P.W. (2000). Morning sickness: a mechanism for protecting mother and embryo. *Q Rev Biol, 75,* 113.

50. Fox, H. (1997). *Pathology of the placenta* (2nd ed.). Philadelphia: W.B. Saunders.

51. Freeman, M. (2000). Feedback control of intercellular signaling in development. *Nature, 408,* 313.

52. Ganapathy, V. (2000). Placental transporters relevant to drug distribution across the maternal-fetal interface. *J Pharmacol Exp Ther, 294,* 413.

53. Garnica, A.D. & Chan, W.Y. (1996). The role of the placenta in fetal nutrition and growth. *J Am Coll Nutr, 15,* 206.

54. Gilbert, S.F. (1996). Cellular dialogues in organogenesis. *Birth Defects Orig Artic Ser, 30,* 1.

55. Goddard, B. (1990). The role of the nurse in the prenatal period. In M.A. Auvenshine & M.G. Enriquez (Eds.). *Comprehensive maternity nursing: Perinatal and women's health.* Boston: Jones & Bartlett.

56. Goldstein, I., Coppel, J.A., & Hobbins, J.C. (1989). Fetal behavior in preterm rupture of the membranes. *Clin Perinatol, 16,* 735.

57. Guthrie, S. (1991). Horizontal and vertical pathways in vertical induction. *Trends Neurosci, 14,* 123.

58. Guyton, A.C. & Hall, J.E. (1996). *Textbook of medical physiology* (9th ed.). Philadelphia: W.B. Saunders.

59. Hamilton, W.J., Boyd, J.D., & Mossman, H.W. (1972). *Human embryology* (4th ed.). Baltimore: Williams & Wilkins.

60. Harper, M.J.K. (1982). Sperm and egg transport. In C.R. Austin & R.V. Short (Eds.). *Reproduction in mammals: Germ cells and fertilization.* Cambridge, England: Cambridge University Press.

61. Harris, T. (1979). Fetal development and physiology. In A. Clark & D. Affonso (Eds.). *Childbearing: A nursing perspective.* Philadelphia: F.A. Davis.

62. Hayashi, R.H. (1987). Abnormalities of placental implantation. In J.P. Lavery (Ed.). *The human placenta: Clinical perspectives.* Rockville, MD: Aspen.

63. Heinrichs, W.L. & Gibbons, W.E. (1989). Endocrinology of pregnancy. In S.A. Brody & K. Ueland (Eds.). *Endocrine disorders in pregnancy.* Norwalk, CT: Appleton & Lange.

64. Henson, M.C. & Castracane, V.D. (2000). Leptin in pregnancy. *Biol Reprod, 63,* 1219.

65. Hertig, A.T. (1967). The overall problem in man. In K. Benirschke (Ed.). *Comparative aspects of reproductive failure.* New York: Springer-Verlag.

66. Hill, L.M., Kislak, S. & Runco, C. (1987). An ultrasonic view of the umbilical cord. *Obstet Gynecol Surv, 42,* 82.

67. Hill, L.M. et al. (1987). Polyhydramnios: ultrasonically detected prevalence and neonatal outcome. *Obstet Gynecol, 69,* 21.

68. Ho, P.C., et al. (1986). Plasma prolactin, progesterone, estradiol, and human chorionic gonadotropin in complete and partial moles before and after evacuation. *Obstet Gynecol, 67,* 99.

69. Holbrook, R.H. & Ueland, K. (1989). Endocrinology of parturition and preterm labor. In S.A. Brody & K. Ueland (Eds.). *Endocrine disorders in pregnancy.* Norwalk, CT: Appleton & Lange.

70. Hollenbach, K.A. & Hickok, D.E. (1990). Epidemiology and diagnosis of twin gestation. *Clin Obstet Gynecol, 33,* 3.

71. Holness, M.J., Munns, M.J., & Sugden, M.C. (1999). Current concepts concentrating the role of leptin in reproductive function. *Mol Cell Endocrinol, 157,* 11.

72. Hubel, C.A. (1999). Oxidative stress in the pathogenesis of preeclampsia. *Proc Soc Exp Biol Med, 222,* 222.

73. Hutchinson-Williams, K.A. & DeCherney, A.H. (1989). Endocrinology of ectopic pregnancy. In S.A. Brody & K. Ueland (Eds.). *Endocrine disorders in pregnancy.* Norwalk, CT: Appleton & Lange.

74. Hutter, H. & Dohr, G. (1998). HLA expression on immature and mature human germ cells. *J Reprod Immunol, 38,* 101.

75. Huxley, R.R. (2000). Nausea and vomiting in early pregnancy: its role in placental development. *Obstet Gynecol, 95,* 779.

76. Jaffe, R. (1998). First trimester utero-placental circulation: maternal-fetal interaction. *J Perinat Med, 26,* 168.

77. Jaffe, R., Jauniaux, E & Hustin, J. (1997). Maternal circulation in the first-trimester human placenta—myth or reality? *Am J Obstet Gynecol, 176,* 695.

78. Jauniaux, E. & Gulbis, B. (2000). Fluid compartments of the embryonic environment. *Human Reprod Update, 6,* 268.

79. Jauniaux, E., et al. (2000). Onset of maternal arterial blood flow and placental oxidative stress: a possible factor in early pregnancy failure. *Am J Pathol, 157,* 3251.

80. Johnson, P.M., Christmas, S.E., & Vince, G.S. (1999). Immunological aspects of implantation and implantation failure. *Hum Reprod, 14,* 26.

81. Jones, K.L. (1996). *Smith's recognizable patterns of human malformation* (5th ed.), Philadelphia: W.B. Saunders.

82. Kam, E.P., et al. (1999). The role of trophoblast in the physiological change in decidual spiral arteries. *Hum Reprod, 14,* 2131.

83. Kaplan, C. (1987). Gross and microscopic abnormalities of the placenta. In J.P. Lavery (Ed.). *The human placenta: Clinical perspectives.* Rockville, MD: Aspen.

84. Kaplan, C. (1993). Placenta pathology for the nineties. *Pathol Annu, 28,* 15.

85. Kaplan, S. & Bolender, D.L. (1998). Embryology. In R.A. Polin & W.W. Fox (Eds.). *Fetal and neonatal physiology* (2nd ed.). Philadelphia: W.B. Saunders.

86. Kaufmann, P. & Scheffen, I. (1998). Placental development. In R.A. Polin & W.W. Fox (Eds.). *Fetal and neonatal physiology* (2nd ed.). Philadelphia: W.B. Saunders.

87. Key, T.C. & Resnik, R. (1988). Obstetric management of the high-risk patient. In G. Burrow & F. Ferris (Eds.). *Medical complications during pregnancy.* Philadelphia: W.B. Saunders.

88. Khong, T.Y. & Pearce, J.M. (1987). In J.P. Lavery (Ed.). *The human placenta: Clinical perspectives.* Rockville, MD: Aspen.

89. Knorr, L.J. (1989). Relieving fetal distress with amnioinfusion. *MCN, 14,* 346.

90. Kilpatrick, S.J. (1997). Therapeutic interventions for oligohydramnios: Amnioinfusion and maternal hydration. *Clin Obstet Gynecol, 40,* 328.

91. Kimber, S.J. & Spanwick, C. (2000). Blastocyst implantation: The adhesion cascade. *Semin Cell Dev Biol, 11,* 77.

92. Kingdom, J. (2000). Development of the placental villous tree and its consequences for fetal growth. *Eur J Obstet Gynecol Reprod Biol, 92,* 35.

93. Kingdom, J.C. & Kaufmann, P. (1997). Oxygen and placental villous development: Origins of fetal hypoxia. *Placenta, 18,* 613.

94. Kingdom, J.C. & Kaufmann, P. (1999). Oxygen and placental vascular development. *Adv Exp Med Biol, 474,* 259.

95. Kiserud, T. (2000). Fetal venous circulation—an update on hemodynamics. *J Perinat Med, 28,* 90.

96. Kliman, H.J. (2000). Uteroplacental blood flow: The story of decidualization, menstruation, and trophoblast invasion. *Am J Pathol, 157,* 1759.

97. Lage, J.M., Mark, S.D. & Driscoll, S.G. (1987). The twin placenta. In J.P. Lavery (Ed.). *The human placenta: Clinical perspectives.* Rockville, MD: Aspen.

98. Lavery, B.S. (1987). The third stage. In J.P. Lavery (Ed.). *The human placenta: Clinical perspectives.* Rockville, MD: Aspen.

99. Lavery, J.P. (1987). Appendages of the placenta. In J.P. Lavery (Ed.). *The human placenta: Clinical perspectives.* Rockville, MD: Aspen.

100. Leppig, K.A., et al. (1987). Predictive value of minor anomalies, Part I: association with major malformations. *J Pediatr, 110,* 531-537.
101. Lessey, B.A., et al. (1992). Integrin molecules in the human endometrium: correlation with the normal and abnormal menstrual cycle. *J Clin Invest, 90,* 188.
102. Lessey, B.A., et al. (1994). Further characterization of endometrial integrins during menstrual cycle and in pregnancy. *Fertil Steril, 62,* 497.
103. Leung, A.K. & Robson, W.L. (1989). Single umbilical artery: A report of 159 cases. *Am J Dis Child, 143,* 108.
104. Liu, J.H. & Rebar, R.W. (1999). Endocrinology of pregnancy. In R.K. Creasy & R. Resnik (Eds.). *Maternal-fetal medicine* (4th ed.). Philadelphia: W.B. Saunders.
105. Lotgering, F.K. & Wallenburg, H.C.S. (1986). Mechanisms of production and clearance of amniotic fluid. *Semin Perinatol, 10,* 94.
106. MacGillvray, I. (1986). Epidemiology of twin pregnancy. *Semin Perinatol, 10,* 4.
107. Machin, G.A. (1996). Some causes of genotypic and phenotypic discordance in monozygotic twin pairs. *Am J Med Genet, 61,* 216.
108. Magann, E.F. & Martin, J.N. (1999). Amniotic fluid volume assessment in singleton and twin pregnancies. *Obstet Gynecol Clin North Am, 26,* 579.
109. Manning, F.A. (1999). General principles and application of ultrasound. In R.K. Creasy & R. Resnik (Eds.). *Maternal-fetal medicine: Principles and practice* (4th ed.). Philadelphia: W.B. Saunders.
110. Mantzoros, C.S. (2000). Role of leptin in reproduction. *Ann N Y Acad Sci, 900,* 174.
111. Martin, C.R. & Gingerich, B. (1976). Uteroplacental physiology. *JOGN, 5*(Suppl), 16s.
112. Mayhew, T.M. & Burton, G.J. (1997). Stereology and its impact on our understanding of human placental functional morphology. *Microsc Res Tech, 38,* 195.
113. McCullough, K. (1988). Neonatal problems in twins. *Clin Perinatol, 15,* 141.
114. McLeskey, S.B., et al. (1998). Molecules involved in mammalian sperm-egg interaction. *Int Rev Cytol, 177,* 57.
115. Merce, L.T., Barco, M.J., & Bau, S. (1996). Color doppler sonographic assessment of placental circulation in the first trimester of normal pregnancy. *J Ultrasound Med, 15,* 135.
116. Miller, D.S., Ballon, S.C., & Teng, N.H. (1989). Gestational trophoblastic diseases. In S.A. Brody & K. Ueland (Eds.). *Endocrine disorders in pregnancy.* Norwalk, CT: Appleton & Lange.
117. Moessinger, A.C. (1983). Fetal akinesia deformation sequence: An animal model. *Pediatrics, 72,* 857.
118. Moessinger, A.C. (1989). Morphological consequences of depressed or impaired fetal activity. In W.P. Smotherman & S.R. Robinson (Eds.). *Behavior of the fetus.* Caldwell, NJ: Telford Press.
119. Moessinger, A.C. et al., (1986). Oligohydramnios-induced lung hypoplasia: the influence of timing and duration of gestation. *Pediatr Res, 20,* 951.
120. Moise, K.J. (1997). Polyhydramnios. *Clin Obstet Gynecol, 40,* 266.
121. Moore, K.L. & Persaud, T.V.N. (1998). *The developing human: Clinically oriented embryology* (6th ed.). Philadelphia: W.B. Saunders.
122. Moore, T.R. & Tipton, E.E. (1997). Amniotic fluid and nonimmune hydrops fetalis. In A. Fanroff & R.J. Martin (Eds.). *Neonatal-perinatal medicine, diseases of the fetus and infant* (6th ed.). Philadelphia: W.B. Saunders.
123. Moriyama, I., et al. (1988). Fetal growth and the placenta-development of the transport function of the human cell membrane and fetal growth. In G.H. Wiknjosastro, W.H. Prakoso, & K. Maeda (Eds.). *Perinatology.* Amsterdam: Elsevier Science.
124. Morrish, D.W., Dakour, J., & Li, H. (1998). Functional regulation of human trophoblast differentiation. *J Reprod Immunol, 39,* 179.
125. Morriss, F.H. & Boyd, R.D.H. (1988). Placental transport. In E. Knobil & J Neill (Eds.). *The physiology of reproduction* (vol. 2). New York: Raven.
126. Muragaki, Y., et al. (1996). Altered growth and branching patterns in synpolydactyly caused by mutations of HOXD 13. *Science, 272,* 548.
127. Newton, E.R. (1989). The fetus as patient. *Med Clin North Am, 73,* 517.
128. Nielson, T.F., Hagberg, H., & Ljungblad, U. (1989). Placenta previa and antepartum hemorrhage after previous caesarian section. *Gynecol Obstet Invest, 27,* 88.
129. Nordenvall M. & Sandstedt, B. (1990). Placental lesions and maternal hemoglobin levels. *Acta Obstet Gynaecol Scan, 69,* 127.
130. Pacifici, G.M. & Nottoli, R. (1995). Placental transfer of drugs administered to the mother. *Clin Pharmacokinet, 28,* 235.
131. Panesar, N.S. (1999). Human chorionic gonadotropin: a secretory hormone. *Med Hypotheses, 53,* 136.
132. Pauerstein, C.J. (Ed.). (1987). *Clinical obstetrics.* New York: John Wiley.
133. Perrin, E.V.D.K. (1984). Placenta as a reflection of fetal disease. In E.V.D.K. Perrin (Ed.). *Pathology of the placenta.* New York: Churchill Livingstone.
134. Petraglia, F. (1997). Inhibin, activin and follistatin in the human placenta: A new family of regulatory proteins. *Placenta, 18,* 3.
135. Petraglia, F., et al. (1998). Paracrine regulation of human placenta: control of hormonogenesis. *J Reprod Immunol, 39,* 221.
136. Pinjnenborg, R. (1998). The human decidua as a passageway for trophoblast invasion. *Trophoblast Res, 11,* 229.
137. Pinjnenborg, R. (1996). The placentae bed. *Hypertens Preg, 15,* 7.
138. Polzin, W.J. & Brady, K. (1998). The etiology of premature rupture of the membranes. *Clin Obstet Gynecol, 41,* 810.
139. Potter, E.L. (1963). Twin zygosity and placental form in relation to the outcome of pregnancy. *Am J Obstet Gynecol, 87,* 566.
140. Qu, J. & Thomas, K. (1998). Advance in the study of inhibin, activin and follistatin production in pregnant women. *Eur J Obstet Gynecol Reprod Biol, 81,* 141.
141. Ramsey, E.M. & Donner, M.W. (1980). *Placental vasculature and circulation.* Philadelphia: W.B. Saunders.
142. Raz, T. & Shalgi, R. (1998). Early events in mammalian egg activation. *Hum Reprod, 13*(Suppl 4), 133.
143. Redline, R. (1997). Placental pathology. In A. Fanroff & R.J. Martin (Eds.). *Neonatal-perinatal medicine, diseases of the fetus and infant* (6th ed.). Philadelphia: W.B. Saunders.
144. Reynolds, F. & Knott, C. (1989). Pharmacokinetics in pregnancy and placental transfer. *Oxford Rev Reprod Biol, 11,* 389.
145. Roberts, J.M. (2000). Preeclampsia: what we know and what we do not know. *Semin Perinatol, 24,* 24.
146. Robertson, S.A. (1997). Cytokine-leukocyte networks and the establishment of pregnancy. *Am J Reprod Immunol, 37,* 438.
147. Robertson, W.B., et al. (1986). The placental bed biopsy: review of three European centers. *Am J Obstet Gynecol, 155,* 401.
148. Rodesch, F. et al. (1992). Oxygen measurements in endometrial and trophoblastic tissues during early pregnancy. *Obstet Gynecol, 80,* 283.
149. Ross, M.G. & Nijland, M.J. (1997). Fetal swallowing: relation to amniotic fluid regulation. *Clin Obstet Gynecol, 40,* 352.
150. Rutanen, E-M. (1993). Cytokines in reproduction. *Ann Med, 25,* 343.
151. Saito, S. (2000). Cytokine network at the feto-maternal interface. *J Reprod Immunol, 47,* 87.
152. Salas, S.P. (1999). What causes pre-eclampsia? *Baillieres Clin Obstet Gynecol, 13,* 41.

153. Savona-Ventura, C. (1987). Amniocentesis for fetal maturity. *Obstet Gynecol Surv, 42,* 717.

154. Schinzel, A.A., Smith, D.W., & Miller, J.R. (1979). Monozygotic twinning and structural defects. *J Pediatr, 95,* 921.

155. Schlievert, P., Johnson, W., & Galask, R.P. (1977). Amniotic fluid antibacterial mechanisms: New concepts. *Semin Perinatol, 1,* 59.

156. Schorge, J.O., et al. (2000). Recent advances in gestational trophoblastic disease. *J Reprod Med, 45,* 692.

157. Schroder, H.J. & Power, G.G. (1997). Engine and radiator: fetal and placental interactions for heat dissipation. *Exp Physiol, 82,* 403.

158. Schuler-Maloney, D. (2000). Placental triage of the singleton placenta. *J Midwifery Womens Health, 45,* 104.

159. Seppala, M., et al. (1997). Glycodelins as regulators of early events of reproduction. *Clin Endocrinol, 46,* 381.

160. Sibley, C.P., et al. (1998). Mechanisms of maternofetal exchange across the human placenta. *Biochem Soc Trans, 26,* 86.

161. Sibley, C.P. & Boyd, R.D.H. (1998). Mechanisms of transfer across the placenta. In R.A. Polin & W.W. Fox (Eds.). *Fetal and neonatal physiology* (2nd ed.). Philadelphia: W.B. Saunders.

162. Slavkin, H.C. (1998). Regulation of embryogenesis. In R.A. Polin & W.W. Fox (Eds.). *Fetal and neonatal physiology* (2nd ed.). Philadelphia: W.B. Saunders.

163. Smith, S.K. et al. (2000). Angiogenic growth factor expression in placenta. *Semin Perinatol, 24,* 82.

164. Speroff, L., Glass, R.H., & Kase, N.G. (1999). *Clinical gynecologic endocrinology and infertility* (6th ed.). Philadelphia: Lippincott, Williams & Wilkins.

165. Staples, D. (1999). *Physiology in childbearing with anatomy and related biosciences.* Edinburgh: Bailliere Tindall.

166. Strewler, G.J. (2000). The physiology of parathyroid hormone-related protein. *N Engl J Med, 20,* 177.

167. Sunder, S. & Lenton, E.A. (2000). Endocrinology of the periimplantation period. *Baillieres Best Practice Res Clin Obstet Gynaecol, 14,* 789.

168. Taylor, M.J. & Fisk, N.M. (2000). Prenatal diagnosis in multiple pregnancy. *Baillieres Best Pract Res Clin Obstet Gynaecol, 14*(4), 663.

169. Tesarik, J. (1999). Calcium: signaling in human preimplantation development: A review. *J Assist Reprod Genet, 16,* 216.

170. Tharmaratnam, S. (2000). Fetal distress. *Baillieres Best Pract Res Clin Obstet Gynaecol, 14*(1), 155.

171. Thornton, K.L. (2000). Advances in assisted reproductive technologies. *Obstet Gynecol Clin North Am, 27,* 517.

172. Tropper, P.J. & Petrie, R.H. (1987). Placental exchange. In J.P. Lavery (Ed.). *The human placenta: Clinical perspectives.* Rockville, MD: Aspen.

173. Wallenberg, H. (1977). The amniotic fluid: II. *J Perinat Med, 5,* 233.

174. Wallenberg, H. (1977). The amniotic fluid: I. *J Perinat Med, 5,* 193.

175. Walsh, S.W. (1990). Physiology of low-dose aspirin therapy for the prevention of preeclampsia. *Semin Perinatol, 14,* 152.

176. Wassarman, P.M. & Litscher, E.S. (2001). Towards the molecular basis of sperm and egg interaction during mammalian fertilization. *Cells Tissues Organs, 168,* 36.

177. Wigglesworth, J.S. (1984). The placenta in perinatal pathology. In J.S. Wigglesworth (Ed.). *Perinatal pathology.* Philadelphia: W.B. Saunders.

178. Willows, M., et al. (1993). Sperm numbers and distribution within the human fallopian tube around ovulation. *Hum Reprod, 8,* 2019.

179. Wilson, J.G. (1977). Current status of teratology: General principles and mechanisms derived from animal studies. In J.G. Wilson & F.C. Fraser (Eds.). *Handbook of teratology: General principles and etiology.* New York: Plenum.

180. Wright, S.J. (1999). Sperm nuclear activation during fertilization. *Curr Top Dev Biol, 46,* 133.

181. Wysolmerski, J.J. & Stewart, A.F. (1998), The physiology of parathyroid hormone-related protein: An emerging role as a developmental factor. *Ann Rev Physiol, 60,* 431.

182. Yetter, J.F. (1998). Examination of the placenta. *Am Fam Phys, 57,* 1045.

183. Yoshida, Y. & Manabe, Y. (1990). Different characteristics of amniotic and cervical collagenous tissue during pregnancy and delivery: A morphologic study. *Am J Obstet Gynecol, 162,* 190.

184. Zhou, Y. et al. (1993). Preeclampsia is associated with abnormal expression of adhesion molecules by invasive cytotrophoblasts. *J Clin Invest, 91,* 950.

Parturition and Uterine Physiology

During parturition the actions of the myometrium, decidua, fetus, placenta, and membranes must be integrated to achieve birth of the fetus without compromising fetal or placental perfusion. Ulmsten compares the process of parturition to an opera: "Where cervical priming [ripening] is the overture to the grand performance by the cervix and uterus. After training and rehearsals, the cervix and uterus are able to act in concert and produce a successful grand finale, delivery. Yet many players and factors in the parturition orchestra are unknown, and remarkably, the director or conductor who starts the event remains unknown."[137]

This chapter reviews the structure of the uterus and individual myometrial cells; changes during pregnancy; physiology of parturition, with respect to cervical dilatation, initiation of labor, and myometrial contractions; and clinical implications related to pre- and postterm labor onset, labor induction, and dystocia. Maternal pain during labor is discussed in Chapter 14.

UTERUS

The uterus is a major site of physiologic activity during the childbearing years. Alterations in the endometrium occur with the monthly menstrual cycle (see Chapter 2) and during pregnancy (see Chapter 3). Myometrial activity is associated with menstruation, sperm transport, zygote transport, implantation, pregnancy, and parturition. During pregnancy the uterus supports growth and development of the embryo and fetus.[2] At the end of pregnancy, the uterine myometrium must move from a relatively inactive state to produce the strong, synchronous, coordinated contractile forces needed to expel the fetus and placenta. Knowledge of the physiologic changes that bring about this transition in uterine function is incomplete at present but is the focus of much interest and research.

Uterine Structure

The uterine wall consists of three layers: (1) internal endometrium; (2) myometrium; and (3) external serous ep-

ithelial layer. The thin serosa protects the uterus and provides a relatively inelastic base upon which the myometrium develops tension to increase intrauterine pressure. During early pregnancy the endometrial cells enlarge and a hypersecretory state develops with changes in cellular composition as the endometrium is remodeled into the decidua to support implantation, placental development, and fetal nutrition (see Chapter 3).[78]

The myometrium consists of four muscle layers separated by a vascular zone. The muscle layers form a web that supports and protects the developing fetus. The inner layer, below the decidua, is circular and perpendicular to the long axis of the uterus. This layer runs clockwise and counterclockwise in a spiral. The middle layer consists of interconnecting fibers in a figure-eight shape. The outer two layers run parallel to the longitudinal axis of the uterus.[78,113] These muscle layers are composed of smooth muscle cells arranged in interconnected bundles of 10 to 50 partially overlapping cells set in a matrix of collagenous connective tissue and ground substance.[24,41,49] The ground substance transmits the contractile forces from individual myometrial cells along the muscle bundle.[24] Around the bundles of smooth muscle cells are fibroblasts, blood and lymphatic vessels, and nerve cells. The subendothelial myometrium forms the junctional zone where myometrial contractions arise in the nonpregnant uterus.[78] Because the uterine muscle layers have different embryonic origins, they have distinct hormonal responses and thus may respond differentially to uterotonic agonists and antagonists.[12]

The uterus is innervated by adrenergic neurons (postganglionic sympathetic fibers from lumbar and mesenteric ganglia), cholinergic neurons (sparse, primarily innervating the cervix), and peptidergic neurons.[78] Adrenergic fibers are most dense in the area of the fallopian tubes, cervix, and vagina and are relatively sparse in the uterine corpus and fundus.[44] In comparison to other smooth muscle cells, which tend to be richly innervated, the uterus has a relatively low density of nerves to smooth muscles cells.[49] The myometrium normally contracts spontaneously unless this ability is altered by endocrine, paracrine, or apocrine factors. This intrinsic ability is suppressed during pregnancy, then enhanced during labor.[2,97]

The role of the nervous system in myometrial activity is poorly understood. The adrenergic and peptidergic nerves may play a role in suppressing myometrial contractility during pregnancy.[24,49,84] Adrenergic fibers in the uterine wall disappear near term, leaving only those in the cervix and uterine horns.[84] Peptidergic and sympathetic nerves also decrease markedly during pregnancy.[111] Thus control of contractility during pregnancy changes to local control, particularly prostaglandins (PGs) in the decidua and chorion and oxytocin in the myometrium.[111] Communication between myometrial cells during labor occurs primarily via gap junctions (see Gap Junctions).

Uterine Growth

The elastic properties of the uterus support its growth during pregnancy. The uterus increases in weight, length, width, depth, volume, and overall capacity during pregnancy (Table 4-1). Uterine growth begins after implantation. Initially it primarily involves hyperplasia and is influenced by estrogen and growth factors (e.g., insulin-like growth factor 1 [IGF-1], epidermal growth factor, transforming growth factor, β-fibroblast growth factor) and independent of the effects of stretching from the growing embryo.[78,133] This early uterine growth occurs regardless of whether the embryo is implanted in the uterus or at an extrauterine site.[102,113]

Later uterine growth involves hypertrophy and hyperplasia of the myocytes and remodeling of the extracellular matrix, mediated by distention of the uterus by the enlarging fetus.[78] As the uterus grows, the ratio of ribonucleic acid (RNA) to deoxyribonucleic acid (DNA) increases due to increased RNA synthesis and total protein. By 3 to 4 months, the uterine wall has thickened from 10 to 25 mm. With further distention the wall thins to 5 to 10 mm at term. Myometrial smooth muscle fibers increase in length from 50 to 500 μm and width from 5 to 15 μm due to a

progressive increase in actin and myosin content.[102,113] Smooth muscle cell creatinine phosphatase, adenosine triphosphate (ATP), and adenosine diphosphate (ADP) also increase to term.[102]

The height of the uterine fundus reaches the maternal umbilicus by about 20 weeks' gestation and the xiphoid process of the sternum by 8 months. As the fetal head descends into the pelvis ("lightening") late in gestation, the fundal height becomes slightly lower.

After 2 to 4 months' gestation, when the fundus changes from a spherical to an elliptical (cylindrical) shape, distention occurs primarily in a cephalic direction. The shape of the fundus influences intrauterine pressure. In a sphere, tension is a geometric function of the radius of curvature; in a cylinder, tension is a linear function (and thus is lower).[102] In the absence of contractions, intrauterine pressure peaks at midpregnancy, then decreases to less than 10 mmHg of amniotic fluid pressure as the shape of the fundus changes. The pressure remains low until term in spite of the increasing intrauterine volume. Laceration of the internal cervical os or incompetence of the cervix during the period of higher intrauterine pressure may result in "blowout" of the fetal membranes with late spontaneous abortion or preterm birth.[102]

At mid-gestation, contractions of the circular muscles of the uterus are weaker than those of the longitudinal muscles. Contractile strength increases in the circular muscles so that by term these muscles are similar to longitudinal muscles in their contractile ability. The basis for this change is thought to be differences in membranous electrical events, cell-to-cell coupling, and intracellular calcium release.[49]

MYOMETRIUM

The myometrium has two basic properties: contractility and elasticity. Contractility is the ability to lengthen and shorten. Elasticity is the ability to grow and stretch to accommodate the enlarging uterine contents, maintain uterine tonus, and permit involution following delivery.

TABLE **4-1**   **Dimensional Changes of the Uterus during Pregnancy**

	Weight (g)	Length × Weight × Depth (cm)	Capacity (ml)	Total Intrauterine Volume (cm³)
Nonpregnant	50-70	7.5 × 5 × 2.5	10	<300 (early pregnancy)
Term	800-1200	20 × 25 × 22.5	5000	4500

From Resnik, R. (1999). Anatomic alterations in the reproductive tract. In R.K. Creasy & R. Resnik (Eds.). *Maternal-fetal medicine* (4th ed.). Philadelphia: W.B. Saunders.

Myometrial Cell Structure

The contractile units of the uterus are the smooth muscle cells in a connective tissue matrix. Movement of contractile forces along the uterus occurs from transmission of tension generated by individual smooth muscle cells to other smooth muscle cells and the connective tissue matrix.[49] Uterine smooth muscles are unique in that active, synchronous contraction of these muscles occurs only during the birth process.

Myometrial cells contain three types of protein myofilaments (actin, myosin, and intermediate), microtubules, and protein structures called dense bodies. Myosin is a hexamer approximately 160 nm long and a molecular weight of 200 kilodaltons (kDa).[146] Myosin is the principal contractile protein. Myosin is laid down in thick (15 to 18 nm) myofilaments that optimize interaction with actin and generation of force.[24,63,78] Myosin filaments consist of two heavy chains arranged in a head-and-tail structure and two light chains (Figure 4-1). The helical heavy chains unite at one end of the filament to form two globular heads that protrude from the myosin at regular intervals (Figure 4-2).[54] The two light chains are bound to the head in the neck region (see Figure 4-1). The longer light chain (molecular weight 20 kDa) can bind to calcium and magnesium and be phosphorylated; the function of the smaller light chain (molecular weight 17 kDa) is unclear.[24,41,63,78] In addition to the two light chains, the myosin head also contains magnesium adenosine triphosphatase (Mg-ATPase) (an enzyme necessary for the interaction of actin and myosin and subsequent generation of force) sites and an actin binding site where the actin and myosin interact.[24,41,63,78] The helical tail, formed by the heavy chains, transmits the force (tension) generated by the interaction of myosin and actin. Myosin filaments are unidirectional and longer in smooth muscle than in striated muscle. This allows actin to interact with the myosin heads throughout the length of the myosin, increasing the maximum degree of shortening to 5 to 10 times greater than that of skeletal muscle.[24,63,78,99]

Actin is a globular protein monomer (molecular weight 45 kDa) that polymerizes into long, thin (6 to 9 nm) filaments. These filaments originate in and are distributed between dense bodies.[69] Adenosine triphosphatase (ATPase) activity on the myosin head initiates formation of crosslinks or bonds between actin and myosin. The myosin head rotates and as a result pulls on the actin filament, creating tension (force) and a relative spatial displacement (shortening).[63,78,99] Interaction of myosin and actin is illustrated in Figure 4-2.

The exact role of the intermediate fibers is not completely understood. These fibers may be involved in secretion of collagen and extracellular matrix componets.[74] The microtubules, formed by tubulin, are involved in myometrial hyperplasia and hypertrophy during pregnancy. Tubulin is a substrate for G-protein receptor kinase, a substance involved in myosin phosphorylation and downregulation of β_2-adrenoreceptors.[74] The dense protein bodies are scattered throughout the cytoplasm and on the inner surface of the cell membrane and are attached to the poles of the smooth muscle cell by intermediate (10 nm thick) filaments. The dense bodies and their filaments form a supportive structure for the contractile filaments and a network of actin attachment sites (adhesion plaques).[24,74,78] These structures enable the uterus to enlarge and generate forces sufficient for expulsion of the fetus regardless of the weight or position of the fetus.[63]

In comparison to striated muscle cells, smooth muscle cells are smaller, have a higher ratio of surface area–to–cell volume, and have less myosin. Actin filaments predominate, with approximately 11 to 15 actin filaments per myosin filament versus a 6:1 ratio in skeletal muscle.[24,78] Filaments in smooth muscle occur in random rather than regular bundles throughout the cell, and thus these muscles do not have the striated appearance seen in skeletal muscle. The myofilaments in smooth muscle are oriented obliquely to the long axis of the muscle fibers, which allows the muscle to exert a large force along a short distance at low velocity. This may account for the ability of the myometrium to sustain strong contractions over many hours.[103] The maximal force per area is similar to or greater than that of skeletal muscle.[63] In smooth muscle the pulling force can be exerted in any direction, whereas in skeletal

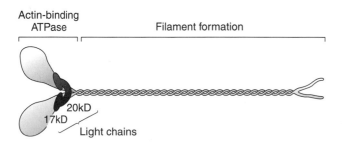

FIGURE **4-1** Schematic representation of smooth muscle myosin showing the globular head region of each 200-kD heavy chain with associated 17- and 20-kD light chain subunits and the filamentous tail region that interacts with similar regions of other myosin molecules to form the thick filament. *ATPase,* Adenosine triphosphatase. (Modified from Adelstein, R. S. & Sellers, J. R. [1996]. Myosin structure and function. In M.S. Barany [Ed.]. *Biochemistry of smooth muscle contraction.* San Diego: Academic Press.)

muscle the force generated and the resultant contraction are aligned with the axis of the muscle fibers.[24,41]

Changes during Pregnancy

Myometrial quiescence during pregnancy is mediated by increases in progesterone, relaxin, nitric oxide (NO), and prostacyclin (PGI$_2$).[78] Uterine blood flow increases during pregnancy as a result of remodeling of the spiral arteries, which results in increased vessel diameter and decreased resistance.[135] (These changes are described in Chapter 3.) The uterus is never completely quiescent; low-frequency, low-amplitude activity occurs even in the nonpregnant state.[24,78,90] The frequency of contractions increases during pregnancy with an increase of approximately 5% per week.[95] Diurnal periodicity has been reported with increased frequency at night (five to six per hour) and lowered frequency in the early afternoon (two to three per hour) near term.[81,95] Initially these contractions tend to be mild, irregular, nonsynchronized, and focal in origin and are generally not felt by the pregnant woman. As pregnancy progresses, contractions become more intense and frequent and more are felt by the woman. With the onset of labor, contractions become regular, coordinated, and intense as individual myometrial cells contract in harmony. The contractile force is about five times greater in the pregnant than in the nonpregnant myometrium. Synchronous contraction of the uterus is dependent on formation of gap junctions.[49,90]

Alterations in the character of uterine contractions are due to structural and functional changes in the myometrium as a result of the extended estrogen-progesterone environment of pregnancy. These changes include the following:

1. *Change in the velocity and timing of action potentials.* In the nonpregnant uterus, action potentials occur at the peak of a contraction at a velocity of about 6 cm/second. In pregnancy the action potential occurs much closer to the beginning of the contraction wave and at 1 to 2 cm/second.
2. *Hypertrophy and hyperplasia of the myometrial cells, with increased contractile proteins, under the influence of estrogen.*
3. *Increased sensitivity of the myometrium to the effects of myosin light-chain kinase phosphorylation*
4. *Alteration in the arrangement of muscle bundles.* In pregnancy these bundles are arranged in closer contact enhancing gap junction formation.
5. *Development of the sarcoplasmic reticulum.* This enhances calcium movement
6. *Increased number of mitochondria and cellular ATP.* This enhances energy production by the myometrial cell.[49,64,73,90,94]

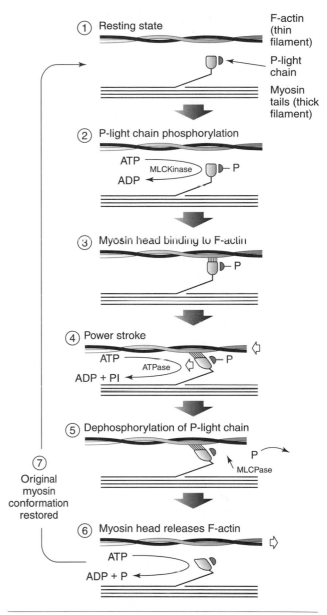

FIGURE **4-2** Mechanisms of smooth muscle contraction and relaxation. (1) Myosin light chain kinase (MLCKinase), activated by calcium-calmodulin complex, phosphorylates P-light chain on the myosin head (2). This results in activation and binding of myosin head with F-actin (3) and adenosine triphosphate (ATP) hydrolysis by myosin adenosine triphosphatase (ATPase). The myosin head undergoes a conformational change while it is bound to the actin filament. Movement of actin filament is powered by adenosine diphosphate (ADP) release and myosin conformational change (4). Myosin light chain phosphatase (MLCPase) phosphorylates the P-light chain (5) resulting in inhibition of both myosin ATPase and binding of the myosin head with F-actin (6). Binding of an ATP molecule to the myosin head results in restoration of the original conformation of myosin (7) resulting in relaxation. (From Nuwayhid, B. & Rahabi, M. [1987]. Beta-sympathomimetic agents: Use in perinatal obstetrics. *Clin Perinatol, 14,* 757.)

Near labor onset the myometrial contractile capacity increases via a process called *myometrial activation* (see Parturition).[21] There is enhanced communication among the cells of the uterus at term, so that the action potential covers the entire uterus in 2 to 3 seconds, resulting in nearly simultaneous contraction of the myometrium. This phenomenon may result from the increased velocity of the action potentials, the closer arrangement of muscle bundles with gap junction formation, and the increased number of muscle cells.[49,95]

CERVIX

During pregnancy the cervix increases in mass, water content, and vascularization. The connective tissue of the uterus (particularly the cervix) undergoes changes in its viscoelastic plasticity so that, by term, "it combines the properties of a rubber band with those of saltwater taffy."[102] Myometrial contractions exert a slow, steady pull on the cervix, resulting in cervical stretching but with little rebound between contractions. This leads to progressive cervical dilatation. In order for the fetus to be expelled, the cervix must first change from a relatively rigid to a soft, distensible structure.

Structure

The cervix is composed primarily of an extracellular connective tissue matrix covered by a thin cellular layer of smooth muscle and fibroblasts that penetrate into the connective tissue matrix.[76,111] Approximately 85% to 90% of the cervix is connective tissue matrix and 10% to 15% is smooth muscle.[24,67,102,142] The amount of smooth muscle varies in the upper (25%), middle (16%), and lower (6%) portions of the cervix. The extracellular matrix is made from substances secreted by the fibroblasts.[4] This matrix consists of a dense network of interlacing collagen and elastin fibers embedded in a gel-like ground substance (proteoglycans).

The collagen fibers form a relatively rigid rod-shaped structure (important during pregnancy to retain the fetus) and impart tensile strength to the cervix.[24] Collagen fibers can be of the cross-striated type I (70%) or the reticular type II (30%). The collagen fibers are arranged in cross-linked triple helices. The cross-linking protects the collagen fibers from being broken down by collagenase and proteases.[76] Elastin is haphazardly arranged parallel to and between collagen fibers, imparting elasticity to the cervical tissue and contributing to the integrity of the tissue.[49,76,142] The elastin-to-collagen ratio is greatest at the internal os.[67] Elastin can stretch in any direction to twice its length and thus may be important in the ability of the cervix to distend in labor and then return to its normal shape after parturition.[76,90,142]

The ground substance (proteoglycans) is composed of glycosaminoglycans attached to a glycoprotein core. The major glycosaminoglycans in the cervix are dermatan sulfate (70%), heparan sulfate (15%), and hyaluronic acid (15%).[24,67,142] These substances are large charged molecules that bind together, attract water, and coil around and lock the collagen fibrils in place.[24]

Changes during Pregnancy

Cervical changes are noted throughout pregnancy. In the nonpregnant cervix, collagen fibers are in bundles forming cable-like structures. During the second trimester the bundles become less dense with thinner and more loosely packed fibers.[76] Hyaluronic acid (which has a high affinity for water) and cervical water content increase.[76] The total collagen increases and is remodeled to maintain cervical integrity. However, the relative amount of collagen decreases 30% to 50% as a result of increases in other proteins and in the water content of the extracellular matrix.[67,142] There is no change in elastin, but its precursor (tropoelastin) increases.[67] Decorin, a dermatan sulfate, increases during later pregnancy and labor.[67,76,110,142] Decorin separates the collagen fibrils, increasing fibril dispersion and disorganization.[67] Smooth muscles cells in the cervix enlarge, then later undergo programmed cell death at term.[67,76]

Fibroblasts, leukocytes, macrophages, and eosinophils proliferate in the cervix during pregnancy. These changes may be important in altering vasopermeability to increase cervical water content and in secretion of proteases for cervical ripening. The fibroblasts are also involved in the metabolism of collagen and glycosaminoglycans.[67,142] Fibronectin, which is different from fetal fibronectin (see Preterm Labor), is also found in the cervix and decreases at labor onset.[67,76] Fibronectin may act as a "biologic glue."[75] Collagenase activity increases threefold, beginning as early as 10 weeks; elastase activity increases toward the end of pregnancy and after parturition.

Cervical Ripening and Dilatation

The rigid cervix of pregnancy must become distensible in order to expel the fetus.[24] Cervical ripening (softening, effacement, and increased distensibility) begins about 4 weeks before delivery and involves changes in collagen, proteoglycans, and smooth muscle with enzymatic degradation of collagen.[102,137,142] Myometrial contractions have little effect on cervical ripening.[24]

Factors involved in the maintenance of cervical integrity during pregnancy and cervical ripening at the end of pregnancy are summarized in Figure 4-3. These include changes in matrix metalloproteinases (MMPs), synthesis of extra-

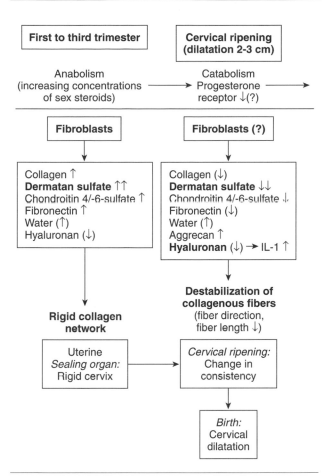

FIGURE 4-3 Biochemical model for cervical ripening during pregnancy. (From Winkler, M. & Werner, R. [1999]. Changes in the cervical extracellular matrix during pregnancy and parturition. *J Perinat Med, 27,* 57.)

cellular matrix proteins, increased collagen turnover, disruption of collagen fibrils, increase in the decorin-to-collagen ratio, increased hyaluronic acid and cervical water content, and infiltration of the cervix by neutrophils and macrophages.[31] These processes are mediated by cytokines such as interleukin-1 (IL-1), interleukin-6 (IL-6), interleukin-8 (IL-8), and tumor necrosis factor–α (TNF-α). IL-1 and TNF-α alter the adhesiveness of vascular epithelium.[142] IL-6 increases PG and leukotriene (LT) production. This dilates cervical blood vessels and enhances movement of neutrophils into the cervix. IL-8 increases neutrophil chemotaxis.[142] NO in the cervix increases near term and may act with PGE_2 to induce cervical vasodilatation and neutrophil infiltration, and may regulate MMP activation.[31,32]

Collagen is degraded by MMPs such as collagenase, elastase, and other nonspecific proteolytic enzymes, resulting in a loss of collagen fibrils. The MMP system is a series of proteins that, with zinc as a cofactor, act in a cascade to degrade collagen.[67] Both MMPs and MMP inhibitors increase during pregnancy. During most of pregnancy these are in balance, but in late pregnancy there is a net increase in MMPs, leading to collagen degradation and cervical ripening.[110] Hyaluronic acid stimulates MMP production in the cervix and neutrophil chemotaxis.[76] Neutrophils and macrophages also secrete MMP. MMP activity is enhanced by IL-1 and IL-8.[10] Hyaluronic acid (which loosely binds collagen fibrils) increases by 50% with labor onset, then decreases rapidly after delivery, accompanied by a decrease in dermatan sulfates, especially decorin (which tightly binds collagen fibrils), and an increase in the water content of the cervix.[67,76] This weakens the structure of the cervix by decreasing the cross bridges between collagen fibers.

A proposed mechanism for the process of cervical ripening and dilatation is illustrated in Figure 4-4. In summary, cervical ripening involves an inflammatory cascade with release of proinflammatory cytokines (e.g., IL-1, IL-6, IL-8, TNF-α), leading to infiltration of the cervix by leukocytes and macrophages, which releases and activates MMP. MMPs alter the synthesis of extracellular matrix proteins, increase collagen turnover, and retention of water.[37] As a result, collagen is degraded and collagen fibers are disrupted and dispersed.

Hormonal control of cervical ripening is a complex process that involves a cascade of changes in estradiol, progesterone, relaxin, PGI_2, PGE_2, and $PGF_{2\alpha}$, mediated NO, and cytokines.[24,31,32,102] Progesterone inhibits collagen breakdown. Alterations in the estrogen-to-progesterone ratio correlate with increased procollagenase activity, collagen degradation, and apoptosis (programmed cell death).[23,67] Increased cervical relaxin may activate collagen peptidase and mediate changes in water and mucopolysaccharide content of the cervix.[24] Uterine activity is enhanced by mechanical stretching of the cervix (Ferguson reflex). This response may be due to the effects of $PGF_{2\alpha}$ and oxytocin release stimulated by cervical stretching.[67]

PGE_2 and $PGF_{2\alpha}$ have a localized influence on cervical softening. PGE_2 action on the cervix is independent of uterine contractile activity and is used to improve cervical inductability (i.e., responsiveness of the cervical tissue) before induction of labor (e.g., when delivery is indicated because of risk factors). PGE_2 dilates small blood vessels in the cervix—increasing leukocyte extravasation—and stimulates neutrophil chemotaxis.[78]

PARTURITION

"Parturition is a multifactorial physiological process that involves multiple interconnected positive feedforward and

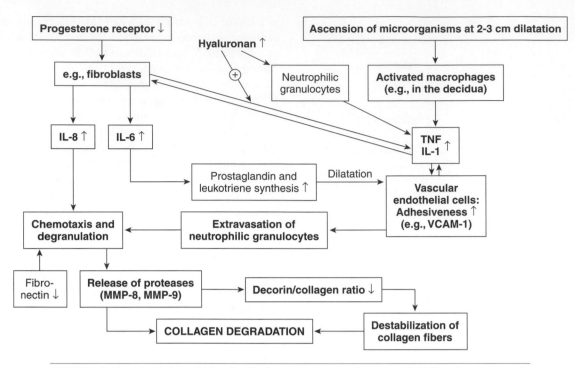

FIGURE **4-4** Hypothetical model for the biochemical changes during cervical dilatation at term. *IL,* Interleukin; *MMP,* matrix metalloproteinase; *VCAM,* vascular cell adhesion molecule. (From Winkler, M. & Werner, R. [1999]. Changes in the cervical extracellular matrix during pregnancy and parturition. *J Perinat Med, 27,* 58.)

negative feedback loops. Each of these loops is connected to others in a carefully time-regulated fashion. When parturition occurs normally, both maternal and fetal processes are involved."[96]

Initiation of Labor

Initiation of labor involves a complex interplay of maternal and fetal factors whose specific interrelationships and significance are still not completely understood. Challis and colleagues have proposed that parturition is divided into four phases: (1) phase 0, *quiescence;* (2) phase 1, *activation;* (3) phase 2, *stimulation;* and (4) phase 3, *involution* (Figure 4-5).[25,28] Phase 0 occurs for 95% of pregnancy. During this phase, progesterone and other uterotonic inhibitors— including PgI$_2$, relaxin, NO, and parathyroid hormone– related peptide (PTHrP)—maintain myometrial quiescence. Casey and MacDonald note that "the physiological investments that must be made to maintain uterine phase 0 are enormous . . . all types of biomolecular systems (neural, endocrine, paracrine, and apocrine), which can call upon multiple cell signaling processes, are implemented and coordinated to impose contractile unresponsiveness on the myometrium, which is ordinarily disposed to spontaneous contractions."[21]

Phase 1, activation, accounts for about 5% of pregnancy.[21] During this phase, levels of uterotonic inhibitors decrease, whereas estrogen and contraction-associated proteins (CAPs) increase. CAPs include gap junction proteins (particularly connexin 43) and myometrial oxytocin receptors, PG receptors (especially PGF receptors), calcium channels, and some sodium channels.[25,28,78] Activation involves an increase in expression of genes that encode CAPs. The fetal genome and maturation of the fetal hypothalamic-pituitary-adrenal system (see Figure 18-10) mediate this process. Fetal and placental corticotrophin-releasing hormone are increased, stimulating production of estrogens and thus changing the hormonal milieu.[28,42,58,60,77,78,83] These changes increase myometrial excitability; responsiveness to uterotonics (e.g., PGs, oxytocin); and electrical coupling.[24,31,32,51,78]

Chwalisz and Garfield describe myometrial activation as part of a conditioning or preparatory stage during which there is activation of uterine contractility, cervical ripening, and activation of fetal membranes (Figure 4-6).[32] The preparatory or activation stage involves interaction of the uterus, cervix, and fetal membranes and involves endocrine, immune and neural control mechanisms.[31,32] Activation has also been called "uterine awakening."[21] Once

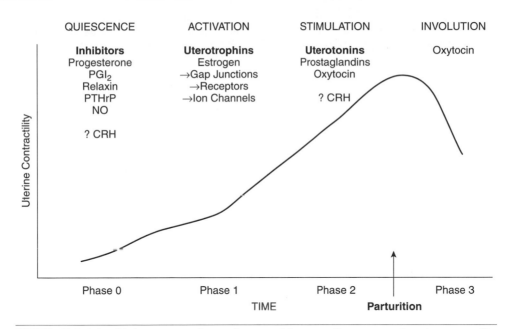

FIGURE **4-5** Relationship between regulators of myometrial contractility, patterns of uterine contractility and time in relation to the onset of parturition. *CRH,* Corticotrophin-releasing hormone; *NO,* nitric oxide; *PGI₂,* prostacyclin; *PTHrP,* parathyroid hormone–related peptide. (From Challis, J.R.G. [1999]. Characteristics of parturition. In R.K. Creasy & R. Resnik [Eds.]. *Maternal-fetal medicine* [4th ed.]. Philadelphia: W.B. Saunders.)

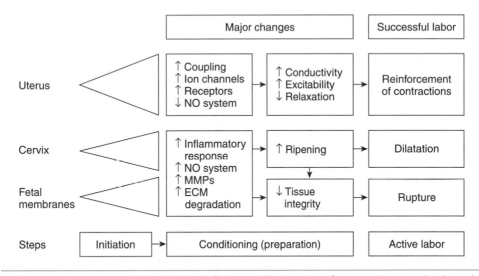

FIGURE **4-6** Proposed model of parturition defining conditioning phase for uterus (myometrium), cervix, and fetal membranes. (From Chwalisz, K. & Garfield, R.E. [1998]. Role of nitric oxide in the uterus and cervix: Implications for the management of labor. *J Perinat Med, 26,* 449.)

myometrial activation has occurred, current tocolytics may not be effective to suppress contractions.[78] During phase 1, myometrial contractions become more regular, with higher frequency and amplitude.[25] The transition from phase 0 to phase 1 is a gradual process over the last few weeks of pregnancy.[21,28]

Phase 2, which accounts for about 0.2% of pregnancy, involves stimulation of the myometrium by uterotonics, primarily PGs and oxytocin, and initiation of coordinated forceful contractions.[21,28] Once labor is initiated, myometrial contraction and relaxation proceed via the enzymatic phosphorylation and dephosphorylation of myosin and subsequent promotion and inhibition of myosin-actin in-

teraction. Phase 3, involution (see Chapter 5), is primarily mediated by oxytocin.[25,28,78]

Thus labor is a phenomenon that depends on complicated interaction between the fetus and mother. A proposed mechanism for the initiation of labor at term is illustrated in Figure 4-7. This interaction factor can be altered by stress, infection, hemorrhage and other factors leading to preterm labor.[69,71,72,83] Endocrine, paracrine and other factors believed to influential in the onset of labor are described in this section. Although knowledge of factors involved in maintaining myometrial quiescence and in myometrial activation has increased significantly in recent years, the exact stimulus for labor onset still remains unknown.[98,101,128]

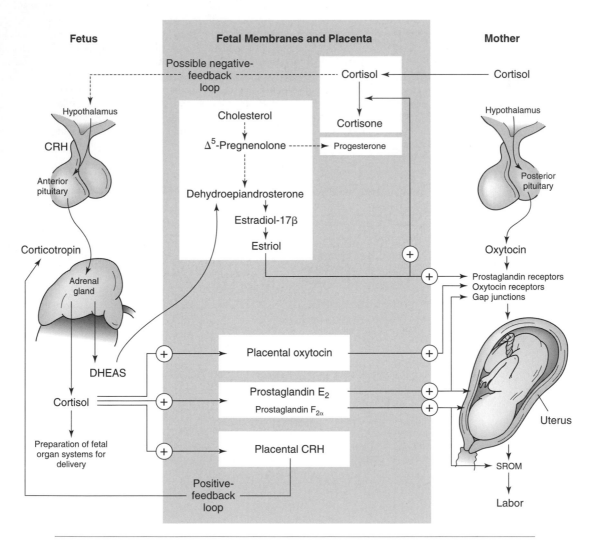

FIGURE **4-7** Proposed mechanism of labor induction at term. *CRH,* Corticotrophin-releasing hormone; *DHEAS,* dehydroepiandrosterone sulfate; *SROM,* spontaneous rupture of membranes; + signs indicate activation or upregulation. (From Norwitz, E.R., et al. [1999]. The control of labor: Current concepts. *N Engl J Med, 341,* 660.)

Corticotrophin-Releasing Hormone

In recent years, there has been much interest in the role of corticotrophin-releasing hormone (CRH) in both term and preterm labor onset.[27,28,42,43,79,82,83,112,118] CRH is a neuropeptide first discovered in 1980 and produced primarily in the hypothalamus and by the placenta during pregnancy. Placental CRH increases before labor onset with increased levels found in the maternal and fetal circulations.[86] Placental CRH concentrations increase up to 50- to 100-fold in the last 6 to 8 weeks of gestation, paralleling the increase in fetal cortisol.[43,82,83] CRH is also produced by the endometrium, decidua, chorion, and amnion. CRH receptors are found on myometrium, and stimulation of these receptors may enhance myometrial contractility. CRH receptors are also found in the decidua and fetal membranes.[43,82]

In the mother, serum CRH (probably primarily from the placenta) increases steadily to 35 weeks, then increases markedly with the onset of labor.[43,82] Before 35 weeks, most of the CRH is neutralized by binding to CRH-binding protein produced in the maternal liver, placenta, decidua, amnion, and chorion.[30,43] Levels of this binding protein decrease 60% after 34 to 35 weeks with an increase in free (physiologically active) CRH to term.[30] In addition, NO inhibits placental CRH production.[132] CRH levels are maximal at the end of labor, decreasing by 50% in the first 20 to 30 minutes after birth and to prepregnancy levels by 1 to 5 days after parturition.[43,82] An inverse relationship between CRH and duration of labor has been reported.[30,132] Levels of CRH in the second trimester have been associated with later preterm or postterm delivery.[10,66,87] CRH levels are increased in pregnancies complicated by pregnancy-induced hypertension and intrauterine growth restriction (IUGR).[27,53,140]

CRH is also involved in increased placental estriol production and increased fetal glucocorticoid production.[79,83] Placental CRH is thought to stimulate fetal ACTH, which in turn stimulates the fetal adrenal cortex to produce glucocorticoids such as cortisol and dehydroepiandrosterone (DHEAS).[83,115,131] DHEAS is needed by the placenta to produce estrogens, particularly estriol. Cortisol stimulates fetal lung maturation (see Chapter 9) and also stimulates further placental CRH production. This is in contrast to the effect of increased cortisol on the hypothalamus, where it has an inhibitory effect. In the placenta, glucocorticoids stimulate CRH receptors and increase CHR production.[43,82,83]

Increased cortisol also stimulates PG synthesis by increasing prostaglandin-H-synthetase-2 (PGHS-2) and decreasing PG catabolism by decreasing 15-hydroxyprostoglandin dehydrogenase (PGDH).[27] PGDH activity in pregnancy may be maintained by activation of glucocorticoid receptors (GRs), which respond to both progesterone or cortisol. Near labor onset the increased cortisol displaces progesterone from the GRs. This inhibits PGDH activity and production.[27]

Progesterone

Progesterone has a major role in controlling the uterus and cervix and suppressing uterine excitement throughout gestation.[51] Progesterone acts by interaction with cell membrane receptors to stimulate cyclic adenosine monophosphate (cAMP), which, along with cyclic guanosine 3'-5'-monophosphate (cGMP), sequesters intracellular calcium in the sarcoplasmic reticulum (SR), thus decreasing contractility.[138] Progesterone works in conjunction with NO to downregulate genes needed to produce the CAPs needed for labor.[31,97]

Antiprogesterone compounds can induce labor in humans at any stage of gestation.[48,49,80] Although human labor is not preceded by a significant fall in maternal serum progesterone, increases in placental estrogen production near term increase the estrogen-to-progesterone ratio with a net estrogenic effect.[22] Localized decreases in progesterone may be caused by increased activity of a progesterone-binding protein induced by increased estrogen near term. Decreased availability of progesterone to the myometrial cells allows estrogen effects to dominate.

Estrogen

Estrogen levels rise beginning at 34 to 35 weeks. Estrogens promote formation of gap junctions; increase oxytocin and estrogen receptors in the myometrium; enhance lipase activity and release of arachidonic acid, thus stimulating PG production; increase binding of intracellular calcium; and increase myosin phosphorylation.[22,24,44,49,57] Estrogen (particularly estriol) production by the placenta (see Chapter 3 and Figure 3-19) is dependent on fetal adrenal precursors. The placenta produces over 90% of the estriol in pregnancy. DHEAS from the fetal adrenal is hydroxylated to 25-OH-DHEAS in the fetal liver. 25-OH-DHEAS is used by the placenta to produce estriol.[57] Increased CRH stimulates ACTH to increased DHEAS output by the fetal adrenal, which leads to increased estrogen in late gestation.[57] Concentrations of estradiol and estrone in amniotic fluid increase 15 to 20 days before onset of either term or preterm labor. Estrone produced locally in the chorion and decidua may influence the intrauterine progesterone-to-estrogen ratio, promote production of stimulatory PG ($PGF_{2\alpha}$), decrease production of inhibitory PG (PGI_2), and promote formation of oxytocin and PG receptors as well as gap junction formation.[24]

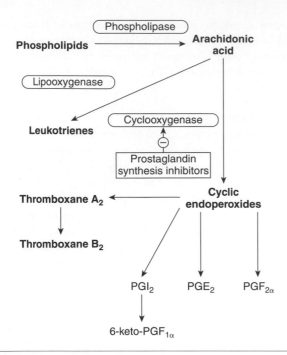

FIGURE **4-8** Metabolism of arachidonic acid and the formation of prostaglandins. (From Holbrook, R.H. & Ueland, K. [1989]. Endocrinology of parturition and preterm labor. In S.A. Brody & K. Ueland [Eds.]. *Endocrine disorders in pregnancy.* Norwalk, CT: Appleton & Lange.)

Prostaglandins

PGs (Figure 4-8 and the box below) are produced in the decidua and fetal membranes and have a central role in the initiation of labor.[7,20,26,62,110,112] PGs bind to the cell membrane, increase the frequency of action potentials, and stimulate actual muscle contraction. Levels of PGE_2 and $PGF_{2\alpha}$ increase before and during labor; mediate labor onset through their role in the formation of gap junctions and activation of the decidua and fetal membranes; and induce contractility by increasing calcium levels in the cytoplasm of myometrial smooth muscle cells.[58] PGE_2 is also involved in ripening of the cervix.[62,137]

The role of the decidua, amnion, and chorion in PG synthesis is summarized in Figure 4-9. The amnion is a major site of PG synthesis with high levels of PGHS and minimal PGDH. The decidua also has high levels of PGHS and minimal PGDH. PGDH predominates in the chorion, located between the amnion and decidua.[26,110,112,114] PGHS is found in two forms. One form is always present for normal homeostasis; the other form is generated by macrophages and can be induced by cytokines, growth factors, and glucocorticoids.[75] Activity of this latter form increases with both term and preterm labor onset.[26,122] Cyclooxygenases (COX) are enzymes needed for converting arachidonic acid to PGs. COX-I is predominately found in fetal cardiovascular tis-

---

Prostaglandins

Prostaglandins (PGs) are organic compounds that act as intermediaries, exerting their major effect at the subcellular level at or near the site of production. PGs are usually metabolized locally but may enter the blood to be rapidly inactivated by pulmonary and hepatic enzymes. PGs are classified into subgroups based on the configuration of their 5-carbon ring. PGE_2, $PGF_{2\alpha}$, and prostacyclin (PGI_2) are the most important in reproductive processes. During pregnancy, PGs are needed for maternal cardiovascular changes, including preventing hypertension and increasing uteroplacental blood flow, and in cervical ripening and the initiation of labor. PGs are synthesized rapidly, are relatively unstable, and have a short half-life. PGs are formed by enzymatic oxidation of arachidonic acid, a polyunsaturated fatty acid precursor found in an esterified form (glycophospholipid). Formation of PG requires that arachidonic acid be changed to a nonesterified form either directly by cellular phospholipase A_2 or indirectly by phospholipase C. Nonesterified arachidonic acid can be further metabolized by specific microsomal or cytosolic enzymes via several pathways (including cyclooxygenases and lipoxygenases), as illustrated in Figure 4-6.

There are two forms of cyclooxygenase: COX-I and COX-II. COX-1 is normally produced to maintain physiologic homeostasis; COX-II is inductable by exogenous signals such as myometrial activation or infection. PGs and thromboxane A^2 (TXA_2) are formed via the cyclooxygenase pathway under the influence of prostaglandin synthetase and thromboxane synthetase. TXA_2 is a platelet aggregation factor and vasoconstrictor whose actions are balanced by the opposing actions of PGI_2. Nonsteroidal antiinflammatory agents such as aspirin and indomethacin inhibit formation of PGs and TXA_2, which block cyclooxygenase activity. Since PGs mediate the action of the hypothalamus in responding to pyrogens released during an infection, aspirin effectively reduces fever. Arachidonic acid metabolism via the lipoxygenase pathway leads to the production of various acids followed by the formation of leukotrienes (LTs). Leukotrienes are chemotaxic and chemokinetic for leukocytes. PGs act on G-protein coupled receptors tied to different effector systems. There are eight subtypes of PG receptors found in different tissues: TXA_2, PGI_2, PGF, PGD, and four types of PGE receptors.[4,26,62,137]

sues; levels remain constant during pregnancy. COX-II, produced in the fetal membranes and myometrium, increases to term with further marked increase in labor.[138]

PGs act by interacting with cell membrane receptors that are coupled with G-proteins (see the box below) and tied to different effector substances.[4] The myometrium contains all types of PG receptors. Activation of PGF, thromboxane A_2 (TXA_2), PGE_1 (increases intracellular calcium), and PGE_3 receptors (inhibits adenyl cyclase) stimulates contractions. Activation of PGD, PGE_2 (stimulates adenyl cyclase), and PGI_2 receptors inhibits contractions.[4,46] In the amnion the major PG is PGE_2; the decidua produces large amounts of PGI_2 and to a lesser extent $PGF_{2\alpha}$ and PGE_2. The placenta produces PGE_2, PGD_2, PGI_2, and TXA_2. Following delivery, placental TXA_2 may be important in enhancing hemostasis after placental separation.[44]

PGI_2 is produced by the pregnant and the nonpregnant myometrium as well as by the placental vasculature; it helps maintain uterine quiescence.[78] PGI_2 increases in late pregnancy and with uterine distention by the fetus.[78] PGI_2 is a potent vasodilator that inhibits platelet aggregation and protects the vascular epithelium. PGI_2 is important in maintaining blood flow to the placenta and in ensuring adequate uterine blood flow during labor.[24] Suppression of PGI_2 formation leads to vasoconstriction and is thought to have a role in preeclampsia (see Chapter 8). Throboxanes are platelet aggregation factors and potent vasoconstrictors that oppose the action of PGI_2. Increased placental TXA_2 is also implicated in the pathogenesis of preeclampsia because production is blocked by PG synthetase inhibitors (see Figure 4-8).

Oxytocin

Oxytocin is produced not only by the posterior lobe of maternal and fetal pituitary glands, but also by the myometrium, decidua, placenta and fetal membranes.[29,36,45,92,106]

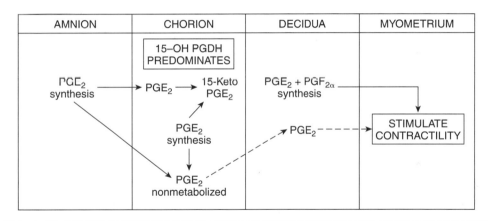

FIGURE **4-9** Compartmentalization of prostaglandin (PG) synthesis and metabolism within the human fetal membranes, decidua, and myometrium in late gestation. (From Challis, J.R.G. [1999]. Characteristics of parturition. In R.K. Creasy & R. Resnik [Eds.]. *Maternal-fetal medicine* [4th ed.]. Philadelphia: W.B. Saunders.)

G-Proteins

Hormones, prostaglandins and other substances act on the myometrium by interacting with specific cell membrane receptors. Many of these receptor are G-protein coupled effectors. Guanosyl triphosphate binding proteins (G-proteins) are membrane-associated proteins with multiple subtypes that help convert extracellular signals into intracellular effects via coupling of receptors to effectors.[100] G-proteins are important in myometrial relaxation and contraction.[42] These proteins couple the receptors to effectors. The main G-protein effectors that convert extracellular signal to intracellular effects are: (1) voltage-dependent ion channels; (2) adenyl cyclase (generates cAMP); phospholipase C (generates inositol 1,4,5-triphosphate [InsP2] and 1,2-diacylglyceride [DAG]); and (4) phospholipase A2 (arachidonic acid production).[46] InsP3 releases calcium from the SR and DAG activates protein kinase C.[46,73,96] Thus some G-proteins increase camp, leading to myometrial relaxation. This type of G-protein increases in pregnancy and decreases with labor onset.[74] Other G-proteins lead to a reduction in cAMP and thus myometrial contraction.[74]

Under the influence of estrogen, the sensitivity of the myometrium to the effects of oxytocin changes markedly during pregnancy. Alterations in myometrial sensitivity to oxytocin are mediated by changes in the density and affinity of oxytocin receptors.[22,43,56,73,93] Oxytocin receptors in the myometrium increase 30- to 100-fold in the first trimester and up to 300-fold by term.[116,150] Oxytocin receptors are also found in the decidua and endometrium, but these decrease during pregnancy.[56,92] Oxytocin receptors are G-protein–coupled receptors whose effects are mediated by phospholipase C, which mediates production of nonesterified arachidonic acid and thus PGs. This increases inositol 1,4,5-triphosphate (InsP3), which increases intracellular calcium and thus myometrial contractility.[4,73,93,107] Binding of oxytocin to receptors on the cell membrane increases the frequency of pacemaker potentials and lowers the threshold for initiation of action potentials. Failed induction and postdate pregnancies are associated with a decreased concentration of oxytocin receptors. Oxytocin is a stimulant that is often used to induce or augment labor. Oxytocin does not work well as a labor stimulant for induction of labor before term, possibly due to the lack of adequate oxytocin receptors. Some but not all women with preterm labor are reported to have an increase in oxytocin receptors.[56]

Relaxin

Relaxin is an insulin-like ovarian hormone produced primarily by the corpus luteum but also by the myometrium, decidua, and placenta. Relaxin levels are greatest during the first trimester but remain detectable in maternal circulation throughout gestation, falling rapidly after delivery.[22,24] Relaxin decreases affinity of myosin light chain kinase for calmodulin and myosin and activates potassium channels. Activation of these channels hyperpolarizes the membrane with uterine relaxation.[78] Relaxin acts synergistically with progesterone in blocking uterine activity and maintaining myometrial quiescence during pregnancy and may suppress oxytocin release.[44] Relaxin enhances cervical ripening and may help regulate gap junction permeability.[149]

Nitric Oxide

NO is produced by the decidua, fetal membranes, placental syncytiotrophoblast, and fetal and placental vascular epithelium.[129] NO is thought to be important in maintaining myometrial quiescence, cervical rigidity, and maternal systemic vasodilatation during pregnancy and in regulating fetal and uteroplacental blood flow.[17,38,51,87,129] Levels of NO are elevated in the myometrium but not in the cervix during pregnancy. NO and progesterone are thought to work together as gene regulators to downregulate the genes needed for CAPs production for parturition.[31,97] NO relaxes

the myometrium and maintains cervical rigidity.[32] Near term, levels of NO decrease in the uterus and increase in the cervix. In the myometrium, NO increases cGMP and thus uterine relaxation.[31,38,75,78,97,109] Therefore a fall in NO is thought to be involved in initiation of labor, whereas an increase in NO is thought to help cervical ripening.[32]

NO synthesis is mediated by nitric oxide synthetase (NOS). NOS isoforms found in the fetal membranes and decidua may have different roles during pregnancy: bNOS enhances uterine quiescence, eNOS is important in uteroplacental and fetal circulation, and iNOS plays a role is cervical ripening.[38,109] Levels of NOS in the uterus decrease near term and disappear in labor.[39,147]

Cytokines and Other Factors

Cytokines such as IL-1, IL-6, IL-8, TNF-α, and transforming growth factor B (TGF-B) play important roles in mediating the events of parturition. IL-1 stimulates PG production by the amnion, deciduas, and myometrium; IL-6 stimulates PG production by the amnion, chorion, and decidua; and IL-8 induces neutrophil chemotaxis and activation.[40,85] TNF-α also stimulates PG production by the amnion and decidua.[40,75] TGF-B is involved in regulating the effects of progesterone on PTHrP, connexin 43, and gap junction formation.[21] Urocortin is a placental peptide similar in structure and function to CRH.[112] Other peptides produced by the placenta and fetal membranes that act as signaling agents include activin A, activin B, and inhibin. Activin A increases in maternal blood during pregnancy and is thought to be produced by the placenta. Activin B increases in amniotic fluid and is found in cord blood. Activin A may stimulate production of uretotonics.[105] Endothelin levels and receptors also increase during pregnancy.[16,38] Endothelin is a peptide that modulates fetoplacental circulation and enhances myometrial contractility by increasing intracellular calcium and myosin light chain phosphorylation.[16,38]

Myometrial Contraction

Myometrial contraction is mediated via interaction of actin and myosin. In smooth muscle such as myometrium, contraction and relaxation are regulated primarily via enzymatic phosphorylation and dephosphorylation of myosin. The key enzyme is myosin light chain kinase (MLCK), the principal control mechanism for smooth muscle contractility.[111] Activity of MLCK is regulated by calcium, calmodulin, and cAMP–mediated phosphorylation, which are in turn influenced by hormones and pharmacologic agents. The mechanisms for myometrial smooth muscle contraction are described below and summarized in Figure 4-10.

Initiation of action potentials in uterine muscle is primarily dependent on the influx of Ca^{2+} across the cell membrane, although other ions such as Na^+ may also be involved. Intracellular calcium is essential for activation of MLCK, and calcium levels increase significantly with contractions. MLCK is associated with the long light chain of myosin and is activated by changes in intracellular calcium. Excitation of the myometrial cell increases concentrations of free calcium in the cytoplasm.[24,49] The calcium may be released from intracellular stores in the sarcoplasmic reticulum. InsP3 mediates this release. Because calcium stores in the sarcoplasmic reticulum are relatively sparse, calcium from other sources (i.e., intracellular membrane-bound calcium vesicles, mitochondrial stores, or extracellular calcium) is also required.[49,63,78]

Mechanisms for transport of extracellular calcium across the cell membrane include: (1) voltage-dependent Ca^{2+} channels activated by electrical charge, (2) ATP-dependent pumps (via Ca,Mg-ATPase), (3) Na^+-Ca^{2+} exchange across the membrane, and (4) receptor-controlled calcium channels (activated by second messengers).[9,111,235] Magnesium may trigger further intracellular calcium release. Voltage-dependent channels allow passage of calcium when the potential across the cell membrane falls to a critical level. In smooth muscles the action potential is carried by calcium, rather than sodium as in nerve cells. Repolarization involves movement of K^+ into the myocyte and inactivation of the calcium channels.[111] These channels are G-protein coupled (see the box on p. 141). Movement of calcium across these channels can be blocked by calcium antagonists or slow channel blockers such as nifedipine. Receptor-operated channels are less specific and are not effectively blocked by calcium antagonists but can be controlled by drugs acting directly on receptors.[78]

Intracellular free calcium levels must be 10^{-6} to 10^{-7} M for MLCK activation.[41,78] Although the amount of free calcium is critical in determining whether or not the muscle

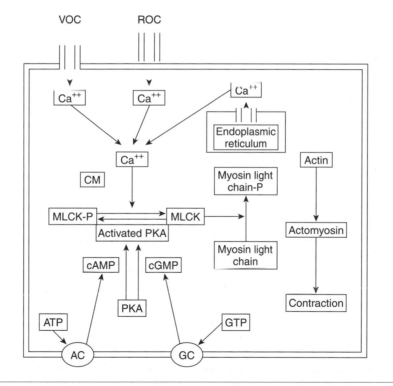

FIGURE **4-10** Biochemistry of myometrial contraction and relaxation. Myosin light chain kinase *(MLCK)* is the central molecule regulating uterine contractility. It is activated by calcium *(Ca⁺⁺)* bound to calmodulin *(CM)*. Cytoplasmic calcium concentration is the result of calcium released from deposits in the endoplasmic reticulum plus the influx of extracellular calcium through channels that are voltage operated or receptor operated. MLCK is deactivated by protein kinase A *(PKA)*, which in turn is activated by cAMP and cGMP. Beta agonists inhibit uterine contractions by activating adenyl cyclase *(AC)* with formation of cAMP, whereas nitric oxide has the same effect by activating guanylate cyclase *(GC)* and increasing production of cGMP. Calcium channel blockers relax muscle by inhibiting calcium influx through voltage-operated channels *(VOCs)*. P, Phosphorus; *ROC*, receptor-operated channel. (From Arias, F. [2000]. Pharmacology of oxytocin and prostaglandins. *Clin Obstet Gynecol, 43*, 457.)

contracts or relaxes, calcium does not act independently. Calcium must first bind with calmodulin, forming a calcium-calmodulin complex, which in turn activates MLCK.[24,63,99] Calmodulin is a cytoplasmic regulatory protein that is activated by increases in unbound intracellular calcium.[24] Calcium binding to calmodulin changes its configuration so calmodulin can modulate the activities of enzymes and protein such as MLCK.[146] Activated MLCK catalyzes phosphorylation (addition of a phosphate group) of the myosin light chain. Phosphorylation activates the ATPase on the myosin head with the release of chemical energy needed for the subsequent binding of myosin and actin (actomyosin). The result is release of ADP and a phosphorus molecule, which changes the configuration of the myosin with flexion of the head on the tail. This flexion pulls on the actin filament and the muscle contracts (see Figure 4-2).[24,63,73,78,99]

Myometrial relaxation occurs when calcium is removed. As soon as intracellular Ca^{2+} levels increase, mechanisms to remove calcium are stimulated.[6] These mechanisms include uptake by the SR, extrusion across the cell membrane, and decreased MLCK sensitivity to calcium.[73] Relaxation involves the action of the enzyme, myosin light chain phosphatase. With removal of the phosphate group from the myosin head, the actin no longer recognizes the myosin. Actin-myosin interaction is inhibited and the muscle cell relaxes.[63] Reduction in MLCK activity due to decreased calcium-calmodulin levels also leads to muscle relaxation, as does inhibition of phosphorylation by increased levels of cAMP and cGMP.[24,73,111] Cyclic AMP and cGMP are second messengers (i.e., they carry the message of a hormone to the site where the hormonal effect is realized) that lower the affinity of myosin for calcium-calmodulin or reduce intracellular calcium by stimulating calcium return to intracellular stores or extrusion across the cell membrane.[49,63,99]

The relative activity of adenyl cyclase (mediates cAMP synthesis) and phosphodiesterase (mediates cAMP breakdown) influence myometrial contractility by altering cAMP levels within the cell. Adenyl cyclase increases intracellular cAMP, which reduces calcium-calmodulin complexes and intracellular calcium levels and thus MLCK (see Figure 4-10). Pharmacologic agents can alter these enzymes. For example, adenyl cyclase is activated by β-adrenergic agonists, resulting in increased cAMP and reduced contractility. Substances that inhibit phosphodiesterase, which normally mediates cAMP breakdown, also result in elevated levels of intracellular cAMP. Therefore substances such as theophylline and α-adrenergic agents also decrease myometrial contractility.[28]

Hormones and pharmacologic agents influence activity of MLCK and cAMP. Oxytocin and $PGF_{2\alpha}$ enhance contractility by increasing intracellular calcium levels and the rate of MLCK phosphorylation. Oxytocin also releases calcium from intracellular stores and inhibits calcium uptake by the sarcoplasmic reticulum, extending actin-myosin interaction and thus muscle contraction. Relaxin increases cAMP, which inhibits MLCK phosphorylation and induces muscle relaxation.

Energy (released from ATP by myosin ATPase) is critical for myometrial contraction. ATP is used for both actin-myosin interaction and ion transport. If adequate oxygen and glucose are not available for ATP formation, as may occur with prolonged labor, the contractile process will be inhibited. The myosin head contains Mg-ATPase sites where ATP is hydrolyzed, converting chemical energy to mechanical force. Transport of calcium back across the cell membrane may be mediated by cell membrane Ca,Mg-ATPase. Oxytocin inhibits this enzyme, thus enhancing contractility.[63]

PGs and oxytocin promote release of calcium from intracellular pools or prevent uptake of calcium into these pools. This promotes contractility. On the other hand, agents that inhibit myometrial activity (e.g., progesterone, relaxin, PGI_2, and β-agonists) promote calcium sequestration or extrusion (via cAMP-dependent enzymes) and thus myometrial relaxation.[24,28]

In summary, control of myometrial activity is dependent on enzymatic phosphorylation of myosin by MLCK to allow interaction of actin and myosin. Hormonal, biochemical, and physical factors mediate MLCK activity, uterine activity, and myometrial structural and functional alterations. Before onset of labor, the myometrium undergoes activation, with decreases in substances that maintain uterine quiescence and increases in CAPs (Figures 4-5 and 4-6) that enhance uterine contractility.

Coordination of Uterine Contractions

Electrical and contractile activity in smooth muscle cells is controlled by myogenic, neurogenic, and hormonal control systems.[24,48] Myogenic activity, the spontaneous activity of the myometrium that occurs in the absence of any neural or hormonal input, includes the intrinsic excitability of the muscle cell, the ability of the muscle to contract spontaneously, and the mechanisms that produce rhythmic contractions. Neurogenic and hormonal control systems are superimposed on the muscle's inherent myogenic properties to initiate, augment, and suppress myometrial activity.[24,48] Myogenic control is dominated by hormonal influences, especially those of estrogen and progesterone, which influence myogenic characteristics through their generally opposing actions.[50] Estrogen increases and progesterone decreases the potential for contraction. Neurogenic control is not critical, since labor can occur in women with spinal injury (see Chapter 14), although the length of labor may be altered.

Coordination of contractions occurs by coupling of myometrial cells via electrical (e.g., gap junctions) and chemical (e.g., PGs, oxytocin) mechanisms.[6] Polarization and depolarization of the cell membranes moves the electrical signals across the myometrium.[2] These electrical signals are generated by movement of calcium through ion channels into the myometrial cell. Action potentials propagate rapidly throughout the uterus, initiating movement of calcium into the cells. These intracellular calcium waves propagate more slowly than the action potentials, gradually increasing the number of bundles involved in the contraction.[149]

Spontaneous cycles of activity in myometrial cells are characterized by: (1) slow, rhythmic fluctuations in the magnitude of electrical potential across the cell membrane (pacemaker potential); (2) spikes of electrical activity that occur in bursts at the crests of slow waves (action potentials) and become synchronous at parturition (a single spike can initiate a contraction; multiple spikes are needed to maintain forceful contractions); and (3) prepotential-like pacemaker potentials associated with initiation of action potentials.[49]

Pacemaker potential in the human uterus is not well understood. Specific pacemaker cells have not been identified.[63] The pacemaker potential depolarizes the cell membrane to a critical threshold. This triggers a change in the Na^+, Ca^{2+}, and K^+ conductance (action potential). The action potential increases membrane permeability to calcium and release of intracellular calcium stores.[49,63] As long as extracellular K^+ concentrations are high, action potentials increase in frequency. When maximum ion concentrations are reached within the cell, ionic stability is restored by active outward transport of Na^+ and Ca^{2+} intracellular uptake of calcium, and recapturing of intracellular K^+ The muscle cell returns to a resting state. Specific cells located near the fallopian tubes were once thought to initiate action potentials and myometrial contractions. Investigations have not supported this hypothesis.[49] Although it is likely that a cell initiating depolarization will be located in the fundus near the uterotubal junction, any myometrial cell is now thought to have pacemaker potential and be able to generate spontaneous activity.[49,102,111]

As action potentials are conducted to neighboring myometrial cells, groups of cells contract, leading to what is perceived by the woman as a uterine contraction. Coordination of uterine contractions occurs when all myometrial cells contract nearly simultaneously. Coordination and synchronization of contractions is mediated by the low-resistance gap junctions between myometrial cells. These junctions allow propagation of the action potential between cells and thus throughout the uterus.

Gap Junction Formation

Smooth muscle bundles normally separated from each other within connective tissue may come into closer approximation to form intercellular gap junctions (or low-resistance bridges or intercellular communication channels). Gap junctions allow transfer of current-carrying ions and exchange of second messengers between the cytoplasm of adjacent cells.[73,78] Thus gap junctions are the site where the action potential is propagated from cell to cell.[134] Increased gap junction interaction is associated with improved propagation of electrical impulses, increased conduction velocity, and coordinated contractility of the myometrium.[48,49,63]

Gap junctions proteins are called *connexins*. There are three forms of these membranes spanning proteins found in myocytes. Connexin 43 (Cx43) increases to term and is maximal during labor. Increased Cx43 is associated with decreased electrical resistance and thus myometrial contractility.[78,111] Connexin 26 (Cx26) increases in early pregnancy, then decreases before labor. Cx26 may help maintain uterine quiescence and inhibit controactions.[78,111] Levels of the third connexin (Cx45) are low throughout pregnancy.[78] Connexins within the cell membranes of adjacent smooth muscle cells align to create symmetric openings (gap junctions) between their cytoplasm. Each opening or pore contains multiple channels; each channel consists of six connexins aligned symmetrically in a hexametric structure with six connexins in the adjacent cell.[78,94,134] These pores are separated by a narrow gap and provide a pathway for transport of ions, metabolites, and second messengers.[24] Gap junctions can be open or closed, thus controlling intercellular communication.[63] Increased permeability across the junctions increases synchrony of electrical conduction and muscular contraction and subsequently more effective labor.

The number and size of gap junctions increase markedly during gestation to approximately 1000 per cell during labor.[49] Gap junctions are absent or infrequent in nonpregnant myometrium and decline markedly within 24 hours of delivery.[24,49] An increase in gap junctions has been reported in women in preterm labor; delay in the formation of gap junctions is associated with prolonged pregnancy.[24,49]

Estrogen stimulates gap junction formation by stimulating synthesis of connexins. One way progesterone functions to inhibit labor and maintain the pregnancy may be by inhibition of estrogen-enhanced connexin synthesis.[49] Some PGs stimulate whereas others inhibit gap junction formation, either directly or indirectly via estrogen and progesterone activities.[49] Gap junction formation is also inhibited or decreased by indomethacin, relaxin, isoxsuprine, and isoproterenol; oxytocin has little effect.[63] Lack of adequate concentrations of gap junctions decreases the effectiveness of oxytocin; as a result, oxytocin may not be effective with women experiencing pre- or postterm labor. Increased intracellular calcium reduces coupling, and increased cAMP in the uterus decreases gap junction permeability.[48,49] One mechanism by which relaxin, PGI_2, and β-agonists are thought to inhibit myometrial contractility is by increasing intracellular cAMP, which uncouples gap junctions, thus preventing synchronous uterine activity.[48]

Physiologic Events during a Uterine Contraction

A normal uterine contraction spreads downward from the cornus within about 15 seconds. Although the actual contractile phase begins slightly later in the lower portion of the uterus, functional coordination of the uterus is such that the contraction peak is attained simultaneously in all portions. The intensity of the contraction decreases from the cornus downward and is essentially absent in the cervix.

Resting baseline tonus in labor is at an intrauterine pressure of approximately 10 to 12 mmHg, which may increase to 30 mmHg with hypertonia.[102] Uterine contractions can be palpated abdominally with intrauterine pressure greater than 10 to 20 mmHg and perceived by the woman at 15 to 20 mmHg (Figure 4-11).[90] During early first stage, intrauterine pressure increases 20 to 30 mmHg above resting values, increasing to greater than 50 mmHg in the active phase and to 100 to 150 mmHg during a Valsalva maneuver with maximal expulsive efforts.[90] A laboring woman generally perceives pain at pressures greater than 25 mmHg or more, although this varies with individual thresholds. Thus the duration of a contraction assessed from palpation or patient perception will be shorter than the actual contraction, and the duration between contractions will seem longer.[90]

Page and colleagues define *hyperactive labor* as pressure greater than 50 mmHg at the peak or contractions closer than 2 minutes apart and *hypoactive labor* as generation of peak pressures less than 30 mmHg or an interval greater than 5 minutes between contractions.[1,2] Women exhibit marked individual variation in the intensity, frequency, and duration of contractions. Position and the use of oxytocin, analgesics, and anesthesia may also influence contractions.[90]

CLINICAL IMPLICATIONS FOR THE PREGNANT WOMAN AND HER FETUS

Labor and delivery place additional stressors on the maternal-fetal unit, which may be further increased in high-risk situations. Alterations in the physiologic processes of parturition can have a significant impact on the well-being of the mother, fetus, and neonate. Knowledge of these processes is critical in understanding the basis for nursing care and therapies to initiate or inhibit labor and the etiologic factors in dystocia and pre- or postterm labor onset.

Maternal Position during Labor

Position during labor is influenced by cultural factors, obstetric practices, place of delivery, technology, and the preference of the mother and health care providers.[68,88] Maternal position during labor influences the characteristics and effectiveness of uterine contractions, fetal well-being, maternal comfort, and course of labor.[1,13,59,88,89,117,120]

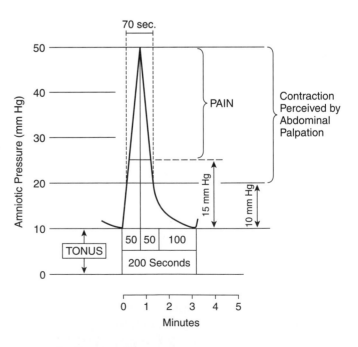

FIGURE **4-11** Correlation between abdominal palpation and intrauterine pressure tracing. (Data from Caldeyro-Barcia, R. *Second World Congress F.I.G.O.* Montreal: Libraire Beauchemin, Ltd.)

Historically a variety of positions have been used for labor and delivery. Delivery positions currently used in many U.S. institutions include lithotomy, lateral (Sims), semi-sitting, dorsal (or modified lithotomy), and occasionally kneeling.[116] Although lithotomy has often been used routinely, primarily for the comfort and convenience of the person delivering the infant, this position has no physiologic advantages and may interfere with expulsive efforts. Therefore alternative positions are currently being used in many settings.

Several positions have advantages or disadvantages from an anatomic and physiologic standpoint. During the first stage of labor, upright positions, such as sitting, standing, squatting, and kneeling, allow the abdominal wall to relax, and the influence of gravity causes the uterine fundus to fall forward. This directs the fetal head into the pelvic inlet in an anterior position and applies direct pressure to the cervix, which helps stimulate and stretch the cervix. Feedback from the cervix to the myometrium may stimulate more intense contractions and shorten labor.[68] The lateral recumbent position reduces pressure on maternal blood vessels and promotes venous return and cardiac output, thus increasing uterine perfusion and fetal oxygenation.[89] Side-lying may be effective during labor with a posterior fetus, by allowing the weight of the uterus and fetus to tip away from the back and permitting application of counterpressure over the lumbosacral area.[118]

Position at delivery should optimize alignment for fetal descent and maximize the capacity of the pelvis and efficiency of maternal expulsive efforts.[116] Squatting enhances engagement and descent of the fetal head and increases maternal pelvic diameters. In this position the upper portion of the symphysis pubis is compressed and the bottom part separated slightly. This results in an outward movement and separation of the innominate bones and backward movement of the lower sacrum. The pelvic outlet increases 28% with increased transverse (1 cm) and anteroposterior (0.5 to 2 cm) diameters. Thigh pressure against the abdomen during squatting may also promote fetal descent and correction of unfavorable fetal positions. Sitting or semi-sitting (30-degree angle) may have similar advantages.[68,130]

Dorsal and supine positions have been associated with adverse effects on maternal hemodynamics and fetal status and with the supine hypotension syndrome.[116,130] A supine position is a disadvantage during engagement and descent of the fetal head because this position does not optimize fetal alignment, maximize pelvic diameter, or maximize efficiency of maternal expulsive efforts.[68]

Most studies of maternal position during labor have compared the effects of two positions, so findings vary with the positions used. A recent Cochrane Review of 18 studies of maternal positioning during second-stage labor concluded that any upright or lateral position as compared to a supine or lithotomy position decreased the length of the second stage, need for forceps, episiotomy, severe pain, and abnormal fetal heart rate patterns; increased the risk of blood loss (particularly with use of birthing chairs or stools); and slightly increased the risk of perineal tears.[35,37,59,139] In the supine position, contractions were more frequent but less intense than in the side-lying position. The use of the supine position during the first stage of labor compromised effective uterine activity, prolonged labor, and increased use of drugs to augment labor.[117] Placing a woman in the side-lying position increased the intensity and decreased the frequency of contractions and promoted greater uterine efficiency.[24,28,130] Frequency and intensity of contractions and uterine activity increased with sitting or standing.[13] Upright positions (e.g., standing, sitting, squatting, kneeling) (as opposed to supine ones) were associated with more regular and intense contractions and shorter duration of first and second stages and total labor.[68] The lateral recumbent position (as opposed to sitting) led to more intense, less frequent contractions and greater uterine efficiency during the first stage.[119,120] Squatting has been found to be the most effective position for pushing.[54,121,145]

Positional effects appear as soon as the maternal position is changed and last as long as the position is maintained.[118,119] Changes are more marked with spontaneous than with induced labor and do not seem to be affected by parity or fetal position. Alternating positions after the woman has maintained one position for a period of time can enhance the effectiveness of contractions. If the woman prefers a supine position, alternating this position with standing or side-lying can increase the efficiency of contractions.[119]

Although many studies have not found specific alterations in fetal status associated with maternal position, positions that increase the efficiency of contractions and decrease the duration of labor may reduce fetal stress.[13,119,120] For example, semi-sitting positions during delivery may shorten the length of the second stage and reduce fetal acidosis.[13,116]

Maternal comfort is also an important consideration. Many women prefer lateral or standing positions to supine.[89] Position preferences may change during labor. A woman may prefer sitting or walking during early labor but semirecumbent or side-lying with pillow support as labor progresses. Roberts and colleagues summarize factors to consider in selecting a position conducive to labor progress and maternal comfort: "potential mechanical advantage of the position; the associated hemodynamic alterations and subsequent uteroplacental perfusion; the position of the fetus; the parturient's perception of her contractions, discomfort, and fatigue; and obstetrical indications for confinement to bed for continuous fetal monitoring, medication, or care."[118, p.115]

Maternal Pushing Efforts during the Second Stage

There have been increasing concerns regarding the effects of bearing down (i.e., prolonged Valsalva maneuver) and the Valsalva maneuver on maternal hemodynamics and fetal status.[5,14,68,116,141,148] A long Valsalva push increases maternal intrathoracic and intraabdominal pressure and decreases cardiac output, uterine blood flow, and blood in the intervillous space and thus fetal oxygenation.[3,103] Yeates and Roberts conclude that fetal outcome is probably affected more by maternal position and sustained maternal bearing down than by duration of the second stage per se.[148] Maternal hypotension and fetal hypoxia may develop more rapidly with supine position or epidural anesthesia.[141] Maternal hemodynamic changes with bearing down and the Valsalva maneuver are mediated by sympathetic discharge and catecholamine release, which also increase maternal discomfort and, in combination with maternal acidosis, may decrease uterine activity.[116]

Investigations have compared the effects of open-glottis pushing (based on involuntary maternal urges to push) with those of the Valsalva maneuver accompanying directed bearing down.[5,14,47,48,124,136,144,145] With long Valsalva pushing, there were less frequent expulsive contractions and a trend toward a longer second stage.[5] Bearing down that lasts more than 5 to 6 seconds was associated with decreased maternal blood pressure and placental blood flow, alterations in maternal and fetal oxygenation, decreased fetal pH and PO_2, increased fetal PCO_2, an increased incidence of fetal heart rate pattern changes, and delayed recovery of the fetal heart rate with fetal asphyxia. [5,14,15,47,124,144,145] Open-glottis pushing was not associated with changes in maternal blood pressure (probably because intrathoracic pressure elevations were not sustained) or increased fetal pH.[5] Spontaneous involuntary pushing with minimal straining has been associated with fewer episiotomies, forceps deliveries, and second-degree to third-degree perineal tears, and a shorter second stage.[68,1156,124] Roberts suggests that a semirecumbent position with bearing down efforts that are short and in accordance with involuntary urges to push is most conducive to favorable delivery outcomes.[116]

Sleep and colleagues concluded that: (1) directed pushing should be abandoned since no data support this practice and some data suggest it is harmful; (2) supine positions tend to lengthen the second stage, reduce the incidence of spontaneous births, increase fetal heart rate abnormalities, and reduce umbilical cord pH; and (3) arbitrary limits on duration of the second stage should be abandoned if mother and fetus are doing well and labor is progressing.[130]

Preterm Labor

Infants born prematurely are at high risk for health alterations during the neonatal period and for later neurodevelopmental problems. As a result, much effort has been directed toward eliciting the causes for preterm labor and developing intervention strategies to prevent the onset of labor and to terminate uterine contractions that begin prior to term. Preterm labor is defined as the onset of regular contractions with progressive cervical effacement and dilatation before 37 weeks.[18] There is still speculation concerning the specific events leading to onset of labor before term. Preterm labor is probably not initiated by a single etiologic event, but rather by a group of factors that individually or in combination influence the various pathways involved in control of labor onset (see Figure 4-7).

Lockwood and Kuczynski have proposed a conceptual model of preterm labor with four pathways (Figure 4-12): (1) maternal and fetal stress (activation of the maternal or fetal hypothalamic-pituitary-adrenal axis); (2) inflammation (decidual, chorioamniotic, or systemic); (3) decidual hemorrhage; and (4) pathologic uterine distention.[71] Maternal or fetal stress may activate labor via increases in CRH leading to increased estriol production and increased PGs (see Figure 4-7).[22,70,71,72,83] Inflammation activates the cytokine system, leading to increased MMPs and uterotonics.[40,55,58,71,123] Gomez and colleagues suggest that both preterm labor and premature rupture of the membranes (PROM) may be adaptive events that occur when the intrauterine environment is "hostile." If the response to intrauterine infection is secretion of uterotonic agents, preterm labor results; if the response is protease (MMPs) production, PROM results.[58] Decidual hemorrhage activates a proteolytic cascade, whereas uterine overdistension (polyhydramnios or multifetal gestation) or reduction in expansive capacity (uterine anomalies) activates cytokines (see Figure 4-12).[71]

Biochemical markers and other factors associated with preterm birth include genital tract infection, cervicovaginal and amniotic fluid markers, salivary estriol, cervical collagen fluorescence, electromyelogram signals from the lower uterine segment, and cervical changes.[34,60,67,69,75,138] Cervicovaginal markers include bacterial vaginosis and fetal fibronectin. Fetal fibronectin is produced by the fetal membranes and trophoblast and is thought to serve as a "biologic glue" to maintain attachment of the placenta at the chorion-decidua interface.[3,75] Increased levels of fetal fibronectin have been associated with risk of preterm labor and with cervical ripening at term.[67] However, these values have a relatively low positive predictive value in presymptomatic women, as do cervical changes associated with preterm birth risk such as decreased cervical length and funneling (wedge appearance on ultrasound due to

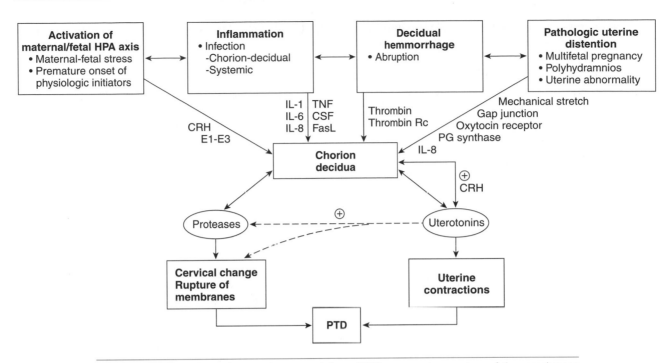

FIGURE **4-12** The major pathways of preterm delivery (PTD) or premature rupture of the membranes (PROM). *CRH,* Corticotrophin-releasing hormone; *E₁,* estrone; *E₃,* estriol; *FasL,* Fas ligand; *IL,* interleukin; *PG,* prostaglandin; *TNF,* tumor necrosis factor. (From Lockwood, C.J. & Kuczynski, F. [1999]. Markers of risk for preterm delivery. *J Perinat Med, 27,* 12.)

protrusion of the fetal membranes into the cervical canal).[34,67]

Altering Uterine Motility and Cervical Ripening

Uterine activity can be controlled directly by blocking or stimulating specific hormonal receptors or altering electro-mechanical coupling, and indirectly via agents that interfere with the synthesis of enzymes and other mediators of myometrial contraction and relaxation.[6] Use of these agents must take into consideration the physiologic properties of as well as the pharmacologic actions on both the cervix and the myometrium. A postterm woman with altered myometrial contractility and an unripe (resistant) cervix needs an agent that increases and coordinates myometrial activity and decreases cervical resistance. On the other hand, agents used for women in preterm labor lead to myometrial relaxation and increase cervical resistance.[6] This section examines pharmacology of labor related to control of cervical ripening, labor induction, and labor inhibition.

Control of Cervical Ripening

Cervical ripening is not dependent on myometrial contractions and occurs in the absence of regular uterine contrac-

tions. PGE₂ (Cervadil, Prepidil) and misoprostol (Cytotec) are currently used most frequently for preinduction cervical ripening.[127,143] Physiologic ripening is under the control of local mediators, in particular PGE₂, whose action is influenced by local mediators. Exogenous PGE₂ induces cervical ripening by relaxing cervical smooth muscle, enhancing enzymatic collagen degradation, and increasing hyaluronic acid and MMP. PGE₂ is more effective than $PGF_{2\alpha}$.[78,104] $PGF_{2\alpha}$ stimulates myometrial contractions but causes no significant changes in cervical resistance.[58,100] Misoprostol is a synthetic PGE analogue that binds to EP₃ and EP₄ receptors and seems to have a greater effect on the cervix than PGE.[4,126] Antiprogesterone agents (RU-486, or mifepristone) have also been evaluated as alternative cervical ripening agents. RU-486 stimulates IL-8 release.[31]

Induction of Labor

Oxytocin (and synthetic forms such as Pitocin and Syntocinon) is usually the drug of choice to initiate uterine activity if the condition of the cervix is favorable.[134] Oxytocin is used for labor augmentation and induction and to promote uterine contraction following parturition. Since oxytocin has little effect on the cervix, an unripe cervix may resist even forceful oxytocin-induced myometrial contractions.

Oxytocin increases myometrial cell membrane spike activity, possibly by altering calcium flux through voltage-dependent calcium channels.[6] Effects of oxytocin on uterine activity depend on the concentration of oxytocin receptors on the myometrial cells, number of available receptors, receptor affinity for oxytocin, and metabolic state of the myometrium.[91] Oxytocin is a potent octapeptide synthesized in the hypothalamus and then transported along the neurons to the posterior pituitary gland via carrier proteins and released episodically. Oxytocin release can also be stimulated by nipple stimulation (similar to the mechanism with suckling described in Chapter 5).[130]

Side effects include uterine hyperstimulation with fetal hypoxia and asphyxia. Maternal water intoxication (due to the antidiuretic activity of oxytocin) may occur at doses above 45 mIU/min.[6,104] The risk of water intoxication is increased if oxytocin is given over a prolonged period of time in a dilute, low-electrolyte solution. This risk may be reduced by using a balanced electrolyte solution when diluting oxytocin and monitoring maternal fluid and electrolyte status.[91,104,142] PGs have also been used to induce or augment labor contractions, but they have not been shown to be more effective and have significant side effects.[100,104]

Inhibition of Labor

Inhibition of uterine contractions is used in the management of preterm labor and to reduce uterine activity in the presence of fetal distress.[6] Uterine activity–inhibiting drugs (tocolytics) are most effective in stopping labor for 48 to 72 hours and thus delay labor so glucocorticoids can be given to enhance fetal lung maturity (see Chapter 9).[22,71] However, tocolytics do not decrease the overall rate of preterm delivery and long-term prophylactic use is not effective.[65,71] Many tocolytic drugs have been investigated, including ethanol, β-adrenergic agonists, magnesium sulfate, and PG synthetase inhibitors.[6,18,22,34,56,62,138] Characteristics of currently used drugs are summarized as follows and in Table 4-2. Use of one agent is unsuccessful in 20% to 40% of cases.[18] Because each group of drugs has a different action, combinations of drugs tend to enhance their effectiveness since they act synergistically.[18,61]

Magnesium sulfate is the tocolytic with the fewest side effects.[71] Magnesium affects smooth muscle excitation, excitation-contraction coupling, and the contractile apparatus by modulating calcium uptake, binding, and distribution in the cell; competitive blocking of Ca^{2+} influx across the cell membrane; and activation of adenyl cyclase and cAMP.[18] Magnesium regulates the voltage-gated calcium channels to prevent them from opening in response to the action potential.[138] Magnesium sulfate acts on the myometrium, primarily by competitive antagonism to control calcium entry into

the cell, reducing intracellular Ca^{2+} levels and thus contractility.[6,61,62] Magnesium sulfate is effective in inhibiting preterm labor and is being used more often.[9] Maternal and neonatal side effects are summarized in Table 4-2.

β-Adrenergic agonists (β-sympathomimetics) have been widely used. They are effective in postponing delivery for 24 to 48 hours but do not significantly reduce the rate of preterm birth or alter neonatal mortality or morbidity.[138] Drugs that have been used for inhibition of preterm labor include ritodrine, terbutaline, fenoterol, isoxsuprine, salbutamol, hexoprenaline, and orciprenaline.[9,18,62,65] β-Adrenergic agonists act to relax myometrial cells by triggering intracellular formation of cAMP. These effects are mediated by β_2-receptors on the outer membrane of the myometrial cell.

Interaction of the β-adrenergic agonist and the β_2-receptor catalyzes the formation of cAMP from ATP by activating adenyl cyclase on the inner surface of the cell membrane. Cyclic AMP phosphorylates a protein kinase that decreases the affinity of medium light chain kinase for the calcium-calmodulin complex, thus promoting relaxation. cAMP also decreases intracellular calcium, possibly by interfering with the Na,K-ATPase exchange pump.[9,18,61]

The myometrium contains α- and β-receptors. If PGs or oxytocin stimulates the α-receptors, the uterus contracts. Stimulation of the β-receptors inhibits uterine contraction. Two subtypes of β-receptors may be present in the same organ or on the same cell. β_1-Receptors dominate in the heart, small intestine, and adipose tissue; β_2-receptors predominate in the smooth muscle of the uterus, blood vessels, and bronchioles.[99] Since β-adrenergic agonists are not specific for β_2- or β_1-receptors, use of these agents is associated with a variety of side effects (see Table 4-2).

Prolonged use of β-adrenergic agents results in desensitization (also called *downregulation* or *refractoriness*) and the need to increase dosage to achieve the same therapeutic effect. Desensitization is a multistep process and is thought to result from an agonist-stimulated decrease in the number of β-receptors with a reduction in the effect of the agonist on intracellular processes and myometrial relaxation.[18,99] The first step in desensitization is inactivation of the receptor by phosphorylation, which is mediated by a cAMP-independent protein kinase activated by catecholamines. This is followed by uncoupling of the regulator protein and adenyl cyclase. The β-receptors then become sequestered in vesicles within the membrane. Phosphorylation is reversed and the receptor reactivated and recycled back to the outer membrane where it recouples with adenyl cyclase.[99] Discontinuing β-adrenergic agonists with use of an alternative agent allows the myometrial cell to recover responsiveness so these agents can be used later.

TABLE **4-2** Tocolytic Agents

Tocolytic Agent	Dosage and Administration	Contraindications	Maternal Side Effects	Fetal and Neonatal Side Effects
Betamimetic	Terbultaline: .25 mg subcutaneous every 20 minutes to 3 hours (hold for a pulse >120) Ritodrine: Initial dose of 50-100 μg/min increase by 50 μg/minutes every 10 minutes until contractions cease or side effects develop. Maximum dose is 350 μg/min	Cardiac arrhythmias Poorly controlled thyroid disease Poorly controlled diabetes mellitus	Cardiac or cardiopulmonary arrhythmias, pulmonary edema, myocardial ischemia, hypotension, tachycardia Metabolic: Hyperglycemia, hyperinsulinemia, hypokalemia, antidiuresis, altered thyroid function Physiologic: Tremor, palpitations, nervousness, nausea and vomiting, fever, hallucinations	Fetal: Tachycardia, hyperinsulinemia, hyperglycemia, myocardial and septal hypertrophy, myocardial ischemia Neonatal: Tachycardia, hypoglycemia, hypocalcemia, hyperbilirubinemia, hypotension, intraventricular hemorrhage
Magnesium sulfate	4-6 g bolus for 20 minutes, then 4-6 g per hour	Myasthenia gravis	Flushing, lethargy, headache, muscle weakness, diplopia, dry mouth, pulmonary edema, cardiac arrest	Lethargy, hypotonia, respiratory depression, demineralization with prolonged use
Calcium channel blockers	30 mg loading dose, then 10-20 mg every 4-6 hours	Cardiac disease Renal disease (use with caution) Maternal hypotension (<90/50) Avoidance of concomitant use with MgSO$_4$	Flushing, headache, dizziness, nausea, transient hypotension	None noted as yet
Prostaglandin synthetase inhibitors	Indomethacin: Loading dose of 50 mg rectally or 50-100 mg orally, then 25-50 mg orally every 4 hours for 48 hours Ketorolac: Loading dose of 60 mg intramuscularly, then 30 mg intramuscularly every 6 hours for 48 hours Sulindac: 200 mg orally every 12 hours for 48 hours	Significant renal or hepatic impairment Active peptic ulcer disease Coagulation disorders or thrombocytopenia NSAID-sensitive asthma Other sensitivities to NSAIDs	Nausea, heartburn	Constriction of ductus arteriosus, pulmonary hypertension, reversible decrease in renal function with oligohydramnios, intraventricular hemorrhage, hyperbilirubinemia, necrotizing enterocolitis

From Hearne, A.E. & Nagey, D.A. (2000). Therapeutic agents in preterm labor: Tocolytic agents. *Clin Obstet Gynecol, 43,* 789.
NSAID, Nonsteroidal antiinflammatory drug.

Calcium antagonists (calcium channel blockers) are organic compounds such as nifedipine, nicardipine, and verapamil that act on the cell membrane to inhibit the influx of extracellular calcium through membrane potential-dependent channels.[61,138] These agents are less effective in blocking influx through receptor-operated channels that are less specific for calcium.[6,18] Calcium antagonists may also act by altering calcium-calmodulin binding and inhibiting actin-myosin interaction.[62] Oxytocin receptor antagonists (atosiban) have been investigated for labor inhibition.[56,138] These agents, which are still investigational drugs, act directly by blocking oxytocin receptors and indirectly by altering PG synthesis in the decidua.[138]

PG synthetase inhibitors include nonsteroidal antiinflammatory agents such as indomethacin, Ketorolac, and Sulindac. These agents block PG synthesis probably by interfering with cyclooxygenase, the enzyme that regulates the production of PGs from arachidonic acid.[6,18,22,138] Since PGs are important in both initiation of myometrial activity and cervical ripening, the potential of this group of agents has generated considerable interest. Although their effectiveness has been documented, concerns remain over the potential risk for premature closure of the fetal ductus arteriosus and other side effects such as pulmonary hypertension and alterations in renal function.[6,9,61,62] The concern about ductal closure is that PG synthetase inhibitors act on both COX-I (found primarily in fetal cardiovascular tissues) and COX-II (found in the myometrium and fetal membranes).[138] The risk for premature ductal closure is dose dependent and seems greatest in fetuses over 35 weeks' gestation and with long-term therapy.[9,18,62]

Dystocia

Dysfunctional labor can result from problems in the powers (alteration in myometrial function and contraction patterns), passage (obstruction of fetal descent by the maternal bony pelvis or soft tissues), or passenger (fetal malposition or abnormal development).[63] Functional dystocia due to alterations in the physiologic function (powers) results in inadequate contractility and failure of the cervix to dilate. The cellular and molecular basis for weak or ineffective myometrial contractions includes lack of adequate stimulation, depression or the presence of some form of strong inhibitory control, or a combination of these events (Table 4-3).[48]

Stimulation or inhibition of myometrial activity is influenced by myogenic, neurogenic, and hormonal control systems. Dystocia secondary to alterations in myogenic properties arises from factors such as modifications in intracellular ion concentration (as a result of an inadequate supply of energy or calcium) with depression or absence of myometrial contractility, closure or inadequate function of

gap junctions with modifications in the propagation of electrical events, and poor synchronization of contractions across the uterus. Abnormalities in gap junction structure or function may arise from alterations in regulatory hormones or their receptors. Dystocia can also arise secondary to alterations in neurogenic control (overstimulation by inhibitory neurons or understimulation by excitatory neurons) or in the hormonal control systems. These latter alterations arise directly from inadequate levels of hormones or their receptors or indirectly from alterations in gap junction function or structure.[48]

Supportive interventions with women experiencing dystocia are directed toward preventing or reducing maternal fatigue, providing calories for energy, maintaining hydration, monitoring fluid and electrolyte status, and maintaining fetal homeostasis. Energy (ATP) is essential for labor progression. If adequate calories and ATP are not available, ketoacidosis may develop. With inadequate ATP the effectiveness of uterine contractions is further impeded. Women with dystocia whose labor is not progressing and

TABLE **4-3** **Possible Reasons for Dystocia**

MYOGENIC: INTRINSIC FACTORS

Inadequate depolarization
    Ionic disturbance (local)
        Insufficient stimulation or excessive inhibition by hormonal or neural mechanisms
        Lack of stimulatory receptors or redundant intrinsic inhibitory systems
Deficient propagation of electrical events
    Lack of development of gap junctions
    Suppression of channel opening in gap junctions
Incomplete muscle development
Unsatisfactory energy supply for muscle cells and fatigue

NEUROGENIC: NERVE FACTORS

Depressed neural output by excitatory neurons
Continued dominance by inhibitory nerves
    Failure of inhibitory nerves to degenerate

HORMONAL: HUMORAL FACTORS

Inadequate steroid ratios (estrogen-to-progesterone)
    Progesterone dominance
    Failure of steroid hormones and their receptors to control synthesis of necessary proteins, membrane receptors, gap junctions, and so on
Hormonally regulated closure of gap junction channels
Elevated levels of inhibitory prostaglandins, relaxin, and so on
Failure of stimulatory prostaglandins to increase sufficiently

From Garfield, R.E. (1987). Cellular and molecular basis for dystocia. *Clin Obstet Gynecol, 30*, 3.

who are exhausted may be provided with a period of medicated therapeutic rest.[48]

Postterm Labor

Postterm labor (onset of labor after 42 weeks or 294 days) occurs in 4% to 14% of all pregnancies; 2% to 3% exceed 43 weeks.[114] Fetal and neonatal morbidity increases after 42 weeks, often as a result of the effects of prolonged gestation or placental morphology and functional ability. Postterm pregnancies are associated with an increased frequency of both IUGR and macrosomia, fetal distress, meconium aspiration, congenital anomalies, and intrauterine death.[11,93]

A specific postmaturity syndrome has been described by Clifford.[33] This syndrome is characterized clinically by three progressive stages of alterations in the infant's skin: (1) maceration accompanied by loss of vernix caseosa with dry, wrinkled, parchment-like skin; (2) meconium staining of the skin and amniotic fluid; and (3) yellow staining of the skin (caused by conversion of the meconium to bilirubin).

Factors that may result in failure of initiation of spontaneous labor and postdate gestation are as follows: (1) lack of the normal increase in estrogen near term, perhaps due to anencephaly and associated adrenal hypoplasia, deficiency in placental sulfatase (necessary for production of estrogen), or fetal adrenal hypoplasia; (2) decreased adrenocortical function, leading to reduction in cortisol levels (cortisol promotes hydroxylation of progesterone, reduction in progesterone levels, and increases in estrogen precursors); and (3) decreased fetal adrenocorticotropic factors such as CRH and ACTH, which stimulate fetal cortisol and estrogen precursor production, perhaps related to delayed maturation of the fetal brain.[11,114] The result is delay in myometrial activation with failure of oxytocin receptor, PG receptor, or gap junction development, or delay in cervical ripening.[114]

SUMMARY

An understanding of physiologic processes during the intrapartum period is essential for recognition of the effects of parturition on the pregnant woman and the fetus and in optimizing maternal, fetal, and neonatal outcome. This knowledge provides the basis for assessment of functional and dysfunctional labor patterns and maternal responses to pharmacologic agents used to alter or control uterine activity, for recognition of preterm and postterm labor, and for nursing interventions such as positioning during the first and second stages of labor. Recommendations for clinical practice related to parturition and uterine physiology during parturition are summarized in Table 4-4.

TABLE **4-4** **Recommendations for Clinical Practice Related to Parturition and Uterine Physiology**

Recognize usual changes in the uterine size and shape during pregnancy (p. 131 and Table 4-1).

Know the usual changes in the myometrium during pregnancy and their bases (pp. 133-134).

Recognize factors involved in the initiation of labor and know how these may be altered (pp. 136-142).

Understand the physiologic basis for myometrial contraction and factors that may alter muscular contraction (pp. 142-144 and Table 4-3).

Assess contractions and document their characteristics (p. 146).

Monitor energy and oxygen needs of the laboring woman (pp. 144, 152).

Understand the basis for cervical ripening and dilatation and factors that may alter this process (pp. 134-135).

Avoid use of the supine position for prolonged periods during the first stage of labor (pp. 146-147).

Alternate supine and side-lying positions for a woman who prefers supine positions during the first stage (pp. 146-147).

Promote use of upright positions in first-stage (especially early) labor (pp. 146-147).

Assist the woman in selecting a position conducive to labor progress and maternal comfort (pp. 146-148).

Try side-lying position with a posterior fetus (p. 147).

Assist the woman in selecting a position at delivery to optimize alignment for fetal descent and maximize capacity of the pelvis and efficiency of maternal expulsive efforts (p. 148).

Avoid directed pushing and the Valsalva maneuver during the second stage (p. 148).

Teach the woman to use open-glottis pushing (p. 148).

Avoid supine positions during the second stage (p. 148 and Chapter 8).

Recognize factors that increase the risk of preterm labor (pp. 148-149 and Figure 4-12).

Understand the basis for pharmacologic agents used to control cervical ripening (p. 149).

Understand the basis for pharmacologic agents used for induction or augmentation of labor (pp. 149-150).

Monitor the woman for side effects of agents used to induce or augment labor (pp. 149-150).

Understand the basis for pharmacologic agents used to inhibit labor (pp. 150-151 and Table 4-2).

Monitor the woman for side effects of agents used to inhibit labor (Table 4-2).

Recognize and monitor for factors that can lead to dystocia (pp. 152-153 and Table 4-3).

Monitor the woman with postterm labor for fetal distress (p. 153).

REFERENCES

1. Abitbol, M.N. (1985). Supine position in labor and associated fetal heart rate changes. *Obstet Gynecol, 65,* 481.
2. Akerlund, M. (1997). Contractility in the nonpregnant uterus. *Ann N Y Acad Med, 828,* 213.
3. Anderson, H.F. (2000). Use of fetal fibronectin in women at risk for preterm delivery, *Clin Obstet Gynecol, 43,* 746.
4. Arias, F. (2000). Pharmacology of oxytocin and prostaglandins. *Clin Obstet Gynecol, 43,* 453.
5. Barnett, M. & Humenick, S. (1982). Infant outcomes in relation to second stage labor pushing. *Birth, 9,* 221.
6. Baxi, L.V. & Petrie, R.H. (1987). Pharmacologic effects on labor: Effects of drugs on dystocia, labor and uterine activity. *Clin Obstet Gynecol, 30,* 19.
7. Bennett, P.R. (1990). Mechanisms of parturition: The transfer of PGE_2 and 5-hydroxyeicosatetraenoic acid across fetal membranes. *Am J Obstet Gynecol, 162,* 683.
8. Benedetto, C., et al. (1994). Corticotrophin-releasing hormone increased prostaglandin $F_{2\alpha}$ activity on human endometrium in vitro. *Am J Obstet Gynecol, 171,* 126.
9. Besinger, R.E. & Niebyl, J.R. (1990). The safety and efficacy of tocolytic agents for the treatment of preterm labor. *Obstet Gynecol Surv, 45,* 415.
10. Bisits, A. (1998). Corticotrophin releasing hormone: a biochemical predictor of preterm delivery in a pilot randomized trail of the treatment of preterm labor. *Am J Obstet Gynecol, 178,* 862.
11. Brody, S.A. (1994). Endocrinology of postdate pregnancy. In S.A. Brody & K. Ueland (Eds.). *Endocrine disorders in pregnancy.* Norwalk, CT: Appleton & Lange.
12. Brosens, J.J. (1995). Uterine junctional zone: function and disease. *Lancet, 346,* 558.
13. Caldeyro-Barcia, R. (1979). The influence of the maternal position on time of spontaneous rupture of membranes, progress of labor, and fetal head compression. *Birth Family J, 6,* 7.
14. Caldeyro-Barcia, R. (1979). The influence of maternal bearing-down efforts during second stage on fetal well being. *Birth Family J, 6,* 17.
15. Caldeyro-Barcia, R., et al. (1981). The bearing down efforts and their effect on fetal heart rate, oxygenation and acid-base balance. *J Perinat Med, 9(6),* 3.
16. Cameron, I.T., et al. (1995). Endothelin expression in the uterus. *J Steroid Biochem Mol Biol, 53,* 209.
17. Cameron, I.T. & Campbell, S. (1998). Nitric oxide in the endometrium. *Hum Reprod Update, 4,* 565.
18. Caritis, S.N., Darby, M.J., & Chan, L. (1988). Pharmacologic treatment of preterm labor. *Clin Obstet Gynecol, 31,* 635.
19. Casey, M.L. & MacDonald, P.C. (1986). The initiation of labor in women: Regulation of phospholipid and arachidonic acid metabolism and of prostaglandin production. *Semin Perinatol, 10,* 270.
20. Casey, M.L. & MacDonald, P.C. (1988). Biomolecular processes in the initiation of parturition: Decidual activation. *Clin Obstet Gynecol, 31,* 533.
21. Casey, M.L.& MacDonald, P.C. (1997). The endocrinology of parturition. *Ann N Y Acad Sci, 828,* 273, 277.
22. Castracane, V.D. (2000). Endocrinology of preterm labor. *Clin Obstet Gynecol, 43,* 717.
23. Challis, J.R., et al. (1988). Placental, membrane and uterine interactions in the control of birth. In C.T. Jones (Ed.). *Research in perinatal medicine (VI): Fetal and neonatal development.* Ithaca, New York: Perinatology Press.
24. Challis, J.R. & Lye, S.J. (1994). Parturition. In E. Knobil & J. Neill (Eds.). *The physiology of reproduction* (2nd ed.). New York: Raven.

25. Challis, J.R. & Gibb, W. (1996). Control of parturition, *Prenat Neonat Med, 1,* 283.
26. Challis, J.R., et al. (1997). Prostaglandins and parturition. *Ann N Y Acad Sci, 828,* 254.
27. Challis, J.R., et al. (1999). Prostaglandin dehydrogenase and the initiation of labor. *J Perinat Med, 27,* 26.
28. Challis, J.R. (1999). Characteristics of parturition. In R.K. Creasy & R. Resnik (Eds.). *Maternal-fetal medicine* (4th ed.). Philadelphia: W.B. Saunders.
29. Chibbar, R., et al. (1993). Synthesis of oxytocin in amnion, chorion, and decidua may influence the timing of human parturition. *J Clin Investig, 91,* 185.
30. Chrousos, G.P. (1999). Reproductive placental corticotrophin-releasing hormone and its clinical implications. *Am J Obstet Gynecol, 180(1),* 249S.
31. Chwalisz, K. & Garfield, R.E. (1997). Regulation of the uterus and cervix during pregnancy and labor: Role of progesterone and nitric oxide. *Ann N Y Acad Sci, 828,* 238.
32. Chwalisz, K. & Garfield, R.E. (1998). Role of nitric oxide in the uterus and cervix: implications for the management of labor. *J Perinat Med, 26,* 448.
33. Clifford, S.H. (1954). Postmaturity and placental dysfunction: Clinical syndrome and pathologic findings. *J Pediatr, 44,* 1.
34. Colombo, D.J. & Iams, J.D. (2000). Cervical length and preterm labor. *Clin Obstet Gynecol, 43,* 735.
35. Crawley, P., et al. (1991). Delivery in an obstetric birth chair: a randomized controlled trial. *Br J Obstet Gynaecol, 98,* 667.
36. Cummiskey, K.C. & Dawood, M.Y. (1990). Induction of labor with pulsitile oxytocin, *Am J Obstet Gynecol, 163,* 1868.
37. DeJong, P.R., et al. (1997). Randomized trial comparing the upright and supine position for the second stage of labour. *Br J Obstet Gynaecol, 104,* 567.
38. Di Iorio, R., et al. (1998). New peptides, hormones, and parturition. *Gynecol Endocrinol, 12,* 429.
39. DiIulio, J.L., et al. (1996). Human placental and fetal membrane nitric oxide synthetase activity during, during, and after labor at term. *Reprod Fert Dev, 7,* 1505.
40. Dudley, D.J. (1999). Immunoendocrinology of preterm labor: The link between corticotrophin releasing hormone and inflammation. *Am J Obstet Gynecol, 180(1),* 251S.
41. Egarter, C.H. & Husslein, P. (1992). Biochemistry of myometrial contractility. *Baillieres Clin Obstet Gynecol, 6,* 755.
42. Emanuel, R.L., et al. (1994). Corticotrophin-releasing hormone levels in human plasma and amniotic fluid during gestation. *Clin Endocrinol, 40,* 257.
43. Eadalti, M., et al. (2000). Placental corticotrophin-releasing factor. An update. *Ann N Y Acad Sci, 900,* 89.
44. Fuchs, A.R. & Fuchs, F. (1984). Endocrinology of human parturition: A review. *Br J Obstet Gynaecol, 91,* 948.
45. Fuchs, A.R., et al. (1991). Oxytocin secretion and human parturition: pulse frequency and duration increase during spontaneous labor in women. *Am J Obstet Gynecol, 165,* 1515.
46. Fuchs, A.R. (1995). Plasma membrane receptors regulating myometrial contractility and their hormonal modulation, *Semin Perinatol, 19,* 15.
47. Fuller, B.F., et al. (1993). Acoustical analysis of maternal sounds during the second stage of labor. *Applied Nurs Res, 6,* 7.
48. Garfield, R.E. (1987). Cellular and molecular basis for dystocia. *Clin Obstet Gynecol, 30,* 3.
49. Garfield, R.E., Blennerhassett, M.G., & Miller, S.M. (1988). Control of myometrial contractility: Role and regulation of gap junctions. *Oxf Rev Reprod Biol, 10,* 436.

50. Garfield, R.E., et al. (1995). Role of gap junctions and nitric oxide in control of myometrial contractility. *Semin Perinatol, 19,* 41.

51. Garfield, R.E., et al. (1998). Control and assessment of the uterus and cervix during pregnancy and labour. *Hum Reprod Update, 4,* 673.

52. Goland, R.S., et al. (1993). Elevated levels of umbilical cord plasma corticotrophin-releasing hormone in growth-retarded fetuses. *J Clin Endocrinol Metab, 77,* 1174.

53. Goland, R.S., et al. (1995). Concentration of corticotrophin-releasing hormone in the umbilical cord blood of pregnancies complicated by preeclampsia. *Reprod Fert Dev, 7,* 1227.

54. Golay, J., et al. (1993). The squatting position for the second stage of labor: effects on labor and on maternal and fetal well-being. *Birth, 20,* 73.

55. Goldenberg, R.L., et al. (2000). Intrauterine infection and preterm delivery. *N Engl J Med, 342,* 1500.

56. Goodwin, T.M. & Zograbyan, A. (1998). Oxytocin receptor antagonists. Update. *Clin Perinatol, 25,* 859.

57. Goodwin, T.M. (1999). A role for estriol in human labor, term and preterm. *Am J Obstet Gynecol, 180*(1), 208S.

58. Gomez, R., et al. (1997). Pathogenesis of preterm labor and premature rupture of the membranes associated with intraamniotic infection. *Infect Dis Clin North Am, 11,* 135.

59. Gupta, J.K. & Nikodem, V.C. (2000). Women's position during second stage of labour (Cochrane Review). In *The Cochrane Library* (Issue 4). Oxford: Update Software.

60. Hayashi, R.H. & Mozurkewich, E.L. (2000). How to diagnose preterm labor: A clinical dilemma. *Clin Obstet Gynecol, 43,* 768.

61. Hearne, A.E. & Nagey, D.A. (2000). Therapeutic agents in preterm labor: tocolytic agents. *Clin Obstet Gynecol, 43,* 787.

62. Holbrook, R.H. & Ueland, K. (1989). Endocrinology of parturition and preterm labor. In S.A. Brody & K. Ueland (Eds.). *Endocrine disorders in pregnancy.* Norwalk, CT: Appleton & Lange.

63. Huszar, G. (1989). Physiology of the myometrium. In R.K. Creasy & R. Resnik (Eds.). *Maternal-fetal medicine: Principles and practice.* Philadelphia: W.B. Saunders.

64. Izumi, H., et al. (1990). Gestational changes in mechanical properties of skinned muscle tissues of human myometrium. *Am J Obstet Gynecol, 163,* 638.

65. Katz, V.L. & Farmer, R.M. (1999). Controversies in tocolytic therapy. *Clin Obstet Gynecol, 42,* 802.

66. Korebrits, C., et al. (1998). Maternal corticotrophin releasing hormone is increased with impending preterm birth. *J Clin Endocrinol Metab, 83,* 1585.

67. Leppert, P.C. (1995). Anatomy and physiology of cervical ripening. *Clin Obstet Gynecol, 38,* 267.

68. Liu, Y.C. (1989). The effects of the upright position during childbirth. *Image J Nurs Sch, 21*(Spring), 14.

69. Lockwood, C.J. (1994). Recent advances in elucidating the pathogenesis of preterm delivery, the detection of patients at risk, and preventative therapies. *Curr Opin Obstet Gynecol, 6,* 7.

70. Lockwood, C.J. (1999). Stress-associated preterm delivery: the role of corticotrophin-releasing hormone. *Am J Obstet Gynecol, 180*(1), 264S.

71. Lockwood, C.J. & Kuczynski, E. (1999). Markers of risk for preterm delivery. *J Perinat Med, 27,* 5.

72. Lockwood, C.J. (1999). Stress-associated preterm delivery: the role of corticotrophin-releasing hormone, *Am J Obstet Gynecol, 180*(1), S264.

73. Lopez Bernal, A. et al. (1995). Parturition: activation of stimulatory pathways or loss of uterine quiescence? *Adv Exp Med Biol, 395,* 435.

74. Lopez Bernal, A. (2000). Preterm Labour. *Ballieres Best Pract Res Clin Obstet Gynaecol, 14,* 133.

75. Lu, G.C. & Goldenberg, R.L. (2000). Current concepts on the pathogenesis and markers of preterm births. *Clin Perinatol, 27,* 263.

76. Ludmir, J. & Sehdev, H.M. (2000). Anatomy and physiology of the uterine cervix. *Clin Obstet Gynecol, 43,* 433.

77. Lye, S.J. (1997). Initiation of parturition, *Anim Reprod Sci, 42,* 495.

78. Lye, S.J. (1999). Myometrial physiology and parturition. In C.H. Rodeck & M.J. Whittle (Eds.). *Fetal medicine: Basic science and clinical practice.* London: Churchill-Livingstone.

79. MacGregor, J.A., et al. (1995). Salivary estriol as a risk assessment for preterm labor: a prospective trial. *Am J Obstet Gynecol, 173,* 1337.

80. MacKenzie, L.W. & Garfield, R.E. (1985). Hormonal control of gap junctions in the myometrium. *Am J Physiol, 248,* C296.

81. Main, D.M., et al. (1991). Extended longitudinal study of uterine activity among low-risk women. *Am J Obstet Gynecol, 165,* 1317.

82. Majzoub, J.A. & Karalis, K.P. (1999). Placental corticotrophin-releasing hormone: function and regulation. *Am J Obstet Gynecol, 180,* 242S.

83. Majzoub, J.A., et al. (1999). A central theory of preterm and term labor: putative role for corticotrophin releasing hormone. *Am J Obstet Gynecol, 180*(1), S232.

84. Marshall, J.M. (1981). Effects of ovarian steroids and pregnancy on adrenergic nerves of uterus and oviduct. *Am J Physiol, 240,* C165.

85. Mazor, M., et al. (1998). Cytokines in human parturition. *Gynecol Endocrinol, 12,* 421.

86. McLean, M., et al. (1994). Plasma beta-endorphin and CRH during labour. *Eur J Endocrinol, 131,* 167.

87. McLean, M., et al. (1995). A placental clock controlling the length of human pregnancy. *Nature Med, 1,* 460.

88. Mendez-Bauer, C. & Newton, M. (1986). Maternal position in labor. In E. Phillip, J. Barnes, & M. Newton (Eds.). *Scientific foundations of obstetrics and gynecology.* London: Heinemann.

89. Mendez-Bauer, C., et al. (1975). Effects of standing position on spontaneous uterine contractility, and other aspects of labor. *J Perinat Med, 3,* 89.

90. Miller, F.C. (1983). Uterine motility in spontaneous labor. *Clin Obstet Gynecol, 26,* 78.

91. Miller, F.C. & Mattison, D.R. (1989). Oxytocin for induction of labor. In S.A. Brody & K. Ueland (Eds.). *Endocrine disorders in pregnancy.* Norwalk, CT: Appleton & Lange.

92. Miller, F.D., et al. (1993). Synthesis of oxytocin in amnion, chorion, and decidua: a potential paracrine role for oxytocin in the onset of human parturition. *Reg Peptides, 45,* 247.

93. Molnar, M., et al. (1999). Oxytocin activates mitogen-activated protein kinase and upregulates cyclooxygenase-2 and prostaglandin production in human myometrial cells. *Am J Obstet Gynecol, 181,* 42.

94. Monga, M. & Sanborn, B.M. (1999). Uterine biology and the control of myometrial contraction, In R.K. Creasy & R. Resnik (Eds.). *Maternal-fetal medicine* (4th ed.). Philadelphia: W.B. Saunders.

95. Moore, T.R. (1995). Patterns of human uterine contractions: implications for clinical practice. *Semin Perinatol, 19,* 64.

96. Nathanielsz, P.W. (1998). Comparative studies on the initiation of labor. *Eur J Obstet Gynecol Reprod Biol, 78,* 127.

97. Norman, J. (1996). Nitric oxide and the myometrium. *Pharmacol Ther, 70,* 91.

98. Norwitz, E.R., et al. (1999). The control of labor: current concepts. *N Engl J Med, 341,* 660.

99. Nuwayhid, B. & Rahabi, M. (1987). Beta-sympathomimetic agents: Use in perinatal obstetrics. *Clin Perinatol, 14,* 757.

100. O'Brien, W.F. (1995). The role of prostaglandins in labor and delivery. *Clin Perinatol, 22,* 973.

101. Olson, D.M., et al. (1995). Control of human parturition. *Clin Perinatol, 19,* 52.

102. Page, E.W., Villee, C.A., & Villee, D.B. (1981*). Human reproduction: Essentials of reproductive and perinatal medicine* (3rd ed.). Philadelphia: W.B. Saunders.

103. Paine, L.L. & Tinker, D.D. (1992). The effect of maternal bearing-down efforts on arterial umbilical cord pH and length of the second stage of labor. *J Nurs Midwifery, 37,* 61.

104. Payton, R.G. & Brucker, M.C. (1999). Drugs and uterine motility. *J Obstet Gynecol Neonatal Nurs, 28,* 628.

105. Petralglia, F., et al. (1996). Peptide signaling in human placenta and membranes: apocrine, paracrine, and endocrine mechanisms. *Endocrin Rev, 17,* 156.

106. Petraglia, F., et al. (1997). Placental stress factors and human parturition. *Ann N Y Acad Sci, 828,* 230.

107. Phaneuf, S., et al. (1993). Oxytocin-stimulated phosphoinositide hydrolysis in human myometrial cells: involvement of pertussin toxin–sensitive and –insensitive G-proteins. *J Endocrinol, 136,* 497.

108. Rajab, M.R., et al. (1990). Changes in active and latent collagenase in human placenta around the time of parturition. *Am J Obstet Gynecol, 163,* 499.

109. Ramsay, B., et al. (1996). Nitric oxide synthetase activities in human myometrium and villous trophoblast throughout pregnancy. *Obstet Gynecol, 87,* 249.

110. Rechberger, T., et al. (1993). Collagenase, its inhibitors, and decorin in the lower uterine segment in pregnant women. *Am J Obstet Gynecol, 168,* 1598.

111. Reimer, R.K. & Heymann, M.A. (1998). Regulation of uterine smooth muscle function during gestation. *Pediatr Res, 44,* 615.

112. Reis, F.M., et al. (1999). Putative role of placental corticotrophin-releasing factor in the mechanisms of human parturition. *J Soc Gynecol Investig, 6,* 109.

113. Resnik, R. (1999). Anatomic alterations in the reproductive tract. In R.K. Creasy & R. Resnik (Eds.). *Maternal-fetal medicine* (4th ed.). Philadelphia: W.B. Saunders.

114. Resnik, R. & Calder, A. (1999). Post-term pregnancy. In R.K. Creasy & R. Resnik (Eds.). *Maternal-fetal medicine* (4th ed.). Philadelphia: W.B. Saunders.

115. Riley, S.C., et al. (1991), The localization and distribution of corticotrophin-releasing hormone in the human placenta and fetal membranes through gestation. *J Clin Endocrinol Metab, 72,* 1001.

116. Roberts, J. (1980). Alternative positions for childbirth. Part II: Second stage of labor. *J Nurse Midwifery, 25,* 13.

117. Roberts, J.E. (1989). Maternal positioning during the first stage of labour. In I. Chalmers, M. Enkin, & M.J.N.C. Keirse (Eds.). *Effective care in pregnancy and childbirth.* Oxford, England: Oxford University Press.

118. Roberts, J., Malasanos, L. & Mendez-Bauer, C. (1981). Maternal positions in labor: Analysis in relation to comfort and efficiency. *Birth Defects, 17*(6), 97.

119. Roberts, J., Mendez-Bauer, C., & Wodell, D. (1983). The effects of maternal position on uterine contractility and efficiency. *Birth, 10*(4), 243.

120. Roberts, J., et al. (1984). Effects of lateral recumbency and sitting on the first stage of labor. *J Reprod Med, 29,* 477.

121. Romond, J.L. & Baker, I.T. (1985). Squatting in childbirth: a new look at an old tradition. *J Obstet Gynecol Neonatal Nurs, 14,* 406.

122. Sadovsky, V. (1999). Human parturition is associated with enhanced expression and activity of cyclooxygenase-2. *Am J Obstet Gynecol, 180,* 2S.

123. Saji, F. et al. (2000). Cytokine production in chorioamnionitis. *J Reprod Immunol, 47,* 185.

124. Sampselle, C.M. & Hines, S. (1999). Spontaneous pushing during birth: Relationship to birth outcomes. *J Nurs Midwifery, 44,* 36.

125. Sanborn, B.M. (2000). Relationship of ion channel activity to control of myometrial calcium. *J Soc Gynecol Investig, 7,* 4.

126. Sanchez-Ramos, L. et al. (1998). Labor induction with prostaglandin E$_1$, misoprostol compared with dinoprostone vaginal insert: A randomized trial. *Obstet Gynecol, 91,* 401.

127. Sanchez-Ramos, L. & Kaunitz, A.M. (2000). Misoprostol for cervical ripening and labor induction: A systematic review of the literature. *Clin Obstet Gynecol, 43,* 473.

128. Schwartz, L.B. (1997). Understanding human parturition. *Lancet, 350,* 4792.

129. Sladek, S.M., et al. (1997). Nitric oxide and pregnancy. *Am J Physiol, 272*(2), R441.

130. Sleep, J., Roberts, J. & Chalmers, I. (1989). Care during the second stage of labour. In I. Chalmers, M. Enkin, & M.J.N.C. Keirse (Eds.). *Effective care in pregnancy and childbirth.* Oxford, England: Oxford University Press.

131. Smith, R., et al. (1998). CRH directly and preferentially stimulates dehydroepiandroesterone sulfate secretion by human fetal adrenal cortical cells. *J Clin Endocrinol Metab, 83,* 2916.

132. Smith, R. (1999). Corticotrophin-releasing hormone and the feto-placental clock: An Australian perspective. *Am J Obstet Gynecol, 180,* 269S.

133. Strauss, J. & Coutifaris, C. (1999). The endometrium and myometrium: regulation and dysfunction. In S.S.C. Yen, R.B. Jaffe, & R.L. Barbieri (Eds.), *Reproductive endocrinology* (4th ed.). Philadelphia: W.B. Saunders.

134. Stubbs, T.M. (2000). Oxytocin for labor induction. *Clin Obstet Gynecol, 43,* 489.

135. Thaler, I., et al. (1990). Changes in uterine blood flow during human pregnancy. *Am J Obstet Gynecol, 162,* 121.

136. Thomas, A.M. (1993). Pushing techniques in the second stage of labour. *J Adv Nurs, 18,* 171.

137. Ulmsten, U. (1989). Prostaglandins in high-risk obstetrics. In S.A. Brody & K. Ueland (Eds.). *Endocrine disorders in pregnancy.* Norwalk, CT: Appleton & Lange.

138. Vause, S. & Johnson, T. (2000). Management of preterm labor. *Arch Dis Child Fetal Neonatal Ed, 83,* F79.

139. Waldenstrom, U. & Gottvall, K. (1991). A randomized trial of a birthing stool or conventional semirecumbent position for second-stage labor. *Birth, 18,* 5.

140. Warren, W.B., et al. (1995). Corticotrophin-releasing hormone and pituitary-adrenal hormones in pregnancies complicated by chronic hypertension. *Am J Obstet Gynecol, 172,* 661.

141. Weaver, J.B., Pearson, J.F., & Rosen, M. (1977). Response to a Valsalva maneuver before and after an epidural. *Anesthesia, 32,* 148.

142. Winkler, M. & Werner, R. (1999). Changes in the cervical extracellular matrix during pregnancy and parturition. *J Perinat Med, 27,* 45.

143. Witter, F.R. (2000). Prostaglandin E$_2$ preparations for preinduction cervical ripening. *Clin Obstet Gynecol, 43,* 469.

144. Woolley, D. & Roberts, J. (1995). Second stage pushing: A comparison of Valsalva-style with mini-pushing. *J Perinat Ed, 4*(4), 37.

145. Woolley, D. & Roberts, J. (1996). A second look at the second stage of labor. *J Obstet Gynecol Neonatal Nurs, 25,* 415.

146. Word, R.A. (1995). Myosin phosphorylation and the control of myometrial contraction/relaxation. *Semin Perinatol, 19,* 2.

147. Yallampalli, C., et al. (1993). Nitric oxide inhibits uterine contractility during pregnancy but not during delivery. *Endocrinology, 133,* 1899.

148. Yeates, D.A. & Roberts, J.E. (1984). A comparison of two bearing down techniques during the second stage of labor. *J Nurse Midwifery, 29*(1), 3.

149. Young, R.C. (2000). Tissue-level signaling and control of uterine contractility: the action potential-calcium wave hypothesis. *J Soc Gynecol Investig, 7,* 146.

150. Zeeman, G.G., et al. (1997). Oxytocin and its receptor in pregnancy and parturition: current concepts and clinical applications. *Obstet Gynecol, 89,* 874.

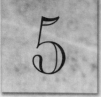

CHAPTER 5
Postpartum Period and Lactation Physiology

The postpartum period is a time of restoration and return to the nonpregnant state. This period is generally defined as the 6-week period beginning with delivery of the placenta. Although some women may experience involution of the reproductive organs as early as 4 weeks after delivery, it may take 10 to 12 weeks for some structures and systems to heal or return to their prepregnancy state. The postpartum period is characterized by significant anatomic, physiologic, and endocrinologic changes as the woman recovers from the stresses of labor and delivery and lactation is initiated. In addition, all of the anatomic and physiologic changes that occurred during the 9 months of pregnancy are reversed for the most part within a 6-week period. Many of these changes occur within the first 10 to 14 days following delivery. This places additional stresses on the woman, who at the same time is undergoing major psychologic, social, and role changes as she attaches to and assumes responsibility for care of her new infant and incorporates him or her into the family system.

The focus of this chapter is on the hormonal and involutional changes associated with return of the reproductive system to its nonpregnant state and on the anatomic, physiologic, and endocrinologic changes involved in the initiation and maintenance of lactation and production of milk. The physiologic and anatomic changes within other body systems as they return to the nonpregnant state are described in Chapters 7 to 19.

INVOLUTION OF THE REPRODUCTIVE ORGANS

The reproductive system (i.e., uterus, cervix, vagina, and breasts in the nonlactating woman) gradually returns to its nonpregnant state during the 6-week postpartum period. This process is referred to as *involution*.

Uterus

Immediately following delivery of the placenta, the uterus weighs about 1000 g and lies with its anterior and posterior walls in close approximation in midline about halfway between the umbilicus and symphysis pubis. Over the next 12 hours the fundus of the uterus rises to the level of the umbilicus (or slightly above or below), followed by a gradual decrease in height over the subsequent 2 to 3 days. By 24 hours postpartum, the uterine size is similar to its size at 20 weeks.[60,76] The height of the fundus usually decreases by about 1 cm per day so that by 3 days the fundus lies 2 to 3 fingerbreadths below the umbilicus or slightly higher in multigravidas. By 5 to 6 days, the uterus weighs about 500 g and is 4 to 5 fingerbreadths below the umbilicus. Magnetic resonance imaging (MRI) studies of involution found that the mean length of the uterine corpus was 13.8 cm at 30 hours postpartum versus 5 cm at 6 months.[96] Generally the uterus has descended into the true pelvis by 10 days, and the fundus can no longer be palpated abdominally. The size of the uterus gradually decreases over the next month so that by 6 weeks the uterus has returned to its nonpregnant location and weighs approximately 60 to 80 g (slightly more than a nulliparous uterus). Involution is slower in multiparous women and following multiple gestation, infection, polyhydramnios, delivery of a large infant, or retention of placental or membrane fragments. Uterine involution has also been shown to be related to delivery mode and feeding choice: the uterus was longer and wider at 3 months in mothers delivered by cesarean section and shorter in women who breastfed.[63]

Involution of the uterus involves three processes: (1) contraction of the uterus, (2) autolysis of myometrial cells, and (3) regeneration of epithelium.[54] Immediately following delivery, contractions of the uterine myometrium compress the blood vessels supplying the placental site, causing hemostasis. At the placental site, only part of the basal portion of the decidua is left. During the first 12 to 24 hours, these contractions ("afterpains") are relatively strong, gradually diminishing in intensity and frequency over the next 4 to 7 days. Postpartal uterine contractions tend to be stronger and to persist for a longer period in multiparous women. Contractions can also be stimulated by oxytocin release associated with suckling.

Under the influence of estrogens, the myometrium undergoes hypertrophy and hyperplasia during pregnancy with increases in cell cytoplasm and size. Following delivery excess intracellular proteins (especially actin and myosin) and cytoplasm within the myometrial cells are eliminated by autolysis with degradation by proteolytic enzymes and macrophages. As a result, the size of individual myometrial cells is markedly reduced without a significant reduction in the total number of cells.

Initially the endometrium resembles a large desquamating wound. The upper portion of the spongy endometrial layer is sloughed off with delivery of the placenta. Regeneration of the uterine epithelial lining begins 2 to 3 days postpartum with differentiation of the remaining decidua into two layers (a superficial layer and a basal layer). The superficial layer of granulation tissue, which provides a barrier to infection, is formed as leukocytes invade the remaining decidua. This layer gradually degenerates, becoming necrotic, and is sloughed off in lochia. The basal layer, which contains the fundi of the uterine endometrial glands, remains intact and is the source of the new endometrium. Regeneration of the endometrium (except at the placental site) occurs by 2 to 3 weeks. By about 16 days, this layer is similar to the nonpregnant endometrium in the proliferative phase of the menstrual cycle except for remnants of hyalinized decidua with areas of leukocyte infiltration.[76] The new endometrium forms from proliferation of the fundi of the endometrial glands and the interglandular connective tissue stroma.[76,14]

Healing at the placental site occurs more slowly over 6 to 7 weeks. Following delivery the placental site is a raised rough area 4 to 5 cm in diameter and consists of many thrombosed vascular sinusoids. The large blood vessels that supplied the intervillous spaces are invaded by fibroblasts and their lumen is obscured. Some of these vessels recanalize later but with smaller lumina. The placental site heals by exfoliation without leaving a scar. This occurs with upward growth of the fundi of the endometrial glands in the decidua basalis under the placental site, with simultaneous growth of endometrial tissue from the margins of the site.[14]

Lochia

The process of involution and restoration of the endometrium is reflected in the characteristics of postpartum vaginal discharge (loss or lochia). Lochia varies in amount and color as healing occurs. Three forms of lochia are observed: rubra, serosa, and alba. The pattern of lochia has generally bee reported as follows. Lochia rubra is seen during the first 2 to 4 days after delivery and contains blood from the placental site; pieces of amnion and chorion; and cellular elements from the decidua, vernix, lanugo, and

meconium. As a result, lochia rubra is dark red or brownish and has a fleshy odor. Lochia serosa is a pinkish-brown discharge seen from day 3 or 4 through about day 10.[67] Lochia serosa contains some blood, wound exudate, erythrocytes, leukocytes, cervical mucus, microorganisms, and shreds of degenerating decidua from the superficial layer. Lochia alba initially appears about 10 to 14 days and lasts until 3 to 6 weeks postpartum. This form of lochia is whitish-yellow in color since it contains primarily leukocytes along with decidual cells, mucus, bacteria, and epithelial cells.

However, Sherman and colleagues recently described three patterns of lochia with a mean duration of 36 ± 7.5 (range of 17 to 151) days.[82] The most common phase was the classic phase described above of rubra → serosa → alba, with a mean length of the rubra phase of 12.1 ± 6.7 days. This pattern was seen primarily in breastfeeding mothers. The next most common phase also proceeded rubra → serosa → alba, but the rubra phase was prolonged (mean 24.8 ± 5 days), with short serosa and alba phases. This pattern was associated with short or no breastfeeding and with increased parity. The third and least common pattern, which may be a variant of the second phase, was rubra (mean 5.5 ± 2.5 days) → serosa/alba → rubra → serosa/alba, with similar duration of each phase.[82] Another study of vaginal loss (all fluids lost from the vagina postpartum) reported a median time of 21 days (range of 10 to 42 days) with a predominance of rubra.[49]

Most women produce a total of 150 to 400 ml of lochia (average 225 ml).[54,61] The amount of lochia is greater in multiparous women and increases with activity; decreased flow is seen at night or with lying down and following cesarean delivery. Women who breastfeed tend to have less lochia (probably due to more rapid healing secondary to hormonal influences), although flow may increase temporarily during feeding.

Cervix and Vagina

Immediately following a vaginal delivery, the cervix hangs into the vagina and is thin, bruised, and edematous with multiple lacerations. Over the next 12 to 18 hours, the cervix shortens and becomes firmer ("forming up") and, as measured by MRI, has a mean length of 5.6 cm by 30 hours (vs. 2.9 cm by 6 months).[96] During the first 2 to 3 days, the cervix is dilated 2 to 24 cm and two fingers can be inserted into the cervical os. By one week the os barely accommodates one finger; by 10 to 12 days a finger can barely be inserted into the internal os but no further. By 4 weeks the external os is a small transverse slit characteristic of multiparous women.[54,61] Even by 6 weeks, there may still be evidence of stromal edema and round cell infiltrates, which may persist to 3 to 4 months.[76] Reconstruction of the cervix, which was significantly remodeled prior to birth (see Chapter 4), begins immediately after birth. This process may be mediated by transforming growth factor–β (TGF-β) and other cytokines.[93] A two- to three-fold increase in mRNA for components of proteoglycans (ground substance) and collagen is seen in the first few days after birth.[93] These substances are needed to restore the cervical structure altered during cervical ripening and delivery.

After a vaginal delivery the vagina is edematous and relaxed, with decreased tone and absence of rugae. The vagina gradually decreases in size and regains tone, although never returning to its prepregnancy state. By 3 to 4 weeks, rugae have begun to reappear, and edema and vascularity have decreased. The vaginal epithelium is generally restored by 6 to 10 weeks postpartum.[60,76] Decreased lubrication of the vagina during this period can lead to discomfort with sexual intercourse, as can an episiotomy site.

Episiotomies are commonly used (in 65% of vaginal deliveries and 80% of primiparas) in the United States to prevent tearing of the fascia and muscle during delivery.[6] This technique is controversial and associated with postpartum problems such as pain, infection, alterations in urination, third-degree lacerations, and dyspareunia.[6,94] Alternative strategies to avoid an episiotomy, such as perineal massage and positioning to enhance perineal stretching, are advocated, although their effectiveness has been questioned.[8,11] Although initial healing occurs in 2 to 3 weeks, the episiotomy site may take 4 to 6 months to heal completely. In a recent study the median time for perineal comfort (including walking and standing) was reported as one month (range, 1 to 6 months) with 20% of women reporting discomfort for more than 2 months. A longer period of discomfort was reported after forceps delivery or spontaneous vaginal tears, but there were no differences in women without or with episiotomies (without forceps).[1] Delayed perineal healing is seen more often in women with episiotomies (7.7%) than those without (2.2%).[53]

Breasts

The breasts or mammary glands undergo marked changes during pregnancy with development of alveolar tissue and the ductile system in preparation for lactation. Following delivery, further anatomic and physiologic changes occur in women who choose to breastfeed (see "Physiology of Lactation"). In women who do not breastfeed, involution occurs. Distention and stasis of the vascular and lymphatic circulation result in primary engorgement by 2 to 4 days following delivery. Secondary engorgement due to distention of the lobules and alveoli with milk may be seen as lactation is established. Without stimulation by suckling and

removal of milk, secretion of prolactin decreases and milk production ceases. Glandular tissue gradually returns to a resting state over the next few weeks. Since new alveoli formed during pregnancy never totally disappear, the breasts do not completely return to their prepregnant state.

The treatment of engorgement varies depending on whether or not the woman is lactating. Suckling or manual expression of milk provides relief to the lactating woman but is not indicated in the nonlactating woman since these maneuvers increase milk production. Heat is used with lactating women to promote milk flow, whereas cold is used with nonlactating women to reduce flow.[61]

Sexual Function and Activity

The postpartum period is characterized by alterations in sexual activity and function for many women and their partners. Trauma to the reproductive organs, postpartum anatomic and physiologic problems, lochia flow, the presence and stress of the new baby, leaking or engorged breasts, fatigue, and psychologic factors can modify sexual function. Vaginal lubrication is altered for up to 6 months after delivery due to reduction of estrogen following removal of the placenta.[89] Prolactin and oxytocin may also alter vaginal lubrication in the lactating woman. Masters and Johnson reported that orgasms in women for the first few months following birth tended to be shorter and less intense with greater latency of response and decreased vasocongestion of the labia majora and minora and vaginal lubrication.[51] These alterations, along with decreased tone in the perineal muscles, may result in more painful and less fulfilling intercourse. An episiotomy or a laceration, which may take 4 to 6 more months to completely heal depending on the extent of the wound, can also increase discomfort during intercourse. In a recent study the median time for reported comfort during intercourse was 3 months (range, 1 to >12 months), with 20% reporting discomfort for more than 6 months. No differences were found between women with and without episiotomies.[1]

Many cultures have taboos against resumption of sexual intercourse and other activities during the postpartum period (and sometimes for longer periods). In the United States the timing for resumption of intercourse by individual couples varies from shortly after delivery to several months. The timing for resumption of sexual intercourse should be based on maternal physical restoration (cessation of bleeding and absence of perineal discomfort) and the psychologic readiness of both partners.[40] Interventions include counseling regarding postpartum sexual function, encouraging alternate forms of sexual intimacy, recommending vaginal lubricants, and teaching Kegel exercises to strengthen the perineal muscles.

ENDOCRINE CHANGES

Endocrine changes after delivery primarily occur secondary to removal of the placenta with its hormones and to changes in prolactin secretion. Removal of placental hormones alters the physiologic function of many body systems, thus initiating return of those systems to their nonpregnant state. The rate at which placental hormones disappear from the maternal system depends on the half-life of the particular substance in maternal plasma and involves two components.[89] The "first half-life" involves removal of a substance from blood and is relatively short, resulting in rapid clearance of hormones from maternal plasma. The second component involves removal of substances from extravascular compartments and generally takes longer. The longer this "second half-life" is, the longer that substances remain in maternal plasma postpartum.[89] For example, human placental lactogen (hPL) generally disappears by 1 to 2 days, whereas human chorionic gonadotropin (hCG) can be detected for 3 to 4 weeks.[89] Pregnancy-associated proteins (PAPs) disappear within a few days after delivery. Other proteins such as α-fetoprotein are present in maternal plasma for several weeks or longer, suggesting that these substances are derived from maternal as well as placental sources.[53,89] In general, most peptide hormones, enzymes, and other circulating proteins of placental origin reach nonpregnant levels by 6 weeks postpartum. Endocrine changes in lactating and nonlactating women are summarized in Figure 5-1.

Estrogens and Progesterone

Since the placenta is the major source of estrogens and progesterone, these hormones tend to disappear rapidly following delivery. Plasma estradiol (with a first half-life of 20 minutes and second half-life of 6 to 7 hours) reaches levels that are less than 2% of pregnancy values by 24 hours. By 1 to 3 days, estradiol levels are similar to those found during the follicular phase of the menstrual cycle (less than 100 pg/ml), and unconjugated estriol is undetectable.[89] Estrogen levels fall further to day 7 after delivery then gradually increase to follicular phase levels over the next few weeks. Although the first and second half-lives of progesterone are quite short, progesterone levels do not fall as rapidly as estradiol levels because the corpus luteum continues progesterone secretion during the first days following delivery.[89] Generally, progesterone levels similar to those found in the luteal phase of the menstrual cycle (2 to 25 ng/ml) are reached by 24 to 48 hours and follicular phase levels (less than 1 ng/ml) by 3 to 7 days.[89] Ovarian production of estrogens and progesterone is low during the first 2 weeks, maintaining low levels of these hormones. Levels of estradiol and progesterone gradually increase with

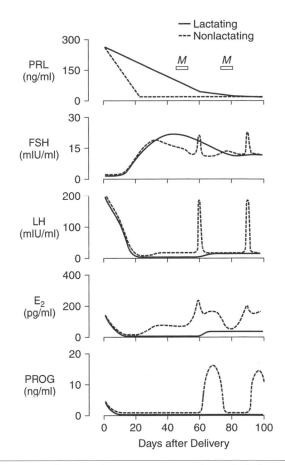

FIGURE **5-1** Changes in serum concentrations of pituitary and gonadal hormones in lactating and nonlactating women in the puerperium. In the top graph, the *M* boxes refers to menses in the nonlactating women. Changes in hormone levels associated with these menstrual periods are seen in the other graphs for the non-lactating woman. The lactating woman is still lactating and not menstruating. The elevated luteinizing hormone (LH) immediately postpartum is due to cross-reaction with assays of human chorionic gonadotropin and the estradiol (E_2) and progesterone (PROG) are of placental origin. *FSH,* Follicle-stimulating hormone; *PRL,* prolactin. (From Rebar, R.W. [1999]. The breast and the physiology of lactation. In R.K. Creasy & R. Resnik [Eds.]. *Maternal-fetal medicine* [4th ed.]. Philadelphia: W.B. Saunders. Based on Rolland, R., et al. [1975]. The role of prolactin in the restoration of ovarian function during the early postpartum period in the human female. Part I: A study during physiological lactation. *Clin Endocrinol, 4,* 15.)

resumption of gonadotropin secretion by the pituitary and ovarian cycling.[46]

Pituitary Gonadotropin

The pituitary-hypothalamic-ovarian axis (see Chapter 2), along with production of pituitary gonadotropin, follicle-stimulating hormone (FSH), and luteinizing hormone (LH), is suppressed during pregnancy. Serum levels of FSH and LH remain very low during the first 2 weeks postpartum in both lactating and nonlactating women, then gradually increase over the next few weeks with resumption of pituitary function by 4 to 6 weeks. The basis for the initially sluggish pituitary response is unknown. Tulchinsky suggests that this phenomenon may be related to: (1) suppression of the pituitary-hypothalamic axis by the high levels of circulating estrogens during pregnancy, (2) need for time to reestablish adequate stores of FSH and LH leading to a delay in secretion of gonadotropin-releasing hormone (GnRH) by the hypothalamus, and (3) inhibition of LH release by hCG (which can be found for up to 2 weeks postpartum) and prolactin.[46,89]

Prolactin

Prolactin is a single-chain peptide hormone secreted in pulses by the anterior pituitary gland. Serum levels of prolactin increase during pregnancy (from 5 to 10 ng/ml to 140 to 200 ng/ml), although its effects are suppressed by estrogen.[7,30] During pregnancy, prolactin is one of several hormones acting synergistically to promote development of the mammary alveoli and duct system. Prolactin release from the pituitary is suppressed by prolactin-inhibiting factor (PIF) from the hypothalamus. Prolactin levels are similar in nonlactating females and males and vary diurnally with an increase during sleep. Prolactin levels increase with stress, anesthesia, surgery, exercise, nipple stimulation, and sexual intercourse.[43]

The onset of labor is associated with a decrease in prolactin followed by an increase immediately after delivery that peaks at about 3 hours postpartum.[77] The increase postpartum is not due to an increase in the number of pulses but rather to increased prolactin in each pulse.[75] Secretion of prolactin postpartum is triggered by suckling. In nonlactating women, prolactin levels fall into the high end of the nonpregnant range by 7 to 14 days.[89] Patterns of prolactin secretion associated with lactation are described in Physiology of Lactation.

Oxytocin

Oxytocin is an octapeptide hormone produced in the hypothalamus and stored and secreted by the posterior pituitary gland. The uterus becomes increasingly sensitive to oxytocin throughout pregnancy, probably as a result of increasing estrogens that mediate an increase in oxytocin receptors. The placenta may contain a catabolic enzyme to maintain lower levels during pregnancy.[89] Oxytocin stimulates electrical and contractile activity in the myometrium (see Chapter 4) and is critical in the ejection of milk during lactation. Thus putting the infant to breast immediately after delivery may enhance uterine involution.[64]

RESUMPTION OF MENSTRUATION AND OVULATION

The postpartum period tends to be a period of relative infertility for many women. Resumption of menstruation and ovulation varies among individual women regardless of whether or not the woman is lactating. Resumption of ovulation is associated with an increase in plasma progesterone. Although for most women the initial menstrual cycle following delivery is anovulatory, up to 25% of these cycles may be preceded by ovulation.[89] In addition, an estimated two thirds of women ovulate before their first menses; however, 47% of these cycles have a defective luteal phase, reducing the chance of conception.[10] The sooner menstruation returns following delivery, the more likely that the cycle will be anovulatory. Anovulatory cycles are more frequent in lactating women, who are more likely to ovulate before return of menses than are nonlactating women.[10]

The cause of the postpartum amenorrhea is not completely understood but is likely related to the decreased gonadotropin secretion (possibly as a result of a transient pituitary insensitivity to LH-releasing factor) for the first 2 to 3 weeks postpartum.[76] The period of amenorrhea seen in lactating women is due to low ovarian function due in part to suckling induced alterations in GnRH production and release.[75,98]

In nonlactating women, menstruation generally begins by 6 to 10 weeks postpartum, with 50% of the first cycles anovulatory.[91] Ovulation rarely occurs before 25 to 26 days and has been reported in only 6% of woman before 6 weeks. The average time to the resumption of menstruation and first ovulation in nonlactating women has been reported as 45 ± 3.8 (range of 25 to 72) days. Vorherr reported that in nonlactating women, 40% experienced a resumption of menses by 6 weeks, 65% by 12 weeks, and 90% by 24 weeks postpartum; 15% resumed ovulation by 6 weeks, 40% by 12 weeks, and 65% by 24 weeks.[91] Recent studies have reported that menses resumes in most nonlactating women between 7 and 9 weeks, with 45% by 45 days and more than 90% by 12 weeks.[10,55,76,89] In women taking bromocriptine for lactation suppression, ovulation may resume as early as 23 to 28 days.[38]

Lactation is associated with a delay in resumption of menstruation and ovulation.[12] Lactating women experience anovulation for varying lengths of time, with up to 80% of these woman reported to have anovulatory first cycles.[91] Anovulation is related to increased production of prolactin by the anterior pituitary gland. Prolactin reduces the sensitivity of the pituitary to the effects of GnRH from the hypothalamus, reducing FSH and LH secretion. Prolactin also lowers the sensitivity of ovarian follicles to

LH and FSH.[89] Hyperprolactinemic states (i.e., during lactation or with infertility-associated abnormalities) tend to inhibit the LH surge and ovulation.

Ovulation usually does not occur in lactating women prior to 10 weeks following delivery but may occur as early as 35 days.[10,89] Vorherr noted that menses returned in 15% of these women by 6 weeks, 45% by 12 weeks, and 85% by 24 weeks. By 6 weeks, 5% of lactating women had resumed ovulation, with 25% ovulating by 12 weeks, and 65% by 24 weeks.[91] The resumption of menstruation and ovulation in lactating women is influenced by the length of time that they lactate. Campbell and Gray found that 45% of women breastfeeding 0 to 12 weeks had ovular cycles (ovulation preceding resumption of menses) versus 67% of women breastfeeding for 13 to 24 weeks, 75% of women breastfeeding for 25 to 48 weeks, and 100% of women breastfeeding more than 49 weeks.[10] Howie and colleagues reported that the average time to return of menstruation in lactating women was 30 to 36 weeks, with an average time to first ovulation of 17 weeks in woman who breastfed for 3 months and 28 weeks in woman breastfeeding for 6 months.[34] Women who lactated for less than 1 month tended to follow the pattern of nonlactating women for resumption of menstruation and ovulation. Duration of amenorrhea is longer in women who exclusively breastfeed than in those who combine breastfeeding and bottle feeding; the longer a woman breastfeeds, the more likely she is to ovulate before resumption of menses.[87] Longer periods of lactational amenorrhea and anovulation are also seen in women who have more total time breastfeeding per day and more total infant suckling time, who maintain night feedings longer, and who introduce supplements most gradually.[33,34,87] Suckling may prevent GnRH release from the hypothalamus and thus the normal pituitary LH surge probably via a prolactin-mediated effect of breast stimulation.[87] Although pulsatile secretion of LH is seen by 8 weeks postpartum, levels are low and of variable frequency with no preovulatory surge. With regular suckling, LH remains supressed.[64]

Therefore lactation, although associated with decreased fertility, may not be a reliable method for preventing pregnancy. Approximately 5% to 15% of breastfeeding amenorrheic women become pregnant unintentionally.[87] The most important factors to reduce the risk of pregnancy during breastfeeding in women using the *lactational amenorrhea method* (LAM) of birth control are initiation of breastfeeding as soon as possible after birth and "complete" breastfeeding (i.e., on demand at least five to six times per day with more than 10-minute sessions, or more than 65 minutes per day with no sup-plementation).[87] Complete breastfeeding is associated with less than 2% of unwanted pregnancies in the first 6 months after delivery.[13,24,45,50] Some investigators feel that even with occasional supplementation, protection can be achieved if adequate frequency and duration are maintained.[10] However, the problem is often that introduction of supplements (liquid or solid feedings) is associated with decreased frequency and duration of breastfeeding.

STRUCTURE OF THE MAMMARY GLANDS

The breasts or mammary glands are modified exocrine glands consisting of epithelial glandular tissue with an extensive system of branching ducts surrounded by adipose tissue and separated from the pectoralis major muscles of the chest and the ribs by connective tissue. The breasts are highly innervated with rich vascular and lymphatic systems. The basic glandular unit is the alveolus, which consists of clusters of epithelial secretory cells (the site of milk production) around a lumen, into which the ductules terminate. Myoepithelial cells surrounding the secretory cells form smooth muscle contractile units responsible for ejecting milk from the lumen of the alveoli into the ductules.[43,97] The structure of milk production and ejection portions of the mammary glands is illustrated in Figure 5-2.

The branching ductule system from the alveoli gradually merges into larger lactiferous or mammary ducts. At the base of the nipple (mammary papilla), the ducts dilate, forming ampullae, or lactiferous sinuses. The lactiferous sinuses are surrounded by fibromuscular tissue and provide an area for milk storage. The ends of the lactiferous sinuses constrict as the duct system enters the nipple. The breast consists of 15 to 20 lobes arranged in spokes around the nipple and separated from each other by connective tissue. Each lobe terminates in a lactiferous duct that opens onto the nipple and from which milk is ejected. A lobe consists of 20 to 40 lobules, each containing 10 to 100 alveoli with their respective ductules.[43] Figure 5-3 illustrates the mammary alveolus. The ducts and alveoli are surrounded by a stroma of fibroblasts, adipocytes, blood vessels, plasma cells (B lymphocytes capable of producing immunoglobulins, especially secretory immunoglobulin A [IgA]), and a few nerves.[64,85] Stomal cells produce lipoprotein lipase needed for lipid synthesis.[66] The areolar area around the nipple contains small sebaceous glands (tubercles of Montgomery) that provide nipple lubrication and antisepsis. Washing the nipple with soap can remove these protective secretions and lead to drying and cracking of the nipples and increase the risk of infection.

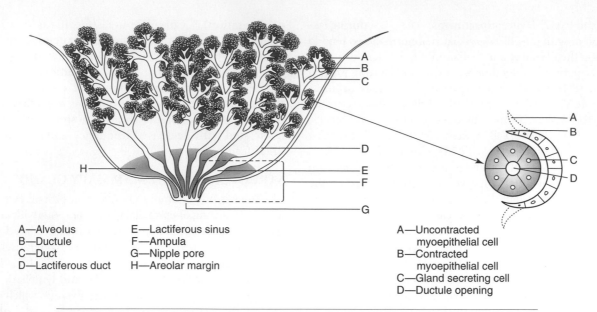

A—Alveolus
B—Ductule
C—Duct
D—Lactiferous duct

E—Lactiferous sinus
F—Ampula
G—Nipple pore
H—Areolar margin

A—Uncontracted
　　myoepithelial cell
B—Contracted
　　myoepithelial cell
C—Gland secreting cell
D—Ductule opening

FIGURE **5-2** Functional unit of milk production: lobular and alveolar systems. (From Applebaum, R.M. [1975]. The obstetrician's approach to the breasts and breastfeeding. *J Reprod Med, 14*[3], 100.)

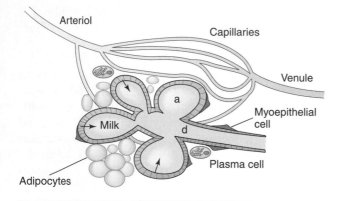

FIGURE **5-3** Model of mammary alveolus *(a)* with surrounding supporting structures that include a ductule *(d)* through which milk is ejected by contraction of the myoepithelial cells, vasculature, and a rich stroma composed of fibroblasts and adipocytes, some of them depleted of fat during lactation, and plasma cells. (From Neville, M.C. [1999]. Physiology of lactation. *Clin Perinatol, 26,* 252.)

PHYSIOLOGY OF LACTATION

Lactation is a complex physiologic process involving integration of neuronal and endocrine mechanisms. Lactation can be divided into five phases: embryogenesis, mammogenesis (mammary growth during puberty and pregnancy), lactogenesis (initiation of milk secretion), galactopoiesis (maintenance of established milk secretion), and involution with cessation of lactation.[64,89] These phases are summa-

rized in Table 5-1. Hormonal influences on lactation are summarized in Table 5-2.

Embryogenesis

Mammary growth begins during fetal life. The mammary or milk ridges appear in the fourth week. Much of this ridge regresses, but remnants in the thoracic area thicken to form a primordial mammary bud. A primitive breast bud appears around 18 to 19 weeks after conception. The bulb-shaped bud composed of epithelial tissue arises from the epidermis. The bud forms 15 to 25 secondary buds, which will form the ductule system in the mature breast. This bud extends into the surrounding mesenchyme where mammary fat pads are developing. The secondary buds elongate, invading the mammary fat pad. Initially the ducts are solid but later canalize to form a rudimentary ductile system.[64,75] Occasionally the newborn may have transient secretions from the breast in the first few days after birth, probably due to the high prolactin levels present in the newborn.

Mammogenesis

Mammogenesis involves mammary growth after birth that accelerates at puberty with further development and maturation of the breasts. During childhood, before the onset of menses, further (minimal) development of the ductile system is seen, mediated by estrogen and growth hormone. Labioalveolar development accelerates after the onset of menses with development of terminal duct lobular units

TABLE **5-1** Stages of Mammary Development

DEVELOPMENTAL STAGES	HORMONAL REGULATION	LOCAL FACTORS	DESCRIPTION
Embryogenesis	???	Fad pad necessary for ductal extension	Epithelial bud develops in 18- to 19-week fetus, extending a short distance into mammary fat pad with blind ducts that become canalized; some milk secretion may be present at birth. Anatomic development
Mammogenesis Puberty:			
Before onset of menses	Estrogen, GH	IGF-1, HGF, TGF-β, ???	Ductal expansion into the mammary fat pad; branching morphogenesis
After onset of menses	Estrogen, progesterone, PRL?	Herregulin, ???	Lobular development with formation of TDLU
Pregnancy	Progesterone, PRL, hPL		Alveolus formation; partial cellular differentiation
Lactogenesis	Progesterone withdrawal, PRL, glucocorticoid	Not known	Onset of milk secretion: Stage I: Mid-pregnancy Stage II: Parturition
Galactopoiesis (stage III lactogenesis)	PRL, oxytocin	FIL	Ongoing milk secretion
Involution	Withdrawal of prolactin	Milk stasis (FIL???)	Alveolar epithelium undergoes apoptosis and remodeling and gland reverts to prepregnant state

From Neville, M.C. (1999). Physiology of lactation. *Clin Perinatol, 26,* 253.
???, Additional factors unknown; *FIL,* feedback inhibitor of lactation *GH,* growth hormone; *HGF,* hyperglycemic glyconeolytic factor; *hPL,* human placental lactogen; *IGF,* insulin-like growth factor; *PRL,* prolactin; *TGF,* transforming growth factor; *TDLU,* terminal duct lobular unit.

TABLE **5-2** Hormonal Contributions to Breast Development

		FUNCTION	
HORMONE	ORIGIN	BEFORE AND DURING PREGNANCY	AFTER DELIVERY
Prolactin (PRL)	Anterior pituitary	Serum levels rise but estrogen suppresses its effect during pregnancy	Stimulates alveolar cells to produce milk (is probably of primary importance in initiating lactation but of secondary importance in maintaining lactation); may also cause lactation infertility by suppressing release of FSH and LH from pituitary or by causing ovaries to be unresponsive to gonadotropins; levels rise in response to various psychogenic factors, stress, anesthesia, surgery, high serum osmolality, exercise, nipple stimulation, and sexual intercourse
Prolactin-inhibiting factor (PIF)	Hypothalamus	Suppresses release of PRL into blood; release stimulated by dopaminergic impulses (i.e., catecholamines)	Suppresses release of PRL from anterior pituitary; agents that increase PRL by decreasing catecholamines and thus PIF include phenothiazides and reserpine
Oxytocin	Posterior pituitary	Generally no effect on mammary function; sensitivity of myoepithelial cells to oxytocin increases during pregnancy	Causes myoepithelial cells to contract, leading to "milk ejection"; release is inhibited by stresses such as fear, anxiety, embarrassment, distraction; also causes uterine contraction and postpartum involution of the uterus

Adapted from Worthington-Roberts, B.S. & Williams, S.R. (1989). *Nutrition in pregnancy and lactation* (4th ed.). St. Louis: Mosby.

Continued

TABLE **5-2**   Hormonal Contributions to Breast Development—cont'd

| | | FUNCTION | |
HORMONE	ORIGIN	BEFORE AND DURING PREGNANCY	AFTER DELIVERY
Estrogen	Ovary and placenta	Stimulates proliferation of glandular tissue and ducts in breast; probably stimulates pituitary to secrete PRL but inhibits PRL effects on breasts	Blood level drops at parturition, which aids in initiating lactation; not important to lactation thereafter
Progesterone	Ovary and placenta	With estrogen, stimulates proliferation of glandular tissue and ducts in breast; inhibits milk secretion	Blood levels drop at parturition, which aids in initiating lactation; probably unimportant to lactation thereafter
Growth hormone	Anterior pituitary		May act with PRL in initiating lactation but appears to be most important in maintaining established lactation
Adrenocorticotropic hormone (ACTH)	Anterior pituitary	Blood levels gradually increase during pregnancy; stimulates adrenal to release corticosteroids	High level is believed necessary for maintenance of lactation
Human placental lactogen (hPL)	Placenta	Like growth hormone in structure; stimulates mammary growth; associated with mobilization of free fatty acids and inhibition of peripheral glucose utilization and lactogenic action	
Thyroxine	Thyroid	Normally no direct effect on lactation	Appears to be important in maintaining lactation either through some direct effect on the mammary glands or by control of metabolism
Thyrotropin-releasing hormone	Hypothalamus	Normally no effect on lactation	Stimulates release of PRL; can be used to maintain established lactation

Adapted from Worthington-Roberts, B.S. & Williams, S.R. (1989). *Nutrition in pregnancy and lactation* (4th ed.). St. Louis: Mosby.

and alveoli formation under the influence of estrogen, progesterone, and probably prolactin.[64] The breasts undergo additional changes during pregnancy and after delivery in order to support lactation. Breast changes begin soon after conception. The weight of the breast increases by about 12 oz during pregnancy. External changes include increases in size and areolar pigmentation. The tubercles of Montgomery enlarge and become more prominent, and the nipples more erect. The myoepithelial cells hypertrophy. The skin over the breasts appears thinner; the blood vessels are more prominent, and there is a twofold increase in blood flow to the breast.

During the first trimester the ductule system proliferates and branches under the influence of estrogen. The glandular tissues of the alveoli proliferate under the influ-

ence of hPL, hCG, and prolactin; lobular formation is enhanced by progesterone (Figure 5-4). Growth hormone and adrenocorticotropic hormone (ACTH) act synergistically with prolactin and progesterone to promote mammogenesis. Concurrently breast interstitial tissue becomes infiltrated with lymphocytes, plasma cells, and eosinophils. During the second and third trimesters there is further lobular growth with formation of new alveoli and ducts and dilation of the lumina. Ductile arborization with development of extensive lobular clusters begins at mid-gestation. Secretory material similar to colostrum accumulates in the lumina beginning in the second trimester.[42,68,97]

During the third trimester the epithelial cells of the alveoli differentiate into secretory cells capable of milk production and release. Fat droplets accumulate in the secre-

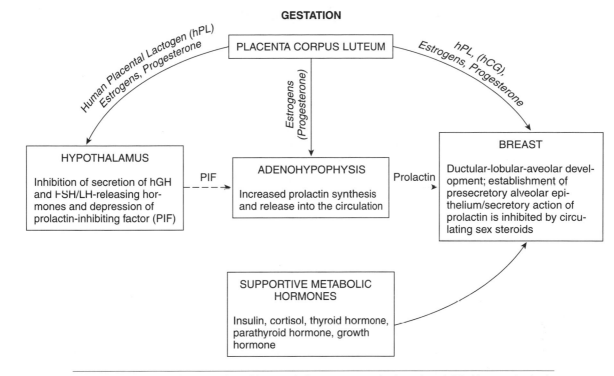

GESTATION

FIGURE **5-4** Hormonal preparation of breast during pregnancy for lactation. *hCG,* Human chorionic gonadotropin; *hGH,* human growth hormone. (Modified from Vorherr, H. [1974]. *The breast.* New York: Academic Press, by Lawrence, R.A. & Lawrence, R.M. [1999]. *Breastfeeding: A guide for the medical profession* [5th ed.]. St. Louis: Mosby.)

tory cells. Progressive dilation of the breast results from the increase in secretory cells and distention of the alveoli with colostrum.[43] Following birth the alveolar epithelial cells continue to proliferate with synthesis of milk under the influence of increased levels of prolactin and the stimulus of suckling. Initial synthesis of milk components is preceded by an increase in required enzymes within the secretory cells.

Lactogenesis

Lactogenesis, or initiation of milk production, involves a complex neuroendocrine process with interaction of several hormones. Lactogenesis can be divided into two stages. The initial stage (lactogenesis I) is from midpregnancy to term as the mammary glands become competent to secrete milk. Only small amounts of milk are secreted, however, as a result of the inhibitory effects of the placental hormones. The second stage (lactogenesis II) begins at birth and takes about 4 days to complete. Sometimes the next phase of lactation, galactopoiesis, is included in lactogenesis as stage III. With birth, milk protein and lactose synthesis and secretion increase rapidly along with immunoglobulins and other proteins.[5] The major increase in milk volume is

not until after 2 or 3 days postpartum. In addition, the tight junctions between mammary cells close to prevent backflow of milk components.[64]

The predominant hormone in control of lactation is prolactin, which acts synergistically with growth hormone, insulin, cortisol, thyrotropin-releasing hormone, thyroid hormones, and parathyroid hormone (see Table 5-2 and Figure 5-5). Growth hormone and insulin are important for survival of alveolar cells and for stimulating glucose entry in the mammary epithelial cells to accelerate lipogenesis. Glucocorticoids may enhance many of the enzymes needed for milk synthesis.[72,75]

Prolactin Patterns in Lactating Women

Milk production and release are controlled primarily by the effect of suckling on prolactin release via a complex neuroendocrine process. Suckling stimulates prolactin release from the anterior pituitary (Figure 5-6). Suckling also stimulates sensory nerve endings in the nipple and areola, sending impulses to the hypothalamus via the spinal cord. As a result, hypothalamic secretion of prolactin-inhibiting factor is suppressed, and adenohypophysis secretion of prolactin increases. Prolactin levels increase toward the end of

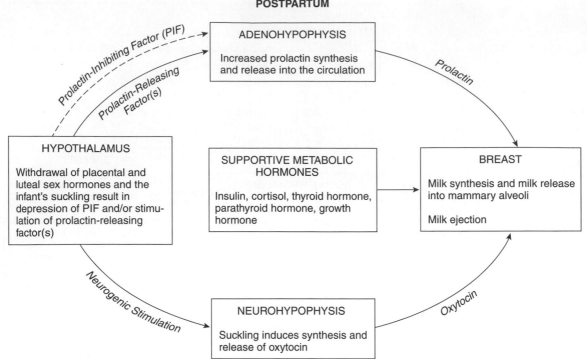

FIGURE **5-5** Hormonal preparation of the breast postpartum for lactation. (Modified from Vorherr, H. [1974]. *The breast.* New York: Academic Press; and Lawrence, R.A. & Lawrence, R.M. [1999]. *Breastfeeding: A guide for the medical profession* [5th ed.]. St. Louis: Mosby.)

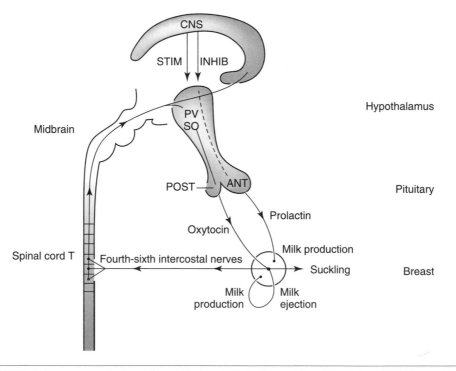

FIGURE **5-6** The neuroendocrine reflexes that are initiated by suckling. Stimulatory (STIM) as well as inhibitory (INHIB) influences leading to milk production are shown. *PV,* Paraventricular nucleus; *SO,* supraoptic nucleus; *T,* thoracic region. (From Tulchinsky, D. [1994]. Postpartum lactation and resumption of reproductive function. In D. Tulchinsky & A.B. Little [Eds.]. *Maternal-fetal endocrinology* [2nd ed.]. Philadelphia: W.B. Saunders.)

a feeding, increasing the volume, fat, and protein content of milk in the next feeding.[89]

Prolactin is important in generating milk for subsequent feedings. Decreased frequency of feedings or bottle supplementation decreases milk production. The daily regulation of the volume of milk secreted is thought to be mediated by the milk protein feedback inhibitor of lactation (FIL). If milk is not completely removed from the breast, FIL accumulates over time in the lumen of the mammary gland. FIL can inhibit synthesis and secretion possibly by decreasing sensitivity of cells to prolactin.[64,71,95] The role of FIL is not completely understood, and there may be other factors such as a stretch response mediating milk synthesis and secretion.[58,81,95] If frequency of suckling is increased, within certain time constraints, milk production will again increase. During early lactation, increasing the frequency of feedings is especially important in establishing adequate milk production. This can often be accomplished by demand feeding. Increasing maternal fluid intake does not significantly increase milk production.[20] For mothers of preterm or other infants who cannot yet tolerate enteral feedings, increasing the frequency of breast pumping can help to establish and maintain the mother's milk supply. Hopkinson and colleagues found that optimal milk production in mothers of preterm infants was associated with five or more milk expressions per day and pumping duration exceeding 100 min/day.[32]

Prolactin acting synergistically with insulin and cortisol, in particular, stimulates the alveolar secretory cells to produce milk proteins and fat. If prolactin is absent, milk secretion will not occur. However, lactation will not begin unless preceded by a fall in plasma estrogens (removing a blocking effect and allowing breast tissue to respond to prolactin) and progesterone (which may have an inhibitory effect on production of α-lactalbumin and consequently lactose).[89] The number of prolactin receptors on breast tissue increases markedly following delivery. The decrease in hPL following removal of the placenta may also facilitate prolactin action, since hPL competes with prolactin for the same breast tissue receptors.[89] Bromocriptine mesylate, a substance used to suppress lactation, acts by decreasing the number of specific prolactin receptors.

Three patterns of prolactin secretion are seen in lactating women.[69] During the first week following delivery, basal prolactin levels are high and increase only slightly with suckling. From approximately 2 weeks to 3 months, baseline levels are 2 to 3 times higher. With suckling, prolactin levels increase 10 to 20 times. After 3 months, baseline prolactin levels are similar to those of nonlactating women and do not rise significantly with suckling (Figure 5-7).[43,69,90] Thus levels of prolactin are not proportional to milk volume. In lactating women, prolactin levels are highest with more frequent suckling and after the last feeding in the day (maintaining the normal diurnal increase in prolactin seen in both males and females).[16]

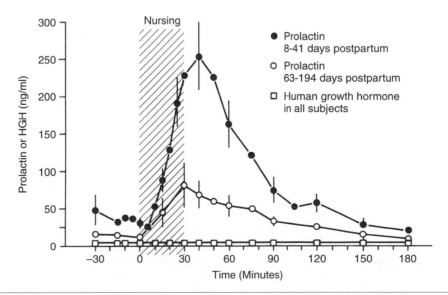

FIGURE **5-7** Plasma prolactin and human growth hormone (hGH) concentrations (mean ±SE) during nursing in days 8 to 41 and 63 to 194 postpartum. (From Noel, G.L., Suh, H.K. & Frantz, A.G. [1974]. Prolactin release during nursing and breast stimulation in postpartum and nonpostpartum patients. *J Clin Endocrinol Metab, 38,* 413. Copyright by The Endocrine Society.)

Galactopoiesis

Galactopoiesis (sometimes called stage III lactogenesis) is the maintenance of established milk secretion. This phase of lactation is dependent on establishment of periodic suckling, removal of milk, and an intact hypothalamic-pituitary axis regulating prolactin and oxytocin levels.[43] Other hormones enhancing galactopoiesis include growth hormone, corticosteroids, thyroxine, and insulin (see Figure 5-5). Prolactin seems most critical during initiation of lactation and less so with long-term maintenance of lactation. Oxytocin stimulates propulsion of milk through the duct system (let-down reflex).

Oxytocin and the Let-Down Reflex

The let-down (or milk ejection) reflex is a complex neuroendocrine process important for movement of milk along the duct system to the nipple. Suckling stimulates sensory nerve endings in the nipple and areola. These impulses travel via afferent neural pathways in the spinal cord to the mesencephalon and hypothalamus, stimulating oxytocin release from the posterior pituitary gland (see Figure 5-6). Oxytocin stimulates contraction of the myoepithelial cells surrounding the alveoli. Contraction of these cells shortens and widens the ducts, enhancing milk flow to the nipples.[64] As a result, milk is ejected into the duct system and propelled to the lactiferous ducts and sinuses. With suckling, the nipple and much of the areolar are drawn into the infant's mouth, forming a teat. Milk is removed by the stripping action of the infant's tongue against the hard palate. Smooth muscle and elastic fibers in the areola and nipple form a sphincter to prevent milk loss when the infant is not suckling.[64] Oxytocin also stimulates uterine contractions and involution. The let-down reflex can also be triggered by thinking of the infant, infant crying, and orgasm. Anxiety, stress, pain, and fatigue can reduce the let-down reflex and decrease the amount of milk released to the infant.[43,77] This reflex is also inhibited by ethanol consumption.[12]

Involution

Upon cessation of lactation, and removal of the suckling stimulus for prolactin secretion, involution of the breasts occurs over several months. This process involves increased secretion of lactoferrin, opening of the tight junctions between the alveolar cells (see "Lactogenesis"), apoptosis of the mammary epithelium, and changes in secretory proteases.[47,64,95] The protein FIL and stretch responses, discussed previously, also play a role in the cessation of milk synthesis and secretion. Stretch responses may be mediated by ATP release and increased entry of calcium into the cells.[71,81] The breasts never return to their prelac-

tation size due to retention of many of the new labioalveolar structures.

Milk Production and Composition

The components of milk are synthesized in the secretory cells of the alveoli (protein, fat, lactose) or extracted from maternal plasma (vitamins, minerals) by these same cells. The individual components of milk then pass into the alveolar lumen where the final milk is constituted. The secretory cells proceed through several stages as milk is produced, moving from a resting state to a secretory state and back to a resting state.[43] Milk synthesis occurs at very low levels much of the time, but is most active during infant suckling. The secretory cells change from a cuboidal to clublike appearance immediately before milk secretion, reflecting cellular uptake of water.[97]

Proteins, lactose, and fats synthesized within the microsomal fraction of the cell are packaged into vesicles that migrate through the cytoplasm to the apex of the secretory cells. These substances are then released into the alveolar lumen via either apocrine or merocrine secretion. Merocrine secretion involves release of materials, such as newly synthesized proteins, through the cell apex without significant loss of cytoplasm. Apocrine secretion also involves expulsion of secretory material such as fat droplets from the cell apex.[43] The fat droplets move through the cytoplasm of the secretory cell to the cell apex, projecting into the alveolar lumen. The droplets are secreted into the lumen accompanied by pieces of cell membrane and surrounding cytoplasm.

Mechanisms for Milk Secretion

Five routes have been identified for secretion of substances across the mammary epithelium: exocytosis, milk fat secretion, membrane (direct movement), transcytosis, and paracellular routes (Figure 5-8).[64,65] Whey proteins, casein, lactose, citrate, and calcium are secreted by exocytosis, sequestered in the Golgi apparatus, and then transported via secondary vesicles to the alveolar lining where the vesicular contents are extruded. Milk fat is secreted in milk fat globules (Figure 5-9). These globules have an inner core of triglycerides, cholesterol esters, and retinyl esters surrounded by phospholipids, proteins, cholesterol, and enzymes in a loose network called the *fat-milk-globule–membrane*.[78,92] The membrane also contains some growth factors, lipid-soluble hormones and leptin, and it may contain lipid-soluble drugs. (Leptin is a protein product of the *obese [ob] gene* that appears to play a role in many reproductive processes, including fertility, maternal adaptation pregnancy, and placental-fetal physiology.[84]) The fat-milk-globule–membrane prevents the individual fat globules

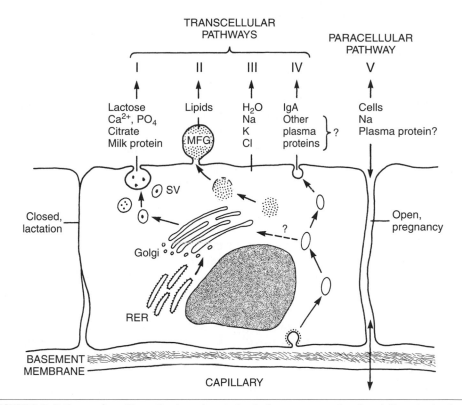

FIGURE **5-8** Pathways for milk synthesis and secretion in the mammary alveolus. *I.* Exocytosis of milk protein and lactose in Golgi derived secretory vesicles. *II.* Milk fat secretion via milk fat globule. *III.* Secretion of ions and water across apical membrane. *IV.* Transcytosis of immunoglobulins. *V.* Paracellular pathway for plasma components and leukocytes. *MFG,* Milk fat globule; *RER,* rough endoplasmic reticulum; *SV,* secretory vesicle. (Modified from Neville, M.C. [1990]. The physiological basis of milk secretion. Part I: Basic physiology. *Ann NY Acad Sci, 586,* 1.)

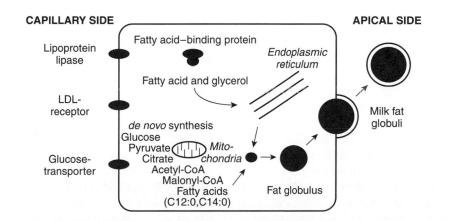

FIGURE **5-9** Formation of milk fat globule in the mammary alveolus. Substrates for milk fat synthesis are lipoprotein lipids taken up after hydrolysis by lipoprotein lipase activity or binding to low-density-lipoprotein (LDL) receptor, as well as glucose taken up by a glucose transporter. Fatty acids are taken up from the circulation together with those synthesized de novo from glucose can be reesterified and incorporated into milk fat globules, which are surrounded by the milk-fat-globule–membrane. (From Rodriguez-Palmero, M., et al. [1999]. Nutritional and biochemical properties of human milk. Part II. *Clin Perinatol, 26,* 336.)

from coalescing into large globules that would be difficult for infants to digest. The membrane route involves the direct movement of ions (e.g., sodium, potassium, chloride), water, and glucose across the apical cell membrane. Transcytosis is the mechanism for movement of intact proteins from the interstitial space into milk. This mechanism is used for immunoglobulins, especially IgA, phospholipids, insulin, growth factors, probably albumin, and possibly transferrin.[35,64,70,81,87]

These first four mechanisms are all active during milk production and are unidirectional (blood to milk). The final mechanism, the paracellular route, is open only during pregnancy, mastitis, and involution. The paracellular route allows plasma components, intact proteins, leukocytes, and degraded cells to pass bidirectionally between the mammary cells. During lactation this route is closed because tight junctions (gasket-like structures) join the cells together and prevent substances moving from the milk back to the mother.[64] However, immune cells can reach milk by diapedesing through these junctions, which seal tightly behind them, leaving no permanent opening.[64] During pregnancy, with mastitis, or during involution, these junctions are open and "leaky," allowing substances to move bidirectionally. In mastitis this helps to provide antiinflammatory components and to clear the end products of the infectious process. During involution, this route allows degraded components to be removed.[64,68] If these junctions are open during lactation, increased sodium and chloride are found in breast milk. Thus increases in these components suggest a problem.[62]

Composition of Human Milk

The initial substance produced by the alveolar secretory cells is colostrum. Colostrum appears early in the second trimester and is present during the first few days following delivery. Colostrum is a transparent yellow substance (the yellow color comes from its high carotene content). Colostrum is higher in protein than mature milk due to increased concentrations of globulins, and lower in carbohydrate, fat, and calories (mean of 67 versus 75 kcal/dl). A transitional form of milk gradually replaces colostrum after the first few days. This milk contains greater quantities of fat, lactose, and calories than colostrum and is replaced by mature milk over the first 1 to 2 weeks as lactation is established.[40,97] As lactation progresses, volume, potassium, lactose, and fat content increase whereas protein, secretory IgA, lactoferrin, sodium, carotenoids, and chloride content decrease.[39,78,85]

Although the composition of human milk varies with the stage of lactation, gestation, and amount of milk secreted, the overall content of human milk is fairly consistent.[43,97] The vitamin and fat content of human milk is related to maternal nutrition; the content of other substances is generally independent of maternal nutrition. Human milk has over 200 known constituents.[43] The primary components of mature human milk are fats (3% to 5%), proteins (0.8% to 1.2%), carbohydrates (6.8% to 7.2%), water (87%), vitamins, and minerals (0.2%).[75] Each 100 ml of human milk contains 60 to 75 kcal/dl.[75] The average volume of milk increases during lactation from about 500 ml/day at 1 week, to 750 to 850 ml/day (and up to 1200 ml) by 6 months.[43,64] Increases in milk volume of 5% to 15% are seen in women with very low body fat. This is thought to be due to the decreased milk fat content and caloric density, which leads to increased infant suckling stimulation.[9,64] Volume is also increased with multiple infants due to increased suckling stimulation. Concentrations of substances contained in colostrum, mature human milk, and cow's milk are listed in Table 5-3.

Milk fat, protein, and lactose are synthesized in the secretory cells of the alveoli. Water, electrolytes, and water-soluble compounds cross the alveolar membrane via diffusion through water-filled pores or active transport.[43] Human milk is isosmotic with plasma. Lactose appears in high concentrations in human milk and is the major osmotic component. In order for milk to maintain isosmolarity with plasma, concentrations of other ions—sodium and chloride, in particular—must remain proportionately lower.

Substances such as calcium, amino acids, glucose, magnesium, and sodium are actively transported across the milk-blood barrier. This barrier is analogous in many ways to both the blood-brain barrier and the placental barrier. The milk-blood barrier is a lipid membrane barrier with water-filled pores consisting of tissue layers that separate the lumen of the alveoli from maternal capillary blood. This barrier consists of the capillary epithelium and basement membrane, interstitial space, myoepithelial cells, and alveolar cell basement membrane.

The total mineral content of human milk (including sodium, potassium, chloride, calcium, and magnesium) is generally stable at any stage of lactation and is not closely related to maternal nutrition. As lactation continues, absorption of iron and zinc decreases regardless of maternal nutritional status or milk content. Calcium is taken up by the alveoli from maternal blood. Much of this calcium comes from maternal bone stores so that the calcium content of milk is generally not affected by maternal nutritional intake.

Human milk also contains vitamins, iron, and trace minerals derived from maternal blood.[43,78] In general, if maternal nutrition is adequate, the vitamin and trace

TABLE **5-3**   Approximate Composition of Human Colostrum, Mature Human Milk, and Cow's Milk

Component	Human Colostrum (dl)	Mature Human Milk (dl)	Cow's Milk (dl)
Water (g)	87	87	87
Total solids (g)	13	13	13
Protein (g)	7.9	1.1	3.5
Fat (g)	1.3	4.5	3.7
Lactose (g)	3.2	6.8	4.9
Ash (i.e., mineral content) (g)	0.6	0.2	0.7
Protein (% of total protein)			
Casein	—	40	82
Whey	—	60	18
Major whey proteins (mg)			
α-Lactalbumin	333	263	40
Lactoferrin	384	168	—
Lyzozyme	34	42	
Albumin	36	52	23
IgA	354	142	40
MINERALS (mg)			
Na	92	15	58
K	55	55	138
Cl	117	43	103
Ca	31	33	123
Mg	4	4	12
P	14	15	100
Fe	0.09	0.15	0.10
VITAMINS (mg)			
A	89	53	34
C	4400	4300	1600
D		0.03	0.06
Riboflavin	30	43	157
Nicotinic acid	75	172	85
Thiamin	15	16	42

From Rebar, R.W. (1999). The breast and the physiology of lactation. In R.K. Creasy. & R. Resnik (Eds). *Maternal-fetal medicine* (4th ed.). Philadelphia: W.B. Saunders.

mineral components will meet minimal requirements. Water-soluble vitamins pass readily from maternal blood to breast milk, and levels reflect maternal diet. Minimal amounts of fluoride pass into breast milk so supplementation may be needed if the infant does not receive this mineral from the water supply.[97] Although the iron content of human milk is significantly less than that of cow's milk, a much greater proportion of the iron is absorbed, facilitated by lactose and ascorbic acid. Zinc levels are similar in human and cow's milk; however, the bioavailability of zinc in human milk is increased due to the presence of a zinc-binding ligand that facilitates intestinal absorption.

Because levels of protein, calcium, sodium, potassium, phosphorus, and other ions are lower in human than in cow's milk, the potential renal solute load is also lower (about one third that of cow's milk) and thus puts less stress on the kidneys (see Chapter 10). Human milk is also rich in immunologic substances that protect the infant from infections (especially gastrointestinal and respiratory infections) and provides some protection against the development of allergies—both by reducing exposure of the infant to cow's milk allergens and by providing secretory IgA, which reduces intestinal absorption of potentially antigenic proteins before gut closure (see Chapter 12) at 6 to 9 months. Cellular components of human milk include sloughed epithelial cells, macrophages, neutrophils, and lymphocytes. The antiallergic and antiinfectious properties of human milk are discussed in Chapter 12. Other components of human milk include enzymes, growth factors, and even naturally occurring benzodiazepines that may have a sedative effect.[67,75,85]

Fat Synthesis and Release

The largest portion of calories in human milk comes from fat. The major constituents of milk fat are triglycerides (98%); palmitic and oleic acids are the main triglycerides.[48,66] Other lipids found in human milk include free fatty acids, cholesterol (0.5%), phospholipids (0.7%), and glycolipids.[48] In comparison with cow's milk, human milk has greater concentrations of linoleic acid (an essential fatty acid) and cholesterol, with fewer short-chain saturated fatty acids.[36,45] The higher cholesterol may benefit the infant by enhancing synthesis of myelin in the central nervous system and stimulating development of the enzyme system essential in later life for cholesterol degradation. Human milk also contains a lipase that initiates fat digestion before the time milk enters the infant's intestine, enhancing release of energy and fat digestion and absorption.

Fats vary in concentration during the day, over a feeding, between breasts, and over time, as well as between women.[43,66] The concentration of fat in human milk shows marked diurnal variation, with lowest levels at night (perhaps due to altered fat concentration with relative inactivity and the horizontal position) and highest levels in the late afternoon and evening.[43] In addition, within a given feeding the fat content is highest at the end of a feeding (hindmilk), perhaps facilitating infant satiety.[28,39] Fat concentration is also increased during weaning.[43] Severe maternal caloric restriction alters the fatty acid composition, as, to some extent, do alterations in the type of fat consumed by the mother. The major proportion of milk fat is derived from maternal circulating lipids (from diet) and stores (especially of polyunsaturated fatty acids). These changes are buffered somewhat by use of lipid stores, especially in well-nourished women.[27,78,97] For example, if the maternal diet is altered to include more polyunsaturated fatty acids, her milk will also contain more polyunsaturated fats. Fatty acid and some vitamin (A, carotene, niacin, B_{12}, and D) concentrations are the only components of milk affected appreciably by maternal dietary varaitions.[78] Some fat is also synthesized from glucose, and this synthesis may be increased in women with low-fat, high-carbohydrate diets.[52,78]

Milk fat is synthesized in the endoplasmic reticulum (Figure 5-9) from precursors available within the secretory cell or obtained from maternal blood. Short-chain fatty acids are synthesized from acetate, whereas long-chain fatty acids are obtained from maternal plasma. Triglycerides are either obtained from maternal plasma or synthesized from intracellular carbohydrates (primarily glyceride and glucose). Two enzymes (lipoprotein lipase and palmitoyl-CoA transferase) involved in the production and utilization of triglycerides are stimulated by prolactin. Lipoprotein lipase acts in the capillaries to catalyze the lipolysis and uptake of triglyceride (and its component fatty acids and glycerol) into the secretory cell. Palmitoyl-CoA transferase is involved in intracellular synthesis of triglyceride from glyceride.[36,37,97]

Fatty acids are esterified in the endoplasmic reticulum to form triglycerides. The triglycerides accumulate and coalesce to form larger fat droplets surrounded by a membrane rich in phospholipids and cholesterol. As fat droplets increase in size, they migrate to the apex of the secretory cell and are released into the alveolar lumen via apocrine secretion. Occasionally small bits of cytoplasm may also enter the fat globule.[52]

Carbohydrate Synthesis and Release

The major carbohydrate found in human milk is lactose. Other carbohydrates found in small quantities include glucose, glucosamines, nucleotide sugars, and nitrogen-containing oligosaccharides. The oligosaccharides enhance development of intestinal bacterial flora and prevent bacterial adhesion, thus reducing the risk of gastrointestinal infections. (Immunologic properties of human milk are discussed in Chapter 12.[99]) Lactose promotes growth of lactobacilli in the infant's intestine and facilitates synthesis of B-complex vitamins. As lactose is metabolized, lactic and acetic acid are produced and increase intestinal acidity to help protect the infant from intestinal infection by reducing growth of enteropathic organisms. The acidic environment enhances absorption of calcium, phosphorus, and magnesium.[42,97]

Lactose is synthesized in the secretory cell's Golgi apparatus from glucose and galactose. The glucose is obtained from maternal circulating blood glucose. Production of lactose from glucose and galactose is catalyzed by galactosyl transferase, which in turn is catabolized by α-lactalbumin (a whey protein). The availability of α-lactalbumin is the rate-limiting step in the production of lactose. During pregnancy, progesterone inhibits this enzyme. Following delivery, reduction in progesterone and estrogens along with the concomitant increase in prolactin result in increased production of α-lactalbumin and therefore lactose.[43,97]

The concentration of lactose in human milk is constant and independent of maternal nutritional status. The amount of water in the milk is regulated by the quantity of lactose. Lactose acts as an osmotic compound to pull water into the Golgi apparatus.[75] Thus lactose is a critical factor in controlling the volume of milk produced. If less lactose is available, less milk will be produced so that the lactose concentration remains constant. The lactose synthesized in the Golgi apparatus attaches to protein and is released from the surface of the secretory cell into the alveolar lumen via merocrine secretion.

Protein Synthesis and Release

Milk protein consists of whey proteins and casein. The major whey protein is α-lactalbumin. Other whey proteins include lactoferrin, β-lactoglobulin, lysozyme, serum albumin, and immunoglobulins (IgA, IgG, and IgM).[39,43] The concentrations of whey protein and casein in human milk are in a 60:40 ratio versus the 20:80 ratio seen in cow's milk. Whey protein is easily digested, forming soft, flocculent curds. Casein, the predominant cow's milk protein, is less easily digested and forms tough, rubbery curds. Casein requires greater energy expenditure to digest, and digestion is more likely to be incomplete. Some casein is needed, however, to enhance the absorption of minerals by keeping them in solution in the gut. Casein may also promote the growth of beneficial gut flora and inhibit adherence of pathogenic organisms.[39]

Protein content decreases slowly during the first 6 months of lactation. Colostrum has three times as much protein as mature milk due to the addition of several amino acids, antibodies such as secretory IgA, and lactoferrin (see Chapter 12). All of the essential amino acids are present in colostrum. Although the total protein content of human milk is less than half that of cow's milk, the infant has adequate nitrogen for growth of new cells as a result of increased nonprotein nitrogen in the form of urea, free amino acids, amino sugars, choline, creatinine, nucleic acids, and other substances.[21]

In addition the free amino acid content is specific to the unique physiologic characteristics of the human newborn.[73,74] For example, human milk has lower levels of methionine and increased cystine. As a result, the breast-fed infant is less dependent on the enzyme cystathionase, an enzyme which develops late in fetal life. Human milk also has less tyrosine and phenylalanine. Because the enzymes that catabolize these amino acids also develop later, low levels prevent excessive concentrations of these substances in young infants. Human infants do not synthesize taurine well, and levels of taurine are higher in human as compared with cow's milk. Taurine is involved in bile acid conjugation and as a neurotransmitter and modifier in the brain and retina.[43,97] Glutamic acid and glutamine levels are elevated and enhance zinc absorption and serve as precursors to brain glutamate.[43]

The major milk proteins—casein, α-lactalbumin (whey), and β-lactalbumin (whey)—are derived primarily from synthesis in the secretory cells from amino acids. All the essential and some of the nonessential amino acids come from maternal plasma. Other nonessential amino acids are synthesized in the alveolar secretory cells.[86] A small amount of protein (primarily the proteins found in colostrum) is derived from maternal plasma. Prolactin acting in conjunction with insulin and cortisol induces the production of milk proteins by the ribosomes of the endoplasmic reticulum of the secretory cell.

Synthesis of milk proteins is similar to synthesis of other proteins by the body. Prolactin induces synthesis of messenger and transfer ribonucleic acid (tRNA). Messenger RNA (mRNA) transmits the genetic information to the ribosomes. This information is interpreted by tRNA to utilize specific amino acids to assemble appropriate sequences of polypeptide chains to form the specific milk proteins.[43] The milk proteins are then released from the secretory cell into the alveolar lumen via apocrine secretion.

Human milk also contains other nonprotein nitrogen components and other protein factors. These components are used to synthesize nonessential amino acids; enhance gut maturation, growth, and nutrient absorption; or contribute to the immunologic properties of human milk (see Chapter 12). Examples of protein factors include peptide hormones, growth factors, enzymes, epidermal growth factor (regulates intestinal mucosal growth), carnitine (needed for brain lipid synthesis), nucleic acids, and nucleotides (for growth and immunologic capacity).[19,23,26,29,43]

Preterm versus Term Milk

The milk of women who deliver before 32 to 33 weeks differs from that of women who deliver at term (see Table 11-20).[44,79,80,88] Preterm breast milk has a higher protein content (up to 2.4 g/dl) during the first month.[43] Nitrogen content of preterm milk is 15% to 20% higher than that of term milk.[4,31,88] In addition, the energy density of preterm milk has been reported to be higher over the first month in some studies.[3,15,43] Other investigators have reported either no differences or marked variability in caloric density among individual women.[2,31] Preterm milk contains similar or slightly lower levels of lactose; is higher in sodium, potassium, chloride, iron, and possibly magnesium during the first month; and has similar or slightly higher levels of calcium and phosphorus as compared with term milk (see Table 11-20).[5,22,25,43,83] Levels of other minerals such as zinc and copper are also slightly higher in preterm milk.[56] Preterm milk contains higher levels of vitamin E, niacin, vitamin B_{12}, vitamin A, and pantothenic acid than term milk.[78] Use of human milk for feeding low-birth-weight infants is discussed in Chapter 11.

TABLE 5-4   Extra Daily Nutrient Allowances for Lacatation over Baseline

NUTRIENT	NONPREGNANT AND NONLACTATING	LACTATING	INCREASE
Energy (kcal)	2100	2700	500
Protein (g)	40	65	25
Retinol (μg)	800	1300	500
Vitamin D (μg)	7.5	10	3
Vitamin E (mg)	8	11	3
Vitamin C (mg)	60	100	40
Riboflavin (mg)	1.3	1.8	0.5
Nicotinic acid (mg)	14	20	6
Vitamin B$_6$ (mg)	2.0	2.5	0.5
Folate (μg)	40	280	240
Thiamin (mg)	1.1	1.6	0.5
Calcium (mg)	800	1200	400
Iron (mg)	18	18	18
Zinc (mg)	15	25	10

From Lawrence, R.A. & Lawrence, R.M. (1999). *Breastfeeding: A guide for the medical profession* (5th ed.). St. Louis: Mosby.)

NUTRITION DURING THE POSTPARTUM PERIOD AND LACTATION

Maternal nutritional requirements during the postpartum period for nonlactating women are generally similar to those for nonpregnant women. However, these women do need adequate protein, vitamins, and minerals to promote healing and restoration. Some women may also need iron supplementation to replenish body stores. Other women may have increased energy requirements to meet the demands and added responsibility of the new infant.

As with pregnancy, there are specific maternal physiologic changes associated with lactation that influence nutritional requirements. These changes include an increased demand for nutrients, redistribution of blood to increase the supply of nutrients and precursors to the mammary glands, increased metabolic rate, and increased cardiac output with increased blood flow to the liver and gastrointestinal system (to meet increased demands for specific nutrients and precursors).[43] Maternal diet must be altered to meet the demands of lactation. The two components that are most affected by lactation are maternal protein intake and energy production.

During lactation the maternal basal metabolic rate increases. Approximately 900 kcal of energy are required to produce a liter of milk.[18,86] Thus it has been estimated that women need a minimum of 750 kcal/day to support lactation (150 kcal for synthesis and secretion of milk and 600 kcal to provide for the energy content of the milk).[43,97] These calories come from maternal fat stores and caloric intake. During the initial 3 months of lactation, women use the 2 to 4 kg of body fat stored during pregnancy to pro-

vide about 200 to 300 kcal/day, or one third of the additional calories needed each day. The additional 500 kcal is supplied by maternal diet. Increased caloric intake is needed after 3 months (when pregnancy fat stores are depleted), in undernourished women, or if the mother is nursing more than one infant.[97]

Protein intake is generally increased to 65 g/day.[43] Inadequate protein intake may reduce the volume of milk produced.[75] Intake of water-soluble vitamins is increased, as are calcium (1200 mg), retinol (1300 μg); vitamins D (10 μg) and E (11 μg), and folate (280 μg).[43] Maternal calcium status is altered during lactation, with decreased bone mineral stores (especially in the axial skeleton), increased bone mineral turnover, and decreased urinary calcium excretion (see Chapter 16).[73,75] Changes in nutritional requirements during lactation are summarized in Table 5-4 .

SUMMARY

The postpartum period is a time of rapid and complex change as the woman recovers from labor and delivery and undergoes reversal of the anatomic, physiologic, and endocrine changes of pregnancy. For most women these changes occur almost unnoticed, yet they provide the background for the new mother's physical function and sense of well-being and may influence the adaptation of the woman to her infant and new role. Understanding of the physiologic basis of lactation is essential in intervening appropriately to support the lactating woman and in assisting with problems. Clinical recommendations related to postpartum involutional changes are summarized in Table 5-5.

TABLE **5-5** **Recommendations for Clinical Practice Related to Involutional Changes and Lactation**

Recognize and monitor the progress of normal involutional changes for each of the reproductive organs (pp. 158-160).

Teach postpartum women the physiologic and anatomic changes to expect during the postpartum period (pp. 158-160).

Monitor the fundus and ensure that the uterus remains contracted (pp. 158-159).

Know the factors associated with afterpains and institute interventions to promote maternal comfort (p. 158).

Observe for signs of altered or delayed involution (pp. 158-160).

Monitor color and characteristics of lochial flow (p. 159).

Counsel women and their partners regarding changes in vaginal tone and lubrication postpartum (p. 160).

Counsel women regarding actions to increase vaginal lubrication and perineal tone (p. 160).

Counsel women and their partners regarding resumption of sexual activity (p. 160).

Encourage alternative forms of sexual intimacy during the postpartum period (p. 160).

Recognize breast engorgement and implement interventions appropriate for breastfeeding and nonbreastfeeding women (p. 160).

Teach women interventions to reduce the risk of infection (pp. 160, 163, 172).

Counsel women regarding the expected timing for resumption of menstruation and ovulation (pp. 162-163).

Counsel women regarding methods of family planning (pp. 162-163).

Counsel women who are breastfeeding regarding the potential risks of using lactation as a method of fertility control (p. 163).

Counsel women who use lactation as a method of fertility control strategies to reduce the risk of unplanned pregnancy (p. 163).

Teach women the physiology of lactation and milk production (pp. 163-175).

Encourage frequent breastfeeding on demand to assist women in establishing their milk supply (p. 169).

Assist women who are pumping to increase their milk volume by increasing the frequency of pumping (p. 169).

Teach breastfeeding women nipple and breast care (p. 163).

Counsel women regarding factors that promote or interfere with the let-down reflex (p. 170).

Counsel women to abstain from or limit alcohol intake during lactation (p. 160 and Chapter 6).

Know the composition of human milk and the factors that influence composition and volume (pp. 172-175).

Know the advantages and limitations of human milk for preterm infants (p.175 and Chapter 11).

Encourage early initiation of breastfeeding after delivery and use of demand feeding (pp. 167, 172).

Encourage women to ensure that their infants consume hindmilk or that this milk is included in pumped milk (p. 174).

Counsel lactating women regarding nutritional requirements and effects of their nutritional status on milk production (pp.172-176).

Assess nutritional status and counsel women regarding nutritional needs postpartum (p. 176).

REFERENCES

1. Abram, S., et al. (1990). Recovery after childbirth: A preliminary prospective study. *Med J Aust, 152,* 9.
2. Anderson, G.H., Atkinson, S.A., & Bryan, M.H. (1981). Energy and macronutrient content of human milk during early lactation from mothers giving birth prematurely and at term. *Am J Clin Nutr, 34,* 258.
3. Arrata, W.S.M. & Chatterton, R.T. (1974). Human lactation: Appropriate and inappropriate. *Obstet Gynecol Ann, 3,* 443.
4. Atkinson, S.A., Anderson, G., & Bryan, M.H. (1980). Human milk: Comparison of nitrogen composition of milk from mothers of premature infants. *Am J Clin Nutr, 33,* 811.
5. Atkinson, S.A., Radde, I.C., & Anderson, G.H. (1983). Micromineral balances in premature infants fed their own mothers' milk or formula. *J Pediatr, 102,* 99.
6. Banta, H. & Thackers, S. (1982). Risks and benefits of episiotomy: A review. *Birth, 9,* 25.
7. Bigg, L.A., Lein, A., & Yen, S.S. C. (1977). Pattern of circulating prolactin levels during human gestation. *Am J Obstet Gynecol, 129,* 454.
8. Bromberg, M. (1986) Presumptive maternal benefits of routine episiotomy. *J Nurse Midwifery, 31,* 121.
9. Butte, N.F., et al. (1995). Human milk intake and growth faltering of rural Mesoamerindian infants. *Am J Clin Nutr, 55,* 1109.
10. Campbell, O.M.R. & Gray, R.H. (1993). Characteristics of postpartum ovarian function in women in the United States. *Am J Obstet Gynecol, 169,* 55.
11. Chalmers, I., et al. (1989). *Effective care in pregnancy and childbirth.* Oxford, England: Oxford University Press.
12. Cobo, E. (1973). Effect of different doses of ethanol on the milk-ejecting reflex in lactating women. *Am J Obstet Gynecol, 113,* 819.
13. Cooney, K.A., et al. (1996). An assessment of the nine-month lactational method (MAMA-9) in Rwanda. *Stud Fam Plann, 27,* 102.
14. Cunningham, F.G. & Whitridge, W.J. (1997). *Williams obstetrics* (20th ed.). Stamford, CT: Appleton & Lange.
15. De Curtis, M., Senterre, J., & Rigo, J. (1986). Carbohydrate derived energy and gross energy absorption in preterm infants fed human milk or formula. *Arch Dis Child, 61,* 867.
16. Delvoye, P., et al. (1977). The influence of the frequency of nursing and of previous lactation experience on serum prolactin in lactating mothers. *J Biosoc Sci, 9,* 447.
17. Demmelmair, H., et al. (1998). Metabolism of U13C-labeled linoleic acid in lactating women. *J Lipid Res, 39,* 1389.
18. Dewey, K.G. (1997). Energy and growth requirements during lactation. *Ann Rev Nutr, 17,* 19.

19. Donovan, S.M. & Dole, J. (1994). Growth factors in milk as mediators of infant development. *Ann Rev Nutr, 14,* 147.

20. Dusdieker, L.B., et al. (1985). Effect of supplemental fluids on human milk production. *J Pediatr, 106,* 207.

21. Garza, C., et al. (1987). Special properties of human milk. *Clin Perinatol, 14,* 11.

22. Georgieff, M.K. (1999). Nutrition. In G.B. Avery, A.B. Fletcher & M.G. Macdonald (Eds.). *Neonatology: Pathophysiology and management of the newborn* (5th ed.). Philadelphia: J.B. Lippincott.

23. Gil, A. & Uauy, R. (1995). Nucleotides and related compounds in human and bovine milk. In R.G. Jensen (Ed.). *Handbook of milk composition.* San Diego: Academic Press.

24. Gray, R.H., et al. (1990). Risk of ovulation during lactation. *Lancet, 1,* 25.

25. Gross, S.J., et al. (1980). Nutritional composition of milk produced by mothers delivering preterm. *J Pediatr, 96,* 641.

26. Grosvenor, C.E., Picciano, M.F., & Baumrucker, C.R. (1993). Hormones and growth factors in milk. *Endocr Rev, 14,* 710.

27. Guthrie, H.A., Picciano, M.F., & Sheehen, D. (1977). Fatty acid patterns of human milk. *J Pediatr, 90,* 39.

28. Hall, B. (1979). Uniformity of human milk. *Am J Clin Nutr, 32,* 304.

29. Hamosh, M. (1995). Enzymes in human milk. In R.G. Jensen (Ed.). *Handbook of milk composition.* San Diego: Academic Press.

30. Hendrick, V., Altshuler, L.L., & Suri, R. (1998). Hormonal changes in the postpartum and implications for postpartal depression, *Psychosomatics, 39,* 93.

31. Hibberd, C.M., et al. (1982). Variation in the composition of breast milk during the first 5 weeks of lactation. *Arch Dis Child, 57,* 658.

32. Hopkinson, J.M., Schanler, R.J., & Garza, C. (1988). Milk production by mothers of premature infants. *Pediatrics, 81,* 815.

33. Howie, P.W., et al. (1982). Fertility after childbirth: Infant feeding patterns, basal prolactin levels and post-partum ovulation. *Clin Endocrinol, 17,* 315.

34. Howie, P.W., et al. (1982). Fertility after childbirth: Post-partum ovulation and menstruation in bottle and breastfeeding mothers. *Clin Endocrinol, 17,* 323.

35. Hunker, W. & Kraehenbuhl, J.P. (1998). Epithelial cell transcytocis of immunoglobulins. *J Mammary Gland Biol Neoplasia, 2,* 287.

36. Jensen, R.G. & Jensen, G.L. (1992). Specialty lipids for infant nutrition: I. Milks and formulas. *J Pediatr Gastroenterol Nutr, 15,* 232.

37. Jensen, R.G., Bitman, J., & Carlson, S.E. (1995). Human milk lipids. In R.G. Jensen (Ed.), *Handbook of milk composition.* San Diego: Academic Press.

38. Kremer, J.A., et al. (1989). Return of gonadotropic function in postpartum women during bromocriptine treatment. *Fertil Steril, 51,* 622.

39. Kunz, C., et al. (1999). Nutritional and biochemical properties of human milk, part I: general aspects, proteins, and carbohydrates. *Clin Perinatol, 26,* 307.

40. Kyndely, K. (1978). The sexuality of women in pregnancy and postpartum: A review. *J Obstet Gynecol Neonatal Nurs, 7,* 28.

41. Larson, B.L. & Smith, V.R. (1974). *Lactation* (vols. 1-3). New York: Academic Press.

42. Larson, B.L. (1978). *Lactation* (vol. 4). In *The mammary gland/human lactation/milk synthesis.* New York: Academic Press.

43. Lawrence, R. A. & Lawrence, R.M. (1999). *Breastfeeding: A guide for the medical profession* (5th ed.). St Louis: Mosby.

44. Lepage, G., et al. (1984). The composition of preterm milk in relation to the degree of prematurity. *Am J Clin Nutr, 40,* 1042.

45. Lewis, P.R., et al. (1991). The resumption of ovulation and menstruation in a well-nourished population of women breastfeeding for an extended period of time. *Fertil Steril, 55,* 529.

46. Liu, J.H. & Yen, S.S.C. (1989). Endocrinology of the postpartum state. In S.A. Brody & K. Ueland (Eds.), *Endocrine disorders in pregnancy.* Norwalk, CT: Appleton & Lange.

47. Lund, L.R., et al. (1996). Two distinct phases of apoptosis in mammary gland involution: proteinase-independent and -dependent pathways. *Development, 121,* 181.

48. Madden, J.D., et al. (1997). Analysis of secretory patterns of prolactin and gonadotropin during twenty-four hours in a lactating women before and after resumption of menses. *Am J Obstet Gynecol, 132,* 436.

49. Marchant, S., et al. (1999). A survey of women's experienced vaginal loss from 24 hours to three months after childbirth (the BliPP Study). *Midwifery, 15,* 72.

50. Marcu, G., et al. (1993). Breast-feeding and natural family planning. *Rev Med Chir Soc Med Nat, 97,* 243.

51. Masters, W.H. & Johnson, V.E. (1966). *Human sexual response.* Boston: Little, Brown.

52. Mather, I.H. & Keenan, T.W. (1998). Origin and secretion of milk lipids. *J Mammary Gland Biol Neoplasia, 3,* 261.

53. McGuinness, M., Norr, K., & Nacion, K. (1991). Comparison between different perineal outcomes on tissue healing. *J Nurse Midwifery, 36,* 192.

54. McKensie, C.A., Canaday, M.E., & Carroll, E. (1982). Comprehensive care during the postpartum period. *Nurs Clin North Am, 17,* 23.

55. McNeilly, A.S., et al. (1983). Fertility after childbirth: Pregnancy associated with breastfeeding. *J Endocrinol, 18,* 167.

56. Mendelson, R.A., Anderson, G.H., & Bryan, M.H. (1982). Zinc, copper and iron content of milk from mothers of preterm infants. *Early Hum Dev, 6,* 145.

57. Mepham, T.B. (1987). *Physiology of lactation.* Philadelphia: Open U Press.

58. Millar, I.D., et al. (1997). Mammary protein synthesis is acutely regulated by the cellular hydration state. *Biochem Biophys Res Commun, 230,* 351.

59. Miyake, A., et al. (1978). Pituitary LH response to LHRH during the puerperium. *Obstet Gynecol, 51,* 37.

60. Monheit, A., Cousins, L., & Resnick, R. (1980). The puerperium: Anatomical and physiologic readjustments. *Clin Obstet Gynecol, 23,* 973.

61. Moore, M.L. (1983). *Realities in childbearing* (2nd ed.). Philadelphia: W.B. Saunders.

62. Morton, J.A. (1994). The clinical usefulness of breast milk sodium in the assessment of lactogenesis. *Pediatrics, 93,* 802.

63. Negishi, H., Kishida, T., & Yamada, H. (1999). Changes in uterine size after vaginal delivery and cesarean section determined by vaginal sonography in the puerperium. *Arch Gynecol Obstet, 263,* 12.

64. Neville, M.C. (1999). Physiology of lactation. *Clin Perinatol, 26,* 251.

65. Neville, M.C. & Neifert, M.R. (1983). *Lactation: physiology, nutrition and breastfeeding.* New York: Plenum.

66. Neville, M.C. & Picciano, M.F. (1997). Regulation of milk lipid synthesis and composition. *Ann Rev Nutrition, 17,* 159

67. Newburg, D.S. (1996). Oligosaccharides and glycoconjugates of human milk. *J Mammary Gland Biol Neoplasia, 1,* 271.

68. Nguyen, D. & Neville, M.C. (1998). Tight junction regulation in the mammary gland. *J Mammary Gland Biol Neoplasia, 3,* 227.

69. Noel, G.L., Suh, H.K., & Frantz, A.G. (1974). Prolactin release during nursing and breast stimulation in postpartum and nonpostpartum patients. *J Clin Endocrinol Metab, 38,* 13.

70. Olliver-Bousquet, M. (1998). Transferrin and prolactin transcytosis in the lactating mammary epithelial gland, *J Mammary Gland Biol Neoplasia, 3,* 303.

71. Peaker, M & Wilde, C.J. (1996). Feedback control of milk secretion from milk. *J Mammary Gland Biol Neoplasia, 1,* 307.

72. Powers, N.G. (1999). Slow weight gain and low milk supply in the breastfeeding dyad. *Clin Perinatol, 26,* 399.

73. Prentice, A. (2000). Maternal calcium metabolism and bone mineral status. *Am J Clin Nutr, 71*(Suppl), 1312S.

74. Rassin, D.K. (1990). Quality of human milk versus milk formulas: Protein composition. In N.M. Van Gelder, R.F. Butterworth & B.D. Drugan (Eds.). *Neurology and neurobiology* (Vol. 58). New York: Wiley-Liss.

75. Rebar, R.W. (1999). The breast and the physiology of lactation. In R.K. Creasy. & R. Resnik (Eds.). *Maternal-fetal medicine* (4th ed.). Philadelphia: W.B. Saunders.

76. Resnik, R. (1999). The puerperium. In R.K. Creasy. & R. Resnik (Eds.). *Maternal-fetal medicine* (4th ed.). Philadelphia: W.B. Saunders.

77. Rigg, L.A. & Yen, S.C. (1977). Multiphasic prolactin secretion during parturition in human subjects. *Am J Obstet Gynecol, 128,* 215.

78. Rodriguez-Palmero, M., et al. (1999). Nutritional and biochemical properties of human milk: II. Lipids, micronutrients, and bioactive factors. *Clin Perinatol, 26,* 335.

79. Schandler, R.J. (1996). Human milk fortification for premature infants. *Am J Clin Nutr, 64,* 249.

80. Schanler, R.J., Hurst, N., & Lau, C. (1999). The use of human milk in breastfeeding premature infants. *Clin Perinatol, 26,* 379.

81. Shennan, D.B. & Peaker, M. (2000). Transport of milk constituents by the mammary gland. *Physiol Rev, 80,* 925.

82. Sherman, D., et al. (1999). Characteristics of normal lochia. *Am J Perinatol, 16,* 399

83. Shulman, R.J., et al. (1996). Early feeding in preterm infant increases lactase activity. *Pediatr Res, 39,* 320A.

84. Smith-Kirwin, S.M., et al. (1998). Leptin expression in human mammary epithelial cells in breast milk. *J Clin Endocrinol Metab, 83,* 1746.

85. Telmo, E. & Hansen, L.A. (1996). Antibodies in milk. *J Mammary Gland Biol Neoplasia, 1,* 243.

86. Thomson, A.M., Hytten, F.E. & Billewicz, W.Z. (1970). The energy cost of human lactation. *Br J Nutr, 24,* 565.

87. Tommaselli, G.A., et al. (2000). Using complete breastfeeding and lactational amenorrhea as birth spacing methods. *Contraception, 61,* 253.

88. Tsang, R.C., et al. (1993). *Nutritional needs of the preterm infant.* Baltimore: Williams & Wilkins.

89. Tulchinsky, D. (1994). Postpartum lactation and resumption of reproductive function. In D. Tulchinsky & A.B. Little (Eds.). *Maternal-fetal endocrinology* (2nd ed.). Philadelphia: W.B. Saunders.

90. Tyson, J.E. (1977). Mechanisms of puerperal lactation. *Med Clin North Am, 61,* 153.

91. Vorherr, H. (1974). *The breast.* New York: Academic Press.

92. Wendrinska, A., et al. (1993). Effect of a milk fat globule membrane fraction on cultured mouse mammary cells. *Biochem Soc Trans, 21,* 220S.

93. Westergren-Thorsson, G., et al. (1998). Differential expressions of mRNA for proteoglycans, collagens, and transforming growth factor-beta in the human cervix during pregnancy and involution. *Biochim Biophys Acta, 1406,* 203.

94. Wilcox, L.S., et al. (1989). Episiotomy and its role in the incidence of perineal lacerations in a maternity center and a tertiary hospital obstetric service. *Am J Obstet Gynecol, 160,* 1047.

95. Wilde, C.J., et al. (1995). Autocrine regulation of milk secretion by a protein in milk. *Biochem J, 306,* 51.

96. Willms, A.B., et al. (1995). Anatomic changes in the pelvis after uncomplicated vaginal delivery: evaluation with serial MR imaging. *Radiology, 195,* 91.

97. Worthington-Roberts, B.S., Vermeersch, J., & Williams, S.R. (1989). *Nutrition during pregnancy and lactation.* St. Louis: Mosby.

98. Zinaman, M.G., et al. (1995). Pulsitile GnRH stimulates normal cyclic ovarian function in amenorrheic lactating postpartum women. *J Clin Endocrinol Metab, 60,* 2088

99. Zopf, D. & Roth, S. (1996). Oligosaccharide anti-infective agents. *Lancet, 347,* 1017.

Pharmacology and Pharmacokinetics during the Perinatal Period

Pharmacologic therapy for the pregnant women, fetus, neonate, and lactating woman is one of the most challenging in health care. Pharmacologic treatment during pregnancy is unique in that a drug taken by one person (pregnant woman) may significantly affect another (embryo or fetus).[27] Maternal handling of drugs can be altered by the normal physiologic changes of pregnancy, such as increased plasma volume, altered gastrointestinal (GI) motility, and changes in plasma components and renal function. These changes influence plasma levels, half-lives, and distribution and elimination of many drugs, and may increase the risk of subtherapeutic or toxic drug levels.

Fetal drug exposure may be inadvertent (secondary to maternal treatment) or intended (treatment of fetus via treatment of mother). For many years it was believed that the placental barrier shielded the fetus from many drugs and other potentially harmful substances. However, the placenta provides little protection for the fetus from many drugs. The placenta and fetus are able to metabolize some agents; however, gestational age and maturation of hepatic enzyme systems influence the efficiency of these processes. Many maternal drugs are present in the fetus in lower levels than seen in the mother, but some drugs may be found at higher levels in the fetus. Fetal effects of maternal drugs can range from no effect to pregnancy loss to teratogenesis with structural or functional changes, to alterations in later growth and development.

Pharmacologic therapy of the neonate is complex because hepatic metabolism and renal elimination change rapidly over the first weeks after birth. This challenge is magnified in preterm infants in whom maturation of hepatic and renal systems is changing based on both postconceptional age and postbirth age. This can lead to significant changes in drug handling, sometimes within a few days or weeks. Many drugs also cross the blood-milk barrier in the lactating women and have the potential to affect the infant. However, drugs generally reach breast milk in significantly lower quantities than drugs reach the fetus across the placenta.

Pharmacokinetics refers to the processes involved in drug absorption, distribution, metabolism, and biotransformation and excretion (Figure 6-1). Site of absorption depends on route of administration (e.g., oral, intramuscular, intravenous, topical, inhaled). Drugs are carried in the blood either bound to plasma proteins or as free drug. Protein-bound drugs provide a reservoir for future use, whereas free drug is the active component available to interact with the target cell. Biotransformation occurs primarily in the liver with a series of enzymatic reactions to convert the drug into more polar (water-soluble) compounds. Intermediary steps in biotransformation may result in active metabolites. For example, codeine is demethylated to morphine and theophylline is methylated to caffeine.[19] Biotransformation also takes place in the lungs, intestinal mucus, and kidneys. Biotransformation occurs in two phases. Phase I (nonsynthetic reactions) takes place primarily in the microsomes, although some occur in the mitochondria and cytosol. Phase I reactions modify the activity of a drug. Phase I enzymes include the cytochrome P450 (CYP450) monooxygenase system. Phase II (synthetic) reactions require ATP and, except for glucuronidation, are extramicrosomal.[19] Phase II reactions generally inactivate the drugs by converting them to more polar substances. Table 6-1 provides examples of drugs metabolized by various phase I and phase II reactions. Not all drugs undergo hepatic metabolism prior to elimination; some drugs are excreted directly via the kidneys (Table 6-2)

The term *drug* is used generically in this chapter to refer to prescription and nonprescription pharmacologic agents, herbal agents, and vitamins, as well as drugs of abuse. In addition the principles that govern placental transfer of drugs are also applicable to transfer of chemicals, food additives, and environmental agents.[47] Definitions of common terms used in pharmacokinetics are summarized in the box on p. 182.

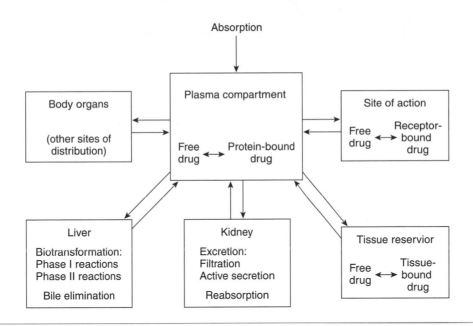

FIGURE **6-1** Schema of possible disposition of drugs throughout various compartments in the body. (From Chemtob, S. [1998]. Basic pharmacologic principles. In R.A. Polin & W.W. Fox [Eds.]. *Fetal and neonatal physiology* [2nd ed.]. Philadelphia: W.B. Saunders.)

TABLE **6-1**   Biotransformation Reactions

REACTION	EXAMPLES OF DRUG SUBSTRATES
PHASE I (NONSYNTHETIC REACTIONS)	
Oxidation	Phenytoin, phenobarbital, ibuprofen, acetaminophen, morphine, codeine, diazepam, cimetidine
Reduction	Prontosil, chloramphenicol, ethanol
Hydrolysis	Acetylsalicylic acid, indomethacin
PHASE II (SYNTHETIC REACTIONS: CONJUGATIONS)	
Glucuronide conjugation	Morphine, acetaminophen
Glycine conjugation	Salicylic acid
Sulfate conjugation	Acetaminophen, α-methyldopa
Glutathione conjugation	Ethacrynic acid
Methylation	Dopamine, epinephrine
Acetylation	Sulfonamides, clonazepam

Adapted from Chemtob, S. (1998). Basic pharmacologic principles. In R.A. Polin & W.W. Fox (Eds.). *Fetal and neonatal physiology* (2nd ed.). Philadelphia: W.B. Saunders.

TABLE **6-2**   Sites of Drug Metabolism and Elimination

SITE	DRUG EXAMPLES
NONRENAL (PRIMARILY HEPATIC)	
	Acetaminophen, amphotericin, barbiturates, caffeine, chloral hydrate, clindamycin, codeine, diazepam, hydralazine, meperidine, morphine, phenytoin, propanolol, theophylline
RENAL	
Glomerular filtration rate	Aminoglycosides, digoxin, vancomycin
Tubular excretion (secretion)	Cephalosporins, digoxin, furosemide, penicillins, thiazides, tolazoline
Tubular reabsorption	Aminoglycosides, caffeine
RENAL AND NONRENAL	
	Ampicillin, cefoperazone, chloramphenicol, digoxin, penicillin G, phenobarbital

From Nagourney, B.A. & Aranda, J.V. (1998). Physiologic differences of clinical significance. In R.A. Polin & W.W. Fox (Eds.). *Fetal and neonatal physiology* (2nd ed.). Philadelphia: W.B. Saunders.

Definitions of Selected Terms Used in Pharmacokinetics

Pharmacokinetics is the study of drug disposition over time and includes absorption, distribution, metabolism, and excretion.

Volume of distribution (Vd) is the distribution of a drug in the body. The greater the Vd is, the longer it will take the drug to be cleared from the body. Drugs can be distributed in body water and fat compartments, or bound to plasma proteins or tissue.

Half-life is the time for blood concentration of a drug to decline by 50%. There may be two half-lives calculated for drugs given intravenously: the initial or distribution half-life and the terminal or elimination half-life.

Oral bioavailability is the ability of a drug taken orally to reach the systemic circulation. A drug with high oral bioavailability moves readily from the GI tract to the systemic circulation.

Protein binding is the percentage of the drug that is normally bound to plasma proteins. The two main drug-binding proteins are albumin and α1-acid glycoprotein.

Free drug is the fraction of drug that is unbound in plasma. Free drug can move across the placenta or blood-milk barrier; bound drug cannot.

Clearance is the amount of a drug that is cleared from the plasma by hepatic and renal systems in a given unit of time. Hepatic and renal clearance can be calculated separately.

Molecular weight (MW) is the weight of the drug in daltons. The smaller the MW is, the more readily a substance can cross cell membranes. Very small substances (MW less than 100 to 200 daltons) may be able to move though pores in the cell membrane.

pKa is the pH at which a drug is 50% ionized. Ionized drugs do not cross cell membranes (including the placenta and the blood-milk barrier) as readily.

PHARMACOKINETICS DURING PREGNANCY

Drug Use during Pregnancy

A survey of drug utilization by 14,000 pregnant women in 22 countries found that 86% of these women took some medication during pregnancy, with an average of 2.9 medications (range, 1 to 15) being used.[66] Other studies have reported that one third to two thirds of pregnant women took at least one prescribed drug (other than vitamins and iron) during pregnancy, with an average of 1.3 to 4 over-the-counter drugs.[55,70,109] The most common prescribed drugs were antimicrobial agents, antiemetics, tranquilizers, and analgesics. Nonsteroidal antiinflammatory drugs, laxatives, antiemetics, antacids, antinausea agents, antihistamines, and cough and cold preparations were the most frequent over-the-counter drugs.[70,109] The use of prescribed and over-the-counter drugs during pregnancy has decreased in recent years; use of drugs of abuse has increased.[16,70,109]

Adherence to prescribed drug regimens is a problem during pregnancy, with up to 50% of women either not taking a prescribed drug or stopping before receiving a full course of the drug.[17] Problems with adherence stem primarily from concerns about teratogenic effects. Most women overestimate the teratogenic risks of common agents.[60,61] For example, in a recent study women personally estimated that the risk of having a baby with a birth defect was 25% (which is the risk associated with a potent teratogen such as thalidomide). After counseling, however, they more correctly estimated the risk at 5%.[60] The background risk of a birth defect for the general population is 5%. However, the risk may be higher or lower for an individual woman depending on factors such as her health status, teratogen exposures, and genetic makeup.

Evidence regarding effects and effectiveness of most pharmacologic agents during pregnancy is limited.[66,108] Several principles have been identified to guide drug therapy during pregnancy: (1) avoid medications in the first trimester whenever possible; (2) anyone prescribing drugs for a woman of childbearing age must consider a potential pregnancy before prescribing; (3) women receiving long-term drug therapy require counseling before pregnancy of the potential implications and risks; (4) a necessary treatment should not be stopped without good reason; (5) drugs may have altered effects during pregnancy (e.g., the increased metabolism of methicillin or increased renal elimination of digoxin may result in decreased levels, resulting in the need for higher doses); (6) use single action, short-acting medications rather than long-acting or combination drugs; (7) use the lowest effective dose of the safest available medication; (8) use drugs only if the benefits outweigh the risk; (9) use alternate routes of administration if available (i.e., topical or inhaled rather than systemic agents); (10) select drugs that have a history of use during pregnancy without adverse effects, rather than "latest" drug; and (11) use doses at the low end of the normal dose range while recognizing that for some drugs (e.g., digoxin, phenytoin, lithium), the woman's usual dose may need to be increased due to increased volume of distribution (Vd) and clearance of these agents during pregnancy.[66,108] These principles also apply to all women of childbearing age and to

TABLE **6-3**   Influence of Pregnancy on Physiologic Aspects of Drug Disposition

PHARMACOKINETIC PARAMETER	CHANGE IN PREGNANCY
ABSORPTION	
Gastric emptying	Increased
Intestinal motility	Decreased
Pulmonary function	Increased
Cardiac output	Increased
Blood flow to skin	Increased
DISTRIBUTION	
Plasma volume	Increased
Total body water	Increased
Plasma proteins	Decreased
Body fat	Increased
METABOLISM	
Hepatic metabolism	Increased or decreased
Extrahepatic metabolism	Increased or decreased
Plasma proteins	Decreased
EXCRETION	
Renal blood flow	Increased
Glomerular filtration rate	Increased
Pulmonary function	Increased
Plasma proteins	Decreased

Adapted from Reed, M.D. & Blumer, J.L. (1997). Pharmacologic treatment of the fetus. In A.A Fanaroff & R.J. Martin (Eds.). *Neonatal-perinatal medicine: Diseases of the fetus and infant* (6th ed.). Philadelphia: W.B. Saunders.

preconceptional and interconceptional use of drugs, since approximately half of all pregnancies are unplanned and critical developmental processes occur before most women realize they are pregnant.[66,108]

Alterations in Drug Absorption, Distribution, Metabolism, and Excretion during Pregnancy

Maternal responses to drugs during pregnancy are influenced by both maternal physiology and the presence of the placental-fetal unit.[70] Variations in handling of specific drugs by the pregnant woman may occur due to effects of the normal physiologic changes of pregnancy on drug absorption, distribution, metabolism, and excretion (Table 6-3). The presence of the placental-fetal compartment also can alter maternal kinetics.[70,80] For example, many antibiotics are lipid-soluble and may readily cross the placenta and become sequestered in the fetal compartment and thus be unavailable to the mother. This can lead to lower maternal levels.

Pharmacokinetic data on specific drugs during pregnancy is minimal since pregnant women are excluded from drug trials. As a result, many drugs are not labeled for use in pregnancy, because the effects of the drug on the fetus are unknown.[62,130] This is protective for the fetus but may also limit benefits to the pregnant women from these drugs. The net result of changes in drug handling during pregnancy depends on the individual drug, with both increases in levels (with need for a lower dose or less frequent dosing) and decrease in levels (with a need for a higher dose or more frequent dosing) seen for various substances.[69]

Little analyzed data on pharmacokinetics of drugs in pregnancy from studies published between 1963 and 1997 and found that across all agents (1) drug oral bioavailability decreased in 47% of studies of different agents; (2) Vd increased in 39%, with no change in 48%; (3) peak plasma levels decreased in 33%, with no change in 57%; (4) steady-state plasma levels decreased in 45%, with no change in 45% (5) half-life decreased in 41%, with no change in 44%; (6) clearance increased in 55%, with no change in 34%; and (7) protein binding decreased in 86%.[69] Little noted that many studies had significant methodologic problems such as small sample sizes, varying compositions of control groups, and variations in dosing methods. Many studies did not report data for individual pharmacokinetic parameters.[69] Therefore during pregnancy, there are considerable variations in the direction of pharmacokinetic changes among different drugs. This increases the complexity for the practitioner in choosing a specific pharmacologic agent and monitoring its effects.

Drug Absorption

The GI, pulmonary, and peripheral blood flow changes during pregnancy can alter absorption of drugs from the lungs, gut, and skin. The hyperventilation that occurs in pregnancy can increase the rate of drug uptake across the alveoli.[70] As a result, the pulmonary system may have a greater role in drug and metabolite excretion during pregnancy.[85] Alveolar uptake of inhalation agents is also influenced by changes in cardiac output, which leads to increased pulmonary blood flow and thus increased alveolar uptake.[63] As a result, doses of volatile anesthetics (e.g., halothane, isoflurane, methoxyflurane) need to be decreased to compensate for these changes in the pregnant women.[70]

Absorption of oral medications is influenced by gastric acidity, gastric motility, presence of bile acids or mucus, nausea and vomiting of pregnancy, and intestinal transit time. During pregnancy there is decreased gastric acid (hydrochloric acid [HCl]) secretion, delayed gastric and intestinal emptying time, increased mucus, and decreased intestinal motility. Decreased gastric motility can increase the oral bioavailability of slowly absorbed drugs such as digoxin by prolonging transit time, and it can decrease peak plasma levels of rapidly absorbed drugs.[102] These factors altering GI function in pregnancy may initially delay, then prolong absorption of oral medications. Peak plasma levels and the time to peak levels may also be later than normal.[80] Changes in pH affect ionization, and absorption of drugs.[63,70] For example, decreased gastric pH decreases the rate at which weak acids (e.g., aspirin) are absorbed and increases absorption of weak bases (e.g., narcotic analgesics).[63,87] Decreased GI motility and delayed gastric emptying may alter initial absorption of oral antibiotics and lead to unpredictable patterns of intestinal absorption. Increased cardiac output and peripheral blood flow may increase the rate of absorption of drugs from the stomach and small intestine.[69] Iron chelates with some drugs taken concurrently, preventing absorption.[102] However, even with these changes in GI function, the clinical effect for most drugs is not significant. This is because therapeutic windows are usually wide enough for drugs administered orally that these factors do not significantly alter therapeutic effects.[85,89]

The increased extracellular water and peripheral blood flow to the skin during pregnancy may enhance absorption and alter distribution of topical agents.[105] For example, topical and vaginal preparations with iodine are not recommended during pregnancy because of the increased absorption of iodine. Iodine is of concern because it is actively transported across the placenta to the fetus, whose thyroid gland has a high avidity for this substance (Chapter 18).[77,105] Decreases in blood flow to the lower extremities in late pregnancy may alter absorption of drugs given intramuscularly.[63]

Drug Distribution

The distribution of drugs within the body depends on many factors, including the amount of body water, which affects Vd; degree to which a drug is bound to plasma proteins or body tissues; and the presence of the fetal-placental unit. For many drugs the Vd is increased during pregnancy because of the increased plasma volume, blood volume, cardiac output, and total body water.[41,80,85] The increased plasma and blood volumes may result in decreased drug levels in the central compartment.[21,121] Elevated blood and plasma volumes during pregnancy increase the volume for distribution, which may reduce serum levels of drugs and necessitate larger loading doses. Increases in total body water during pregnancy affect primarily water-soluble (polar) drugs that tend to stay in the extracellular space. Because of changes in the Vd, some pregnant women may notice that their prepregnancy dose

of a drug taken chronically, such as digoxin or phenytoin, may not achieve the same therapeutic effect during pregnancy.[102] Concentrations of lipophilic drugs are influenced more by changes in protein and tissue binding than Vd.[102]

The Vd for lipophilic drugs is increased during pregnancy because of the accumulation of fat, which may serve as a reservoir for some drugs via tissue binding.[69,102] Some lipid-soluble drugs (e.g., caffeine, diazepam, thiopental) have a prolonged half-life in the pregnant women, whereas polar drugs (e.g., oxazepam, ampicillin) tend to have a shorter half-life.[38] Tissue binding is a mechanism by which a drug is removed from circulation and stored in tissue such as hair, bone, teeth, and adipose tissue. This mechanism can result in storage of significant quantities of a drug, since tissue storage sites may need to be saturated before there is sufficient free drug to be effective at receptor sites. When the drug is discontinued, tissue deposits may give up their stores slowly, resulting in persistent drug effects. Since lipid-soluble drugs are stored in adipose tissue, increased adipose tissue during pregnancy can lead to a slight decrease in the amount of free lipid-soluble drugs such as sedatives and hypnotics and persistence of drug effects ("hangover") after the drug has been discontinued. Factors reducing maternal serum drug levels increase the risk of subtherapeutic drug levels.

Drugs in plasma are either unbound (free) or bound to plasma proteins, primarily albumin or α1-acid glycoprotein. The reduction in plasma proteins, especially albumin, during pregnancy may increase plasma levels of free (active) drug. Albumin is the major binding protein for acidic drugs such as salicylates, anticonvulsants, nonsteroidal antiinflammatory agents, and some neutral drugs such as warfarin and diazepam.[70] Serum albumin levels fall during pregnancy, increasing the unbound or free drug fraction. Total plasma drug concentration stays the same during pregnancy, but the unbound fraction of albumin-bound drugs is greater; therefore the drug may be cleared faster.[70] Thus increases in free drug do not necessarily lead to an increase in plasma levels of that drug if the increase in free drug is balanced by more rapid hepatic biotransformation or renal elimination.[70] However doses of some drugs that are bound to albumin, such as many antiepileptic drugs, may need to be altered during pregnancy. In addition, free fatty acids and steroid hormones, both of which are increased in pregnancy, may compete with drugs for albumin bindings sites, further increasing levels of unbound drug.[41,80] The decrease in albumin coupled with increases in free fatty acids and steroid hormones are most prominent in late pregnancy. This change can result in unpredictable transient increases in free levels of some drugs, such as phenytoin, valproate acid, sulfisoxazole, theophylline, and phenobarbitol as well as the potential for more rapid elimination leading to subtherapeutic maternal levels.[102,136]

α1-Acid glycoprotein is the major protein for binding basic drugs such as local anesthetics, most opioids, and beta-blockers.[102] Levels do not change significantly in pregnancy, although there may be decreased binding of some basic drugs.[80,85,102]

Alterations in protein bindings during pregnancy not only influence availability of free drug for the mother and to cross the placenta, but may also alter the fetal-to-maternal drug ratios, thus further altering placental transfer. Drugs whose biotransformation is hepatic blood flow–limited (e.g., propanolol, lidocaine) are rapidly eliminated in their first pass through the liver, regardless of whether they are bound or unbound.[80] Therefore, even with the decreased protein binding in pregnancy, hepatic clearance and total drug concentration generally are not significantly altered, although concentrations of free drug, Vd, and half-life may increase.[80] Conversely, with drugs whose hepatic biotransformation is independent of hepatic blood flow (e.g., warfarin, phenytoin), only the unbound fraction is removed by the liver. For these drugs, total drug concentrations may be lower than usual, with a decreased half-life and greater fluctuations in peak and trough levels.[80]

Hepatic Drug Metabolism

The hepatic changes during pregnancy can alter biotransformation of drugs by the liver and clearance of drugs from the maternal serum. Drugs that are primarily (greater than 70%) metabolized in their first pass through the liver (high extraction ratio) are usually cleared rapidly by the liver, since clearance of these drugs is dependent on hepatic blood flow.[102] Hepatic elimination of drugs with high extraction ratios is generally unchanged in pregnancy. Drugs with low (less than 30%) first-pass hepatic clearance (low extraction ratio) are more dependent on liver enzyme systems.[102] The rate of elimination of these drugs (e.g., theophylline, caffeine, diazepam) is related to free drug levels and tends to be decreased in pregnancy with increased half-lives.[102] Hepatic elimination of other drugs—including many antibiotics, pancuronium, phenytoin, and paracetamol—is increased in the pregnant woman.

Some liver enzymatic processes may be slowed during pregnancy, delaying drug metabolism and degradation. The cytochrome P450 (CYP450) monooxygenase system is a group of enzymes essential for hepatic metabolism of drugs. The enzymes of this system are indicated by the prefix CYP (cytochrome) followed by a series of numbers and letters (e.g., CYP1A2, CYP3A4, CYP2D6). CYP3A4, CYP2D6, and CYP2C19 activity is increased in pregnancy.

However, CYP1A2, which is responsible for hepatic elimination of about half of all drugs, is decreased.[69] Some extrahepatic enzymes, particularly cholinesterase, are also decreased, which may alter the woman's response to neuromuscular agents.[126,130] For example, the decrease in pseudocholinesterase during pregnancy has been enough to impair breakdown of suxamethonium with subsequent prolonged paralysis after anesthesia in some women.[102] Although hepatic blood flow is unaltered during pregnancy, the 35% decrease in the proportion of cardiac output delivered to the liver may slow hepatic clearance of drugs from the blood. In general, slowly metabolized drugs that are cleared primarily by the liver tend to be cleared more slowly in pregnancy due to decreased enzymatic activity and the net decrease in liver blood flow. This may also increase the length of time potentially teratogenic intermediary metabolites remain in circulation.[87]

Clearance and metabolism of drugs by the liver during pregnancy may be influenced by the increased steroid hormones that stimulate hepatic microsomal enzyme activity. For example, progesterone may induce enzyme activity for phenytoin clearance, whereas progesterone and estradiol alter hepatic elimination of caffeine and theophylline by competitive inhibition of microsomal oxidase.[70,80] Estrogens have cholinergic effects and may interfere with clearance of drugs such as rifampin that are excreted into the biliary system.[70,80] Smoking and alcohol may also induce hepatic enzymes.[102]

Renal Drug Excretion

Many drugs are excreted primarily by the kidneys. Thus the increased glomerular filtration rate (GFR) in pregnancy alters renal excretion of drugs, especially water-soluble drugs such as penicillin G, digoxin, aminoglycosides, lithium, and pancuronium. These drugs are eliminated more rapidly, leading to lower and potentially subtherapeutic blood and tissue levels.[64,69,85,111] In many cases the changes are not clinically significant enough to require alteration in drug dose.[94] However, this is not always the case. For example, pregnant women with paroxysmal atrial tachycardia may experience an increased frequency of attacks even though maintained on their usual doses of digoxin. These women may require up to a 50% increase in their digoxin dose during pregnancy.

Alterations in Drug Absorption, Distribution, Metabolism, and Excretion during the Intrapartum and Postpartum Periods

Drug handling is further altered during the intrapartum period. GI absorption may decrease to a greater extent.[80] Gastric emptying is reported to decrease further during labor; however, this may be secondary to use of opiate agents such as meperidine and pentazocine.[80,97] Administration of antacids to decrease the risk of acid aspiration with anesthesia can alter ionization by altering gastric pH, prolonging gastric emptying, or complexing with drugs, reducing their absorption.[80] Cardiac output increases in the intrapartum period further increase the Vd and may transiently alter hepatic and renal blood flow.[97] Blood flow to the lower extremities may be reduced, especially if the woman is in a supine position. This may result in a slower and more unpredictable rate of absorption of drugs given intramuscularly into the buttocks or thigh.[97] Plasma nonesterified fatty acids rise during labor and may compete for albumin binding sites, with an increase in free drug levels.[97] Both supine positioning and oxytocin may reduce renal blood flow and delay renal excretion of drugs and drug metabolites during labor.[80] Most analgesics and anesthetics used in labor will cross to the fetus once entering maternal circulation. The clinical effects depend on the timing of the dose, half-life, drug physicochemical characteristics, and maternal and fetal drug metabolism and excretion.[10]

During the immediate postpartum period the pattern of pharmacokinetics and drug distribution is similar to that of late pregnancy and remains so until the pregnancy-induced physiologic alterations of each system return to nonpregnant status.[20] During this transition, drug handling by the woman may remain altered to some extent for some drugs. Transfer of drugs to nursing infants is discussed later in this chapter in Drugs and Lactation.

Transfer of Drugs across the Placenta

Dancis has suggested that in thinking of placental transfer one should: "Ask not whether a maternal [substance] crosses the placenta. Ask rather, how, how much, and how fast. Ask also as to fetal need."[25] There are few compounds, endogenous or exogenous, that are unable to cross the placenta in detectable amounts given sufficient time and sensitivity of detection.[16,25,63,85] Drugs with similar physiodynamic properties can differ in placental transfer.[92] Nau and Plonait suggest that if no other information is available and a group of drugs is not known to have teratogenic effects, a comparison of lipid solubility, molecular weight (MW), ionization, and degree of protein binding might assist the clinical selection of an appropriate drug for more efficient transfer (fetal drug therapy) or least efficient transfer (limited fetal exposure).[92] For example, drugs that are lipid soluble, have an extremely low (50 daltons) or low (51 to 599) MW, and are nonionized with low protein binding in maternal plasma cross the placenta more rapidly and in higher concentrations than drugs that are water soluble (polar), have a high MW (greater than 600), and are ionized and highly bound to protein in maternal plasma.

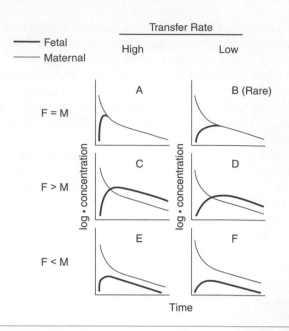

FIGURE **6-2** Simulation of maternal and fetal plasma concentrations time curves from various transplacental pharmacokinetic models. Examples of drugs that fit each curve are in Table 6-4. (From Nau, H. & Plonait, S.L. [1998]. Physiochemical and structural properties regulating placental drug transfer. In R.A. Polin & W.W. Fox [Eds.]. *Fetal and neonatal physiology* [2nd ed.]. Philadelphia: W.B. Saunders.)

Patterns of Transfer Kinetics

Three major patterns of transfer pharmacokinetics are seen: (1) complete transfer (drugs that rapidly equilibrate between mother and fetus, with blood flow the rate limiting step; (2) exceeding transfer (levels are higher in the fetus than in the mother); and (3) incomplete transfer (levels are higher in the mother than the fetus).[96] These patterns are illustrated in Figure 6-2. Examples of drugs with each pattern are listed in Table 6-4.

There is a great deal of variability even among drugs with similar pharmacokinetic characteristics. However, in general, complete transfer tends to be seen with drugs that have a high pKa and MW less than 600 daltons, whereas incomplete transfer is seen with drugs that have a high pKa and MW greater than 600. Strongly ionized drugs generally have incomplete transfer, although exceptions occur. For example, ampicillin and methicillin are strongly ionized but have lipophilic side groups, so they have a complete transfer pattern.[97] Valproate and salicylates are ionized at the normal (physiologic) pH level but rapidly cross the placenta.[70] There is no consistent relationship between the ionization of weak bases and transfer pattern.[96]

TABLE **6-4** **Examples of Drugs with Transplacental Kinetics***

MODEL A OR B	MODEL C	MODEL D	MODEL E	MODEL F

Some barbiturates:
  Thiopental
  Pentobarbital
  Secobarbital
Antipyrine
Promethazine
Ritodrine
Magnesium sulfate
Thiamphenicol
  digoxin
	Some
	  benzodiazepines:
	  Diazepam
	  Lorazepam
	  Desmethyldiazepam
	  Oxazepam
	Valproate
	Salicylate
	Nalidixic acid
	Nicotine
	Urea
	Some penicillins:
	  Ampicillin
	  Penicillin G
	  Methicillin
	  Azidocillin
		Ascorbate
		Colistimethate†
		Furosemide
		Meperidine
		Some
		  cephalosporins:
		  Cephalothin
		  Cefazolin
		  Cephapirin
		  Cephalexin
		Some
		  aminoglycosides:
		  Gentamycin
		  Kanamycin
			Amide-type local
			  anesthetic agents:
			  Lidocaine
			  Bupivacaine
			Some β-adrenoceptor
			  blockers:
			  Propanolol
			  Sotalol
			  Labetalol
			Dexamethasone
			Cimetidine
			Ranitidine
			Methadone
			Some sulfonamides‡
				Heparin
				Quaternary ammo-
				  nium compounds:
				  Tubocurarine
				  Succinylcholine
				  Vecuronium
				  Pancuronium
				  Fazadinium
				  Alcuronium
				Elementary ions:
				  Fenoterol
				  Chlorthalidone
				  Etozolin (ozolinone)
				  Dicloxacillin
				  Erythromycin
				  Nitrofurantoin

From Nau, H. & Plonait, S.L. (1998). Physiochemical and structural properties regulating placental drug transfer. In R.A. Polin & W.W. Fox (Eds.). *Fetal and neonatal physiology* (2nd ed.). Philadelphia: W.B. Saunders.

*According to models A through F in Figure 6-2. Differentiation between models A and B, C and D, and E and F is often uncertain because of incomplete data on the initial phase of drug distribution across the placenta. Model B is rarely applicable.

†Polypeptide antibiotic, with a molecular weight of 1200 daltons.

‡First and second trimester.

Factors Influencing Placental Transfer

Placental transfer is influenced by the following: (1) maternal and fetal drug handling; (2) surface area of the placenta; (3) diffusing distance between maternal and fetal blood; (4) physicochemical characteristics of the drug; (4) gradients (drug concentration, electropotential [normally 20 mV], and pH) between mother and fetus; (5) degree of binding of a substance to hemoglobin or other proteins in maternal and fetal circulations; (6) concentrations of binding proteins and protein binding gradients between mother and fetus; (7) permeability of the placental barrier (primarily the syncytiotrophoblast); (8) and rates of maternal and fetal blood flow through the intervillous space and villi (Table 6-5).[9,45,75,86,89,96,102]

Diffusing distance and surface area. Most drugs cross the placenta by diffusion. Diffusion of a substance across the placenta can be expressed as follows:

$$\text{Diffusion} = \frac{\text{Substance characteristics} \times \text{Surface area} \times}{\text{Distance}} \frac{\text{Concentration gradient}}{\text{Distance}}$$

Increased surface area for exchange, increased concentration gradient, and decreased diffusing distance enhance transfer across the placenta.[9] With increasing gestation and placental growth, efficiency of the placenta transfer increases as a result of the increased surface area. As the placenta matures, the distance between maternal and fetal blood decreases due to thinning of the syncytial trophoblast and connective tissue and to increases in the size and number of capillaries in the villi (see Chapter 3). Thus more drug passes to the fetus in the third trimester than in the first trimester. Transfer may be reduced with decreased surface area (small placenta, placental infarcts) or increased diffusing distance (placental edema, infection).[36]

Although most drugs cross by diffusion, some drugs may be transferred across the placenta by nutrient carriers, including amino acid, glucose, or monoamine carriers. Various transporters are located along the brush border facing maternal blood in the intervillous space and on the syncytiotrophoblast basal membrane (facing the fetal connective tissue matrix and blood vessels in the villi) to facilitate movement of nutrients and other physiologic substances across the placenta.[9,35,85,115] Nonphysiologic substances—such as some drugs, environmental pollutants, and toxins—if structurally similar to nutrients, may compete for these transporters. The drugs that seem to be particularly able to use this method to cross the placenta include amphetamines, cocaine, cannabinoids, and nicotine and other substances from cigarettes.[35,36] By successfully combining with nutrients for these transporters, nutrient transfer is reduced and fetal growth and development altered.

TABLE **6-5**   Factors Influencing the Distribution of Drugs and Other Substances in the Fetus

FACTOR	POSSIBLE INFLUENCES
Type of drug	Factors that increase transfer include lipid solubility, low molecular weight (less than 600 daltons for non-soluble and less than 100 daltons for polar substances), non-ionized, and unbound.
Amount of drug	Transfer is increased by greater maternal-to-fetal gradient, especially for drugs transferred by diffusion.
Membrane permeability	Diffusion of substances increases with increasing gestation and greater placental efficiency. Some drugs have greater affinity for specific fetal tissues (e.g., tetracycline in teeth, warfarin in bones, phenytoin in the fetal heart [because this is a highly lipid organ in the fetus, whereas in adults the central nervous system has a high lipid content owing to myelin sheaths], streptomycin in the otic nerve).
Fetal body water compartment	Drug distribution and dilution change as the total body water compartment decreases with increasing gestation. With an increased volume of distribution peak volumes of drugs are reduced, but excretion is delayed.
Fetal circulation	Maternal and fetal blood flow rates will influence transfer. Upon reaching the fetal circulation, drugs may be shunted by the ductus venosus past the liver (thus missing an opportunity for detoxification), with highest concentrations of these substances in blood going to the heart and upper body.
Serum protein binding	Protein binding of a drug in the maternal system limits the amount of free drug available for transfer to the fetus. Binding of drugs to macromolecules in the fetal circulation may increase the maternal-to-fetal transfer by maintaining a concentration gradient from the mother to the fetus.
Receptor function	Functional ability of receptors on cell membranes increases with gestation, leading to increased specificity to respond to or exclude certain drugs.
Placental enzymes	Enzymes produced by the placenta (e.g., insulinase) may detoxify drugs and reduce transfer to the fetus.
Gestational age	Many of the factors identified above are altered with advancing gestation and maturity of the fetus and placenta. The size and efficiency of the placental exchange area increase with increasing gestational age.
Fetal pH during labor	The fetal pH is usually 0.1 to 0.15 units below that of the mother. A decrease in the fetal pH may increase the transfer of acidophilic agents from the mother to fetus. Hypoxia alters blood flow and thus drug distribution, metabolism, and excretion. For example, with hypoxia, blood flow to the liver and kidneys may be reduced with preferential flow to the brain. Albumin binding of drugs may also be reduced, resulting in more free drug in the fetal circulation.

Physicochemical characteristics and concentration gradients. Physicochemical characteristics that influence movement across the placenta include lipid solubility, MW, degree of ionization, and protein binding. These characteristics can increase, decrease, or prohibit movement of potentially harmful drugs and other substances from maternal-to-fetal circulation.[24,75,92] For example, placental transfer may be increased or enhanced if a substance is lipid soluble (e.g., diazepam, lipoproteins, most sedatives) or nonionized (e.g., phenobarbital), has a MW less than 600 daltons (e.g., propylthiouracil), or lacks significant binding to albumin (e.g., ampicillin).[1,10] A substance will have reduced, slower, or no transport across the placenta if it has a certain charge or molecular configuration (e.g., heparin) or certain size (e.g., heparin, IgM), is altered or bound by enzymes within the placenta (e.g., amines, insulin), or is firmly and highly bound to the maternal red blood cell (e.g., carbon monoxide) or plasma proteins (e.g., dicloxacillin).

Lipid-soluble substances cross the placenta more readily than water-soluble substances, because cell membranes are made primarily of lipids that enhance diffusion. Lipid-soluble substances dissolve in the lipid membranes of the tissues separating maternal and fetal blood. Polar substances cross slowly unless they have low MW. Figure 6-3 illustrates several models for transplacental passage of different types of drugs and drug metabolites.

The exact MW limit for placental transfer is unknown, although substances up to a MW of 5000 daltons are known to cross the placenta; substances with MW over 7500 probably have minimal transfer unless a specific carrier exists for that substance. Insulin (with an MW over 6000) does not cross the placenta, due to its size and configuration but also due to effects of placental insulinase enzymes.[96] Substances

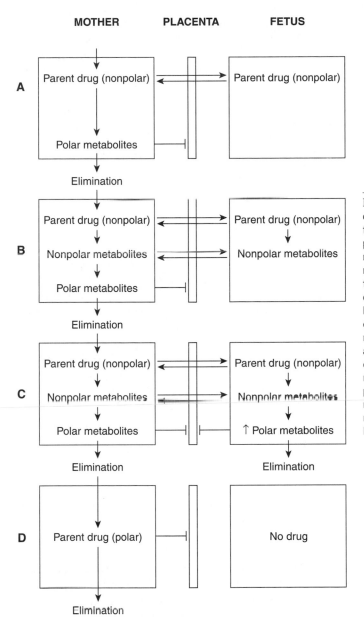

FIGURE **6-3** Schematic representation of different possibilities of drug and drug metabolite transfer between mother and fetus. **A,** The parent drug is nonpolar and readily crosses the placenta to reach the fetus. Polar metabolites are formed in the mother, but do not cross the placenta and are eliminated by maternal renal mechanisms. **B,** Nonpolar metabolites are formed in the mother and cross the placenta readily in both directions: maternal-fetal and fetal-maternal. Further metabolism to polar metabolites and subsequent elimination occur only in the mother. **C,** The nonpolar parent drug and nonpolar metabolites equilibrate across the placenta between mother and fetus. Polar metabolites formed on either side of either placental membrane do not cross the placenta. They are eliminated by the mother, but may accumulate in the fetus. **D,** The parent drug administered to the mother in so polar that it does not cross the placenta but is eliminated unchanged by maternal renal mechanisms. (From Krauer, B. & Krauer, F. [1977]. Drug kinetics in pregnancy. *Clin Pharmacokinet, 2,* 174.)

with higher MW tend to cross more slowly and are influenced by maternal concentrations; for example, if maternal concentrations are high, the substance is more likely to cross.[74] These substances may also cross via active transport if a carrier is present. For example, immunoglobulin G (IgG) with a MW of 150,000 daltons is actively transported across the placenta (see Chapter 12).[9,36,128] Water-soluble substances with MW lower than 100 diffuse readily; those with MW higher than 100 diffuse more slowly.[102] Small lipid-soluble substances (MW less than 600) cross rapidly and are blood flow dependent; those with a MW over 600 cross more slowly.[85] However, MW is of limited value clinically since most drugs have MWs below 600. Exceptions include thyroid hormones (MW 889) insulin (MW greater than 6000), heparin (MW 20,000 to 40,000), and low-MW heparin (MW 3000 to 5000).[96]

Maternal-to-fetal concentration or electrochemical gradients also influence transfer. The maternal-fetal pH gradient influences transfer of drugs and can result in "ion trapping," with higher concentrations of some drugs in the fetus than mother. Nonionized substances cross the placenta more efficiently than ionized substances.[102] Normally the fetus and amniotic fluid are slightly more acidotic than the mother by 0.1 to 0.15 pH units.[96,102] As a result of this difference, basic drugs may accumulate in the fetus and amniotic fluid with levels higher than in the mother. In the mother a weak base tends to remain nonionized in her plasma and cross the placenta rapidly. As this weak base comes into contact with the more acidic fetal blood, the drug becomes more ionized, increasing the flow gradient from mother to fetus. The now-ionized drugs will not be able to return across the placenta to the mother as readily, thus becoming trapped in the fetus.[70,96] For example, most opioids are weak bases that may accumulate in the fetus, which is one reason that effects of these drugs may persist in the neonatal period.[102] The opposite effect is seen with acidic drugs: that is, these drugs are more likely to be ionized in the mother and thus not cross the placenta as readily.[80] For nonionized, lipophilic drugs, the rate-limiting step for placental transfer is blood flow; for polar drugs, the rate-limiting step is diffusion.[70] Hypoxia and acidosis in the fetus can influence transplacental passage of drugs. For example, local anesthetics are weak bases whose degree of ionization depends on pH. If the fetus becomes acidotic, ionization of these drugs increases with accumulation ("ion trapping") in the fetus and neonate.[96]

Drug metabolites also cross the placenta to the fetus and vice versa. The majority of fetal drug elimination is by transfer back to the mother across the placenta. However, some elimination may occur by fetal metabolism, placental metabolism, or excretion into amniotic fluid.[36] This transfer is also based on physicochemical characteristics, primarily ionization and lipid solubility. Most drug metabolites are polar, since polarity enhances biliary and renal elimination. Once polar substances are transferred to the fetus, elimination back across the placenta is slow and may result in accumulation in the fetus or amniotic fluid.[63] In addition the fetus may metabolize a drug producing polar metabolites (see Figure 6-3). These metabolites can also become trapped and accumulate in the fetus or be excreted into amniotic fluid and reswallowed by the fetus. Examples of drugs that tend to concentrate in amniotic fluid are the β-lactams, such as penicillin G, dicloxacillin, and amiodarone.[80,102]

If a drug is transferred slower than the maternal elimination rate, then a significant portion of the drug may be eliminated by the mother before it can be transferred to the fetus.[120] A single dose of a drug given to the mother by intravenous administration tends to cross more quickly to the fetus until concentrations are equalized. As the mother clears the drug from her blood, transfer is reversed as the drug crosses from fetus back to mother.[120] With drugs given repeatedly to reach steady-state concentrations in the mother, protein binding and fetal drug elimination are more critical in determining fetal exposure.[109,120]

Protein binding. Drugs that are protein bound in mother or fetus do not cross the placenta. Therefore plasma protein gradients between mother and fetus can also influence transfer. For example, only 20% of ampicillin is bound to proteins, thus increasing the amount of free drug that can cross to fetus, and resulting in decreased maternal levels. Protein binding of methicillin is 40% and that dicloxacillin is 96%. Therefore dicloxacillin would be an appropriate choice to treat maternal infections, but not to treat intrauterine or fetal infection.[20] Decreased maternal levels of aminoglycosides are also seen.

Maternal albumin levels fall during pregnancy and are about 15% lower than the those in the fetus at term; α1-acid glycoprotein levels in the fetus are only about 37% of maternal levels.[85,96] Albumin (or fetal albumin macromolecule) bound drugs may be more highly bound in the fetus, whereas α1-acid glycoprotein drugs are more highly bound in the mother.[85] Binding to proteins in the fetus may increase transfer of the drug by maintaining a concentration gradient across the placenta. Plasma protein binding and thus concentrations of drugs in the mother versus the fetus changes with increasing gestational age for some drugs. The decreased maternal albumin with increasing gestation increases the amount of free drug in the mother available for placental transfer. For example, diazepam binds to albumin. Albumin binding of diazepam is low in the fetus in the first half of gestation. However, in late gestation, as maternal serum albumin levels decrease, more free diazepam is present in maternal serum and, since this is a lipophilic drug, readily crosses the placenta. Thus, by term, fetal diazepam levels are greater than maternal levels (Table 6-6).[92] This may increase the risk of neonatal hyperbilirubinemia since diazepam competes with bilirubin for albumin binding (see Neonatal Pharmacokinetics).

Placental blood flow. The rate of maternal blood flow to and through the intervillous space and fetal blood flow to and through the villi influence placental transfer, particularly of nonionized, lipophilic substances such as anticonvulsants, alcohol, and opioid derivatives. Contractions decrease transfer so drugs that cross rapidly and are given during a contraction may demonstrate decreased transfer to the fetus.[102] In addition to uterine contractions, factors that may alter uteroplacental blood flow include maternal position; anesthesia; nicotine and other drugs; emotional or physical stress; and degenerative changes within the placenta that are seen with hypertension, prolonged pregnancy, diabetes, or renal disease.[45,72,86,88]

Route of administration. The route of administration can also affect placental transfer. For example, nalbuphine that is given intramuscularly results in fetal blood levels that are 80% of maternal venous levels; if it is given intravenously, fe-

TABLE **6-6**   Fetal and Maternal Protein Binding and Total Concentration Ratios of Selected Drugs during Late Human Gestation

DRUG	PRIMARY BINDING PROTEIN	BOUND IN MOTHER (%)	BOUND IN FETUS (%)	FETUS/MOTHER TOTAL PLASMA CONCENTRATION RATIO
Betamethasone	AGP	60	41	0.33
Bupivacaine	AGP	91	51	0.27
Diazepam	ALB	97	98.5	1.6
Lidocaine	AGP	64	24	0.66
Mepivacaine	AGP	55	36	0.71
N-desmethyl diazepam	ALB	95	97	1.7
Phenobarbital	ALB	41	36	1.0
Phenytoin	ALB	87	82	1.0
Salicylate	ALB	43	54	1.2
Valproic acid	ALB	73	88	1.7

From Nau, H. & Plonait, S.L. (1998). Physiochemical and structural properties regulating placental drug transfer. In R.A. Polin & W.W. Fox (Eds.). *Fetal and neonatal physiology* (2nd ed.). Philadelphia: W.B. Saunders.
ALB, Albumin; *AGP*, α1-acid glycoprotein.

tal levels are three to six times greater than maternal levels.[10,70,96] Peak drug concentrations in the fetus (and the infant, if delivered after maternal administration) do not necessarily occur at the same time as in the mother. For example, meperidine peaks at 30 to 50 minutes in the mother, but 90 minutes to 3 hours after maternal administration in the fetus as a result of transfer kinetics across the placenta.[10] Therefore meperidine levels are highest in the infant if given to the mother 90 minutes to 3 hours before delivery; on the other hand, fentanyl is higher in the neonate than mother if given shortly before delivery.[10] Therefore it is reasonable to give meperidine if birth is expected within the hour.

Antibiotics are some of the most commonly prescribed drugs in pregnancy. Since antibiotics cross the placenta primarily by simple diffusion, rate-limiting factors include maternal-fetal concentration gradients, MW, and other physicochemical characteristics of the drug, placental surface area, diffusing distance, and the degree to which the drug is bound to maternal plasma proteins (see Table 6-5). A general pattern of antibiotic distribution to the fetus has been described.[43] After an intravenous dose, peak maternal serum concentrations are seen within 15 minutes then fall exponentially. Peak umbilical cord values are seen in 30 to 60 minutes followed by an exponential fall. Peak amniotic fluid levels are seen in 4 to 5 hours. This lag results from slow excretion in fetal urine due to fetal renal immaturity.[20,56,114]

Placental Metabolism of Drugs

The placenta has many enzyme systems, including various peptidases that can metabolize drugs, thus influencing transfer of specific substances from mother to fetus or fetus to mother. Several isoforms of the CYP450 system are found in the placenta, although at levels about half of those seen in the liver.[102] The primary CYP450 isoform seen in the placenta are CYP1A1/1A2, although other isoforms have also been reported.[9,39,85,97,103] Expression of placental CYP1A1 increases with exposure to PCBs or maternal cigarette smoking.[9,95]

Fetal Drug Therapy

Planned fetal drug exposure may occur as a method of treating fetal disorders by administration of drugs to the mother. The most common fetal treatment is administration of one full course of glucocorticoids to induce surfactant synthesis and reduce the risk of respiratory distress syndrome in preterm infants (see Chapter 9). Not all glucocorticoids are equally effective, because some are metabolized by the maternal-fetal-placental unit and thus rendered inactive. Inactivation of betamethasone and dexamethasone is limited, so these glucocorticoids are more effective in enhancing surfactant synthesis than drugs such as hydrocortisone, which are rapidly metabolized in the placenta.[128] Glucocorticoids may also be given to treat inborn errors of adrenal metabolism. Glucocorticoids suppress fetal androgen production and may prevent development of ambiguous genitalia in female fetuses if begun by 8 to 10 weeks gestation.[117,128] Drugs may also be given to the mother to treat other inborn errors of metabolism, fetal cardiac arrhythmias, congestive heart failure, and infection.[100]

Administration of antibiotics to the mother with the purpose of protecting the fetus is probably reasonably effective for protection of the GI (swallowing of amniotic fluid) and renal (adequate blood flow) systems. The fetal circulation shunts blood away from the lungs, however, which limits delivery of antibiotics to the respiratory tract for protection against congenital pneumonia in the presence of chorioamnionitis. Since amniotic fluid levels of antibiotics are dependent on excretion of the drug in fetal urine, therapeutic levels of antibiotics in amniotic fluid are attained only with a live fetus. This limits the effectiveness of this treatment for chorioamnionitis after intrauterine death.[20,56,114] An example of a preventive fetal drug therapy is the use of folic acid for prevention of neural tube defects (see Chapter 14).

SUMMARY

The impact of maternal physiologic alterations and fetal drug transfer can be illustrated by examining pharmacokinetics and distribution of several drug classes, namely antibiotics and anticonvulsants. Serum levels and the half-life of many antibiotics are reduced during pregnancy, primarily because of a more rapid excretion associated with the increased GFR. For example, renal clearance of ampicillin and cefuroxime (in ml/minute) is 394 and 198, respectively, in nonpregnant women versus 613 and 287 during pregnancy.[102] Most cephalosporins have a shorter half-life in late pregnancy, except for cefoperazone, which is excreted in bile rather than by the kidneys, so it has a similar half-life in pregnant and nonpregnant women.[26]

The increased GFR augments renal clearance of antibiotics, thus further reducing serum levels. Most antibiotics are lipid soluble and readily cross the placenta. As a result of these alterations, dosages of some antibiotics may need to be increased or the dosing interval reduced.[20,43,83,118] Maternal antibiotic levels must be carefully monitored to ensure that the mother is receiving an adequate therapeutic dose and to avoid maternal or fetal toxicity. With most local infections the reduction in maternal serum concentrations probably does not alter therapeutic efficacy of the antibiotic. Pregnant women with acute infections or who need high serum concentrations require much higher doses than nonpregnant women.[83]

Only about 20% of ampicillin is protein bound, increasing the level of free drug that readily crosses into the fetal compartment. As a result, fetal and amniotic fluid levels are elevated and maternal serum and plasma levels decreased. The Vd and renal clearance are increased and the half-life of ampicillin reduced in the pregnant woman.[56,110] Decreased maternal serum and plasma levels of aminoglycosides are also found in some women, increasing the likelihood of subtherapeutic levels. For example, Weinstein and colleagues reported that 40% of pregnant women required twice the recommended dose of gentamicin to achieve therapeutic levels.[116] Cord blood levels of gentamicin are about half of maternal levels and are often subtherapeutic.[56] If aminoglycosides are used, blood levels (risk of subtherapeutic levels) and maternal renal function (risk of nephrotoxicity) require careful monitoring.

Higher maternal serum levels and lower fetal and amniotic fluid levels are seen with the use of antibiotics with increased protein binding such as methicillin (40%) and dicloxacillin (96%). As a result, a drug such as dicloxacillin would be appropriate for treating a maternal infection but not effective in treating an intrauterine infection.[20,130] Dicloxacillin and erythromycin (base or stearate) have limited placental transfer, so fetal levels are low. Maternal absorption, serum levels, and tissue levels of erythromycin may be somewhat erratic and unpredictable.[56,130] Higher concentrations of antibiotics are found in the fetus and amniotic fluid after bolus administration versus continuous drip infusion to the mother and after multiple versus single doses.[20]

A major factor affecting the pregnant epileptic is the effect of the usual physiologic changes of pregnancy on the metabolism of antiepileptic drugs (AEDs). These changes are summarized in Table 6-7. As a result of these changes, the apparent plasma clearance of AEDs decreases with subtherapeutic plasma concentrations and increased risk of seizures. In general the pregnant woman on AEDs needs to have the dosages of her medication(s) increased by 30% to 50% above prepregnant levels.[2] These changes occur predominantly during the second half of pregnancy and reverse by 6 weeks postpartum.[30] As the physiologic alterations of pregnancy are reversed following delivery, drug levels may fluctuate rapidly, leading to toxicity. Monitoring of drug levels must include evaluation of free (unbound) drug, since this parameter is better correlated with seizure activity than total drug levels.[2,30] Drug levels are monitored regularly during pregnancy to ensure therapeutic dosages, with monitoring con-

TABLE **6-7**   **Effects of Pregnancy on Metabolism of Antiepileptic Drugs**

PREGNANCY CHANGE	EFFECT
Hemodilution	Increased volume of distribution
Decreased protein binding and concentrations of serum proteins/unit of volume	Increased unbound (free) drug
	Increased availability of drugs for placental transfer
Placental transfer	Similar cord and maternal blood levels of drugs
Impaired gastrointestinal absorption	Decreased absorption of phenytoin
Altered hepatic metabolism	Increased metabolism of primidone, carbamazepine, and phenytoin
Altered renal function	Increased renal excretion of phenobarbital

tinuing after delivery until drug levels have stabilized.[98] Phenytoin, phenobarbital, and primidone have also been associated with teratogenic effects (see Teratogenesis) and may interfere with folic acid and vitamin K metabolism, increasing the risk of neural tube defects (see Chapter 14) and hemorrhagic disease of the newborn (see Chapter 7). Therefore the fetus and infant must also be monitored carefully. Pregnant women on AEDs can enroll in the Antiepileptic Drug Pregnancy Registry at Massachusetts General Hospital/Harvard Medical School ([888] 233-2334); the program follows pregnancy outcomes in women on different AEDs to determine which is the safest drug.

PHARMACOKINETICS IN THE FETUS
Drug Distribution, Metabolism, and Excretion in the Fetus

Distribution, metabolism, and elimination of drugs are altered in the fetus. Factors that influence the effects of drugs in the fetus include individual drug characteristics, dosage and duration of use of the drug, genetic makeup of the mother and fetus (genetic susceptibility), maternal handling and elimination of the drug, timing in relation to stage of embryonic or fetal development, maternal physiology, and placental transfer.[102] Placental transfer is affected by drug physicochemical characteristics (described in the previous section), blood flow, maturation, and metabolic activity.

Fetal Drug Distribution

Fetal drug distribution is influenced by individual drug characteristics, specificity of individual agents for certain fetal tissues, and receptor function. Some drugs have a greater affinity for specific fetal tissue that are not the agents' expected target tissue. Examples include the high affinity of tetracycline for fetal teeth, warfarin for the fetal bones, and phenytoin for fetal heart tissue. Receptor function of fetal cells increases with increasing gestational age. Receptors become more specific in their ability to respond to or exclude certain drugs, whereas in the embryo and young fetus, these receptors are less discriminating in excluding drugs, increasing the likelihood of teratogenic effects. Other factors influencing drug distribution in the fetus are gestational age, degree of serum protein binding, and fetal body water compartment. The fetus has lower levels of serum proteins, increasing the amount of free drug. Fetal proteins may bind some drugs with greater affinity (salicylates) than in the mother and others (ampicillin, benzyl penicillin with less affinity).[70] Levels of $\alpha 1$-acid glycoprotein are up to three times lower in the fetus than in the mother.[80] Even as proteins increase with advancing gestational age, levels of free drug tend to remain high because of the lowered protein binding affinity. The fetus has an in-

creased Vd due to increased total body water. This results in a reduction in peak volume of drugs, but also wider distribution of drugs in the body and delayed excretion. Factors influencing distribution of drugs and other substances within the fetus are summarized in Table 6-5.

Fetal Drug Metabolism and Elimination

Once a drug reaches the fetal circulation the drug can: (1) be metabolized by the fetal liver, (2) bypass the fetal liver via the ductus venosus to enter specific fetal tissues or body compartments, (3) be eliminated by the fetal kidney into amniotic fluid (and perhaps be reswallowed in that fluid by the fetus), or (4) return to the maternal circulation via the umbilical arteries and placenta.[47] Drugs and metabolites in amniotic fluid may diffuse across the fetal membranes and decidua to maternal blood or be swallowed by the fetus. Swallowed drugs or their metabolites are reabsorbed into the fetal blood from the gut and cleared via the placenta. Some such as cocaine are deposited in meconium. Drug metabolites are also excreted by the liver into bile and thus into meconium. Polar metabolites may accumulate in amniotic fluid, reaching levels higher than in either mother or fetus.[14] Examples of drugs that may accumulate in amniotic fluid are ampicillin, amoxicillin, cefuroxime, and cefalothin.[96] Metabolites of some drugs that the fetus is exposed to in the third trimester may also be found in fetal hair.[120] Because most metabolites are more polar than the original drug, substances that cross the placenta to the fetus may not return across the placenta to the mother as readily (see Figure 6-3, *C*). Therefore these substances can accumulate in fetal tissues and at levels that may be higher than in the mother.[70]

Fetal hepatic metabolism. By the end of the first trimester, the fetal liver can oxidize some substances via the CYP450 system[9,14,102,103] (phase I biotransformation) (see Table 6-1). Before 8 to 9 weeks, CYP450 enzymes are found in extrahepatic tissue, primarily the fetal adrenal.[39] The major fetal isoform is CYP3A7, a form found primarily in the fetal liver, although it can also be found in the placenta and endometrium; some CYP3A7 is also found in low levels in the adult liver. CYP3A7 accounts for about 50% of the total fetal CYP450 content and is involved in steroid metabolism.[103] Fetal CYYP3A7 has a lower catalytic activity than in adults; levels decrease markedly after birth.[96,103] Other isoforms reported in the fetal liver (although in low quantities) include CYP1A1 (involved in metabolism of endogenous toxins), CYP2E1 (found by the second trimester and involved in prenatal alcohol metabolism), CYP1B1, CYP3A4, CYP2D6, CYP2CB, and CYP3A5.[9,39,85,95,103] Even by term, CYP450 enzyme activity is about half that of adults.[102]

Phase II hepatic biotransformation reactions (see Table 6-1) mature at different rates. Glucuronyl transferase activity is low at term, so substances dependent on this mechanism (such as salicylates or lorazepam) for elimination are metabolized three to four times more slowly than in the adult.[102] On the other hand, morphine can be glucuronidated in the first trimester, whereas sulfate conjugation is well developed at birth. Sulfation activity increases with gestational age and, in infancy, activity exceeds that of adults.[102,103]

Lipophilic drugs are more dependent on hepatic metabolism for elimination than are polar substances. The reduced hepatic metabolism in the fetus may be an advantage because drug metabolites are polar and thus tend to cross back to the mother slowly. Lipophilic drugs that remain in that form for longer periods are more likely to cross back to the mother for eliminataion.[102] Phase I metabolites from the CYP450 system generally slowly cross the placenta to the mother for elimination. Phase II metabolites are more polar, an advantage after birth since these are primarily eliminated by biliary excretion or renal elimination. In the fetus these metabolites have decreased placental transfer, so they tend to accumulate in the fetus and amniotic fluid.[102,103]

Fetal hepatic metabolism of drug is limited by a decreased first-pass effect, since much of the blood coming to the fetus from the placenta via the umbilical vein bypasses the liver through the ductus venosus. Biochemically, the left and right lobes of the fetal liver function independently of each other. The more highly oxygenated umbilical vein blood supplies the left lobe, whereas less oxygenated portal vein blood supplies the right lobe. CYP450 activity is higher in the right lobe.[102,103]

Thus the fetal liver has the ability to metabolize drugs but at a decreased rate due to lower enzyme activity. Metabolism of drugs by the fetal liver may not be a advantage since the intermediary metabolites in these reactions may be toxic, and since they tend to be more polar and are cleared more slowly than the original drug, thus prolonging exposure.[103,120] For example, heroin is a lipophilic drug that readily crosses the placenta, where it is converted by the fetal liver to morphine and other metabolites. These substances are less lipid soluble that heroin and may be "trapped" on the fetal side of the placenta.[36]

Fetal renal elimination. Although polar substances cross the placenta slowly, they are rapidly eliminated by the fetal kidney into amniotic fluid. These drugs may be recycled as the fetus swallows amniotic fluid.[102] Since renal blood flow is low (about 5% of cardiac output), renal elimination in general is not a significant mechanism in the fetus.[85]

NEONATAL PHARMACOKINETICS

Absorption, distribution, metabolism, and excretion of drugs are developmentally different in newborns than in adults. Pharmacokinetic changes in the neonate are dependent on both gestational age and postbirth age. Changes in absorption, distribution, metabolism, and elimination of drugs occur at different rates; there may be marked individual differences as well as day-to-day differences.[107] Postbirth age changes are especially marked in the first month. In terms of pharmacokinetics, the neonatal time is the "period of life when most profound and rapid physiologic changes occur."[51]

There are relatively few pharmacokinetic studies for most agents used in neonates. The majority of studies involve relatively heterogeneous samples (in terms of age, weight, disease state) of infants being treated with the specific drug rather than randomized studies.[51] Alterations in drug absorption, distribution, hepatic metabolism, and renal elimination in the neonate affect pharmacokinetics of many drugs used in the neonatal period. Often an individual drug is influenced by multiple pharmacokinetic factors. For example the prolonged diuretic response to furosemide seen in newborns is due to both an increased plasma half-life (which is eight times greater than in adults and may be up to 24 hours in infants less than 3 weeks of age), and an increase in Vd (four times greater than adults), probably because of decreased protein binding.[52] Drug half-lives are almost always longer in the fetus and neonate than in older individuals (Table 6-8). Physiologic differences affecting drug pharmacokinetics in neonates are summarized in Table 6-9.

TABLE **6-8** **Comparative Plasma Half-lives of Miscellaneous Drugs in Newborns and Adults**

Drug	Plasma Half-Life (Hours) in Newborns	Plasma Half-Life (Hours) in Adults
Acetaminophen	3.5	2.2
Phenylbutazone	21-34	12-30
Indomethacin	7.5-51	6
Meperidine	22	3.5
Phenytoin	21	11-29
Carbamazepine	8-28	21-36
Phenobarbital	82-199	24-140
Caffeine	100	6
Theophylline	30	6
Chloramphenicol	14-24	2.5
Salicylates	4.5-11.5	2.7
Digoxin	52	31-40

Data from Aranda, J.V., et al. (1980). Drug monitoring in the perinatal patient: Uses and abuses. *Ther Drug Monit, 2,* 39; Morselli, P.L., et al. (1980). Clinical pharmacokinetics in newborns and infants: Age-related differences and therapeutic implications. *Clin Pharmacokinet, 5,* 485; and Morselli, P.L. (1976). Clinical pharmacokinetics in neonates. *Clin Pharmacokinet, 1,* 81.

TABLE **6-9**   Physiologic Differences of Clinical Significance for Neonatal Drug Therapy

PHYSIOLOGIC DIFFERENCE	CLINICAL SIGNIFICANCE
PRETERM	Receives multiple drugs
	Susceptible to averse drug reactions
BODY COMPOSITION	
Increased body water	↑ AVd, ↑ drug dose, ↑ dosing interval
Decreased body fat	↓ AVd, ↓ drug dose
Maturational changes	↓ Total body water with ↑ PNA
PLASMA PROTEINS	
Decreased binding	↑ Unbound drug, potential toxicity
	Potential displacement of bilirubin
	Potential displacement of other drugs
GI FACTORS	
Gastric acid secretion	↓ Drug absorption
Large surface area	↑ Drug absorption
Decreased motility	↑ Drug absorption
Enzymatic activity	Deconjugation → ↑ drug reabsorption
	↓ Activity → ↓ drug absorption
Maturational changes	Requires therapeutic drug monitoring
SKIN	
Immature epidermis	↑ Absorption of substances
	Percutaneous drug administration
Maturational changes	↓ Drug absorption with ↑ PNA
BIOTRANSFORMATION	
Slower rate	↓ Drug metabolism and elimination
Individual variability	Requires close drug levels monitoring
Alternate pathways	Theophylline metabolizes to caffeine in a newborn
Maturational changes	Drug doses vary by gestational age and PNA
RENAL ELIMINATION	
Decreased GFR	↓ Drug clearance, ↑ dosing intervals
Decreased RBF	↓ Drug clearance, ↑ dosing intervals
Decreased tubular function	↓ Drug elimination
Maturational changes	Requires therapeutic drug monitoring
DISEASE STATES	
Patent ductus arteriosus	↑ AVd → ↑ drug dose, ↓ clearance
Asphyxia	Hypoxia → ↓ renal, hepatic, and GI function
Hepatic dysfunction	↓ Biotransformation
Renal failure	↓ Excretion
DRUGS	
Indomethacin	↓ RBF, ↓ GFR
Tolazoline	↓ RBF, ↓ GFR
Phenobarbital	Induces hepatic microsomal activity

From Nagourney, B.A. & Aranda, J.V. (1998). Physiologic differences of clinical significance. In R.A. Polin & W.W. Fox (Eds.). *Fetal and neonatal physiology* (2nd ed.). Philadelphia: W.B. Saunders.

AVd, Apparent volume of distribution; *GFR*, glomerular filtration rate; *GI*, gastrointestinal; *PNA*, postnatal age; *RBF*, renal blood flow.
↑, Increased; ↓, decreased; →, results in.

Drug Absorption
Oral Agents

Absorption of oral medications in the neonate is altered by the following: (1) decreased bile salts and pancreatic enzymes; (2) slower gut transit time due to delayed gastric emptying and decreased motility; (3) mucus in the stomach; (4) differences in gastric and duodenal pH; (5) high levels of β-glucuronidase in the duodenum; and (6) intestinal surface area.[13,19,56,90] These alterations are more pronounced in preterm and intrauterine growth–restricted (IUGR) infants.[19,90] Decreased bile salts and pancreatic enzymes can result in poorer absorption of lipid-soluble substances such as vitamin K, or drugs that must be hydrolyzed for absorption, such as chloramphenicol. Slower gut transit time due to delayed gastric emptying and decreased motility initially delays then prolongs absorption. Mucus in the stomach may also delay absorption. Differences in gastric and duodenal pH may partially or totally inactivate some drugs. β-Glucuronidase in the small intestine unconjugates some substances that have been metabolized (conjugated) in the liver.[13,19,56,90] Absorption of oral drugs by the neonate is also influenced by the drug's physicochemical characteristics. Drugs such as phenytoin, acetaminophen, and chloramphenicol are absorbed slowly and erratically, whereas penicillin and ampicillin are absorbed more efficiently than in adults because of the higher gastric pH in the neonate.[92] Other drugs such as theophylline, digoxin, and diazepam have oral absorption patterns that are more similar to those in adults.[87]

Gastric and duodenal pH influences drug solubility and ionization. An acid pH increases the absorption of acidic drugs (low pKa) because these drugs tend to stay in a non-ionized, lipid-soluble form. A higher pH enhances alkaline drug absorption and slows absorption of acidic drugs.[13] Gastric pH is higher for the first 12 to 24 hours after birth, then decreases following establishment of feeding. Preterm infants who are less than 32 weeks' gestational age have decreased gastric acid secretion with a more alkaline pH and thus poorer absorption of weak acids and bases.[19,90] Delayed gastric emptying, for up to 6 to 8 hours in immature infants, may delay absorption and reduce the time and level of peak drug concentration.[107]

The neonate's duodenum has higher levels of β-glucuronidase, an enzyme that deconjugates drugs (e.g., indomethacin, chloramphenicol) that the liver has metabolized to glucuronide conjugates. These drugs reenter the blood via the enterohepatic circulation (see Chapter 17) and must be remetabolized by the liver. This increases the half-life and prolongs activity of these drugs.[90] Intestinal absorption of drugs, gut transit time, and motility depend on perfusion and food intake. Better GI absorption occurs with drugs of low MW that are nonionized and lipid soluble.[90] An ill infant who is not being fed may have further impairment of gut function and erratic absorption of oral medications. Intestinal surface area is decreased with genetic disorders such as cystic fibrosis and disorders such as necrotizing enterocolitis, thus reducing absorption.[90]

Intramuscular and Rectal Absorption

The infant's small muscle mass and alterations in peripheral perfusion influence intramuscular medications. Decreased muscle mass may limit use of intramuscular administration in very-low–birth-weight (VLBW) infants.[87] Drugs given intramuscularly may have slower, more erratic absorption, depending on the infant's gestational age and health status. In the first few days after birth, muscle blood flow is decreased, slowing absorption.[87,107] Infants with respiratory problems or low cardiac output have decreased peripheral perfusion, leading to even slower and more erratic absorption of drugs given intramuscularly.[13,107] On the other hand, rectal administration may be more effective in neonates than in adults.[56,107]

Skin Absorption

Percutaneous absorption of substances occurs via the cells of the stratum corneum (transepidermal route) or via the hair follicle–sebaceous gland complex (transappendageal route). The major pathway is most likely transepidermally, with diffusion of a substance through the stratum corneum and epidermis into the dermis and microcirculation. In addition, the subepidermal circulation is readily accessible, enhancing rapid absorption. Preterm infants have greater skin absorption because their skin is thinner than the term infants. VLBW infants have minimum to no stratum corneum and higher dermal water content.[13,87,90]

Neonates are at increased risk for toxic reactions from absorption of topically applied substances for the reasons listed in Table 6-10. Skin metabolism is also different in neonates, so drugs applied topically may result in the release of metabolites different from those that would occur if the drugs were given by other routes. This increases the risk of toxicity.[131] Occlusion of the skin (e.g., placement against the mattress) permits more complete absorption, with longer contact enhancing absorption of the substance. In preterm infants, percutaneous absorption occurs even more rapidly and completely as a result of the marker increased skin permeability.[59] Topical analgesic agents are more easily absorbed, increasing the risk of toxicity (see Chapter 13). Permeability of these agents, such as EMLA cream (lidocaine and prilocaine) is further increased in preterm infants in the first few weeks after birth.[90]

TABLE **6-10**   Factors Placing Neonates at Risk for Toxic Reactions Secondary to Absorption of Topically Applied Substances

Increased permeability of the skin
Increased surface area-to-body weight ratio
Lower blood pressure
Variable skin blood flow patterns
Greater proportion of body weight being made up of brain and liver
Incomplete kidney development resulting in changes in drug excretion
Different body compartment ratios
Increased total body water content
Elevated ratio of intracellular to extracellular water
Decreased adipose tissue

From West, D., Worobec, S., & Solomon, L. (1981). Pharmacology and toxicology of infant skin. *J Invest Dermatol, 76,* 147.

The history of neonatal practice demonstrates the problems with the use of topical agents.[15,16,23,59,99,115,126] For example, central nervous system (CNS) damage has been encountered with the use of hexachlorophene to prevent coagulase-positive staphylococci colonization.[15,18] Practices can lead to detrimental effects if not monitored carefully. Topical application of povidone-iodine (Betadine) yields significantly elevated levels of iodine in blood plasma if not removed completely from the skin after completion of invasive procedures (e.g., chest tube insertion, percutaneous line insertion).[99] Gentle cleansing of the skin with water reduces this risk.

Isopropyl alcohol is also absorbed through the skin. Alcohol use can result in dry skin, skin irritation, and skin burns. The concentration of the solution, duration of exposure, and condition of the exposed skin determine the effects of alcohol use. Tissue destruction occurs with the de-esterifying of the skin and the disruption of the cell structure. Exposure, pressure, and decreased perfusion can contribute to the development of burns from alcohol, complicating fluid management and providing portals for infection.[18]

Drug Distribution

The distribution of drugs is influenced by the infant's large extracellular fluid space, increased total body water, decreased fat, and decreased plasma protein content and binding.[42] The blood-brain barrier is less well developed, which may result in increased amounts of drugs (especially lipid-soluble substances) reaching and being deposited in the brain. The greater total body water and lower fat content in neonates increases the apparent Vd, especially for water-soluble substances.[90,118] The Vd is further increased with decreasing gestational age, since more immature infants have a greater total body water percentage.

The altered Vd in the neonate may reduce peak volumes of drugs and delay excretion. Factors that alter total body water alter drug distribution by increasing (congestive heart failure, patent ductus arteriosus, syndrome of inappropriate antidiuretic hormone secretion) or decreasing (diuretic use) extracellular water.[19,87] Because of the increased extracellular water, higher doses per kilogram may be needed in the neonate for water-soluble drugs distributed in extracellular fluid.[13] For example, an increased Vd is seen with drugs such as theophylline, caffeine, phenobarbital, phenytoin, digoxin, and aminoglycoisides.[90,118] VLBW infants may need higher loading doses and an increased dosing interval of some drugs because of their even greater apparent Vd and immature hepatic and renal function.

Decreased fat in the newborn, especially preterm and IUGR infants, decreases the apparent Vd for lipophilic drugs.[90] Body fat content increases from 1% to 3% at 28 weeks' gestation to 15% to 28% by term, thus increasing the deposition and distribution of lipid-soluble drugs with increased gestational age.[19,90] In addition neonatal adipose tissue is over 50% water (versus approximately 25% in adults), further altering tissue distribution of lipid-soluble drugs.[19]

Protein binding is lower in the neonate due to decreased concentrations of binding proteins; altered binding affinity; and increased levels of nonesterified fatty acids and bilirubin, which compete for protein binding sites.[107] The major drug-binding proteins are albumin, which generally binds acidic drugs, and $\alpha 1$-acid glycoprotein, which along with lipoproteins generally binds basic drugs.[92] Levels of both albumin and $\alpha 1$-acid glycoprotein are low in the neonate, resulting in increased free drug levels of substances such as theophylline, digoxin, phenytoin, and many analgesic compounds.[13,19,87,90,118]

In addition to lower plasma protein levels, the newborn tends to have fewer binding sites and a lower affinity of these sites for drugs such as phenobarbital, phenytoin, penicillin, and theophylline. As a result, the newborn tends to saturate protein binding sites at lower drug concentrations with increased free drug, longer half-lives, and risk of toxicity.[90] However, increased levels of free drug can also lead to lower drug levels since the free drug may be more rapidly eliminated by the kidneys.[19,90]

Protein bindings of drugs may also be reduced by acidosis, free fatty acids, maternal drugs from placental transfer prior to birth, and indirect bilirubin. Drugs and bilirubin compete with each other for binding sites. Bilirubin is displaced from albumin by sulfonamides, ceftriaxone, and chloral hydrate, leading to increased free indirect bilirubin levels. However, bilirubin is more likely to displace drugs than to be displaced. Drugs that may be displaced from albumin by bilirubin include ampicillin, penicillin, phenobarbital, and phenytoin, leading to higher free drug concentrations of these agents.[90] Other drugs, such as furosemide and indomethacin, when given together, compete against each other for albumin binding sites.[90]

Hepatic Drug Metabolism

Neonates and infants have immature organ systems, especially the lungs (see Chapter 9), kidney (see Chapter 10), and liver (see Chapter 11), which are typical routes for drug excretion. The large surface-to-mass ratio and high metabolic rate of the neonate and infant affect drug metabolism.

Liver enzyme systems necessary for metabolism of many drugs are depressed in the newborn. In the mature liver, oxidation and conjugation result in water-soluble drugs that are readily excreted into bile. In the fetus, depression of these processes is an advantage, since lipid-soluble metabolites are more readily transferred across the placenta so they can be handled by the maternal system. The liver smooth endoplasmic reticulum (SER) is the location of many hepatic microsomal enzymes. The neonatal liver has little SER, and activities of many microsomal enzymes are reduced or undetectable at birth, interfering with drug metabolism.[87] As a result, drug metabolism may be markedly altered with slower biotransformation and elimination and increased individual varability.[90] The reduced levels of hepatic microsomal enzymes extend the half-life of drugs dependent on them for metabolism and increase the risk of drug intolerance.

Phase I (see Table 6-1) reactions are reduced in the fetus and newborn, impairing degradation and increasing half-lives of drugs such as phenytoin, phenobarbital, diazepam, mepivacaine, lidocaine, theophylline, phenylbutazone, salicylate, indomethacin, furosemide, and sulfa drugs.[19,87] Both microsomal enzyme (e.g., CYP450 system, NADPH-cytochrome reductase) and extramicrosomal enzyme (e.g., deaminases, esterases) activity are decreased in the newborn, with a rapid increase in activity over the first few weeks after birth.[13,19,107] Levels of CYP1A1, the isoform responsible for degradation of over half of all drugs, has low activity until 4 to 5 months after birth.[95] As a result, alternative pathways of biotransformation are seen for some drugs in the neonate. For example, methylxanthine metabolism is different in neonates versus adults. In the neonate, theophylline is metabolized to caffeine in infants; whereas in adults caffeine is metabolized to theophylline that is excreted with little further metabolism in the urine.[90]

Within 2 to 3 weeks of age, liver enzyme systems are maturing at varying rates, with activity eventually exceeding adult rates in some cases (CYP2D6).[103] Maturation of some enzyme activity may be very rapid; that is, within days activity may change from 20% of adult levels to two to four times higher than adult levels; other systems mature more slowly. There are marked variations in maturation rates of processes for specific drugs and within individual infants. This increases the risk of both under- and overdosing.[19,87] Maturation is correlated with both postconceptional age and postbirth age. Activity may also be altered if the infant was exposed in utero to inducing agents such as heroin, methadone, or phenobarbital.[87]

Phase II reactions (see Table 6-1), particularly glucuronidation, are also altered in the newborn. Glucuronic acid conjugation, needed for metabolism of drugs such as morphine, acetaminophen, phenytoin, sulfonamides, chloramphenicol, salicylic acid, and indomethacin, is reduced at birth and does not reach adult levels until 24 to 30 months.[13,87] Other phase II reactions (sulfate and glycine conjugation) are somewhat decreased but more similar to those in adults.[13,87,90] Methylation reactions may be more important in infants than in adults for drugs such as theophylline.[13,90] Decreased hydrolysis and increased Vd may prolong the effect of local anesthetic agents.[87] Ligandin (carrier protein Y) needed for hepatocyte uptake of substances including bilirubin and many drugs is low for 5 to 10 days after birth, further altering hepatic clearance of some drugs.[13]

Immaturity of liver enzyme systems can delay metabolism and clearance of drugs and increase their serum levels and half-lives. For example, chloramphenicol is eliminated by the kidney after conjugation in the liver. The hepatic glucuronyl transferase system responsible for conjugation of this drug is immature in the neonate (especially in preterm infants), and free (unconjugated) chloramphenicol is eliminated by glomerular filtration, which is reduced in neonates. The result is higher and prolonged peak serum chloramphenicol concentrations. Half-life of chloramphenicol is approximately 20 hours in the neonate and longer in preterm infants, falling to about 10 hours by 21 days (versus 4 to 5 hours in adults).[67] This results in increased risk of toxicity ("gray baby syndrome") with aplastic anemia, shock, and cardiovascular collapse.[6,83]

Renal Drug Excretion

Because of the decreased hepatic metabolism in neonates, the infant is more reliant on renal elimination. However, renal elimination is reduced compared to adults and correlated with both postconceptional and postbirth ages. Alterations in renal function in neonate can markedly alter the infant's ability to eliminate drugs and drug metabolites, increasing the half-life and risk of toxic effects and the need for longer dosing intervals. Any pathologic event that alters renal function (e.g. congestive heart failure, respiratory distress syndrome, hypovolemia, ischemia, or hypoxemia) further compromises the ability of the infant to eliminate drugs.[5,43] Renal processes involved in drug handling are GFR, tubular secretion, and tubular reabsorption. Tubular reabsorption plays a small role in renal handling of aminoglycosides and caffeine but otherwise has minimal influence in the neonate.[52]

The GFR is significantly lower in the neonate than in adults (see Chapter 10), although partially compensated by an increase in tubular reabsorption. The reduced GFR delays clearance of drugs that are eliminated by the kidneys, leading to prolonged half-lives and longer dosing intervals.[13,52] For example, clearance of indomethacin and many aminoglycosides is 10% to 30% lower than in adults.[87] The GFR is particularly low in the first week after birth, increasing susceptibility to nephrotoxic drugs such as aminoglycosides.[43] Plasma half-lives of many drugs used in the neonate—including penicillin, aminoglycosides, penicillin, methicillin, furosemide, barbiturates, and digoxin—vary inversely with creatinine clearance (which is a measure of GFR).

Renal maturation progresses at variable rates after birth depending on gestation and postconceptional ages. The increased half-life of drugs such as digoxin, vancomycin, and indomethacin correlate with both postconceptional and postbirth age and may be significantly lower in preterm infants.[52] Drug levels must be carefully and regularly monitored. Use of drugs such as vancomycin in combination with indomethacin (which decreases GFR) can further decrease vancomycin elimination.[90] Renal elimination of drugs is further altered in preterm infants who are less than 34 weeks' gestational age. In these infants, GFR increases at birth, but then tends to plateau or increase slowly until 34 weeks, when nephron maturation is complete (see Chapter 10). As a result, some antibiotics are given less frequently to VLBW infants. Serum half-lives of antibiotics change rapidly over the first few weeks after birth as renal function matures.[50] Therefore dosages of these drugs or dosing intervals may need to be increased.[5,125]

Elimination of drugs by tubular secretion is reduced in the neonate for the first 6 months as a result of decreased renal blood flow to the peritubular area, shorter tubular length, decreased energy for carriers, and reduced number of carriers to transport drugs from the blood into the tubule.[52] This affects drugs such as penicillin G and other drugs of its class, which are therefore more dependent on GFR instead for clearance in early infancy. In older children and adults, tubular secretion is the most important mechanism for penicillin excretion (versus GFR in neonates). As a result, penicillin clearance is nearly one fifth of that of adults, and penicillin blood levels may persist for three times as long. Urine flow rates can also influence elimination of drugs such as chloramphenicol, phenobarbital, and theophylline by decreasing the concentration gradient due to formation of dilute urine or reducing the time for drug diffusion.[52]

SUMMARY

Specific physiologic alterations that influence handling of antibiotics by the neonate include changes in the Vd, liver and renal function, and protein binding. The functional immaturity of the neonate's body systems alters drug distribution and pharmacokinetics and renders the infant more susceptible to adverse reactions. The ability to metabolize and excrete a given agent varies with gestational age, health status, and postbirth age. Individual infants often have unique responses to drugs, so infants with similar gestational and postbirth ages may vary in their ability to metabolize and excrete a specific drug.

The Vd is altered in the neonate because of the increased total body water and increased proportion of extracellular water. As a result, peak volumes of some drugs are reduced and excretion delayed. Immaturity of liver enzyme systems can delay metabolism and clearance of drugs. The reduced GFR seen in neonates increases serum concentrations and prolongs the half-life of many drugs and may result in longer dosing intervals. Doses of some drugs, such as digoxin, may be higher due to an increased Vd, reducing plasma levels. Doses may also need to be altered because of increased or decreased sensitivity of neonatal tissue to some drugs. For example, the neonate needs a higher dose per kilogram of dopamine than an adult, possibly because of decreased sensitivity of the infant's myocardium to dopamine, incomplete sympathetic innervation, and decreased norepinephrine stores.[118] Digoxin doses are also higher in the neonate due to increased Vd, more rapid elimination, and decreased sensitivity of the myocardium to both therapeutic and toxic effects.[118]

Because of these physiologic limitations, serum concentrations and drug dosages of drugs such as aminoglycosides, phenytoin, phenobarbital, digoxin, and theophylline must be carefully monitored. Monitoring of peak and trough levels of drugs such as aminoglycosides (e.g., gentamicin) is particularly important, since levels associated with toxicity are close to therapeutic levels. Peak (highest drug concentration) plasma levels are measured approximately 30 minutes after administration, whereas trough (lowest drug concentration) levels are measured immediately before an ordered dose. If peak levels are not within therapeutic ranges (i.e., subtherapeutic or in the toxic range), the dose should be altered. Trough levels can be used to determine how frequently a drug should be given. Drug doses cannot be determined on infant size alone, but must also take into account postbirth age, maturity, and health status.

CLINICAL IMPLICATIONS FOR THE PREGNANT WOMEN, FETUS, AND NEONATE

Teratogenesis

Drugs administered to the mother during pregnancy can affect the fetus in a variety of ways ranging from no effect to major structural or functional deficits. Drugs administered during labor affect the fetus primarily by exaggerating the degree of fetal asphyxia and influencing the rate and quality of infant recovery from birth, adaptation to extrauterine life, and neurobehavioral status.

A teratogen is any substance, organism, physical agent, or deficiency state present during gestation that is capable of inducing abnormal postnatal structure or function (biochemical, physiologic, or behavioral) by interfering with normal embryonic and fetal development. [28] Fewer than 30 drugs are proven teratogens, and of these fewer are in current clinical use.[58] Table 6-11 list examples of drugs that are known human teratogens. Drugs are not the only teratogens; other teratogens include environmental toxins, chemicals, ionizing radiation, infectious agents (e.g., bacteria, viruses, protozoa), and excess or deficient nutrients.

It is often difficult to prove teratogenesis. To detect a defect due to a specific agent, an increase in a specific anomaly or group of anomalies over what would be expected by chance must be documented. Thalidomide was recognized as a teratogen sooner than some other agents because it

TABLE 6-11   Drugs Associated with Congenital Malformations in Humans

Drug	Fetal Growth	Postnatal Growth	Mental Retardation	CNS	CV	MS	UG	Eye and Ear	Thyroid
ANTIMICROBIALS									
Tetracycline						X			
Streptomycin								X	
Quinine								X	
ANTINEOPLASTICS									
Methotrexate	X	X		X		X			
Busulfan, chlorambucil, cyclophosphamide	X	X		X		X	X	X	
CNS DRUGS									
Cocaine				X	X				
Lithium					X				
Thalidomide						X			
ANTICONVULSANTS									
Phenytoin		X	X			X		X	
Barbiturates			X		X	X			
Trimethadione			X		X	X	X	X	
Valproic acid		X		X		X			
Carbamazepine				X		X			
STEROID HORMONES									
Androgens							X		
Diethylstilbestrol							X		
Estrogen, progestins							X		
OTHER									
Iodine, propylthiouracil									X
Warfarin		X				X		X	
Alcohol		X	X		X	X	X	X	
Tobacco smoking	X	X							
Isotretinoin, vitamin A			X	X		X		X	

Adapted from Aranda, J.V., Hales, B.F., & Reider, M.J. (1997). Developmental pharmacology. In Fanaroff, A.A. & Martin, R.J. (Eds.). Neonatal-perinatal medicine. Diseases of the fetus and infant (6th ed.). Philadelphia: W.B. Saunders.
CNS, Central nervous system; CV, cardiovascular system; MS, musculoskeletal system; UG, urogenital system.

produced significant malformations, with small doses given once or twice in early pregnancy with a malformation rate of 20% to 30%.[62] Documentation of teratogenesis is often difficult to do in a single location, especially with rare anomalies. Koren et al note the following:

> Most congenital malformations occur rarely, and many teratogens, even when known to be associated with an increase risk of a given malformation, do not affect the great majority of exposed fetuses. In fact, very few drugs increase the malformation rate by a factor of more than two (isotretinoin and thalidomide are two such drugs). If, for example, the risk of malformations in a given population is 3%, then at least 220 pregnancies with a specific exposure and a similar number of control pregnancies will be required to show a risk that is increased by a factor of 2.5 with a power of 80%.[62]

Other common methodologic issues in establishing teratogenesis, in addition to sample size, are recall bias in retrospective studies, use of nonrandomized observational studies, limitations in voluntary reporting, issues in choosing the right animal model, and the effects of maternal disease.[62,130] An example of the difficulty with recall bias occurred with Bendectin in which women whose infants had defects recalled taking this drug, which was commonly used, in early pregnancy. Subsequent studies did not confirm a link between this and malformations.[82,93] Maternal pharmacologic therapy may be administered for an illness that itself leads to a defect or malformations or may produce maternal symptoms requiring treatment with a specific drug; several agents may interact with each other so that the combination is teratogenic rather than either individual drug; or the mother may be talking multiple drugs for different problems.[562] Problems with human studies include difficulty studying cause and effect, lack of random sampling, lack of control over dosing and timing, and expense.

Animal studies can also be problematic. Drug studies with animals may involve administration of large doses that exceed the usual therapeutic dose in humans. Selecting the appropriate animal model can be difficult. Drug kinetics and metabolism may differ between different species and between humans and animals.[62] For example, thalidomide, a potent teratogen in humans, did not produce limb reduction anomalies in the animal models used to study the drug before its release; subsequently, similar anomalies were seen in macaque monkeys. On the other hand, benzodiazepines cause oral clefts in some animal models but not in humans given clinically appropriate doses. Similarly, salicylates cause cardiac defects in some animal species but not humans.[82] Dicke has noted: "We will never be in a position to state that an environmental agent has no teratogenic potential. The most we can say is that an agent poses no measurable risk."[28]

Principles of Teratogenesis

General principles that govern the action of teratogens include:[28,31,131,132]

1. *Susceptibility to a teratogenic agent is dependent upon the genotype of the embryo and the manner in which the agent interacts with environmental factors.* The genetic makeup of the developing embryo is the environmental programmer to which the teratogenic agent is introduced. This programming means that the genes and extrinsic factors interact in varying degrees with varied responses in different individuals and species. Since individual sensitivity is dependent upon the biochemical and morphologic makeup of that particular individual, data from animal models and sometimes even from studies on other individuals cannot always be applied. For example, individuals with a gene mutation that reduces levels of an enzyme needed to detoxify anticonvulsant drugs such as phenytoin are at greater risk of having a child with defects.[54]

2. *Susceptibility to teratogenic agents is dependent on the timing of the exposure and the developmental stage of the embryo.* A basic precept of biology is that the more immature an organism is, the more susceptible that organism is to change. This suggests that there is a critical period where teratogenic events have the greatest impact. As discussed in Chapter 3, the period of greatest susceptibility is during the first trimester, when cell differentiation and organogenesis are occurring. Structural and functional maturation continues after birth, and therefore many systems remain susceptible to alterations in later development. Sometimes the specific period of vulnerability can be identified; for example, the hypoplastic limb defects seen with thalidomide occur with exposure at 20 to 36 days after fertilization.[79,119]

Malformations resulting from incomplete morphogenesis within an organ usually originate before organ structure is complete. The exact time at which a specific defect occurs cannot be determined; it can be said only that a defect occurred at some time *before* a particular point. For example, anencephaly must occur before closure of the anterior neural tube (25 to 26 days); meningomyelocele before closure of the posterior neural tube (27 to 28 days); cleft palate before fusion of the maxillary palatal shelves (10 weeks); cleft lip before closure of the lip (36 days); tracheoesophageal fistula before separation of the foregut into the trachea and primitive esophagus (30 days); ventricular septal defect before closure of the ventricular septum (6 weeks); transposition of the great vessels before directional development of the aorticopulmonary septum (34 days); diaphragmatic hernia before closure of the pleuroperitoneal canal

(6 weeks); omphalocele before or during return of the gut to the abdomen (10 to 10.5 weeks); and imperforate anus before perforation of the anal membrane (8 weeks).

3. *Teratogenic agents act in specific ways on cells or tissues to cause pathogenesis.* Unfavorable factors within the environment are able to trigger changes in developing cells that alter their subsequent development. These changes are not specific to the type of causative factor, and initial changes may result in a variety of alterations within the embryo. These early changes may not be discernible because they occur subcellularly at the molecular level. Pathogenesis is the visible sign of cellular damage and may occur from cell necrosis or by secondary interference with cellular interactions—that is, by induction, adhesion, and migration; reduced biosynthesis of macromolecules; or accumulation of foreign materials, fluids, or blood.

4. *The final manifestations of abnormal development are death, malformation, growth retardation, and functional disorders.* For the early embryo a teratogenic event will most likely result in death. Once organogenesis begins, teratogenic events lead to malformation in the organs or organ systems. The insult might also make the embryo more susceptible to death or general cell necrosis, resulting in a reduced cell mass and slower overall rate of growth. Functional defects may be induced throughout infancy and childhood.

Before conception, damage can occur to the chromosomes of one or both parents, or they may have inherited defective genes from their parents. Alterations in spermatogenesis; in seminal fluid or sperm transport in the male; or in oogenesis or the environment of the vagina, cervix, or uterus of the female may also alter development.[124]

The preembryonic stage (conception to 14 days) is a time of little morphologic differentiation in specific organ systems. Exposure to teratogens during this period usually has an all-or-nothing effect; that is, either the damage is so severe that the zygote is aborted or there are no apparent effects. However, this may be the time that syndromes affecting multiple organ systems arise. Teratogens or environmental disturbances may interfere with implantation of the blastocyst or cause death and early abortion. However, most congenital anomalies probably do not arise during this period, possibly due to the lack of cell differentiation, at least in the early part of this period. Many cells within the inner cell mass are not yet programmed to become specific structures. Thus damage to a few cells does not alter development if the preembryo is able to produce sufficient cells to restore the lost volume.[133] If a teratogen is potent or the dosage

is high, the effect is death or possibly mitotic disjunction during cleavage, with chromosomal alterations that subsequently cause malformation syndromes rather than local defects.[53] If only a few cells are damaged, development continues, although the genetically programmed schedule may be delayed.[84]

The period of organogenesis (15 to 60 days after conception) is a period of extreme sensitivity to teratogens; it is the period when many congenital malformations develop. Insults early in this period (15 to 30 days) are likely to result in death if the embryo is damaged. Early events in organ formation are generally most sensitive to extraneous forces, although in some systems (e.g., the sensory organs), critical periods occur during relatively late stages. The more specialized the metabolic requirements of a group of cells, the more sensitive they are to deprivation and damage.[84,133]

From 11 weeks to term, the fetus becomes increasingly resistant to damage from toxic agents. The ability to produce major structural deviations is reduced as organ systems become organized. Once the definitive form and relationships within a system are established, gross anatomic defects are no longer possible. However, histogenesis continues postnatally and the function of most organ systems can still be altered.[84,133] Defects can occur at the microscopic level, or functional abilities can be altered, resulting in physiologic defects and delayed growth. Insults during late fetal life and early infancy can lead to dysfunction such as brain damage or deafness, prematurity, growth restriction, stillbirth, infant death, or malignancy.

5. *Access to the embryo by environmental teratogens depends on the nature of the agent.* There are several routes by which agents reach the embryo or fetus. Agents such as ultrasound, ionizing radiation, and microwaves pass directly through maternal tissue without modification. Chemical agents or their metabolites reach developing tissues indirectly via transmission across the placenta. Whether these agents reach toxic or teratogenic concentrations depends on maternal dosage, rate of absorption, and maternal homeostatic capabilities as well as physical properties of the agent and the placenta. Pathogenic organisms may also reach the fetus by an ascending route via the vaginal canal and cervix.

6. *As the dosage increases, manifestations of deviant development increase.* There appears to be a threshold at which embryotoxicity occurs and damage is initiated. When the effect threshold is exceeded, cell damage or death exceeds restoration. For example, diagnostic x-rays with a dose lower than 5 rads (dosage for most common procedures) is not thought to have teratogenic effects. Exposure to 5 to

10 rads is of concern, whereas exposure to more than 10 rads (e.g., with radiation therapy) is associated with significant risk.[54] Sometimes the specific threshold cannot be determined, as is the case with alcohol. Different types of embryotoxicity exist for different thresholds. A given teratogenic effect may be induced by a variety of agents. For example, a specific defect may result from infection, drugs, genetic alteration, an environmental toxin, or a combination of these factors.[28,31,1132,133]

Proposed mechanisms of teratogenesis include the following:

1. *Gene mutation.* Mutation is the basis of heritable developmental defects and is the result of a change in the sequence of nucleotides. If the change appears in the germinal cell line, it is likely to be heritable. A mutation in a somatic cell will be passed to daughter cells but cannot be transferred to the next generation. Gene mutations can result in biochemical or structural disorders or later development of malignancies (see Chapter 1).

2. *Chromosome breaks and nondisjunction.* These alterations lead to excesses, deficiencies, or rearrangements of chromosomes, or parts of chromosomes and can be transmitted to offspring. For example, sperm of men exposed to radiation or chemotherapy have increased numbers of chromosomal aberrations for at least 3 to 4 months (chemotherapy) to up to 36 months (ionizing radiation).[124]

3. *Mitotic interference and cell death.* Interference with mitosis can result from inhibition of deoxyribonucleic acid (DNA) synthesis, prevention of spindle formation, or failure of chromosome separation. For example, aminopterin and methotrexate inhibit an enzyme needed during the cell cycle (see Chapter 1), leading to cell death during the S (DNA synthesis) phase.[54] Viruses and other infectious agents may also interfere with mitosis.

4. *Altered nucleic acid integrity or function.* These alterations occur secondary to biochemical changes that interfere with nucleic acid replication, transcription, natural base incorporation, or ribonucleic acid (RNA) translation and protein synthesis. Since processes such as protein synthesis are essential for survival of the embryo, interference usually results in death rather than malformation. Diethylstilbestrol (DES) acts on estrogen-responsive tissue by altering RNA, protein, and DNA synthesis with development of columnar epithelium not normally found in the vaginal area. This "foreign" tissue is at risk for later malignant degeneration.[54]

5. *Lack or excess of precursors, substrates, or coenzymes needed for biosynthesis.* These deficiencies result in slowed or altered growth and differentiation and oc-

cur because of dietary deficiencies, placental transfer failure, maternal absorption failure, or the presence of specific analogues or antagonists. Some agents, such as amphetamines, cocaine, cannabis, and nicotine, may occupy receptors for nutrient, thus decreasing transfer of critical substances and altering fetal growth and development.[35,36] Retinoic acid regulates expression of one of the developmental genes involved in craniofacial and axial skeleton development. Excess levels—as occurs with isotretinoin—leads to malformations in these systems.[32] Coumadin inhibits formation of substances needed for proteins to bind to calcium and can alter bone ossification with craniofacial and other skeletal anomalies.[54]

6. *Altered energy sources.* As a result of interference with energy pathways (glucose sources, glycolysis, citric acid cycle, terminal electron transport systems), the energy needs of the rapidly proliferating and synthesizing tissues of the embryo are not met. For example, biotin deficiency—seen with an inborn error of metabolism—decreases activity of a mitochondrial biotin-dependent enzyme.[54]

7. *Enzyme and growth factor inhibitions.* Inhibition of critical enzymes interferes with cell functioning, cellular repair, differentiation, and growth. Inadequate folic acid increases the risk of neural tube defects, especially if the deficiency occurs in women with an enzyme defect in folic acid metabolism. Thalidomide may inhibit angiogenesis and thus limb growth by decreasing critical growth factors such as insulin-like growth factor-I and fibroblast growth factor.[79,119] Inhibition of alcohol dehydrogenases, needed to detoxify alcohol, alters retinoic acid metabolism similarly to action of isotretinoin (which leads to similar craniofacial and skeletal defects).[54]

8. *Osmolar imbalance.* These imbalances lead to pathogenesis by causing edema that impinges upon the embryo.

9. *Altered membrane characteristics.* These changes can result in abnormal membrane permeability and lead to osmolar imbalances and edema.

10. *Altered cell and neuronal migration or CNS organization.* These processes are influenced by neurotransmitters, especially monoamines (dopamine, serotonin, and norepinephrine). Inborn errors of metabolism—especially those involved with amino acid metabolism—alter CNS organization. Drugs, such as cocaine, that increase or reduce levels of neurotransmitters may alter migration or later organization of cortical neurons (see Chapter 14).[36,106,131,132]

The ultimate result of any of these mechanisms is an organ with too few normally functioning cells. Cells needed for normal differentiation are lacking, thus disturbing

TABLE **6-12**   Successive Stages in the Pathogenesis of a Developmental Defect*

Mechanisms	Pathogenesis	Common Pathways	Final Defect
Initial types of changes in developing cells or tissues after teratogenic insult: Mutation (gene) Chromosomal breaks, nondisjunction, and so on Mitotic interference Altered nucleic acid integrity or function Lack of normal precursors, substrates, and so on Altered energy sources Changed membrane characteristics Osmolar imbalance Enzyme inhibition	Ultimately manifested as one or more types of abnormal embryogenesis Excessive or reduced cell death Failed cell interactions Reduced biosynthesis Impeded morphogenetic movement Mechanical disruption of tissues	Too few cells or cell products to effect localized morphogenesis or functional maturation Other imbalances in growth and differentiation	

From Wilson, J.G. (1977). Current status of teratology: General principles and mechanisms derived from animal studies. In J.G. Wilson & F.C. Fraser (Eds.). *Handbook of teratology: General principles and etiology.* New York: Plenum.

*Beginning with the initial types of changes in developing cells or tissues (the mechanisms) and continuing to the final defect: One or more mechanisms are initiated by the teratogenic cause from the environment. This leads to changes in the developmental system which become manifested as abnormal embryogenesis. This in turn leads into pathways that are often characterized by too few cells or cell products to effect normal morphogenesis or functional maturation. The suggestion that this is a single or common pathway for all developmental defects is conjecture.

development.[28] Table 6-12 summarizes the successive stages in the pathogenesis of a developmental defect.

Drugs and Lactation

Drugs cross into breast milk across the milk-blood barrier via mechanisms similar to those described for movement of substances across the placenta. Many pharmacologic agents and environmental pollutants (as well as alcohol, nicotine, and other abused drugs) can be found in human milk, although usually at levels lower than those in the mother. In a study of 14,000 pregnant or breastfeeding women, an average of 3.3 drugs were taken during the course of breastfeeding.[22] Another study of 838 breastfeeding mothers reported a mean of 1.2 drugs, with over 70% of the women taking more than one prescribed drug.[49] Others reported that 90% to 99% of breastfeeding mothers took prescribed medications in the first week after delivery and 17% to 25% at 4 months, with 5% on chronic pharmacologic therapy.[71] Often breastfeeding is interrupted or discontinued for maternal therapy even though there are relatively few maternal medications that are not compatible with breastfeeding.[10,29] Even if the mother is on drugs with potential risks, strategies to minimize infants' exposure can be often used so that the mother can decide to continue breastfeeding if she chooses.[10] In general, serious side effects in infants are uncommon. For example, an incidence of 11% of minor reactions (e.g., drowsiness, diarrhea, irritability) have been found in infants of mothers on prescribed narcotics, antibiotics, antihistamines, and analgesics.[12,49]

The use of any pharmacologic agent in the breastfeeding woman should be carefully evaluated. Most drugs enter breast milk in some quantity. Often little is known about side effects of less commonly used agents. Table 6-13 provides examples of specific drugs contraindicated (or with relative contraindications) during lactation. Other drugs should still be used with caution and only as absolutely needed in the lactating woman, with careful monitoring of both infant and mother. The nurse and the mother should be aware of potential hazards of any drug, for both mother and infant, since drugs other than those listed in Table 6-13 may cause side effects in the infant. There are many reviews of drug use during breastfeeding and concerns or potential hazards of specific agents.[2,16,24,37,40,104]

Drugs taken by a nursing mother reach infants in much smaller amounts than drugs from the pregnant woman reach the fetus.[10,71] Figure 6-4 illustrates transfer of milk from mother to infant. Drugs from the pregnant woman to the fetus move directly from maternal blood to fetal blood, whereas drugs from the nursing mother to infant pass from mother's blood into milk and then to the infant's gut. In the infant's gut the drug may be destroyed or absorption reduced due to limitations is GI absorption in infants, especially in the early months. In addition, there are more tissue layers

TABLE **6-13**   **Drugs Contraindicated in Nursing Mothers**

ANTIMETABOLITES

Azathiopine
Cyclophosphamide
Doxorubicin
Methotrexate

ANTICOAGULANTS

Phenindione

ERGOT ALKALOIDS

Bromocriptine
Ergotamine

GOLD
IODINE-CONTAINING COMPOUNDS

Aminodarone
Potassium iodide
Povidone iodine (extensive topical use)
Oral contraceptives (relative contraindications)*

PSYCHOACTIVE DRUGS

Lithium
Phenobarbital

RADIOPHARMACEUTICALS
(RELATIVE CONTRAINDICATION)†
RECREATIONAL CHEMICALS

Amphetamines
Cocaine
Ethanol
Heroin
Marijuana
Phencyclidine (PCP)
Nicotine (cigarette smoking)

*Recommended to avoid in malnourished mothers and in women in the first 6 weeks postpartum
†Contraindicated until cleared from maternal system and breast milk.

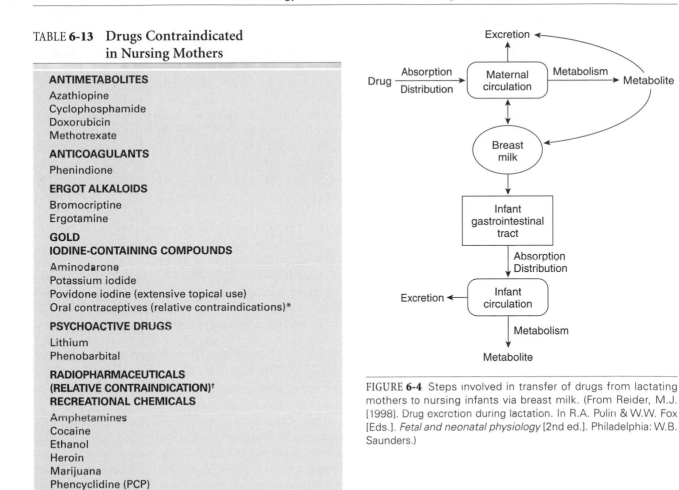

FIGURE **6-4** Steps involved in transfer of drugs from lactating mothers to nursing infants via breast milk. (From Reider, M.J. [1998]. Drug excretion during lactation. In R.A. Polin & W.W. Fox [Eds.]. *Fetal and neonatal physiology* [2nd ed.]. Philadelphia: W.B. Saunders.)

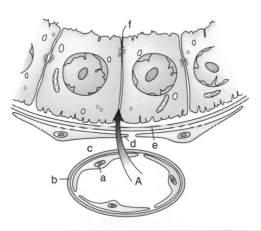

FIGURE **6-5** Milk-blood barrier of mammary gland alveolus. The arrow *(A)* shows passive diffusion of material in lumen of blood vessel into lumen of alveolus. All nonionized molecules must cross the endothelial cell of the blood vessels *(a)*, basement membrane of blood vessel *(b)*, interstitial breast space *(c)*, myoepithelial cell of alveolus *(d)*, basement membrane alveolus *(e)*, and intra-alveolar space *(f)*. (From George, D.I. & O'Toole, T.J. [1983]. A review of drug transfer to the infant by breast-feeding: Concerns for the dentist. *J Am Dent Assoc, 106,* 204.)

between maternal blood and milk than between maternal and fetal blood across the placenta. This increases the diffusing distance and reduces the efficiency of transfer. Calculated doses received by the infant of maternal drug range from 0.1% to 0.5% of the standard therapeutic doses tolerated by infants without toxicity.[28] Therefore some drugs that are not recommended during pregnancy may pose little risk during lactation.[1,110]

Factors influencing the amount and rapidity of drug excretion into milk include drug dosage and duration; route of administration; drug physicochemical characteristics; blood level in maternal circulation; oral bioavailability; protein binding in maternal circulation; maternal physiology and drug handling; blood-milk barrier (Figure 6-5); and infant physiology, drug handling, and maturity (see Table 6-9). Other infant factors to consider include the age of the infant, drug oral bioavailability, amount of milk intake, and record of the drug's use as a therapeutic agent in infants.[48,67,110] Characteristics of drug most likely to cross into milk are agents that are lipid soluble, have low MW, have a long half-life in the mother, have low protein binding, are given to the mother in large doses, or are used for chronic conditions or used long term so that plasma levels are maintained at steady-state conditions.[10,48,71,89]

Infant drug exposure can be calculated by the milk-to-plasma ratio of a drug, percentage of maternal dose, infant dosage (drug concentration in milk times the volume of milk ingested), and estimated infant serum concentration (using oral bioavailability/clearance in the infants).[12,48,71] The milk-to-plasma (M/P) ratio is the most common index and ranges from 0.01 to 6.5 (averaging 0.5 to 1 for most drugs used during lactation).[27] This value may be calculated as a single value, but the M/P_{AUC} (where AUC is the area under the curve), which is based on concentration time curves, provides a better estimate of the ratio over a dosing interval.[12] Highly lipid-soluble and water-soluble substances with MW lower than 200 daltons generally have an M/P ratio near 1. High M/P ratios (greater than 1) are seen with weak bases and actively transported substances; a low M/P ratio (less than 1) is generally found with drugs that are weak acids or highly protein bound substances.[67] Drugs with a low (less than 1) M/P ratio and high maternal and infant clearance rates generally have low risk of infant side effects.[29] M/P and M/P_{AUC} ratios are available in several resources.[8,40]

Most drugs cross by passive or facilitated diffusion from higher to lower concentrations. Some low-MW drugs may also cross via membrane pores, while other substances such as immunoglobulins may pass between alveolar cells.[101] The blood-milk barrier consists of the maternal capillary epithelium, mammary alveolar cell membrane, intracellular structures (including protein micelles and lipid vesicles), and the apical membrane of the mammary alveolar cell (see Figure 6-5). The alveolar cell is a lipid barrier that reduces transfer of water-soluble and ionized drugs.[48] Therefore, lipid-soluble drugs cross into milk more readily than water-soluble drugs, although this is somewhat influenced by MW. Concentration of drugs in milk may change with time from birth or during a feeding. For example, drugs such as diazepam and phenobarbital that are highly lipid-soluble may be more concentrated in hindmilk which has four to five times greater lipid content than foremilk.[8] Lipid content is higher in mature milk versus colostrum; thus concentrations of lipid-soluble drugs may be reduced initally.[48,71]

Low MW substances such as ethanol rapidly diffuse across the tissue layers between maternal blood and milk. Water-soluble drugs with a MW less than 200 daltons can move across the blood-milk barrier via water-filled membrane pores.[48,71] Larger molecules (greater than 200) cannot pass through these pores, are transferred more slowly since they must first dissolve in the outer lipid membrane of the alveolar cell, diffuse across the cell, then dissolve in the apical membrane to reach milk.[48] Substance with MWs larger than 800, such as insulin and heparin, generally do not cross into milk or do so very minimally.[10] Larger substances may cross in the first 4 to 10 days after delivery due to larger gaps between alveolar cells during this time.[10,48]

The major milk protein (α-lactalbumin) does not significantly bind drugs. One of the main serum drug-binding proteins (α1 acid-glycoprotein) is not present in milk. Therefore the major milk drug-binding proteins are albumin and lactoferrin, which have markedly decreased binding compared to plasma proteins.[12] Drugs that are highly bound in maternal blood are less likely to cross, since plasma levels of free drug are lower. Free drug levels may be increased in the mother in the first 5 to 7 weeks postpartum as the lower albumin levels of pregnancy gradually return to nonpregnant vlaues.[71]

Milk pH (mean of 7.1 to 7.2, with a range of 6.7 to 7.4) is lower than blood pH.[8,48] Weak acids are highly ionized in maternal plasma and less likely to cross into milk. Weak bases, however, tend to be transferred and are at equal or higher concentrations in milk than in maternal plasma.[71] Colostrum has a mean pH of 7.45, so it is more likely to have higher levels of basic drugs than mature milk.[10] Ion trapping may occur in milk. Weak bases are generally nonionized and readily cross into milk. As these drugs encounter the low milk pH, they become ionized. This creates a gradient toward movement of more of the drug into milk and reduces the ability of the drug to return across the blood-milk barrier to maternal blood.[48,71,89] Drugs with a pKa higher than 7.2 are most likely to be sequestered in milk.[81]

Steady-state concentrations of drugs in the infant are influenced by drug oral bioavailability, dose, and infant clearance. Drugs given to the mother via methods other than oral administration often have a low oral bioavailability. Drugs with high oral bioavailability (1 to 5) may be sequestered in milk at high levels. Drugs with low oral bioavailability (less than 1) have only minimal milk tranfer.[71] This reduces infant exposure, since the infant receives these drugs via milk into the gut. The amount of drugs reaching the nursing infant is also influenced by non-steady-state conditions. Milk is supplied on a continuous basis during sucking, so milk drug concentrations at time of feeding tend to reflect maternal plasma levels at that time. Concentrations of drugs in milk are independent of volume of milk.[89]

Drugs may also affect lactation via either central or peripheral mechanisms to increase or reduce milk output.[29,55,101] Central mechanisms include increased or decreased oxytocin, prolactin, or CNS dopamine release. Increased dopamine depresses prolactin. Peripheral mechanisms act directly on the breast to alter milk production. Exogenous substances that increase milk production include thyrotropin-releasing hormone; metoclopramide; and psychotropic agents such as reserpine, imipramine, and phenothiazine derivatives that interfere with dopamine release.[29] Nicotine and estrogens (i.e., the older lactation suppressants such as Tace and Deladumone) may depress lactation.

Use of combination oral contraceptives by lactating women is controversial, with many differing opinions. Estrogen containing oral contraceptives suppress lactation probably through inhibition of prolactin by estrogen. These agents have been associated with decreases in milk production, shorter overall length of time of breastfeeding, and slower infant weight gain.[121] The effects of combined agents on breast milk production are most prominent in the first 4 to 6 weeks postpartum.[10,29,33,127] As a result, the World Health Organization recommends no hormonal contraception in the first 6 weeks postpartum and no noncombined oral contraceptives from 6 weeks to 6 months.[136]

Minimizing Infant Drug Exposure

A drug with a high dose may be safe if given after feeding or before the infant's longest predictable sleep period. However, a normally safe drug may be problematic if given in a high dose or over a long duration.[29] Most data on drug levels in milk are with mature milk, with minimal data on milk from mothers of preterm infants. These infants may be at greater risk for adverse effects from exposure to drugs in breast milk due to their immature hepatic and renal function. In addition, these infants are more likely to absorb large macromolecules across their immature ("open") gut (see Chapter 12).[8] Although the major concern is that the infant will receive a pharmacologically significant concentration of drug, other possible effects are allergic sensitivities and altered gut flora with antibiotics.[29]

Suggestions from Anderson (and others) for reducing the effects of drugs in breast milk on the infant include the following:

1. Using a short-acting form of the drug to reduce the risk of accumulation.
2. Using alternative forms of drugs within the same drug class that pass more poorly into milk, have shorter half-lives or can be given via alternate routes (topical or inhaled).

3. Using single components rather than compound drugs (e.g., a decongestant for allergy rather than a multisymptom drug, especially since liquid forms may contain alcohol).
4. Feeding the infant before taking the medication, thus avoiding feeding during peak plasma levels, which tend to occur 1 to 3 hours after a maternal oral dose.
5. Using preparations that can be given at longer intervals (once versus three to four times/day).[4,10,11,29,40,67,71,101]

If the mother is on a chronic drug with potential for elevated infant plasma levels, drug levels may need to be monitored periodically. Monitor the infant closely (growth pattern, sleep patterns, activity, alertness, behaviors, responsiveness, and general health).[4] Breastfeeding may need to be temporarily discontinued with use of previously expressed milk or formula while the mother is on the medication for diagnostic procedures or drugs with a high potential for toxicity which can be given once. The timing for reinstitution of breastfeeding varies with the toxicity of the agent. For mild toxicity, resumption of nursing may be as soon as 1 to 2 maternal half-lives (50% to 75% elimination); for high toxicity, it may be necessary to wait for 4 to 5 maternal half-lives (94% to 97% elimination) or longer.[4,10,71,101] Rarely breastfeeding may need to be discontinued if a highly toxic drug is necessary for maternal health such as chemotherapy.

Effects of Drug Exposure in Utero

The fetus is a passive recipient of all drugs entering the mother's system. Drug use in pregnancy is common. From laxatives and antacids to cocaine and heroin, all of these substances are chemicals that may have an effect on the fetus and newborn. Medications are not "approved" for use in pregnancy; rather, medications are "presumed safe" for use in pregnancy. Some classes of drugs are more significant to CNS development and function after birth than are others. Drugs known to produce significant CNS effects are ethanol, narcotics, and cocaine.

Neonatal Abstinence Syndrome

The fetus is not immune from developing chemical dependency. Neonatal abstinence syndrome (NAS) refers to particular withdrawal behaviors (CNS hypersensitivity, respiratory distress, autonomic dysfunction, and GI disturbances) observed in neonates exposed to dependency-producing drugs in utero.[58] NAS is seen most commonly with opiates such as heroin and methadone. After birth the neonate who has been exposed to ethanol, barbiturates, cocaine, and narcotics in utero exhibits withdrawal symptoms (neonatal withdrawal syndrome). The timing and severity of withdrawal are based on the type of drug, the mother's drug dosage, the length of time since the mother's last dose, the duration of exposure, the neonate's degree of immaturity, and the neonate's general health status. Symptoms usually appear within 72 hours after birth but can be seen as late as 2 to 4 weeks of age. The neonate's withdrawal responses may last from 6 days to 8 weeks.

The responses to drug withdrawal are similar to those in the adult, but because of the nature of neurologic organization, the implications are more severe in neonates. Neonatal abstinence syndrome includes both physiologic and behavioral responses. The Finnegan scale has been developed to aid observation and measurement of the responses to neonatal abstinence. Interventions are initiated based on the severity of withdrawal as assessed by the Finnegan scale. Withdrawal may be treated pharmacologically with drugs such as phenobarbital, morphine, or diazepam.[58]

Cocaine

Cocaine is a central and peripheral stimulant that produces its effects by preventing the reuptake of monoamines such as dopamine, norepinephrine, and serotonin, resulting in increased levels of these neurotransmitters at the neuronal junction. The excess monoamines result in prolonged neuronal activation, leading to characteristic neurobehavioral responses (binding to central receptors) and cardiovascular and motor effects (binding to peripheral receptors located in tissues innervated by the sympathetic nervous system).[7,57,73,134] Monoamines have a trophic role in CNS cell proliferation, neural migration, and organization. Thus exposure to elevated levels of monoamines may alter CNS organization, increasing the risk for later alterations in arousal and attention.[68,78]

The actions of cocaine are similar to those of amphetamines, causing intense sympathetic nervous system activity. Cocaine produces vasoconstriction, tachycardia, and elevation of blood pressure in addition to a sense of excitement and euphoria. Cocaine is lipid-soluble, easily crossing the placenta. In the fetus, it produces increased motor activity and tachycardia; cocaine crosses the fetal blood-brain barrier. Cocaine competes with nutrients for monoamine transporters in the placenta.[35,36] By successfully combining with nutrients for these transporters, cocaine reduces nutrient transfer, which can lead to fetal growth restriction. In the first and second trimesters, cocaine may also be transported across the placental membranes. Levels of cocaine are high in amniotic fluid, resulting in a reservoir that prolongs fetal exposure.[134]

Because cocaine is a potent vasoconstrictor, blood flow to the placenta is reduced and associated with a high incidence of abruptio placentae. Blood flow to the fetus through the placenta is also curtailed. In addition, the umbilical arteries constrict in response to cocaine.[134] The resultant placental ischemia has been attributed as the cause of low birth weight (LBW), decreased body length, and smaller head circumference found among infants of cocaine-abusing mothers. Cocaine also increases uterine irritability and results in contractions. Cocaine may have teratogenic effects via damage to developing tissue either by vascular disruption and placental vascular insufficiency or production of reactive oxygen species during biotransformation of cocaine in the liver by P450 enzymes.[7]

After birth, cocaine does not produce withdrawal behaviors, per se, but its effect appears to be related to an alteration of neurobehavioral organization that probably results from its direct influence on the developing brain. In addition, cocaine may cause cerebral infarcts. Neonates exposed in utero to cocaine are irritable, tremulous, and difficult to soothe and have rapid respiratory and heart rates; these infants exhibit excessive motor activity, altered sleep-wake patterns, poor feeding and feeding intolerance, and diarrhea.[7] The half-life of cocaine is longer in the fetus and neonate than in the adult since the enzyme systems governing the drug's metabolism are not mature, and cocaine may persist in the neonate for several days after birth.[120] Cocaine passes easily into breast milk; active use of cocaine by a lactating mother may produce severe reactions and possibly death in the neonate. Cocaine has been found in breast milk as late as 36 hours after maternal use.[120]

SUMMARY

Drug therapy of the pregnant woman, fetus, neonate, and lactating woman is a complex health challenge. Both pregnant women and neonates have alterations in drug absorption, distribution, metabolism, and elimination that increase the risk of subtherapeutic or toxic levels of individual drugs. An understanding of the principles influencing transfer of drug across the placenta and into breast milk is critical to reducing risk in the fetus and young infant. Drug therapy of the lactating women generally poses fewer risks to the infants than therapy of the pregnant women. However, the use of any pharmacologic agent for either the pregnant and breastfeeding woman must be carefully evaluated and drugs used with caution. Neonates present a unique challenge for pharmacologic therapy mainly because of their physiologic immaturity but also because their systems continue to undergo maturation during early infancy, so drug handling can change within a relatively short period of time. Recommendations for clinical practice related to perinatal pharmacology are listed in Table 6-14. The box on p. 209 lists on-line resources for information about drugs in pregnancy and lactation.

TABLE **6-14** **Recommendations for Clinical Practice Related to Perinatal Pharmacology**

Know the effects of physiologic alterations during pregnancy on pharmacokinetics (pp. 183-186 and Table 6-3).

Recognize the effects of altered gastrointestinal and hepatic function during pregnancy on drug absorption and metabolism (pp. 183-185).

Recognize the effects of altered body water, fat, and plasma proteins on drug distribution and binding during pregnancy (pp. 184-185).

Recognize the effects of altered renal function on drug elimination during pregnancy (p. 185).

Counsel women regarding the side effects of drugs and potential toxicity to mother, fetus, and neonate (pp. 182-183, 200-204).

Monitor and evaluate maternal responses to drugs (pp. 183-186).

Monitor and evaluate maternal responses to drugs taken prior to pregnancy for evidence of subtherapeutic doses (pp. 184, 192-193).

Know or verify the usual doses for medications given during pregnancy (pp. 183-186).

Recognize the effects of maternal physiologic adaptations on the pharmacokinetics of antibiotics (pp. 192-193).

Counsel women regarding the side effects of drugs used to treat specific chronic conditions and potential toxicity to the woman and fetus (pp. 192-193 and Table 6-7).

Counsel women with chronic disorders, regarding the impact of their disorder and its pharmacologic treatment during pregnancy and of treatment alternatives (pp. 183-186, 192-193).

Know the factors that influence distribution of drugs and other substances in the fetus (pp. 193-194 and Table 6-5).

Recognize critical periods of development and principles of teratogenesis (pp. 200-203 and Chapter 3).

Recognize risks associated with fetal exposure to drugs and other environmental agents during pregnancy (pp. 202-203).

Provide appropriate counseling and health teaching to promote optimal fetal development and health (pp. 200-204 and Chapter 3).

Provide counseling and health teaching to reduce exposure of the fetus to adverse environmental influences (pp. 200-204 and Chapter 3).

Counsel women regarding the use of drugs or exposure to other environmental agents during pregnancy (pp. 200-204).

Know the effects of neonatal physiology on pharmacokinetics (pp. 194-200 and Table 6-9).

Recognize the effects of immature gastrointestinal and hepatic function in the neonate on drug absorption and metabolism (pp. 196-198).

Recognize the effects of altered body water, fat, and plasma proteins on drug distribution and binding in the neonate. (pp. 197-198).

Recognize the effects of maturation of liver enzyme systems on drug metabolism and risks of side effects in the neonate (p. 198).

Recognize the effects of immature renal function on drug elimination and risks of side effects in the neonate (pp. 198-199).

Know or verify the usual doses for drugs given during the neonatal period (pp. 199-200).

Recognize the side effects of drugs and potential toxicity to the neonate (pp. 194-200).

Monitor and evaluate neonatal responses to drugs, including peak and trough and serum levels (pp. 197-198).

Know the factors that place neonates at risk for toxic responses to topically applied substances (pp. 196-197 and Table 6-10).

Provide care to reduce the risk of topically applied substances (pp. 196-197).

Counsel women regarding the use of medications during lactation (pp. 204-207).

Recognize the risk associated with use of pharmacologic agents in breastfeeding women (pp. 200-204 and Table 6-13).

Know the drugs that are contraindicated in nursing mothers (Table 6-13).

Evaluate the need for use of specific drugs and counsel women regarding side effects (pp. 200-204 and Table 6-13).

Monitor and evaluate maternal and neonatal responses to drugs taken by the breastfeeding woman (pp. 204-207).

Institute interventions as appropriate to reduce the risks associated with specific drugs (p. 207).

Assess infants for signs of intrauterine drug exposure from maternal substance abuse (pp. 207-208).

Resources for Information on Teratogens and Drugs during Lactation

American Academy of Pediatrics Statement on Transfer of Drugs and Other Chemicals into Breast Milk: www.aap.org/policy/00026.html

Lactation Study Center (Ruth Lawrence): (716) 275-0088

March of Dimes Resource Center: (888) 633-4637 in the United States and Canada; 001-914-997-4765 internationally; www.modimes.org/HealthLibrary2/RC/Default.htm

Organization of Teratology Information Services: www.otispregnancy.org/home.html (links to teratology information services in each state and in Canada)

Thomas Hale's Breastfeeding Pharmacology Page: neonatal/ttuhsc.edu/lact/

REFERENCES

1. Ala-kokko, T.I., et al. (1992). Placental function and principles of drug transfer. *Acta Anesthesiol Scand, 37,* 47.
2. Aminoff, M.J. (1999). Neurologic disorders. In R.K. Creasy & R. Resnik (Eds.). *Maternal-fetal medicine: Principles and practice* (4th ed.). Philadelphia: W.B. Saunders.
3. American Academy of Pediatrics, Committee on Drugs. (1994). Transfer of drugs and other chemicals into human milk. *Pediatrics, 93,* 137.
4. Anderson, P.O. (1991). Drug use during breast-feeding. *Clin Pharm, 10,* 594-624.
5. Anker, J.N. (1996). Pharmacokinetics and renal function in preterm infants. *Acta Paediatr, 85,* 1393.
6. Aranda, J.V., Hales, B.F., & Reider, M.J. (1997). Developmental pharmacology. In A.A. Fanaroff & R.J. Martin (Eds.). *Neonatal-perinatal medicine. Diseases of the fetus and infant* (6th ed.). Philadelphia: W.B. Saunders
7. Askin, D.F. & Diehl-Jones, B. (2001). Cocaine: effects on the fetus and neonate. *J Perinat Neonatal Nurs, 14*(4), 83.
8. Atkinson, H.C., Begg, E.J., & Darlow, B.A. (1988). Drugs in human milk: clinical pharmacokinetic considerations. *Clin Pharmacokinet, 14,* 217-240.
9. Audus, K.L. (1999). Controlling drug delivery across the placenta. *Eur J Pharm Sci, 8,* 161.
10. Auerbach, K.G. (1999). Breastfeeding and maternal medication use. *J Obstet Gynecol Neonatal Nurs, 28,* 554.
11. Banta-Wright, S. (1997). Minimizing infant exposure to and risks from medications when breastfeeding. *J Perinat Neonat Nurs, 11*(2), 71-84.
12. Begg, E.J. & Atkinson, H.C. (1991). Partitioning of drugs into human milk. *Ann Acad Med Singapore, 20,* 51.
13. Besunder, J.R., Reed, M.J., & Blumer, J.L. (1988). Principles of drug biodisposition in the neonate: A critical evaluation of the phamacokinetic-pharmacodynamic interface. Part I. *Clin Pharmacokinet, 14,* 189.
14. Bourget, P., Roulot, C., & Fernandez, H. (1995). Models for placental transfer studies of drugs. *Clin Pharmacokinet, 28,* 161.
15. Bressler, R., et al. (1977). Hexachlorophene in the newborn nursery: A risk-benefit analysis and review. *Clin Pediatr, 16,* 342.
16. Briggs, G., Freeman, R.K., & Yaffe, S.J. (2001). *Drugs in pregnancy and lactation* (6th ed.). Philadelphia: Lippincott, Williams & Wilkins.
17. Butters, L. (1990). Awareness among pregnant women of the effect on the fetus of commonly used drugs. *Midwifery, 6,* 146.
18. Champagne, S., Fussell, S., & Scheifele, D. (1984). Evaluation of skin antisepsis prior to blood culture in neonates. *Infection Control, 5,* 489.
19. Chemtob, S. (1998). Basic pharmacologic principles. In R.A. Polin & W.W. Fox (Eds.). *Fetal and neonatal physiology* (2nd ed.). Philadelphia: W.B. Saunders.
20. Chow, A.W. & Jewesson, P.J. (1985). Pharmacokinetics and safety of antimicrobial agents during pregnancy. *Rev Infect Dis, 7,* 287.
21. Colie, C.F. (1996). Medications in pregnancy. *Curr Opin Obstet Gynecol, 8,* 398.
22. Collaborative Group on Drug Use in Pregnancy. (1992). Medication during pregnancy: An intercontinental cooperative study. *Int J Gynecol Obstet, 39,* 185.
23. Curley, A., et al. (1971). Dermal absorption of hexachlorophene in infants. *Lancet, 2,* 296.
24. Daffos, F. (1989). Access to the other patient. *Semin Perinatol, 13,* 252.
25. Dancis, J. (1981). Placental transport of amino acids, fats and minerals. In *Placental transport.* Mead Johnson Symposium on Perinatal and Developmental Medicine (No. 18). Evansville, IN: Mead Johnson.
26. Dashe, J.S. & Gilstrap, L.C. (1997). Antibiotic use in pregnancy. *Obstet Gynecol Clin North Am, 24,* 618.
27. Dickason, E.J., Schult, M.O., & Morris, E.M. (1978). *Maternal and infant drugs and nursing interventions.* New York: McGraw-Hill.
28. Dicke, J.M. (1989). Teratology: Principles and practice. *Med Clin North Am, 73,* 567.
29. Dillon, A.E., Wagner, C.L., Wiest, D., & Newman, R.B. (1997). Drug therapy in the nursing mother. *Obstet Gynecol Clin N Am, 24,* 675-696.
30. Donaldson, J.O. (1999). Neurologic complications. In G.N. Burrow & T.P. Duffy (Eds.). *Medical complications during pregnancy.* Philadelphia: W.B. Saunders.
31. Doyle, D.K. (1986). Teratology: A primer. *Neonatal Network, 4,* 24.
32. Epstein, C.J. (1995). The new dysmorphology: Application of insights from basic developmental biology tot he understanding of human birth defects. *Proc Natl Acad Sci, 92,* 8566.
33. Erwin, P.C. (1994). To use or not to use combined hormonal oral contraceptives during lactation. *Fam Planning Perspect, 26,* 26.
34. Ganapathy, V., et al. (1999). Drugs of abuse and placental transport. *Adv Drug Del Rev, 38,* 99.
35. Ganapathy, V. (2000). Placental transporters relevant to drug distribution across the maternal-fetal interface. *J Pharmacol Exp Ther, 294,* 413.
36. Garland, M. (1997). Pharmacology of drug transfer across the placenta. *Obstet Gynecol Clin N Am, 25,* 21-42.
37. Giacoia, G.P. & Catz, C.S. (1988). Drug therapy in the lactating mother: How to decide whether to prescribe or proscribe. *Postgrad Med, 83,* 211.
38. Guay, J., Grenier, Y., & Varin, F. (1998). Clinical pharmacokinetics of neuromuscular relaxants in pregnancy. *Clin Pharmacokinet, 34,* 483.
39. Hakkola, J., et al. (1998). Xenobiotic-metabolizing cytochrome P450 enzymes in the human feto-placental unit: Role in intrauterine toxicity. *Crit Rev Toxicol, 28,* 35.
40. Hale, T.W. (1998). *Medications and mother's milk* (7th ed.). Amarillo, TX: Pharmasoft Medical.
41. Hedstrom, S. & Martens, M.G. (1993). Antibiotics in pregnancy. *Clin Obstet Gynecol, 36,* 886.
42. Heiman, G. (1998). Basic pharmacologic principles. In R.A. Polin & W.W. Fox (Eds.). *Fetal and neonatal physiology* (2nd ed.). Philadelphia: W.B. Saunders.
43. Heisler, D. (1993). Pediatric renal function. *Int Anaesthesiol Clin, 31,* 103.
44. Hekkola, A. & Erkkola, R. (1994). Review of β-lactam antibiotics in pregnancy: The need for adjustment of dosing schedules. *Clin Pharmacokinet, 27,* 49.
45. Hill, E.P. & Longo, L.D. (1980). Dynamics of maternal-fetal nutrient transfer. *Fed Proc, 39,* 239.
46. Hill, H.R. (1987). Biochemical, structural, and functional abnormalities of polymorphonuclear leukocytes in the neonate. *Pediatr Res, 22,* 375.
47. Hill, R.M. & Stern, L. (1979). Drugs in pregnancy: Effects on the fetus and newborn. *Drugs, 17,* 182.
48. Howard, C.R. & Lawrence, R.A. (1999). Drugs and breastfeeding. *Clin Perinatol, 26,* 447.
49. Ito, S., et al. (1993). Prospective follow-up of adverse reactions in breastfed infants exposed to maternal medication. *Am J Obstet Gynecol, 168,* 1393.

50. Jacobs, N.M. (1991). Antibacterial therapy. In T.F. Yeh (Ed.). *Neonatal therapeutics* (2nd ed.). St. Louis: Mosby.

51. Jacqz-Aigrain, E. & Burtin, P. (1996). Clinical pharmacokinetics of sedatives in neonates. *Clin Pharmacokinet, 31*, 423.

52. John, E.G. & Guignard, J.P. (1998). Development of renal excretion of drugs during ontogeny. In R.A. Polin & W.W. Fox (Eds.). *Fetal and neonatal physiology* (2nd ed.). Philadelphia: W.B. Saunders.

53. Jones, KL. (1996). *Smith's recognizable patterns of human malformation* (5th ed.). Philadelphia: W.B. Saunders.

54. Jones, K.L. (1999). Effects of therapeutic, diagnostic, and environmental agents. In R.K. Creasy & R. Resnik (Eds.). *Maternal-fetal medicine* (4th ed.). Philadelphia: W.B. Saunders.

55. Kazilo, O., et al. (1988). Information on drug use in pregnancy from the viewpoint of a regional drug information centre. *Eur J Clin Pharmacol, 35*, 447.

56. Kearns, G.L. & Reed, M.D. (1989). Clinical pharmacokinetics in infants and children: a reappraisal. *Clin Pharmacokinet, 17*(Suppl), 29.

57. Keller, R.W. & Snyder-Keller, A. (2000). Prenatal cocaine exposure. *Ann N Y Acad Sci, 909*, 217.

58. Kenner, C. & Amlung, S. (2000). Nursing management of substance-dependent neonates. Online self-study course. Available online at www.nann.org/public/articles/details.cfm?id=84.

59. Kopelman, A.E. (1973). Cutaneous absorption of hexachlorophene in low-birth-weight infants. *J Pediatr, 82*, 972.

60. Koren, G. et al. (1989). Perception of teratogenic risk by pregnancy women exposed to drugs and chemicals during the first trimester. *Am J Obstet Gynecol, 160*, 1190.

61. Koren, G. & Pastuszak, A. (1990). Prevention of unnecessary pregnancy termination by counseling women on drug, chemical and radiation exposure during the first trimester. *Teratology, 41*, 657.

62. Koren, G., Paturszack, A. & Ito, S. (1998). Drugs in pregnancy. *N Engl J Med, 228*, 1128.

63. Krauer, B. & Krauer, F. (1977). Drug kinetics in pregnancy. *Clin Pharmacokinet, 2*, 167.

64. Kuller, J.M. (1990). Effects on the fetus and newborn of medications commonly used during pregnancy. *J Perinat Neonatal Nurs, 3*, 73.

65. Landers, D.V., Green, J.R. & Sweet, R.L. (1983). Antibiotic use during pregnancy and the postpartum period. *Clin Obstet Gynecol, 26*, 391.

66. Larrimore, W.L. & Petrie, K.L. (2000). Drug use during pregnancy and lactation. *Prim Care, 27*, 35-53.

67. Lawrence, R. & Lawrence, R.M. (1999). *Breastfeeding: A guide for the medical profession* (5th ed.). St Louis: Mosby.

68. Levitt, P., Reinose, B. & Jones, L. (1998). The critical impact of early cellular environment on neuronal development. *Prevent Med, 27*, 180-183.

69. Little, B.B. (1999). Pharmacokinetics during pregnancy: evidence-based maternal dose formulation. *Obstet Gynecol, 93*(5, Pt 2), 858.

70. Loebstein, R., Lalkin, A & Koren, G. (1997). Pharmacokinetics changes during pregnancy and their clinical relevance. *Clin Pharmacokinet, 33*, 328.

71. Logsdon, B.A. (1997). Drug use during lactation. *J Am Pharm Assoc (Wash), NS37*, 407.

72. Longo, L.D. (1982). Some physiological implications of altered utero-placental blood flow. In A.H. Moawad & M.D. Lindheimer (Eds.). *Uterine and placental blood flow.* New York: Masson Publishing.

73. Malanga, C.J. & Kosofsky, B.E. (1999). Mechanisms of action of drugs of abuse on the developing fetal brain. *Clin Perinatol, 26*, 17.

74. Malek, A. et al. (1996). Human placental transport of oxytocin. *J Maternal-Fetal Med, 5*, 245.

75. Martin, C.R. & Gingerich, B. (1976, September-October). Utero-placental physiology. *JOGN 5*(Suppl.), 16s.

76. Matheson, I., Kristensen, K. & Lunde, P.K.M. (1990). Drug utilization in breast-feeding women: A survey in Oslo. *Eur J Clin Pharmacol, 38*, 453.

77. Mattison, D.R. (1990). Transdermal drug absorption during pregnancy. *Clin Obstet Gynecol, 33*, 718.

78. Mayes, L.C. (1999). Developing brain and in utero cocaine exposures: effects on neural ontogeny. *Dev Psychopathol, 11*, 685.

79. Miller, M.T. & Stromland, K. (1999). Teratogen update: thalidomide: a review with focus on ocular findings and new potential uses. *Teratology, 60*, 306.

80. Mitani, G.M., et al. (1987). The pharmacokinetics of antiarrhythmic agents in pregnancy and lactation. *Clin Pharmacokinet, 12*, 253.

81. Mitchell, J.L. (1999). Use of cough and cold preparations during breastfeeding. *J Hum Lact, 15*, 347.

82. McKeigue, P.M., et al. (1994). A meta-analysis of epidemiologic studies. *Teratology, 50*, 27.

83. Moellering, R.C. (1979). Special consideration of the use of antimicrobial agents during pregnancy, postpartum and in the newborn. *Clin Obstet Gynecol, 22*, 373.

84. Moore, K.L. & Persaud, T.V.N. (1998). *The developing human: clinically oriented embryology* (6th ed.). Philadelphia: W.B. Saunders.

85. Morgan, D.J. (1997). Drug disposition in mother and foetus. *Clin Exp Pharmacol Physiol, 24*, 869.

86. Morris, F.H. & Boyd, R.D.H. (1988). Placental transport. In E. Knobil & J Neill (Eds.). *The physiology of reproduction* (vol. 2). New York: Raven Press.

87. Morselli, P.L. (1989). Clinical pharmacology of the perinatal period and early infancy. *Clin Pharmacokinet, 11*,13.

88. Mowad A.H. & Lindheimer, M.D. (1982). *Uterine and placental blood flow.* New York: Masson Publishing.

89. Murray, L. & Seger, D. (1994). Drug therapy during pregnancy and lactation. *Emerg Med Clin North Am, 12*, 129.

90. Nagourney, B.A. & Aranda, J.V. (1998). Physiologic differences of clinical significance. In R.A. Polin & W.W. Fox (Eds.). *Fetal and neonatal physiology* (2nd ed.). Philadelphia: W.B. Saunders.

91. Nation, R.L. (1980). Drug kinetics in childbirth. *Clin Pharmacokinet, 5*, 340.

92. Nau, H. & Plonait, S.L. (1998). Physiochemical and structural properties regulating placental drug transfer. In R.A. Polin & W.W. Fox (Eds.), *Fetal and neonatal physiology* (2nd ed.). Philadelphia: W.B. Saunders.

93. Neutel, C.L. & Johnson, H.L. (1995). Measuring drug effectiveness by default: the case of Bendectin. *Can J Public Health, 68*, 66.

94. Nice, F.J. (1989). Can a breast-feeding mother take medication without harming her infant? *MCN, 14*, 27.

95. Oesterheld, J.R. (1998). A review of developmental aspects of cytochrome P450. *J Child Adolesc Psychopharmacol, 8*, 161.

96. Pacifici, G.M. & Nottoli, R. (1995). Placental transfer of drugs administered to the mother. *Clin Pharmacokinet, 28*, 235.

97. Pasanen, M. (1999). The expression and regulation of drug metabolism in the human placenta. *Adv Drug Del Rev, 38*, 81.

98. Patterson, R.M. (1989). Seizure disorders in pregnancy. *Med Clin North Am, 73*, 661.

99. Pyati, S.P., et al. (1977). Absorption of iodine in the neonate following topical use of providone iodine. *J Pediatr, 91*, 825.

100. Reed, M.D. & Blumer, J.L. (1997). Pharmacologic treatment of the fetus. In A.A. Fanaroff & R.J. Martin (Eds.). *Neonatal-perinatal medicine. Diseases of the fetus and infant* (6th ed.). Philadelphia: W.B. Saunders.

101. Reider, M.J. (1998). Drug excretion during lactation. In R.A. Polin & W.W. Fox (Eds.). *Fetal and neonatal physiology* (2nd ed.). Philadelphia: W.B. Saunders.

102. Reynolds, F. & Knott, C. (1989). Pharmacokinetics in pregnancy and placental transfer. *Oxford Rev Reprod Biol, 11,* 389.

103. Ring, J.A. et al. (1999). Fetal hepatic drug elimination. *Pharmacol Ther, 84,* 429.

104. Rivera-Calimlim, L. (1987). The significance of drugs in breast milk: pharmacokinetic considerations. *Clin Perinatol, 14,* 51.

105. Robert, E. & Scialli, A.R. (1994). Topical medications during pregnancy. *Reprod Toxicol, 8,* 197.

106. Roe, V.A. (1999). Antimicrobial agents: pharmacology and clinical application in obstetric, gynecologic, and perinatal infections. *J Obstet Gynecol Neonatal Nurs, 28,* 639.

107. Routledge, P.A. (1994). Pharmacokinetics in children. *J Antimicrob Chemother, 34* (Suppl A), 19.

108. Rubin, P. (1998). Drug treatment during pregnancy. *BMJ, 317,* 1503-1506.

109. Rurak, D.W., Wright, M.R. & Axelson, J.E. (1991). Drug disposition and effects in the fetus. *J Dev Physiol, 15,* 33.

110. Sagraves, R. (1997). Drugs in breast milk: a scientific explanation. *J Pediatr Health Care, 11,* 230.

111. Schneider, H. (1994). Drug treatment in pregnancy. *Curr Opin Obstet Gynecol, 6,* 50.

112. Schick, J.B. & Milstein, J.M. (1981). Burn hazard of isopropyl alcohol in the neonate. *Pediatrics, 68,* 587.

113. Schroeder, H.J. (1995). Comparative aspects of placental exchange functions. *Eur J Obstet Gynecol Reprod Biol, 63,* 81.

114. Schwartz, R.H. (1981). Considerations of antibiotic therapy during pregnancy. *Obstet Gynecol, 58*(Suppl), 95s.

115. Shuman, R.M., Leech, R.W. & Alvord, E.C. (1974). Neurotoxicity of hexachlorophene in the human: I. A clinicopathologic study of 248 children. *Pediatrics, 54,* 689.

116. Sibley, C.P., et al. (1998). Mechanisms of maternofetal exchange across the human placenta. *Biochem Soc Trans, 26,* 86.

117. Speiser, P.W., et al. (1990). First trimester prenatal treatment and molecular genetic diagnosis of congenital adrenal hyperplasia (21-hydroxylase deficiency). *J Clin Endocrinol Metab, 70,* 838.

118. Steinberg, C. & Notterman, D.A. (1994). Pharmacokinetics of cardiovascular drugs in children: inotropes and vasopressors. *Clin Pharmacokinet, 27,* 345.

119. Stephens, T.D., et al. (2000). Mechanism of action in thalidomide teratogenesis. *Biochem Pharmacol, 59,* 1489.

120. Szeto, H.H. (1993). Kinetics of drug transfer to the fetus. *Clin Obstet Gynecol, 36,* 246.

121. Tankeyoon, M., et al. (1984). Effects of hormonal contraceptives on milk volume and infant growth. *Contraception, 30,* 505.

122. Tarask, C.L. & Kosofsky, B.E. (2000). Developmental considerations of neurotoxic exposures. *Neurol Clin, 18,* 541

123. Trange, J.M., Kluza, R.B., & Kearns, G.L. (1984). Pharmacokinetics for pediatric nurses. *Pediatr Nurs, 10,* 267.

124. Trasler, J.M. & Doerksen, T. (1999). Teratogen update: paternal exposures-reproductive risks. *Teratology, 60,* 161.

125. Van den Anker, J.N. (1996). Pharmacokinetics and renal function in preterm infants. *Acta Paediatr, 85,* 1393.

126. Vesell, E.S. (1997). Clinical pharmacotherapeutics. In. S.J. Yaffe & J.V. Aranda (Eds.). *Pediatric pharmacology: Therapeutic principles in practice.* Philadelphia: W.B. Saunders.

127. Voora, S. & Yeh, T.F. (1985). Drugs in breast milk. In T.F. Yeh (Ed.). *Drug therapy in the newborn and small infant.* Chicago: YearBook Medical Publishers.

128. Ward, R.M. (1993). Drug therapy of the fetus. *J Clin Pharmacol, 33,* 780.

129. Weinstein, A.J., Gibbs, R.S. & Gallager, M. (1976). Placental transfer of clindamycin and gentamicin in term pregnancy. *Am J Obstet Gynecol, 124,* 688.

130. Weller, T.M. & Rees, E.N. (2000). Antibacterial use in pregnancy. *Drug Saf, 22,* 335.

131. West, D., Worobec, S., & Solomon, L. (1981). Pharmacology and toxicology of infant skin. *J Invest Dermatol, 76,* 147.

132. Wilson, J.G. (1973). Mechanisms of teratogenesis. *Am J Anat, 136,* 129.

133. Wilson, J.G. (1977). Current status of teratology: General principles and mechanisms derived from animal studies. In J.G. Wilson & F.C. Fraser (Eds.). *Handbook of teratology: General principles and etiology.* New York: Plenum.

134. Woods, J.R. (1998). Maternal and transplacental effects of cocaine. *Ann N Y Acad Sci, 846,* 1.

135. World Health Organization. (2000). *Improving access to quality care in family planning. Medical eligibility criteria for contraceptive use* (2nd ed.). WHO/RHR/00.2. Available online at www.who.int/reproductive-health/publications/RHR_00_2_medical_eligibility_criteria_second_edition/medical_eligibility_criteria_table_of_contents.en.htm.

136. Wright, L.L. & Catz, C.S. (1998). Drug distribution during fetal life. In R.A. Polin & W.W. Fox (Eds.). *Fetal and neonatal physiology* (2nd ed.). Philadelphia: W.B. Saunders.

CHAPTER 7

Hematologic and Hemostatic Systems

The hematologic system encompasses blood and plasma volume, the constituents of plasma, and the formation and function of blood cellular components. The lineages of the various blood cells are summarized in Figure 7-1. Hemostasis involves mechanisms that result in the formation and removal of fibrin clots. Pregnancy and the neonatal period are associated with significant changes in these processes, increasing the risk for anemia and alterations in hemostasis such as thromboembolism and consumptive coagulopathies. This chapter examines alterations in the hematologic system and hemostasis during the perinatal period and their implications for the mother, fetus, and neonate.

MATERNAL PHYSIOLOGIC ADAPTATIONS

The significant changes in the hematologic system and hemostasis during pregnancy have a protective role for maternal homeostasis and are important for fetal development. These changes are also critical in allowing the mother to tolerate blood loss and placental separation at delivery. The maternal adaptations also increase the risk for complications such as thromboembolism, iron deficiency anemia, and coagulopathies.

Antepartum Period

Most hematologic parameters, including blood and plasma volume, cellular components, plasma constituents, and coagulation factors, are altered during pregnancy. These changes are reflected in progressive changes in many common hematologic laboratory values. As a result, it is essential to recognize the normal range of laboratory values and usual patterns of change during pregnancy and to evaluate findings in conjunction with clinical data and previous values in order to distinguish between normal adaptations and pathologic alterations (Table 7-1).

Changes in Blood and Plasma Volume

Among the most significant hematologic changes during pregnancy are increases in blood and plasma volume (Figure 7-2). These changes result in the hypervolemia of pregnancy, which is in turn responsible for many of the alterations in blood cellular components and plasma constituents. Circulating blood volume increases by 30% to 40% (approximately 1½ L), with a usual range of 30% to 50%.[39,124,159,176] Changes in individual women may range from a minimal change to a twofold increase.[49,106] The increased blood volume is due to an increase in plasma volume that is followed by an increase in the total red blood cell (RBC) volume. Blood volume changes begin at 6 to 8 weeks, peak at 30 to 34 weeks at values about 1200 to 1500 ml higher than in nonpregnant women, then reach a plateau or decrease slightly to term.[18,24,106]

Plasma volume increases by 40% to 50% (range, 30% to 60%) or about 1250 ml above nonpregnant values.[135,164] This change begins at 6 to 10 weeks and increases rapidly during the second trimester, followed by a slower but progressive increase that reaches its maximum at 28 to 32 weeks.[106] Although decreases in plasma volume after 36 weeks have been reported in older studies, the decline was probably related to the supine position of the woman during measurement, with compression of the pelvic veins by the enlarged uterus and sequestering of fluid in the lower extremities. This fluid was not fully accounted for in the volume measurements, and it seemed as if the plasma volume had declined when in fact it had not.[18,39,63,92] The enlarged plasma volume is accommodated by the vasculature of the uterus, breasts, muscles, kidneys, and skin. The increased volume leads to hemodilution with a net decrease in RBC volume and total circulating plasma proteins.

Plasma volume, placental mass, and birth weight are positively correlated.[92] Fetal growth correlates more closely with maternal plasma volume increases than with changes in RBC volume. Alterations in the usual increase in plasma volume are associated with pregnancy complications. A greater than normal increase in plasma volume has been observed in multiparous women (probably related to a tendency for higher-weight infants) and with maternal

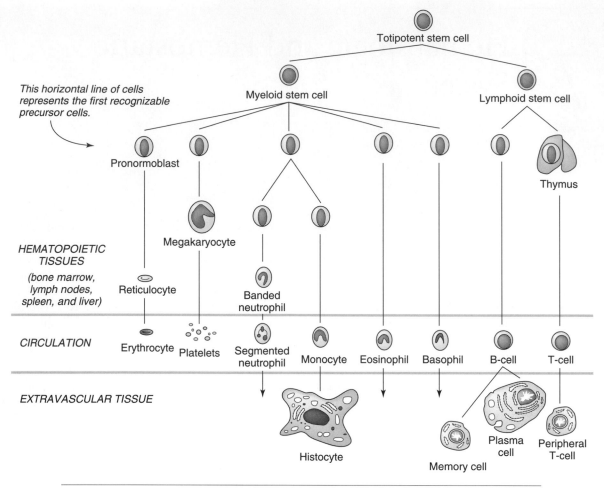

This horizontal line of cells represents the first recognizable precursor cells.

FIGURE **7-1** Lineage of different types of blood cells. (From Dixon, L.B. [1997]. The complete blood count: Physiologic basis and clinical usage. *J Perinat Neonat Nurs*, 11[3], 4.)

TABLE **7-1** Normal Laboratory Values in Nonpregnant and Pregnant Women

	NONPREGNANT	PREGNANT
GENERAL SCREENING ASSAYS		
Hemoglobin	12-16 g/dl	11-13 g/dl
Packed cell volume (PCV)	37%-45%	33%-39%
Red blood cell count (RBC)	4.2-5.4 million/mm^3	3.8-4.4 million/mm^3
Mean corpuscular volume (MCV)	80-100 fl	70-90 fl
Mean corpuscular hemoglobin (MCH)	27-34 fl	23-31 fl
Mean corpuscular hemoglobin concentration (MCHC)	32-35 fl	32-35 fl
Reticulocyte count	0.5%-1%	1%-2%
SPECIFIC DIAGNOSTIC TESTS		
Serum iron	50-100 μg/dl	30-100 μg/dl
Unsaturated iron binding capacity	250-300 μg/dl	280-400 μg/dl
Transferrin saturation	25%-35%	15%-30%
Iron stores (bone marrow)	Adequate ferritin	Unchanged
Serum folate	6-16 μg/ml	4-10 μg/ml
Serum vitamin B$_{12}$	70-85 ng/dl	70-500 ng/dl

Adapted from Morrison, J.C. & Pryor, J.A. (1990). Hematologic disorders. In R.D. Eden & F.H. Boehm (Eds.). *Assessment and care of the fetus.* Norwalk, CT: Appleton & Lange.

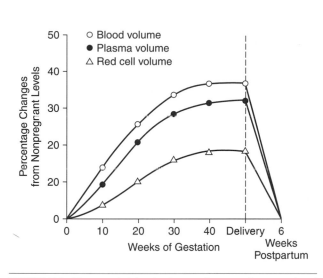

FIGURE **7-2** Changes in blood volume, plasma volume, and red blood cell volume during pregnancy and postpartum. (From Peck, T.M. & Arias, F. [1979]. Hematologic changes associated with pregnancy. *Clin Obstet Gynecol, 22, 788*.)

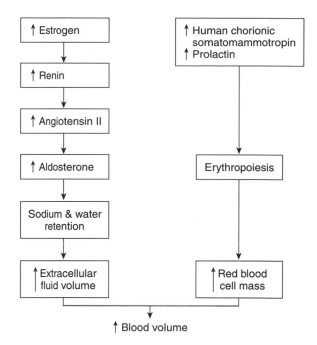

FIGURE **7-3** Possible mechanisms of hypervolemia during pregnancy. (From Gleicher, N. & Elkayam, U. [Eds.]. [1990]. Cardiac problems in pregnancy [2nd ed.]. New York: Alan R. Liss. Reprinted by permission of Wiley-Liss, a division of John Wiley and Sons, Inc.)

obesity, infants large for gestational age, prolonged pregnancy, and multiple gestation.[18,92]

In twin pregnancies, plasma volume increases up to 65% over nonpregnant values, with further elevations seen in women with triplets and other multiple pregnancies.[39,46,63] The lower than expected hematocrit seen in these women may be due to hemodilution from excessive plasma volume and may not indicate a problem with erythropoiesis per se. This increased plasma volume may be the basis for the higher incidence of pulmonary edema reported in women with multiple pregnancy who are treated with β-adrenergic agonists to inhibit preterm labor.[106] The mechanism for pulmonary edema with use of these agents is unclear, but it may occur secondary to maternal cardiovascular alterations with fluid retention and volume overload. Women already in a relative state of volume overload (multiple pregnancy) would be at greater risk.

Preeclampsia has generally been associated with a reduction in the expected increase in plasma and blood volumes (see Chapter 8).[18,124] However, Silver et al. recently reported a decrease in blood volume with women with preeclampsia and proteinuria but not in women with gestational hypertension without proteinuria.[173]

The exact etiology of plasma volume changes in pregnancy is poorly understood.[14] These changes are influenced by hormonal effects and are closely linked with the alterations seen in fluid balance and in the renal and cardiovascular systems (Figure 7-3). Hormonal influences, especially the effects of progesterone, on the vasculature of the venous system lead to decreased venous tone, increased capacity of the veins and venules, and decreased vascular resistance. These changes allow the vasculature to accommodate the increased blood volume. Estrogen and progesterone influence plasma renin activity and aldosterone levels, resulting in retention of sodium and an increase in total body water (see Chapter 10).[92] Most of this extra water is extracellular and available to contribute to the increased plasma volume. Changes in plasma volume have also been linked to a mechanical effect, with the low-resistance uteroplacental circulation acting as an arteriovenous shunt. This shunt provides physical space to accommodate the increased cardiac output and corresponding change in plasma volume.[39,92]

Hypervolemia reduces blood viscosity. Hypervolemia also leads to hemodilution and changes in plasma protein and blood cellular components, which further reduce viscosity. Blood viscosity decreases approximately 20%

TABLE 7-2 Changes in Blood Cellular Components during Pregnancy

COMPONENT	CHANGE	PATTERN OF CHANGE
Red blood cells (RBCs)	Increase 25%-33% (450 ml) with iron; increase 15%-18% (250 ml) without iron	Slow, continuous increase beginning in first trimester; may accelerate slightly in third trimester
Hematocrit	Decreases 3%-5% to 33.8% at term (range of 33%-39%)	Decreases from second trimester as plasma volume peaks
Hemoglobin	Decreases 2%-10% to 12.1-12.5 g/dl (range of 11-13 g/dl) at term	If iron and folate are adequate, little change to 16 weeks; lowest values at 16-22 weeks; slowly increases to term
Reticulocytes	Increase 1%-2%	Gradual increase to third trimester
White blood cells	Increase 8% to 5000-12,000 (up to 15,000 seen)/mm³	Begins in second month; increase involves primarily neutrophils
Eosinophils	Probably increases slightly	Variable
Basophils	Decreases slightly	
Platelets	Probably decrease slightly but within normal adult ranges; usual range 150,000-400,000/mm³	Variable
Erythrocyte sedimentation rate	Increases	Progressive

during the first two trimesters. During the third trimester, viscosity may increase slightly. The decreased viscosity reduces resistance to flow and the cardiac effort needed, thus conserving maternal energy resources.[39]

Changes in Blood Cellular Components

The principal change in blood cellular components during pregnancy is increased RBC volume (Table 7-2). This alteration, in conjunction with changes in plasma volume, is reflected in changes in the hemoglobin and hematocrit.

Changes in Red Blood Cells

The total RBC volume increases during pregnancy, with an average increase in circulating RBC of 25% to 33% (up to 450 ml) in women on iron supplementation and 15% to 18% (up to 250 ml) in women not taking iron.[11,125,176] Changes in RBC volume are due to increased circulating erythropoietin (EPO) and accelerated RBC production.[2] The rise in EPO, which stimulates erythropoiesis, in the last two trimesters is thought to be related to progesterone, prolactin, and human placental lactogen, rather than hypoxemia.[90,164,172] The magnitude of change varies from a moderate rise to 30% to 35% above values seen in nonpregnant women.[39,90] The increase in RBCs reflects the increase in oxygen demands (which rise 15%) during pregnancy.[176]

The increase in erythropoiesis and total RBC volume begins by 10 weeks.[164] The increase occurs at a relatively constant rate, but slower than changes in plasma volume, and may accelerate slightly during the third trimester.[63,90,92] The increased RBC production results in a moderate erythroid hyperplasia of the bone marrow and an increase in the reticulocyte count.[90]

RBC 2,3-diphosphoglycerate (2,3-DPG) increases beginning early in pregnancy and leads to a gradual shift to the right of the maternal oxygen-hemoglobin dissociation curve (see Chapter 9). This results in an increase in the amount of oxygen unloaded in the peripheral tissues, including the intervillous space, which facilitates oxygen transfer from mother to fetus and fetal growth.[28,63,92]

The mean cell diameter and thickness of the RBCs also change, resulting in a cell that is more spherical in shape.[138] Because the increase in plasma volume is three times greater than the RBC volume increase, the net result is a decrease in the total RBC count, hemoglobin, and hematocrit (Table 7-2). Changes in the mean corpuscular volume (MCV) and mean corpuscular hemoglobin volume (MCHV) are related to iron status. In women with adequate iron, the MCV and MCHV are relatively stable; in iron-deficiency women, these values may decrease.[106,176]

The hemoglobin and hematocrit decrease from the second trimester on as plasma volume peaks. In a group of pregnant women with adequate iron and folate, the hemoglobin was relatively stable until 16 weeks, fell to its lowest point at 16 to 22 weeks, then increased slowly to

BASIS FOR CHANGE	INTRAPARTUM CHANGES	POSTPARTUM CHANGES
Erythropoietin stimulated by human placental lactogen, progesterone, and prolactin Hemodilution	Slight increase due to slight hemo-concentration; 50% of increased RBCs lost at delivery	RBC production ceases temporarily; remainder of increased RBCs lost via normal catabolism Returns to nonpregnant levels by 4-6 weeks as a result of RBC catabolism
Hemodilution; total body hemo-globin increases by 65-150 g	Slight increase as a result of stress and dehydration	Initial decrease; stabilizes at 2-4 days; nonpregnant values by 4-6 weeks
Increased RBC production		Increase slightly; nonpregnant values by 4-6 weeks
Estrogen	Increase to 25,000-30,000/mm^3	Decrease to 6000-10,000/mm^3; normal values by 4-7 days
	Disappear from peripheral blood	By 3 days return to peripheral blood
?Hemodilution	20% decrease with placental separation	Increase by 3-5 days with gradual return to nonpregnant levels
Increased plasma globulin and fibrinogen	Increases	Initially 55-80 mm/hr; peaks 1-2 days postpartum

term.[18] Total body hemoglobin increases 85 to 150 g in pregnancy, whereas net hemoglobin decreases. Even with adequate iron supplementation, the hemoglobin decreases about 2 g/dl to a mean of about 11.6 g/dl in the second trimester as a result of hemodilution.[93] At term the hemoglobin averages 12.1 to 12.5 g/dl, with a range of 11 to 13 g/dl (versus a mean of 14 $\pm$2 for nonpregnant females).[17] The Centers for Disease Control and Prevention (CDC) suggest values of 11 (first and second trimesters) and 10.5 g/dl (third trimester) as the lowest acceptable values for screening pregnant women.[37] The mean hematocrit is 33.8% (range, 33% to 39%) at term.[106,125,138] The World Health Organization (WHO) recommends that the hemoglobin not fall below 11 at any point in pregnancy; others have suggested that it not fall below 10.[111,125] A high hematocrit in a pregnant woman may indicate a low plasma volume and a relative hypovolemia.[111,125] Changes in the hemoglobin and hematocrit in pregnant women with and without iron supplements are illustrated in Figure 7-4.

Changes in White Blood Cells

Total white blood cell (WBC) volume increases slightly during early pregnancy beginning in the second month and levels off during the second and third trimesters (see Table 7-2). The total WBC count in pregnancy varies with individual women, ranging from 5000 to 12,000/mm^3, with values as high as 15,000/mm^3 reported.[106,124] The increased WBC count is due to a neutrophilia with an elevation in mature leukocyte forms. A slight shift to the left may occur with occasional myelocytes and metamyelocytes seen on the peripheral smear.[106] Changes in other WBC forms are minimal (see Table 7-2), with a possible slight increase in eosinophils and slight decrease in basophils and no systematic changes in monocytes.[106] Alkaline phosphatase activity of the leukocytes rises during pregnancy, falling several days before to delivery. Changes in leukocytes accompanying pregnancy are similar to changes that occur with physiologic stress, such as vigorous exercise, with return to the circulation of mature leukocytes that were previously shunted out of the circulatory system.[949] The basis for these changes is unclear but is probably related to hormonal changes.[106] The neutrophil count normally increases slightly with the estrogen peak during the menstrual cycle. In women who become pregnant, the neutrophils continue to increase after fertilization, peaking around 30 weeks then remaining stable to term.

The total lymphocyte count is unchanged, as are numbers of circulating B and T lymphocytes. Some studies suggest that T-cell function and numbers of natural killer cells are decreased (see Chapter 12), possibly mediated by the effects of estrogen.[176]

Changes in Platelets

Older reports regarding changes in platelets during pregnancy were conflicting: platelets were reported to increase,

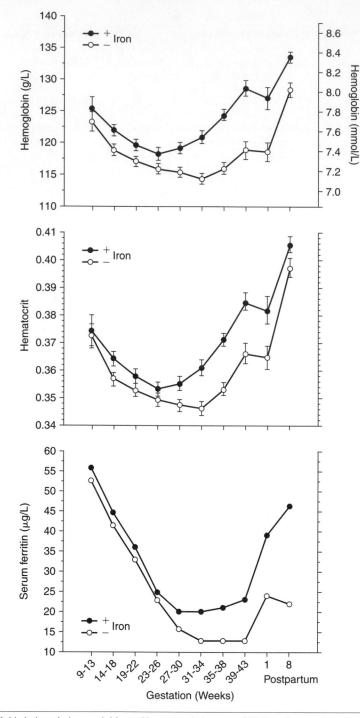

FIGURE 7-4 Variations in hemoglobin and hematocrit (mean ±SEM) and serum ferritin (median) in normal pregnancy and postpartum in placebo-treated and iron-treated women taking 66 mg ferrous iron daily. From Milman, N. et al. [1999]. Iron status and iron balance during pregnancy: A critical reappraisal of iron supplementation. *Acta Obstet Gynecol Scand,* 78, 752.

decrease, or stay the same.[84,106,129] Recent reports demonstrate a slight decrease in platelet count, probably due to hemodilution, and an increase in platelet aggregation during the last 8 weeks of pregnancy, suggesting a low-grade activation and consumption of platelets.[84,106] In healthy pregnant women, platelet counts have generally not been reported at values below lower limits for normal nonpregnant women.[106] Mild to moderate thrombocytopenia (less than 150,000/mm³) has been reported at term in 6% of healthy pregnant women who have no other evidence of idiopathic thrombocytopenic purpura (ITP).[106,129] The acceptable range for platelet values in pregnancy is 150,000 to 400,000/mm³.

Changes in Plasma Components

Many components of plasma—including plasma proteins, electrolytes, serum iron, lipids, and enzymes—change during pregnancy (Table 7-3). Total plasma proteins decrease 10% to 14%, with much of the change occurring in the first trimester. Although there is an absolute increase in albumin concentration during the first trimester, there is a relative decrease due to increased blood volume and hemodilution. Decreased albumin leads to a net decrease in colloid osmotic (oncotic) pressure, reducing the normal forces counteracting edema formation.[16] Although edema formation in pregnancy is primarily due to alterations in venous hydrostatic pressure, decreased oncotic pressure from decreased albumin is an important contributory factor.[16]

Globulin concentration demonstrates both absolute and relative increases, leading to progressive falls in the albumin-to-globulin ratio. Both α- and β-globulin increase progressively during pregnancy, whereas γ-globulin decreases slightly. Fibrinogen also demonstrates both absolute and relative increases of 50% to 80%.[16,49] The erythrocyte sedimentation rate (ESR) increases progressively during pregnancy, probably due to the elevation in plasma globulin and fibrinogen levels. Alterations in other plasma proteins are summarized in Table 7-3.

The alterations in plasma proteins alter protein binding of substances such as calcium, drugs, and anesthetic agents. Because many drugs are transported in the blood bound to albumin, doses of some drugs may need to be altered during pregnancy (see Chapter 6). Increased binding of substances such as calcium reduces the level of free calcium in the maternal plasma. As a result, calcium must be actively transported across the placenta to the fetus (see Chapter 16).

Decreases in serum electrolytes (anions, cations, and buffer base) reduce plasma osmolarity from 290 to 280 mOsm/L during the first trimester.[16] These changes are due to both hypervolemia and the effects of respiratory system alterations, particularly hyperventilation with increased CO_2 loss (see Chapter 9).[39]

Serum iron decreases during pregnancy, especially after 28 weeks and in women not receiving adequate iron.[18] Iron needs during pregnancy are summarized in Table 7-4. Serum ferritin (1μg/L serum ferritin is equal to 8 mg of stored iron in the adult) is a more precise indicator of reticuloendothelial iron stores. Serum ferritin levels in pregnancy are 15 to 150 ng/ml.[63] In women without iron supplementation, serum ferritin levels fall until 30 to 32 weeks and then stabilize. The greatest decrease in serum ferritin is between 12 and 25 weeks due to the rapid expansion of maternal RBC volume during this time (Figure 7-4).[2,182] With supplemental iron, serum ferritin levels stabilize by 28 weeks or slightly earlier, and may even rise near term.[18,90,111] Decreases in serum ferritin in early pregnancy are due to mobilization of iron stores for maternal hemoglobin synthesis; later decreases are due to increased fetal iron uptake. In multiparous women the decrease in serum ferritin occurs earlier and may be greater.[18]

Levels of serum lipids rise with marked elevations in cholesterol and phospholipids. Cholesterol is an essential precursor for steroid hormone production by the placenta; phospholipids are major components of cell membranes. The rise in serum lipids begins in the first trimester, increasing to 40% to 60% at term (see Table 7-3). Increases in serum alkaline phosphatase are due to increased placental production. As a result, alkaline phosphatase levels are not useful in evaluating liver disorders during pregnancy. Serum cholinesterase activity decreases by 30%. Increased cholinesterase activity may lead to longer periods of paralysis if substances such as succinylcholine are used during surgical procedures.[16]

Changes in Coagulation Factors and Hemostasis

Pregnancy has been called an acquired hypercoagulable state, reflecting an increased risk for thrombosis and consumptive coagulopathies such as disseminated intravascular coagulation (DIC). Hemostatic changes during pregnancy are thought to result in an ongoing low-grade activation of the coagulation system, beginning as early as 11 to 15 weeks. This state of compensated intravascular coagulation is characterized by thrombin formation and local consumption of clotting factors in which component synthesis equals or exceeds consumption.[20,84,159,174]

Intra- and extravascular fibrin deposits are found in the uteroplacental circulation, intervillous spaces, and placental

TABLE 7-3 Changes in Plasma Components during Pregnancy

COMPONENT	CHANGE	TIMING	BASIS	SIGNIFICANCE
Total plasma proteins	↓ 10%-14%	First trimester	Estrogen/progesterone	↓ Colloid osmotic pressure (edema formation)
				Altered protein binding of calcium, drugs, and so on
Albumin	Total: 144 g Serum: 3.5 g	First trimester	Estrogen/progesterone Hemodilution	See above
Fibrinogen	↑ 50%-80%	First to third trimesters	Estrogen/progesterone	Alterations in hemostasis
Globulin	↑	First to third trimesters	Estrogen/progesterone	↓ Erythrocyte sedimentation rate
Alpha and beta globulin	↑	Progressive throughout pregnancy		↓ Erythrocyte sedimentation rate
				See individual globulins
				Facilitate transport of carbohydrates and lipids to placenta and fetus
Gamma globulin	↓	Third trimester		Transplacental passage of IgG
Thyroxin-binding globulin	↑	First trimester		↑ Plasma T₃ and T₄
α₁-Antitrypsin	Doubles			Protects lungs from deported trophoblast tissue
α₂-Macroglobulin	↑ 20%			Anti-plasmin effect, which may predispose to disseminated intravascular coagulation
Total serum lipids	↑ 40%-60%	Continuous to term	Human placental lactogen and altered metabolism	
Cholesterol	↑ 40%	Continuous to term		Essential precursor for steroid hormones (e.g., estrogen, progesterone)
Phospholipids	↑ 37%	Continuous to term		Major component of cell membranes needed for maternal and fetal growth
β-Lipoprotein	↑ Up to 180%	First trimester		Possible ↑ risk of thrombosis
Serum electrolytes	↓ 5-10 mg/L			↓ plasma osmolarity
Serum ferritin	↓ 30%	To 30-32 weeks, then reaches a plateau	Hemoglobin synthesis (early) Fetal uptake (late)	Reflects decreasing iron stores
Transferrin	↑ 70%	Linear rise	Altered liver function	Facilitates Fe absorption and transport
Iron-binding capacity	↓ 15%			

bed. Tissue factor (which initiates clotting via the extrinsic system) is found in amniotic fluid, the decidua, and endometrial stroma.[116] Circulating high-molecular-weight, soluble fibrin-fibrinogen complexes—which are indicative of uteroplacental fibrin formation—also increase. During pregnancy, smooth muscle and elastic tissue within the uterine spiral arteries are replaced by a fibrin matrix (see Chapter 3). These changes allow for expansion of the vessels to accommodate increased blood flow to the placenta and to facilitate collapse of the terminal portion of the vessel with placental separation.[84,176] Increased (20% to 200%) fibrinogen, thrombin generation, and inhibition of fibrinolysis during pregnancy may interact to ensure integrity of uteroplacental vessels.[116] During late pregnancy, accumulation of mural thrombi in the vessel walls decreases the diameter of the lumen, reducing blood flow, which may result in the placental infarcts and small areas of ischemia often seen at term.[84]

Contact factors (XII, prekallikrein, and high-molecular-weight kininogen) involved in initiation of the clotting cascade are all elevated.[84] (Table 7-5 summarizes the properties of major factors.) Factor VIII complex doubles; factors I (fibrinogen), VII, IX, and X; and von Willebrand factor (vWF) antigen are increased.[62,80,116,176] Factor II is reported to be either slightly elevated or to remain stable (Figure 7-5).[106,174] Factors XI and XIII are reported to decrease or increase and then decrease.[132] A concurrent increase in fibrinogen and decrease in factor XIII (fibrin stabilizing factor) alters the process of clot stabilization and subsequent lysis during pregnancy.[84] Changes in coagulation factors during pregnancy are reflected in the activated partial thromboplastin time (APTT) and prothrombin time (PT), which decrease slightly.

Endogenous anticoagulants protein C and antithrombin are unchanged, whereas protein S may be decreased by up to 40% during pregnancy.[60,116] Thrombin-antithrombin

TABLE 7-4 Iron Requirements for Pregnancy

REQUIRED FOR	AVERAGE (mg)	RANGE (mg)
External iron loss	170	150-200
Expansion of red blood cell mass	450	200-600
Fetal iron	270	200-370
Iron in placenta and cord	90	30-170
Blood loss at delivery	150	90-310
Total requirement	980	580-1340
Requirement less red blood cell expansion	840	440-1050

From Kilpatrick, S.J. & Laros, R.K. (1999). Maternal hematologic disorders. In R.K. Creasy & R. Resnik (Eds.). *Maternal-fetal medicine* (4th ed.). Philadelphia: W.B. Saunders.

TABLE 7-5 Coagulation Factors

NUMBER	NAME	FUNCTION
I	Fibrinogen	Fibrin precursor
II	Prothrombin	Thrombin precursor (vitamin K)
III	Tissue factor thromboplastin and calcium to activate X	Tissue factor formed in plasma or tissues that reacts with VII
IV	Calcium ions	Activator of enzyme activity in all stages of coagulation
V	Plasma accelerator globulin	Accelerates conversion of prothrombin to thrombin
VII	Proconvertin	Reacts with III and calcium to activate X (vitamin K)
VIII	Antihemophilic globulin	Reacts with IX, calcium, and phospholipid to activate X
IX	Plasma thromboplastin component (PTC)	Reacts with VIII, calcium, and phospholipid to activate X (vitamin K)
X	Stuart-Prower factor	Accelerates conversion of prothrombin to thrombin (vitamin K)
XI	Plasma thromboplastin	Contact factor for tissue factor thromboplastin
XII	Hageman factor	Contact factor for initiation of clotting cascade
XIII	Fibrin stabilizing factor	Maintain firm fibrin clot
	High-molecular-weight kininogen (HMWK)	Contact factor that reacts with prekallikrein and XI
	Prekallikrein	Contact factor that reacts with HMWK and XI
	Protein C, protein S	Coagulation inhibitors of V and VIII (vitamin K)
	Antithrombin	Coagulation inhibitor of thrombin, II, X, and other factors
	Plasminogen	Fibrinolytic; plasmin precursor

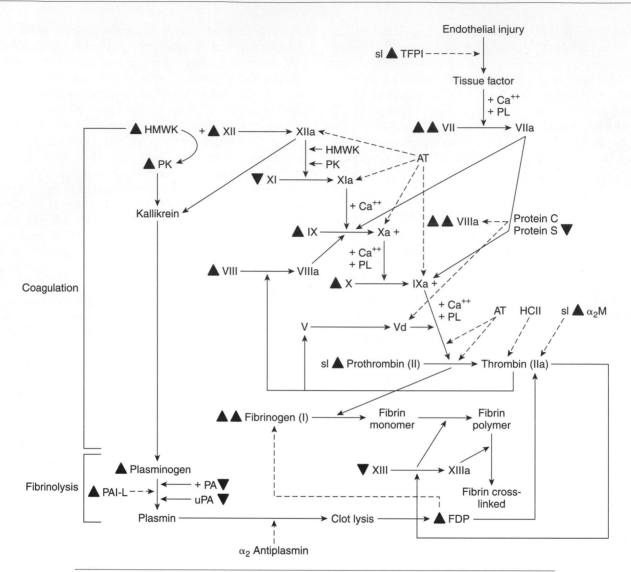

FIGURE 7-5 Alterations in coagulation and fibrinolysis during pregnancy. Coagulation involves a series of enzymatic reactions (coagulation cascade) to convert substrates to active products. Coagulation is initiated by endothelial damage and release of tissue factor (TF). TF is a glycoprotein bound to cell membranes and found on epithelial, stromal, and perivascular cells. With tissue damage or vascular disruption, TF and plasma factor VII, in the presence of calcium, produce VIIA. The tissue factor–factor VIIA complex then activates factors XI and X, leading to formation of thrombin from prothrombin. Thrombin acts as an enzyme in the formation of fibrin from fibrinogen. Fibrin is an insoluble protein consisting of dense interlacing threads that entrap platelets and erythrocytes. Fibrinolysis is accomplished by activation of plasmin from plasminogen via intrinsic (contact factors) or extrinsic (tissue plasminogen activator) substances. Lysis of the fibrin clot produces fibrin-fibrinogen degradation products (FDP) or fibrin split products (FSP), which can interfere with further clotting by impairing platelet aggregation and thrombin formation. The maintenance of normal hemostasis is also dependent on the presence of naturally occurring coagulation inhibitors (e.g., antithrombin, protein C). α_2M, α_2-macroglobulin; *AT*, antithrombin; *Ca*, calcium; *FDP*, fibrin-fibrinogen degradation products; *HCII*, heparin cofactor II; *HMWK*, high-molecular-weight kininogen; *PAI-1*, plasminogen activator inhibitor-1; *PK*, prekallikrein; *PL*, phospholipid; *sl*, slight; *TFPI*, tissue factor pathway inhibitor; *t-PA*, tissue plasminogen activator; *u-PA*, urokinase plasminogen activator. Dashed line denotes inhibitory action. ↑ and ↓ denote changes during pregnancy.

complexes increase, indicating increased thrombin generation.[116] Tissue factor inhibitor (TFP1) and α_1-macroglobulin increase slightly.[116] In addition, a fetal anticoagulant, dermatan sulfate–like proteoglycans (DSPG), is found in maternal serum. DSPG is released by the placenta, catalyzes thrombin, and is inhibited by heparin cofactor II; DSPG disappears from maternal serum by about 5 days after birth.[4]

Fibrinolytic activity increases during the first two trimesters, then decreases to term.[12] Inhibitors of fibrinolysis produced by the placenta can be found in maternal plasma.[150] Type-1 plasminogen activator inhibitor (PAI-1) is another inhibitor of fibrinolysis. PAI-1 is produced by the decidua and increases two- to threefold during pregnancy.[62,116]

The net effect of changes in hemostasis during pregnancy is increased activity of most coagulation factors and a lowering of factors that inhibit coagulation. The result is a hypercoagulable state that promotes clot formation, extension, and stability.[84,116] The hypercoagulable state of pregnancy is balanced to some extent by changes in plasminogen. Plasminogen is elevated and tissue plasmin inhibitors are decreased, which helps retain the dynamic equilibrium between clotting and clot lysis and thus overall hemostatic balance during pregnancy.[6,44,84] The increased tendency toward coagulation during pregnancy may also be partly balanced by pregnancy-specific proteins (PSPs), which act similarly to heparin to facilitate neutralization of thrombin by antithrombin. Many clotting factors are synthesized by the liver and influenced by estrogen and many of the changes seen in pregnancy are similar to those seen with oral contraceptives.[101,159,174] Figure 7-5 summarizes hemostatic changes during pregnancy.

Intrapartum Period

Changes in the hematologic system and hemostasis are crucial in preparing the pregnant woman to tolerate the normal blood loss at delivery and prevent significant bleeding with placental separation. The amount of blood loss with delivery averages up to 500 ml (vaginal delivery) or 1000 ml (cesarean section or a vaginal delivery of twins), with minimal changes in blood pressure or pulse.[16,25,63,159] This loss at delivery may be underestimated by up to 50%.[86,121] Blood loss at delivery and in lochia over the first few postpartum days account for about half of the increased RBC volume acquired during pregnancy.[159]

Changes in Hematologic Parameters

Hemoglobin levels tend to increase slightly during labor due to hemoconcentration. The degree of hemoconcentration is related to increases in erythropoiesis (as a stress response), muscular activity, and dehydration.[49,159] Leukocyte alkaline phosphatase activity increases with the onset of labor. Increases in this enzyme are often associated with inflammatory responses. The WBC count increases during labor and immediately postpartum to values up to 25,000 to 30,000/mm³. This increase is primarily due to an increase in neutrophils and may represent a response to stress.[159] Circulating eosinophils decrease and may disappear.[176] Changes in hematologic parameters are summarized in Table 7-2.

Changes in the hematologic system can complicate diagnosis of infection during this period. The usual increase in WBC count may include release of immature neutrophils, which is similar to findings associated with bacterial infection. The ESR also rises and is therefore less useful. In addition, the laboring woman may experience a relative tachycardia, dehydration, and elevated temperature.

Changes in Hemostasis

The coagulation system undergoes further activation during the intrapartum period both before and after placental separation. The placenta and decidua are rich in thromboplastin, and exposure or release of this tissue factor during placental separation will activate coagulation via the extrinsic system (see Figure 7-5). Concentrations of clotting factors increase during labor. PT shortens significantly, especially during the third stage of labor with clotting at the placental site. Levels of fibrinogen and plasminogen may also decrease as a result of their increased utilization after placental separation.[84] Factor VIII complex increases during labor and delivery. Factor V increases after placental separation, which contributes to activation of clotting via the extrinsic system.

Fibrinolytic activity decreases further during labor and delivery, enhancing formation of clots at the placental site following separation.[16,84] This promotes development of a hemostatic endometrial fibrin mesh over the wound. About 5% to 10% of the total body fibrin is deposited at this site.[84]

Levels of fibrin-fibrinogen degradation products (FDP) increase after delivery. This change increases the risk of coagulation disorders in the immediate postpartum period by interfering with formation of firm fibrin clots.[16,84] The number of platelets falls about 20% with placental separation due to clotting at the placental site. Platelet activation and fibrin formation are maximal at delivery (Figure 7-6).[74] Thus the hypercoagulable state of pregnancy is further magnified during the intrapartum period. This state protects the woman from hemorrhage and excessive blood loss at delivery by providing for rapid hemostasis following removal of the placenta.

Postpartum Period
Changes in Blood Volume

The decrease in blood and plasma volume during the immediate postpartum period corresponds to the amount of blood loss with delivery. This loss usually accounts for over half of the RBC volume accumulated during pregnancy.[39] During the first few days after delivery, plasma volume decreases further as a result of diuresis. After 3 to 4 days, mobilization of interstitial fluid leads to a slight increase in plasma volume. This hemodilution decreases hemoglobin, hematocrit, and plasma protein by the end of the first postpartum week (Figure 7-7).[39] The volume change may contribute to circulatory embarrassment in women with cardiac problems (Chapter 8). Plasma volume continues to decrease after the first week, reaching nonpregnant values by 6 to 8 weeks or earlier.

Accurate and consistent assessment of blood loss is essential at delivery and postpartum. Blood losses during these periods are reported to be both under- and overestimated. Unit and product-specific standards for estimating losses increase accuracy of these assessments.[86,121]

Changes in Hematologic Parameters

Increased RBC production ceases early in the postpartum period due to suppression of EPO.[39] Mean hemoglobin levels decrease slightly in the first 24 hours after delivery, then plateau for 4 days, followed by a slow rise to day 14.[164] Hematocrit values follow a similar pattern. A 500-ml blood loss such as occurs with vaginal delivery will usually result in a 1-g reduction in hemoglobin. The hematocrit returns to nonpregnant levels by 4 to 6 weeks following usual RBC destruction. The reticulocyte count is increased by the end of pregnancy, with a further increase during the first 1 to 2 postpartum days, followed by a rapid decrease. The initial increase may be a result of EPO stimulation because of decreased RBC oxygen carrying capacity from blood loss at delivery.[164] Levels of fetal hemoglobin (HbF) return to nonpregnant values by about 8 weeks.[176]

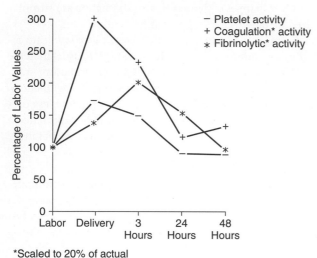

FIGURE **7-6** Platelet, coagulation, and fibrinolytic activity in labor, delivery, and postpartum. Hemostasis activity is calculated from β-thromboglobulin, platelet factor 4 (platelet), fibrinopeptide A (clotting), and fibrin-fibrinogen degradation product (fibrinolysis) values. (From Gerbasi, F.R., et al. [1990]. Changes in hemostasis during delivery and the immediate postpartum period. *Am J Obstet Gynecol, 162,* 1158.)

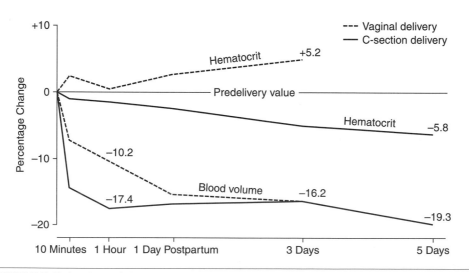

FIGURE **7-7** Estimations of changes in blood volume and hematocrit following vaginal and cesarean births. Values are expressed as percent changes from values immediately before delivery. (From Metcalfe, J. & Ueland, K. [1980]. Heart disease and pregnancy. In N.O. Fowler [Ed.]. *Cardiac diagnosis and treatment* [3rd ed.]. Hagerstown, MD: Harper & Row.)

Excess circulating hemoglobin is catabolized, and the iron released is stored in the reticuloendothelial system. During the first 2 weeks, there is little change in serum ferritin levels, with a decrease in transferrin and increase in serum iron, and marked decrease in C-reactive protein.[164] Serum ferritin levels increase by 5 to 8 weeks to levels seen early in pregnancy.[125] This increase occurs regardless of whether or not the woman received supplemental iron during pregnancy and is more marked after vaginal delivery.[18,63,93,125]

The WBC count, which increases in labor and immediately postpartum, falls to 6000 to 10,000/mm³, then returns to normal values by 6 days.[106,164] Eosinophils, which tend to disappear from the peripheral blood during delivery, return by 3 days postpartum; basophils and monocytes remain unchanged.[176] The number of platelets, which falls following placental separation, increases beginning at 3 to 4 days and gradually returns to nonpregnant levels. It is unclear if this change is due to stimulation of platelet production, or secondary to changes in blood volume.[164] Postpartum changes are summarized in Table 7-2.

Changes in Hemostasis

Fibrinolytic activity is maximal for the first 3 hours after delivery, although it may return to normal ranges as early as 1 hour after delivery.[74] Return to normal activity reflects removal of the fibrinolytic inhibitors produced by the placenta. Secondary increases in fibrinogen, factor V, and factor VIII complex occur during the first week, followed by a return to predelivery levels by 3 to 5 days, and a slow decrease to nonpregnant levels.[84] Clotting factors, which increase during labor, slowly decrease, reaching their lowest levels by 7 to 10 days. Factors VII and X return to normal levels by 2 weeks. The hemostatic system has usually returned to nonpregnant status 3 to 4 weeks postpartum.[84] Changes in the flow velocity and diameter of the deep veins may take up to 6 weeks to return to prepregnant levels.[80] Thus the postpartum period continues to be a time of increased risk for thromboembolism.

CLINICAL IMPLICATIONS FOR THE PREGNANT WOMAN AND HER FETUS

The changes in the hematologic system and in hemostasis during pregnancy are important for maternal and fetal homeostasis but also increase the woman's need for iron and other nutrients and place her at risk for developing anemia, thromboembolic disorders, and coagulopathies. This section examines maternal-fetal implications related to hypervolemia, hemodilution, and the hypercoagulable state along with implications for women with pathophysiologic states affecting the hematologic system.

Hypervolemia of Pregnancy

The increased blood and plasma volume during pregnancy results in a physiologic hypervolemia that allows the woman to tolerate many of the changes associated with pregnancy and delivery and helps to: (1) meet the demands of an enlarged uterus and hypertrophied vascular system while maintaining normal systemic blood pressure; (2) allow the woman to tolerate blood loss at delivery; (3) protect the woman from impaired venous return and hypotension with position changes late in the third trimester (when a significant proportion of her fluid volume may be sequestered within the venous system of the lower extremities) and thus reduce the risk of supine hypotension; (4) enhance maternal-fetal exchange of gases and nutrients; and (5) increase cutaneous blood flow by four- to sevenfold, thus assisting with heat dissipation via the skin.[16,18,39,63,159]

The increased RBC volume helps offset hemodilution and maintain blood oxygen-carrying capacity and availability of oxygen for the fetus. The increased volume allows for adequate blood flow within the expanding uteroplacental circulation, thus ensuring adequate nutrient availability for the fetus throughout gestation. These changes alter evaluation of hematologic variables in the pregnant woman (see Table 7-1).

Iron Requirements during Pregnancy

Iron stores in nonpregnant women are generally marginal due to menstrual blood, and thus iron, loss. The usual menses loss is 12 to 15 mg of elemental iron (1 ml blood is equal to 0.5 mg of iron).[106] Most women have a daily iron intake of about 9 mg/day, below the recommended 12 to 18 mg.[136] Worldwide, an estimated 20% of fertile women have iron reserves greater than 500 mg, the minimum iron requirement in pregnancy; 40% have reserves between 100 and 500 mg; and 40% have reserves less than 100 mg.[136] In the U.S., pregnant women have an average of 300 mg of iron stored at the beginning of pregnancy. This means that in order to meet the iron demands of pregnancy, they must absorb an additional 500 to 700 mg (or 2 to 8 mg/day more than normal).[122] The WHO estimates that 35% to 75% (mean, 56%) of women in developing countries and 15% of women in industrialized nations are anemic during pregnancy.[198]

Iron requirements increase during pregnancy by about 1 g over the usual body iron stores of 2 to 2.5 g in adult women.[83] Table 7-4 summarizes how this additional iron is used during pregnancy. The need for iron begins early in the second trimester and peaks in the second half of pregnancy (increasing from an additional 0.8 mg/day in early pregnancy to 7.5 mg/day by term).[44,122,136]

The amount of iron needed by the fetus and placenta and to replace usual maternal losses is an obligatory requirement that is met regardless of the cost to maternal iron stores.[18] Even if the mother is iron-deficient and anemic, the fetus will usually not suffer, since the placenta continues to transport iron to meet fetal needs. If adequate iron is not available for synthesis of additional RBCs, the maternal RBC volume will not increase to the usual levels and the hematocrit and hemoglobin will decrease further as plasma volume increases.[18,49,106]

Prophylactic iron supplementation in pregnancy continues to be controversial.[1,94,135,170,185,188] Although intestinal iron absorption increases in the second half of pregnancy (probably as a compensatory mechanism in response to increased iron demand), dietary sources and maternal stores alone may not be adequate to meet the increased demands of pregnancy. Iron stores affect iron absorption. Women who have good iron stores have minimal increases in absorption during the first trimester, then increase absorption during the second trimester. By later pregnancy, iron stores may be exhausted and iron needs met primarily from absorption.[122] Barrett et al suggest that if a woman has good iron stores prior to pregnancy and a diet high in bioavailable iron, most of these women will not develop anemia if they are not supplemented.[15] However, iron stores in young, healthy nonpregnant women may be marginal to nonexistent.[36] Iron supplementation increases iron reserves, hemoglobin levels, and decreases the risk of iron deficiency anemia during pregnancy and postpartum, even in women with good iron stores at the beginning of pregnancy.[2,136,170] Even with adequate nutrition, 10% to 20% of pregnant women will develop an iron deficiency.[45,179] The Institute of Medicine's (IOM) general recommendations for iron supplementation during pregnancy are 30 mg ferrous iron (which is provided by 150 mg ferrous sulfate, 300 mg ferrous gluconate, or 100 mg ferrous fumarate) daily beginning at 12 weeks along with a well-balanced diet.[93] The need for iron can also be met with supplementation of 60 to 85 mg/day of elemental iron from 20 weeks.[94,106,136] Iron supplementation is needed if serum ferritin levels are less than 12 μg/L. However, due to the high cost of screening, iron supplementation is generally used routinely with all women.[94] Iron supplementation does not prevent or correct the normal decline in hemoglobin seen in pregnancy but can prevent depletion of stores, the first stage of iron deficiency anemia.[18,93] No significant side effects have been reported with use of routine iron supplementation.[85,169]

Fetal Iron Requirements

Fetal and neonatal iron content is 75 mg/kg. The majority (75%) of fetal iron is found in hemoglobin, with about 7 mg/kg in tissues and 10 mg/kg stored in the liver and spleen. The stored iron doubles during the last few weeks of gestation.[150]

The fetus has been called an "efficient parasite" in terms of iron transport across the placenta.[150] Iron passes rapidly against a concentration gradient from mother to fetus via transferrin. Iron bound to maternal serum transferrin will not cross the placenta. The maternal transferrin releases its iron in the intervillous space. The iron is taken up by transferrin receptors located on the surface of syncytiotrophoblast cells.[2] Iron is transported across the placenta to fetal blood and attaches to fetal serum transferrin. Fetal transferrin is synthesized by the fetal liver after about 29 to 30 days of gestation.[18,150]

By the end of pregnancy, 90% of the mother's transferrin-bound iron is delivered to the placenta.[125] Poor maternal iron stores are associated with increased placental transferrin receptors to enhance uptake of iron.[2]

With fetal growth the rate of iron transfer across the placenta increases. Thus transport of iron from mother to fetus is greatest during the last few months of gestation (up to 4 mg/day at term). Serum iron and ferritin levels in cord blood are higher than in maternal blood and have been related to maternal hemoglobin or ferritin in most but not all studies.[2,70,88] Cord blood serum ferritin levels are lower (but usually still within normal limits) in infants of iron-deficient mothers, reflecting lower fetal iron stores. These infants are reported to have reduced iron stores and an increased risk of anemia in the first year.[2,43,111]

Fetal Oxygenation and Growth

Increased levels of 2,3-DPG in the pregnant woman shift her oxygen-hemoglobin dissociation curve to the right (see Chapter 9). This reduces the affinity of maternal hemoglobin for oxygen, favors release of oxygen in the intervillous space, and facilitates transfer to the fetus. Alterations in placental function that occur with maternal disorders such as preeclampsia, chronic renal disease, diabetes, and severe anemia can decrease oxygen transfer across the placenta. The fetus may develop chronic hypoxia, with stimulation of EPO production, increased erythropoiesis, polycythemia, and increased neonatal morbidity. Poorer fetal growth and an increased placenta-to-birth weight ratio is reported in women with iron deficiency anemia.[77]

Severe Anemia and Pregnancy

The most common anemias encountered in pregnancy are iron deficiency anemia, megaloblastic anemia of pregnancy (folic acid deficiency), sickle cell disorders, and β-thalassemia.[63] Anemias caused by iron or folate deficiency are due to underproduction of RBCs and are associated with decreased reticulocytes. The normal hematologic changes along with altered nutritional needs during pregnancy increase the risk for these nutritional anemias. Sickle cell anemia and β-thalassemia are caused by increased RBC destruction and loss and thus are associated with increased reticulocytes in the peripheral blood.[63] Changes in the hematologic system may influence the course of these disorders during pregnancy and alter fetal outcome.

In women with severe anemia (hemoglobin less than 6 to 8 mg/dl), maternal arterial oxygen content and oxygen delivery to the fetus are decreased. The fetus attempts to adapt through increased uterine and fetal blood flow, redistribution of blood within the fetal organs, increased RBC production (to increase the total oxygen-carrying capacity), and a decrease in the diffusing distance for oxygen across the placenta.[18]

Because fetuses have predominantly fetal hemoglobin, they cannot readily increase the availability of oxygen to the tissues by further altering the affinity of hemoglobin for oxygen. Although the fetus adapts, the cost may be high, with decreased growth and an increased mortality due to the lack of an adequate oxygen supply and nutrients.[21] Severe maternal anemia (especially with a maternal PaO_2 less than 70 torr) has also been associated with congenital anomalies, low birth weight, and preterm birth and placental hyperplasia (more than 900 g), perhaps as a compensatory response to fetal anoxia.[18,106,107,138]

Iron Deficiency Anemia

The most common cause of anemia during pregnancy is iron deficiency anemia.[111] Generally this form of anemia is preventable or easily treated with iron supplements. Hematologic changes in pregnancy can make diagnosis of iron deficiency difficult.[63] Total iron binding capacity and serum iron often fall during pregnancy, as well as with iron deficiency anemia. A useful test for iron deficiency in the pregnant woman is serum ferritin levels, which correlate well with iron stores during pregnancy.[18,63] Serum ferritin levels lower than 12 μg/L with a low hemoglobin indicate iron deficiency, which can be treated with ferrous sulfate until the hemoglobin returns to levels normal for the stage of gestation.[93]

In general, even with significant maternal iron deficiency, the fetus will often be protected and receive adequate stores at cost to the mother. If the mother is severely iron deficient and anemic, the fetus may be affected with decreased RBC volume, hemoglobin, iron stores, and cord ferritin levels and increased risk of iron deficiency in infancy.[6,7,39,63] Maternal hemoglobin levels of less than 10.4 g/dl are associated with a risk of low birth weight and preterm infants and increased perinatal mortality.[2,93,107,136] Maternal anemia before midpregnancy has been associated with an increased risk of preterm birth.[168,203]

Megaloblastic Anemia

Megaloblastic anemia in the nonpregnant woman is usually due to folic acid or vitamin B_{12} deficiency. Folic acid deficiency is the most common cause of megaloblastic anemia encountered during pregnancy.[63] Vitamin B_{12} deficiency with pregnancy is rare because: (1) stores of vitamin B_{12} are normally large (most women have a 2- to 3-year store in their liver), so deficient states take years to develop; (2) vitamin B_{12} is used for chromosome replication, so a deficiency usually leads to infertility; and (3) vitamin B_{12} deficiency is usually due to pernicious anemia, a disorder seen primarily in older women.[63] Vitamin B_{12} deficiency in pregnancy most often occurs with a vegan diet. Vitamin B_{12} deficiency may be misdiagnosed in a pregnant woman, since serum vitamin B_{12} levels fall with the expanded plasma volume and consequent hemodilution. In addition, the alterations in plasma proteins during pregnancy interfere with vitamin B_{12} assays.[63]

Folate demands increase threefold during pregnancy. Since folic acid is essential for DNA synthesis and cell duplication, folate is needed for growth of the fetus and placenta as well as for maternal RBC production.[111] Folate requirements increase throughout pregnancy and are higher in multiple pregnancy.[63] Maternal serum folate levels fall during pregnancy, and women with an inadequate dietary intake need supplements. The recommended dietary intake of folate in pregnancy is 600 μg of dietary folate equivalent per day.[13] The changes in folate metabolism during pregnancy are due to decreased serum folate and RBCs, increased plasma clearance, increased urinary excretion, and altered histidine metabolism.[133]

Severe folic acid deficiency has been associated with fetal malformations, preeclampsia, abruptio placentae, prematurity, and low birth weight, although the causal association between these events is questionable.[63] Maternal folate deficiency increases the risk of neural tube defects (NTDs).[38,50,133] Supplementation is recommended for all women of childbearing age. Supplementation should begin prior to pregnancy since NTDs occur early in the first trimester (see Chapter 14). Later in pregnancy, the fetus has higher levels of folate and elevated folate-binding protein, which protects against fetal folate deficiency; even with low maternal folate levels, neonatal cord levels are usually within normal limits.

Sickle Cell Anemia

Sickle cell anemia is a disorder of beta-chain structure of the hemoglobin molecule. A woman with sickle cell anemia normally has a lower hemoglobin level (7 to 8 g/dl) and oxygen-carrying capacities, to which her system has adjusted. Pregnancy places both the woman and her infant at greater risk for complications. As plasma volume increases during pregnancy, the woman may become slightly more anemic. In addition, she often experiences an increase in frequency and severity of sickling attacks. Sickle cell crises are triggered by physical or emotional stress, which may be caused by infection, trauma, hypoxia, and pregnancy. Crises in pregnancy may be related to the hypercoagulable state, increased susceptibility to infection, or vascular stress.[156] The rapid hemodynamic changes postpartum will often precipitate crises, especially if associated with a long or difficult labor and delivery.[106]

In women with sickle cell anemia, tissue deoxygenation or acidosis triggers structural changes in the sickle hemoglobin (HbS), so the RBCs take on a half-moon or sickle appearance. The sickled cells can obstruct blood flow in the microvasculature. The areas most susceptible to obstruction are those characterized by slow flow and high oxygen extraction such as the spleen, bone marrow, and placenta. Obstruction leads to venous stasis, further deoxygenation, platelet aggregation, hypoxia, acidosis, further sickling, and eventually infarction.[63,106]

Fetal and neonatal mortality are increased, with a higher incidence of prematurity, stillbirth, intrauterine growth restriction (IUGR), and neonatal death. The increased fetal wastage is due to placental infarction and fetal hypoxia. Fetal hypoxia results from decreased oxygen transport due to the abnormal biochemistry of the maternal hemoglobin and the loss of functional placental tissue for gas and nutrient exchange caused by infarctions associated with maternal sickling crises.[63,106]

β-Thalassemia

Thalassemia is a disorder in the synthesis of either the alpha or beta peptide chains of the hemoglobin molecule. This leads to alterations in the RBC membrane and decreased RBC life span. β-Thalassemia minor is the most frequently encountered thalassemia during pregnancy. Females with thalassemia major (Cooley anemia) usually die in childhood or adolescence; those who survive are often amenorrheic and infertile.[63,106,156]

Women with β-thalassemia minor are mildly anemic but generally healthy otherwise. There is controversy as to whether or not this disorder is associated with increased maternal or infant morbidity.[63] Laboratory values normally associated with β-thalassemia minor, which indicate a mild hypochromic microcytic anemia, may lead to the diagnosis of iron deficiency. Parenteral iron supplementation therapy is potentially dangerous in that β-thalassemia is associated with increased iron absorption and storage and a susceptibility to iron overload. Iron therapy can increase morbidity in these women unless a true iron deficiency

state (as diagnosed by bone marrow aspiration) is present.[63] However, Letsky has noted that oral iron supplementation during pregnancy is not necessarily contraindicated in all women with β-thalassemia minor.[11]

Thromboembolism and Pregnancy

The hypercoagulable state of pregnancy is crucial in protecting the mother against excessive blood loss with delivery and placental separation. However, the hypercoagulable state is also a disadvantage because it significantly increases the risk of thromboembolic disorders (TEDs) during pregnancy and postpartum.

The risk of TED increases up to sixfold during pregnancy (0.6 to 3 in 1000 pregnant women).[54] TED is the greatest single cause of maternal mortality in developed countries.[71] The risk increases with parity and age and is 3 to 16 times higher among women with cesarean than among those with vaginal births. Pulmonary embolism occurs in 1 in 2000 pregnancies and is a major cause of maternal mortality.[84] Pulmonary emboli usually result from dislodged deep venous thrombi in the lower extremities.

The three factors (Virchow triad) that predispose to thromboembolic disorders (stasis, altered coagulation, and vascular damage) are all present or potentially present during pregnancy.[80] During pregnancy, increased venous capacitance leads to increased distensibility, decreased flow in the lower extremities, and venous stasis. By late pregnancy the velocity of venous blood flow in the lower extremities has been reduced by half, and venous pressure has risen an average of 10 mmHg.[84] The blood flow velocity decreases by early in the second trimester, with a nadir from 34 weeks to term that does not return to prepregnant values until 6 or more weeks after delivery. In addition, the diameter of the major leg veins increases, more so on the left than the right. During pregnancy, 85% of deep vein thromboses occur on the left (versus 55% in nonpregnant women).[11] This is because of compression of the left iliac vein by the right iliac and ovarian veins.[11,17] About two thirds of TEDs occurs during the antepartum period, and one third postpartum.[17]

The hypercoagulable state during pregnancy increases the risk of clot formation. If a clot develops, the decreased fibrinolytic activity impedes fibrin removal and clot lysis. An increase in the incidence of TEDs is seen during the third trimester, when fibrinolytic activity decreases. Finally, the potential for localized vascular damage and release of tissue thromboplastin exists with delivery and particularly with cesarean section. Thus the risk of TED is higher in women following surgical intervention. TED is also increased with obesity and with increased parity and maternal age.[71] Once a thrombus develops, it is more likely that it will extend if the predisposing factors persist over time, as occurs with pregnancy.

Women with a history of a TED either prior to or during pregnancy have an increased risk of developing a similar disorder in subsequent pregnancies. Women with a history of TED during a previous pregnancy have a recurrence risk of 5% to 30%.[54,174] Other women at increased risk are those with anemia, artificial heart valves, or PIH (due to exaggeration of the hypercoagulable state) and those who undergo operative deliveries. Ambulation soon after delivery decreases venous stasis and the risk of TED.

Pregnant women with TEDs present with a clinical dilemma in terms of treatment. Coumarin derivatives (warfarin sulfate) inhibit vitamin K–dependent coagulation factors. These agents cross the placenta, whereas vitamin K–dependent coagulation factors do not, impairing fetal coagulation and increasing the risk of fetal and neonatal hemorrhage.[132,174] The risk of fetal bleeding and intracranial hemorrhage is especially high during labor. Warfarin has been associated with an increased risk of abortion and with a specific syndrome of fetal anomalies, involving the face, eyes, bones, and central nervous system, if given in the first 11 to 13 weeks of gestation.[80] These abnormalities may be due to inhibition of vitamin K–dependent proteins (osteocalcins) involved in bone development.

Heparin is considered the drug of choice for TED in pregnancy because its molecular weight prevents placental transfer or excretion in breast milk.[174] Heparin is more costly and difficult to regulate than other anticoagulants and is associated with complications such as maternal osteoporosis, thrombocytopenia, and hemorrhage and an increased incidence of prematurity and stillbirth. If used on an outpatient basis, heparin must be self-administered via subcutaneous injections.[49] The newer low-molecular-weight heparin (LMWH) has the advantages of more predictable anticoagulant properties, fewer side effects, longer half-life, and increased bioavailability, so it can be administered once a day rather than more frequently.[64,80,143] LMWH is produced by enzymatic or chemical breakdown of the heparin molecule. Although LMWH is a shorter and lighter molecule, it is still too large to cross the placenta.[143] LMWH is not yet licensed for use in pregnancy, although use has been reported.[143] In addition, there are several ongoing clinical trials of use with women at risk for TED.

Heparin doses often need to be increased as pregnancy progresses, particularly during the third trimester. Changes in heparin requirements have been related to increasing plasma volume and renal clearance and to the presence of a placental heparinase enzyme. Heparin doses may need to be decreased in women who develop significant alterations in renal function or in whom plasma volume changes are reduced.[54,132]

Heparin treatment is usually stopped during labor and delivery, then resumed in the early postpartum period. An alternative approach is to use heparin during the first trimester and late third trimester, switching to warfarin in the intervening interval. This approach is often used with women who have artificial heart valves or mitral valve disease, conditions associated with a significant risk of arterial emboli, for which heparin is often not an effective anticoagulant.[54] Warfarin control is often more difficult during pregnancy because of the increase in plasma volume and changes in hemostasis.[80] It is also used during the postpartum period. Warfarin is excreted in breast milk in very small amounts. Although many feel that with careful monitoring the use of warfarin by women who are breast-feeding is safe, this is an area of controversy.[80]

Coagulopathies during Pregnancy

Pregnancy is characterized by increases in fibrinolytic activity and plasminogen, plasminogen activators in the uterus, and an ongoing low-grade activation of the coagulation system within the uteroplacental circulation. As a result, events such as extravasation of blood into the myometrium or rupture of blood vessels in the area can activate the fibrinolytic system and lead to a consumptive coagulopathy.[16] The risk of coagulopathies such as DIC is higher during pregnancy, particularly in association with abruptio placentae, preeclampsia, intrauterine fetal death, amniotic fluid embolism, and septic abortion.[11,53,168] These events result in one or more of the processes commonly associated with intravascular coagulation: release of tissue thromboplastin, endothelial injury, or shock and stasis.[11] Many of these complications trigger the formation of tissue thromboplastin or endotoxin, thus inducing thrombin formation.[168] The resulting activation of the coagulation pathway (see Figure 7-5) leads to depletion of fibrinogen and increased fibrinolytic activity.[84]

DIC arises from inappropriate activation of normal clotting processes within the circulation with intravascular consumption of procoagulant proteins, clotting factors and platelets, formation of fibrin clots within the vascular bed, and activation of fibrinolysis. As a result, the normal balance between the coagulation and fibrinolytic systems is disrupted.[11] Consumption of the clotting factors can lead to hemorrhage and shock. As clots are formed and fibrin is deposited in the microcirculation, further cell (tissue) injury may occur, triggering further coagulation and eventual depletion of plasma clotting factors. These fibrin clots may also cause intravascular obstruction and infarction. Activation of clotting also activates the fibrinolytic system, which leads to formation of fibrin-fibrinogen degradation products (FDP) or fibrin split products (FSP). These

TABLE 7-6 Recommendations for Clinical Practice Related to Changes in the Hematologic System of Pregnant Women

Recognize usual hematologic values and patterns of change during pregnancy and postpartum (pp. 216-225 and Tables 7-1 to 7-4).

Recognize that isolated laboratory values must be evaluated in light of clinical findings and previous values (pp. 216-225 and Table 7-1).

Assess maternal nutritional status in relation to iron, folate, and vitamins, and provide nutritional counseling (pp. 225-227).

Monitor hematocrit and hemoglobin values throughout pregnancy (pp. 216-217, 225-227).

Know the patterns of change in plasma and blood volume during pregnancy and the postpartum period (pp. 213-216, 223-224).

Monitor and counsel women with cardiac problems, paying particular attention to periods when blood and plasma volume increases significantly (pp. 213-216, 223-224 and Chapter 8).

Monitor women on tocolytic therapy regarding pulmonary edema with particular attention to women with greater increases in plasma volume (p. 215).

Monitor for and teach pregnant woman to recognize the signs of thromboembolism and consumptive coagulopathy (pp. 228-230).

Recognize risk factors for the development of thromboembolism (p. 228).

Ambulate women soon after delivery to reduce the risk of thromboembolism (pp. 228-229).

Recognize risk factors for development of consumptive coagulopathies (p. 229).

Evaluate maternal responses to prescribed drugs for signs of subtherapeutic levels or side effects (p. 219 and Chapter 6).

Counsel women regarding the effects of plasma volume increases and decreased plasma proteins on drug levels during pregnancy (p. 219 and Chapter 6).

Recognize factors that may alter signs of infection during the intrapartum and early postpartum period (pp. 223, 225).

Note the timing of cord clamping (pp. 234-236).

fibrin degradation products further inhibit coagulation and decrease platelet function.[22,187]

SUMMARY

The hematologic and hemostatic systems undergo significant alterations during pregnancy that promote maternal adaptation but also influence interpretation of laboratory values and increase the risk of thromboembolic insults and coagulopathies. Because of the significant risks associated with these events, appropriate measurement, observation, data gathering, and evaluation are essential. Changes in the hematologic system during pregnancy are also critical for fetal homeostasis. Maternal hypervolemia promotes delivery of oxygen and nutrients to the fetus, and changes in albumin concentration may influence the availability of both nutrients and potentially harmful substances. The fetus can, in turn, affect maternal status, as is the case with iron metabolism and needs. Clinical recommendations for nurses working with pregnant women based on changes in the hematologic system are summarized in Table 7-6.

DEVELOPMENT OF THE HEMATOLOGIC SYSTEM IN THE FETUS

The hematologic system arises early in gestation and along with the primitive cardiovascular system is one of the earliest systems to achieve some functional capacity. The hematologic system is critical for the well-being of the fetus through transport of nutrients and oxygen and removal of waste products. Fetal RBCs, WBCs, and platelets are often found in the maternal circulation. Fetomaternal transfusion occurs in an estimated 50% of pregnancies, although this generally involves a small volume.[26,144] RBCs can pass as early as 4 to 6 weeks. Later, antigens on these cells may stimulate maternal antibody production against the fetal cells, which can lead to fetal anemia, neutropenia, or thrombocytopenia.[32,34]

Formation of Blood Cells

Blood cells develop from stem cells derived from mesenchymal tissues. Stem cells first appear in the yolk sac and at about 6 weeks migrate to the developing liver, thymus, lymph nodes, and bone marrow. Hematopoiesis in the fetus can be divided into three periods: mesoblastic, hepatic, and myeloid (Figure 7-8). In all sites, primitive cells arise first, followed by definitive cells. Embryonic and fetal hematopoietic stem cells are pluripotent cells that can reproduce and repopulate in adults better than adult stem cells. Thus these fetal cells have greater potential for transplant with lower risk of graft failure.[51,177]

During the mesoblastic period (from 14 to 19 days to a peak at 6 weeks), blood cells are formed in blood islands in the secondary yolk sac. The secondary yolk sac arises at 12 to 15 days and is a site of early protein synthesis, nutrient transfer, and hematopoiesis. Peripheral cells in

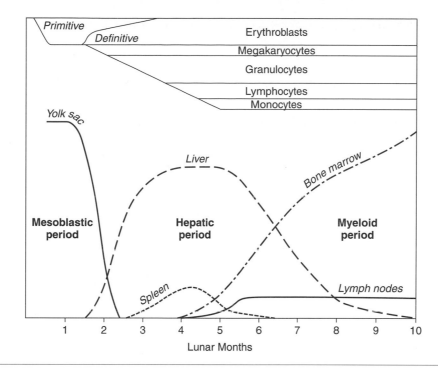

FIGURE **7-8** Stages of hematopoiesis in the embryo and fetus. (From Wintrobe, M. [1981]. *Clinical hematology* [8th ed.]. Philadelphia: Lea & Febiger.)

these islands form primitive blood vessels; central cells develop into hematoblasts (primitive RBCs).[150] Although only RBCs and macrophages are produced in the yolk sac, the yolk sac stem cells are all multipotential.[53,82] Blood formation in the yolk sac disappears by the third month.[127,55] Another site of early blood formation during this period is the ventral aspect of the aorta in the periumbilical area. Hematopoiesis occurs in this area until about 40 days.[182]

The hepatic period begins during the fifth to sixth week, immediately after the onset of circulation during weeks 4 to 5. This period peaks from 6 to 18 weeks. Thus, from 3 to 5 months the liver is the major source of fetal blood cells, although some blood formation continues in this site through the first week after birth. Liver mass increases 40-fold after liver hematopoiesis begins, and at 11 to 12 weeks, hematopoietic cells make up 60% of the liver.[51] The predominant cells produced by the liver are normoblastic erythrocytes, although megakaryocytes, granulocytes, and lymphocytes are also produced. Hematopoiesis can be detected in the spleen and thymus during the third month and shortly thereafter in the lymph nodes. Blood formation in the spleen, initially producing erythrocytes and later lymphocytes, declines after 4 to 5 months.[202]

The thymus and lymph nodes become seeded with stem cells by the fourth month.[167] These structures are primarily involved in lymphopoiesis but are also involved in maturation and activation of the immature WBCs that develop from myeloid stem cells.[150,167]

The myeloid period begins at about 8 weeks, with eventual production of all types of blood cells.[51] The bone marrow is the major site for blood production after 6 months' gestation. Centers for blood formation arise in mesenchymal tissues and invade cavities produced during bone formation (see Chapter 16). Initially bone marrow produces granulocytes and megakaryocytes. After liver erythropoiesis declines, bone marrow erythropoiesis increases. The major area of blood production is the fatty marrow in the core of the long bones. Large fat cells are not found in fetal marrow as they are in adults, suggesting that fetal marrow is functioning at full hematopoietic capacity.

The long bones of the fetus and newborn are cartilaginous, and their relative marrow volume is smaller than in older individuals. As a result, the only way the fetus or newborn can significantly increase production of blood cells is by either reactivation or persistence of extramedullary hematopoiesis in the abdominal viscera, such as the liver and spleen. This extramedullary erythropoiesis is responsible for much of the hepatosplenomegaly seen in infants with erythroblastosis fetalis.[61]

Fetal and postbirth hematopoiesis are mediated by hematopoietic growth factors and cytokines, including stem cell factors, interleukin-3 (IL-3), EPO, macrophage colony stimulating factor (M-CSF), granulocyte-colony stimulating factor (G-CSF), thrombopoietin, and possibly insulin and insulin-like growth factor (Figure 7-9).[51,175] During fetal life the placenta is a source of cytokines. These cytokines probably play a role in growth and maturation of many tissues, including those of the gut, eye, and kidneys.[60] Hematopoietic growth factors are either non–cell-lineage or cell-lineage specific. Non–cell-lineage-specific growth factors—such as IL-3 and granulocyte-macrophage colony stimulating factor (GM-CSF)—stimulate a variety of progenitor cells. Cell-lineage-specific growth factors stimulate differential maturation of granulocytes (G-CSF), monocytes (M-CSF) or erythrocytes (EPO).[100,165,197] G-CSF and M-CSF are being

evaluated for treatment of neonatal sepsis; EPO is being evaluated for treatment of anemia of prematurity. EPO and other growth factors also appear to be important in development of other systems (including cardiovascular, gastrointestinal, and brain) both before and after birth.[98]

Development of Red Blood Cells

Fetal RBC production is independent of the mother.[146] The initial RBCs are primitive nucleated megaloblasts that appear at 3 to 4 weeks, followed by normative megaloblastic erythropoiesis at 6 weeks. The primitive cells contain embryonic hemoglobin and are not dependent on EPO. The definitive fetal RBC contains primarily HbF and is regulated by EPO.[51,52] By 10 weeks the latter cells constitute 90% of the RBC volume. The early cells are large nucleated cells with increased deformability. With increasing gestation, hemoglobin, hematocrit, and total RBC count increase, whereas the number of nucleated RBCs, MCV, cell diame-

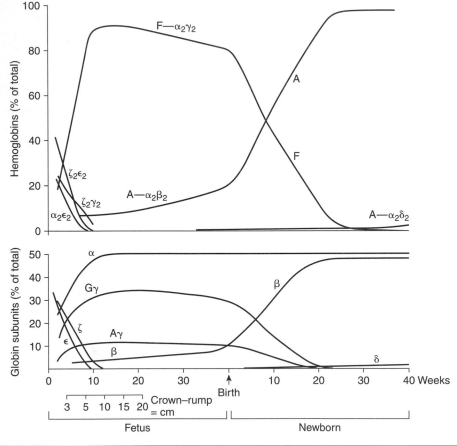

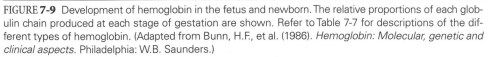

FIGURE 7-9 Development of hemoglobin in the fetus and newborn. The relative proportions of each globulin chain produced at each stage of gestation are shown. Refer to Table 7-7 for descriptions of the different types of hemoglobin. (Adapted from Bunn, H.F., et al. (1986). *Hemoglobin: Molecular, genetic and clinical aspects*. Philadelphia: W.B. Saunders.)

ter, MCHV, reticulocytes, and proportion of immature cell forms decrease.[150]

EPO does not cross the placenta, so fetal erythropoiesis is endogenously controlled.[146,194] Fetal EPO increases from 19 weeks to term and is produced primarily in the liver rather than in the kidneys, with increasing amounts from the kidneys from 20 weeks to term associated with renal maturation.[49,104,146,152] It is not clear what causes the shift from liver to renal EPO production.[74] From 32 weeks on, and perhaps earlier, the fetus reacts to hypoxia with increased EPO production.[150]

EPO inhibits the death of erythroid precursors and stimulates development and differentiation of these precursors. EPO levels are elevated with fetal hypoxia, anemia and placental insufficiency and in infants of insulin-dependent diabetic women.[51]

Development of White Blood Cells and Platelets

Formation of WBCs begins in the liver at 5 to 7 weeks, followed by the spleen (8 weeks), thymus (10 weeks), and lymph nodes (12 weeks). Significant numbers are not produced until the myeloid period. Initially erythropoiesis is greater than granulopoiesis; however, by 10 to 12 weeks granulopoiesis predominates, and by 21 weeks the adult ratio of granulopoiesis to erythropoiesis is seen.[202] Circulating granulocytes increase rapidly during the third trimester. At birth, numbers of WBCs are equal to or greater than those found in adults. Eosinophils appear by 10 weeks, increasing to 5% of total marrow cells by 21 weeks. Basophils also appear by 10 weeks, but levels remain low. Macrophage levels peak at 10 to 16 weeks; monocyte levels peak by 12 to 16 weeks.[202]

T lymphocytes can be detected by 7 weeks and B lymphocytes by 8 weeks. Lymphocytes are formed in the fetal liver and lymphoid plexuses initially, then in the thymus (7 to 10 weeks) and spleen and bone marrow (10 to 12 weeks).[98] The numbers of circulating lymphocytes increase rapidly to peak at 20 weeks (10,000 mm^3), then decline to 3000/mm^3 by term.[150] Megakaryocytes are found at 5 to 6 weeks in the yolk sac and by 8 weeks in the liver and circulation. Platelets increase from a mean of 187,000/mm^3 at 15 weeks to a mean of 274,000 by term.[186]

Formation of Hemoglobin

Hemoglobin synthesis begins around 14 days. Several forms of hemoglobin (Hb) are found in the embryo and fetus (see Figure 7-9). All forms have two alpha or alpha-like globulin chains (controlled by genes on chromosome 16) and two beta-like globulin chains (controlled by genes on chromosome 11). Two pairs of polypeptide chains form the different hemoglobin forms (Table 7-7). The primitive embryonic varieties formed in the yolk sac are Gower 1 (seen at less than 5 weeks' gestational age), followed by Gower 2 and Hb Portland (seen between 5 and 10 to 12 weeks).[51,152] The predominant hemoglobin from 10 to 12 weeks to term is HbF, which consists of a pair of alpha chains and a pair of gamma chains. Adult hemoglobin (HbA), which consists of pairs of alpha and beta chains, appears after 6 to 8 weeks and increases rapidly after 16 to 20 weeks.[159] By 30 to 32 weeks, 90% to 95% of the hemoglobin is HbF. After this point, the amount of HbF begins to slowly decline to 84% at 34 weeks and 60% to 80% by term.[157] Simultaneously, levels of HbA increase along with the total body hemoglobin mass.[150] The switch from fetal to adult hemoglobin synthesis is related to postconceptional, not postbirth, age. Synthesis of HbA and HbF is not significantly affected by intrauterine transfusions or exchange transfusions after birth.

All forms of hemoglobin have similar functions but vary in their oxygen affinity.[51] HbF has a greater affinity for oxygen because HbF does not bind 2,3-DPG as effectively as does HbA. Increased affinity facilitates oxygen transfer

TABLE 7-7 Human Hemoglobins Expressed during Development

Hemoglobin (Hb)	Globulin Chain Composition	Stage of Expression	Primary Site of Production
Hb Gower 1	Zeta$_2$ epsilon$_2$	Embryonic	Yolk sac
Hb Gower 2	Alpha$_1$ epsilon$_2$	Embryonic	Yolk sac
Hb Portland	Zeta$_2$ gamma$_2$	Embryonic	Yolk sac
HbF	Alpha$_2$ ^{A} gamma$_2$ or alpha$_2$^{G} gamma$_2$	Fetal	Liver
HbA$_2$	Alpha$_2$ delta$_2$	Adult	Bone marrow
HbA	Alpha$_2$ beta$_2$	Adult	Bone marrow

From Luchtman-Jones, L., Schwartz, A.L. & Wilson, D.B. (1997). Hematological problems in the fetus and neonate. In A.A. Fanaroff & R.J. Martin (Eds.). *Neonatal-perinatal medicine: Diseases of the fetus and infant* (6th ed.). St. Louis: Mosby.

across the placenta but reduces oxygen release to the tissues. Fetal hemoglobin has several other unique properties. HbF is more resistant to acid elution and can be oxidized to methemoglobin more readily, increasing the susceptibility of newborns to methemoglobinemia.

The resistance of fetal hemoglobin to acid elution is the basis for tests such as the Kleihauer-Betke techniques used to detect fetal cells in maternal blood. These tests may be unreliable as a measure of fetal cells if maternal HbF is elevated or with ABO incompatibility. In the presence of ABO incompatibility, fetal cells may be destroyed by maternal antibody and cleared from the mother's circulation. Altered levels of HbF are seen in women with sickle cell anemia, thalassemia minor, hydatidiform mole, and leukemia and in a pregnancy-induced elevation of HbF. Fetal cells may still be identified, since with elevated maternal HbF there tend to be many cells with varying amounts of HbF and the fewer fetal cells have consistently high HbF concentrations.[61]

Development of the Hemostatic System

The hemostatic and fibrinolytic systems develop simultaneously. Most coagulation proteins are present in measurable quantities by 5 to 10 weeks' gestation.[67] Fetal blood demonstrates clotting ability by 11 to 12 weeks.[84] Fibrinogen synthesis in the liver begins at 5 weeks. Fibrinogen can be found in the plasma by 12 to 13 weeks, reaching adult values by 30 weeks.[179] The placenta is rich in tissue thromboplastin and is thus able to respond rapidly to insults with initiation of the clotting cascade.[84] This helps to protect the fetus from significant blood loss. Vitamin K levels are 30% of adult values by the end of the second trimester and 50% by term.[179]

Fibrinolytic activity can also be demonstrated at 12 to 13 weeks. The whole blood clotting time in the fetus is relatively short, and the fetus is in a hypercoagulable state during the first and second trimesters. Fibrinolytic activity in the fetus is increased even though levels of blood plasminogen are low, due to increased tissue plasminogen activator (tPA) or decreased inhibitor or both.[84] The elevated fibrinolytic activity may help to protect and maintain the extensive fetal capillary circulation within the placental villi.

NEONATAL PHYSIOLOGY

The neonate experiences significant alterations in the hematologic system and hemostasis. Among the more striking differences are the structural and functional alterations in the neonatal RBC and the potential impact of HbF on oxygen delivery to the tissues. Variations are also seen in blood volume and blood cellular components and in hemostasis parameters. These alterations increase the risk for anemia, thromboembolism, and coagulopathies in the neonate.

Transitional Events

A major transitional event for the neonate is removal of the placental circulation with clamping of the umbilical cord. The timing of umbilical cord clamping influences the amount of placental transfusion and subsequent plasma and RBC volume of the neonate. At term, fetal blood volume is approximately 70 to 80 ml/kg and placental blood volume 45 ml/kg of fetal weight.[115] At 30 weeks, about 50% of this volume is in the fetal circulation, increasing to two thirds by term.[192] Blood volume in normal neonates is around 90 ml/kg, varying from 80 to 100 ml/kg depending on the direction and magnitude of blood transfer between the fetus and placenta at birth.[114,150,192]

The umbilical arteries constrict at birth in response to the increasing PaO_2. Therefore blood does not flow from the infant into the placenta via these vessels. The umbilical vein remains dilated, however, so blood flows from the placenta to the infant via gravity.[41,206] If the newly delivered infant is kept at or below the level of the placenta, transfer of blood from the placenta to the fetus will occur during the first 3 minutes after birth. If the newborn is significantly elevated above the placenta, blood in the umbilical vein can flow back into the placenta.[41]

The timing of cord clamping and the position of the infant in relation to the placenta influence placental transfusion. Yao and Lind reported that if the infant's position was maintained at the level of the introitus (± 10 cm) until the cord was clamped, or held 40 cm below the introitus for no more than 30 seconds, the infant received a placental transfusion of approximately 80 ml.[199,201] The amount of placental transfusion was negligible if the infant was held 50 to 60 cm above the introitus.

With the infant held at the level of the introitus or slightly below, if the cord is clamped 30 to 60 seconds after delivery, placental transfusion increases the newborn's blood volume by 15% to 20%; clamping at 60 to 90 seconds results in a 25% increase; and clamping at 3 minutes produces a 50% to 60% increase.[114,199,301] No disadvantage was found for term infants placed on the mother's abdomen with delay of clamping until cessation of pulsations ("intermediate" transfusion).[115]

There is little consensus on when to clamp the umbilical cord. Early (before 30 to 40 seconds) versus late (after 3 minutes) clamping can result in a 30% difference in blood volume and RBC mass.[153,192] A recent survey of nurse-midwifery practice examined early (before 1 minute and primarily immediately), intermediate (between 1 and 3 minutes), and late (after 3 minutes or cessation of cord pulsation) clamping in healthy and distressed newborns.[134] The reported practices with healthy newborns were 26.1% early, 35% intermediate, and 33.1% late clamping; for distressed newborns, early clamping was the predominant (89%) practice. About 87% of the nurse-midwives surveyed placed the infant on the mother's abdomen after delivery.[134]

The timing at which the umbilical cord is clamped and the magnitude of placental transfusion have physiologic and clinical effects on many body systems. The significance of these changes in healthy infants is unclear; however, concerns have recently been raised that cords are being clamped too early, depriving infants of blood that has an important role in opening the lungs, increasing pulmonary perfusion,

enhancing lung fluid clearance, and improving oxygen delivery to the infant's tissues.[135,137,192] Potential benefits of later rather than immediate cord clamping have recently been described.[95,137,140,141,142,191,192,201] Mercer and Skovgaard note that early cord clamping may interfere with completion of normal physiologic transition at birth, resulting in a 25% to 30% decrease in blood volume.[135] Table 7-8 summarizes the effects on infants of placental transfusion with late versus early clamping. Late clamping is associated with increased initial total blood volume, which may be important for initial transition. However, by 3 days after birth, differences in blood volume between early- and late-clamped infants are actually slight as a result of the usual fluid shifts

TABLE **7-8** **Effects of Placental Transfusion on Neonatal Adaptation after Birth**

Alteration	Late or Early Clamping*	Basis for Change
VOLUME EFFECTS		
↑ Atrial pressure	Late	Increased blood volume; may enhance closure of fetal shunts or lead to transient excess volume
↑ Systolic blood pressure	Late	Increased blood volume; may enhance cardiovascular transition or lead to transient excess volume
↑ Central venous pressure	Late	Increased blood volume; may enhance cardiovascular transition or lead to transient excess volume
↑ Pulmonary artery pressure	Late	↑ Pulmonary vascular resistance as a result of distention of pulmonary capillary-venous bed; may enhance cardiopulmonary transition
↓ Peripheral blood flow	Early	↓ Volume and compensatory mechanisms
↑ Effective renal blood flow and urinary output	Late	↑ Glomerular filtration rate as a result of systolic BP changes
Hypovolemia	Early	↓ Blood volume; altered cardiopulmonary transition; ↓ oxygen-carrying capacity
EFFECTS ON HEMATOCRIT		
↑ Hematocrit	Late	RBC volume; may enhance oxygen-carrying capacity or lead to risk of transient polycythemia or hyperbilirubinemia
Transient polycythemia	Late	↑ RBC volume; hemoconcentration in first 24 or so hours because of compensatory fluid shifts
↓ Hematocrit	Early	↓ RBC volume and oxygen-carrying capacity
↓ Iron stores	Early	↓ RBCs, less iron from degraded RBCs
RESPIRATORY EFFECTS		
↓ Pulmonary blood flow	Early	Inadequate filling of pulmonary vascular system, limiting lung expansion and thus ↓ oxygen supply
↓ Lung compliance (first 6 hours)	Late	Higher cardiac load and pulmonary and capillary filling
↑ PaO$_2$, PCO$_2$	Early	↓ Transudation of fluid at alveolar-capillary interface
↑ PaO$_2$	Late	Enhanced oxygen carrying capacity and cardiopulmonary transition
↑ Respiratory distress syndrome (?)	Late	↓ Lung compliance and ↓ FRC
↓ Respiratory distress syndrome (?)	Late	Improved oxygen carrying capacity

Data compiled from references 73,95,105,115,130,135,137,140,141,142, 153,191,192, and 201.
*Definitions of late versus early clamping varied among studies reported.
BP, Blood pressure; *FRC,* functional residual capacity; *RBC,* red blood cell.

after birth with a decrease in plasma volume.[150] Papagno noted that late clamping or clamping after cessation of pulsation was associated with a transient polycythemia peaking at up to 12 hours after birth, with a return to normal ranges by 24 to 36 hours. No adverse effects of this transient polycythemia were noted.[153] Iron stores at 3 months of age are not influenced by the timing of cord clamping.[73]

In preterm infants, early cord clamping has often been recommended because of concerns about hyperbilirubinemia, due to the increased volume of RBCs, and respiratory distress. Respiratory distress may result from movement of excess plasma volume that cannot be accommodated in the vascular compartment into extravascular spaces, including areas around the lungs, with a decrease in lung compliance and functional residual capacity.[114] However, if these infants' cords are clamped too early, they may be hypovolemic, with reduction in RBCs and thus decreased oxygen-carrying capacity, oxygen delivery, and pulmonary blood flow, limiting lung expansion.[192] Wardrop argues for optimizing placentofetal transfusion in preterm infants in order to enhance lung expansion, reduce need for later transfusions and thus blood donor exposure, and increase autologous stem cells (especially rich in blood of infants 25 to 31 weeks of age), which have long-term hematologic and immunologic benefits.[192] Recent studies suggest that there may be benefits to avoiding immediate cord clamping in preterm infants.[95,105,130,142] For example, Kinmond et al. compared immediate cord clamping of preterm infants with clamping that employed a 30-second delay, holding the infant 20 cm below the introitus.[105] The infants with the delayed clamping had increased pack cell volume and no differences in blood pressure or peak bilirubin levels, required fewer transfusions, and had higher arterial-alveolar oxygen tension ratios, suggesting a decrease in right-to-left shunting.

There are groups of infants for whom increased placental transfusion may not be warranted and for whom very late cord clamping or milking of the cord is questioned. For example, hydropic infants are already fluid overloaded and may not tolerate additional volume. Placental transfusion in the erythroblastotic infant may increase the load of maternal antibodies, which destroy fetal and neonatal RBCs. Even though these infants are often anemic, administration of packed cells after birth may be more appropriate than attempting to increase RBCs by placental transfusion. Earlier clamping may also be appropriate for infants at risk for polycythemia, such as infants of diabetic mothers (IDM) or severely growth-retarded infants. With multiple births, early cord clamping of the first infant is recommended to protect the unborn fetuses because the circulations of these infants may communicate via the placenta. Earlier clamping may also be warranted in the severely asphyxiated infant so that resuscitative efforts can be initiated promptly; however, in these infants, hypovolemia and reductions in their oxygen-carrying capacity must also be avoided.

Changes in Hematologic Parameters

Hematologic parameters differ in neonates as compared with adults and change rapidly during the first week after birth. Considerable variation may be noted between individual infants and within the same infant over time.[206] General values for hematologic parameters in preterm and full-term neonates are summarized in Table 7-9. Values for

TABLE **7-9** Normal Hematologic Values in Newborns

Value	Gestational Age (Weeks) 28	34	Full-Term Cord Blood	Day 1	Day 3	Day 7	Day 14
Hb (g/dl)	14.5	15.0	16.8	18.4	17.8	17.0	16.8
Hematocrit (%)	45	47	53	58	55	54	52
Red blood cells (mm³)	4.0	4.4	5.25	5.8	5.6	5.2	5.1
MCV (μ³)	120	118	107	108	99	98	96
MCH (pg)	40	38	34	35	33	32.5	31.5
MCHC (%)	31	32	31.7	32.5	33	33	33
Reticulocytes (%)	5-10	3-10	3-7	3-7	1-3	0-1	0-1
Platelets (1000s/mm³)			290	192	213	248	252

From Klaus, M.H. & Fanaroff, A.A. (2001). *Care of the high risk neonate* (5th ed.). Philadelphia: W.B. Saunders.
MCH, Mean corpuscular hemoglobin; *MCHC,* mean corpuscular hemoglobin concentration; *MCV,* mean corpuscular volume.

infants of varying gestational and postbirth ages can be found in neonatology texts.[10,120]

Blood Volume

Blood volume averages about 80 to 100 ml/kg in term infants and 90 to 105 ml/kg in preterm infants. Variations in blood volume at birth are due primarily to placental transfusion and gestational age. The higher blood volume of the preterm infant is due to increased plasma volume. Plasma volume decreases with gestation.[147]

Red Blood Cells

RBC counts are 4.6 to 5.2 million/mm^3 at birth, increasing by about 500,000 in the initial hours after birth, then falling to around 5.2 million/mm^3 by the end of the first week.[150] Nucleated RBCs are seen in most newborns during the first 24 hours, perhaps as a response to the stresses of delivery, disappearing by 4 days in term infants and by 1 week in most preterm infants. Increased numbers of nucleated RBCs are found in more immature infants (and may persist beyond the first week) and in infants with Down syndrome or congenital anomalies.[150] Nucleated RBCs are also seen in the neonate as an acute stress response to asphyxia, with anemia, and following hemorrhage. In older individuals, these cells are rare and associated with abnormal erythropoiesis.[206] The ESR is decreased in neonates due to alterations in plasma viscosity, protein content, and hematocrit.[127] The RBC of the neonate differs from that of the adult.[127,128,162,169] These differences and their implications are summarized in Table 7-10.

Hemoglobin and Hematocrit

Hemoglobin levels are higher in newborns, ranging from 13.7 to 20.1 g/dl, with most in the 16.6 to 17.5 g/dl range.[150] Hemoglobin levels increase by up to 6 g/dl within the first hours after birth. This increase results from a shift in fluid distribution after birth—with a decrease in plasma volume and a net increase in RBCs—and partially compensates for placental transfusion.[113]

The hemoglobin concentration decreases by the end of the first week to values similar to cord blood levels. Higher hemoglobin levels are seen in infants with severe hypoxia

TABLE 7-10   Characteristics of Neonatal Red Blood Cells and Their Implications

RBC Characteristic	Clinical Implication
Macrocytosis with increased mean cellular diameter and mean corpuscular volume	More susceptible to damage in small capillaries; increased RBC turnover
Increased permeability to sodium and potassium	Increased risk of cell lysis as a result of osmotic changes
Altered enzyme activity with increased glucose utilization	Risk of hypoglycemia, especially in infants with low glucose stores or altered glucose metabolism with a tendency toward polycythemia (i.e., cases of IDM, SGA)
Increased ATP utilization	Higher energy (glucose) needs and oxygen consumption
Decreased survival time (80 to 100 days for term infants and 60 to 80 days for preterm infants versus 35 to 50 days in ELBW infants versus 120 days for adults)	Increased RBC turnover rate; proportionately greater amounts of bilirubin produced
Increased receptor sites for substances such as insulin and digoxin	Insulin receptor sites facilitating increased glucose uptake; digoxin sites contributing to greater tolerance for digoxin
Increased fetal hemoglobin and less adult hemoglobin	Increased affinity of hemoglobin for oxygen with less ready release to tissues
Increased RBC count at birth (4.6 to 5.2 million/mm^3, falling to 3 to 4 million/mm^3 by 2 to 3 months of age)	Increased RBC turnover rate and bilirubin production
Increased phospholipid, cholesterol, and total lipid content	Increased risk of lipid peroxidation and hemolysis (cholesterol may provide protection against hemolysis)
Decreased catalase glutathione peroxidase	Increased susceptibility to oxidative injury and decreased RBC life span
Increased fragility, decreased deformability, and increased variety and frequency of morphologic abnormalities	Increased susceptibility to damage, especially in microcirculation; increased RBC turnover
Increased free intracellular iron	May lead to decreased RBC survival

Data compiled from references 41, 61, 127, 128, and 196.
ATP, Adenosine triphosphate; *ELBW*, extremely low birth weight; *IDM*, infant of a diabetic mother; *RBC*, red blood cell; *SGA*, small for gestational age.

and in some IUGR and postterm infants, possibly as a compensatory mechanism to increase oxygen availability to the tissues. Lower hemoglobin levels are found in preterm infants. An elevation of either the reticulocyte count or the number of nucleated RBCs above normal values in any infant, regardless of the hemoglobin level, suggests a compensatory response and may indicate anemia.[150]

Cord blood at term contains 50% to 80% HbF, 15% to 40% HbA, and less than 1.8% hemoglobin A_2 (a minor normal adult form). A fourth type, Hb Bart (less than 0.5%), is seen in small amounts in some infants. Cord blood hemoglobin levels vary with gestational age.[150] Preterm infants have a greater percentage of HbF than term infants.

HbF does not bind 2,3-DPG as readily as does HbA, shifting the oxygen-hemoglobin dissociation curve of the fetus and newborn to the left (see Chapter 9). Increased concentrations of HbF are seen in infants that are small for gestational age (SGA) and other infants who have experienced chronic hypoxia in utero, probably due to a delay in the normal switch to synthesis of HbA at about 32 weeks.[61,179] Alterations in HbF are not seen in infants with acute intrapartal hypoxia, since the more recent onset of this condition does not allow the infant sufficient time to compensate.[150] The increased HbF seen in infants with trisomy 13 during the first 2 years of life is also thought to be due to a delay in HbA synthesis. Decreased HbF is seen in infants with Down syndrome.[152] Increased HbA is found in infants with erythroblastosis fetalis due to rapid destruction of older RBCs containing HbF and replacement by new cells containing higher concentrations of HbA.[150]

Hematocrit levels at birth normally range from 51.3% to 56%. The hematocrit increases in the first few hours or days due to the movement of fluid from intravascular to interstitial spaces. The hematocrit falls again to levels near cord blood values by the end of the first week.[41,145]

Changes in 2,3-DPG

Although 2,3-DPG levels at birth in term infants are similar to those in adults, the 2,3-DPG of infants is less stable than that of adults. Concentrations of 2,3-DPG may fall the first week, then increase by the time the infant is 2 to 3 weeks of age.[127] The P_{50} (the PO_2 at which 50% of the hemoglobin is saturated with oxygen) is decreased at birth but gradually increases during the first week of life.[206] This change in the P_{50} is due primarily to an increase in 2,3-DPG rather than in the percentage of Hb F. In comparison with term infants, the preterm infant has a lower P_{50}, decreased concentrations of 2,3 DPG, and increased

amounts of Hb F. Therefore, in the initial few weeks after birth, the functioning DPG fraction in the preterm infant is significantly reduced.[56,96,206]

Erythropoietin

EPO levels are higher at birth in term infants than in preterm infants. After the first day, EPO is not found in the plasma of healthy term infants until 4 to 6 weeks of age.[166] The return of EPO coincides with the resumption of bone marrow activity and RBC production (see Physiologic Anemia of Infancy). EPO disappears from the plasma for longer periods in the preterm infant. In the preterm infant the liver is still the main site of EPO production. Hepatocyte production of EPO in response to hypoxic stimulation is only 10% of that seen by renal cells. In addition, the liver requires more prolonged hypoxic stimulation to produce EPO. In preterm infants, this increases the risk of anemia, but it may also protect from polycythemia.[51,146]

Elevated levels of EPO are found at birth in infants with Down syndrome, IUGR, or anemia secondary to erythroblastosis fetalis and those born to women with diabetes or PIH. In the first 24 hours, EPO is elevated in infants with severe anemia or cyanotic congenital heart defects.[150] The increased levels in the latter group result from low arterial oxygen saturations, which stimulate continued production of EPO. EPO is also thought to be important in maturation of the gut and neurodevelopment.[98,99]

Reticulocytes

The reticulocyte count is elevated at birth, ranging from 3% to 7% (absolute values of 200,000 to 400,000/μL) in term infants and up to 8% to 10% (absolute values of 400,000 to 500,000/μL) in preterm infants.[41] The reticulocyte count decreases markedly to 0% to 1% (absolute values of 0 to 50,000/μL) by 1 week of age.[41]

Iron and Serum Ferritin

Maturity, birth weight, and hemoglobin level determine iron status of the neonate. Cord serum ferritin levels at term are five times higher than maternal values and rise further in the first 24 hours with RBC catabolism and release of hemoglobin iron.[18] Cord hemoglobin and serum ferritin levels are inversely related. At birth the serum folate level of the neonate is three times higher than that in maternal blood. Stores in preterm infants are lower and more rapidly depleted in the first months due to rapid growth.

White Blood Cells

The WBC count ranges from 10,000 to 26,000/mm³ in term infants and from 6000 to 19,000/mm³ in preterm infants. The number of cells increases during the first 12 to 24 hours, then gradually decreases to the level of 6000 to 15,000/mm³ (mean of 12,000/mm³) by 4 to 5 days in both term and preterm infants.[150] The initial increase in WBCs may be due to displacement of cells from the margins of larger vessels and is similar to changes seen in adults following strenuous exercise. The stress of labor and delivery may result in similar changes in the newborn.[84]

Initially up to 60% of the WBCs may be neutrophils with a variety of immature forms. During the first 3 to 4 days, the neutrophil count is higher in preterm than in term infants. By the fourth day, both groups generally stabilize, with neutrophil counts ranging from 2000 to 6000/mm³, although individual variations can be seen in otherwise healthy infants.[12,139] Immature forms of neutrophils (e.g., bands, metamyelocytes, myelocytes) may be seen in healthy neonates during the first 2 to 3 days.[126] The number of monocytes increases slightly during the first 12 hours, then gradually decreases.

Eosinophil counts in the neonate show great individual variation, with reported values ranging from 19 to 851 cells/mm³ in term infants in the first 12 hours and increasing during the first 4 to 5 days of life to 100 to 2500 cells/mm³.[12,61,181] On the other hand, Burrell reported a progressive increase in eosinophils during the initial 3 to 5 weeks, especially in preterm infants who may have an absence of eosinophils in the first 24 hours after birth.[30] Eosinophilia (more than 700/mm³) is more common in preterm infants during the first few weeks, with 75% having values above 700/mm³.[181] Disappearance of eosinophils from the peripheral circulation has been noted before death.[30]

Alterations in Hemostasis

Neonatal hemostasis is altered and characterized by a low reserve capacity.[109] Values for all components are related to gestational age and change gradually after birth, necessitating use of postbirth- and gestational age–dependent reference tables for accurate assessment of individual parameters.[5,67,109]

Platelets

In term and healthy preterm infants, platelet counts are similar to those in adults, ranging from 150,000 to 450,000/mm³. Preterm infants tend to have values slightly lower than term infants, but still within normal range.[23,41,57,109] Platelet counts increase by the end of the first month in both term infants and preterm infants. Higher levels may persist for the first 3 months in preterm infants. Platelet counts below 150,000/mm³ are abnormal in neonates.[57,61,179] Neonatal megakaryocytes are small and

generate fewer platelets than in adults. The normal (i.e., similar to adult values) platelet count in neonates is probably due to the increased proliferative rate by these smaller cells.[175]

Neonatal platelets have a decreased functional reserve capacity and hypoactive response to stimuli in the first few days. By 5 to 9 days, adult activity is noted in both term and preterm infants.[23,72,161] Platelet aggregation and adhesion—as well as release of substances that enhance the clotting cascade—may also be altered. Platelet hypoactivity in neonates may serve as a protective mechanism against the increased tendency toward thrombosis in these infants.[150] However, if the infant is ill or immature, these limitations increase the risk of bleeding and coagulopathy. Coagulation in the neonate may be impaired by maternal drugs such as aspirin that alter platelet aggregation and factor XII (contact factor) activity. Thrombocytosis has been seen by 2 weeks in offspring of polydrug users, which may persist for several months.[31]

Coagulation

Vitamin K–dependent clotting factors II (prothrombin), VII, IX, and X are reduced to less than 70% of adult values at birth and in the early weeks after birth.[9,66,67] This reduction is greater in preterm infants, since concentrations of vitamin K–dependent factors are dependent on gestational age. Contact factors involved in the initiation of the clotting cascade (XI, XII, prekallikrein, and high-molecular-weight kininogen) are also reduced to less than 50% to 70% of adult values in preterm infants.[4,9] Neonatal fibrinogen levels are similar to those in adults or slightly increased at birth.[5] Factors V, VIII, and XIII and von Willebrand factor levels are greater than 70% of adult values or are indistinguishable from adult values.[9,67,181] As a result of these changes, thrombin generation is 50% of adult capacity resulting in resistance to heparin and an increased risk of hemorrhage.[109] Activity of factors involved in the clotting cascade in the neonate are illustrated in Figure 7-10. Activity is further diminished with decreasing gestational age and in severely ill neonates.

Inhibitors of coagulation are also altered. Levels of antithrombin (a protease inhibitor that neutralizes activated clotting factors) and heparin cofactor II (HCII) are at 50% of adult values.[6,7,67] Protein C and S (inhibitors of factors VII and V and the vitamin K–dependent factors) are decreased to less than 30% of adult values.[67] Protein C is found in a fetal form in neonatal circulation. Protein S is found primarily in a free form (versus protein bound as in adults) in neonates because of absence of its binding

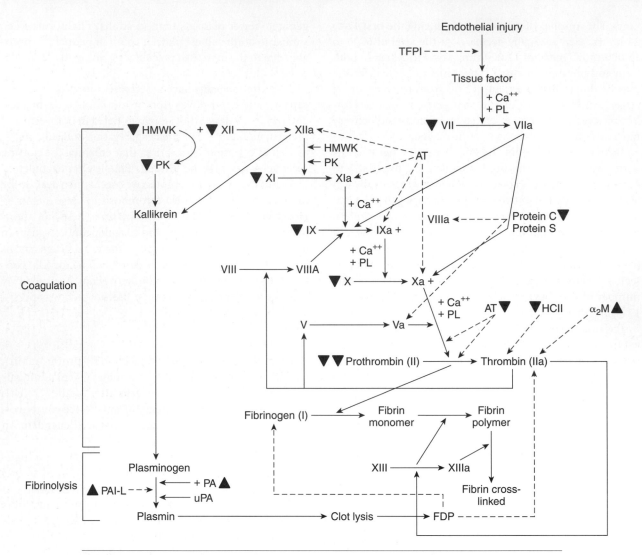

FIGURE **7-10** Alterations in coagulation and fibrinolysis in the neonate. $_{\alpha}2M$, α_2-macroglobulin; *AT,* antithrombin; *Ca,* calcium; *FDP,* fibrin-fibrinogen degradation products; *HCII,* heparin cofactor II; *HMWK,* high-molecular-weight kininogen; *PAI-1,* plasminogen activator inhibitor-1; *PK,* prekallikrein; *PL,* phospholipid; *sl,* slight; *TFPI,* tissue factor pathway inhibitor; *t-PA,* tissue plasminogen activator; *u-PA,* urokinase plasminogen activator. Dashed line denotes inhibitory action. ▲ and ▼ denote changes in the newborn. See Figure 7-5 for a summary of the physiology of coagulation.

protein. This is an advantage for the neonate, because the increased levels of free protein S result in net activity that is 75% of adult values even though absolute values are closer to 25% of adult levels.[67] Levels of another inhibitor, α_1-macroglobin, are elevated to twice adult values, which may help to compensate for the decreased antithrombin and HCII.[6,7,67] Possible mechanisms for these alterations in

coagulation include decreased factor synthesis, accelerated clearance (due to the accelerated basal metabolic rate), and activation and increased consumption of coagulation components at birth.[4,5,67] These changes increase the risk for hypercoagulable states and thrombi formation.[84,179] Inhibition of thrombin is slower in the newborn, but the total capacity is similar to the adult capacity due to increased binding of thrombin by the elevated α_1-macroglobulin and by a circulating fetal anticoagulant (dermatan sulfate–like proteoglycans) that probably arises from the placenta.[4] Edstrom et al note that "thrombin generation in neonates is similar to that in adults receiving therapeutic doses of warfarin or heparin."[67, p.243]

PT, thrombin clotting time (TT), and APTT are prolonged, more so with decreasing gestational age. However, specific values for these tests vary between laboratories and with differences in cord versus neonatal samples, reagents used, and assay conditions. Reference values are available for term and preterm infants of varying postbirth ages.[5,67] PT greater than 17 seconds at any gestation or PTT greater than 45 to 50 seconds in a term infant is of concern. PTT is generally not a useful parameter in preterm infants. PTT measures all coagulation factors except VII and XIII and is abnormal if any one factor is 20% to 40% of normal. PTT is influenced unduly by decreases in the contact factors, such as are seen in many healthy preterm infants.[1] Despite the prolonged APTT, PT, and TT, newborn whole blood clotting times are slightly shorter than adult values (mean of 80 $\pm$5.1 in term infants).[8] The mechanism for this paradoxical finding is unknown, but it may represent a slight overbalance of the tendency toward thrombosis (decreased antithrombin and proteins C and S) in comparison with the physiologic hypocoagulability (low levels of factors II, VII, IX, and X) as well as increased vWF levels and function and the increased size and number of RBCs.[4,8,17]

Fibrinolysis

Activity of the fibrinolytic system is increased at birth. In addition, clearance of collagen debris, fibrin, and injured cells is delayed secondary to immaturity of the reticuloendothelial activating system and low levels of fibronectin (glycoprotein involved in clearance of debris from tissue injury and inflammation).[145] Alterations in healthy preterm infants are similar to or slightly less than those in term newborns. However, activity of the fibrinolytic mechanism may be significantly depressed in some infants—especially preterm infants with severe respiratory distress syndrome (RDS) and asphyxiated infants—for at least the first 24 hours after birth and possibly longer. Plasminogen levels are 58% of adult values at birth and are decreased even further in SGA infants and some preterm infants, increasing the risk for hemostatic disorders.[5,6,39,67] Levels of plasminogen activator inhibitor (PAI-1) and tPa are twice adult levels, decreasing by 5 days; PAI-1 increases again after 5 days to twice adult values by 6 months.[6,7,67]

CLINICAL IMPLICATIONS FOR NEONATAL CARE

Alterations in the hematologic system and hemostasis in the neonate have a significant impact on neonatal adaptations to extrauterine life. These alterations, along with the changes that occur during the first few months of life, can influence interpretation of laboratory test results, lead to alterations such as physiologic anemia or hemorrhagic disease of the newborn, and increase the risk of thromboembolism and consumptive coagulopathies. This section discusses these implications and two areas of controversy related to the hematologic system: the role of vitamin K and decisions regarding transfusion of preterm infants.

Factors Influencing Hematologic Parameters

Factors that influence blood values and their interpretation in the neonate include the timing, site, and amount of blood sampled; placental transfusion; and infant growth rate.[61,150] The timing of blood sampling in relation to changes in hemoglobin and hematocrit during the first week of postnatal life and effects of placental transfusion are discussed earlier in this chapter. The detection of hemolysis can be more difficult due to the unique characteristics of the neonate's hematologic system.[61,206]

Site of Sampling

The site of sampling can result in significant variations in values. Capillary hemoglobin values average 2 to 4 g/dl higher than venous values (with differences up to 8 g/dl reported); arterial values average 0.5 g/dl above venous values and are probably of less clinical significance.[61,160,184] Hematocrits, hemoglobins, and RBC counts from heel capillaries are 5% to 25% higher than venous or arterial values.[41] Differences are greatest with decreasing gestational age. The neonate's hematocrit does not reflect RBC mass as accurately as in an adult, with a correlation of .63 versus .78 in adults.[51] Poorer correlations are reported in ill and preterm infants who are growing rapidly and thus have increased circulating blood volumes.

Both sampling site and physical activity can alter WBC counts. A mean capillary difference of $+1.8 \times 10^9$/L has been found in neutrophil counts between capillary and arterial samples.[184] Using simultaneously drawn blood samples, arterial WBC counts were reported to be 75% of venous or capillary values.[40,41] These differences may be due to the pulsatile nature of arterial flow that moves larger cells to the periphery.[41] Intense crying or other exercise such as chest physiotherapy has been associated with an increase in WBC counts of up to 146% and a shift to the left in the differential count, with the appearance of more immature forms of WBCs in the peripheral circulation.[11] No differences were noted in platelet counts between umbilical artery catheter, venipuncture, and capillary heel stick samples.[184]

Differences between capillary and venous blood samples are due to poor circulation and venous stasis in the peripheral circulation. Differences between arterial and venous samples are thought to be due to passage of plasma to the interstitial spaces in the capillary bed with later return to circulation via the lymphatic system.[184] Capillary and venous differences are more marked with decreasing gestational age; after a large placental transfusion; and in infants with acidosis, hypotension, or severe anemia.[61] Prewarming of the heel before drawing blood, obtaining a good blood flow, and discarding the initial few drops of blood reduce the magnitude of capillary and venous differences.[150] The site of sampling is critical in interpreting hematologic values in the neonate and should be recorded for all samples. Unfortunately, site-related differences are most marked in those infants for whom accurate determination of hematologic values is most critical.[150]

Iatrogenic Losses

Hematologic parameters are also influenced by iatrogenic losses. In the first 6 weeks after birth, infants in intensive care nurseries had a mean iatrogenic blood loss equivalent to 22.9 ± 10 ml of packed cells; 46% of these infants had cumulative losses that exceeded their circulating RBC mass at birth.[61] Iatrogenic blood losses were greater in ill than in healthy preterm infants (26.9 ± 9 ml versus 14.6 ± 5 ml). In very-low-birth-weight (VLBW) infants, these losses were equivalent to a significant proportion of their circulating RBC mass (32.2 to 45.5 ml/kg in the preterm infant). A recent study reported significant overdraws of blood (19% ± 1.8% above that required by the lab) for laboratory testing of neonatal intensive care unit (NICU) infants.[112] The greatest overdraws were in the smallest and most critical infants. Removal of 1 ml of blood from a 1000-g infant is estimated to be equivalent to removing 70 ml from the average adult.[61] Accurate determination of true anemia versus "anemia" due to blood loss is often dependent on accurate recording of the amount of blood that has been previously drawn for sampling.[61]

Growth Influences

Rapid weight gain results in an obligatory increase in total blood volume that often precedes any change in RBC mass. The ensuing hemodilution can lead to a static or falling hemoglobin even with active erythropoiesis as evidenced by reticulocytosis.[12,151] The correlation between RBC mass and hemoglobin is low during the first 6 weeks due to the effects of this hemodilution, so hemoglobin levels do not accurately reflect RBC mass.[206]

Alterations in Hemoglobin-Oxygen Affinity

The increased affinity of hemoglobin for oxygen is an advantage to the fetus in facilitating oxygen transfer across the placenta but may be a liability for the neonate. Preterm infants who have higher levels of Hb F and lower concentrations of 2,3-DPG are more vulnerable. With increased affinity, oxygen is unloaded less rapidly and efficiently in the peripheral tissues. Therefore the newborn may be less able to respond to hypoxia by significantly increasing oxygen delivery to the tissues.[151,196] The newborn is also lacking in some of the protective responses seen in adults. For example, in adults, but not in neonates, hypoxia tends to stimulate increased production of 2,3-DPG, a response that further facilitates oxygen release to the tissues.[150]

The measurement of arterial hemoglobin saturation (SaO_2) by pulse oximetry is generally as reliable in neonates (who have high levels of HbF) as it is in adults (whose hemoglobin is predominantly HbA).[27,158] This occurs because pulse oximetry is a direct measure of percent saturation, whereas calculating saturation from PaO_2 requires knowledge of the percent concentrations of HbA and HbF in the blood.[55] Pulse oximetry works on the principle of light absorbance. The light absorbed by the hemoglobin molecule is absorbed primarily by the heme portion (which is similar in both HbA and HbF) and not by the globulin chains (which are different in HbA and HbF). Infants with HbF can have a high SaO_2 (greater than 85%) even with a low PaO_2; therefore, infants on pulse oximeters must also have their PaO_2 levels regularly evaluated. Even if an infant is well saturated, PaO_2 levels must be kept within normal ranges, since this is the driving force for movement of oxygen from the blood to the tissues. In preterm infants with a higher percentage of HbF, a PaO_2 of 41 to 53 is often high enough to provide an SaO_2 of 88% to 92%.[57]

Since the P_{50} (see Chapter 9) of preterm infants is lower than that of term infants, the progressive shift to the right of the oxygen-hemoglobin dissociation curve is more gradual in pre-term infants and related to postconceptional rather than postbirth age.[18,150] As a result, the oxygen-unloading capacity in the preterm infant who has not been transfused is reduced for at least the first 3 months.[206] In some circumstances the shift to the left in the oxygen-hemoglobin dissociation curve may be an advantage to the infant by helping to maintain oxygen delivery with severe hypoxemia and low cardiac output.[178]

Vitamin K and Hemorrhagic Disease of the Newborn

The newborn has reduced levels of all the vitamin K–dependent clotting factors (II, VII, IX, X) at birth, leading to a physiologic hypoprothrombinemia. The reduction in these factors is the consequence of poor placental transport of vitamin K to the fetus as well as lack of intestinal colonization by bacteria that normally synthesize vitamin K.[159] It is unclear why vitamin K levels are low in the fetus. It may be a mechanism to control levels of other (noncoagulation) vitamin K–dependent proteins, or ligandins, for cutaneous receptor enzymes that regulate growth in the fetus. Since normal fetal growth is carefully regulated within a narrow range, vitamin K levels may be kept low to prevent growth dysregulation.[96]

Neonatal vitamin K deficiency is characterized by low plasma vitamin K_1 (phylloquinone), low liver K_1, and a near absence of K_2 (menaquinone), the major vitamin K component in the liver.[96,205] Unless the infant is given vitamin K at birth, the deficiency intensifies in the first few days after birth as maternally acquired vitamin K is catabolized (half-life is about 24 hours). This decline is more marked in infants who are breastfed, have a history of perinatal asphyxia, or are born to mothers on coumarin derivative anticoagulants. Neonatal liver stores are one fifth those of adults because placental transport of K is low. In addition, neonatal stores are composed of K_1, which has a rapid turnover, especially with a diet such as breast milk that is low in vitamin K.[205] Stores gradually increase in the first month, more rapidly in infants who are formula fed rather than breastfed. This is due both to the increased levels of vitamin K in formula (40 to 50 versus less than 5 μg/L) and differences in intestinal colonization. Formula-fed infants are colonized with bacteria that can produce K_2, whereas lactobacillus, the primary organism colonizing the intestine of breastfed infants, cannot.

Because this decline in vitamin K after birth leads to a bleeding tendency in some newborns, prophylactic vitamin K is given after birth to prevent hemorrhagic disease of the newborn (HDN). HDN involves bleeding from the gastrointestinal tract, umbilical cord, or circumcision site; oozing from puncture sites; and generalized ecchymosis. Three forms of HDN have been described: early, classic, and late.[87,205] The early form occurs within 48 hours of birth and is seen primarily in infants of women on medications such as antiepileptic drugs, warfarin, and antibiotics. The classic form is seen at 2 to 6 days as the vitamin K deficiency intensifies. The preva-

lence of the classic form is 0.4 to 1.7 per 100 if no intramuscular (IM) vitamin K is given.[81] Laboratory findings include reduction in the vitamin K–dependent clotting factors, decreased prothrombin activity, and prolonged clotting and PTs.[81,82,87,205]

A late form of HDN is occasionally seen at 2 to 12 weeks in infants who do not receive vitamin K at birth and are subsequently breast fed or infants who received oral vitamin K, especially if a small oral dose was given without follow-up.[87] This form is also sometimes seen in infants with gastrointestinal disorders leading to fat malabsorption.[81] Prophylactic vitamin K may also be given to preterm and ill infants who are on prolonged antibiotic therapy (particularly with use of third-generation cephalosporins). Antibiotics may significantly reduce the normal intestinal bacterial flora essential for vitamin K synthesis and compete for vitamin K in the liver.

Vitamin K is not required for the synthesis of clotting factors per se but rather for the conversion of precursor proteins synthesized in the liver to activated proteins with coagulant properties.[56] This process (posttranslational γ-carboxylation) is needed for calcium binding, which is critical for activation of these factors. The hypoprothrombinemia commonly present at birth is secondary to decreased levels of the precursor proteins.[150] Term neonates respond to prophylactic vitamin K administration at birth by achieving normal or near normal PTs, although actual values of individual clotting factors may not reach adult values for several weeks or more. The response in preterm infants is less predictable, with minimal response to vitamin K seen in some VLBW infants due to an inability of the immature liver to synthesize adequate amounts of the precursor proteins.[150]

The need for routine vitamin K prophylaxis in all newborns has been questioned, especially with publication of a report that IM vitamin K increased the risk of childhood cancer.[79,154] Subsequent studies have not confirmed this relationship.[131,149,155,187,204] A difficulty with some of these studies is that in many of them routine IM vitamin K was not the usual practice and infants were selected to get vitamin K because of high risk factors; studies of routine IM usage show no increased risk.[68,155,189] In countries where routine use of IM vitamin K was eliminated or oral forms used, the incidence of HDN increased.[154,204] It is likely that many newborns do not need vitamin K at birth. Classic HDN usually occurs in infants without specific risk factors.[205] Therefore it is difficult to identify which infants need this prophylaxis and which do not, and clinical and research evidence clearly demonstrate the risk of hemorrhage in some infants.

The effectiveness of oral vitamin K has not been established. Concerns about oral vitamin K include unpredictable absorption, regurgitation of part or all of the dose and aspiration.[205] Zipursky suggests that the oral form may prevent classic HDN, but not the late form.[205] IM dosing leads to higher, more predictable plasma K levels. Vitamin K levels are higher at 3 months in infants who have received IM versus oral vitamin K.[205] This may be due to a "depot" effect; that is, the IM dose is slowly released from the site of injection for up to 6 weeks after the initial dose.[117]

Vitamin K–dependent clotting factors may be further reduced in infants of women taking antiepileptic drugs (AEDs) such as phenobarbital and phenytoin diphenylhydantoin (Dilantin) during pregnancy. These agents, especially diphenylhydantoin, tend to concentrate in the fetal liver and inhibit the action of vitamin K in the formation of precursor proteins for factors II, VII, IX, and X.[26] Women on AEDs are often given vitamin K in the last weeks of pregnancy to reduce the risk of neonatal bleeding. Vitamin K–dependent clotting factors may also be reduced in infants of women on anticoagulants (warfarin) and chronic antibiotic therapy, especially antituberculosis medications (e.g., isoniazide, rifampin). In addition to receiving the usual dose of vitamin K following birth, these infants must be assessed for signs of bleeding throughout the neonatal period.

Blood Transfusions

Decisions regarding whether or not to transfuse an infant, especially a preterm infant, are often difficult. The advantages of transfusion must be balanced against the consequences and potential risks. Risks of transfusion include infection, metabolic and cardiovascular complications, hypothermia, and graft-versus-host disease.[21]

The major risk from infection arises from blood contaminated with hepatitis B, human immunodeficiency virus (HIV), and cytomegalovirus. Careful screening of donors and blood prior to administration has reduced the risk of infection. Metabolic complications include hypoglycemia (from stimulation of insulin secretion and rebound hypoglycemia due to the high glucose load of transfused citrate-phosphate-dextrose [CPD] or acid-citrate-dextrose [ACD] blood), hyperkalemia (due to transfusion of nonviable cells in blood stored over 5 days), and hypocalcemia (with the use of blood preserved with the anticoagulant citrate, which combines with ionized calcium in the infant's blood). Cardiovascular complications include volume overload, arrhythmias, and thromboembolism. Rapid transfusion and volume expansion may increase the risk of intraventricular hemorrhage in VLBW

infants. Hypothermia can result from transfusion of unwarmed or inadequately warmed blood. Graft-versus-host disease is an immunologic reaction seen in 0.1% to 1.0% of transfused infants. The risk of graft-versus-host disease can be reduced with irradiation of blood prior to administration.[160] With assessment and monitoring, most complications are preventable.

Following transfusions, particularly exchange transfusions with adult blood, there may be rapid alterations in the oxygen-hemoglobin dissociation curve. These changes are influenced by the characteristics of the blood utilized for the exchange. For example, blood stored over 5 days, especially ACD blood, is characterized by a significant decrease in 2,3-DPG and an increased oxygen-hemoglobin affinity.[206] Transfusion with this type of blood may further impair the infant's oxygen-unloading capacity to the tissues.

On the other hand, use of fresh heparinized blood or CPD blood stored for less than 5 days leads to a rapid shift in the P_{50} to adult values.[61] This shift is an advantage to the infant because it improves oxygen release to the tissues; however, it may result in rapid changes in PaO_2, increasing the risk of retinopathy of prematurity (ROP). Following an exchange transfusion or after multiple transfusions, a portion of the infant's HbF will have been replaced by HbA, which has a greater ability to unload oxygen. This change can lead to a rapid improvement in the amount of oxygen delivered to the tissues at a given PaO_2 and possible hyperoxia.

Neonatal Polycythemia and Hyperviscosity

Factors that increase RBC production or decrease neonatal blood volume can lead to polycythemia and hyperviscosity. Neonatal polycythemia is generally defined as a venous hematocrit greater than 65% or hemoglobin greater than 22 g/dl.[76,113,145,193] In general, infants with polycythemia have increased RBC mass and normal plasma volume, leading to increased total blood volume.[106] Hyperviscosity can occur with hematocrits below 65%, although rarely with those below 60% since blood viscosity is not only proportional to the hematocrit but also influenced by increases in mean cell volume and decreases in deformability.[106] Polycythemia and hyperviscosity arises from prenatal, intrapartal, and postbirth factors.

Infants who experience chronic hypoxia prior to birth—including infants with IUGR and cyanotic heart disease; those born at high altitudes or to mothers who smoke or have hypertension syndromes, and possibly infants of diabetic mothers (especially with poor maternal diabetic control during pregnancy)—respond to decreased tissue oxygenation by increasing EPO production.[106] Polycythemia is also sometimes seen in infants with trisomy 13, 18, or 21; congenital adrenal hyperplasia; and Beckwith-Wiedemann syndrome.[193] EPO increases erythropoiesis and fetoplacental blood volume. Infants with acute hypoxemia during the intrapartum period may also develop polycythemia due to fluid shifts from the intravascular to interstitial space and hemoconcentration.

The amount of placental transfusion may rapidly alter the newborn's blood volume, leading to a rise in hematocrit and risk for polycythemia and hyperviscosity in some infants. Fluid moves from the intravascular to the interstitial space, further increasing RBC volume.[145] Fluid transudation within the lungs can produce respiratory distress, and the increased RBC mass leads to hypoglycemia (due to the high glucose utilization of the neonatal RBC) and hyperbilirubinemia.

Infant with a Hemoglobinopathy

Disorders such as thalassemia and sickle cell anemia rarely cause difficulty in the neonatal period because of the neonate's increased levels of HbF (which consists of two alpha and two gamma chains) in relation to HbA (two alpha and two beta chains). The neonate with a higher proportion of HbF has an increased number of gamma chains, fewer beta chains, and similar percentage of alpha chains to those of the adult. Thus disorders of beta-chain structure (sickle cell anemia) or synthesis (β-thalassemia) do not manifest themselves until the infant is 1 to 2 months of age and usually not before 6 months.[148,152] On the other hand, alpha-chain disorders such as α-thalassemia will usually be apparent in the neonate, depending on the clinical severity and number of affected genes. Since alpha-chain production is controlled by two pairs of genes, infants may have one to four affected genes, with clinical manifestations ranging from silent thalassemia (one affected gene) to fetal death usually before 30 weeks (four affected genes). A few infants with four affected genes have survived because they were recognized and treatment begun in utero or they were born prematurely.[148,152]

Infant at Risk for Altered Hemostasis

High-risk neonates are at increased risk for both thromboembolism and consumptive coagulopathies such as DIC as a result of the imbalance between procoagulant, anticoagulant, and fibrinolytic factors.[181] The preterm infant, in particular, is at risk for hemostatic problems as a result of significant decreases in clotting factors, platelet function, and factors protecting against excessive clot formation. Although clotting factors are also decreased in term infants, these infants, unless severely ill, generally do not have impaired hemostasis, since only 20% to 30% of most coagulation factors are normally needed for clot formation. Thus, even with the significant alterations in concentrations of procoagulant, anticoagulant, and fibrinolytic factors, these factors are still at physiologic levels in the neonate.[17,181]

The most common cause of bleeding due to impaired hemostasis in the neonate is DIC. The increased risk for this disorder is secondary to decreased levels of antithrombin and protein C, which normally protect against accelerated coagulation by neutralizing or inhibiting activated clotting factors. Other limitations that make the newborn more susceptible to DIC are a decreased capacity of the reticuloendothelial system to clear intermediary products of coagulation (which stimulate further coagulation and consumption of clotting factors), difficulty in maintaining adequate perfusion of small vessels (resulting in local accumulation of clotting factors and delayed clearance), hepatic immaturity (with delay in compensatory synthesis of essential clotting factors), and vulnerability to pathologic problems known to initiate DIC.[84] Even in preterm infants, the major risks for bleeding disorders or thrombosis are not the infant's physiologic limitations per se but rather the presence of other pathologic problems (for DIC) and trauma or indwelling lines (for thrombosis).[66]

Respiratory distress, sepsis, necrotizing enterocolitis, and other severe diseases are all associated with one or more of the processes that usually lead to intravascular coagulation: (1) release of tissue thromboplastin (sepsis; severe perinatal asphyxia; and other hypoxic-ischemic events such as severe RDS, necrotizing enterocolitis, and CNS hemorrhage), (2) endothelial injury (viral infections), and (3) shock and venous stasis (severe disease that promotes local accumulation of clotting factors and decreased clearance by the liver of activated factors).[66,84]

Altered hemostasis in the ill VLBW infant—with release of tissue thromboplastin secondary to ischemic events in the germinal matrix microcirculation—may increase the risk of both intraventricular hemorrhage and extension of earlier hemorrhages.[84] Fibrinolytic activity in the periventricular area and germinal matrix is increased, leading to more rapid destruction of fibrin clots that might prevent further hemorrhage.

Thrombosis is also a risk during the neonatal period. The three factors that predispose to thromboembolism (stasis, altered coagulation, and vascular damage) are present in some neonates. Infants with polycythemia and hyperviscosity have alterations in blood flow with increased platelet adhesion as well as thrombi formation in the microcirculation, especially in the bowel, kidneys, and extremities. This may explain the increased risk of renal vein thrombosis in infants of diabetic women, who also have a high incidence of polycythemia.[145,181] The infant with shock or perinatal asphyxia also has altered flow with hypotension and stasis.[61] Vascular damage can occur prior to birth within placental vessels in association with maternal complications such as PIH or secondary to trauma from indwelling catheters.[66,151] Thrombotic lesions are frequent findings with umbilical artery catheters (UACs).[61] UACs act as foreign bodies along which fibrin is deposited and thrombi form. Infants with these catheters require close observation for vasospasm or emboli formation, especially in the extremities or buttocks.

The newborn is also at risk for thrombi caused by alterations in hemostasis such as the shorter whole blood clotting time, increased levels of factors V and VIII, and altered function along with decreased levels of major naturally occurring anticoagulants (antithrombin and proteins C and S).[84] Antithrombin levels are further reduced in SGA infants, increasing their risk of thrombosis. The neonatal period is also characterized by decreased fibrinolytic activity, so that once clots develop the infant is less able to remove fibrin and lyse the clots.

Physiologic Anemia of Infancy

Both term infants and preterm infants experience a decline in hemoglobin during the first few months after birth. This process has been termed *physiologic anemia of infancy* in term infants because the infant tolerates the change without any clinical difficulties. Preterm infants experience a similar phenomenon that leads to anemia of prematurity (see next section). Physiologic anemia of infancy results from postnatal suppression of hematopoiesis (Figure 7-11).

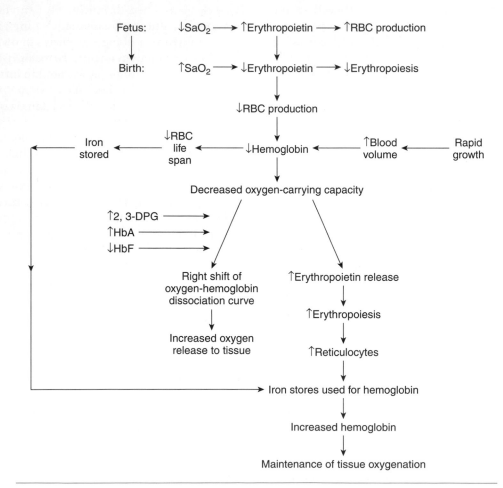

FIGURE **7-11** Physiologic anemia of infancy.

Hematopoiesis is controlled by EPO, which increases when oxygen delivery to the tissues is reduced. This hormone stimulates the bone marrow to increase production of RBCs. The low fetal arterial oxygen tension stimulates EPO release, which leads to production of RBCs.[146]

At birth the arterial oxygen saturation rapidly increases, EPO disappears from the plasma, and production of new RBCs is reduced. Because of the shorter life span of neonatal RBCs, the turnover of these cells is more rapid. Iron released from the destroyed cells is stored in the reticuloendothelial system. With rapid expansion of blood volume due to the infant's rapid growth, hemoglobin levels progressively decrease to 2 to 3 months of age in the term infant.

Although the decrease in hemoglobin reduces the oxygen-carrying capacity of the blood in early infancy, this is balanced by the gradual shift to the right in the oxygen-hemoglobin dissociation curve caused by increasing concentrations of 2,3-DPG and HbA. As a result, the actual amount of oxygen capable of being released to the tissues increases. Eventually hemoglobin levels fall to a point where tissue oxygen needs stimulate EPO and resumption of erythropoiesis (see Figure 7-11).

In the term infant the lowest hemoglobin level (11.4 ± 0.9 g/dl) is reached at 8 to 12 weeks, then slowly increases by 4 to 6 months[61,160] Administration of iron during this period will not increase the hemoglobin to the level necessary to stimulate erythropoiesis nor diminish the rate of hemoglobin decrease.[206] With resumption of erythropoiesis, the reticulocyte count increases to 2% to 8%, followed by a decrease to 1% to 2% after 5 to 6 months. Total body hemoglobin levels also rise. Blood hemoglobin levels may not increase significantly if RBC production only keeps up with growth and the increase in blood volume. In older individuals the combination of increased production of RBCs (as evidenced by a reticulocytosis) with no change in hemoglobin levels would indicate either hemorrhage or hemolysis. However, during early infancy the infant is growing so rapidly that, although total body hemoglobin is increasing, blood hemoglobin values decrease because of hemodilution.[150,206]

Once erythropoiesis is resumed, iron stores are used to produce new RBCs. The reticuloendothelial system of the term infant has adequate iron stores at this point for another 6 to 12 weeks. After this time, hemoglobin levels will again decrease if adequate iron (about 1 mg/kg/day) is not available from dietary sources or as a supplement (see "Iron Supplementation").[178,206]

The resumption of EPO production and erythropoiesis may be delayed in infants who have had exchange transfusion or multiple blood transfusions during the first few weeks after birth. These infants have increased HbA, which releases oxygen more readily to the tissues, providing less stimulation for EPO production.[206] Infants with hemolytic disorders due to isoimmunization may experience a late and often severe anemia that is not physiologic but the result of continued hemolysis. Infants with severe hemolysis who never required an exchange transfusion are at greatest risk for this form of late anemia because of the presence in the infant's blood of maternal antibodies that continue to hemolyze the infant's RBCs. Maternal antibodies are normally removed during an exchange transfusion, reducing the risk of late anemia. The normal hemoglobin decrease after birth is often not seen in infants with cyanotic heart disease, who maintain higher EPO levels (because of their low PaO_2 levels), and thus higher hemoglobin levels in an attempt to increase oxygen delivery to their tissues.

Anemia of Prematurity

Preterm infants also experience a decline in hemoglobin during the first few months after birth secondary to postnatal suppression of hematopoiesis; this decline is similar to that described in "Physiologic Anemia of Infancy" (Figure 7-11). However, preterm infants experience a greater decline in hemoglobin (to 7 to 10 g/dl) and their hemoglobin levels remain low for a longer period of time.[89] This phenomenon, termed *anemia of prematurity,* is a normocytic, normochromic anemia characterized by low EPO.

Anemia of prematurity is seen most often in infants of less than 32 weeks' gestational age. Lowest hemoglobin levels are seen in the most immature infants. These levels may be as low as 7 to 8 g/dl even without significant loss from blood draws.[146,147] The hemoglobin nadir is reached by 3 to 12 weeks and hemoglobin levels remain low for 3 to 6 months.[145,147] The decrease in hemoglobin cannot be prevented by nutritional supplements (i.e., iron, vitamin B_{12}, vitamin E) and is not associated with hematologic abnormalities.[150,180] The lower hemoglobin values in preterm infants are due to decreased iron stores, an altered response of EPO along with a net decrease in RBC mass, RBC survival time and marrow erythroid elements, and rapid postnatal growth and concomitant increase in circulating blood volume.[150,206] Preterm infants do not increase serum EPO levels in the face of hypoxia as occurs in term infants and older individuals. This may be because EPO production in the preterm infant occurs primarily in the liver. Hepatocytes require a more prolonged hypoxic stimulus to produce EPO. Hepatic production of EPO in response to hypoxic stimulation is only 10% of that seen in renal cells.[51,146] However, once EPO is released, the erythroid progenitor cells respond readily.[60,146] The drop in hemoglobin may be intensified in sick infants who have had repeated blood sampling.

Although administration of iron does not prevent anemia of prematurity, once erythropoiesis resumes, the infant uses the stored iron. In preterm infants or infants who experienced early blood losses, iron stores are reduced and may be depleted by 2 to 3 months of age. Therefore iron supplementation is critical to ensure adequate stores for RBC production once erythropoiesis is resumed (see Iron Supplementation).

Infants with anemia of prematurity may be symptomatic or asymptomatic. Clinical findings include tachycardia, tachypnea, lethargy, poor feeding, fatigue with feeding, poor weight gain (less than 25 g/day), pallor, increased serum lactate, increased oxygen requirements, and episodes of apnea or bradycardia.[19,97,103,190] The correct time to transfuse the preterm infants has been an area of controversy. The major reason for transfusion in preterm infants is iatrogenic blood loss rather than diminished erythropoiesis.[29] In one study, all infants who had total blood draws of more than 30 ml required transfusion, whereas fewer than half of those with total losses of less than 30 ml required transfusion.[171] In recent years, most institutions have implemented restrictive transfusion guidelines to reduce the numbers of transfusions and donor exposures without increasing length of stay or morbidity.[20,146,195] These guidelines designate specific hematocrits, which vary with infant age and clinical status at which to transfuse.[20,98,123,146,195] Donor exposure has also been reduced by use of small-volume RBC transfusions with multiple aliquots from the same unit.[91,98] Use of restrictive guidelines has reduced the number of transfusions and donor exposures in extremely low-birth-weight infants by 70% to 80% in the past decade.[98,123]

Administration of recombinant human erythropoietin (rHuEPO) has been used to maintain the hematocrit level in VLBW infants. Recent studies examining the use of rHuEPO have recently been reviewed.[60,146] rHuEPO is reported to increase the hematocrit and reticulocyte count and reduce the need for blood transfusions in preterm infants by 20% to 40%.[60,146] Many uncertainties remain over cost, efficacy, dosing regimens, and long-term effects. rHuEPO seems most cost effective in infants who weigh less than 800 to 1000 grams.[198] Early administration (within the first 1 to 2 weeks) after birth has generally been reported to increase the hemoglobin, hemat-ocrit, and reticulocytes but not reduce the number of transfusions.[59,60] However, a recent study suggested that early administration of rHuEPO accompanied by iron supplementation may reduce the number of transfusions.[34] Late use (after 21 days) reduces the number of late transfusions but not early ones.[60] Some early studies reported decreased neutrophils, but most studies to date have shown no significant short- or long-term side effects with either early or late dosing.[60,146] Since there are EPO receptors in the fetal and neonatal small intestine, EPO may play a role in maturation of the gut.[110] Human milk contains EPO.[108] The enteral effectiveness of rHuEPO is being investigated, with possibly decreased necrotizing enterocolitis reported.[14,110]

Iron Supplementation

Iron supplementation is generally begun before the point of depletion to maintain and build up the infant's iron stores. The American Academy of Pediatrics recommends that breastfed infants receive iron by 6 months of age, usually in the form of iron fortified infant cereal. Formula-fed infants should be fed with an iron fortified formula for the first 12 months.[46] Preterm infants should receive iron by 2 months of age or by the time of reaching 2000 g or being discharged.[46] Supplementation may be in the form of drops or in fortified cereal or formula. Breast milk is low in iron, although the available iron is more readily absorbed.

Very early administration of iron has generally not been recommended in preterm infants due to the association of early iron administration and anemia in these infants. Iron acts as a catalyst in nonenzymatic oxidation of unsaturated fatty acids, especially in the absence of adequate levels of an antioxidant such as vitamin E, resulting in RBC lipid peroxidation and hemolysis. This risk occurs primarily in the first few weeks, when supplemental iron is not needed by the body and vitamin E levels are often low because of stress and poor fat absorption. A recent study reported that iron supplementation begun when enteral feedings were established in VLBW infants (who did not receive rHuEPO) may reduce iron deficiency and the number of late transfusions.[69]

MATURATIONAL CHANGES DURING INFANCY AND CHILDHOOD

Most of the maturational changes in the hematologic system occur during the first 6 to 12 months. The most significant changes are related to the decline in hemoglobin, with the resulting physiologic anemia of infancy, accumulation of higher concentrations of 2,3-DPG, and shift of the oxygen-hemoglobin dissociation curve to the left. An awareness of these changes in infancy is necessary for an appropriate evaluation and treatment of anemia and hypoxia.

Changes in Hematologic Parameters

Blood volume values per unit weight are higher than adult values for the first month or two, increasing the risk of hypovolemia.[150] The mean RBC corpuscular volume and mean diameter decrease rapidly during the first week, followed by a gradual decrease to diameters similar to those of adult cells by 3 to 4 months, declining further to lower than adult by 4 to 6 months, then increasing to adult volumes by about 1 year.[41] RBC fragility also decreases and is similar to that of adults by 3 months.[140] During the first 2 to 3 months, blood and total body hemoglobin levels decrease secondary to decreased RBC production, resulting in the physiologic anemia of infancy discussed previously.

EPO production reaches adult levels by 10 to 16 weeks and the switch from hepatic to renal EPO production is probably completed by several months of age.[51] Differences between capillary and venous hemoglobin levels persist until 3 months of age.[150] The hematocrit decreases to around 30% by 2 months, then increases to 35% by 1 year and to adult values in adolescence. Reticulocyte levels reach adult values by 2 years. Serum ferritin levels rise after birth and remain high for 4 to 6 weeks, with a mean of 356 ng/ml. After this time, levels fall to 30 ng/ml (versus 39 in females and 140 in male adults) by 6 months and remain stable until early to mid-adolescence.[18,150]

With the occurrence of hypoxia, congestive heart failure, or other physiologic stressors, the liver and spleen in early childhood can resume active hematopoiesis and serve as alternate sites for RBC production.[118] During early childhood, blood cells are found in the bones of the tibia, femur, ribs, sternum, and vertebrae rather than in the axial skeleton as seen in adults.[167] Blood tissue in long bones is gradually replaced by adipose tissue beginning at 3 years. By puberty the red marrow in these bones is found only in the upper ends of the humerus and femur and has disappeared by adulthood.[48] Production of WBCs in the thymus ceases in early childhood.[50] Megakaryocytes reach adult size by 2 years.[175]

Activity of coagulation factors gradually increases during infancy and early childhood with the gradual evolution of hemostasis to adult parameters by adolsecence.[4] Some values approach adult levels by 2 weeks to 12 months depending on the individual factor. However vitamin K–dependent factors remain 15% to 20% below adult values until childhood.[4] Levels of antithrombin, HCII, and protein S reach adult ranges by 6 months, protein C does not reach adult values until early childhood.[67] α_1-Macroglobulin is twice adult values at 6 months and remains high throughout childhood.[4] Contact factors also reach adult levels by 6 months.[5] During childhood, bleeding times remain longer than in adults.[4]

Changes in Oxygen-Hemoglobin Affinity

During the first 3 months after birth, the P_{50} gradually increases, and by 4 to 6 months the P_{50} and the oxygen-hemoglobin dissociation curve is similar to that of the adult.[206] From 8 to 11 months, the curve may actually be shifted slightly to the right of the adult curve due to increased blood organic phosphates along with changes in the concentrations of HbA and 2,3-DPG.[150] HbF concentrations decrease 3% to 4% per week during the first 6 months. By 4 months, HbF accounts for only 5% to 10% of the hemoglobin. Levels of HbF gradually decrease to adult levels (less than 2%) by 2 to 3 years. HbA_2 concentrations increase to adult levels of 2% to 3% by 5 to 6 months.[152]

The gradual shift of the oxygen-hemoglobin dissociation curve during the first 6 months after birth is determined by the relative proportions of HbF to HbA and concentrations of 2,3-DPG. Infants with similar concentrations of Hb F may have different P_{50} values if they have significantly different levels of 2,3-DPG. Similarly, infants with similar levels of 2,3-DPG may have different P_{50} values if concentrations of HbF are significantly different. Thus an infant with elevated levels of HbA and low levels of 2,3-DPG may have a P_{50} that is similar to that of another infant with high levels of HbF and 2,3-DPG.[21,61,150] This seeming paradox is explained by what Delivoria-Papadopoulos and colleagues called the *functioning DPG fraction:* the gradual decrease in affinity of hemoglobin for oxygen during the first 6 months after birth correlates with a fraction derived from multiplying the total RBC 2,3-DPG content by the percentage of HbA.[56] Thus the two critical factors in determining the position of the oxygen-hemoglobin dissociation curve during infancy are the amounts of HbA and 2,3-DPG. The rate of postnatal decline in fetal hemoglobin concentrations is generally not affected by persistent cyanosis secondary to cyanotic heart disease.[150]

SUMMARY

The hematologic and hemostatic systems undergo significant alterations during the neonatal period. Because of these changes, the infant is at risk for anemia, thromboembolic

TABLE 7-11 Recommendations for Clinical Practice Related to the Hematologic System in Neonates

Monitor for physiologic effects of early or late cord clamping (pp. 234-236 and Table 7-8).

Know normal parameters for hematologic values in the preterm and term neonate and patterns of change during the neonatal period (pp. 236-241 and Table 7-9).

Recognize changes in hematocrit during the first few days post birth that are due to fluid shifts (versus changes indicating pathologic processes) (pp. 234-236).

Monitor for problems for which the newborn is at increased risk owing to alterations in the neonate's red blood cells (p. 237 and Table 7-10).

Recognize the effects of sampling site and physical activity (especially crying) on hematologic values (pp. 241-242).

Record the sampling site and infant activity each time blood is drawn (pp. 241-242).

Prewarm heel before drawing blood and discard first few drops (p. 242).

Record the amount of blood drawn and other iatrogenic blood loss (p. 242).

Evaluate the amount of iatrogenic blood loss in light of infant's blood volume (p. 242).

Ensure that vitamin K is given following birth (pp. 243-244).

Monitor for signs of hemorrhagic disease of the newborn, especially in infants of mothers on anticonvulsants, anticoagulants, or chronic antibiotic therapy and in infants on long term antibiotic therapy (pp. 243-244).

Recognize laboratory and clinical signs associated with anemia in preterm and term neonates and with anemia of infancy (pp. 246-248).

Recognize laboratory and clinical signs associated with hemolysis in the neonate (pp. 246-248).

Monitor for clinical signs of anemia, anemia of prematurity, and hemolysis (pp. 246-248).

Recognize and monitor for signs of bleeding and disseminated intravascular coagulation, especially in infants at risk (pp. 245-246).

Recognize transfusion complications (p. 244).

Monitor PO_2 values regularly in infants on pulse oximetry and maintain within normal limits (pp. 242-243).

Monitor PO_2 and for hyperoxia in infants following transfusions (especially with fresh blood, after multiple or exchange transfusions) (p. 244).

Recognize and monitor for signs of thromboembolism in infants with indwelling lines or who are hypotensive, polycythemic, or in shock (pp. 245-246).

Recognize and monitor infants at risk for polycythemia and hyperviscosity (pp. 244-245).

Ensure that term and preterm infants receive iron supplementation at recommended time points (p. 248).

---

insults, and coagulopathies. Many of the changes in the hematologic system encountered in the neonate occur progressively over time. Therefore gestational and post-birth age as well as health status must be considered in evaluating and managing individual infants. Clinical recommendations for nurses working with neonates based on changes in the hematologic system are summarized in Table 7-11.

REFERENCES

1. Allen, L. (1997). Pregnancy and iron deficiency: unresolved issues. *Nutr Rev, 55*, 91.
2. Allen, L.H. (2000). Anemia and iron deficiency: effects on pregnancy outcome. *Am J Clin Nutr, 71*(Suppl), 1280S.
3. Alur, P., et al. (2000). Impact of race and gestational age on red blood cell indices in very low birth weight infants. *Pediatrics, 106*, 306.
4. Andrew, M. (1995). Developmental hemostasis: relevance to hemostatic problems during childhood. *Semin Thromb Hemost, 21*, 341.
5. Andrew, M. (1997). The relevance of developmental hemostasis to hemorrhagic disorders of newborns. *Semin Perinatol, 21*, 70.
6. Andrew, M., et al. (1987). Development of the human coagulation system in the full-term infant. *Blood, 70*, 165.
7. Andrew, M., et al. (1988). Development of the human coagulation system in the preterm infant. *Blood, 72*, 1651.
8. Andrew, M., et al. (1990). Evaluation of an automated bleeding time device in the newborn. *Am J Hematol, 35*, 275.
9. Andrew, M., et al. (1990). Development of the hemostatic system in the neonate and young infant. *Am J Pediatr Hematol Oncol, 12*, 95.
10. Ansell, P. (1996). Childhood leukaemia and intramuscular vitamin K: findings from a case control study. *BMJ, 313*, 204.
11. Arafeh, J.M.R. (1997). Disseminated intravascular coagulation in pregnancy: an update. *J Perinat Neonat Nurs, 11*(3), 30.
12. Arias, F., et al. (1979). Whole blood fibrinolytic activity in normal and abnormal pregnancies and its relation to placental concentrations of urokinase inhibitors. *Am J Obstet Gynecol, 133*, 624.
13. Bailey, L.B. & Gregory, J.F. (1999). Folate metabolism and requirements, *J Nutr, 129*, 779.
14. Balin, A., et al. (1999). Erythropoietin, given enterally, stimulates erythropoiesis in premature infants. *Lancet, 353*, 1849.
15. Barrett, J.F.R., et al. (1994). Absorption of nonheme iron from food during normal pregnancy. *Br Med J, 309*, 78.
16. Bassell, G.M. & Marx, G.F. (1981). Physiologic changes of normal pregnancy and parturition. In E.V. Cosmi (Ed.). *Obstetrical anesthesia and perinatology.* New York: Appleton-Century-Crofts.
17. Bennhagen, R. & Holmberg, L. (1989). Protein C activity in preterm and fullterm newborns. *Acta Paediatr Scand, 78*, 31.
18. Bentley, D.P. (1985). Iron metabolism and anemia in pregnancy, *Clin Hematol, 14*, 613.
19. Bitano, E.M., et al. (1992). Relationship between determinants of oxygen-delivery and respiratory abnormalities in preterm infants with anemia. *J Pediatr, 120*, 292.
20. Bitano, E.M. & Curran, T.R. (1995). Minimizing donor blood exposure in the neonatal intensive care unit. Current trends and future prospects. *Clin Perinatol, 22*, 657.

21. Blajchman, M.A., Sheridan, D., & Rowls, W.E. (1985). Risks associated with blood transfusion in the newborn infant. *Clin Obstet Gynecol, 28,* 403.

22. Blake, P.G., Martin, J.N., & Perry, R.C. (1993). Disseminated intravascular coagulation, idiopathic thrombocytopenic purpura, and hemoglobinopathies. In R.A. Knuppel & J.E. Drukker (Eds.). *High risk pregnancy: A team approach* (2nd ed.). Philadelphia: W.B. Saunders.

23. Blanchette, V.S. & Rand, M.L. (1997). Platelet disorders in newborn infants: diagnosis and management. *Semin Perinatol, 21,* 53.

24. Blank, J.P., et al. (1984). The role of red blood cell transfusion in the premature infant. *Am J Dis Child, 138,* 831.

25. Bonnar, J. (2000). Massive obstetrical hemorrhage. *Ballieres Clin Obstet Gynecol, 16,* 1.

26. Bowman, J.M., Pollock, J.M., & Penston, L.E. (1986). Fetomaternal transplacental hemorrhage during pregnancy and post delivery. *Vox Sang, 51,* 117.

27. Brouillette, R.T. & Waxman, D.H. (1997). Evaluation of the newborn's blood gas status. *Clin Chem, 43,* 215.

28. Brown, E.G., et al. (1990). The relationship of maternal erythrocyte oxygen transport parameters to intrauterine growth retardation. *Am J Obstet Gynecol, 162,* 223.

29. Brown, M.S. & Keith, J.F. (1999). Comparison between two and five doses a week of recombinant human erythropoietin for anemia of prematurity: a randomized trial. *Pediatrics, 104,* 210.

30. Burrell, J.M. (1952). A comparative study of the circulating eosinophil levels in babies. *Arch Dis Child, 27,* 337.

31. Burstein, Y., et al. (1977). Thrombocytosis and increased platelet aggregates in newborn infants of polydrug users. *J Pediatr, 94,* 895.

32. Calhoun, D.A. (2000). Hematologic aspects of the maternal-fetal relationship. In R. Christensen (Ed.). *Hematologic problems of the neonate.* Philadelphia: W.B. Saunders.

33. Calhoun, D.A. & Christensen, R.D. (2000). Human developmental biology of granulocyte colony-stimulating factor. *Clin Perinatol, 27,* 559.

34. Carnielli, V.P. (1998). Iron supplementation enhances response to high doses of recombinant human erythropoietin in preterm infants. *Arch Dis Child Fetal Neonatal Ed, 79,* F44.

35. Cavil, J.L. (1995). Iron and erythropoiesis in normal subjects and in pregnancy, *J Perinat Med, 23,* 47.

36. Cavil, J.L. (2000). Iron requirements in adolescent females. *J Nutr, 12*(Suppl), 440S.

37. Centers for Disease Control and Prevention. (1989). CDC criteria for anemia in children and childbearing women. *MMWR, 38,* 400.

38. Centers for Disease Control and Prevention. (1991). Use of folic acid for prevention of spina bifida and other neural tube defects. *MMWR, 40,* 531

39. Chesley, L.C. (1972). Plasma and red cell volumes during pregnancy. *Am J Obstet Gynecol, 112,* 440.

40. Christensen, R. & Rothstein, G. (1979). Pitfalls in the interpretation of leukocyte counts of newborn infants. *Am J Clin Pathol, 72,* 608.

41. Christensen, R.D. (2000). Expected hematologic values for term and preterm neonates. In R. Christensen (Ed.). *Hematologic problems of the neonate.* Philadelphia: W.B. Saunders.

42. Christensen, R.D., et al. (2000). A practical approach to evaluating and treating neutropenia in the neonatal intensive care unit. *Clin Perinatol, 27,* 577.

43. Colomer, J., et al. (1990). Anaemia during pregnancy as a risk factor for infant iron deficiency: report from the Valencia Infant Anaemia Cohort (VIAC) Study. *Pediatr Perinat Epidemiol, 4,* 196.

44. Comeglio, P., et al. (1996). Blood clotting activation during normal pregnancy. *Thromb Res, 84,* 199

45. Committee on Iron Deficiency. (1988). Iron deficiency in the United States. *JAMA, 203,* 407.

46. Committee on Nutrition, American Academy of Pediatrics. (1985). Nutritional needs of low birth weight infants. *Pediatrics, 75,* 976.

47. Cornellison, M., et al. (1997). Prevention of vitamin K deficiency bleeding: efficacy of different multiple oral dose schedules of vitamin K. *Eur J Pediatr, 156,* 126.

48. Corrigan, J.J. (1989). Neonatal coagulation disorders. In B.P. Alter (Ed.). *Perinatal hematology.* Edinburgh, Scotland: Churchill Livingstone.

49. Cunningham, F.G. & Whitridge, W.J. (1997). *Williams obstetrics* (20th ed.). Stamford, CT: Appleton & Lange.

50. Czeizel, A.E., et al. (1992). Prevention of the first occurrence of neural-tube defect by periconceptional vitamin supplementation. *N Eng J Med, 327,* 1832.

51. Dame, C. & Juul, S. (2000). The switch from fetal to adult erythropoiesis. *Clin Perinatol, 27,* 507.

52. Dati, F., et al. (1998). Relevance of markers of hemostasis activation in obstetrics/gynecology and pediatrics. *Semin Thromb Hemost, 24,* 443.

53. De Boer, K., et al. (1989). Enhanced thrombin generation in normal and hypertensive pregnancy. *Am J Obstet Gynecol, 160,* 95.

54. De Swiet, M. (1985). Thromboembolism. *Clin Haematol, 14,* 643.

55. Deckardt, R. & Steward, D.J. (1984). Noninvasive arterial oxygen saturation versus transcutaneous oxygen tension monitoring in the preterm infant. *Critical Care Medicine, 12,* 935.

56. Delivoria-Papadopoulous, M., Roncevic, N.P., & Oski, F.A. (1971). Postnatal changes in oxygen transport of term, preterm, and sick infants: The role of 2,3-DPG and adult hemoglobin. *Pediatr Res, 5,* 235.

57. Del Vecchio, A. & Sola, M.C. (2000). Performing and interpreting the bleeding time in the neonatal intensive care unit. *Clin Perinatol, 27,* 643.

58. Dixon, L.B. (1997). The complete blood count: physiologic basis and clinical usage, *J Perinat Neonat Nurs, 11*(3), 1.

59. Donato, H., et al. (2000). Effect of early versus late administration of human recombinant erythropoietin on transfusion requirements in premature infants: results of a randomized placebo-controlled, multicenter trial. *Pediatrics, 105,* 1066.

60. Doyle, J.J. (1997). The role of erythropoietin in the anemia of prematurity, *Semin Perinatol, 21,* 20.

61. Doyle, J.J., Schmidt, B., Blanchette, V. & Zipursky, A. (1999). Hematology. In G.B. Avery, M.A. Fletcher, & M.G. Macdonald (Eds.). *Neonatology-pathophysiology and management of the newborn* (5th ed.). Philadelphia: J.B. Lippincott.

62. Duerbeck, M.B., et al. Platelet and hemorrhagic disorders associated with pregnancy: a review. Part I. *Obstet Gynecol Sur, 52,* 575.

63. Duffy, T.P. (1999). Hematologic aspects of pregnancy. In G.N. Burrows & T.P. Duffy (Eds.). *Medical complications during pregnancy* (5th ed.). Philadelphia: W.B. Saunders.

64. Dulitzki, M., et al. (1996). Low-molecular-weight heparin during pregnancy and delivery: preliminary experience with 41 pregnancies. *Obstet Gynecol, 97,* 380.

65. Economides, D.L., et al. (1999). Inherited bleeding disorders in obstetrics and gynaecology. *Br J Obstet Gynaecol, 106,* 5.

66. Edstrom, C.S. & Christensen, R.D. (2000). Evaluation and treatment of thrombosis in the neonatal intensive care unit. *Clin Perinatol, 27,* 623.

67. Edstrom, C.S., Christensen, R.D., & Andrew, M. (2000). Developmental aspects of blood hemostasis and disorders of coagulation and fibrinolysis in the neonatal period. In R. Christensen (Ed.). *Hematologic problems of the neonate.* Philadelphia: W.B. Saunders.

68. Ekeland, H. (1991). Late haemorrhagic disease in Sweden 1987-1989. *Acta Paediatr, Scand, 80,* 966.

69. Franz, A.R., et al. (2000). Prospective randomized trial of early versus late enteral iron supplementation in infants with birth weight of less than 1301 grams. *Pediatrics, 106,* 700.

70. Gaspar, M.J., et al. (1993). Relationship between iron status in pregnant women and their babies. *Acta Obstet Gynecol Scand, 72,* 534.

71. Gates, S. (2000). Thromboembolic disease in pregnancy. *Curr Opin Obstet Gynecol, 12,* 117.

72. Gatti, L., et al. (1996). Platelet activation in newborns detected by flow cytometry. *Biol Neonate, 70,* 322.

73. Geethanath, R.M., et al. (1997). Effect of timing of cord clamping on the iron status of infants at 3 months, *Indian Pediatr, 34,* 103.

74. Gerbasi, F.R., et al. (1990). Changes in hemostasis during delivery and the immediate postpartum period. *Am J Obstet Gynecol, 162,* 1158.

75. Gilstrap, L.G. & Gant, N.F. (1990). Pathophysiology of pre-eclampsia. *Semin Perinatol, 14,* 147.

76. Glader, B.E. (1989). Recognition of anemia and red blood cell disorders during infancy. In B.P. Alter (Ed.). *Perinatal hematology.* Edinburgh, Scotland: Churchill Livingstone.

77. Godfrey, K.M., et al. (1991). The effect of maternal anaemia and iron deficiency on the ratio of fetal weight to placental weight. *Br J Obstet Gynaecol, 98,* 886.

78. Goldenberg, R.L. (1996). Plasma ferritin and pregnancy outcome. *Am J Obstet Gynecol, 175,* 1356.

79. Golding, J., et al. (1992). Childhood cancer, intramuscular vitamin K and pethidine given during labour. *Br Med J, 307,* 341.

80. Greer, F.G., et al. (1991). Vitamin K status of lactating mothers, human milk, and breast-feeding infants. *Pediatrics, 88,* 751.

81. Greer, F.R. (1995). Vitamin K deficiency and hemorrhage in infancy. *Clin Perinatol, 22,* 759.

82. Greer, I.A. (1997). Epidemiology, risk factors, and prophylaxis of thromboembolism in obstetrics and gynecology. *Ballieres' Clin Obstet Gynecol, 11,* 403.

83. Hallberg, L. (1988). Iron balance in pregnancy. In H. Berger (Ed.). *Vitamins and minerals in pregnancy and lactation.* New York: Raven.

84. Hathaway, W.E. & Bonnar, J. (1987). *Hemostatic disorders of the pregnant woman and newborn infant.* New York: Elsevier.

85. Hemminki, E. & Rimpela, U. (1991). Iron supplementation, maternal packed cell volume, and fetal growth. *Arch Dis Child, 66,* 422.

86. Higgins, P.G. (1982). Measuring nurses' accuracy of estimating blood loss. *J Adv Nurs, 7,* 157.

87. Hogenbirk, K. (1993). The effect of formula versus breast feeding and exogenous vitamin K_1 supplementation on circulating levels of vitamin K_1 and vitamin K-dependent clotting factors in newborns. *Eur J Pediatr, 152,* 72.

88. Hokama, T., et al. (1996). Iron status of newborns born to iron deficient anaemic mothers. *J Trop Pediatr, 42,* 75.

89. Holland, B.M., Jones, J.G. & Wardrop, C.A.J. (1987). Lessons from the anemia of prematurity. *Hematol Oncol Clin North Am, 1,* 355.

90. Howells, M.R., et al. (1986). Erythropoiesis in pregnancy. *Br J Haematol, 64,* 595.

91. Hume, H. (1997). Red blood cell transfusions for preterm infants: the role of evidence-based medicine. *Semin Perinatol, 21,* 8.

92. Hytten, F. (1985). Blood volume changes in normal pregnancy. *Clin Hematol, 14,* 601.

93. Institute of Medicine. (1990). *Nutrition during pregnancy.* Washington, DC: National Academy Press.

94. Institute of Medicine. (1993). *Iron deficiency anemia: guidelines for prevention, detection, and management among U.S. children and women of childbearing age.* Washington, DC: National Academy Press.

95. Ibraham, H., et al. (2000). Placental transfusion: umbilical cord clamping and preterm infants. *J Perinat, 20,* 351.

96. Israels, L.G., et al. (1997). The riddle of vitamin K_1 deficit in the newborn. *Semin Perinatol, 21,* 90.

97. Izraeli, S., et al. (1993). Lactic acid as a predictor for erythrocyte transfusion in healthy preterm infants with anemia of prematurity. *J Pediatr, 122,* 629.

98. Juul, S.E. (1999). Erythropoiesis in the neonate. *Curr Probl Pediatr, 29,* 129.

99. Juul, S. (2000). Nonerythropoietic roles of erythropoietin in the fetus and neonate. *Clin Perinatol, 27,* 527.

100. Juul, S.E. (2000). Nonhematopoietic aspects of hematopoietic growth factors in the fetus and newborn. In R. Christensen (Ed.). *Hematologic problems of the neonate.* Philadelphia: W.B. Saunders.

101. Kelleher, C.C. (1990). Clinical aspects of the relationship between oral contraceptives and abnormalities of the hemostatic system. *Am J Obstet Gynecol, 163,* 392.

102. Kenny, L. & Baker, P.N. (1999). Maternal pathophysiology in pre-eclampsia. *Ballieres Best Prac Res Clin Obstet Gynaecol, 13,* 59.

103. Keyes, W.G., et al. (1989) Assessment of the need for transfusion of premature infants and the role of hematocrit, clinical signs and erythropoietin level. *Pediatrics, 84,* 412.

104. Khoury, S.T. & Khoury, M.J. (1993). Erythropoietin production by the kidney. *Semin Nephrol, 13,* 79.

105. Kinmond, S., et al. (1993). Umbilical cord clamping and preterm infants: a randomized trial. *Br Med J, 306,* 172.

106. Kilpatrick, S.J. & Laros, R.K. (1999). Maternal hematologic disorders. In R.K. Creasy & R. Resnik (Eds.). *Maternal-fetal medicine* (4th ed.). Philadelphia: W.B. Saunders.

107. Klebanoff, M.A., et al. (1991). Anemia and spontaneous preterm birth. *Am J Obstet Gynecol, 101,* 1447.

108. Kling, P.J., et al. (1998). Human milk as a potential enteral source of erythropoietin. *Pediatr Res, 43,* 216.

109. Kuhne, T. & Imbach, P. (1998). Neonatal platelet physiology and pathophysiology. *Eur J Pediatr, 157,* 87.

110. Ledbetter, D.J. & Juul, S.E. (2000). Erythropoietin and the incidence of necrotizing enterocolitis in infants with very low birth weight, *J Pediatr Surg, 35,* 178.

111. Letsky, E.A. (1995). Erythropoiesis in pregnancy. *J Perinatal Med, 23,* 39.

112. Lin, J.C., et al. (2000). Phlebotomy overdraw in the neonatal intensive care nursery, *Pediatrics, 106,* e19.

113. Lindeman, R. & Haga, P. (2000). Evaluation and treatment of polycythemia in the neonate. In R. Christensen (Ed.). *Hematologic problems of the neonate.* Philadelphia: W.B. Saunders.

114. Linderkamp, O. (1982). Placental transfusion: Determinants and effects. *Clin Perinatol, 9,* 559.

115. Linderkamp, O.L., et al. (1992). The effects of early and late cord-clamping on blood viscosity and other hemorrheological parameters in full-term neonates. *Acta Pediatr, 81,* 745.

116. Lockwood, C.J. (1999). Heritable coagulopathies in pregnancy. *Obstet Gynecol Surv, 54,* 754.

117. Loughnan, P.M. & MacDougall, P.N. (1996). Does intramuscular vitamin K1 act as an unintended depot preparation? *J Pediatr, 32,* 251.

118. Lowrey, G.H. (1986). *Growth and development of children.* Chicago: Year Book.

119. Lu, Z.M. (1991). The relationship between maternal hematocrit and pregnancy outcome. *Obstet Gynecol, 77,* 190.

120. Luchtman-Jones, L., Schwartz, A.L., & Wilson, D.B. (1997). Hematological problems in the fetus and neonate. In A.A. Fanaroff & R.J. Martin (Eds.). *Neonatal-perinatal medicine, diseases of the fetus and infant* (6th ed.). St. Louis: Mosby.

121. Luegenbiehl, D.L., et al. (1990). Standardized assessment of blood loss. *MCN, 15,* 241.

122. Lynch, S.R. (2000). The potential impact of iron supplementation during adolescence on iron status in pregnancy. *J Nutr, 120*(Suppl), 448S.

123. Maier, R.F., et al. (2000). Changing practices of red blood cell transfusion in infants with birth weights less than 1000 g. *J Pediatr, 136,* 220.

124. Manga, M. (1999). Maternal cardiovascular and renal adaptations to pregnancy. In R.K. Creasy & R. Resnik (Eds.). *Maternal-fetal medicine* (2nd ed.). Philadelphia: W.B. Saunders.

125. Mani, S. & Duffy, T.P. (1995). Anemia of pregnancy. *Clin Perinatol, 22,* 593.

126. Manroe, B.L., et al. (1979) The neonatal blood count in health and disease. I. Reference values for neutrophil cells. *J Pediatr, 95,* 89.

127. Matovcik, L.M. & Mentzer, W.C. (1985). The membrane of the human neonatal red cell. *Clin Hematol, 14,* 203.

128. Matovcik, L.M., et al. (1986). The aging process of the human neonatal erythrocyte. *Pediatr Res, 20,* 1091.

129. Matthews, J.H., et al. (1990). Pregnancy-associated thrombocytopenia: Definition, incidence and natural history. *Acta Haematol, 84,* 24.

130. McDonnell, M. & Henderson-Smart, D.J. (1997). Delayed umbilical cord clamping in preterm infants: a feasibility study. *J Paediatr Child Health, 33,* 208.

131. McKinney, P.A., et al. (1998). Case-control study of childhood leukaemia and cancer in Scotland: findings for neonatal intramuscular vitamin K. *Br Med J, 316,* 173.

132. McPhedren, P. (1999). Venous thromboembolism during pregnancy. In G.N. Burrows & T.P. Duffy (Eds.). *Medical complications during pregnancy* (5th ed.). Philadelphia: W.B. Saunders

133. Medical Research Counsel Vitamin Study Research Group. (1991). Prevention of neural tube defects. Results of the Medical Research Counsel Vitamin Study, *Lancet, 338,* 131.

134. Mercer, J.S., Nelson, C.C. & Skovgaard, R.L. (2000). Umbilical cord clamping: beliefs and practices of American nurse-midwives. *J Midwifery Womans Health, 45,* 58.

135. Mercer, J.S. & Skovgaard, R.L. (2002). Neonatal transitional physiology: a new paradigm. *J Perinat Neonatal Nurs, 15*(4), 56.

136. Milman, N., et al. (1999). Iron status and iron balance during pregnancy. A critical reappraisal of iron supplementation. *Acta Obstet Gynecol Scand, 78,* 749.

137. Morley, G. & Morley, G.M. (1998). Cord closure: can hasty clamping injure the newborn? *OBG Management, 7,* 29.

138. Morrison, J.C. & Pryor, J.A. (1990). Hematologic disorders. In R.D. Eden & F.H. Boehm (Eds.). *Assessment and care of the fetus.* Norwalk, CT: Appleton & Lange.

139. Mouzinho, A., et al. (1994). Revised reference ranges for circulating neutrophils in very-low-birth-weight neonates. *Pediatrics, 94,* 76.

140. Nelle, M., et al. (1993). Effect of Leboyer delivery on blood viscosity and other hemorrhagologic parameters in term neonates. *Am J Obstet Gynecol, 69,* 189.

141. Nelle, M., et al. (1995). Effect of Leboyer childbirth on cardiac output, cerebral and gastrointestinal blood flow velocities in full term neonates. *Am J Perinatol, 12,* 212.

142. Nelle, M., et al. (1994). Effect of red blood cell transfusion on cardiac output and blood flow velocities in cerebral and gastrointestinal arteries in premature infants. *Arch Dis Child, 71,* F45.

143. Nelson-Piercy, C. (1997). Hazards of heparin: allergy, heparin-induced thrombocytopenia, and osteoporosis. *Ballieres' Clin Obstet Gynecol, 11,* 489.

144. Nicholaides, K.H. & Mibashan, R.S. (1989). Fetal red blood cell isoimmunization. In B.P. Alter (Ed.). *Perinatal hematology.* Edinburgh: Churchill Livingstone.

145. Oh, W. (1986). Neonatal polycythemia and hyperviscosity. *Pediatr Clin North America, 33,* 523.

146. Ohls, R.K. (2000). The use of erythropoietin in neonates. *Clin Perinatol, 27,* 681.

147. Ohls, R.K. (2000). Evaluation and treatment of anemia in the neonate. In R. Christensen (Ed.). *Hematologic problems of the neonate.* Philadelphia: W.B. Saunders.

148. Olivieri, N.F. (1997). Fetal erythropoiesis and the diagnosis and treatment of hemoglobin disorders in the fetus and child. *Semin Perinatol, 21,* 63.

149. Olsen, J.H., et al. (1994). Vitamin K regimens and incidence of childhood cancer in Denmark. *Br Med J, 308,* 895.

150. Oski, F.A. & Naiman, J.L. (1982). *Hematologic problems in the newborn* (3rd ed.). Philadelphia: W.B. Saunders.

151. Oski, F.A. (1979). Clinical implications of the oxygen-hemoglobin dissociation curve in the neonatal period. *Crit Care Med, 7,* 412.

152. Palis, J. & Segel, G.B. (1998). Developmental biology of erythropoiesis. *Blood Rev, 12,* 106.

153. Papagno, L. (1998). Umbilical cord clamping. An analysis of a usual neonatological conduct. *Acta Physiol Pharmacol Ther Latinoam, 48,* 224.

154. Passmore, S.J., et al. (1998). Case-control studies of relation between childhood cancer and neonatal vitamin K administration. *Br Med J, 316,* 178.

155. Passmore, S.J., et al. (1998). Ecologic studies of relation between hospital policies on neonatal vitamin K administration and subsequent occurrence of childhood cancer. *Br Med J, 316,* 184.

156. Perry, K.J. & Morrison, J.C. (1990). The diagnosis and management of hemoglobinopathies during pregnancy. *Semin Perinatol, 14,* 90.

157. Pert, K.G., et al. (1998). Quantitative correlation between globulin mRNAs and synthesis of fetal and adult hemoglobin during hemoglobin switchover in the perinatal period. *Pediatr Res, 43,* 504.

158. Pologe, J.A. & Raley, D.M. (1987). Effects of fetal hemoglobin on pulse oximetry. *J Perinatol, 7,* 324.

159. Pritchard, J.A. (1965). Changes in blood volume during pregnancy and delivery. *Anesthesiology, 26,* 393.

160. Pritchard, S.L. & Rogers, P.C.J. (1987). Rationale and recommendations for the irradiation of blood products. *CRC Crit Rev Oncol Hematol, 7,* 115.

161. Rajasekhar, D., et al. (1994). Neonatal platelets are less reactive than adult platelets to physiological agonists in whole blood, *Thromb Hemost, 72,* 957.

162. Ramos, J.L.A., et al. (1990). Red cell enzymes and intermediates in AGA term newborns, AGA preterm newborns and SGA preterm newborns. *Acta Paediatr Scand, 79,* 32.

163. Ray, J.G. & Chan, W.S. (1999). Deep vein thrombosis during pregnancy and the puerperium: a meta-analysis of the period of risk and the leg of presentation. *Obstet Gynecol Surv, 54,* 265.

164. Richter, C., et al. (1995). Erythropoiesis in the perinatal postpartum period. *J Perinatal Med, 23,* 51.

165. Rondini, G. & Chirico, G. (1999). Hematopoietic growth factor levels in term and preterm infants. *Curr Opin Hematol, 6,* 192.

166. Ruth, V., et al. (1990). Postnatal changes in serum immunoreactive erythropoietin in relation to hypoxia before and after birth. *J Pediatr, 116,* 950.

167. Sallah, S. (1997). Inhibitors to clotting factors. *Ann Hematol, 75*, 1.

168. Scholl. T.O., et al. (1992). Anemia vs iron deficiency: increased risk of preterm delivery in a prospective study. *Am J Clin Nutr, 55*, 985.

169. Scholl, T.O. (1999). High third-trimester ferritin concentrations: associations with very preterm delivery, infection, and maternal nutritional status. *Obstet Gynecol, 93*, 156.

170. Scholl, T.O. & Reilly, T. (2000). Anemia, iron, and pregnancy outcome. *J Nutr, 130*(Suppl), 443S.

171. Shannon, K.M., et al. (1995). Recombinant human erythropoietin stimulates erythropoiesis and reduces erythrocyte transfusions in very low birth weight preterm infants. *Pediatrics, 95*, 1.

172. Sibai, B.M. & Frangieh, A. (1995). Maternal adaptation in pregnancy. *Curr Opin Obstet Gynecol, 7*, 420.

173. Silver, H.M., et al. (1998). Comparison of total blood volume in normal, preeclamptic, and nonproteinuric gestational hypertensive pregnancy by simultaneous measurement of red blood cell and plasma volumes. *Am J Obstet Gynecol, 179*, 87.

174. Sipes, S.L. & Weiner, C.P. (1990). Venous thromboembolic disease in pregnancy. *Semin in Perinatol, 14*, 103.

175. Sola, M.C. (2000). Fetal megakaryocytopoiesis. In R. Christensen (Ed.). *Hematologic problems of the neonate*. Philadelphia: W.B. Saunders.

176. Stables, D. (1999). *Physiology in childbearing with anatomy and related biosciences*. Edinburgh, Scotland: Balliere Tindall.

177. Stevens, K. (1997). Umbilical cord blood transplants: treatment for selected hematologic and oncologic diseases. *J Perinat Neonat Nurs, 11*(3), 19.

178. Stockman, J.A. & Oski, F.A. (1978). Physiologic anaemia of infancy and anaemia of prematurity. *Clin Hematol, 7*, 3.

179. Stockman, J.A. (1990). Fetal hematology. In R.D. Eden & F.H. Boehm (Eds.). *Assessment and care of the fetus*. Norwalk, CT: Appleton & Lange.

180. Strauss, R.G. (1986). Current issues in neonatal transfusion. *Vox Sang, 51*, 1.

181. Sullivan, S.E. (2000). Eosinophilia in the neonatal intensive care unit. *Clin Perinatol, 27*, 603.

182. Tanindi, S., et al. (1995). The normalization period of platelet aggregation in newborns. *Thromb Res, 80*, 57.

183. Thornburg, K.L., et al. Hemodynamic changes in pregnancy. *Semin Perinatol, 24*, 11.

184. Thurlbeck, S.M. & McIntosh, N. (1987). Preterm blood counts vary with sampling site. *Arch Dis Child, 62*, 74.

185. U.S. Preventative Services Task Force. (1993). *Routine iron supplementation during pregnancy*. Washington, DC: U.S. Preventative Services Task Force.

186. Van den Hof, M.C. & Nicolaides, K.H. (1990). Platelet count in normal, small, and anemic fetuses. *Am J Obstet Gynecol, 162*, 735.

187. Vander, A., Sherman, J., & Luciano, D. (2000). *Human physiology: The mechanism of body function* (8th ed.). New York: McGraw-Hill.

188. Viteri, F.E. (1997). Iron supplementation for the control of iron deficiency in populations at risk. *Nutr Rev, 55*, 195.

189. VonKries, R., et al. (1996). Vitamin K and childhood cancer: a population based case-control study in lower Saxony, Germany. *Br Med J, 313*, 199.

190. Wardrop, C., et al. (1978). Nonphysiological anemia of prematurity. *Arch Dis Child, 53*, 855.

191. Wardrop, C.A., Holland, B.M. & Jones, J.G. (1995). Consensus on red cell transfusion. *Br Med J, 311*, 965.

192. Wardrop, C.A. & Holland, B.M. (1995). The roles and vital importance of placental blood to the newborn infant. *J Perinat Med, 23*, 139.

193. Werner, E.J. (1995). Neonatal polycythemia and hyerviscosity. *Clin Perinatol, 23*, 693.

194. Widness, J.A., et al. (1991). Lack of maternal to fetal transfer of 125-labelled erythropoietin in sheep. *J Dev Physiol, 15*, 139.

195. Widness, J.A., et al. (1996). Changing patterns of red blood cell transfusion in very low birth weight infants. *J Pediatr, 129*, 689.

196. Wimberley, P.D. (1982). Fetal hemoglobin, 2,3-diphosphoglycerate and oxygen transport in the newborn premature infant. *Scand J Clin Lab Invest, 160*(Suppl), 1.

197. Wolfe, M. & Wandstrat, T.L. (1996). Hematopoietic growth factors: part I. *Neonat Net, 15*(6), 7.

198. World Health Organization. (1992). *The prevalence of anaemia in women: a tabulation of available information* (2nd ed). Geneva: World Health Organization.

199. Yao, A.C. & Lind, J. (1969). Effect of gravity on placental transfusion. *Lancet, 2*, 505.

200. Yao, A.C., Moinian, M., & Lind, J. (1969). Distribution of blood between the infant and placenta at birth. *Lancet, 2*, 871.

201. Yao, A.C. & Lind J. (1982). *Placental transfusion*. Springfield, IL: Charles C Thomas.

202. Yoder, M.C. (2000). Embryonic hematopoiesis. In R. Christensen (Ed.). *Hematologic problems of the neonate*. Philadelphia: W.B. Saunders.

203. Zhou, L.M., et al. (1998). Relation of hemoglobin measured at different times in pregnancy to preterm birth and low birth weight in Shanghai, China. *Am J Epidemiol, 148*, 998.

204. Zipursky, A. (1996). Vitamin K at birth. *Br Med J, 313*, 179.

205. Zipursky, A. (1999). Prevention of vitamin K deficiency bleeding in newborns. *Br J Haematol, 104*, 430.

206. Zipursky, A. (1987). Hematology of the newborn infant. In L. Stern & P. Vert (Eds.). *Neonatal medicine*. New York: Masson.

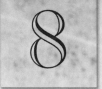

Cardiovascular System

The circulatory system is the transport system that supplies body cells with substrates absorbed from the gastrointestinal tract and oxygen from the lungs and returns carbon dioxide to the lungs for disposal; other by-products of metabolism are routed to the kidneys for elimination. The cardiovascular system (CVS) is also involved in the regulation of body temperature and the distribution of hormones and other substances that regulate cellular functioning.

During pregnancy the maternal cardiovascular system must meet the demands of both the mother and the dynamically changing fetus. The constant ebb and flow of nutrients and by-products via the uteroplacental system creates a sensitive interdependence between the mother and the fetus. At birth the infant undergoes significant changes in the CVS that may, if altered, compromise extrauterine existence and postnatal adaptation. This chapter examines alterations in the CVS during the perinatal period and implications for the mother, fetus, and neonate.

MATERNAL PHYSIOLOGIC ADAPTATIONS

Pregnancy is associated with physiologically significant but reversible changes in maternal hemodynamics and cardiac function. These changes are mediated by increased levels of circulating estrogens; progesterone; prostaglandins (PG), especially PGE_1 and PGE_2; and other vasoactive substances, as well as by the increased load on the cardiovascular system. The increased circulating maternal blood mass, fetal nutritional requirements, and placental circulatory system demands place increased demands on the maternal cardiovascular system. In most women these demands are met without compromising the mother. However, when superimposed upon an existing disease state, in which hemodynamics are already compromised, pregnancy may prove to be a dangerous situation for maternal homeostasis.

Conversely, if maternal hemodynamics do not change, adverse effects on the uteroplacental circulation can lead to fetal compromise, which may be manifested as fetal malformations (including congenital heart disease), in-

trauterine growth restriction (IUGR), or pregnancy loss. Therefore the maternal cardiovascular system must achieve a balance between fetal needs and maternal tolerance.

During the second stage of labor, expulsive efforts lead to an increase in muscle tension and intrathoracic and intraabdominal pressure, all of which affect the functioning of the heart and the hemodynamics of the system. Intraabdominal pressure is abruptly decreased upon delivery and blood pools in the abdominal organs, thereby affecting cardiac return. Blood loss during delivery may also affect hemodynamics.

Antepartum Period

The major hemodynamic changes that occur during pregnancy are outlined in Table 8-1. Cardiovascular and hemodynamic changes are due to hormonal influences, changes in other organ systems, and mechanical forces. The hemodynamic changes are partly the result of hormonal influences as well as of the development of the placental circulation and alterations in systemic vascular resistance. These changes include modifications in total blood volume, plasma volume, red blood cell (RBC) volume, and cardiac output. Anatomic changes such as the upward displacement of the diaphragm by the gravid uterus shift the heart upward and laterally. There is slight cardiac enlargement on radiograph, and the left heart border is straightened. The size and positioning of the uterus, the strength of the abdominal muscles, and the configuration of the abdomen and thorax determine the extent of these changes.[58]

Hemodynamic Changes

Hemodynamic alterations in pregnancy include changes in blood volume, cardiac output, heart rate, systemic blood pressure, vascular resistance, and distribution of blood flow. Stroke volume, heart rate, and cardiac output increase significantly, whereas systemic vascular resistance, pulmonary vascular resistance (PVR), and colloid osmotic pressure decrease.[51] Changes in blood, plasma, and RBC volume are discussed further in Chapter 7.

255

TABLE **8-1** **Physiologic Changes of Pregnancy on the Cardiovascular System**

Parameter	Modification	Magnitude	Time of Peak Increase or Decrease
Oxygen consumption (VO_2)	Increase	+20% to 60%	Term
Oxygen delivery (DO_2)	No change to increase	700 to 1400 ml/min	Term
Blood volume:			
Plasma*†	Marked increase	+45% to 60%	32 weeks
Red blood cells	Increase	+25% to 32%	30 to 32 weeks
Total body water	Increase	+6-8 L	Term
Resistance changes:			
Systemic circulation	Decrease	−20%	16 to 34 weeks
Pulmonary circulation	Decrease	−34%	34 weeks
Blood pressure (SVR × CO):†			
Systolic	Slight or no decrease		
Diastolic	Decrease	10 to 15 mmHg	24 to 32 weeks
Myocardial contractility:			
Chronotropism (HR)	Increase	+20% to 30%	28 to 32 weeks
Intropism (SV)	Increase	+11% to 32%	Term
Cardiac output (HR × SV)	Increase	+30% to 50%	28 to 32 weeks
Uteroplacental circulation	Increase	Greater than 1000%	Term

Adapted from Gei, A.F. & Hankins, G.D. (2001). Cardiac disease and pregnancy. *Obstet Gynecol Clin North Am, 28,* 469.
*Correlates positively with the number of fetuses.
†Position dependent (e.g., lower for systolic and diastolic in left lateral decubitus position).
CO, Cardiac output; *HR,* heart rate; *SV,* stroke volume; *SVR,* systemic vascular resistance.

Total blood volume. Total blood volume (TBV) is a combination of plasma volume and RBC volume, each of which increases during pregnancy. Circulating blood volume increases by 30% to 40%, beginning as early as the sixth week of gestation. The usual range of TBV increase is 30% to 50%, although wide individual variations are reported.[148] TBV increases rapidly until midpregnancy and then more slowly during the latter half. A plateau or slight decline in circulating volume may occur during the last few weeks of gestation.[71,126, 148,152,159,166,176,199] Figure 7-2 illustrates changes in total blood volume and its component parts, plasma volume, and RBC volume.

The rise in blood volume correlates directly with fetal weight, supporting the concept of the placenta as an arteriovenous shunt of the maternal vascular compartment. Although the degree of hypervolemia varies from woman to woman, subsequent pregnancies in the same woman result in similar increases in circulating volume. Twin and other multiple pregnancies, however, result in greater increases in blood volume, imposing substantially greater demands on the cardiovascular system.[166,176]

Red blood cell volume. RBC production and thus volume increases throughout pregnancy to a level 25% to 33% higher than nonpregnant values (approximately 250 to 450 ml).[148] Intravascular expansion is mainly due to an increase in plasma volume; therefore hemodilution occurs. This physiologic anemia of pregnancy is reflected in a lower hematocrit and hemoglobin (see Table 7-2). This cannot be prevented with iron supplementation; however, women who are provided exogenous sources of iron do have higher hemoglobin levels in the third trimester than women not receiving supplements (see Figure 7-4).[71,111] Changes in RBC volume are due to increased circulating erythropoietin and accelerated RBC production. The rise in erythropoietin in the last two trimesters may be stimulated by progesterone, prolactin, and human placental lactogen.[148,187,213] Changes in RBC volume are described further in Chapter 7.

Plasma volume. About 75% of the TBV increase is in plasma volume. Plasma volume increases by 40% to 50% (range, 30% to 60%), or about 1250 ml above nonpregnant values.[187] This change begins at 6 to 10 weeks and increases rapidly during the second trimester, followed by a slower but progressive increase that reaches its maximum at 28 to 32 weeks.[126] Alterations in blood and plasma volume are influenced by hormonal effects, mechanical factors (blood flow in uteroplacental vessels), and changes in the renal system and fluid and electrolyte homeostasis (see Chapters 7 and 10 and Figure 7-3). Fluid balance changes are probably mediated by changes in the renin-angiotensin-aldosterone system, with increased sodium and water retention.[148]

Plasma renin activity and blood aldosterone levels are increased due to the action of estrogens, progesterone, and prostaglandins. An increase in plasma renin activity enhances sodium retention, thereby stimulating aldosterone secretion. Progesterone inhibits the action of aldosterone on the renal tubular cells, thus contributing to sodium retention and an increase in total body water. The degree of fluid retention is influenced by the increased distensibility of the vascular system and the uterine vein capacity present during pregnancy.[50,71]

Fluid distribution. Fluid distribution changes depending on body position. Supine positioning produces the lowest central blood volume, with a decrease being noted after being supine for 1 hour. This is probably due to the trapping of blood in the legs and pelvis as the gravid uterus creates a mechanical impedance to blood flow through the inferior vena cava. This causes an increase in venous pressure in the lower extremities and a sharp rise in hydrostatic pressure in the microcirculation, with subsequent leakage of fluid from the vascular bed into the interstitium. The result is edema of the feet and ankles. Venous distensibility contributes to the decreased venous return to the heart.[52,125,159]

Cardiac output. Cardiac output is the product of heart rate times stroke volume and is one of the most significant hemodynamic changes encountered during pregnancy. Cardiac output increases by 1 L/min by 8 weeks, a 22% increase over the prepregnant value.[31] Cardiac output continues to rise more slowly until the third trimester to values, as measured in the left lateral recumbent position, 30% to 50% greater than in nonpregnant women.[18,31,32,50,70,148,156,194,222,271] In some women the increased cardiac output may exceed 50%.[35] A slight decline in cardiac output may be seen in late pregnancy due to the decrease in stroke volume near term.[69] The increase in cardiac output is associated with an increase in venous return and greater right ventricular (RV) output, especially in the left lateral position.[64,147,227] Changes in cardiac output during pregnancy in supine and left lateral positions are illustrated in Figure 8-1.

The increased cardiac output is due to changes in both stroke volume and heart rate. Changes in heart rate and stroke volume are reported by 5 weeks' and 8 weeks' gestation, respectively.[13,31,148,194] The rise in cardiac output early in pregnancy is due primarily to an increase in stroke vol-

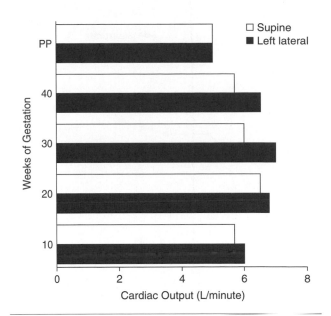

FIGURE **8-1** Cardiac output measured in the left lateral and supine positions during uncomplicated pregnancies. *PP,* Postpartum. (From Caulin-Glaser, T. & Setano, J.F. [1999]. Pregnancy and cardiovascular disease. In G.N. Burrow & T.P. Duffy [Eds.]. *Medical complications during pregnancy* (5th ed.), as adapted from Capeless E.L. & Clapp J.F. [1989]. Cardiovascular changes in early phases of pregnancy. *Am J Obstet Gynecol, 161,* 1449; Ueland, K. & Hansen J.M. [1969]. Maternal cardiovascular dynamics. II: Posture and uterine contractions. *Am J Obstet Gynecol, 103,* 1; and Robson S.C., et al. [1989]. Serial study of factors influencing changes in cardiac output during human pregnancy. *Am J Physiol, 256,* H1060.)

ume (30% increase).[32] As pregnancy advances, the heart rate continues to increase (by 10 to 20 beats per minute), becoming a more dominant factor in determining cardiac output.[148] Stroke volume declines during the latter stages of pregnancy, and may return to values that are within the normal nonpregnant range.[37,30,70,148,152,156,238] Figure 8-2 compares the changes in heart rate and stroke volume over gestation.

During pregnancy (especially the third trimester), the resting cardiac output fluctuates markedly with changes in body position.[148,163,232] For example, a change from the left lateral recumbent position to supine can lead to a 25% to 30% decrease in cardiac output.[9] In the supine position, there is a greater decline in cardiac output than that experienced in the sitting or lateral recumbent position. The compression of the inferior vena cava by the uterus in the third trimester results in a decreased venous return and a markedly decreased cardiac output (20% to 30%). Heart rate changes do not necessarily occur with positional

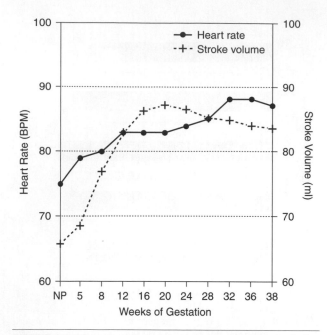

FIGURE **8-2** Alteration of stroke volume and heart rate during pregnancy. Stroke volume increases maximally during the first half of gestation. There is a slight decrease in stroke volume toward term. The mild increase in heart rate begins early in gestation and continues until term. (Adapted from Robson, S.C., et al. [1989]. Serial study of factors influencing changes in cardiac output during human pregnancy. *Am J Physiol, 256,* H1060, by Manga, M. [1999]. Maternal cardiovascular and renal adaptations to pregnancy. In R.K. Creasy & R. Resnik [Eds.]. *Maternal-fetal medicine.* Philadelphia: W.B. Saunders.)

changes; therefore these changes in cardiac output are more likely due to a decrease in stroke volume. There is also no decrease in blood pressure, probably due to an increase in peripheral vascular resistance.[121,125,148,232,238]

The slight decline in cardiac output in the last couple of weeks of pregnancy is more pronounced in the supine position than in the sitting or lateral recumbent position.[69] This lower value is actually less than levels seen 6 to 8 weeks postpartum. This decline in cardiac output is another indication of compression of the inferior vena cava by the gravid uterus and is seen even in the sitting position. Tamponade leads to a decreased venous return even in those women with well-established collateral circulation.[70,71,97,152,232,238]

Twin, triplet, and other multiple pregnancies have a greater increase in cardiac output than do singletons. The peak is greater, and the decline in cardiac output seen in late pregnancy is smaller. The cardiac output at 20 weeks' gestation is higher than that encountered in a singleton pregnancy and remains higher for the remainder of gestation. The maximum cardiac output in multiple pregnancy is also increased by about 15% to 20%.[70,152]

The increase in cardiac output during pregnancy is not related to the metabolic requirements of the mother or the fetus, nor to the increase in maternal body mass (which is approximately 13%).[196] At the time the increase in cardiac output occurs, the fetus is relatively small. When fetal growth is accelerated (late in gestation), there is an actual decline in maternal cardiac output. There is, however, a progressive increase in maternal oxygen consumption, which may be due to the rising metabolic needs of the fetus as well as the demands of the maternal heart and respiratory muscles. However, this increase in oxygen consumption begins at the end of the first trimester and therefore does not help to explain the increase in cardiac output seen earlier.

The increased oxygen requirements are most likely the result of the contractility-promoting influences of estrogen and progesterone and the development of the placental circulation. The placenta functions much like an arteriovenous shunt, with a concomitant decrease in peripheral vascular resistance. Therefore, despite the increase in cardiac output, there is a decrease in mean blood pressure due to a decrease in diastolic pressure. The concomitant increase in blood volume (either in time or magnitude) probably explains the increase in cardiac output. Both begin to rise as early as 6 to 8 weeks of gestation, peaking toward the end of the second trimester, around 30% to 50% higher than prepregnant levels.[70,152,167,196]

Changes in uterine blood flow might also contribute to the increased cardiac output. Uterine blood flow increases from 50 ml/min at 10 weeks' gestation to 500 to 600 ml/min by term. The progressive rise in uterine blood flow, however, does not parallel the resting maternal cardiac output changes. Therefore uterine blood flow can account for only a portion of the increase in cardiac output seen by 20 weeks.

Steroid hormones and prolactin may cause changes in hemodynamics by directly affecting the myocardium. Estrogens may alter the actomyosin-adenosine triphosphatase (ATPase) relationship in the myocardium, thereby increasing the contractility of the heart and altering the stroke volume. This same effect can be seen when oral contraceptives are used.[152]

Heart rate. Heart rate is the determinant of cardiac output that has the widest range (60 beats per minute to 200 beats per minute in women of childbearing age). The wide range provides stability to the circulatory system under a variety of circumstances (e.g., rest to maximal exercise). Heart rate can be altered in order to maintain blood pressure if changes in vascular resistance or stroke volume are encountered. However, an increased heart rate is insufficient to increase cardiac output; it must be accompanied by an increase in venous return. Both heart rate and venous return are increased in pregnancy, contributing to the increase in cardiac output seen throughout gestation.[163]

The maternal heart rate increases progressively during pregnancy, averaging 10 to 20 beats per minute (10% to 20% increase) over the nonpregnant state.[138] This increase in heart rate is seen as early as 5 weeks' gestation and peaks by 32 weeks (see Figure 8-2).[41] Since stroke volume decreases near term, the elevated cardiac output late in the third trimester can probably be attributed primarily to heart rate changes.[148]

At term the heart rate may return to near baseline levels in some women. Maternal position affects heart rate; heart rate is higher in a sitting or supine position and slightly lower in the lateral recumbent position. Twin pregnancies have an earlier acceleration in heart rate, with a maximum increase 40% above the nonpregnant level near term.[30,58,171]

The increased heart rate results in an elevated myocardial oxygen requirement, which is probably not important in women without cardiac disease, but may become significant in pregnant women with underlying cardiovascular pathology. Beyond this, the increased resting heart rate decreases the maximal work capacity by diminishing the output increment that can be achieved during maximal exercise.[163]

Stroke volume. Stroke volume is determined by preload, contractility, and afterload. Stroke volume increases progressively during the first and second trimesters, to a peak value of approximately 30% above nonpregnant values.[163] Stroke volume peaks and plateaus by about 20 weeks, decreasing slightly to term (see Figure 8-2).[227] Before 20 weeks' gestation, stroke volume is the primary factor responsible for the increased cardiac output. The changes in stroke volume are presumably due to increased ventricular muscle mass and end-diastolic volume changes.[69,148] The left ventricular (LV) pressure volume curve is shifted to the right as a result of the Frank-Starling mechanism and the hypervolemia of pregnancy.[164]

Blood pressure. Although there are substantial increases in both blood volume and cardiac output during pregnancy, these changes are not associated with increases in either venous or arterial pressure.[163] In fact, blood pressure, especially diastolic pressure, begins to fall in the first trimester. The early decrease is probably due to a lag in compensation for changes in peripheral vascular resistance.[13,148] The diastolic blood pressure decrease reaches a nadir at 24 to 32 weeks and then gradually returns to nonpregnant baseline values by term (Figure 8-3).[37,148] Serial observations in a sitting or standing position show that as women advance through their preg-

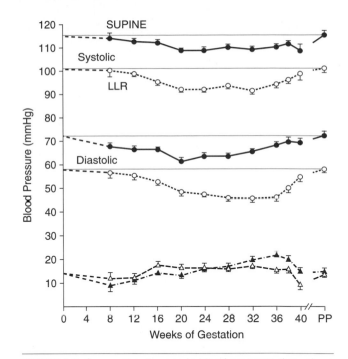

FIGURE **8-3** Sequential changes in blood pressure throughout pregnancy with subjects in supine and left lateral recumbent (LLR) positions. The change in systolic (open triangles) and diastolic (closed triangles) blood pressures produced by movement from the left lateral recumbent to the supine position is illustrated in the bottom part of the figure. (From Wilson, M., et al. [1980]. Blood pressure, the renin-aldosterone system, and sex steroids throughout normal pregnancy. *Am J Med, 68,* 97.)

nancies, systolic blood pressure remains either stable or decreases slightly, whereas diastolic pressure decreases markedly.[37,142] The magnitude of blood pressure changes varies from study to study and the position of the woman during measurement, but the diastolic decrease averages 10 to 15 mmHg.[37,142] As a result of these changes, pulse pressure increases in the third trimester. The reduction in blood pressure may be secondary to the vasodilatory effects of nitric oxide that increases in pregnancy as well as hormonal factors that mediate a decrease in peripheral vascular resistance.[13,169,252]

Both age and parity have significant effects on blood pressure during pregnancy. As parity increases (regardless of age), both the systolic and diastolic blood pressures decrease, with the greatest difference being between nulliparas and primiparas. As maternal age advances (greater than 35 years), systolic pressure remains unchanged. Diastolic pressure, however, gradually increases with age.

Techniques and differences in the diastolic measurement point also influence blood pressure measurement. Therefore it is important to use a consistent method and maternal position to evaluate blood pressure. Conventional blood pressure techniques often lack standardization in terms of use of appropriate cuff size, equipment calibration, rounding off (to nearest 5 to 10 mmHg versus the recommended 2 mmHg), and method.[27,100,171] Measurement of the diastolic pressure to the point of muffling (Korotkoff phase IV) results in measurements 13 mmHg greater than if measured to the point of disappearance (Korotkoff phase V).[100,148] Phase V measurements are closer to intraatrial pressure and easier to detect.[232] The use of phase IV versus V has been the subject of much controversy in obstetric care. However, a recent study reported no clinically significant differences in outcome in a prospective trial of women with diastolic hypertension in late pregnancy.[28]

Differences are also seen in intraatrial versus manual versus 24-hour automated cuff diastolic measurements.[39,148] Ambulatory automated 24-hour blood pressure measurements have been used with women with "white-coat" hypertension (i.e., increased blood pressure during an office visit to their primary care provider, but normal blood pressure at other times), in early recognition of preeclampsia, and for prognostic assessment of hypertension in late pregnancy.[91,99,100] These measurements have had variable clinical usefulness, with a need for additional study.[100]

Venous pressures during pregnancy also do not change significantly. Given the large increase in blood volume during pregnancy, an increase in venous pressure would be expected. The increased vascular capacitance and compliance seen during pregnancy can explain this lack of change. These changes are probably due to the effects of progesterone and endothelial-derived relaxant factor on blood vessel smooth muscle and collagen.[4] Venous pressure below the uterus is increased, which may be caused by the increased capacitance encountered in the large pelvic veins and the veins distal to the uterus.[164] The latter may affect venous return to the heart—especially in the upright position—due to regional pooling. Late in gestation the gravid uterus may also contribute to reduced venous return and pooling in all positions except the lateral recumbent position. The ability to sustain venous return is crucial in determining maternal exercise capacity (see Exercise during Pregnancy).[163]

Systemic vascular resistance. Changes in cardiac output during pregnancy are accomplished without an increase in arterial pressures because of the marked decrease in systemic vascular resistance (SVR), especially in peripheral vessels.[34,227] SVR (mean arterial pressure divided by cardiac output) is decreased during pregnancy and parallels the decrease in blood pressure.[242] SVR decreases by 5 weeks and

usually reaches its lowest level by 16 to 34 weeks, then progressively increases to term (Figure 8-4).[148]

This decreases is due in part to remodeling of the maternal spiral arteries (see Chapter 3) and the addition of the low-resistance uteroplacental circulation, which receives a large proportion of cardiac output.[35] The decline in resistance is not limited to the uteroplacental circulation; rather, it is seen throughout the body.[71,138] The decreased SVR is also due to progesterone and vasoactive prostaglandins and may also be influenced by endothelial-derived relaxant factors (e.g., nitric oxide) that enhance vasodilation.[34,65] The decrease in SVR may be the stimulus for changes in heart rate and stroke volume, and thus cardiac output, in early pregnancy.[148] Decreased systemic and renal vascular tone occur very early in pregnancy and precede changes in blood volume.[34] The hormonal activity of pregnancy also has a role in the reduction of systemic vascular resistance—with reduction of SVR also seen with use of oral contraceptives—and contributes to changes in regional blood flow. Along with this, the increased heat production by the fetus results in vasodilatation of vessels (especially in heat-losing areas such as the hands) and further reductions in resistance.[71]

Regional blood flow. Much of the increased maternal cardiac output is distributed to the uteroplacental circuit. The increase in cardiac output above the needs of the uteroplacental circulation leads to increased flow to other organ systems, particularly the mammary glands, skin, and kidneys. This creates a reservoir that can be tapped as pregnancy progresses.

Mammary blood flow is probably increased.[148] Clinically increased flow is evident by the engorgement that occurs early in pregnancy and the dilatation of veins on the

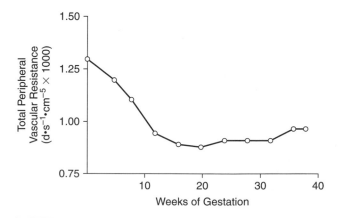

FIGURE **8-4** Total peripheral vascular resistance drops dramatically over the course of pregnancy. (From Thornburg, K.L., et al. [2000]. Hemodynamic changes in pregnancy. *Semin Perinatol, 24,* 12.)

surface of the breasts. This dilatation is usually accompanied by a sensation of heat and tingling.[156] The effect of pregnancy on coronary artery blood flow is unknown. With the increased workload of the LV (because of the increased cardiac output, blood volume, fetal growth, uterus enlargement, and body weight gain), it can be assumed that the coronary blood flow is increased to meet the cardiac myometrial demands. Hepatic and cerebral blood flow are not significantly altered during pregnancy.[70,169] Absolute blood flow to the liver does not change significantly, but the percentage of the cardiac output perfusing the liver decreases.[144]

Uterine blood flow. The decline in uterine vascular resistance allows blood flow to the uterus to increase during gestation. At 10 weeks' gestation the blood flow is approximately 50 ml/min, increasing to 200 ml/min by 28 weeks and 500 to 600 ml/min at term. Thus by term the uterus is receiving between 10% and 20% of the total cardiac output.[77,135,148] Because the uterine vascular bed is widely dilated with minimal or no autoregulation, uterine oxygen consumption and fetal oxygenation are maintained by increased oxygen extraction rather than by increases in blood flow. Studies demonstrate that fetal oxygenation can be maintained in this fashion until uterine blood flow decreases by 50%.[135,144]

The uterine spiral arteries undergo marked changes during pregnancy (see Chapter 3) that disrupt their muscular and elastic elements (Figure 8-5). As a result, the uteroplacental arteries are almost completely dilated and are no longer responsive to circulating pressor agents or influences of the autonomic nervous system.[119,192]

Renal blood flow. Renal blood flow (RBF) increases 35% to 60% by the end of the first trimester and then decreases from the second trimester to term (Chapter 10).[76,148,227] The decline in flow is probably due to the gravid uterus impeding flow through the vena cava.[138] The percentage of the cardiac output perfusing the kidneys does not change and remains around 18%.[142] The glomerular filtration rate (GFR) increases 40% to 50% over nonpregnant levels and is due in large part to the increased RBF. The decrease in renal vascular resistance may be mediated by nitric oxide, prostacyclin (PGI_2), and atrial natriuretic factor.[133,138]

Skin perfusion. Skin perfusion increases significantly during pregnancy, with a slow but steady rise in perfusion up to 18 to 20 weeks' gestation. This slow rise is followed by a sharp increase between 20 and 30 weeks, with no significant increase after that. This increased flow is measurable for up to 1 week postpartum.[122,138] Clinically this increased flow can be indicated by an increase in skin temperature and clammy hands, which are the result of dermal capil-

lary dilatation. Vascular spiders and palmar erythema can be seen in many women during pregnancy (see Chapter 13). This vasodilatation may facilitate the dissipation of excessive heat created by fetal metabolism. Increased peripheral flow can also be seen in the mucous membranes of the nasal passages, explaining the nasal congestion that is common in pregnancy.[138,169]

Extremity blood flow. Studies examining extremity blood flow (forearm and leg) have provided inconclusive and conflicting data. Some studies have indicated that there is a progressive rise in blood flow in both the hands and feet during pregnancy. These changes begin early in gestation and continue up to 6 to 8 weeks postpartum. The flow in twin pregnancies is somewhat higher after the thirtieth week than it is in single pregnancies.[83]

Pulmonary vascular blood flow. Pulmonary vascular blood flow increases secondary to increased circulating blood volume and increased cardiac output. This can be demonstrated on roentgenogram by increased vascular markings. PVR is decreased, probably in response to hormonal stimulation, and is reflected in a lowered mean pulmonary artery pressure.

Oxygen Consumption

Oxygen consumption is a reflection of metabolic rate. During pregnancy there is a progressive increase in rest-

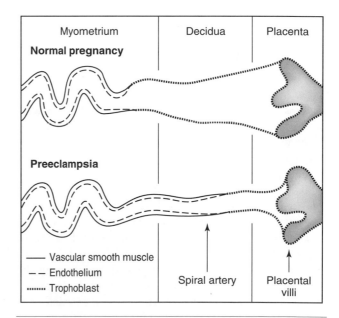

FIGURE **8-5** Trophoblast invasion into the spiral arteries in the placental bed in normal pregnancy and in preeclampsia. (From VanWijk, M.J. (2000). Vascular function in preeclampsia. *Cardiovasc Res, 47,* 39.)

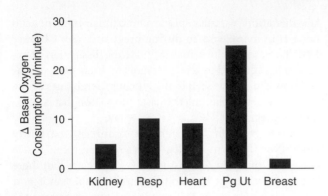

FIGURE **8-6** The maximal increase in basal oxygen consumption (ml/min) during pregnancy. *Pg Ut,* Pregnant uterus. (From Thornburg, K.L., et al. [2000]. Hemodynamic changes in pregnancy. *Semin Perinatol, 24,* 12.)

ing oxygen consumption, with a peak increase of 20% to 30% by term (Figure 8-6). This increase in oxygen consumption is due to the increased metabolic needs of the mother and the growing fetus.[227] Oxygen consumption increases gradually over gestation, whereas cardiac output increases dramatically in the first and second trimesters. Because the resting cardiac output increases before there is a significant rise in maternal oxygen consumption, the arteriovenous oxygen difference is small in early pregnancy and increases as oxygen consumption increases in the later phases of pregnancy. This provides the uterus with well-oxygenated blood flow during the first trimester, before the completed development of the feto-placental circulation.[227]

Physical Changes

The physiologic hypervolemia of pregnancy results in alterations in the cardiac silhouette, chamber size, pressures, and electrocardiogram (ECG). These changes—along with the hemodynamic alterations—lead to changes in the physical findings encountered during cardiovascular assessment of the pregnant woman (Figure 8-7 and Table 8-2).

The heart and blood vessels undergo remodeling during pregnancy.[227] Cardiac ventricular wall muscle mass increases by 10% to 15% in the first trimester, whereas end-diastolic volume increases in the second and third trimesters.[28,37,148,205,227] These changes increase compliance, augmenting stroke volume and maintaining the ejection fraction, although the exact role of the increased cardiac mass and contractility in increasing cardiac output during pregnancy is unclear.[28,80,81,148,155,227] Increases in left atrial diameter parallel increases in blood volume, beginning in the first trimester and peaking around 30 weeks.[148] Thus the pregnant woman has a physiologi-

cally dilated heart with increased contractility.[227] This physiologic dilation occurs without significant changes in the ejection fraction.[148]

The exact mechanism underlying changes in blood vessels is also unclear, but the result is an increase in aortic size, aortic compliance, venous blood volume, and venous compliance.[227] Compliance of the entire vasculature is increased due to softening of the collagen and smooth muscle hypertrophy.[148]

The pregnant woman often experiences reduced exercise tolerance, tiredness, and dyspnea (see Chapter 9). Hyperventilation is common, and basilar rales may give the impression of heart failure. These rales, however, are a normal development during gestation and are caused by the compression and atelectasis of the lower portions of the lungs by the enlarging uterus.

As the uterus grows, the diaphragm is displaced upward and the heart shifts to a more horizontal position (see Figure 8-7). The LV point of maximum impact is easily palpated and may be shifted to the left. A RV impulse can usually be palpated at the middle- to lower-left sternal border; this is the pulmonary trunk. Difficulty in localizing this point may be caused by the enlarged breast tissue.

The arterial pulse is full, becoming sharp and jerky between 12 and 15 weeks. This finding remains until 1 week after delivery. Jugular vein pulsations are more readily seen, as vein distention appears around 20 weeks' gestation. A venous hum may be associated with the rapid downward flow through the jugular veins. This is indicative of a rapid circulation and high cardiac output state.[59,94]

Edema of the ankles and legs is a frequent finding during the latter part of pregnancy (see Chapter 13). As maternal age increases, edema is more common. An increase in capillary permeability and the fall in colloid osmotic pressure in the plasma, along with the increase in femoral venous pressure, are implicated in edema formation.[168] Thigh-high support hose have been found to significantly reduce this edema by increasing SVR and reducing venous pooling.

Heart sounds. Auscultation of the heart reveals an exaggerated split and loudness of both components of the first heart sounds (mitral and tricuspid valve closure). These changes can be heard for the first time between 12 and 20 weeks and continue into the postpartum period (2 to 4 weeks).[59] Nearly 90% of pregnant women will have a louder and more widely split first sound that is best heard at the left sternal border between the third and fifth intercostal spaces. This change is primarily due to the earlier closure of the mitral valve.[59,71,138,148]

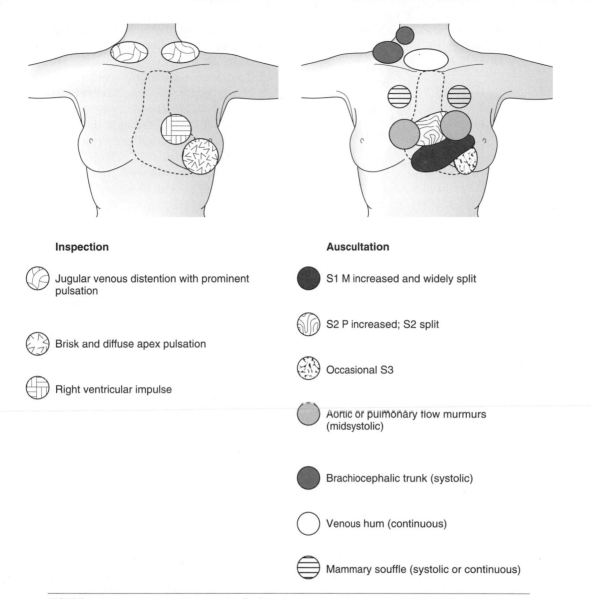

Inspection

Jugular venous distention with prominent pulsation

Brisk and diffuse apex pulsation

Right ventricular impulse

Auscultation

S1 M increased and widely split

S2 P increased; S2 split

Occasional S3

Aortic or pulmonary flow murmurs (midsystolic)

Brachiocephalic trunk (systolic)

Venous hum (continuous)

Mammary souffle (systolic or continuous)

FIGURE **8-7** Normal cardiac examination findings in the pregnant woman. *M,* Mitral; *P,* pulmonary; *S1,* first sound; *S2,* second sound. (From Gei, A.F. & Hankins, G.D. [2001]. Cardiac disease and pregnancy. *Obstet Gynecol Clin North Am, 28,* 472.)

There are no significant changes in the aortic and pulmonic elements of the second heart sound during the first 30 weeks of gestation. During the last 10 weeks, persistent splitting that does not vary with respiration may be heard. This change may be due to the reduced diaphragmatic movement secondary to uterine size.[59,71,138,168] A loud third heart sound is heard in up to 90% of pregnant women.[148]

Most (92% to 95%) women demonstrate a systolic murmur, particularly during the last two trimesters, that is in-

dicative of the increased cardiovascular load.[59,138] This is considered an innocent murmur that is usually short and heard in early to mid-systole. Such murmurs are best auscultated along the left sternal border in the third intercostal space, although some are more prominent along the lower-left sternal border at the apex or aortic area. These murmurs have a musical quality and represent audible vibrations caused by ejection of blood from the RV into the pulmonary trunk or from the LV into the brachiocephalic arteries at the point of branching from the aortic

TABLE **8-2**   Effect of Pregnancy on Cardiac Evaluation Methods

PARAMETER	MODIFICATIONS
Chest radiography	Apparent cardiomegaly (enlarged transverse diameter
	Enlarged atrium (lateral view)
	Increased vascular markings
	Straightening of left-sided heart border
	Postpartum pleural effusion (right-sided)
Electrocardiography	Rate:
	Right axis deviation
	Right branch bundle block
	ST-segment depression of 1 mm on left precordial leads (14%)
	Rhythms:
	Q wave in lead III*
	T-wave inversion in III,* V2 and V3 (14%)
	Intervals:
	Small decrease of PR and QT (heart rate dependent)
	Axis:
	Rotation of ± 15 degrees (QRS axis)
Echocardiogram	Trivial tricuspid regurgitation (43-945 at term)
	Pulmonary regurgitation (945 at term)
	Increased left atrial size by 12% to 14%
	Increased left ventricle end-diastolic dimensions by 6% to 10%
	Inconsistent increase in left ventricle thickness
	Mitral regurgitation at term (28%)
	Pericardial effusions (40% postpartum)

From Gei, A.F. & Hankins, G.D. (2001). Cardiac disease and pregnancy. *Obstet Gynecol Clin North Am, 28,* 473.
*Decrease or normalize with deep inspiration.

arch.[59,71,168] A systolic precordal murmur due to functional tricuspid regurgitation may also be heard.[4] Systolic murmurs louder than grade 2/4 or any diastolic murmur require further investigation.[4] A third heart sound, venous hum, or mammary soufflé may be misinterpreted as a diastolic murmur.[71,168]

About 14% of women have murmurs of mammary vessel origin.[59] Of these, 70% are continuous, whereas the other 30% are heard only during diastole. They are more common in lactating women but can be auscultated during pregnancy as well. Often unilateral, these murmurs are best heard at the second to fourth intercostal space lateral to the left sternal border. They can be changed or obliterated by varying the pressure applied by the stethoscope. The mammary soufflé is an indication of the increased blood flow in the mammary vessels. The murmur disappears after the termination of lactation.[59,71,168]

Electrocardiograph and echocardiograph changes. Changes in the ECG occur as the position of the heart shifts with the enlarging uterus and elevated diaphragm.[37] These changes are usually minor and are summarized in Table 8-2. A small Q wave and inversion of the P wave are not uncommon. T-wave and ST-segment changes can also be seen.[168,208] With descent of the fetus into the pelvis in late pregnancy, a right axis shift may be noted.[208] As the heart size increases, the incidence of arrhythmias—usually in the form of supraventricular tachycardias—increase. Benign arrhythmias that were present before pregnancy may intensify or progress.

Echocardiography demonstrates an increase in left end-diastolic dimensions during the second and third trimesters. This is probably due to the expanded blood volume and increased filling during diastole. The increased stroke volume that accompanies this added volume maintains the end-systolic dimensions of the LV at nonpregnant levels. These findings are supported by cardiac catheterization data. The right ventricular diastolic pressure is slightly increased over the nonpregnant values. On the other hand, the RV systolic pressure is just below the nonpregnant values (25 to 30 mmHg). This is probably due to the diminished mean pulmonary artery pressure and decreased PVR.[71,148,200] Changes in the echocardiogram during pregnancy are summarized in Table 8-2.

These changes in clinical signs and symptoms during pregnancy may lead to inappropriate diagnosis of heart disease. A complete cardiac history; careful physical assessment; and an understanding of the changes, differential diagnosis, and norms related to pregnancy should limit cardiac referrals to those women who warrant specialized evaluation and monitoring.

Intrapartum Period

During the intrapartum period the repetitive, forceful contractions of the uterus as well as pain, anxiety, and apprehension can have an effect on the cardiovascular system.[2,97,138] Significant hemodynamic changes can be attributed to the pain and anxiety associated with labor and delivery (see Chapter 14), especially in primiparous women. This is probably due to the release of catecholamines and the increased systemic vascular tone. Each

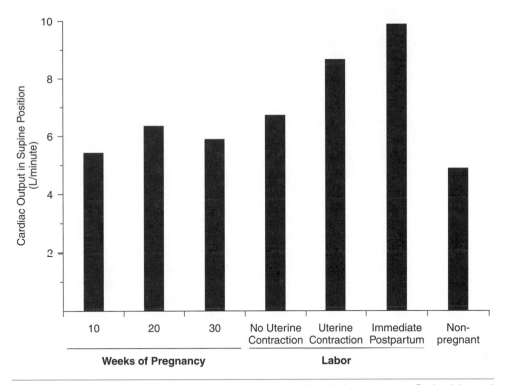

FIGURE **8-8** Cardiac output values measured in the supine position during pregnancy. During labor and delivery, cardiac output is approximately 13% above prelabor values (increasing by almost 50% with contractions) and is higher still immediately after delivery. (From McAnulty, J.H., Metcalfe, J., & Ueland. K. [1995]. Cardiovascular disease. In G.N. Burrow & T.F. Ferris [Eds.]. *Medical complications during pregnancy* [4th ed.]. Philadelphia: W.B. Saunders.)

contraction contributes approximately 300 to 500 ml of additional volume to the circulation.[37,221] This results in a significant increase in cardiac output (Figure 8-8), with a cumulative effect over the course of labor. A progressive rise in cardiac output is seen during the first stage of labor. Cardiac output rises further during the second stage and peaks immediately after delivery.[148,193] Cardiac output increases 12% to 31% above pregnancy values during the first stage and is up to 50% greater in the second stage of labor.[37,148,232] These increases in cardiac output may be due to hemodynamic changes during a contraction that lead to an improved venous return, transient tachycardia, and an increased circulating volume. The increase in pulmonary arterial-venous oxygen difference also supports this hypothesis, suggesting that there is a sudden influx of blood from the maternal vascular bed into the systemic circulation.[97,234]

Other factors that contribute to the increase in cardiac output include sympathetic nervous system stimulation by pain and anxiety, position, method of delivery, and anesthesia.[37] Hendricks and Quilligan noted a 50% to 61% increase in cardiac output in women experiencing pain and anxiety alone.[97] This change was accompanied by a rise in

both systolic and diastolic blood pressures and heart rate. Thus the increase in sympathetic tone due to pain, anxiety, and muscular activity is an important factor in the increased cardiac output during contractions. Pain and anxiety can be reduced by psychoprophylactic strategies as well as analgesia and anesthesia. Epidural or spinal anesthesia result in a sympathetic blockade that can lead to decreased blood pressure, hypotension and decreased uteroplacental perfusion if maternal intravascular volume is not maintained.

Supine positioning results in lower cardiac output, increased heart rate, and decreased stroke volume.[232] Movement from the supine to the lateral decubitus position leads to an increase in cardiac output, a decrease in pulse rate, and an increase in stroke volume.[232,236]

In general, both systolic and diastolic blood pressure increase during contractions, returning to baseline levels between contractions. Oxygen consumption gradually increases up to 100%.[152] Heart rate changes are variable, with increases or decreases occurring. Systemic vascular resistance does not change.[152] Labor may lead to an increase in not only the number but also the variety of arrhythmias.

Arrhythmias seen during labor may include premature ventricular contractions, atrial premature beats, premature nodal contractions, sinus bradycardia, sinus tachycardia, and supraventricular tachycardia.[168]

Postpartum Period

Delivery of the fetus, placenta, and amniotic fluid results in dramatic maternal hemodynamic alterations that can result in cardiovascular instability during the immediate postpartum period. These changes are due to the loss of blood at delivery and the body's compensatory mechanisms. On average, 500 ml (10%) of blood is lost in vaginal deliveries and 1000 ml (15% to 30%) with cesarean sections. Despite this amount of blood loss, cardiac output is significantly elevated above prelabor levels for 1 to 2 hours postpartum.[175] Immediately after delivery, cardiac output is 60% to 80% higher than prelabor levels (see Figure 8-8). However, within 10 to 15 minutes there is a sharp decline that stabilizes at prelabor values by 1 hour.[97,148,152,193,234]

Several factors may contribute to this transient increase in maternal cardiac output. These include reduction in gravid uterus pressure and improved venacaval blood flow, autotransfusion of uteroplacental blood back into maternal circulation, and decreased systemic vascular resistance and vascular capacitance due to contraction of the muscular uterus and absence of placental blood flow.[138] Mobilization of extracellular fluid also improves venous return to the heart. The increased return to the heart contributes to the higher central venous pressure seen postpartally. Maternal hypervolemia acts as a protective mechanism for excessive blood loss at delivery (see Chapter 7).

During the first week after delivery, there is a decrease in the sodium compartment space by 2 liters. This results in a 3-kg weight loss. Diuresis in order to dissipate the increased extracellular fluid occurs between day 2 and day 5. Without the diuresis of mobilized extracellular fluid, increased pulmonary wedge pressures and pulmonary edema can result.[58,138] The latter may be encountered in women with preeclampsia or heart disease who do not undergo normal diuretic patterns. Wedge pressures eventually normalize once diuresis occurs.[138]

Stroke volume and thus cardiac output remain elevated for at least 48 hours after delivery.[185] This increase is probably due to increased venous return with loss of uterine blood flow and mobilization of interstitial fluid (see Chapter 10).[185] Cardiac output decreases by 30% by 2 weeks postpartum then gradually decreases to nonpregnant values by 6 to 12 weeks in most women and perhaps up to 24 weeks in some women.[33,34,82,193]

Most of the other cardiovascular system changes resolve by 6 to 8 weeks postpartum. Left atrial size and heart rate reach prepregnancy values by 10 days postpartum and LV size by 4 to 6 months.[148] The audible vibrations caused by ejection of blood from the RV into the pulmonary trunk or from the LV into the brachiocephalic arteries at the point of branching from the aortic arch usually disappear by postpartum day 8. For approximately 20% of women, the systolic murmur persists beyond 4 weeks postpartum. The intensity of the murmur does, however, decrease by day 8, even if it does not disappear.[59,71,168]

CLINICAL IMPLICATIONS FOR THE PREGNANT WOMAN AND HER FETUS

The effects of pregnancy on the cardiovascular system can result in alterations in the ability of the woman to carry on the activities of daily living, exercise, or be comfortable in various positions. Because the maternal circulatory system is the lifeline for the fetus to receive oxygen and nutrients, hemodynamic alterations can affect the well-being of the fetus. Some of the changes experienced are exaggerations of normal and have little impact on the fetus; however, disease states may result in significant growth alterations or potentiate hypoxic episodes.

Arrhythmias

Many pregnant women experience rhythm disruptions that become more intense during the second and third trimesters. It is unclear how much of the reported increase is due to an actual change in frequency with pregnancy versus due to closer monitoring.[37] Most of these arrhythmias are benign and are not indicative of heart disease. The woman may describe skipped beats, momentary pressure in the neck or chest, or extra beats. These are usually representative of premature ventricular contractions and require no further treatment. Extra systoles or supraventricular tachycardia may also be seen in some women.[208]

The increase in arrhythmias is probably due to increased sympathetic nervous system activity and not due to structural defects.[37] Occasionally cardiac problems may present during pregnancy, so arrhythmias should be evaluated and managed in a manner similar to that in nonpregnant women. Awareness of the increased heart rate can be uncomfortable for some women. True tachycardia, such as paroxysmal atrial tachycardia or paroxysmal atrial fibrillation, may be evident for the first time during pregnancy. This may be frightening for the woman. Taking a deep breath or coughing may result in a slowing or conversion of the heart rate into a more normal pattern.[94]

Supine Hypotensive Syndrome

Orthostatic stress generated by changes in position (from recumbent to sitting to standing) is associated with acute

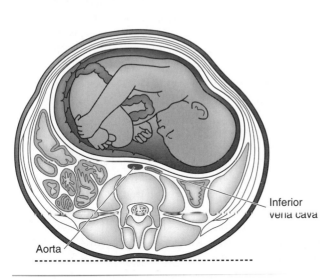

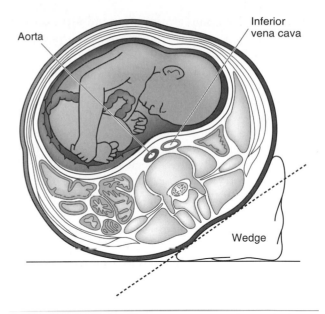

FIGURE 8-9 The pregnant uterus compressing the aorta and the inferior vena cava (aortocaval compression). Patient in supine position. (From Cohen, W.R., Acker, D.B., & Friedman, E.A. [Eds.]. [1989]. *Management of labor* (2nd ed.]. Rockville, MD: Aspen.)

FIGURE 8-10 Uterine displacement with wedge under hip to relieve aortocaval compression. (From Cohen, W.R., Acker, D.B., & Friedman, E.A. [Eds.]. [1989]. *Management of labor* (2nd ed.). Rockville, MD: Aspen.)

hemodynamic changes. Blood pools in dependent vessels, which reduces venous return and decreases cardiac output and blood pressure with increasing orthostatic stress. Heart rate and systemic vascular resistance increase; mean arterial pressure changes, however, are not significant. In situations where orthostatic stress is not compensated, the uteroplacental circulation may be compromised and fetal distress experienced.[66]

The gravid uterus is also associated with a significant amount of caval blood flow obstruction in the supine position. Approximately 90% of gravid women experience obstruction of the inferior vena cava in the supine position. Late in pregnancy, but before the fetal presenting part becomes engaged, the uterus is mobile enough to fall back against the inferior vena cava in both the supine and lateral recumbent positions (Figures 8-9 and 8-10). This results in vena caval tamponade. Vascular compression may also be applied to the aorta and its branches. In most women, paravertebral collateral circulation develops during pregnancy. This, along with the dilated utero-ovarian circulation, permits blood flow from the legs and pelvis to bypass the vena cava.[124,125,138]

Usually the fall in cardiac output due to a posture change is compensated for by an increase in peripheral resistance. This allows systemic blood pressure and heart rate to remain unchanged. However, about 8% of pregnant woman in the supine position may experience a significant decrease in heart rate and blood pressure, leading to symptoms of weakness, lightheadedness, nausea, dizziness, or syncope. This is referred to as supine hypotensive syndrome of pregnancy and is usually corrected when position is changed.[125,148,162,179]

Initially it was felt that the symptoms were due to the occlusion of the vena cava by the uterus. More recently it has been suggested that failure to develop adequate collateral circulation may result in a 25% to 30% drop in cardiac output and symptomatology when in the supine position for longer than a few minutes.[16,124,125,130,179]

Exercise during Pregnancy

The current health and fitness awareness in the United States has brought about many questions regarding exercise during pregnancy. Exercise has significant benefits for the mother and fetus.[45,145] Regular aerobic exercise done two to three times per week maintains or improves maternal fitness during pregnancy.[134] Fit women have been shown to have shorter labors and fewer perinatal complications.[90,188] Concerns regarding exercise during pregnancy include the effects on the fetus and mother, including the risks of hyperthermia (see Chapter 19) and increased cardiac workload. Further exploration of these areas is still needed as are differences between women who train and those who do not.

Physiologic responses to exercise include increased oxygen consumption, redistribution of blood, altered venous pooling, and changes in cardiac output and stroke volume. Both exercise and pregnancy increase oxygen consumption and the need for energy substrate by different tissues. Blood flow is redistributed during exercise, moving blood away from the viscera and to the skin and skeletal muscles. This leads to a reduction in utero-ovarian blood flow. Greater intensity and duration of exercise is associated with increased redistribution of blood from the uterus to the skin and muscles.[93] The limitation in substrate delivery to the fetus could potentially have adverse effects resulting in fetal hypoxia; however, to cause such changes, the reduction in uterine blood flow has to exceed 50%. However in healthy pregnant women, these occurrences would be rare, being most likely during very strenuous and prolonged exercise.[44,49,144,152,158]

Therefore under normal conditions there is probably enough oxygen available to the uterus to meet and exceed uterine and fetal demands. Compensatory mechanisms help to maintain oxygen availability during maternal exercise.[93] The decrease in placental blood flow is significantly less than the decrease in uterine blood flow.[93] Blood flow is selectively distributed to the placenta, at the expense of the myometrium.[93,152] Regular sustained exercise during pregnancy has been reported to increase placental villous size and volume.[113] The significance of this change is uncertain.

Maternal hematocrit rises during exercise. This increases maternal oxygen-carrying capacity, and there is a smaller reduction in oxygen availability–to–blood flow ratio.[152] Uterine oxygen uptake increases during exercise in order to maintain a stable oxygen consumption level.[93,152] Maternal ventricular performance is maintained with exercise. In response to strenuous exercise in early pregnancy, the LV adapts by increasing its contractile reserve; in late pregnancy, it adapts by increasing preload reserve.[240]

Along with the redistribution of weight that occurs with the anterior displacement of the uterus, the progressive enlargement of the fetus and uterus can lead to alterations in venous blood return. The woman may experience dizziness due to poor venous return and resultant orthostatic hypotension. Altered cardiac return may modify blood flow to the uterus and place the fetus at risk for hypoxia. Therefore certain positions and activities may need to be modified in exercise regimens.

Pregnancy increases the workload of the heart, although in most pregnancies the cardiac reserve is adequate to meet these demands. During early pregnancy, exercise is associated with further increases in stroke volume and cardiac output. As pregnancy progresses, the cardiac output changes with exercise are lower.[46] These changes in later pregnancy may be due to increased peripheral pooling rather than a progressive decline in circulatory reserve as pregnancy progresses.[152] Decreased exercise tolerance with fatigue and dyspnea is also noted in later pregnancy. Changes in cardiac output, stroke volume, and heart rate with exercise in late pregnancy are illustrated in Figure 8-11.

Exercise results in changes in epinephrine, norepinephrine, glucagon, cortisol, prolactin, and endorphin levels. Maternal exercise is also associated with a significant increase in circulating catecholamines. The placenta, under normal circumstances, is very efficient in metabolizing the catecholamines, and only 10% to 15% reach the fetus. Elevated catecholamine levels could have an additional restrictive effect on the fetal circulation.[158]

The usual fetal response to maternal exercise is an increase in heart rate by 5 to 25 beats per minute.[90,188] This increase may be due to decreased placental blood flow, stimulation of maternal vasoactive hormones, or exercise-induced uterine contractions.[90,188] These changes are consistent and are independent of either gestational age or intensity of maternal exercise. Immediately after exercise and during the next 5 minutes, fetal heart rate (FHR) remains elevated regardless of the type of exercise. Within 15 minutes, FHR drops to preexercise values in women engaged in mild to moderate exercise activities. For women engaged in strenuous activities, the FHR does not return to baseline for up to 30 minutes.[42,55,90,158,188] The elevated FHR seen following exercise may also be a normal physiologic response to compensate for short periods of mild hypoxia.

In a few women, transient fetal bradycardia has been reported after strenuous exercise, possibly due to a rapid increase in catecholamines. These episodes of bradycardia did not compromise fetal outcome.[11] An initial response of tachycardia may lead to bradycardia if hypoxia becomes prolonged and vagal stimulation occurs. There is also the possibility that these brief occurrences are within the normal realm of fetal reflex responses to major maternal hemodynamic and hormonal events.[158] In most situations, fetal bradycardia was mild (100 to 119 beats per minute). Fetal reserve should be assessed if any abnormalities are suspected, and maternal cardiac as well as fetoplacental reserve should be the basis for determining exercise and work levels and activities during pregnancy.[158]

Regular exercise during pregnancy has many benefits including maintenance of fitness; improved cardiovascular function; control of blood pressure; decreased backaches, fatigue, and shortness of breath; shorter labors; decreased clot formation and varicosities; psychologic feelings of wellness; prevention of excessive weight gain and fat deposition; decreased leg cramps; decreased leg edema; and more rapid postpartum recovery.[48,90,93,152,188] Fetal benefits

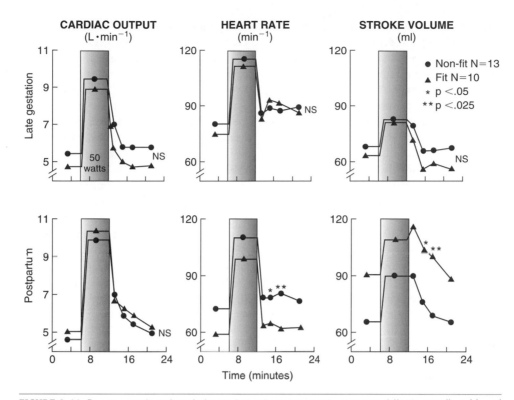

FIGURE 8-11 Pregnancy alterations in hemodynamic responses to exercise. Effects usually achieved with physical training in nonpregnant women (depicted in lower panels) include a relatively greater increase in stroke volume and a relatively lesser increase in heart rate with moderate exercise when fit women are compared to nonfit women. In late pregnancy (upper panels) these differences are not seen. One explanation may be that the stroke volume response to training is blunted by limitation of venous return to the heart due to vena cava obstruction by the pregnant uterus in late gestation. (From Morton, M.J., et al. [1985]. Exercise dynamics in late gestation: Effects of physical training. *Am J Obstet Gynecol, 152,* 91.)

may include better growth, improved stress tolerance, and enhanced neurobehavioral maturation, with a leaner body composition at 5 years of age.[48] Women with conditioning before pregnancy demonstrate improved metabolic effects with exercise during pregnancy than unconditioned women.[43] Mild to moderate aerobic exercise (to 50% to 85% of maximum) has not been demonstrated to increase spontaneous abortions, but does decrease length of labor, number of cesarean births, fetal fat mass (and thus mean birth weight), and number of episodes of fetal distress.[5,43,47,90,251] Maternal risks of exercise include musculoskeletal injury, risk of cardiovascular complications, hypoglycemia, and uterine contractions.[93] Exercise is contraindicated in women with complications such as preterm labor and uterine bleeding.

American Academy of Obstetrics and Gynecology recommendations can be used as guidelines for activity in pregnancy.[4] Moderate exercise three to four times a week is a good guideline for pregnant women to follow and is preferable to intermittent activity.[4] Women should maintain the level of aerobic exercise done before pregnancy and avoid increasing the level during pregnancy.[5] Suggested activities include swimming, biking, aerobic walking, stretching, and normal walking if the women cannot tolerate aerobic exercise. Swimming and other aquatic exercise have particular benefits during pregnancy. Changes in heart rate and vital capacity are less while stroke volume is increased during exercise in water. Hydrostatic pressure moves extravascular fluid back into the vascular space, reducing fluid retention and enhancing diuresis.[93] The water reduces thermal changes with exercise by acting as a thermoregulatory buffer around the woman.[93]

Vigorous exercise should not be performed in hot, humid weather or during a period of febrile illness, and body temperature should never exceed 40° C.[4] Jumping, jerky movements, or deep flexion or extension of joints should be avoided because of the joint instability that occurs during pregnancy. Gradual changes in position should be undertaken to avoid orthostatic stress and hypotension. Heart rate should be self-monitored during peak activity and should not exceed 70% of maximum. Heart rate and respiratory rate should return to resting rates within 15 minutes after exercise. Strenuous activity should be limited to 15 minutes. Caloric intake needs to be high enough to meet not only the demands of exercise but also of pregnancy.[4]

Competitive activities are generally discouraged. Studies on elite athletes with high-intensity exercise during pregnancy are limited, but there is some evidence of an increase in low-birth-weight infants.[90] Maternal anatomic changes (weight gain, relaxation of ligaments and joints, progressive lordosis, and changes in center of gravity) of pregnancy usually interfere with standard training routines in these athletes by the second trimester.[90]

At no time should exercise be continued if pain or contractions are experienced. The primary health care provider should be contacted if bleeding, dizziness, shortness of breath, palpitations, faintness, tachycardia, back pain, pubic pain, or difficulty in walking is experienced. Women designated as high risk for preterm labor need to receive special counseling regarding not only appropriate activity levels but also signs and symptoms of labor.[4]

Multiple Pregnancy

The woman with a multiple pregnancy is subject to a higher risk of morbidity and mortality. There is an increased production of estriol, progesterone, and human placental lactogen (hPL) that results in an increased volume expansion and weight gain. Whereas plasma volume is increased by about 50% in single pregnancies, in twins there is an increase of up to 65%, with further elevations seen in women with higher order multiples. There is also a higher RBC volume, increased hemodilution of iron and folate, and an exaggerated physiologic anemia. Whether the hemodilution is due to a greater increase in total body volume or a greater demand for iron or folic acid is unclear; however, it is probably some combination of the two.[168,252]

The increase in maternal cardiac output in twin pregnancies is also greater than that found in singletons. The average increase is approximately 0.4 L/min higher at term in twins versus singletons. Beyond this, however, heart rate, stroke volume, and mean circulation time are similar in single and multiple pregnancies.[37,168,252] The change in cardiac output suggests decreased cardiovascular reserve.[27]

Characteristic changes in blood pressure with multiple pregnancy include a lowered diastolic pressure at 20 weeks (74% of women with twins have a diastolic pressure less than 80 mmHg), which is followed by a greater rise in diastolic pressure between midpregnancy and delivery (95% experience a rise in diastolic pressure of 15 mmHg or more).

Mothers with twins are at greater risk for preterm labor, preeclampsia, placenta previa, placental abruption, anemia, hyperemesis gravidarum, and postpartum hemorrhage. The length of labor is similar in twin and single pregnancies, although with twins the active phase is longer and the latent phase is shorter. Labor may be more difficult, possibly due to uterine overdistention and an increased incidence of malpresentation. Blood loss is about double that in a single delivery, and hemorrhage is more frequent due to uterine atony and sudden decompression of the overdistended uterus. There is also a slightly higher incidence of vasa praevia and placenta previa, increasing the possibility of hemorrhage at delivery. The risk of preeclampsia is five times greater in twin than in single pregnancies. This is probably due to the larger placental mass that is to be found with twin pregnancies.[2,168]

Cardiac Disease and Pregnancy

Cardiac disease affects about 1% of pregnant women.[37] This incidence is slowly increasing as improved management and technical capabilities for both the mother and fetus make it possible to sustain pregnancy in those who previously would have been advised to terminate or avoid pregnancy. Corrective surgery for infants and children with congenital heart disease has increased the number of these women who are now of childbearing age. In addition, the incidence of heart disease increases in women who wait until their thirties or forties to have children.[248]

Pregnancy brings about profound alterations in the cardiovascular system. These hemodynamic changes can result in death or disability to women who have underlying heart disease. Many early symptoms of cardiac disease, such as fatigue, dyspnea on exertion, dependent edema, presyncope (due to pressure on the inferior vena cava) and palpitations are normal findings in pregnancy.[212] Thus the diagnosis of cardiac disease may be delayed in women who present with symptoms of cardiac disorders for the first time during pregnancy.

Some cardiac diseases may actually benefit somewhat from the increase in cardiac output, decrease in systemic vascular resistance, and increased heart rate. On the other hand, cardiac diseases associated with fixed lesions do not tolerate the volume increase because the stenotic area cannot accommodate the increased flow. The increased heart rate shortens the diastolic filling time, thereby preventing adequate filling of the heart. This combined with the decrease in systemic vascular resistance may result in a drop in blood pressure.[248]

When blood volume reaches its peak at midpregnancy, the potential for congestive heart failure increases. At delivery this risk is further increased by the 20% increase in blood volume. Acute pulmonary edema may occur. Applying pressure to the abdomen can slow the blood return to the heart and facilitate cardiovascular stabilization. If the heart is unable to compensate for the decrease in systemic vascular resistance, the blood pressure falls. This may increase fatigue and contribute to episodes of dizziness and syncope as well as reduce uterine blood flow. Maintenance of blood pressure can be attempted by administration of chronotropic and alpha pressor agents. Epidural and spinal anesthesia may further decrease systemic vascular resistance and should be used with caution in these patients.[248]

Pregnancy is particularly dangerous for women who have cardiac lesions, such as Eisenmenger syndrome, primary pulmonary hypertension, Marfan syndrome, and hemodynamically significant mitral stenosis (Table 8-3). The

TABLE 8-3 Risk for Maternal Mortality with Cardiac Disease

MATERNAL MORTALITY	CARDIAC DISORDER
25% to 50% Mortality	Pulmonary hypertension Marfan syndrome with aortic involvement Aortic coarctation with valvular involvement
5% to 15% Mortality	Aortic stenosis Mitral stenosis with NYHA Class III/IV Uncorrected tetralogy of Fallot Marfan syndrome without aortic involvement Aortic coarctation without valvular involvement Previous myocardial infarction Prosthetic value Mitral stenosis with atrial fibrillation
0% to 1% Mortality	Ventricular septal defect Atrial septal defect Corrected tetralogy of Fallot Mitral stenosis with NYHA class I/II Persistent ductus arteriosus Bioprosthetic valve

Adapted from American College of Obstetricians and Gynecologists (1992, June). *Cardiac disease in pregnancy* (ACOG technical bulletin no. 168). Washington, DC: American College of Obstetricians and Gynecologists *NYHA*, New York Heart Association.

presence of a cardiac lesion involving pulmonary hypertension during pregnancy carries a risk of maternal mortality somewhere between 30% and 50%. Pregnancy may also aggravate preexisting cardiac conditions such that damage is extensive and recovery to prepregnancy levels is not possible. In addition, pregnancy may result in maternal heart disease (e.g., peripartal cardiomyopathy).[37,49,152,208,212,222]

The fetus must also be monitored closely during pregnancy in a woman with cardiac disease. Fetal well-being and growth are dependent upon a continuous flow of well-oxygenated blood to the uterus. When this supply is reduced or interrupted or oxygenation is decreased, the fetus is at risk for altered growth and development and for increased mortality.[153] In addition, the fetus is at increased risk of being born with a congenital heart defect if either parent has congenital heart disease. If the mother is the affected parent, she adds an environmental risk as well as a genetic risk for her infant.[152]

All of these factors and the risk to the mother and fetus should be discussed in depth with couples before pregnancy. This preconception counseling allows the potential problems and treatment options to be explored and the woman's current health status to be characterized. It is generally recommended that surgical correction or palliative procedures are done before pregnancy, followed by several months to a year of recovery time.[208]

Obstructive Lesions

These lesions are basically stenotic in nature. The main concern is an obstruction of flow causing an elevation of pressure proximal to the obstructive lesion and a decrease in flow distal to the stenotic area. Pulmonary stenosis without septal defect, coarctation of the aorta, aortic stenosis, mitral stenosis, and tricuspid stenosis are included in this group. Mitral stenosis and mitral regurgitation are presented as examples.

Mitral stenosis. This lesion is caused almost exclusively by rheumatic fever. The stenotic valve restricts cardiac output, resulting in fatigue, which is the most common symptom. The obstruction of left atrial outflow leads to pressure elevations in the left atrium, pulmonary veins, and pulmonary capillaries, causing severe pulmonary congestion. Risk of death is greatest in the third trimester and postpartum.[208]

The increased blood volume, cardiac output, and heart rate of pregnancy, along with the fluid retention, may lead to an increase in symptoms. Signs of pulmonary congestion usually occur by 20 weeks and stabilize by 30 weeks.[37] The increase in cardiac output, plasma volume, and heart rate peak during this time, decreasing diastolic filling time in the LV and increasing the pressure gradient across the mitral valvue.[37] An exacerbation may occur at the time of delivery if there is prolonged tachycardia. The first 24 hours after delivery is a time of increased vulnerability in these women due to intravascular fluid shifts.[37]

Management should include avoidance of the supine position and prophylaxis against rheumatic fever during the pregnancy and against endocarditis during labor and delivery. If severe mitral stenosis is diagnosed, mitral commissurotomy is advised before conception. If symptoms develop during the course of pregnancy, activity restrictions to reduce the strain on the heart, sodium intake restrictions, diuretics, and digitalis may be considered. If symptoms of pulmonary congestion persist despite medical therapy, surgical intervention (either a balloon valvuloplasty or valve replacement) may be necessary. If thromboembolism occurs, anticoagulation therapy with subcutaneous heparin is needed.[37,151,208]

Mitral regurgitation. Mitral regurgitation may be due to rheumatic fever; however, there are numerous other conditions that can lead to its development. Prolapse of the mitral valve during systole allows for regurgitation of blood back into the left atrium. Fatigue is the result. If severe, pulmonary congestion can occur. These women have a propensity for atrial fibrillation and left atrial thrombus formation.[222] Individuals with mitral regurgitation may be asymptomatic for extended periods of time. In the woman with mild regurgitation, pregnancy is usually well tolerated, and the development of congestive failure is rare. Prophylactic antibiotics are warranted.[37]

Mitral valve prolapse. Mitral valve prolapse (MVP) is one of the most common congenital heart lesions. MVP is found in 2% to 10% of women of childbearing age.[37] Most women with MVP are asymptomatic and tolerate pregnancy well; in fact, there is evidence that pregnancy may actually improve hemodynamics and symptoms in some women. Although rare, complications associated with MVP (arrhythmias, infective endocarditis, and cerebral ischemic events) may result in serious complications during pregnancy.

MVP can be both a primary disease function and a secondary pathology associated with connective tissue diseases or cardiac disease that reduces the size of the LV.[57] The latter includes syndromes such as Marfan syndrome, pseudoxanthoma elasticum, and osteogenesis imperfecta.

The hemodynamic changes of pregnancy can reduce the clinical signs of MVP by decreasing audible murmurs (usually a late systolic murmur associated with a click), possibly by increasing the LV end-diastolic volume and favorably realigning the mitral valve complex. The decrease in peripheral vascular resistance relieves the mitral insufficiency, thereby reducing the murmur. Once these parameters return to normal in the postpartum period, the auscultatory findings of MVP return. These changes are also reflected on echocardiography.[183]

In most situations, pregnancy is tolerated well in women with MVP, with good maternal and fetal outcomes. However, there have been anecdotal reports of women experiencing transient thromboembolic ischemia and left hemiparesis and endocarditis.[57] However it is more likely that the woman will experience an increase in palpitations, arrhythmias, or chest pains that may require medical intervention with the use of beta-blockers. Whether prophylactic antibiotics to prevent bacterial endocarditis are necessary in all pregnant women with MVP remains controversial. Current recommendations suggest that antibiotics should be used in patients in whom MVP is complicated by mitral insufficiency.[57]

Left-to-Right Shunts

Left-to-right shunts are characterized by recirculation of oxygenated blood through the lungs, bypassing the peripheral circulation. This can occur through an atrial septal defect (ASD), ventricular septal defect (VSD), or a patent ductus arteriosus (PDA). Most patients born with these defects either have experienced closing of the defect on its own during childhood or have had corrective surgery to reduce the defect. A residual defect may remain, however.[152]

The magnitude of the left-to-right shunt is dependent upon the ratio of resistance in the systemic and pulmonary vascular circuits. During pregnancy both circuits have a decline in resistance (Table 8-1) so that there is usually no significant change if shunting occurs. If pulmonary vascular disease exists, the normal fall in PVR may not occur. It is rare that cyanosis occurs with these defects unless significant pulmonary hypertension or RV failure develops. Pregnancy does not seem to precipitate these events, however.[152]

Atrial septal defect. An atrial septal defect (ASD) is one of the most common defects seen in adults and therefore in pregnancy. ASDs are usually asymptomatic but may become symptomatic for the first time in pregnancy.[37] The most common complications are arrhythmias and heart failure; however, arrhythmias usually do not appear until the woman is in her forties.[49]

The hypervolemia of pregnancy increases the left-to-right shunt through the ASD, thereby creating an additional burden on the RV. This additional load is usually tolerated well by most women, although up to 15% fetal loss has been reported.[37] The additional load is not well tolerated; RV failure occurs, leading to marked peripheral edema, atrial arrhythmias, pulmonary hypertension, and paradoxic systemic emboli across the septal defect.[49,152]

Ventricular septal defect. A VSD can occur either as an isolated lesion or in conjunction with other congenital cardiac anomalies (tetralogy of Fallot, transposition of the great vessels, or coarctation of the aorta). The size of the defect determines the degree of shunting, tolerance to the additional burden of pregnancy, and prognosis. Small defects are usually tolerated well; large VSDs often lead to congestive failure, arrhythmias, or the development of pulmonary hypertension. A large VSD is often associated with some degree of aortic regurgitation, which contributes to the possibility of congestive failure.

Patent ductus arteriosus. A PDA is usually identified in the early neonatal period or during infancy. Surgical correction is usually done at that time. Therefore it is uncommon to find this type of defect in childbearing women. However, if it does exist, it is usually well tolerated during gestation, labor, and delivery. If the PDA is complicated by pulmonary hypertension, the prognosis is poorer.

Right-to-Left Shunts

Right-to-left shunts are characterized by shunting of blood from the systemic venous circulation to the arterial circulation without oxygenation. Right-to-left shunting occurs through an ASD, VSD, or PDA when the PVR rises so that it exceeds the systemic vascular resistance or when an obstruction to RV outflow exists. These women present with cyanosis, clubbing of the fingers, and RV hypertrophy. Conditions include Eisenmenger syndrome, tetralogy of Fallot, and primary pulmonary hypertension.

Eisenmenger syndrome. This syndrome combines the presence of a congenital left-to-right shunt with progressive pulmonary hypertension that leads to shunt reversal or bidirectional flow. It is more commonly associated with VSD or PDA. During pregnancy the decreased systemic vascular resistance increases the degree of right-to-left shunting, which reduces pulmonary perfusion, leading to hypoxemia and maternal and fetal compromise. Systemic hypotension leads to decreased RV filling pressures, which may be insufficient to perfuse the pulmonary bed, where high PVR exists. The result may be the onset of sudden and profound hypoxemia. Hemorrhage or complications of conduction anesthesia (hypovolemia) may precipitate hypoxemia and lead to death during the intrapartum period.[49,208]

The mortality rate for pregnant women with Eisenmenger syndrome can be as high as 50% when pulmonary hypertension is associated with a VSD.[14] Because of this high mortality rate, pregnancy termination is usually recommended. If gestation continues, hospitalization, continuous oxygen administration, and the use of pulmonary vasodilators are recommended. Even if the woman survives, fetal mortality is up to 50% in women with cyanosis.[37,208] During labor it is essential to maintain an adequate fluid load, and the placement of a pulmonary artery catheter is often warranted to monitor fluid status. Maintaining a preload edge to protect against unexpected blood loss may risk tipping the scales toward pulmonary edema.[49]

Tetralogy of Fallot. This defect is the most common cause of right-to-left shunting; it includes a combination of VSD, pulmonary valve stenosis, RV hypertrophy, and rightward displacement of the aortic root. PVR is normal. Surgical correction usually occurs during infancy, although there may be residual shunting following correction. Pregnancy outcome is relatively good for those individuals who have undergone surgical correction.[12,137,208] In pregnant women with uncorrected VSDs, the decrease in systemic vascular resistance leads to worsening right-to-left shunting. This can be complicated by intrapartum blood loss, leading to systemic hypotension. Therefore careful monitoring of fluid status is warranted.[49,208]

Pulmonary artery hypertension. Severe pulmonary hypertension associated with pregnancy carries a 50% maternal mortality rate and a 40% fetal mortality rate if the mother survives. Significant pulmonary hypertension is a contraindication to pregnancy, and pregnancy should be prevented or termination recommended if it occurs. If termination is not possible, physical activity should be curtailed and supine positioning avoided during late gestation. Careful monitoring of oxygenation and fluid status at the time of labor and delivery is essential in order to identify problems early and intervene appropriately.[152]

Marfan Syndrome

Marfan syndrome is an autosomal dominant disorder of connective tissue whose clinical manifestations include skeletal, ocular, and cardiovascular abnormalities. Aortic dilatation is one of these manifestations. Complications that can result include aneurysm formation and rupture, aortic dissection, and aortic regurgitation. Structural changes in the aortic wall due to high estrogen levels predispose pregnant women to aortic dissection. Rupture usually occurs in the third trimester or in the first stages of labor. If there is no preexisting cardiovascular disease, the risk of maternal death is relatively low.[46,49,178,208]

Counseling regarding the risk of inheritance and the potential maternal complications should be given preconceptually if possible. If pregnancy occurs and abortion is not desired, the use of oral propranolol to decrease pulsatile pressure on the aortic wall is indicated. If a surgical delivery is performed, the generalized connective tissue weakness must be taken into consideration and the use of retention sutures may be necessary.[49]

Hypertension

Hypertension is the most common complication of pregnancy, complicating 7% to 13% of all pregnancies.[13,23,140] Hypertension during pregnancy is classified as chronic hypertension, preeclampsia-eclampsia, preeclampsia superimposed on chronic hypertension, and gestational hypertension. Definitions of each form are in Table 8-4.

Chronic hypertension occurs in 1% to 5% of pregnant women Maternal-fetal complications of chronic hypertension include superimposed preeclampsia, abruptio placentae, stroke, preterm delivery, still birth, low birth weight, and neonatal loss.[140] Perinatal mortality is two to four times higher.[140] Recognition of chronic hypertension in women whose prepregnancy blood pressure is unknown may be more difficult in pregnancy, because these women have the usual physiologic decrease in blood pressure in early pregnancy.[140]

Nonpregnant women with chronic hypertension generally have decreased renal plasma flow (RPF) and GFR, with an exaggerated excretion of sodium in response to a salt load. During early pregnancy, RPF and GFR increase, but the total increase by late pregnancy is less than in normotensive pregnant women. With increased blood pressure, fluid moves from the vascular to the extravascular spaces, and the blood becomes hemoconcentrated with further reductions in RPF and GFR. The pregnant woman with chronic hypertension also has a 20% to 30% decrease in sodium excretion. Vasoconstriction may reduce uteroplacental perfusion, with alterations in fetal growth.[13,23]

Preeclampsia

Preeclampsia is a hypertensive, multisystem disorder characterized by hypertension and proteinuria that complicates 3% to 5% of all pregnancies.[61,100] Other features may include central nervous system irritability and, at times, coagulation or liver function abnormalities. Changes in different organ systems with preeclampsia are summarized in Table 8-5. Women with preeclampsia may develop seizures (eclampsia) or a variant with abnormal liver function and thrombocytopenia known as the *HELLP syndrome.* The term *HELLP* comes from this syndrome's characteristic clinical findings: hemolysis (H), elevated liver enzymes (EL), and a low platelet (LP) count.

Preeclampsia is characterized by decreased perfusion to all organ systems secondary to vasospasm; increased sensitivity to pressors, including angiotensin II; and decreased plasma volume due to loss of fluid from the vascular space. Factors predisposing to preeclampsia are conditions in which oxygen demand is increased (multiple pregnancy, molar pregnancy, or an edematous placenta) or that with decreased oxygen transfer (primipara, microvascular disease, chronic hypertension, diabetes, collagen disorders, or abnormal placentation).[55,101,189,246] The net result of these factors is a direct or relative placental hypoperfusion. This suggests altered uteroplacental perfusion as an early event in the pathogenesis of preeclampsia. In addition, many of these factors are also associated with increased fetal antigen load (i.e., multiple pregnancy, hydrops, molar pregnancy or other increased placental mass), supporting the theory of an immunologic basis for preeclampsia.[206]

The exact pathogenesis of preeclampsia is unclear, but research in recent years has pointed to inadequate remodeling of maternal uterine spiral arteries as an early pathogenic event. Endothelial disruption and release of

TABLE 8-4 Classification of Hypertensive Disorders of Pregnancy

CLASSIFICATION	DEFINITION AND DIAGNOSTIC CRITERIA
Preeclampsia	Hypertension with proteinuria Hypertension: blood pressure >140 mmHg systolic or 90 mmHg diastolic after 20 weeks' gestation in a woman normotensive before 20 weeks' gestation Proteinuria: 300 mg/L protein in a random specimen or and excretion of 300 mg/24 hours Hypertension with other systemic symptoms of preeclampsia in the absence of protienuria is highly suspicious of preeclampsia
Chronic hypertension	Blood pressure 140/90 mmHg or greater before the twentieth week of gestation or, if only diagnosed during pregnancy, persisting 6 weeks after pregnancy
Preeclampsia superimposed on chronic hypertension	Highly likely in women who develop new proteinuria or with preexisting hypertension and protienuria protienuria who develop sudden increases in blood pressure or proteinuria, thrombocytopenia, or increases in hepatocellular enzymes
Gestational hypertension	Development of hypertension without other signs of preeclampsia

Adapted from National High Blood Pressure Education Program. (2000). Report of the national high blood pressure education program working group on high blood pressure in pregnancy. *Am J Obstet Gynecol, 183,* 1.

vasoactive substances and cytokines accompany this change.[13,34,55,61,189,246,166] Normally extravillous trophoblast cells from the placenta migrate into the uterine spiral arteries in both the decidua and myometrium. The fetal trophoblast cells remodel the maternal spiral arteries so that little vascular smooth muscle tissue, neural elements, and elastic matrix are left. The spiral arteries become large, flaccid uteroplacental vessels establishing a low-resistance circuit that enhances blood supply to the fetus and placenta. This remodeling process is described in Chapter 3.

In preeclampsia the remodeling is confined of the decidual portion of the blood vessels (see Figure 8-5), with 30% to 50% of the vessels in the myometrium left intact.[73,153] In these vessels the adrenergic nerve supply is also intact.[189] The cause of this failure is unknown, but it may have a genetic or immunologic basis.[61,189]

HLA-G expression, which helps protect the fetal tissue from the maternal immune system (see Chapter 12), may be decreased or abnormal in the extravillous trophoblast in women who develop preeclmapsia.[54] This may lead to an inappropriate maternal inflammatory response to the invading trophoblast (i.e., the maternal arteries recognize the trophoblast as foreign because of the altered HLA-G and defend against it).[61,189] An immunologic basis is supported by the increased incidence of classic preeclampsia in primiparous women or multiparous women with new partners.[230] A similar lack of spiral artery change is seen without preeclampsia in some forms of IUGR and in some women with preterm labor. Development of preeclampsia seems to require decreased placental perfusion, with oxidative stress and endothelial activation. This may be due to genetic factors or maternal disease that alters maternal antioxidant enzymes or increases sensitivity to oxidative stress.[212]

Plasma lipoproteins, nonesterified fatty acids, and small dense low-density lipoproteins are elevated in women with preeclampsia.[225] These provide increased substrate for lipid peroxidation.[55] Decreased placental perfusion may also increase lipid peroxidation with

TABLE 8-5   Findings and Clinical Manifestations of Preeclampsia

VASCULATURE OR SYSTEM	FINDINGS	CLINICAL MANIFESTATIONS
Cardiovascular	Increased cardiac output (CO) and systemic vasoconstriction Increased hydrostasis present High CO and HTN	Systemic hypertension (HTN) Generalized edema Increased hemolysis
Uteroplacental	Uteroplacental insufficiency Decidual ischemia Decidual thrombosis	Increased vascular hemolysis Fetal somatic growth deficiency Fetal hypoxemia and distress Abruptio placentae; placental infarcts Thrombocytopenia
Renal	Decreased renal blood flow and glomerular filtration rate Endothelial damage High angiotensin II responsiveness to tubular vasculature Cerebral motor dysfunction	Proteinuria; elevated creatinine and decreased creatinine clearance; oliguria Elevated uric acid Renal tubular necrosis and renal failure
Cerebrovascular	High cerebral perfusion pressure with regional edema Cerebral edema Regional ischemia	Generalized grand mal seizures (e.g., eclampsia) Cerebral hemorrhage Coma Central blindness Loss of appetite
Hepatic	Ischemic and hepatic cellular injury Mitochondrial injury	Elevated liver enzymes Intracellular fatty deposition
Hematologic	Intravascular hemolysis Decidual thrombosis, release of fibrin degradation products	Schistocyte burr cells Elevated free hemoglobin and iron-decreased haptoglobin levels Thrombocytopenia Antiplatelet antibodies

From Shah, D.M. (2002). Hypertensive disorder of pregnancy. In A.A. Fanaroff & R.J. Martin (Eds.) Neonatal and perinatal medicine, diseases of the fetus and infant (7th edition; p. 266). St Louis: Mosby.

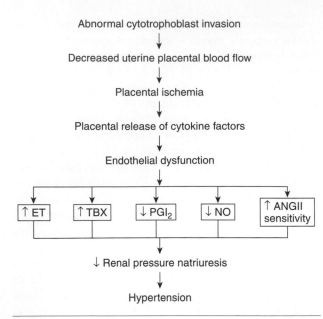

Abnormal cytotrophoblast invasion
↓
Decreased uterine placental blood flow
↓
Placental ischemia
↓
Placental release of cytokine factors
↓
Endothelial dysfunction
↓

| ↑ ET | ↑ TBX | ↓ PGI$_2$ | ↓ NO | ↑ ANGII sensitivity |

↓
↓ Renal pressure natriuresis
↓
Hypertension

FIGURE **8-12** Potential mechanisms whereby chronic reductions in uteroplacental perfusion may lead to hypertension. *ANG II*, Angiotensin II; *ET*, endothelin; *NO*, nitric oxide; *PGI$_2$* prostacyclin; *TBX*, thromboxane. (From Granger, J.P., et al. [2001]. Pathophysiology of pregnancy-induced hypertension. *Am J Hypertens, 14*, 183S.)

release of oxygen radicals without adequate counteracting antioxidant enzymes.[61] This damages maternal vascular endothelium and activation of neutrophils and macrophages (inflammatory response).

The results of the failure of spiral artery remodeling are decreased uteroplacental perfusion, placental ischemia, and alterations in maternal vascular endothelium (Figure 8-12).[55,191] Placental ischemia stimulates release of cytokines that disrupt endothelial function by inducing structural and functional changes in endothelial cells, enhancing endothelin production and a decrease in acetylcholine-induced vasodilation.[55,86,239] The endothelium is a single layer of epithelium lining the blood vessels and in direct contact with blood.[110] The endothelium releases factors to maintain vascular tone, enhance permeability, control plasma lipids, inhibit white blood cell adhesion and migration, inhibit platelet activation and aggregation, and inhibit smooth muscle proliferation and migration (to prevent atherosclerotic changes).[261,266] Normally antithrombic, antiproliferative, vasodilating substances (e.g., nitric oxide, prostacyclin or PGI$_2$) are in a homeostatic balance with vasoconstrictive, prothrombic, proliferative factors (e.g., thromboxane A$_2$, endothelin, platelet-activating factor, superoxide, angiotensin II).

During pregnancy the most important mediators of vasodilation and hemostatic balance within the uteroplacental circuit are nitric oxide and PGI$_2$.[66] The balance within the uteroplacental circulation normally favors vasodilation (Figure 8-13, *A*). In women with preeclampsia, this balance is disrupted (Figure 8-13, *B*). Markers of endothelial dysfunction found in women with preeclampsia include alteration in the procoagulant/anticoagulant ratio; increased fibronectin; enhanced platelet activation; and alterations in vasomediators such as nitric oxide, endothelin, prostaglandins, and cytokines.[55,223,216]

Nitric oxide production is normally increased in pregnancy and is thought to play a major role in renal vasodilation and perfusion.[9] In women with preeclampsia, nitric oxide synthetase, needed for nitric oxide production is reduced, although various studies report nitric oxide levels to be increased, decreased, or unchanged.[55,162,241] Prostacyclin production is also decreased with preeclampsia.[62] Endothelin synthesis is stimulated by endothelial damage.[54] Most studies show an increase in endothelin in women with preeclampsia. Endothelin may mediate the decreased renal perfusion and increased arterial blood pressure with preeclampsia.[55] Altered remodeling of maternal uterine vasculature may leave it more sensitive to the effects of the angiotensin II, a potent vasoconstrictor, which is elevated during pregnancy.[110]

Low-dose aspirin has been used to prevent preeclampsia. The reduced placental production of prostacyclin (vasodilator) versus thromboxane A$_2$ (vasoconstrictor)—which leads to thromboxane dominance—increases the risk for platelet aggregation and endothelial damage in the placenta as well as other maternal organs. Aspirin inhibits platelet thromboxane A$_2$ but not prostacyclin. Although early studies suggested a benefit, more recent, larger randomized clinical trials do not demonstrate significant findings, except perhaps in women with increased blood pressure at study entry.[10,52,95,116,211,249] Low-dose aspirin may still have a role with high-risk nulliparous women.[98] Another preventative strategy that has been tested recently is calcium supplements. Research to date suggests that these may be beneficial if the woman has a low calcium intake but not if her calcium intake is adequate. Antioxidants and magnesium are also being investigated.[13]

SUMMARY

The cardiovascular changes associated with pregnancy are significant, although well tolerated by most women. Maternal and fetal risks occur when underlying cardiovascular or pulmonary disease processes are compounded with the changes incurred during pregnancy. Cardiovascular problems increase maternal morbidity and mortality and

Normal Pregnancy

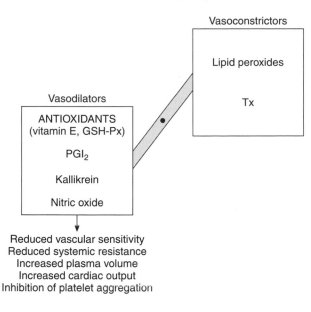

Preeclampsia

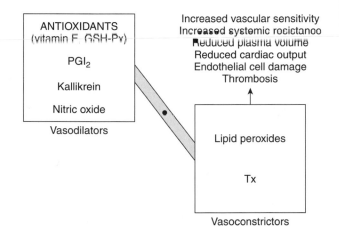

FIGURE **8-13** During normal pregnancy there is a dominance of the effects of vasodilator substances over those of vasoconstrictors, leading to vasodilation and inhibition of platelet aggregation. In preeclampsia there is an imbalance of increased lipid peroxides and thromboxane (Tx) and decreased prostacyclin (PGI_2), vitamin E (an antioxidant), and other vasodilators (e.g., GSH-Px [glutathione peroxidase]). (Adapted by Salas, S.P. [1999]. What causes preeclampsia? *Ballière's Clin Obstet Gynecol, 13,* 48, from Wallenburg, H.C.S. [1988]. Prevention of hypertensive disorders in pregnancy. *Clinical and experimental hypertension in pregnancy.* B7, 121-137; and Wang X.X., et al. [1991]. Maternal levels of prostacyclin thromboxanes, vitamin E, and lipid peroxidases throughout normal pregnancy *Am J Obstet Gynecol, 165,* 1690-1694.)

can compromise the health and well-being of the fetus. Careful assessment and ongoing monitoring of cardiovascular status throughout the prenatal, intrapartum, and postpartum periods are essential for early identification and prompt intervention, thereby improving maternal and neonatal outcome. Table 8-6 summarizes clinical implications related to the cardiovascular system during pregnancy.

DEVELOPMENT OF THE CARDIOVASCULAR SYSTEM IN THE FETUS

The cardiovascular system is the first system in the embryo to begin to function. The need for substrates to support the rapid growth and development of the embryo necessitates the early development of a system that transports nutritional elements and metabolic by-products to and from the cells of the body. Initially the embryo is small enough that diffusion of nutrients can meet the demands of the cells; however, this is short lived because of the exponential growth of the embryo. Blood can be seen circulating through the embryonic body as early as the end of the third week.[16,159] Each of the developing regions of the embryo requires different amounts of circulatory support at various times throughout gestation; therefore the pattern of vessel development is markedly different from one region to the next, depending on the demand.[35]

TABLE **8-6**   Recommendations for Clinical Practice Related to the Cardiovascular System in Pregnant Women

Recognize usual cardiovascular and hemodynamic patterns of change during pregnancy (pp. 255-266 and Table 8-1).

Assess maternal cardiovascular changes throughout pregnancy (pp. 255-260, 262-264).

Counsel women on normal cardiovascular changes and anticipated symptoms associated with those changes (pp. 262-264).

Counsel women in the third trimester to use the lateral recumbent position (pp. 266-267 and Figures 8-9 and 8-10).

Assess and closely monitor women at risk for and with preeclampsia throughout pregnancy (pp. 274-276).

Encourage moderate exercise on a regular basis during pregnancy (pp. 266-270).

Recommend interval-type exercises rather than long continuous exercise (pp. 268-269).

Provide counseling and regularly evaluate pregnant women who start a progressive exercise program during pregnancy (pp. 266-270).

Teach women self-uterine palpation to assess for uterine contractions during exercise (p. 269).

Advise cessation of exercise if contractions or pain occurs (p. 270).

Discourage exercise in pregnant women with threatened miscarriage, preeclampsia, preterm labor, uterine hemorrhage, or intrauterine growth restriction (pp. 266-270).

Monitor vascular volume status carefully during the intrapartum and postpartum periods (pp. 264-266).

Evaluate blood loss and fundal tone postpartum (p. 266).

Monitor for signs of congestive heart failure in women with cardiac disease, especially at midpregnancy (pp. 270-271).

Assess maternal activity tolerance in women with cardiac disease and discuss management of daily activities (pp. 270-271).

Teach women with cardiac disease the signs and symptoms of cardiovascular decompensation (pp. 270-273).

The cardiovascular system is composed of the heart and the blood vessels. Their development is both independent and contiguous, with the final product being a closed system that continuously circulates a given blood volume. Although considered separately here, development of the two elements of the system (heart and vessels) occurs simultaneously.[16] Major landmarks in the development of the cardiovascular system are summarized in Table 8-7.

Anatomic Development
Development of the Primitive Heart

The cardiovascular system arises from mesenchymal cells known as the angioblastic tissue, which appears early in the third week (Figure 8-14, A). These cells appear as scattered, small masses at the anterior margin of the embryonic disk in front of the neural plate. The cells coalesce to form a plexus of endothelial vessels that fuse to form two longitudinal cellular strands called cardiogenic cords. These cords can be seen ventral to the pericardial coelom at the end of the third week. These cords canalize to form two thin-walled tubes—the endocardial heart tubes. As the embryo undergoes lateral folding, the tubes come into proximity and fusion occurs in a cranial-to-caudal direction (Figure 8-14, A through C). Fusion results in a single tube that will eventually form the endocardium.[35,159]

At this stage the mesenchymal tissue around the endocardial tube thickens to form the myoepicardial mantle. Cardiac jelly, a gelatinous connective tissue, separates the simple endothelial tube from the thickened mesenchymal tube, resulting in the appearance of a tube within a tube (see Figure 8-14, C). The inner tube becomes the endothelial lining of the heart (endocardium), and the myoepicardial mantle develops into the myocardium and epicardium (pericardium).[159]

As the head fold occurs, the pericardial cavity and heart rotate on the transverse axis almost 180 degrees to lie ventral to the foregut and caudal to the oropharyngeal membrane. The septum transversum is therefore positioned between the pericardial cavity and the yolk sac, and the heart is now situated in a definitive pericardial cavity.[35,159] The primitive heart, consisting of the endothelial tube and myoepicardial mantle, passes cranially-caudally through the pericardial cavity and is fixed to the pericardial wall only at the venous entrance (caudal end) and at the arterial outlet (cranial end). The cardiac tube begins to beat around 22 days, moving blood from the caudal venous end to the cranial arterial end.

Differentiation of the heart regions begins and alternating dilations and constrictions can be identified (Figure 8-14, D through F). The first areas to appear include the bulbus cordis, ventricle, and atrium. The truncus arteriosus and sinus venosus follow.[159] The truncus arteriosus lies above and is connected to the bulbus cordis. The aortic sac from which the aortic arches arise is included in the truncus arteriosus. The large sinus venosus receives the umbilical, vitelline, and common cardinal veins from the primitive placenta, yolk sac, and embryo, respectively.[35,159]

TABLE **8-7**   Timelines in Normal and Abnormal Cardiac Development

NORMAL TIME	DEVELOPMENTAL EVENTS	MALFORMATIONS ARISING DURING PERIOD
18 days	Horseshoe-shaped cardiac primordium appears.	Lethal mutants
20 days	Bilateral cardia primordia fuse. Cardiac jelly appears. Aortic arch is forming.	Cardia bifida (experimental)
22 days	Heart is looping into S-shape. Heart begins to beat. Dorsal mesocardium in breaking down. Aortic arches I and II are forming.	Dextrocardia
24 days	Atria are beginning to bulge. Right and left ventricles act like two pumps in series. Outflow tract is distinguished from right ventricle.	
Late in week 4	Sinus venosus is being incorporated into right atrium. Endocardial cushions appear. Septum primum appears between right and left atria. Muscular interventricular septum is forming. Truncoconal ridges are forming. Aortic arch I is regressing. Aortic arch III is forming. Aortic arch IV is forming.	Venous inflow malformations Persistent atrioventricular canal Common atrium Common ventricle Persistent truncus arteriosus
Early in week 5	Endocardial cushions are coming together, forming right and left atrioventricular canals. Further growth of interatrial septum primum and muscular interventricular septum occurs. Truncus arteriosus is dividing into aorta and pulmonary artery. Atrioventricular bundle is forming; there is possible neurogenic control of heart beat. Pulmonary veins are being incorporated into the atrium. Aortic arches I and II have regressed. Aortic arches III and IV have formed. Aortic arch VI is forming.	Persistent atrioventricular canal Muscular ventricular septal defects Transposition of the great vessels; aortic and pulmonary stenosis or atresia Aberrant pulmonary drainage
Late in week 5 to early in week 6	Endocardial cushions fuse. Interatrial foramen secundum is forming. Interatrial septum primum is almost contacting endocardial cushions. Membranous part of interventricular septum starts to form. Semilunar valves begin to form.	Low atria septal defects Membranous interventricular septal defects Aortic and pulmonary vascular stenosis
Late in week 6	Interatrial foramen secundum is large. Interatrial septum secundum starts to form. Atrioventricular valves and papillary muscles are forming. Interventricular septum is almost complete. Coronary circulation is becoming established.	High atrial septum defects Tricuspid or mitral valve stenosis or atresia Membranous interventricular septal defects
8 to 9 weeks	Membranous part of interventricular septum is completes.	Membranous interventricular septal defect

Adapted from Carlson, B.M. (1999). *Human embryology and developmental biology* (2nd ed.). St Louis: Mosby.

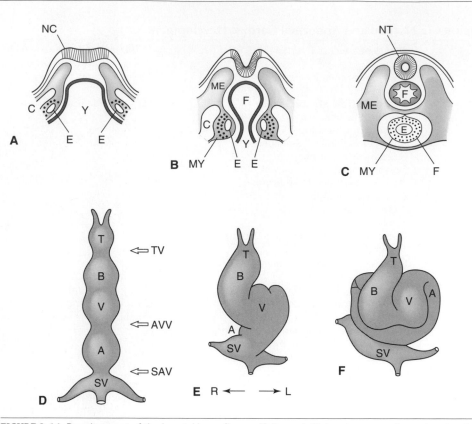

FIGURE **8-14** Development of the heart. Upper figures (**A** through **C**): transverse sections showing that (**A**) fusion of the paired endocardial and myoepicardial tubes (**B**) results in a single straight cardiac tube (**C**). *C,* Coelemic cavity; *E,* endocardial tubes; *F,* foregut; *ME,* mesoderm; *MY,* myocardium; *P,* pericardial cavity; *NC,* neural crest; *NT,* neural tube; *Y,* yolk sac. Lower figures (**D** through **F**): (**D**) simple tubular heart; (**E**) early looping to the left side; (**F**) established looping with definition of unseptated cardiac chambers. The open arrows indicate the valve sites. *A,* atrium; *AVV,* atrioventricular valve; *B,* bulbus cordis, *SAV,* sinoatrial valve; *SV,* sinus venosus; *T,* truncus arteriosus; *TV,* truncal valve. (From Reller, M.D., et al. [1991]. Cardiac embryology: Basic review and clinical correlations. *J Am Soc Echocardiogr,* *4*[5], 519-532.)

During this differentiation stage there is rapid growth of the cardiac tube as well. Because the ends are held fixed and the bulboventricular portion of the tube grows more rapidly (doubling its length from day 21 to day 25) than the surrounding cavity, the tube bends upon itself and forms a U-shaped loop that has its convexity directed forward and to the right. Continued growth results in an S-shaped curve that nearly fills the pericardial cavity (Figure 8-14, *E* and *F*).

The separation of the atrium and sinus venosus from the septum transversum positions the atrium dorsal and to the left of the bulboventricular loop; the sinus venosus lies dorsal to the atrium. The right and left horns of the sinus venosus now partially fuse to form a single cavity that opens into the atrial cavity via the sinoatrial orifice. The heart is still a single tube except at the caudal end, where the remaining unfused portions of the right and left horns of the sinus venosus lie. The three pairs of symmetric veins that return blood to the horns are the placental (umbilical), the yolk sac (vitelline), and the embryo body (cardinal) veins. The vitelline vessels soon develop asymmetrically, with the left vein undergoing retrogression. At 33 to 34 days, the right umbilical vein atrophies and disappears. The left horn of the sinus venosus also becomes much smaller as the veins in the septum transversum rearrange. Eventually the left sinus venosus becomes the coronary sinus.[35,159]

During the rearrangement of vessels, the ductus venosus (DV) is formed. This shunt between the left umbilical vein and the right hepatocardiac channel allows some of the blood from the to bypass the liver sinusoids and flow directly into the heart via the inferior vena cava (see Fetal Circulation) from the placenta. This results in an enlargement of the right horn of the sinus venosus and a change in the position of the sino-atrial orifice. The latter is positioned to the right side of the dorsal surface and is converted

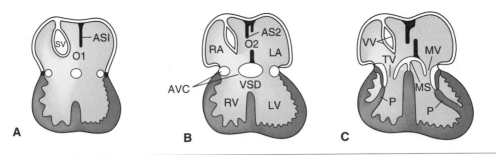

FIGURE **8-15** Changes in cardiac chamber septation. The diagrams represent coronal sections of the heart: **A,** Early stage, commencing atrial and ventricular septation; **B,** atrial ostium primum closed, ostium secundum forming, and ventricular septum incomplete; and **C,** septation complete and membranous septum formed. The atrioventricular valves have been formed by atrioventricular (endocardial) cushion tissue and delamination of myocardium. *AS1,* Atrial septum primum; *AS2,* atrial septum secundum; *AVC,* atrioventricular cushion; *LA,* left atrium; *LV,* left ventricle; *MS,* membranous septum; *MV,* mitral valve; *O1,* atrial ostium primum; *O2,* atrium ostium secundum; *P,* papillary muscles; *RA,* right atrium; *RV,* right ventricle; *SV,* sinus venosus; *TV,* tricuspid valve; *VSD,* ventricular septal defect; *VV,* venous valves. (From Reller, M.D., et al. [1991]. Cardiac embryology: Basic review and clinical correlations. *J Am Soc Echocardiogr, 4*[5], 519-532.)

to a vertical alignment. The margins are now projected into the atrium and compose the right and left venous valves.[35]

The atrium, ventricle, and bulbus cordis continue to expand rapidly, resulting in a change in position. The atrium expands transversely, extending laterally and ventrally, and appears on either side of the bulbus cordis. This results in the atria being deeply grooved. Further growth results in the right and left auricular appendages being formed. At the same time, the bulboventricular sulcus dissipates with the growth of these structures. Eventually the caudal portion of the bulbus becomes part of the ventricle. The ventricle gradually moves to the left and ends up on the ventral surface of the heart. It is at this time that the atrioventricular canal becomes defined.[35]

Septation of the Heart

Septation of the atrioventricular canal, the atrium, and the ventricle begins in the middle of the fourth week and is complete by the sixth week. The changes in shape and position of the heart tube, as described earlier, facilitate the partitioning of these structures. The process of septation takes place while the heart continues to pump and blood continues to move unidirectionally through the tube. The subdivision of the heart into right and left compartments occurs simultaneously in the various regions of the heart; however, all of the processes must be integrated so that normal functional development occurs.

The right horn of the sinus venosus becomes incorporated into the right atrium. Most of the wall of the left atrium is derived from the primitive pulmonary vein. The vein develops to the left of the septum primum and is an outgrowth of the dorsal atrial wall. However, as the atrium expands, the vein is progressively incorporated into the wall of the atrium.[35,159]

Atrioventricular canal. The atrium leads into the ventricle via a narrow atrioventricular canal. During the fourth week the endocardium proliferates to produce dorsal and ventral bulges in the wall of the atrioventricular canal (Figure 8-15). These swellings are the atrioventricular endocardial cushions. Mesenchymal cells invade the swellings, which results in the growth of the cushions toward each other. Fusion of the cushions occurs, leading to right and left atrioventricular canals.[16,159]

Atrium. A thin, crescent-shaped septum (septum primum) begins to grow downward from the roof of the atrium during the fourth week. Initially a large opening exists between the caudal free edge of the septum and the endocardial cushions; this is the foramen primum. This allows oxygenated blood that is returned to the right atrium to pass to the left atrium so that it can be distributed to the systemic circulation. The opening progressively gets smaller and is eventually obliterated when the septum primum fuses with the endocardial cushions.[16] Before the septum primum reaches the atrioventricular cushions, however, a second interatrial communication forms as the result of multiple perforations that coalesce in the upper part of the septum. This is the foramen secundum.[159]

A second, thicker septum (septum secundum) begins to develop just to the right of the septum primum. This septum is also crescent-shaped, but it grows only until it overlaps the foramen secundum. The partition is incomplete, and an oval opening, the foramen ovale, is left.[35,158] The upper portion of the septum primum regresses, whereas the lower segment (attached to the endocardial cushions) remains, serving as a flap valve for the foramen ovale. Atrial septation is illustrated in Figure 8-15. Before birth this valve allows directed blood to move freely from the right to the left atrium. However, flow from the left to the right is prevented by apposition of the thin flexible septum primum to the rigid septum secundum after birth. This results in fusion of the septa and eventual anatomic closure of the foramen ovale.

Ventricles. The interventricular septum consists of muscular and membranous portions. Division of the bulboventricular cavity is first indicated by a sagittal muscular ridge appearing on the floor of the ventricle near the apex; this is the interventricular septum. At first the septum appears to lengthen as a result of the dilation of the lateral halves of the ventricle. Later there is active proliferation of the septal tissue as the muscular portion of the interventricular septum forms.[35,159] Communication between the right and left sides of the ventricle is maintained until the bulbar ridges fuse. This closure is the result of fusion of subendocardial tissue from the bulbar ridges and the atrioventricular cushions.[159]

The membranous portion of the ventricular septum is derived from tissue that extends from the right side of the endocardial cushions. This eventually fuses with the aorticopulmonary septum of the truncus arteriosus and the muscular interventricular septum. Closure of the interventricular foramen results in the pulmonary trunk being in communication with the RV and the aorta with the LV (see Figure 8-15).[159]

Bulbus cordis and truncus arteriosus. Before the interventricular septum has developed completely, spiral subendocardial thickenings appear in the distal part of the bulbus cordis. These are the bulbar ridges, which can be seen during the fifth week of gestation. Initially these ridges are composed of cardiac jelly, but they are later invaded by mesenchymal cells. In the proximal part of the bulbus, the ridges are located on the ventral and dorsal walls, whereas in the distal portion they are attached to the lateral walls. The distal portion of the bulbus is continuous with the truncus arteriosus, which develops truncal ridges that match those of the bulbus cordis. The growth and fusion of these ridges during the eighth week results in the spiral aorticopulmonary septum (Figure 8-16). The spiral effect may be due to the streaming of blood from the ventricles through the truncus during septum development. The result is the creation of two channels: the pulmonary trunk and the aorta. The bulbus cordis is gradually incorporated into the ventricles.[35,159]

Cardiac valves. Part of the septation process involves the development of the cardiac valves. This includes the development of the semilunar valves of the aorta and the pulmonary artery and the atrioventricular valves (tricuspid and mitral valves). The semilunar valves develop from a swelling of subendothelial tissue that appears on each side

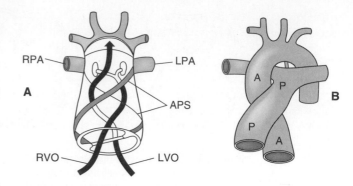

FIGURE **8-16** Septation of the truncus arteriosus. **A,** Diagram showing the aorticopulmonary septum, which separates the systemic arterial flow (solid dark line) from the pulmonary arterial flow (broken line); **B,** the mature pulmonary artery and aorta after septation and separation, showing the persistent spiral relationship. *A,* Aorta; *APS,* aorticopulmonary septum; *LPA,* left pulmonary artery; *LVO,* left ventricular outflow pathway; *P,* pulmonary trunk; *RPA,* right pulmonary artery; *RVO,* right ventricular outflow pathway. (From Reller, M.D., et al. [1991]. Cardiac embryology. Basic review and clinical correlations. *J Am Soc Echocardiogr,* 4[5], 519-532.)

of the ventricular end of the bulbar ridges. These swellings consist of loose connective tissue covered by endothelium. Eventually the swellings become hollowed out and reshaped to form three thin-walled cusps.[35,159]

The atrioventricular valves develop from local proliferation of subendocardial tissue as well as from connective tissue under the endocardium of the atrioventricular canals. These, too, become hollowed out, but on the ventricular side. The atrioventricular valves remain connected to the ventricular wall via muscular strands that are both papillary muscles and chordae tendineae. The mitral valve develops two cusps; the tricuspid has three.[35,159]

Conducting System

The initial pacemaker of the cardiac muscle is located in the caudal part of the left cardiac tube. Because the muscle layers of the atrium and ventricle are continuous, this temporary pacemaker is effective in controlling contractions throughout the primitive heart. Once the sinus venosus develops, the excitatory center (sinoatrial node) is found in the right wall. This node will be incorporated into the right atrium along with the sinus venosus, where it will lie near the entrance of the superior vena cava.[35,159]

Once the sinus venosus is incorporated into the atrium, cells from the left wall of the sinus venosus can be found in the base of the interatrial septum. When combined with cells from the atrioventricular canal, the atrioventricular

(AV) node and the bundle of His are formed. These structures can be identified in embryos early in the second month of gestation.[35,159]

The Purkinje fibers constitute one of the most unusual features of the heart muscle. These cells are responsible for the initiation and propagation of the cardiac impulse and the ensuring of a regular contraction sequence within the organ. Although they are cardiac muscle cells, they are specialized through differentiation for conduction rather than contraction. These cells have fewer fibrils and are larger in diameter than the rest of the cardiac muscle cells. Purkinje cells are located external to the endocardium and run without interruption from the atrium to the ventricle as the atrioventricular bundle.[35]

A fibrous band of connective tissue eventually separates the muscles of the atria and ventricles. This results in the atrioventricular node and bundle of His being the only conductive pathways between the upper and lower halves of the heart.

Blood Vessels

Blood vessels consist of an endothelial lining stabilized by an outer coat of connective tissue. The earliest vessels are derived from angioblastic tissue, which differentiates from the mesenchyme that covers the yolk sac, within the connecting stalk and in the wall of the chorionic sac. The impetus for vascular differentiation seems to be the reduction of nutrients within the yolk sac, which leads to an urgent need for a vascular system to supply nutrients to the cells.[35,159]

Masses of isolated angioblasts come together and form blood islands. Soon spaces can be seen in these islands, around which the angioblasts will arrange themselves. This results in lumen formation and the development of a primitive endothelial layer. The isolated vessels fuse to form a network of channels and extend to adjacent areas either through growth (endothelial budding) or by fusion with other independently formed vessels. Mesenchymal cells surrounding the primitive endothelial vessels differentiate into the muscle and connective layers of the vessels.[159]

Endothelial tissue first appears in the yolk sac wall as isolated cellular cords that develop a lumen. As these vessels join together, a network of endothelial vitelline vessels is formed. By extension and growth the network progressively reaches the embryonic body.[35] Primitive plasma and blood cells are developed from endothelial cells trapped within the vessels of the yolk sac and allantois. Blood formation in the embryo begins in the liver after 3 to 4 weeks (see Chapter 7).[35,159]

The endothelial lining of vessels develops before the circulation. However, once circulation begins, the hemodynamics of blood flow influences the growth of the endothelium and the differentiation of the other parts of the vessel wall. The developing organs and the temporal sequence and metabolic demands of those organs may also influence the differentiation of vessels.[35]

The first vessels seen within the embryonic body seem to form from a diffuse network that runs throughout the embryonic mesenchyme. As tissues and organs differentiate, the regional networks elaborate to meet metabolic demands.[35] The earliest vessels are simple endothelial tubes; differentiation of arteries from veins is not possible. As development continues, the tunica media and tunica adventitia of the definitive arteries and veins arise from mesenchymal tissue.[11,35]

Arteries. The right and left dorsal aortae are the primary embryonic arteries. Initially these vessels are continuations of the endocardial tubes and can be divided into three portions: a short, ventral, ascending portion that supplies blood to the forebrain; a primitive first aortic arch that lies in the mesenchyme of the mandibular arch (pharynx); and a relatively long, descending portion that distributes blood to embryonic body, yolk sac, and chorion via the segmental plexuses, vitelline vessels, and umbilical branches, respectively. The paired dorsal aortae initially run the length of the embryo. As development continues, the two fuse just caudal to the branchial region so that there is only a single midline vessel in the caudal part of the embryo.[16,35]

There are three major arterial branches that run off the dorsal aorta above the level of right and left aortic fusion. The intersegmental arteries are a group of 30 or more vessels that pass between and carry blood to the somites and their derivatives. In the cervical region the first seven intersegmental arteries are connected by a longitudinal anastomosis that forms the vertebral artery. The proximal segments of the first six arteries disappear, and the seventh intersegmental artery becomes the subclavian artery.[16,159]

The somatic arteries also arise from this group of vessels. Eventually the intercostal arteries, lumbar arteries, common iliac arteries, and lateral sacral arteries can be identified.[16,159] The midline branches of the dorsal aorta run to the yolk sac, allantois, and chorion. There are two main groups: the lateral branches and the ventral branches. The ventral or vitelline arteries supply the yolk sac and the gut. These vessels will eventually be reduced to three persisting vessels; the celiac, superior mesenteric, and inferior mesenteric arteries. These vessels service the foregut, midgut, and hindgut, respectively.[16,159] The lateral branches supply the nephrogenic ridge and its derivatives. At first there are several branches, but retrogression results in four vessels remaining in the mature organism. These vessels are the phrenic, suprarenal, renal, and gonadal arteries.[16]

By far the largest of the dorsal aortic vessels are the paired umbilical arteries. These vessels pass through the connecting stalk (umbilical cord) and become continuous with the chorionic vessels in the developing placenta. After delivery the proximal portions of these arteries become the internal iliac and superior vesical arteries. The distal portions are obliterated and become the medial umbilical ligaments.

Aortic arches. The aortic arches are essential in the primitive circulatory system. These vessels arise from the aortic sac and terminate in the dorsal aorta. A total of five pairs develop; however, the third, fourth, and fifth arches are the only ones to contribute to the great vessels. By the end of the eighth week, the adult pattern has been established.[16,159]

Veins. There are three sets of paired veins that drain into the heart of the 4-week-old embryo. These are the vitelline veins, which return blood from the yolk sac; the umbilical veins, which bring oxygenated blood from the chorion; and the cardinal veins, which return blood from the body.

Vitelline veins. The vitelline veins follow the yolk stalk and ascend on either side of the foregut. They then pass through the septum transversum and enter the sinus venosus of the heart. As the primitive liver grows into the septum transversum, the hepatic sinusoids become linked with the vitelline veins. As the right vitelline vein begins to disintegrate, parts are incorporated into the developing hepatic vessels. The portal vein develops from the vitelline-derived vessels that surround the duodenum.

Umbilical veins. The umbilical veins originate as a pair of vessels; however, the right vein and part of the left degenerate so that only a single vessel remains to return blood from the placenta to the fetus. As these vessels degenerate, the DV develops in the liver and connects the remaining umbilical vein with the inferior vena cava. At birth the umbilical vein and the DV are obliterated with the cutting of the umbilical cord and the modifications in the circulation. The remnants of the vessels are the ligamentum teres and ligamentum venosum, respectively.

Cardinal veins. Very early in the embryonic period, the cardinal vessels are the main drainage system. The anterior and posterior cardinal veins bring blood from the cranial and caudal regions and empty into the heart via a common cardinal vein that enters the sinus venosus on each side. By the eighth week the anterior cardinal veins are connected through an anastomosis that allows for shunting of blood from the left vein to the right. This connection becomes the left brachiocephalic vein. The right anterior and right common cardinal veins form the superior vena cava. The posterior cardinal veins are transitional vessels. These vessels service the mesonephric kidneys and disappear when the kidneys degenerate. The subcardinal and supracardinal vessels develop gradually and facilitate perfusion of the mesonephric kidneys. These vessels do not degenerate entirely, as do the posterior cardinal veins.

The inferior vena cava is the result of a series of changes in the embryonic veins of the trunk. The four main segments of the inferior vena cava are derived from the hepatic vein and hepatic sinusoids (hepatic segment), the right subcardinal vein (prerenal segment), the subcardinal and supracardinal anastomosis (renal segment), and the right supracardinal vein (postrenal segment).[159]

Developmental Basis for Common Anomalies

Development of the heart is controlled by a group of cardiac genes and transcription factors that are expressed in a specific sequence. Alterations in these genes or factors or in their sequencing may lead to agenesis or aplasia (failure in development), hypoplasia (incomplete or defective development), dysplasia (abnormal development), malposition, failure of fusion of adjoining parts, abnormal fusion, incomplete resorption, persistence of a vessel, or early obliteration of a vessel and thus cardiac defects.[35] Cardiac defects are seen in 0.8% to 1% of live born infants and 10% of spontaneous abortions.[229] About one fourth of spontaneous abortions with cardiac defects have other noncardiac problems.[35,260] Timing of development of major anomalies is summarized in Table 8-7.

The etiology of most congenital heart defects is unclear. In about 8% of children there is a clear genetic cause; most are associated with obvious chromosomal anomalies (e.g., Down syndrome, trisomy 18, trisomy 13, Klinefelter syndrome, and Turner syndrome). The incidence of cardiac defects is about 40% in infants with Down syndrome and higher in infants with trisomy 13 and 18.[260] Many of the single-gene and other inherited syndromes (e.g., Marfan, Williams, and DiGeorge syndromes) are associated with heart disease, but these syndromes account for only 3% of all congenital heart disease. Environmental factors may also play a role in the etiology of congenital cardiac malformations. Fetal exposure to teratogens through maternal ingestion of drugs such as antiepileptic drugs or warfarin, or alcohol, as well as viral infections (such as rubella), can result in alterations in cardiac development. These variables account for about 2% of known congenital heart disease. Maternal disorders may increase the risk of fetal cardiac defects. For example, the frequency of cardiac defect in infants of women with diabetes mellitus is 2 to 4 times as higher than normal.[229] Systemic lupus erythematosus is associated with fetal heart block (see Chapter 12).

In the remaining 85% of infants, there is no clear cause. There is probably some type of multifactorial inheritance in which there may be a heritable predisposition for cardiac anomalies. This combined with some type of environmental trigger during a vulnerable period results in abnormal development. Implications of selected congenital heart defects are discussed in Clinical Implications for Neonatal Care.

Functional Development
Fetal Myocardium

The fetal myocyte has a small amount of contractile tissue, which is restricted to the subsarcolemmal region. Only 30% of the myocardial tissue consists of contractile mass in the fetus (versus 60% in adults).[227] There are fewer myofibrils and these are arranged in a more random fashion, rather than in a parallel organization as occurs in adults.[74,117] These changes, along with the decreased number of sarcomeres per gram of ventricular muscle, limit the amount of force that the fetus may be able to generate per unit of area.[255] The sarcoplasmic reticulum in the fetal myocardium is reduced and less organized, reducing calcium sequestration and altering calcium transport and thus contractility.[257] Therefore the fetal heart is more dependent on transsarcolemmal calcium movement with lower intracellular concentrations. As a result the fetal myocardium develops less force, with a lower velocity of shortening and reextension.[117]

The fetal myocardium is less compliant than that of the adult, although the relationship between muscle length and force is qualitatively similar. As extrauterine growth occurs, the compliance of both ventricles increases. Right-side pressures are greater than left-side pressures in the fetus, so blood flows from right to left across the foramen ovale from the right atrium to left atrium or across the ductus arteriosus (DA) from the pulmonary artery to aorta.[26,203]

Metabolism is also immature in the fetal myocardium. Carbohydrates are the main energy source in the fetal and neonatal myocardium due to limitations in fatty acid transport.[117,257] However, the fetal heart has an increased ability to utilize anaerobic metabolism.[117]

Myocardial Performance

After birth, when circulation flows in series (Figure 8-17), the stroke volume of the RV equals that of the LV.[72] However, in the fetus, which is not dependent upon the lungs to oxygenate the blood, circulation is arranged in a parallel fashion (see Figure 8-17). This arrangement allows for mixing of oxygenated blood with unoxygenated blood

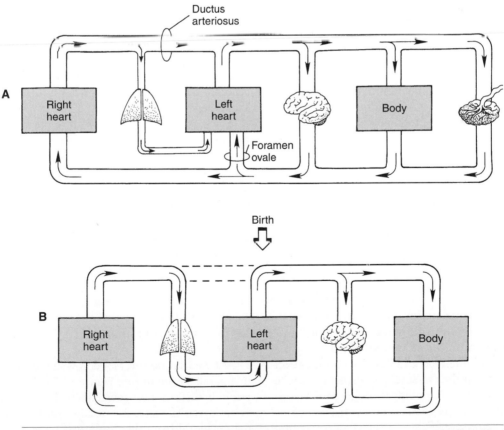

FIGURE **8-17** Comparison of **(A)** fetal (parallel) with **(B)** adult (series) circulatory systems. (Modified from Dawes, G.S. (1968). *Fetal and neonatal physiology*. Chicago: Year Book, by Bloom, R.S. [2002]. Delivery room resuscitation of the newborn. In A.A. Fanaroff & R.J. Martin [Eds.]. *Neonatal and perinatal medicine, diseases of the fetus and infant* [7th ed.]. St. Louis: Mosby.)

at the atrial and great vessel levels. Blood from the RV and LV is mixed in the descending aorta below the DA. The modifications in the circulation that allow for this mixing divert blood from the immature lungs to the placenta, where oxygen–carbon dioxide exchange occurs.[165] Stroke volumes of the two fetal ventricles are not equal. The fetus sends 65% of the venous return to the RV and 25% to the LV; therefore RV stroke volume is 28% greater than that in the LV.[74] As a result of these differences, cardiac output in the fetus is defined as the total output of the RV and LV, or the combined ventricular output (CVO).[74] The RV pumps two thirds of the combined ventricular output.[88]

The fetal resting cardiac output is the highest of any time of life with a CVO of 480 ml/min/kg at term.[88] The high fetal cardiac output may be necessary in order to meet the high fetal oxygen consumption demands. When compared to the adult, fetal oxygen consumption is 1½ to 2 times higher. This may be an adaptive mechanism for the low oxygen tension found in the fetal state.[10] The ability to maintain this high output is due to the elevated heart rate and the cardiac shunts.[88] Changes in fetal cardiac output seem to be directly related to FHR changes, with reduced sensitivity to preload and afterload.[257] A 10% increase in FHR above the resting level is associated with an increase in both right and LV output; a decrease in heart rate results in a decrease in combined ventricular output.[255]

In the fetal heart the RV and LV have stages of filling that are similar to those in the adult; however, the end-diastolic dimensions of the RV are larger than those of the left. There also seems to be a difference in the rate of filling between the ventricles. In the fetus an increase in RV volume or afterload interferes with LV filling. The Frank-Starling relationship is present and a primary regulator of fetal cardiac output.[74] There is little functional reserve, however, because the fetal heart functions at the maximum and interventions such as volume infusion do not significantly increase stroke volume and output.[88,182] "When fetal atrial pressures are increased, there is a diminished capacity to increase myocardial performance, because the length-tension relationship has approached its maximum phase."[74, p.110]

In terms of afterload, the fetal myocardium shortens more slowly when compared with adult tissue. This fetal liability is to be expected given the maturation of the force-generating ability of the myocardium. Arterial pressure is a major component of afterload and has a significant effect on ejection (the higher the pressure, the smaller the stroke volume is). This relationship holds throughout development, although the neonate seems to be less tolerant of increases in arterial pressure.[7,226]

Changes in inotropy (the strength of myocardial contractions) reflect a change in the ability of the myocardium

to contract, and maturational development affects inotropy in the fetus and neonate. One of these changes is related to the availability of calcium and the control of cytosolic calcium. The development of the sarcomeres and their intracellular control mechanisms is integrally tied to this process. Therefore the lower calcium concentrations bathing the sarcomere account for the reduced sarcomere shortening and reextension velocities seen in the fetus and neonate.

Heart rate also affects the strength of contraction in a positive way in the fetus, neonate, and adult. In fetal lambs, however, as heart rate increases, stroke volume decreases. This is most likely due to a decrease in end-diastolic volume that is a natural consequence of the increased heart rate. Conflicting data have been found in studies of the human fetus, although the majority of studies suggest a positive effect on ventricular output. This may be due to additional factors that have inotropic effects.[7]

Fetal Circulation

The fetal circulation (Figure 8-18) is unique in several aspects: (1) presence of intracardiac (foramen ovale) and extracardiac (DV and DA) shunts; (2) high-resistance pulmonary circuit; and (3) low-resistance systemic circuit. The high PVR is a result of the collapsed lungs and the thick medial smooth muscle layer of the pulmonary arteries.[135,203] As a result of the high PVR and collapsed lungs, blood flow to the lungs is low in the fetus, although some is retained to support lung growth and development (see Pulmonary Vasculature).[135]

The high resting tone and PVR in the fetus are thought to be maintained by mechanical factors (compression of small pulmonary arteries by the fluid filled alveolar spaces), the low fetal PO_2, and a balance between vasoconstrictor and vasodilators that favors vasoconstriction. The most important pulmonary vasoconstrictors are probably endothelin, arachidonic acid metabolites, and hypoxia.[17,141,160] PO_2 in the fetal pulmonary circuit is 17 to 20 mmHg.[135]

The communication between the atria (i.e., foramen ovale), along with the DA, allows for equalization of pressures between the atria and the great vessels. Because these pressures are equal, the ventricular pressures are also equal.[259] The low-resistance systemic circuit is also due to the passive nature of umbilical cord and placental blood flow.[259]

As noted previously, blood flow in the fetus is arranged in a parallel fashion (see Figure 8-17). This arrangement results in mixing of oxygenated blood at the atrial and great vessel levels. The fetal shunts allow for this mixing, which diverts blood from the immature lungs to the placenta, where oxygen-carbon dioxide exchange takes place. As a result, 40% to 50% of the fetal cardiac output is directed to-

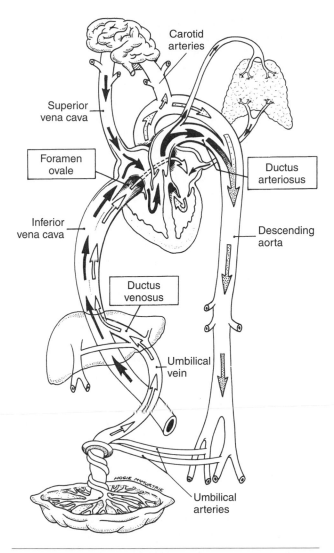

Carotid arteries

Superior vena cava

Foramen ovale

Ductus arteriosus

Inferior vena cava

Descending aorta

Ductus venosus

Umbilical vein

Umbilical arteries

FIGURE **8-18** Fetal circulation. (From Bloom, R.S. [2002]. Delivery room resuscitation of the newborn. In A.A. Fanaroff & R.J. Martin [Eds.]. *Neonatal and perinatal medicine: Diseases of the fetus and infant* [7th ed.]. St. Louis: Mosby.)

across the DV. This is true in the fetal lamb and other animals, but recent studies suggest that the amount may be far less in human infants.[17,127-129] These studies suggest that, at 20 weeks, 30% flows across the DV, decreasing to 18% to 20% by 32 weeks.[17,127,128] Therefore, in late pregnancy, 70% to 80% of the oxygenated blood from the placenta goes first to the liver, reflecting an increased priority of the liver needs near term.[129] With hypovolemia or hypoxemia, more blood is shunted across the DV and thus to the heart.[17,128] Shunting across the DV is also increased in the IUGR infant, even under stable condiitons.[128]

The liver blood supply consists of blood from the UV (80%), portal vein (15%), and hepatic artery (5%).[74] UV blood entering the liver flows to both lobes; portal venous blood is directed primarily to the right lobe.[169] Therefore 95% of the blood flow to the left lobe comes from the UV. The right lobe blood supply comes from the UV (60%), portal vein (30%), and hepatic artery (10%).[74]

The DV is a low-resistance channel that allows a portion of relatively well-oxygenated blood to enter the heart directly. The DV is under tonic adrenergic control and dilates in the presence of nitric oxide, prostaglandins, and hypoxemia.[129] The blood entering the IVC from the UV via the DV joins with the blood that returns from the lower half of the fetal body. The blood that reaches the IVC from the umbilical vein has a greater oxygen content and kinetic energy and so stays in a stream that is separate from the blood returning from the lower body.[21,129] Because of this preferential streaming, DV blood is found along the left dorsal wall of the IVC.[74]

As the IVC blood enters the right atrium, a tissue flap, the eustachian valve, at the junction of the RA and IVC directs blood from the dorsal portion of the IVC (i.e., where the more highly oxygenated blood from the UV streams) toward the foramen ovale.[74] The foramen ovale is formed by the overlap of the septum secundum over the septum primum (see Figure 8-15). Patency of the foramen ovale is maintained by increased blood flow and pressure in the right versus left atrium.[21] The crista dividens (the free edge of the atrial septum) separates the flow into two streams, with 50% to 60% being diverted across the foramen ovale into the left atrium.

In the left atrium the blood from the IVC mixes with the (minimal) pulmonary venous return and passes through the mitral valve into the LV. Thus most of the blood in the LA and LV is the more oxygenated umbilical vein blood. Upon contraction of the heart, this blood is ejected into the ascending aorta to feed the coronary, left carotid, and subclavian arteries. Only 10% continues along the aortic arch into the descending aorta.

The blood flowing along the anterior portion of the IVC consists of hepatic and lower body desaturated blood. This

ward the placenta, with 14% to brain and no more than 10% to 12% to lungs.[21] The remainder is divided among the gastrointestinal tract, kidneys, and the rest of body. The fetal liver is the first organ to receive maternal substances, followed by the heart and brain.

As the blood returns from the placenta to the fetus via the umbilical vein (UV), it passes either into the portal system's microcirculation to later run off into the inferior vena cava (IVC) or into the DV. The DV connects, via the umbilical vein-portal sinus, to the IVC just below the diaphragm (see Figure 8-18). It has long been thought that 40% to 60% of the blood flow from the UV was shunted

blood mixes with blood from the superior vena cava (SVC) and coronary sinus in the right atrium. This blood flow is directed downward across the tricuspid valve and into the RV. Very little of the SVC blood return crosses the foramen ovale to the left atrium. Venous return to the RA is 67% IVC blood (about one third of which is blood from the UV and DV), 37% from the SVC, and 3% from the coronary sinus.[74]

The mixed blood in the right atrium is then ejected into the pulmonary artery, where increased PVR prevents any more than 10% to 12% of the RV blood flow (or about 8% of the CVO) from entering the pulmonary bed.[24,88] Consequently, nearly 60% of the CVO (and 82% to 85% of the RV outflow) is shunted across the DA to enter the descending aorta and the low-resistance systemic circulation.[114,182] Blood flow to the pulmonary bed increases after 30 weeks, perhaps due to growth and thus increased metabolic need of the lungs.[74,114]

The low fetal PO_2 and high levels of circulating prostaglandins (especially PGE_1, PGE_2, and PGI_2) maintain patency of the DA in utero. PGE_2 and PGI_2 are found in the ductal walls. Prostaglandins are normally metabolized in the lungs. Since pulmonary blood flow is so low in the fetus, less are metabolized and therefore levels remains high.

Fetal circulation is not significantly altered by increased intrauterine pressure with uterine contractions in healthy fetal-placental unit. Even with compression of the placental vessels, the vessels are relatively unreactive to short-term changes.[74]

Oxygen Content

The oxygen content of the fetus is lower than that of the neonate, child, or adult. The highest oxygen content is found in the blood returning from the placenta via the umbilical vein, which is 30 to 35 mmHg and 80% to 90% saturated.[74] This falls to 26 to 28 mmHg (saturation, 65%) by the time it reaches the left atrium and mixes with blood from the IVC and pulmonary veins and is ejected into the ascending aorta.

The umbilical return that mixes with the superior vena caval blood (PO_2, 12 to 14 mmHg; saturation, 40%) is reduced to a PaO_2 of 15 to 25 mmHg.[74] This blood is destined for the pulmonary arteries, descending aorta (55% saturated), upper torso, and placenta. Therefore the blood with the highest oxygen content is delivered to the coronary arteries and brain, whereas the blood with the lowest PaO_2 is shunted toward the placenta, where reoxygenation occurs.

Another fetal adaptation to low oxygen tension is the presence of fetal hemoglobin. This specific type of hemoglobin has a high affinity for oxygen even at low oxygen tensions, thereby improving saturation and facilitating transport of oxygen to the tissues. The perfusion rate is greater in the fetus than adult, which helps compensate for the lower oxygen saturations and increased oxygen-hemoglobin affinity.[21] The low oxygen tension in the fetus keeps the pulmonary vasculature constricted and, along with PGE_2, the DA dilated.[21] See Chapters 7 and 9 for a further discussion of fetal hemoglobin and oxygenation.

Fetal Heart Rate

The average baseline FHR in the normal fetus at 20 weeks is 155 beats per minute; at 30 weeks, 144 beats per minute; and at term, 140 beats per minute.[10,167] Variations of 20 beats per minute above or below these levels are considered normal.[10,120,167] This baseline rate is determined by the intrinsic depolarization rate of the sinoatrial node, which is actively inhibited by tonic parasympathetic input. As the parasympathetic system matures with advancing gestational age, the resting heart rate decreases.[10] Changes in FHR reflect changes in fetal oxygenation (see Control of Fetal Circulation).

FHR patterns are classified as baseline (heart rate and variability), which are observed between uterine contractions, periodic changes (seen during uterine contractions) and episodic changes (not associated with uterine contractions).[167] The baseline FHR normally ranges from 110 to 160 beats per minute.

Alterations in fetal heart rate. Fetal tachycardia (baseline over 160 beats per minute for 10 minutes or more) is usually seen with nonasphyxial events that lead to catecholamine release, sympathetic stimulation, or parasympathetic withdrawal. Tachycardia is also sometimes seen with fetal asphyxia, but not as an isolated change (i.e., wider normal FHR variability and no periodic changes).[167] Tachycardia is common in the extremely premature fetus in whom the sympathetic nervous system dominates control of cardiac function. This change in baseline can be mediated by a host of fetal and maternal conditions, of which maternal infection with chorioamnionitis is the most common.[10,120,167]

Other sources of fetal tachycardia may be the use of β-sympathomimetic agents (to inhibit uterine contractions), fetal anemia (Rh isoimmunization), acute fetal blood loss (placental abruption), or abnormal fetal conduction system (Wolff-Parkinson-White disease). Tachycardia may also be a fetal compensatory or recovery response to an acute asphyxial episode or mild hypoxemia and is probably due to a rise in catecholamine levels.[120,167]

Bradycardia is a sustained FHR of less than 110 beats per minute 10 minutes or more. Bradycardia is the initial fetal response to acute asphyxia. Nonasphyxial causes of bradycardia include heart block, changes in cardiac afterload, β-adrenergic agents, hypothermia and head compression. In the last case, vagal nerve stimulation caused by mild cerebral ischemia or increased intracranial pressure seems to explain the bradycardia.[10,120] A few otherwise normal fetuses have a heart rate below 110 that appear to be a normal variant.[167]

Severe bradycardia (below 80 to 100 beats per minute) is the result of acute fetal distress. The fetal hypertension following a hypoxic insult leads to a baroreceptor reflex, which leads to a vagal response and a fall in FHR. The duration and severity of the bradycardia are correlated to the length and severity of the asphyxial event. These events are related to an interruption in blood flow either through decreased umbilical blood flow (cord compression), decreased placental exchange area (abruptio placentae), impaired uterine blood flow (acute maternal hypotension or excessive uterine contractions) a decreased maternal oxygenation (apnea secondary to seizures).[120,167] End-stage bradycardia associated with the second stage of labor is probably a result of a vagal response to head compression as the fetus traverses the birth canal.[167]

Beat-to-beat variability. The time interval between two heart beats in a healthy fetus is seldom the same and may be caused by the interaction of the sympathetic and parasympathetic reflexes or by rapidly oscillating vagal impulses. Baseline variability is fluctuations of 2 cycles/min or greater in the baseline FHR.[167] These fluctuations are irregular in both amplitude and frequency and involve short and long term changes.[167] Normal short-term, and long-term variability is accepted as an indicator of anatomic and functional integrity of the pathways regulating cardiac function. The FHR pathway starts in the cerebral cortex and travels through the midbrain to the vagus nerve and the cardiac conductive system. Fetuses with anomalies, such as anencephaly, demonstrate alterations in variability without the presence of hypoxia.[120] Other factors affecting parasympathetic activity include fetal breathing, fetal movement, and fetal sleep state. The use of local or general anesthetics as well as other maternal drugs (e.g., magnesium sulfate, meperidine) can also affect beat-to-beat variability.[10]

Periodic changes in fetal heart rate. Periodic changes in FHR are associated with uterine contractions or fetal activity. They are usually described either as accelerations or as decelerations that may be early, variable, or late. Early decelerations are the result of a physiologic chain of events that begins with head compression during a uterine contraction; this leads to a reduction in cerebral blood flow, hypoxia, and hypercapnia. Hypercapnia results in hypertension with triggering of the baroreceptors. This results in bradycardia mediated by the parasympathetic nervous system. The fall and rise of the FHR are matched to the rise and fall of the uterine contraction. These changes usually do not exceed 40 beats per minute and are not indicative of fetal distress.[10,120] Early decelerations may be a variant of late reflex decelerations.[167]

Variable decelerations imply an inconsistent time of onset when compared with uterine contractions. The clinical implications are related to the depth and duration of the decelerations. Partial compression or stretching of the umbilical cord with blood flow interruption decreases the blood return to the right heart and causes hypotension. This results in sympathetic nervous system stimulation, catecholamine release, and compensatory fetal tachycardia following the deceleration.[120]

Late decelerations begin characteristically within a few seconds of the peak of a contraction, reach their nadir 20 to 90 seconds later, and have a slow recovery phase. These decelerations mirror the image of the uterine contractions, are repetitive and persistent, and occur with each contraction. Their depth is related to the intensity and frequency of the uterine contraction. These decelerations represent fetal hypoxia and are related to an interruption in oxygen supply at the uteroplacental or myocardial level.[120,167] Two varieties of late decelerations are observed, reflex and nonreflex. Reflex late decelerations are seen secondary to an acute insult, such as decreased uterine blood flow with maternal hypotension, occurs in a previously well-oxygenated fetus. Nonreflex late decelerations occur when the amount of oxygen in blood coming from the placenta cannot support fetal myocardial function and are usually seen with decreased placental reserve with preeclampsia or IUGR.[167]

During contractions the blood in the intervillous space (IVS) is sluggish and stagnant. The transfer of nutrients and waste products is reduced. In situations in which the respiratory reserve (oxygen content) in the IVS is reduced—which can occur with suboptimal replacement between contractions or with contractions that come too frequently—the fetal oxygen supply is diminished. The removal of waste products is also reduced, which can result in lactic acid and carbon dioxide buildup within the fetus. This contributes to the development of fetal acidosis.

The reduced oxygen supply in the fetus leads to stimulation of the carotid and aortic chemoreceptors, resulting in activation of the cardiac centers in the brainstem. The sinoatrial node is affected, and FHR is slowed. If hypoxia is prolonged, fetal myocardium is affected, leading to a further decrease in FHR and hypotension.[74] Recovery will be slower as well. As noted earlier, in the fetus beat-to-beat variability is an indicator of total central nervous system activity; the changes in this variability can be a sign of anything from normal sleep to impending death. Certain drugs as well as catecholamine bursts can also affect the CNS and be reflected in heart rate variability. Therefore this one parameter cannot be used as an independent measure of fetal well-being but can instead provide valuable information when combined with other indicators. Many of these same measures hold true in the neonatal state as well.

Control of Fetal Circulation

Fetal circulation is controlled by neural inputs and humoral factors, such as catecholamines, vasopressin, angiotensin II, and prostaglandins. Baroreflexes in the aortic arch and carotid arteries are sensitive to changes in systemic arterial pressure. Carotid receptor stimulation leads to a mild tachycardia and marked increase in blood pressure, whereas stimulation of aortic chemoreceptors leads to bradycardia and a slight increase in blood pressure.[74] Sympathetic innervation is immature, with parasympathetic (vagal) dominance. Both vagal and sympathetic tone increase with fetal hypoxia.[167] Parasympathetic stimulation has a primary job in maintaining FHR and beat-to-beat variability. The sympathetic nervous system provides a reserve to improve the heart's pumping ability during intermittent stress.[167] Cholinergic fibers develop early in gestation. α-Adrenergic and β-adrenergic fibers also appear early and increase with gestation.[74] If oxygen content of the fetal blood decreases, blood flow to the brain, myocardium, and adrenals increases; pulmonary blood flow and flow to the lower body decreases.[74] Control of fetal circulation is discussed further in the next section.

Fetal Stress Responses

The fetus lives and grows in a relatively hypoxic environment and yet has enough oxygen to meet basal metabolic and growth needs. The integrity of the maternal, fetal, and placental circulations maintains the continual flow of nutrients to meet the demands of the products of conception. If any interruption in flow occurs, the fetus experiences a reduction or loss of available oxygen and nutrient substrates.

Factors affecting oxygen transfer to the fetus can be of environmental, maternal, placental, umbilical, or fetal origin. Substrate consumption by the fetus provides fuel for oxidative metabolism and building materials for tissue growth. When substrate availability or transfer is limited, both processes are in jeopardy. This can occur by reducing arterial oxygen content, restricting uterine blood flow, or reducing umbilical blood flow through cord compression. Maternal hypoxemia reduces only the oxygen supply available to the fetus; however, interruption of uterine or umbilical blood flow interferes not only with oxygen transfer but also with carbon dioxide elimination.[201]

Thus oxygen delivery from the placental circulation to the fetal body can be reduced by either maternal hypoxemia or blood flow disruption. The distribution of blood flow and oxygen to fetal organs is quite different in these two types of stress. During maternal hypoxemia, blood flow is directed to the myocardium, adrenal gland, and cerebral circuits. Blood flow to the skin, lungs, gastrointestinal system, muscles, liver, and kidneys is markedly reduced. Interrupting blood flow, on the other hand, leads to only a moderate increase in blood flow to the myocardium and brain. There is a marked increase in blood flow to the adrenals, however. The pulmonary system does experience a decrease in blood flow, but blood flow to the kidneys, gastrointestinal tract, and peripheral circulation is maintained or increased.[114,201]

Heart rate, blood pressure, and combined ventricular output are affected by hypoxia. Unlike the adult, the fetus responds to hypoxia not with tachycardia but with bradycardia. Along with this, there is a rise in systemic arterial pressure. Which of these responses occurs first is unknown, because both develop slowly over 2 to 3 minutes. The onset of bradycardia is earlier and the duration prolonged if the baseline arterial blood oxygen saturation is lower. The heart rate does return to baseline values when the hypoxemia is prolonged, although when the initial oxygen saturation is lower, recovery from the bradycardia is more protracted.[201]

During umbilical vein occlusion there are insignificant changes in arterial pressure. The onset of bradycardia is delayed and occurs only after the PaO_2 has fallen. In the sudden, complete occlusion of the umbilical cord, however, there is an immediate rise in arterial pressure because of arterial occlusion, and bradycardia is instantaneous.[114,186,201]

The fall in combined ventricular output due to hypoxia is the result of a decrease in LV and RV output. This reduced output is mainly due to the fall in heart rate. Output returns to normal once the FHR is restored to baseline level.[114,201]

In addition to interruptions in oxidative metabolism due to hypoxia or asphyxia on a short-term basis, long-term reductions in oxygenation lead the fetus to shut down oxygen-consuming processes (i.e., growth or behavioral changes). With acute reductions in oxygenation, fetal glucose consumption may fall and glycogen mobilization increase. These alterations ensure a continuous glucose supply to the placenta. If lactate concentrations rise, this may be another substrate source for maintaining the placenta over time.

To maintain the placenta, oxygen-consuming activities such as protein synthesis must be curtailed so as to direct limited resources to more vital functions. Metabolic normality may be maintained by the fetus, which suggests that the fetus is capable of rapid adaptation to limited substrate delivery by decreasing the growth rate. This results in IUGR for the fetus, which can be continued over a protracted period of time. The length of time that normal growth patterns are interrupted can change from being protective to being pathologic for some organ systems. These alterations can influence future extrauterine growth and development.[186]

Along with physiologic changes, behavioral state changes can be seen during acute short-term hypoxemia as well as in sustained acute hypoxemia and graded prolonged hypoxemia. Rapid eye movement (REM) sleep states are decreased with hypoxemia and may be indicative of changes in oxygen consumption. The development of well-defined behavioral states may be delayed in IUGR infants as compared with normal infants.[186]

There is also a reduction in fetal movements with hypoxia. Acute asphyxia may result in a brief increase in extremity movement that falls off quickly if oxygenation is not restored. This cessation in fetal breathing movements and gross body movements can contribute to reducing fetal oxygen consumption. The number and duration of general body movements are decreased in IUGR infants. This is an indication of decreased energy expenditure.[186] Although the fetus is capable of reducing its oxygen needs and compensating for limited substrate availability over a protracted period of time, this may end up being detrimental to organ development and functioning on a long-term basis.

NEONATAL PHYSIOLOGY

The cardiovascular system is designed to deliver adequate oxygen and nutrients to the tissues and remove metabolic by-products at all stages of development. The coordinated functioning of respiratory, cardiovascular, and endocrine systems is essential to meet the cellular metabolic needs, especially in times of stress. During fetal, neonatal, and adult life these processes are quite different, and maturational processes continue after birth.

Transitional Events

At birth the cardiac output is redistributed with increased pulmonary blood flow. Pulmonary and systemic pressure change as PVR decreases and SVR increases. The ventricles begin working in series (see Figure 8-17)—which is the adult configuration—rather than in parallel, and the fetal extracardiac and intracardiac shunts close. With birth, oxygenation is moved from the placenta to the lungs, and air ventilation results in increased oxygen availability, with a concomitant rise in PO₂ levels.

Epinephrine and norepinephrine levels increase rapidly at birth, decreasing to prebirth levels within four hours. The cause of this surge is not completely understood, but it may be related to mild asphyxia with birth, decreased ambient temperature, cord clamping, increased intracranial pressure, or other events during transition.[26] Epinephrine mediates increased cardiac output and myocardial contractility, which are important for changes in myocardial function with birth.[26]

The changeover from fetal to neonatal circulation is linked directly with the development and function of the pulmonary

vasculature and changes in PVR (see Pulmonary Vasculature). At delivery the low-resistance placental circulation is removed, leading to an increase in SVR. The increase in SVR is also due to the increased volume of blood in the arterial system (i.e., blood that no longer has a placenta to return to) so must be accommodated in the systemic circulation as well as the decreasing PVR. The initiation of air breathing leads to lung expansion, an increase in alveolar oxygen concentration, and vasodilation of the pulmonary vascular bed. As vasodilatation occurs, PVR falls rapidly. At birth the PVR falls by almost 80%, resulting in a dramatic increase in pulmonary blood flow and a fall in ductal shunting (Figure 8-19). Before birth the high PVR and low SVR result in 90% of the RV

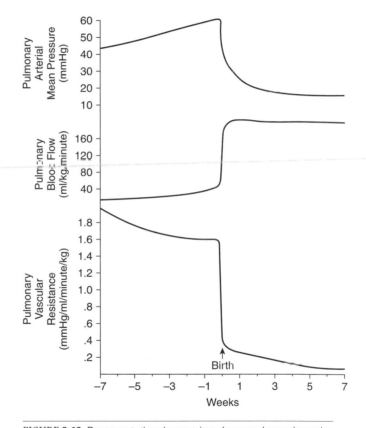

FIGURE **8-19** Representative changes in pulmonary hemodynamics during transition from late term fetal circulation to the neonatal circulation. Pulmonary vascular resistance (PVR) decreases progressively during late gestation due to lung growth and increased cross-sectional area for flow. PVR decreases dramatically at birth due to the vasodilating effect of lung aeration. PVR continues to fall more gradually over the first 6 to 8 weeks of life. Pulmonary blood flow remains at low levels during fetal growth, then increases abruptly with lung expansion and the rapid fall in PVR. Mean pulmonary artery pressure falls rapidly immediately after birth because the pulmonary vasodilation causes PVR to fall more than pulmonary blood flow increases. (From Rudolph, A.M. [1991]. Fetal circulation and cardiovascular adjustments after birth. In A.M. Rudolph, et al. [Eds.]. *Rudolph's pediatrics* [10th ed.]. Norwalk, CT: Appleton & Lange.)

output going through the ductus. After delivery 90% of this flow goes to the pulmonary arteries.[26,74]

Factors decreasing PVR at birth include lung aeration; increasing PO_2; and release of vasodilators such as bradykinin, PGE_1, PGE_2, PGI_2 (prostacyclin), nitric oxide, and endothelial-derived releasing factor (EDRF). Lung aeration and PO_2 are the most critical factors.[161] Lung aeration and increasing PO_2 either alone or together (greatest effect) decrease PVR and increase nitric oxide.[17,203] Lung inflation stimulates pulmonary stretch receptors, leading to a reflexive vasodilation.[74,203] Currently the major pulmonary vasodilators at birth are thought to be nitric oxide and prostacyclin, whose release may be mediated by gaseous expansion of the lungs. Adenosine, bradykinin, and possibly adrenomedullin may also have important roles.[202]

Nitric oxide, a main component of endothelial-derived relaxant factor, is released by the endothelium and stimulated by oxygen.[17] Studies in fetal lambs suggest that both increased PO_2 and rapid increase in pulmonary blood flow (creating shear stress) induce endothelial nitric oxide synthetase (NOS) and thus increase nitric oxide levels with birth.[20] Increased NOS expression with oxygen stimulation develops late in gestation as the pulmonary vasculature become more sensitive to nitric oxide.[135] Pulmonary vasoconstriction in utero is thought to be mediated by inhibition of nitric oxide production by substances such as endothelin type 1.[259] Prostacyclin increases late in gestation and in the early postbirth period. Its action is thought to be stimulated by rhythmic lung distension rather than increased oxygenation.[25,135]

Closure of the Ductus Venosus

The DV is functionally closed within minutes of birth due to cessation of blood flow. Cessation of placental blood flow is mediated by mechanical stimulation with stretching of the umbilical cord and its blood vessels. This enhances initial constriction of the umbilical blood vessels. The rapid increase in PO_2 with initiation of breathing maintains constriction of the umbilical vessels.[74] The DV is obliterated by 1 week in three fourths of term infants and in most by 10 to 14 days.[75,141] The DV remains open longer in preterm infants.[141]

Closure of the Foramen Ovale

Alterations at birth lead to pressure changes within the cardiac chambers and the movement from parallel circulation to in-series circulation. The pressure changes result from the rapid drop in systemic venous return via the IVC and the increase in pulmonary venous return. The left atrial pressure rises, exceeding the right atrial pressure, and the foramen ovale's flap valve closes, separating the two atria.

The foramen ovale may remain patent for up to 9 months in some infants and occasionally into adulthood.[74,169,202]

Closure of the Ductus Arteriosus

The DA begins to close almost immediately after birth but remains patent for several hours to days following delivery. The PVR may remain higher than the systemic vascular bed for a short time following the first breath. This allows for a small right-to-left shunt to remain and for desaturated blood to mix with oxygenated blood in the descending aorta. If the PVR remains high or is increased during the first hours or days after delivery, the right-to-left shunt may become clinically significant, as is seen in persistent pulmonary hypertension of the newborn.

As the SVR continues to increase and stabilize and the PVR continues to fall, the movement of blood across the DA reverses and becomes left to right. For a time, flow is bidirectional, with both right-to-left and left-to-right flow, but then right-to-left flow ceases. Within the first 12 to 14 hours of extrauterine life in most term infants, the DA achieves functional closure through constriction in most term infants.[26] By 96 hours of age, the DA is functionally closed in nearly all term infants.[75,169] The DA remains open for a longer period in preterm infants (see Patent Ductus Arteriosus in the Preterm).

Anatomic closure takes much longer and is usually achieved within 2 to 3 months. During this time, the ductus may be reopened if hypoxia or increased PVR is encountered. This may occur with crying or with pathologic problems. Anatomic closure involves endothelial destruction, proliferation of subintimal tissue, and formation of connective tissues to form a fibrous strand known as the ligamentum arteriosus.[74]

Functional closure of the DA at birth is influenced primarily by oxygen and vasoactive substances (particularly prostaglandins) rather than primarily hemodynamic changes, as is seen with closure of the foramen ovale and DV.[74] Factors favoring DA dilation include PGE_1, PGE_2, PGI_2, hypoxia, and acidosis, whereas factors favoring DA constriction include PGF_2, prostaglandin synthetase, increased PO_2 and pH, and bradykinin.[21,26,169]

Although there is a relative hypoxia present at birth (when compared with adult oxygen levels), within 10 minutes the neonate is hyperoxic, with a PaO_2 of 50 mmHg. This continues to increase over the first hour to approximately 62 mmHg. Arterial oxygen concentrations stabilize between 75 and 85 mmHg over the first 2 days, with a concomitant fall in PVR and improved ventilation-perfusion ratios. The fall in PVR continues for the next several weeks; however, adult circulation is usually achieved within the first 2 days.[10]

PGE$_2$ is thought to be primarily responsible for maintaining the patency of the DA during fetal life. The DA is extremely sensitive to PGE$_2$, and it is the loss of this reactivity that keeps the ductus closed after birth. Just before birth there is a decrease in circulating PGE$_2$ concentrations, possibly due to an increase in pulmonary blood flow that enhances delivery of PGE$_2$ to the lungs for metabolism. This may prepare for or enhance ductal closure at the time the infant converts to air breathing and active ductal constriction occurs.[10,74] The further decrease in PGE$_2$ with birth is related to increased pulmonary blood flow and increased lung metabolic activity as well as removal of the placenta, the main source of PGE$_2$ in the fetus.[74]

Neonatal Myocardium

The myocardium undergoes structural and functional changes during the neonatal period, before achieving maturational properties and capabilities. The major physiologic change in the myocardium is the improved ability to generate force and of the myofibrils to shorten. The weeks following birth bring about a change in ventricular mass, with the left increasing more than the right. However, during this process the RV becomes more compliant. As a result, changes in RV volume have a greater impact on LV filling in the fetus than in the adult.[7,10]

Compliance increases rapidly during the first few days of extrauterine life. Changes in connective tissue content can be seen during this time and may explain the change in compliance, although additional explanations may lie in collagen, extracellular matrix, or matrix attachment site differences between the fetus and the adult.[24]

Pulmonary Vasculature

As noted in the previous section, with transition to extrauterine life, blood flow to the lungs increases eight- to tenfold with the marked decrease in PVR (see Figure 8-19).[223] Failure of PVR to fall at birth can lead to persistent pulmonary hypertension. The high PVR in the fetus is due to a thick muscular coat of medial smooth muscle. This muscle involutes rapidly after birth. Toward the periphery the encircling smooth muscle is less complete and is absent in the most peripheral arteries.[17]

Changes in the pulmonary vasculature after birth occur in two phases (Figure 8-20). The first phase is prominent during the first 24 hours after birth, with dilation and recruitment of nonmuscularized and partially muscularized arteries.[135] The second phase involves further involution from 24 hours of age to 6 to 8 weeks. The partially muscularized arteries become nonmuscularized and the completely muscularized vessels become partially muscularized within thinning of the remaining muscle layer.[135] As a result

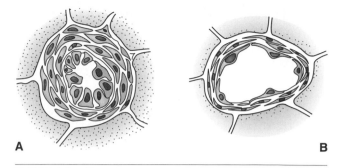

FIGURE 8-20 Changes in the small muscular pulmonary arteries during transition. Muscularized small pulmonary arteries from a near-term gestation fetus **(A)** demonstrate swollen endothelial cells and increased thickness of the muscular layer. Within 24 hours after birth **(B)**, a considerable increase in luminal diameter is noted secondary to flattening of the endothelial cells, spreading of the smooth muscle cell, and an increase in external diameter caused by relaxation of the smooth muscles. These events contribute to the drop in pulmonary vascular resistance after birth. (From Lakshminrushimha, S. & Steinharn, R.H. [1999]. Pulmonary vascular biology during neoantal transition. *Clin Perinatol, 26,* 604.)

of these changes, the vessel lumen size increases, the ability of the pulmonary arteries to constrict decreases, and PVR continues to fall. By 6 to 8 weeks after birth, PVR reaches adult values and the pulmonary vasculature becomes less sensitive to the effects of PO$_2$ changes.[135]

Metabolic Rate and Oxygen Transport

Metabolic rate is measured as oxygen consumption and is much higher in the neonate than in the adult. The neonatal metabolic rate is also higher than that of the fetus because of independent extrauterine functioning and growth requirements. The components of oxygen consumption are related to energy expenditure and include basal metabolic rate, growth, heat production, and physical activity. The growth component is approximately 2% to 3% of the total metabolic rate and is higher in preterm infants. Oxygen consumption in the neonate increases exponentially with physical activity, placement in a nonneutral thermal environment, therapeutic and diagnostic procedures, and increased work of breathing.[256]

The oxygen availability, which is the product of the cardiac output and the arterial oxygen content, is also elevated in the neonate. The estimated delivery of oxygen in the neonate at rest is 75% higher than in the adult. Three major processes impair oxygen availability: ventilation-perfusion mismatching from either intra- or extrapulmonary sources, reduced oxygen-hemoglobin-binding capacity, and reduced cardiac output. Along with these processes, a cardiovascular system that is unable to respond to an increased metabolic demand can result in decompensation.[245]

Endocrine, respiratory, and cardiovascular responses to altered oxygenation are similar to those found in the adult, the major difference being that the neonate functions close to maximum capacity normally and therefore has little reserve to compensate for further demands. Therefore, when impaired oxygen transport results in increased cardiac output (increased heart rate), the maximum is readily reached. Further oxygen demands are associated with an increase in oxygen extraction and a decrease in oxygen saturation.[118,245]

Hypoxemia results in a decrease in oxygen consumption, oxygen availability, and systemic vascular resistance and an increase in oxygen extraction by the tissues. Heart rate and cardiac output increase, since the ability to deliver and release oxygen to the myocardium is essential for the myocardium to respond to the hypoxemia and compensate for impaired oxygen transport.

Isovolemic anemia results in a significant decrease in arterial and mixed venous oxygen content, mean aortic pressure, and systemic vascular resistance. Cardiac output and stroke volume increase regardless of the hemoglobin content; however, heart rate increases are seen only with hemoglobin levels of 6 g/dl or less. If oxygen affinity is reduced, cardiac output and stroke volume increase to a greater degree. These events, once again, occur only when myocardial function is maintained.

Impaired cardiac output results in redistribution of blood flow, with flow directed to the heart and brain preferentially and shunted away from the peripheral organ systems. This is reflected in an increase in vascular resistance in the lower body, with no change in the upper body.

Over the first 2 to 4 months of life, there is a fall in hemoglobin concentration, an increase in HbA, and a rightward shift in the oxygen-hemoglobin dissociation curve (see Chapters 7 and 9). This enables more oxygen to be released to the tissues at the same capillary oxygen tension. However, the increased metabolic demands of extrauterine life (including physical activity) must be accompanied by an increase in the P_{50} to compensate for the total hemoglobin concentration. The pattern of changes during these first 2 to 4 months includes a decline in total hemoglobin (reaching its lowest point at 8 to 12 weeks in term infants); a progressive shift in P_{50} to the right; and an early change in 2,3-diphosphoglycerate (2,3-DPG) (see Chapter 7). There may also be an increase in cardiac output and an increase in oxygen extraction. The latter is adjusted depending on the oxygen consumption, total hemoglobin, and P_{50}. Once hemoglobin levels fall below a critical point, however, cardiac output is unable to compensate for the reduced oxygen availability, necessitating a redistribution in cardiac output.[118]

Myocardial Performance in the Neonate

Myocardial performance is influenced by ventricular preload, myocardial contractility, heart rate, and ventricular afterload. The adaptation to neonatal life is characterized by an increase in heart rate, end-diastolic volume, and inotropic state. This implies that even at rest the neonate is functioning at nearly full capacity with little or no reserve in contractility, preload, or afterload. This functional state is needed to meet the increased vascular loading that occurs with birth. Consequently the newborn heart has less ability to adapt to additional acute pressure (afterload) or volume (preload) stresses.[220]

Preload

Ventricular preload is a measure of end-diastolic volume (EDV). Myocardial fiber length changes with EDV in a predictable manner as described by the Frank-Starling law. According to this law, up to critical length, increased EDV leads to increased fiber length and improved contractility. This leads to increased stroke volume (SV) and CO.

Ventricular preload in the neonate is influenced by the less compliant ventricles. The neonatal heart does function under the Frank-Starling law, but under homeostatic conditions it operates at the upper limit of this law. Compared to the adult heart, the neonatal heart requires a higher filling pressure and this filling pressure is reached at lower volumes. In addition, neonates have a higher CO due to increased metabolism.

The neonatal heart must deal with the increased preload generated by the high volume load at delivery. Moreover, the low compliance of the LV decreases the preload reserve volume. Heart rates in neonates are high, falling during the 6 weeks following delivery. Whether infants can augment cardiac output through further increases in heart rate continues to be debated, as does the effectiveness of inotropic support in the neonate without contractility failure. If increases in afterload or preload are associated with decreased contractility, as with sepsis or asphyxia, inotropic support can improve cardiac output rapidly.[220]

In the fetus and newborn, an increase in RV volume interferes with LV filling. The impact of one chamber on another is also more marked with decreasing compliance. So if there are changes in RV diastolic or loading pressures in the fetus, the LV is compromised and stroke volume is reduced. Once the PVR drops at delivery and throughout the neonatal period, LV filling is enhanced and stroke volume is improved. Therefore neonates are more compromised than adults are if there is an increase in RV preload (i.e., rapid administration of a large fluid bolus) or afterload with specific pathologic conditions (papillary muscle dysfunction or pulmonary hypertension).

Contractility

Myocardial contractility relates to the heart's intrinsic pumping ability, which is dependent on calcium influx in myocardium. Acidosis, hypercarbia, and hypoxia alter cell permeability and the NA-K pump and lead to decreased contractility.

Contractile capabilities are dependent upon the force of contraction, shortening velocity (preload), inotropy, and afterload (load carried at the time of contraction). The maximum shortening of muscle is obtained when there is zero load; however, as the afterload increases, the velocity of muscle shortening decreases. If the load is so great that no external shortening is possible, the contraction is considered isometric. Changing the muscle length can alter the force of the contraction; force development is related to the number of cross-bridges (the greater the number, the greater the force).[7]

An increase in contractility and development of force is part of the maturation process of the myocardium. There is no sudden change in force-generating ability with birth, but rather a slow progression over time as the entire cardiac system matures into adulthood. Most of these maturational processes are related to structural changes in the myocardial anatomy. As myofibril content increases, there is an increase in the number of cross-bridge attachments and therefore greater force generation. The increased organization of the myofibrils may also contribute to the ability to generate forceful contractions. Whether changes in the responsiveness of the contractile apparatus to calcium facilitate any of these changes is currently unclear. Maturation of membrane systems and calcium control may also affect muscle contractions.

The maturational increase in the force-generating ability of the myocardium begins to be seen in late gestation and continues until adulthood. Ventricular filling, pressure development, and ejection in the fetus are similar to those in the neonate and the adult, except that at birth there is a marked increase in combined ventricular output.[74,88] With birth, RV output increases by one third, whereas LV output triples.[88] An increase in pulmonary venous return, improved inotropy (strength of contraction), increased heart rate, and the diastolic and systolic interactions of the right and LVs may contribute to the change in combined ventricular output. LV output increases significantly, during the period when the DA is still patent. The patent DA increases the volume load of the heart, which may initiate a Frank-Starling response.[88,223] Grant et al have suggested that the cause of the doubling of the LV stroke volume seen at birth may be due to release of ventricular constraint (from the chest wall, lungs, and pericardium) with lung aeration and clearance of lung fluid (see Chapter 9), thus increasing ventricular preload.[88]

In the weeks after birth, LV output returns to fetal levels or lower, whereas systolic and end-diastolic pressures continue to rise. Other indicators of the increased birth inotropy also return to fetal baselines. A clear explanation for this is currently not known, although it may have to do with the reaccumulation of reserves after the birth process. Therefore diseases that place an additional demand on the heart to produce more cardiac output in the first days of extrauterine life can result in cardiovascular compromise in the neonate.[7]

Myocardial contractility is altered in the neonate due to the infant's decreased ventricular compliance and reduced contractile mass. As a result, neonates rely more on heart rate than on stroke volume to increase cardiac output. Yet this mechanism is also limited due to parasympathetic domination in the neonate and immaturity of the sympathetic nervous system. In addition the neonate is vulnerable to metabolic and biochemical alterations that can further compromise contractility. Increasing heart rate may only improve cardiac output slightly in the neonate, since cardiac output is near maximum under homeostatic conditions.

Because myocardial contractility in neonates is high during the first week of life, there is little reserve in contractility. This implies that inotropic drugs will do little to improve the contractile state of the normally functioning neonatal heart. One mechanism for this increased inotropic state and the elevated cardiac output is the high level of adrenergic stimulation that occurs around birth. However, the increased cardiac output that remains for several weeks postnatally cannot be explained by continued catecholamine activity. It has been suggested that the postnatal increase in T_3 concentrations may contribute to the increased LV output.[220]

Heart Rate

The baseline heart rate is determined by the intrinsic depolarization rate of the sinoatrial node, which is actively inhibited by tonic parasympathetic input. Myocardial sympathetic innervation is incomplete at birth, with decreased norepinephrine levels during the first 3 weeks. As a result, vagal effects predominate, with limited response to catecholamine stimulation of β-adrenergic receptors. As the parasympathetic system matures, the resting heart rate decreases.[10] Tachycardia (more than 160 beats per minute) is usually seen with events that lead to catecholamine release, sympathetic stimulation, or parasympathetic withdrawal. A higher heart rate is also seen in the extremely premature infant, in whom the sympathetic nervous system dominates control of cardiac function.

Afterload

Ventricular afterload is the resistance against which the heart pumps (i.e., PVR, SVR). Afterload affects contractility. Increased afterload leads to decreased contractility, whereas decreased afterload leads to increased contractility. Even though PVR decreases significantly at birth, PVR remains higher in the neonate than in the adult for 6 to 8 weeks after birth. During this time, PVR gradually decreases to adult values as the medial muscle layer of pulmonary arterioles is restructured (see Pulmonary Vasculature). In addition, neonatal pulmonary vasculature is characterized by increased reactivity of pulmonary arterioles, with a tendency toward vasoconstriction and increased PVR.

The LV end-diastolic volume increases with birth. This probably contributes to the neonatal increase in output via the Frank-Starling relationship. These changes may be due to the circulatory transition that occurs at delivery and the fall in PVR and increased pulmonary venous return. LV filling may be augmented by a decrease in RV afterload. Therefore a fall in pulmonary artery pressure would enhance LV output by decreasing RV afterload, which would improve RV ejection and result in a smaller RV end-diastolic volume. The LV is then able to fill to a larger volume at a comparable filling pressure. This interaction is magnified in the fetus and neonate because of the reduced compliance found in the heart.[7]

Regulation of Fetal and Neonatal Circulation
Central Mechanisms

As in the adult, medullary, hypothalamic, and cerebral cortical activity presumably influence fetal and neonatal cardiovascular functions. The medullary centers appear to influence cardiovascular responses in a variable fashion in the fetus and the newborn; however, higher cortical or hypothalamic activities are associated with an increase in heart rate and hypertension. This stimulation and response are quite different than the baroreflex, which is a peripheral response by the baroreceptors to hypertension that is itself secondary to increased peripheral resistance.

Complex neurohumoral and metabolic responses maintain blood pressure, heart rate, and distribution of blood flow in the fetus and the newborn. These include systemic sensors (stretch receptors and neural and hormonal mediators) as well as local responses that allow an organ to regulate flow. The interaction of the two systems allows the fetus and the newborn to respond to stress events by redistributing blood flow to spare high-priority organs with specific oxygen requirements.

Neural Regulation

Baroreceptors that are sensitive to changes in blood pressure are located in the aortic arch and the carotid sinuses. These sensors cause changes in heart rate and, in the fetus, may be responsible for stabilizing fetal blood pressure, with increasing sensitivity as gestational age advances. Baroreceptor activity has been implicated in the decreasing FHR baseline seen in later gestation as blood pressure rises. In late gestation and in the early postbirth period, the baroreflex is reset.[143] Chemoreceptors can be found in both the peripheral and central nervous systems and may alter FHR in response to hypoxemia and acidosis. Their role in the normal fetus is unclear. Present in the latter half of gestation, they appear to be responsive to changes in pH and carbon dioxide tension and give rise to bradycardia while cardiac output and umbilical blood flow are preserved. Following birth, hypoxia leads to tachycardia and an increase in cardiac output associated with increased respiratory effort.[10,255]

Sympathetic intervention is present and functional in the fetus and newborn, increasing responsiveness with increasing gestational age. Stimulation results in tachycardia, augmented myocardial contractility, and increased systemic arterial blood pressure. Parasympathetic input also increases with advancing gestational age. The major effector is the vagus nerve, which provides an inhibitory effect on FHR. Short-term variability of the FHR is modulated by impulses from the vagus nerve. Studies looking at the relative contributions of the parasympathetic and sympathetic nervous systems seem to indicate that the parasympathetic nervous system matures more quickly than the sympathetic system. Functional balance is achieved in the neonate.[255]

Humoral Regulation

Humoral regulation of the cardiovascular system is related to the impact of catecholamines, vasopressin, renin-angiotensin, and prostaglandins on the heart and vascular bed. Catecholamines are secreted by the adrenal medulla and may be involved in fetal cardiovascular system regulation before the development of the sympathetic nervous system. Fetal myocardium appears to have equal responsiveness to catecholamines when compared with that of the adult.[10,255] As noted earlier, catecholamine levels increase markedly with birth, reaching pharmacologic levels.[143]

Arginine vasopressin is produced by the fetal pituitary gland early in gestation. Although usually undetectable, the concentration of vasopressin increases during hypoxia, hypotension, or hypernatremia. This results in vasoconstriction of the vessels in the musculoskeletal system, skin, and gut while increasing flow to the brain and heart. Prostaglandins may also play a role in augmenting blood flow to the brain during hypoxic episodes. These humoral mechanisms may play a major role in the redistribution of blood flow seen in the fetus during significant hypoxia.[10]

Stimulation of the renin-angiotensin system leads to an increase in FHR, blood pressure, and combined ventricular output. Blood flow to the lungs and myocardium increases; flow to the renal system falls off. Angiotensin II seems to exert a vasotonic effect on the peripheral circulation. These effects may support the fetus during episodes of significant blood loss.[10]

CLINICAL IMPLICATIONS FOR NEONATAL CARE

Cardiovascular disturbances in the neonate include congestive heart failure, cyanosis, murmurs, and arrhythmias. Cardiac malformations occur in 0.8% to 1% of live births and represent about 10% of all congenital malformations. Murmurs that are due to the normal turbulence of transitional circulation (i.e., ductal closure) or physiologic turbulence in the pulmonary artery are considered benign. Gestational age and disease also affect the cardiovascular system and are factors in patent DA and bronchopulmonary dysplasia.

Assessment of Heart Sounds

The neonate heart rate ranges from 120 to 160 beats per minute, with significant state-related variations. Heart rate increases with birth and remains higher for the first hour, although there is marked variability between individual infants.[26] Since heart rate is the most effective method for the neonate to increase CO, cardiorespiratory illness, sepsis, and metabolic problems are often accompanied by tachycardia.

The neonatal heart accounts for 0.75% of body weight in the neonate (versus 0.35 % in adults). On chest roentgenogram the neonatal heart generally occupies about 40% of the field (versus 35% in adults). Because the heart is positioned more transversely, the apical pulse is felt to the left of the sternal border. A visible precordial impulse may be seen along the left sternal border for 4 to 6 hours after birth.[26,96]

Heart sounds are of higher pitch, shorter duration, and greater intensity, and functional murmurs, hums, and clicks may be heard. Murmurs are heard in about one third of healthy infants in the first 24 hours after birth and in two thirds in the first 48 hours.[26] A systolic DA murmur is heard in about 15% of infants while the ductus is still patent, most often around 5 to 6 hours of age.[26] Sinus arrhythmias are common in infants and children. The most common significant arrhythmias in infants are bradycardia and supraventricular tachycardia.[96] Sinus bradycardia

is seen due to the predominant parasympathetic innervation of the sinus node in the neonate.[26] Bradycardia may occur due to vagal stimulation or secondary to hypoxemia or acidosis. Bradycardia may not be well tolerated in infants since heart rate comprises a greater portion of cardiac output than stroke volume. Arrhythmias often do not compromise systemic performance or cardiac output as much in neonates as in older individuals. Abnormal sinus rhythms in infancy may indicate underlying cardiac anomalies that alter reflexive mechanisms for heart rate control.[96]

Cardiac Shunts

Right-to-left cardiac shunts involve shunting of blood from systemic venous circulation to the arterial circulations without oxygenation. These shunts are usually characterized by obstruction to flow on the right side of the heart distal to an abnormal communication. Right-to-left shunting is characteristic of fetal circulation; that is, placental blood moves from the venous circulation to the arterial circulation bypassing the lungs via either the foramen ovale or DA. Pathologic examples of right-to-left cardiac shunts include persistent pulmonary hypertension of the newborn (PPHN), in which the foramen ovale or DA or both remain open; pulmonary stenosis or atresia, in which blood is shunted from right to left via a patent DA, foramen ovale, or VSD; or transposition of the great vessels.

Left-to-right cardiac shunts are characterized by recirculation of oxygenated blood through the lungs, bypassing the peripheral circulation. Examples of left-to-right shunting include a PDA (shunting of blood from the aorta to the pulmonary artery and thus back to the lungs) or a ventricular-septal defect with shunting of oxygenated blood from the LV to the RV and thus back to the lungs.

Cyanosis

Cyanosis is a physical sign characterized by blue-gray mucous membranes, nail beds, and skin. It is the result of deoxygenated hemoglobin in the blood at a concentration of at least 5 g/dl. Hypoxemia is a state of abnormally low arterial blood oxygen concentration. The degree of hypoxemia may or may not correlate with cyanosis, depending on the blood hemoglobin concentration and the ability of the observer to detect cyanosis. The most common causes of cyanosis in the neonate are cardiac disease and pulmonary disease. The ability to be able to distinguish between these two is essential. Therefore, when congenital heart disease is suspected, the degree of hypoxemia must be related to the volume of pulmonary blood flow.[62]

Hypoxemia in these infants is due to right-to-left shunting (diversion of blood from the lungs); therefore ventilation and oxygen delivery do not improve oxygenation. This is the basis for the hyperoxia challenge test. With adequate ventilation and 100% oxygen, the PaO_2 should rise above 150 mmHg. If the PaO_2 does not increase above 100 mmHg, cyanotic congenital heart disease is most likely the cause of the cyanosis. Between 100 and 150 mmHg, cardiac disease is possible but further diagnostic testing needs to be conducted (e.g., echocardiography). Selected congenital anomalies are discussed in the next section to demonstrate these principles.

Persistent Pulmonary Hypertension of the Newborn

PPHN is a syndrome of acute respiratory distress with hypoxemia and acidemia caused by decreased pulmonary blood flow due to elevated PVR. There is central cyanosis associated with right-to-left shunting across the fetal shunts (foramen ovale and DA). This syndrome may represent failure to achieve transition to air breathing or may be secondary to cardiomyopathies, lung hypoplasia (e.g., with congenital diaphragmatic hernia) meconium aspiration syndrome, perinatal asphyxia, or sepsis.[259]

PPHN is a transitional event that is a result of either the failure of pulmonary vessels to dilate or abnormal musculature of the pulmonary arterioles or transient functional defects of the pulmonary bed.[259] This results in inadequate oxygenation secondary to ventilation-perfusion abnormalities. The continued elevation of the PVR and increased right heart pressure, combined with the resulting hypoxemia and acidosis, lead to maintenance of fetal circulatory channels. Blood flow tends to bypass the lungs with right-to-left shunting across the fetal shunts (foramen ovale and/or DA). Therefore pulmonary hypoperfusion, hypoxia, and acidosis develop. This sets up a cyclic, downward spiral, with a negative feedback loop that escalates the problems. Unless aggressive intervention occurs, death as a result of inadequate oxygenation is the result.

This cycle is aggravated by the increased musculature of the pulmonary blood vessels and heightens reactivity of these vessels. Hypoxemia is the greatest stimulus for this vasoconstrictive response. The low fetal PO_2 within these vessels results in constriction and augments the increased PVR created by the increased muscle tissue. As gestational age advances, the constrictor response becomes stronger. The neonatal pulmonary bed is also highly reactive to hypoxic episodes, as compared with the adult. This may be due to the increased medial wall thickness or the lower density of arteries encountered in the newborn versus the adult.

At birth, constriction of the vessels continues if oxygen levels do not rise, so that systemic and pulmonary vascular pressures change. This constriction results in the persis-

tence of fetal circulatory patterns without the benefit of the placenta, the result being hypoxia secondary to transition failure and altered ventilation and perfusion.

PPHN may arise from maladaption of the pulmonary vascular bed at birth. If maladaption occurs, either the normal increase in pulmonary artery compliance does not occur or vasoconstriction occurs during the transition process. Hypoxia for any reason (hypoventilation, upper airway obstruction, or interstitial disease) may contribute to these mechanisms. If acidosis or hypercarbia exists, they may react synergistically to contribute to the increase in PVR. A vicious circle may be set up in which hypoxia leads to reactive vasoconstriction, which in turn leads to increased right-to-left shunting, thereby increasing the degree of hypoxemia and decreasing the normal postnatal transition events that result in pulmonary artery vasodilatation. This results in continued pulmonary vasoconstriction and shunting.

Patent Ductus Arteriosus in the Preterm Infant

There are three general physiologic characteristics of a patent DA: (1) increased flow through the lungs with diastolic volume overload; (2) increased flow through the left atrium, LV, and aorta; and (3) left-to-right shunting to the pulmonary circulation. Blood is shunted from the upper and lower aortic circulations with a large ductus and multiorgan effects.

The preterm infant has less pulmonary arterial muscle and an immature pulmonary parenchyma. The presence of a PDA is associated with interstitial edema and decreased compliance of the lung due to pulmonary edema. Ductal closure results in an increased compliance and a decreased need for ventilatory support (especially end-expiratory pressure). Prolonged ventilatory support due to a PDA increases the risk of BPD, and therefore early intervention is recommended.

Perfusion of peripheral organ systems is dependent upon adequate systolic and diastolic flow. If a large PDA exists, systemic diastolic arterial flow is compromised and may even be reversed in the descending aorta. This can lead to decreased renal perfusion and contribute to the development of volume overload and congestive heart failure. Treatment with furosemide may actually potentiate ductal opening by altering prostaglandin metabolism.

Gastrointestinal effects are also related to a decrease in flow and intestinal ischemia. Preterm infants with intestinal ischemia as a result of a PDA can develop necrotizing enterocolitis. Cerebral ischemia may also occur as blood is diverted from the upper body. Cerebral blood flow changes can also increase the incidence of intraventricular hemorrhage.

A large left-to-right shunt through the PDA increases the left atrial and ventricular volume, leading to enlargement of these two chambers. The increased LV size also increases the myocardial wall stress, which could lead to myocardial ischemia in the preterm infant. If LV compromise exists, inotropic support may be needed until PDA closure is achieved. Treatment includes fluid restriction, ventilatory support, diuretics, prostaglandin inhibitors, and surgical ligation. Early ductal closure may improve outcome and alter the clinical course. In some cases, this may require exposing the infant to the risks of surgery.

Congenital Cardiac Malformations

Most cardiac defects are compatible with intrauterine life and only become significant at birth. Even defects that significantly alter hemodynamics and flow in the fetal heart are often tolerated well since the fetal shunts allow for compensation (see Figure 8-17). The exceptions to this include defects with atrioventricular valve regurgitation and myocardial dysfunction, which tend to be less well tolerated.[74,169] With any severe defect, birth may result in acute compromise as the fetal shunts close. Thus initial management is often directed at maintaining fetal shunts.[74] Table 8-8 classifies congenital

TABLE 8-8   Classification of Congenital Cardiac Disease

CLASSIFICATION	EXAMPLES
Severe cyanosis caused by separate circulation and poor mixing	D-transposition of the great arteries
	D-transposition of the great arteries and ventricular septal defect
	Double outlet right ventricle with subpulmonary ventricular septal defect (Taussig-Bing)
Severe cyanosis caused by restricted pulmonary blood flow	Tetralogy of Fallot
	Double-outlet right ventricle with subaortic ventricular septal defect and pulmonary stenosis
	Tricuspid atresia
	Pulmonary atresia with intact interventricular septum
	Critical pulmonary stenosis
	Ebstein anomaly
	Single ventricle with pulmonary stenosis
	Persistent pulmonary hypertension
Mild cyanosis caused by complete mixing with normal or increased pulmonary blood flow	Total anomalous pulmonary venous connection
	Truncus arteriosus
	Single ventricle without pulmonary stenosis
	Double-outlet right ventricle with subaortic ventricular septal defect
Systemic hypoperfusion and congestive heart failure with mild or no cyanosis	Aortic stenosis*
	Coarctation of the aorta and aortic arch interruption
	Hypoplastic left heart syndrome
	Multiple left heart defects
	Single ventricle with subaortic stenosis or coarctation of the aorta
	Myocardial disease: cardiomyopathy and myocardtis*
	Cardiac tumor*
	Ateriovenous malformation*
	Hypertension*
Acyanosis with no or mild respiratory distress	Normal murmurs
	Pulmonary stenosis
	Ventricular septal defect†
	Atrial septal defect
	Endocardial cushion defect†
	Patent ductus arteriosus†
	Aorticopulmonary window*
	D-transposition of the great arteries
	Ateriovenous malformation
	Hypertension

From Zahka, K.G. & Lane, J.G. (2002). Approach to the neonate with cardiovascular disease. In A.A. Fanaroff & R.J. Martin (Eds.). *Neonatal and perinatal medicine: Diseases of the fetus and infant* (7th ed.). St Louis: Mosby.

*No symptoms with mild forms of disease.

†Congestive heart failure may develop as left-to-right shunt increases with decrease in pulmonary vascular resistance.

cardiac defects by physiologic consequence. Hemodynamic consequences with transition to extrauterine life of selected disorders are described in the following sections.

Total Anomalous Venous Return

In this condition, none of the pulmonary veins connect with the left atrium. Rather, some or all of the pulmonary veins form a confluence or collecting vessel that usually lies posterior to the left atrium. There may be one or more sites of connection between the pulmonary venous collecting vessel or individual pulmonary veins and the systemic venous circuit. Usually the pulmonary veins drain directly or, more commonly, indirectly into the right atrium via one of the normal embryonic channels. The embryonic defect seems to be a failure of development of the common pulmonary vein normally connecting the developing pulmonary venous plexus with the posterior aspect of the left atrium.

The postnatal presentation depends on the degree of obstruction of pulmonary venous drainage. If obstruction is severe, presentation occurs within the first week of life. If obstruction is mild, presentation may not occur until the latter half of the first year. The presence of an intra-arterial communication—either a patent foramen ovale or a true atrial septal defect (ASD)—is necessary to sustain life postnatally. The hemodynamic impact of total anomalous pulmonary venous return does not occur until pulmonary blood flow increases at the time of delivery. Pulmonary edema is the usual result. Oxygenation is interrupted because of edema, right-to-left shunting, and increased pulmonary resistance.

Transposition of the Great Arteries

This defect arises from abnormal septation of the truncus arteriosus so that the aorta arises from the RV and the pulmonary artery from the left. The foramen ovale and DA develop normally and, in a simple transposition, the coronary arteries arise from the aorta. At birth, with closure of the foramen ovale and DA, two separate circulations exist. In one, desaturated blood returning from the body to the RA flows to the RV and out the aorta to the body without being oxygenation. In the other circulation, oxygenated blood from the lungs returns to the LA, then flows to the LV and back to the lungs via the pulmonary artery. Survival at birth is dependent on bidirectional flow via the foramen ovale and DA or the presence of other defects such as an atrial septal defect or VSD. Severe cyanosis develops as the fetal shunts (particularly the DA) close. PGE_2 is given to maintain ductal patency until the infants can be taken to surgery.[74,257]

Truncus Arteriosus

Truncus arteriosus is a single great artery that arises from the base of the heart and supplies the coronary, pulmonary, and systemic arteries. It is thought to result from septation failure. The truncal valve usually resembles a normal aortic valve. In utero, the main consequence of truncus arteriosus is complete mixing of the systemic and pulmonary venous return above the truncal valve. The truncus is usually quite large, and the DA arising from the pulmonary arteries may be smaller than normal. Since blood flow through the heart is normal, the rest of the heart develops normally.

Postnatally the flow of the pulmonary arteries and systemic arteries is a function of the relative resistances in the two circuits. Initially, the pulmonary resistance is high and pulmonary flow will equal or slightly exceed systemic flow. Over the first hours or days of life, however, the pulmonary arteriolar resistance decreases and pulmonary blood flow increases. As the pulmonary venous return increases, the LV must eject an increasing volume load, which eventually leads to congestive failure. Since there is common mixing of systemic and pulmonary venous blood above the truncal valve, the degree of hypoxemia decreases as the pulmonary flow increases so that these infants are only mildly cyanotic until left heart failure and pulmonary edema interfere with oxygen exchange and pulmonary venous desaturation ensues.

Tricuspid Atresia

In tricuspid atresia there is a failure in the development of the right atrioventricular valve; therefore an intraatrial communication is necessary for survival. This communication is usually in the form of a patent foramen ovale. Along with this, there is usually a VSD connecting a large LV cavity with a hypoplastic chamber that is the outflow portion of the RV. The great arteries may be either normally related or transposed. There may also be an atresia.

Fetal growth and development are uncompromised, so the alterations in cardiovascular status must be compatible with normal development. All systemic venous return is diverted across the foramen ovale into the left atrium and LV. If there are no further abnormalities, the entire ventricular volume is ejected into the aorta. If the VSD is large, some of the LV output passes through the VSD into the hypoplastic RV, exiting via the pulmonary artery if the vessels are normally related or via the aorta if transposition is present.

After delivery there is little change in the circulation, but the normal postnatal alterations impose significant liabilities. Neonates with pulmonary atresia or severe pulmonary stenosis continue to depend on the DA for pulmonary blood flow. When the DA begins to close, severe hypoxemia, acidosis, and eventually death follow. In infants with a large VSD and no pulmonary stenosis, the pulmonary blood flow increases as the pulmonary arteriolar resistance drops and congestive heart failure ensues, usually in the first month of life.

Aortic Stenosis/Atresia and Hypoplastic Left Heart Syndrome

Obstruction of LV outflow in the fetus—either by aortic stenosis or aortic atresia—leads to hypertrophy and hyperplasia. LV compliance is decreased with decreased blood flow through the foramen ovale (blood flow may even reverse). RV output is increased as more of the IVC blood flows to the RV and thus across the DA to the lower body. With aortic atresia, all atrial output is via the RV and all systemic blood crosses the DA. Some of this blood follows the normal path via the descending aorta, some via retrograde flow into the ascending aorta to the coronary arteries, upper body, and head.[74,257]

Even if the defect is severe, the fetus does well because of the parallel fetal circulation. At birth the onset of symptoms varies with severity: the more severe the defect, the earlier the onset is. Infants with severe aortic stenosis develop increased left atrial pressure as pulmonary blood flow increases and LV compliance decreases. The foramen ovale closes or remains open with left-to-right shunting of blood from the LA to the RA. Initially systemic blood flow is also partially maintained via the RV and DA. When the ductus closes, all systemic flow is from the LV via the stenotic aorta. Therefore, in these infants, symptoms of poor perfusion and circulatory failure coincide with closing of ductus and are usually seen within the first 24 hours after birth.[74]

In infants with aortic atresia and hypoplastic left heart syndrome, all systemic blood is routed from the RV to the aorta via the DA. Pulmonary blood flow crosses the foramen ovale left to right (LA to RA). Symptoms arise within the first 24 hours if the ductus is narrow or closes at birth. If the ductus remains open, symptoms may not appear for several weeks.[74,257]

Coarctation of the Aorta

This defect involves a constriction in the aorta distal to the left subclavian artery, usually at the junction of the DA and the aortic isthmus between the ductus and the left subclavian artery. There may be tubular hypoplasia of the aortic arch and intracardiac anomalies, and these must be ruled out during evaluation. About one third of infants with this defect also have a VSD.[74]

Since there is normally very little flow across the aortic isthmus in utero, the tubular hypoplasia and narrowing of the arch does not affect fetal growth and development, and blood is shunted across the DA. After birth the constriction in the aorta increases the LV afterload. If a VSD exists, this increased systemic resistance leads to a large left-to-right shunt. As the PVR falls, the left-to-right shunt increases, resulting in a volume as well as a pressure overload of the LV. In addition to congestive heart failure, there is failure

of the blood to pass from ascending to descending aorta if the coarctation is severe. The results are tissue hypoxia, lactic acidosis, and eventual death after the DA closes.

Those neonates with a juxtaductal coarctation but no other associated anomalies have a slightly different hemodynamic makeup. Closure of the DA leads to an acute increase in afterload to the LV, because blood must be pumped through the narrowed segment; before ductal closure, blood was able to circumvent the coarctation via a shelf of tissue at this insertion point. Since no obstruction was present in utero, no collateral vessels have developed. The neonatal myocardium is unable to respond to the increased workload; consequently congestive heart failure with elevation of LV end-diastolic, left atrial, and pulmonary venous pressures follows.[74,257] If the constriction is less severe, the infant may present with decreased femoral pulses and differences between the upper and lower extremities.

Ventricular Septal Defect

VSDs, which comprise the most common congenital heart defect, may be isolated defects or associated with other congenital cardiac defects. The most common site for a VSD is the membranous portion of the septum that lies between the crista supraventricularis and the papillary muscle of the conus when the heart is viewed from the RV side. Less common sites are the area above the crista, the muscular portion of the septum below the tricuspid valve, and the anterior trabecular portion of the ventricular septum near the apex of the RV.

Since the right and left sides of the heart are arranged in a parallel fashion before birth, the presence of a large communication at the ventricular level in addition to the normal ductus connection at the great vessels does not significantly alter the fetal circulation. After birth, however, the hemodynamics depend on the size of the defect and the pulmonary and systemic vascular resistances. If the defect is large, it offers no resistance to flow. The systolic pressure in the ventricles and great vessels is approximately equal and the systemic and PVRs determine the degree of intracardiac shunting. As the PVR gradually falls, the volume of blood in the LV increases. Therefore more blood is ejected through the VSD into the pulmonary artery. When the pulmonary blood flow is about three times greater than the systemic flow, the LV can no longer accommodate the volume load, and congestive heart failure develops. This usually occurs after the first or second week of life. The right atrium and RV are not volume overloaded, but in the presence of a large defect the RV must generate pressures equal to those of the LV, so there is usually RV hypertrophy without significant dilation. Preterm infants often develop symptoms earlier than term infants because PVR is lower in these infants due to decreased muscularization of the pulmonary arteries.[74,257]

If the VSD is small, it does offer resistance to flow, and the pressures in the two ventricles may differ. Infants with this type of defect are a heterogeneous group, with the hemodynamics depending on the size of the hole rather than the PVR. If the defect is very small, the RV and pulmonary artery pressures may be normal and the pulmonary blood flow less than twice the systemic flow. These infants are rarely symptomatic but usually exhibit a murmur.

Tetralogy of Fallot

Tetralogy of Fallot involves a combination of VSD, pulmonary valve stenosis, RV hypertrophy, and rightward displacement of the aortic root. If the VSD is large, right and LV pressures are similar, so the amount of shunting is determined primarily by the degree of pulmonary stenosis to systemic vascular resistance.[74] In the fetus the portion of the CVO from the aorta is increased, as is the diameter of the aorta. Thus blood flow in utero is usually adequate. If the infant has mild to moderate pulmonary stenosis, closure of the DA may not alter pulmonary blood flow enough to reduce PO_2. With severe pulmonary stenosis, closure of the ductus significantly reduces pulmonary blood flow and the infant develops progressive severe cyanosis.[74] PGE_2 infusions are used to maintain ductal patency and pulmonary blood flow until the infant can be taken to surgery.

MATURATIONAL CHANGES DURING INFANCY AND CHILDHOOD

The changes in the heart at birth include a redistribution of workload between the RV and LV. The change to in series circulation results in an increase in cardiac output, with the RV ejecting blood against a lower afterload and the LV ejecting against a higher afterload. The ventricular mass changes in response to these new demands, with the LV wall thickness increasing significantly while the right remains unchanged.

This change in wall thickness is secondary to an increase in cell number and size. Hyperplasia can occur soon after birth, followed by an increase in cell size. Because of the increased workload of the LV, cell replication occurs more rapidly in the left myocardium.[9] Ventricular size and compliance change gradually during infancy and childhood, so cardiac function parallels that of adults by adolescence.[146]

There is little change in heart size for 4 to 6 weeks after birth; then heart size doubles by 1 year. Heart size increases with somatic growth, with a fourfold increase by 5 years and sixfold increase by 9 years. Changes in heart size are due primarily to fat deposition. Changes in heart size are accompanied by descent of the diaphragm, increasing the room for cardiac movement and expansion of the respiratory system. The heart, which is more transverse in the infant, comes to lie more oblique and lower in relation to the ribs. The position of the heart becomes more vertical by 7 years. As a result the apical impulse is lower and nearer the midclavicle line.[96,146]

The cross-sectional area of cardiac muscle fibers increases sevenfold to adulthood. Increased numbers of small blood vessels, whose growth parallels changes in weight and height, accompanies this change. The thickness of great vessel walls doubles between birth and puberty, and their lumens increase to 2½ times normal. By 2 to 3 years of age, the child's cardiac shadow is similar to that of the adult.[146]

The myocardial cells change in size, shape, and architecture following birth. The LV matures more rapidly after birth, which can be seen in myocyte shape changes. The immature cells are rounder and have a smoother surface. As cells mature, their shape becomes increasingly irregular, with identifiable step changes along their lateral borders.[195] The myocytes become longer and acquire a larger cross-sectional area.

Stimulation for these changes may be related to the sympathetic nervous system. During the neonatal period, α-adrenoceptors and circulating norepinephrine levels are higher than at any other stage of development. In tissue cultures, stimulation of α_1-receptors (e.g., with norepinephrine) results in cell growth. Therefore it can be inferred that the presence of increased receptors and stimulant results in induction of myocardial cell growth.[215]

Myofilament and sarcomere changes also occur with maturation. The sarcomere A-I bands are more irregular; the Z band disk is thicker, although more variable; and the M band is absent initially. The myofibrils are more disorganized and often are not oriented in the same direction as the long axis. Instead they are arranged around a large central mass of nuclei and mitochondria, which may persist for weeks following birth. Eventually the myofibrils assume the adult position and are distributed across the cell.

The increase in the proportion of cell volume that contains myofilaments, organizational changes, and modification of the sarcomeres leads to improved contraction ability. Other changes that are indicative of maturation include a postnatal mitochondrial increase, which is most likely in response to metabolic changes in the muscle tissue. Initially there is a dramatic increase in the number of mitochondria; with further maturation the mitochondria become highly ordered in their arrangement. This occurs weeks after delivery. The arrangement facilitates energy transfer to the sarcomere during contraction.

Stroke volume and ventricular EDV increase with age. Stroke volume is 5 to10 ml (1.5 ml/kg) in the infant versus 70 to 90 ml in the adolescent. EDV is 40 ml/m² body surface area (BSA) in infants, increasing to 70 at 2 years of age. Cardiac output falls from 200 ml/kg in the infant to 100 ml/kg in the adolescent (versus 70 to 80 in the adult); absolute cardiac output increases from 0.6 L/min at birth to 6 L/min in adult.[96,146] Infants and young children, like neonates, increase cardiac output primarily by increasing heart rate rather than stroke volume.

Sinus arrhythmias are common in infants and children. The most common significant arrhythmia in children is bradycardia; ventricular tachycardia and ventricular fibrillation are more common in the adult.[96] As collagenous material increases among the fibers of the SA node, the frequency of insignificant arrhythmias decreases.

The cardiac index (cardiac output/m^2 BSA) is 3.5 to 4.5 L/min in the child (slightly higher than in an adult); low cardiac output is less than 2.1 to 2.5 L/min at any age. Right-axis deviation on the ECG is seen for the first few months. LV dominance appears by 3 to 6 months as the LV muscle mass increases, with a net reduction in RV mass. The right and LVs are of equal size by 6 to 10 months. By 7 years the LV is larger than the right, with the LV wall twice as thick as the RV wall (i.e., the adult relationship).[96,146]

Increased P-wave duration, RR interval, and QRS duration and magnitude are observed on the ECG until about 6 years of age. By this age the ECG is similar to that seen in older adolescents.[103]

PVR decreases to adult values by 6 to 8 weeks, and as soon as 3 weeks in some infants. Myocardial response to volume therapy is similar to the response of the adult. This means that the infant can increase stroke volume and cardiac output with fluid challenges or with a moderate increase in afterload. By 1 to 2 years, myocardial function is similar to that of adult.

The pulse rate decreases from birth to late adolescence, and the range of normal pulse becomes narrower. The heart rate ranges from 90 to 140 beats per minute in the toddler, 80 to 110 beats per minute in the preschool child, and 75 to 100 beats per minute in childhood. After about 10 years, heart rate varies by sex, with higher rates in females than in males. Smaller quantitative changes in vital signs may be qualitatively more significant in infants and children than in adults. Gender differences in pulse rate are evident after 10 years, with rates higher in females than in males.[96,148]

Blood pressure—systolic more than diastolic—rises with increasing age. Systolic blood pressure begins to rise after 4 weeks.[116] Increases in systolic blood pressure after puberty are related to changes in height and weight, with a greater change seen in males. Blood pressure levels plateau in females at 15 to 17 years and in males by 20 years.

The rapid growth in heart size between 9 and 16 years is associated with changes in weight and height. The heart reaches adult size by the end of adolescence. A marked increase in heart muscle is also seen with this growth spurt, along with increased length and thickness of blood vessels. These changes—along with the increase in blood pressure and SV and the decrease in HR—may result in the transient sensation of chest fullness or discomfort with palpitations in the adolescent.[146]

SUMMARY

To achieve extrauterine stability, the newborn undergoes significant alterations in cardiovascular status that convert it from a parallel system to an in-series system that must integrate with the respiratory system in order to maintain oxygenation. The complex development of the heart and cardiovascular system places the neonate at greater risk for alterations in normal development that can lead to postnatal compromise affecting multiple systems. Close assessments during the transitional period result in early identification and treatment of cardiovascular disease while promoting normal growth and development. Table 8-9 summarizes recommendations for clinical practice.

TABLE **8-9** **Recommendations for Clinical Practice Related to the Cardiovascular System in Neonates**

Monitor cardiovascular adaptation to extrauterine life (pp. 291-293).	Understand fetal responses to stress and their impact on the functioning of the cardiovascular system (pp. 290-291).
Assess and evaluate the neonate for changes in cardiovascular performance related to those changes (pp. 293-296).	Monitor infants with a patent ductus arteriosus for signs of increasing respiratory distress and congestive heart failure (pp. 298-299).
Conduct a thorough cardiovascular assessment of any infant presenting with a murmur during the transitional period, especially if associated with cyanosis (pp. 297-298).	Evaluate all preterm infants for signs of a patent ductus arteriosus on a serial basis (pp. 298-299).
Provide continuous physiologic monitoring for infants suspected of cardiac disease (pp. 297-302).	Monitor and evaluate infants at risk for persistent pulmonary hypertension (p. 298).
Develop an understanding of the embryonic mechanisms that may result in cardiac congenital anomalies (pp. 284, 299-302).	

REFERENCES

1. Adamson, S.L., et al. (1998). Regulation of umbilical blood flow. In R.A. Polin & W.W. Fox (Eds.). *Fetal and neonatal physiology* (2nd ed.). Philadelphia: W.B. Saunders.

2. Ahn, M.O. & Phelan, J.P. (1988). Multiple pregnancy: antepartum management. *Clin Perinatol, 15*, 55.

3. Alenick, D.S., et al. (1992). The neonatal transitional circulation: a combined noninvasive assessment. *Echocardiography, 9*, 29.

4. American College of Obstetricians and Gynecologists. (1991). Exercise during pregnancy and the postnatal period. In R.A. Mittelmark, R.A. Wiswell & B.L. Drinkwater (Eds.). *Exercise in pregnancy* (2nd ed.). Baltimore: Williams & Wilkins.

5. American College of Obstetricians and Gynecologists. (1994). *Exercise during pregnancy and the postpartum period* (technical bulletin no. 189). Washington, DC: American College of Obstetricians and Gynecologists.

6. Anderson, P.A.W., et al. (1987). In utero right ventricular output in the fetal lamb: The effect of heart rate. *J Physiol (Lond), 387*, 297.

7. Anderson, P.A.W. (1990). Myocardial development. In W.A. Long (Ed.). *Fetal and neonatal cardiology*. Philadelphia: W.B. Saunders.

8. Anderson, P.A.W., et al. (1998). Cardiovascular function during normal fetal and neonatal development and with hypoxic stress. In R.A. Polin & W.W. Fox (Eds.). *Fetal and neonatal physiology* (2nd ed.). Philadelphia: W.B. Saunders.

9. Anversa, P., et al. (1980). Morphometric study of early postnatal development in the left and right ventricular myocardium of the rat. I: Hypertrophy, hyperplasia, and binucleation of myocytes. *Circ Res, 46*, 495.

10. Arnold-Aldea, S.A. & Parer, J.T. (1990). Fetal cardiovascular physiology. In R.D. Eden & F.H. Boehm (Eds.). *Assessment and care of the fetus: Physiological, clinical, and medicolegal principles*. Norwalk, CT: Appleton & Lange.

11. Artal, R., et al. (1984). Fetal bradycardia induced by maternal exercise. *Lancet, 2*, 258.

12. Artal, R. & Wiswell, R. (1986). *Exercise in pregnancy*. Baltimore: Williams & Wilkins.

13. August, P. (1999). Hypertensive disorders in pregnancy. In G.N. Burrow & T.P. Duffy (Eds.). *Medical complications during pregnancy* (5th ed.). Philadelphia: W.B. Saunders.

14. Avila, W.S., et al. (1995). Maternal and fetal outcome in pregnant women with Eisenmenger's syndrome. *Eur Heart J, 16*, 460.

15. Bayliss, C., et al. (1996). Importance of nitric oxide in control of systemic and renal hemodynamics during normal pregnancy: studies on the rate and implications for preeclampsia. *Hypertens Pregnancy, 15*, 147.

16. Beck, F., et al. (1985). *Human embryology* (2nd ed.). Oxford: Blackwell/Year Book Medical Publishers.

17. Belloti, M., et al. (2000). Role of ductus venosus in distribution of umbilical flow in human fetuses during second half of pregnancy. *Am J Physiol, 279*, H1256.

18. Benedetti, T. J. (1990). Pregnancy-induced hypertension. In U. Elkayam & N. Gleicher (Eds.). *Cardiac problems in pregnancy*. New York: Alan R. Liss.

19. Bernheim, J. (1997). Hypertension in pregnancy. *Nephron, 76*, 254.

20. Black, S.M., et al. (1997). Ventilation and oxygenation induce endothelial nitric oxide synthetase gene expression in the lungs of fetal lambs. *J Clin Invest, 100*, 1448.

21. Bloom, R.S. (2002). Delivery room resuscitation of the newborn. In A.A. Fanaroff & R.J. Martin (Eds.). *Neonatal and perinatal medicine, diseases of the fetus and infant* (7th ed.). St. Louis: Mosby.

22. Boldt, T., et al. (1998). Birth stress increases adrenomedullin in the newborn. *Acta Paediatr, 87*, 93.

23. Bolte, A.C., et al. (2001). Pathophysiology of preeclampsia and the role of serotonin. *Eur J Obstet Gynecol Reprod Biol, 95*, 12.

24. Borg, T.K., et al. (1985). Connective tissue of the myocardium. In V.J. Ferrans, G. Rosenquist & C. Weinstein (Eds.). *Cardiac morphogenesis*. New York: Elsevier Science.

25. Brannon, T.S., et al. (1994). Prostacyclin synthetase in ovine pulmonary artery is developmentally regulated by changes in cyclooxygenase-1 gene expression. *J Clin Invest, 93*, 2230.

26. Britton, J.R. (1998). The transition to extrauterine life and disorders of transition. *Clin Perinatol, 25*, 271.

27. Brown, M.A. & Simpson, J.M. (1992). Diversity of blood pressure recording during pregnancy: implications for the hypertensive disorders. *Med J Aust, 156*, 306.

28. Brown, M.A., et al. (1998). Randomized trial of management of hypertensive pregnancies by Korotkoff phase IV or phase V. *Lancet, 352*, 777.

29. Brown, M.A., et al. (1999). The white coat effect in hypertensive pregnancy: much ado about nothing? *Br J Obstet Gynaecol, 106*, 474.

30. Campbell, W.A., et al. (1987). Maternal-fetal reproductive physiology and clinical management. In D.H. Riddick (Ed.). *Reproductive physiology in clinical practice*. New York: Thieme Medical.

31. Capeless, E.L. & Clapp, J.F. (1989). Cardiovascular changes in early phase of pregnancy. *Am J Obstet Gynecol, 161*, 1449.

32. Capeless, E.L. & Cape, J.F. (1989). Cardiovascular changes in early phase of pregnancy. *Am J Obstet Gynecol, 161*, 1440.

33. Capeless, E.L. & Cape, J.F. (1991). When do cardiovascular parameters return to their preconception values? Cardiovascular changes in early phase of pregnancy. *Am J Obstet Gynecol, 165*, 883.

34. Carbillon, L., et al. (2000). Pregnancy, vascular tone, and maternal hemodynamics: a crucial adaptation. *Obstet Gynecol Surv, 55*, 574.

35. Carlson, B.M. (1999). *Human embryology & developmental biology* (2nd ed.). St. Louis: Mosby.

36. Casella, E.S., et al. (1987). Developmental physiology of the cardiovascular system. In R.C. Rogers (Ed.). *Textbook of pediatric intensive care*. Baltimore: Williams & Wilkins.

37. Caulin-Glaser, T. & Setano, J.F. (1999). Pregnancy and cardiovascular disease. In G.N. Burrow & T.F. Ferris (Eds.). *Medical complications during pregnancy* (5th ed.). Philadelphia: W.B. Saunders.

38. Chescheir, N.C. & Seeds, J.W. (1990). Management of hydrops fetalis. In W.A. Long (Ed.). *Fetal and neonatal cardiology*. Philadelphia: W.B. Saunders.

39. Churchill, D. & Beevers, D.G. (1996). Differences between office and 24-hour ambulatory blood pressure measurement during pregnancy. *Obstet Gynecol, 88*, 455,

40. Churchill, D., et al. (1997). Ambulatory blood pressure in pregnancy and fetal growth. *Lancet, 349*, 10.

41. Clapp, J.F. (1985). Maternal heart rate in pregnancy. *Am J Obstet Gynecol, 152*, 659.

42. Clapp, J.F. (1985). Fetal heart rate response to running in midpregnancy and late pregnancy. *Am J Obstet Gynecol, 153*, 251.

43. Clapp, J.F. (1989). Oxygen consumption during treadmill exercise before, during and after pregnancy. *Am J Obstet Gynecol, 161*, 1458.

44. Clapp, J.F. (1991). Maternal exercise performance and early pregnancy outcome. In R.A. Mittelmark, R.A. Wiswell & B.L. Drinkwater (Eds.). *Exercise in pregnancy* (2nd ed.). Baltimore: Williams & Wilkins.

45. Clapp, J.F., et al. (1991). The VO_{2max} of recreational athletes before and after pregnancy. *Med Sci Sports Exercise, 23*, 1128.

46. Clapp. J.F. (1991). The changing thermal response to endurance exercise during pregnancy. *Am J Obstet Gynecol, 105*, 1684.

47. Clapp, J.F. & Little, K.D. (1995). The interaction between regular exercise and selected aspects of women's health. *Am J Obstet Gynecol, 173*, 2.

48. Clapp, J.F. (2000). Exercise during pregnancy. A clinical update. *Clin Sports Med, 19,* 273.

49. Clark, S.L. (1987). Structural cardiac disease in pregnancy. In S.L. Clark, J.P. Phelan & D.B. Cotton (Eds.). *Critical care obstetrics.* Oradell, NJ: Medical Economics Books.

50. Clark, S.L., et al. (1989). Central hemodynamic assessment of normal term pregnancy. *Am J Obstet Gynecol, 161,* 1439.

51. Clark, S., et al. (1989). Central hemodynamic assessment of normal term pregnancy. *Am J Obstet Gynecol, 161,* 1439.

52. CLASP (Collaborative Low-Dose Aspirin Study in Pregnancy) Collaborative Group. (1994). CLASP: A randomized trial of low-dose aspirin for the prevention and treatment of preeclampsia among 9364 women. *Lancet, 343,* 619.

53. Clyman, R.I., et al. (1996). Changes in endothelial cell and smooth muscle cell integrin expression during closure of the ductus arteriosus: an immunohistological comparison of the fetal, preterm newborn, and full term newborn rhesus monkey ductus. *Pediatr Res, 40,* 198.

54. Clyman, R.J. & Heymann, M.A. (1999). Fetal cardiovascular physiology. In R.K. Creasy & R. Resnik (Eds.). *Maternal-fetal medicine* (4th ed.). Philadelphia: W.B. Saunders.

55. Collings, C. & Curret, L. (1985). Fetal heart rate response to maternal exercise. *Am J Obstet Gynecol, 157,* 498.

56. Conrad, K.P. & Benyo, D.F. (1997). Placental cytokines and the pathogenesis of preeclampsia. *Am J Reprod Immunol, 37,* 240.

57. Cowles, T. & Gonik, B. (1990). Mitral valve prolapse in pregnancy. *Semin Perinatol, 14,* 34.

58. Cunningham, F.G & Whitridge, W.J. (1997). *Williams obstetrics* (20th ed.). Stamford, CT: Appleton & Lange.

59. Cutforth, R. & MacDonald, M.B. (1966). Heart sounds and murmurs in pregnancy. *Am Heart J, 71,* 741.

60. Dawes, G.S. (1968). *Foetal and neonatal physiology.* Chicago: Year Book Medical Publishers.

61. Dietl, J. (2000). The pathogenesis of pre-eclampsia: new aspects. *J Perinat Med, 28,* 464.

62. Driscoll, D. (1990). Evaluation of the cyanotic newborn. *Ped Clin N Am, 37,* 1.

63. Duffy, T.P. (1999). Hematologic aspects of pregnancy. In G.N. Burrows & T.P. Duffy (Eds.). *Medical complications during pregnancy* (5th ed.). Philadelphia: W.B. Saunders.

64. Duvekot, J.J., et al. (1993). Early pregnancy changes in hemodynamics and volume homeostasis are consecutive adjustments triggered by a primary fall in systemic vascular tone. *Am J Obstet Gynecol, 169,* 1382.

65. Duvekot, J.J. & Peeters, L.L.H. (1994). Maternal cardiovascular hemodynamic adaptation to pregnancy. *Obstet Gynecol Surv, 49,* 81.

66. Easterling, T.R., et al. (1988). The hemodynamic effects of orthostatic stress during pregnancy. *Obstet Gynecol, 72,* 550.

67. Easterling, T. R. & Benedetti, T. J. (1990). Measurement of cardiac output by impedance technique. *Am J Obstet Gynecol, 163,* 1104.

68. Easterling, T.R., et al. (1990). Maternal hemodynamics in normal and preeclamptic pregnancies: a longitudinal study. *Obstet Gynecol, 76,* 1061.

69. Easterling, T.B., et al. (1990). Maternal hemodynamics in normal and preeclamptic pregnancies: a longitudinal study. *Am J Obstet Gynecol, 76,* 1061.

70. Eliseev, O.M. (1988). *Cardiovascular diseases and pregnancy.* New York: Springer-Verlag.

71. Elkayam, U. & Gleicher, N. (1990). Hemodynamics, exercise and cardiac function during normal pregnancy and the puerperium. In U. Elkayam & N. Gleicher (Eds.). *Cardiac problems in pregnancy: diagnosis and management of maternal and fetal disease* (2nd ed.). New York: Alan R. Liss.

72. Fineman, J.R., et al. (1995). Regulation of pulmonary vascular tone in the perinatal period. *Annu Rev Physiol, 57,* 115.

73. Fisher, S.J. & Roberts, J.M. (1999). Defects in placentation and placental perfusion. In M.D. Linhheimer & J.M. Roberts (Eds.). *Chesley's hypertensive disorders in pregnancy* (2nd ed.). Stamford, CT: Appleton & Lange.

74. Friedman, A.H. & Fahey, J.T. (1993). The transition from fetal to neonatal circulation: normal responses and implications for infants with heart disease. *Semin Perinatol, 17,* 106.

75. Fugelseth, D., et al. (1997). Ultrasonographic study of ductus venosus in healthy neonates. *Arch Dis Child Fetal Neonatal Ed, 77,* F131.

76. Gaboury, C.L. & Woods, L.L. (1995). Renal reserve in pregnancy. *Semin Nephrol, 15,* 449.

77. Gant, N.F. & Worley, B.J. (1989). Measurement of uteroplacental blood flow in the human. In C.R. Rosenfeld (Ed.). *The uterine circulation.* Ithaca, NY: Perinatology Press.

78. Garovic, V.D. (2000). Hypertension in pregnancy: diagnosis and treatment. *Mayo Clin Proc, 75,* 1071.

79. Gei, A.F. & Hankins, G.D. (2001). Cardiac disease and pregnancy. *Obstet Gynecol Clin North Am, 28,* 465.

80. Geva, T., et al. (1997). Effects of physiologic load of pregnancy on left ventricular contractility and remodeling. *Am Heart J, 33,* 53.

81. Gibson, C.J., et al. (1997). Changes in hemodynamics, ventricular remodeling and ventricular contractility during normal pregnancy: a longitudinal study. *Obstet Gynecol, 89,* 957.

82. Gilson, G.J., et al. (1997). Changes in hemodynamics, vascular remodeling, and ventricular contractility during normal pregnancy: a longitudinal study. *Obstet Gynecol, 89,* 957.

83. Ginsburg, J. & Duncan, S.L.B. (1967). Peripheral blood flow in normal pregnancy. *Cardiovasc Res, 1,* 132.

84. Goldman-Wohl, D.S., et al. (2000). Lack of human leukocyte antigen-G expression in extravillous trophoblast is associated with preeclampsia. *Mol-Hum Reprod, 6,* 88.

85. Granger, J.P., et al. (2001). Pathophysiology of hypertension during preeclampsia linking placental ischemia with endothelial dysfunction. *Hypertension, 38,* 718.

86. Granger, J.P., et al. (2001). Pathophysiology of pregnancy-induced hypertension. *Am J Hypertens, 14,* 178S.

87. Grant, D.A. & Walker, A.M. (1996). Pleural and pericardial pressures limit fetal right ventricular output. *Circulation, 94,* 555.

88. Grant, D.A. (1999). Ventricular constraint in the fetus and newborn. *Can J Cardiol, 15,* 95.

89. Gulbert, L., et al. (1993). The trophoblast as a macrophage-cytokine network. *Immunol Cell Biol, 71,* 49.

90. Hale, R.W. & Milne, L. (1996). The elite athlete and exercise in pregnancy. *Semin Perinatol, 20,* 277.

91. Halligan, A., et al. (1993). Twenty-four hour ambulatory blood pressure measurement in a primigravida population. *J Hypertens, 11,* 869.

92. Hart, M.V., et al. (1986). Aortic function during normal human pregnancy. *Am J Obstet Gynecol, 154,* 887.

93. Hartmann, S. & Bung, P. (1999). Physical exercise during pregnancy—physiological considerations and recommendations. *J Perinat Med, 27,* 204.

94. Harvey, W.P. (1975). Alterations of the cardiac physical examination in normal pregnancy. *Clin Obstet Gynecol, 18,* 51.

95. Hauth, J.C., et al. (1993). Low dose aspirin therapy to prevent preeclampsia in women at high-risk. *Am J Obstet Gynecol, 168,* 1083.

96. Hazinski, M.F. & van Stralen, D. (1990). Physiologic and anatomic differences between children and adults. In D.L. Levin & F.C. Morriss (Eds.). *Essentials of pediatric intensive care.* St. Louis: Quality Medical Publications.

97. Hendricks, C.H. & Quilligan, E.F. (1956). Cardiac output during labor. *Am J Obstet Gynecol, 71*, 953.

98. Heyborne, K.D. (2000). Preeclampsia prevention: lessons from the low-dose aspirin therapy trials. *Am J Obstet Gynecol, 183*, 523.

99. Higgins, J.J., et al. (1997). Can 24-hour ambulatory blood pressure measurement predict the development of hypertension in primigravidae? *Br J Obstet Gynaecol, 104*, 356.

100. Higgins, J.R. & de Swiet, M. (2001). Blood-pressure measurement and classification in pregnancy. *Lancet, 357*, 131.

101. Hobel, C.J., et al. (1996). The effect of thigh-length support stockings on the hemodynamic response to ambulation in pregnancy. *Am J Obstet Gynecol, 174*, 1734.

102. Holmes, F.A. (1960). Incidence of the supine hypotensive syndrome in late pregnancy. A clinical study in 500 subjects. *J Obstet Gynaecol Br Emp, 67*, 254.

103. Hosier, D.M. (1978). Changes in the electrocardiogram with age. In T.R. Johnson, W.M. Moore, & J.E. Jeffries (Eds.). *Children are different.* Columbus, OH: Ross.

104. Hutchison, A.A. (1990). Pathophysiology of hydrops fetalis. In W.A. Long (Ed.). *Fetal and neonatal cardiology.* Philadelphia: W.B. Saunders.

105. Hytten, F.F. (1985). Blood volume changes in normal pregnancy. *Clin Haematol, 14*, 601.

106. Hytten, F.F. & Paintin, D.B. (1963). Increase in plasma volume during normal pregnancy. *J Obstet Gynaecol Br Comm, 70*, 402.

107. Hytten, F.F. & Leitch, I. (1971). *The physiology of human pregnancy* (2nd ed.). Oxford: Blackwell Scientific.

108. Hytten, F.E., et al. (1966). Total body water in normal pregnancy. *J Obstet Gynaecol Br Comm, 73*, 553.

109. Hytten, F.E. & Leitch, I. (1971). *The physiology of human pregnancy* (2nd ed.). Oxford: Blackwell Scientific Publications.

110. Imperiale, T.F. & Stollenwerk-Petrulus, A. (1991). A meta-analysis of low-dose aspirin for the prevention of pregnancy induced hypertensive disease. *JAMA, 226*, 261.

111. Institute of Medicine. (1990). *Nutrition during pregnancy.* Washington, DC: National Academy Press.

112. Iwamoto, H.S. (1998). Endocrine regulation of the fetal circulation. In R.A. Polin & W.W. Fox (Eds.). *Fetal and neonatal physiology* (2nd ed.). Philadelphia: W.B. Saunders.

113. Jackson, M.R., et al. (1995). The effects of maternal aerobic exercise on human placental development: placental volumetric composition and surface area. *Placenta, 16*, 179.

114. Jensen, A., et al. (1999) Dynamics of fetal circulatory responses to hypoxia and asphyxia. *Eur J Obstet Gynecol Reprod Biol, 84*, 155.

115. Jibodu, O.A. & Arulkumaran, S. (2000). Intrapartum fetal surveillance. *Curr Opin Obstet Gynecol, 12*, 123.

116. Johnson, T.R. (1978). Changes in the developing cardiovascular system in relation to age. In T.R. Johnson, W.M. Moore, & J.E. Jeffries (Eds). *Children are different.* Columbus, OH: Ross.

117. Jonas, R.A. (1998). Myocardial protection for neonates and infants. *Thoracic Cardiovasc Surg, 46*, 288.

118. Kafer, E.R. (1990). Neonatal gas exchange and oxygen transport. In W.A. Long (Ed.). *Fetal and neonatal cardiology.* Philadelphia: W.B. Saunders.

119. Kam, E.P., et al. (1999). The role of trophoblast in the physiological change in decidual spiral arteries. *Hum Reprod, 14*, 2131.

120. Katz, M., et al. (1990). *Fetal well-being: Physiological basis and methods of clinical assessment.* Boston: CRC Press.

121. Katz, R., et al. (1978). Effects of a natural volume overload state (pregnancy) on left ventricular performance in normal human subjects. *Circulation, 58*, 434.

122. Katz, M. & Sokal, M.M. (1980). Skin perfusion in pregnancy. *Am J Obstet Gynecol, 137*, 30.

123. Kenny, L. & Baker, P.N. (1999). Maternal pathophysiology in preeclampsia. *Baillieres Best Pract Res Clin Obstet Gynaecol, 13*, 59.

124. Kerr, M.G., et al. (1964). Studies of the inferior vena cava in late pregnancy. *Br Med J, 1*, 532.

125. Kerr, M.G. (1965). The mechanical effects of the gravid uterus in late pregnancy. *J Obstet Gynaecol Br Comm, 72*, 513.

126. Kilpatrick, S.J. & Laros, R.K. (1999). Maternal hematologic disorders. In R.K Creasy & R. Resnik (Eds.). *Maternal-fetal medicine* (4th ed.). Philadelphia: W.B. Saunders.

127. Kiserud, T. (2000). Fetal venous circulation—an update on hemodynamics. *J Perinat Med, 28*, 90.

128. Kiserud, T., et al. (2000). Blood flow and degree of shunting through the ductus venosus in the human fetus. *Am J Obstet Gynecol, 183*, 147.

129. Kiserud, T. (2001). The ductus venosus. *Semin Perinatol, 25*, 11.

130. Kjeldsen, J. (1979). Hemodynamic investigations during labor and delivery. *Acta Obstet Gynecol Scand, 89*(suppl), 1.

131. Kleinman, C.S., et al. (1999). Fetal cardiac arrythmias. In R.K. Creasy & R. Resnik (Eds.). *Maternal-fetal medicine* (4th ed.). Philadelphia: W.B. Saunders

132. Kluckow, M. & Evans, N. (2001). Low systemic blood flow in the preterm infant. *Semin Neonatol, 6*, 75.

133. Kolkot, F. (1997). Starvation in the midst of plenty—the problems of volemia in pregnancy and pre-eclampsia. *Nephrol Dial Transplant, 12*, 388.

134. Kramer, M.S. (2000). Regular aerobic exercise during pregnancy. *Cochrane Database Syst Rev 2000, 2*, CD000180.

135. Lakshminrushimha, S. & Steinharn, R.H. (1999). Pulmonary vascular biology during neonatal transition. *Clin Perinatol, 26*, 601.

136. Lee, L.A., et al. (1992). Left ventricular mechanics in the preterm infant and their effect on the measurement of cardiac performance. *J Pediatr, 120*, 114.

137. Lee, W. & Cotton, D.B. (1987). Cardiorespiratory changes during pregnancy. In S.L. Clark, J.P. Phelan & D.B. Cotton (Eds.). *Critical care obstetrics.* Oradell, NJ: Medical Economics Books.

138. Lee, W. & Cotton, D.B. (1990). Maternal cardiovascular physiology. In R.D. Eden and F.H. Boehm (Eds.). *Assessment and care of the fetus: Physiological, clinical, and medicolegal principles.* Norwalk, CT: Appleton & Lange.

139. Lindheimer, M.D. & Katz, A.I. (1985). Hypertension in pregnancy. *N Engl J Med, 313*, 675.

140. Livingston, J.C. & Sibai, B.M. (2001). Chronic hypertension in pregnancy. *Obstet Gynecol Clin North Am, 28*, 447.

141. Loberant, N., et al. (1999). Closure of the ductus venosus in premature infants: findings on real-time gray-scale, color-flow Doppler, and Doppler sonography. *Am J Roentgenol, 172*, 227.

142. Lockitch, G. (1997). Clinical biochemistry of pregnancy. *Crit Rev Clin Lab Sci, 34*, 67.

143. Long, W.A., et al. (1998). Autonomic and central neuroregulation of fetal cardiovascular function. In R.A. Polin & W.W. Fox (Eds,), *Fetal and neonatal physiology* (2nd ed.). Philadelphia: W.B. Saunders.

144. Lotgering, F.K. & Wallenburg, H.C.S. (1986). Hemodynamic effects of caval and uterine venous occlusion in pregnant sheep. *Am J Obstet Gynecol, 155*, 1164.

145. Lotgering, F.R., et al. (1991). Maximal aerobic exercise in pregnant women: heart rate, O_2 consumption, CO_2 production, and ventilation. *J Appl Physiol, 70*, 1016.

146. Lowrey, G.H. (1986). *Growth and development of children.* Chicago: Year Book Medical Publishers.

147. Mabie, W.C., et al. (1994). A longitudinal study of cardiac output in normal human pregnancy. *Am J Obstet Gynecol, 170,* 849.

148. Manga, M. (1999). Maternal cardiovascular and renal adaptations to pregnancy. In R.K. Creasy & R. Resnik (Eds.). *Maternal-fetal medicine* (2nd ed.). Philadelphia: W.B. Saunders.

149. Marsal, K. (1998). Fetal and placental circulation during labor. In R.A. Polin & W.W. Fox (Eds,), *Fetal and neonatal physiology* (2nd ed.). Philadelphia: W.B. Saunders.

150. Martin, R. J., et al. (2001). Respiratory problems. In M.H. Klaus & A. A. Fanaroff (Eds.). *Care of high-risk neonate.* Philadelphia: W.B. Saunders.

151. McAnulty, J.H. (1994). Anesthesia during pregnancy in the patient with heart disease. In J.J. Bonica & J.S. McDonald (Eds.). *Principles and practice of obstetric analgesia and anesthesia.* Philadelphia: Lea & Febiger.

152. McAnulty, J.H., et al. (1995). Cardiovascular disease. In G.N. Burrow & T.F. Ferris (Eds.). *Medical complications during pregnancy* (4th ed.). Philadelphia: W.B. Saunders.

153. Meekins, J.W., et al. (1994). A study of placental bed spiral arteries and trophoblast invasion in normal and severe preclamptic pregnancies. *Br J Obstet Gynaecol, 101,* 669.

154. Mendelson, M.A. (1997). Congenital cardiac disease and pregnancy. *Clin Perinatol, 24,* 467.

155. Mesa, A., et al. (1999). Left ventricular diastolic function in normal human pregnancy. *Circulation, 99,* 511.

156. Metcalfe, J. & Ueland, K. (1974). Maternal cardiovascular adjustments to pregnancy. *Prog Cardiovasc Dis, 16,* 363.

157. Mills, J.L., et al. (1999). Prostacyclin and thromboxane changes predating clinical onset of preeclampsia: a multicenter prospective study. *JAMA, 282,* 356.

158. Mittelmark, R.A. & Posner, M.D. (1991). Fetal responses to maternal exercise. In R.A. Mittelmark, R.A. Wiswell & B.L. Drinkwater (Eds.). *Exercise in pregnancy,* (2nd ed.). Baltimore: Williams & Wilkins.

159. Moore, K.L. & Persaud, T.V.N. (1998). *The developing human: clinically oriented embryology* (6th ed.). Philadelphia: W.B. Saunders.

160. Morin, F.C., et al. (1992). Pulmonary hemodynamics in fetal lambs during development at normal and increased oxygen tension. *J Appl Physiol, 73,* 213.

161. Morin, F.C., et al. (1995). Persistent pulmonary hypertension of the neonate. *Am J Respir Crti Care Med, 151,* 2010.

162. Morris, N.H., et al. (1995). Nitric oxide synthetase activities in placental tissue from normotensive, preeclamptic, and growth retarded pregnancies, *Br J Obstet Gynaecol, 102,* 711.

163. Morton, M.J. (1991). Maternal hemodynamics in pregnancy. In R.A. Mittelmark, R.A. Wiswell & B.L. Drinkwater (Eds.). *Exercise in pregnancy* (2nd ed.). Baltimore: Williams & Wilkins.

164. Morton, M., et al. (1984). Left ventricular size, output, and structure during guinea pig pregnancy. *Am J Physiol, 246,* R40.

165. Morton, M., et al. (1987). In utero ventilation with oxygen augments left ventricular stroke volume in lambs. *J Physiol (Lond), 383,* 413.

166. National High Blood Pressure Education Program. (2000). Report of the national high blood pressure education program working group on high blood pressure in pregnancy. *Am J Obstet Gynecol, 183,* 1.

167. Parer, J.T. (1999). Fetal heart rate. In R.K. Creasy & R. Resnik (Eds.). *Maternal-fetal medicine* (4th ed.). Philadelphia: W.B. Saunders.

168. Parsons, M. (1988). Effects of twins: Maternal, fetal, and labor. *Clin Perinatol, 15,* 41.

169. Patel, C.R., et al. (2002). Fetal cardiac physiology and fetal cardiovascular assessment. In A.A. Fanaroff & R.J. Martin (Eds.). *Neonatal and perinatal medicine, diseases of the fetus and infant* (7th ed.). St. Louis: Mosby.

170. Peeters, L.L.H., et al. (1979). Blood flow to fetal organs as a function of actual oxygen content. *Am J Obstet Gynecol, 135,* 637.

171. Perry, I.J., et al. (1991). Conflicting views on the measurement of blood pressure in pregnancy. *Br J Obstet Gynaecol, 98,* 241.

172. Pivarnik, J.M. (1996). Cardiovascular responses to aerobic exercise during pregnancy and postpartum. *Semin Perinatol, 20,* 242.

173. Poston, L. (1997). The control of blood flow to the placenta. *Exp Physiol, 82,* 377.

174. Poulta, A.M., et al. (1996). Changes in maternal heart dimensions and plasma atrial natriuretic peptide levels in the early puerperium of normal and pre-eclamptic pregnancies. *Br J Obstet Gynaecol, 103,* 988.

175. Pritchard, J.A., et al. (1972). Blood volume changes in pregnancy and the puerperium. II. Red blood cell loss and changes in apparent blood volume during and following vaginal delivery, cesarean section, and cesarean section plus total hysterectomy. *Am J Obstet Gynecol, 84,* 1271.

176. Pritchard, J.A. & Rowland, R.C. (1964). Blood volume changes in pregnancy and the puerperium. III. Whole body and large vessel hematocrits in pregnant and non-pregnant women. *Am J Obstet Gynecol, 88,* 391.

177. Pritchard, J. (1965). Changes in blood volume during pregnancy and delivery. *Anesthesiology, 26,* 393.

178. Pyeritz, R.E. & McKusick, V.A. (1979). The Marfan's syndrome: diagnosis and management. *N Engl J Med, 300,* 772.

179. Quilligan, E.J. & Tyler, C. (1978). Postural effects on the cardiovascular status in pregnancy. *Am J Obstet Gynecol, 130,* 194.

180. Rabinovitch, M. (1998). Developmental biology of the pulmonary vasculature. In R.A. Polin & W.W. Fox (Eds.). *Fetal and neonatal physiology* (2nd ed.). Philadelphia: W.B. Saunders.

181. Ramsey, P.S., et al. (2001). Cardiac disease in pregnancy. *Am J Perinatol, 18,* 245.

182. Rasanen, J., et al. (1996). Role of the pulmonary circulation in the distribution of human fetal cardiac output during the second half of pregnancy. *Circulation, 94,* 1068.

183. Rayburn, W.F., et al. (1987). Mitral valve prolapse: echocardiographic changes during pregnancy. *J Reprod Med, 32,* 185.

184. Redman, C.W. & Sargent, I.L. (2001). The pathogenesis of preeclampsia. *Gynecol Obstet Fertil, 29,* 518.

185. Resnik, R. (1999). The puerperium. In R.K. Creasy. & R. Resnik (Eds.). *Maternal-fetal medicine* (4th ed.). Philadelphia: W.B. Saunders.

186. Richardson, B.S. (1989). Fetal adaptive responses to asphyxia. *Clin Perinatol, 16,* 595.

187. Richter, C., et al. (1995). Erythropoiesis in the perinatal postpartum period. *J Perinatal Med, 23,* 51.

188. Riemann, M.K., et al (2000). Effects on the foetus of exercise in pregnancy. *Scand J Med Sci Sports, 10,* 12.

189. Roberts, J.M & Cooper, D.W. (2001). Pathogenesis and genetics of pre-eclampsia. *Lancet, 357,* 53.

190. Roberts, J.M. & Redman, C.W. (1993). Pre-eclampsia: more than pregnancy-induced hypertension. *Lancet, 341,* 1447.

191. Roberts, J.M. (1999). Pregnancy-related hypertension. In R.K. Creasy & R. Resnik (Eds.). *Maternal-fetal medicine* (4th ed.). Philadelphia: W.B. Saunders.

192. Roberts, J.M. (2000). Preeclampsia: what we know and what we do not know. *Semin Perinatol, 24,* 24.

193. Roberts, S.C., et al. (1989). Hemodynamic changes in the puerperium: a Doppler and M-mode echocardiographic study. *Br J Obstet Gynaecol, 94,* 1028.

194. Robson, S.C., et al. (1989). Serial study of factors influencing changes in cardiac output during human pregnancy. *Am J Physiol, 256,* H1060.

195. Robson, S.C., et al. (1989). Haemodynamic changes associated with caesarean section under epidural anaesthesia. *Br J of Obstet Gynaecol, 96,* 642.

196. Romen, Y., et al. (1991). Physiological and endocrine adjustments to pregnancy. In R.A. Mittelmark, R.A. Wiswell & B.L. Drinkwater (Eds.). *Exercise in Pregnancy* (2nd ed.). Baltimore: Williams & Wilkins.

197. Romero, T.E. & Friedman, W.F. (1979). Limited left ventricular response to volume overload in the neonatal period: A comparative study with the adult animal. *Pediatr Res, 13,* 910.

198. Rosen, K.G. (2001). Fetal electrocardiogram waveform analysis in labour. *Curr Opin Obstet Gynecol, 13,* 137.

199. Rovinsky, J.J. & Jaffin, H. (1965). Cardiovascular hemodynamics in pregnancy. I: Blood and plasma volumes in multiple pregnancy. *Am J Obstet Gynecol, 93,* 1.

200. Rubler, S., et al. (1977). Cardiac size and performance during pregnancy estimated with echocardiography. *Clin Obstet Gynecol, 40,* 534.

201. Rudolph, A.M., et al. (1988). Fetal cardiovascular responses to stress. In G.H. Wiknjosastro, W.H. Prakoso, & K. Maeda (Eds.). *Perinatology.* New York: Elsevier Science.

202. Rudolph, A.M. (1998). Adrenomedullin: its role in perinatal adaptation. *Acta Paediatr, 87,* 235.

203. Rudolph, A.M. (1991). Fetal circulation and cardiovascular adjustments after birth. In A.M. Rudolph & J.I.E. Hollman (Eds.). *Rudolph's pediatrics* (19th ed.). Norwalk, CT: Appleton & Lange.

204. Rudolph, A.M. (2000). Myocardial growth before and after birth: clinical implication. *Acta Paediatr, 89,* 129.

205. Sadaniantz, A., et al. (1996). Long term effects of multiple pregnancy on cardiac dimensions and systolic and diastolic function. *Am J Obstet Gynecol, 174,* 1061.

206. Salas, S.P. (1999). What causes pre-eclampsia? *Baillieres Clin Obstet Gynecol, 13,* 41.

207. Sansoucie, D.A. & Cavaliere, T.A. (1997). Transition from fetal to extrauterine circulation. *Neonatal Netw, 16,* 5.

208. Shabetal, R. (1999). Cardiac disease. In R.K. Creasy & R. Resnik (Eds.). *Maternal-fetal medicine* (4th ed.). Philadelphia: W.B. Saunders.

209. Shah, D.M. (2002). Hypertensive disorder of pregnancy. In A.A. Fanaroff & R.J. Martin (Eds.). *Neonatal and perinatal medicine, diseases of the fetus and infant* (7th ed.). St. Louis: Mosby.

210. Shennan, A., et al. (1996). Lack of reproducibility in pregnancy of Korotkoff phase IV as measured by mercury sphygmomanometry. *Lancet, 347,* 139.

211. Sibai, B.M., et al. (1993). Prevention of pre-eclampsia with low-dose aspirin in healthy nulliparous women. *N Engl J Med, 329,* 1213

212. Sibai, B.M. & Frangieh, A. (1995). Maternal adaptation to pregnancy. *Curr Opin Obstet Gynecol, 7,* 420.

213. Sibai, B.M. & Frangieh, A. (1995). Maternal adaptation in pregnancy. *Curr Opin Obstet Gynecol, 7,* 420.

214. Silver, H.M. (1989). Acute hypertensive crisis in pregnancy. *Med Clin North Am, 73,* 623.

215. Simpson, P. (1985). Stimulation of hypertrophy of cultured neonatal rat heart cells through an α_1-adrenergic receptor and induction of beating through an α_1- and β_1-adrenergic receptor interaction: evidence for independent regulation of growth and beating. *Circ Res, 56,* 884.

216. Sladek, S.M., et al. (1997). Nitric oxide and pregnancy. *Am J Physiol, 272,* R441.

217. Sorenson, K. & Borlum, K. (1986). Fetal heart function in response to short-term maternal exercise. *Br J Obstet Gynaecol, 93,* 310.

218. Sosa, M.E.B. (1999), Nonimmune hydrops fetalis. *J Perinat Neonat Nurs, 12*(3), 33.

219. Soultanakis, H.N., et al. (1996). Prolonged exercise in pregnancy glucose homeostasis, ventilatory and cardiovascular responses. *Semin Perinatol, 20,* 315.

220. Stopfkuchen, H. (1987). Changes of the cardiovascular system during the perinatal period. *Eur J Pediatr, 146,* 545.

221. Sullivan, J.M. & Ramanathan, K.B. (1985). Management of medical problems in pregnancy-severe cardiac disease. *N Engl J Med, 313,* 304.

222. Szekely, P., et al. (1973). Pregnancy and the changing pattern of rheumatic heart disease. *Br Heart J, 35,* 1293.

223. Takahashi, Y., et al. (1996). Changes in left ventricular volume and systolic function before and after the closure of ductus arteriosus in full-term infants. *Early Hum Dev, 44,* 77.

224. Tanel, R.E. & Rhodes, L.A. (2001). Fetal and neonatal arrhythmias. *Clin Perinatol, 28,* 187.

225. Taylor, R.N. & Roberts, J.M. (1999). Endothelial cell dysfunction. In M.D. Linhheimer & J.M. Roberts (Eds.). *Chesley's hypertensive disorders in pregnancy* (2nd ed.). Stamford, CT: Appleton & Lange.

226. Thornburg, K.L. & Morton, M.J. (1983). Filling and arterial pressures as determinants of RV stroke volume in the sheep fetus. *Am J Physiol, 244,* H656.

227. Thornburg, K.L., et al. (2000). Hemodynamic changes in pregnancy. *Semin Perinatol, 24,* 11.

228. Teitel, D.F. (1998). Physiologic development of the cardiovascular system in the fetus. In R.A. Polin & W.W. Fox (Eds.). *Fetal and neonatal physiology* (2nd ed.). Philadelphia: W.B. Saunders.

229. Towbin, J.A. & Belmont, J. (2000). Molecular determinants of left and right outflow tract obstruction. *Am J Med Genet, 97,* 297.

230. Tropin, L.S., et al. (1996). Change in paternity: a risk factor for preeclampsia in multiparas. *Epidemiology, 7,* 240.

231. Ueland, K., et al. (1968). Maternal cardiovascular dynamics. I. Cesarean section under subarachnoid block anesthesia. *Am J Obstet Gynecol, 100,* 42.

232. Ueland, K. & Hansen, J.M. (1969). Maternal cardiovascular dynamics. II. Posture and uterine contractions. *Am J Obstet Gynecol, 103,* 1.

233. Ueland, K., et al. (1969). Maternal cardiovascular dynamics. IV: The influence of gestational age on maternal cardiovascular response to posture and exercise. *Am J Obstet Gynecol, 104,* 856.

234. Ueland, K. & Hansen, J.M. (1969). Maternal cardiovascular dynamics. III: Labor and delivery under local and caudal analgesia. *Am J Obstet Gynecol, 103,* 8.

235. Ueland, K., et al. (1972). Maternal cardiovascular dynamics. VI: Cesarean section under epidural anesthesia without epinephrine. *Am J Obstet Gynecol, 114,* 775.

236. Ueland, K. & Metcalfe, J. (1975). Circulatory changes in pregnancy. *Clin Obstet Gynecol, 18,* 41.

237. Ueland, K. (1976). Maternal cardiovascular dynamics. VII: Intrapartum blood volume changes. *Am J Obstet Gynecol, 126,* 671.

238. Van Engelen, A.D., et al. (1994). Management outcome and follow-up of fetal tachycardia. *J Am Coll Cardiol, 24,* 1371.

239. VanWijk, M.J. (2000). Vascular function in preeclampsia. *Cardiovasc Res, 47,* 38.

240. Veille, J-C. (1996). Maternal and fetal cardiovascular response to exercise during pregnancy. *Semin Perinatol, 20,* 250.

241. Verhaar, M.C. & Rabelink, T.J. (2001). The endothelium: a gynecological and obstetric point of view. *Eur J Obstet Gynecol Reprod Biol, 94,* 180.

242. Villablanca, A.C. (1998). Heart disease during pregnancy. Which cardiovascular changes reflect disease? *Postgrad Med, 104,* 149.

243. Villablanca, A.C. (1998). Heart disease during pregnancy. Which cardiovascular changes are normal or transient? *Postgrad Med, 104,* 183.

244. Vorys, N., et al. (1961). The cardiac output changes in various positions in pregnancy. *Am J Obstet Gynecol, 82,* 1312.

245. Wagner, P.D. (1977). Recent advances in pulmonary gas exchange. *Int Anesthesiol Clin, 15,* 81.

246. Walker, J.J. (2000). Pre-eclampsia. *Lancet, 356,* 1260.

247. Walker, S.P., et al. (1999). The diastolic debate: is it time to discard Korotkoff phase IV in favor of phase V for blood pressure measurements in pregnancy? *Med J Aust, 169,* 203.

248. Walsh, S. (1988). Cardiovascular disease in pregnancy: a nursing approach. *J Cardiovasc Nurs, 2,* 53.

249. Walsh, S.W. (1990). Physiology of low dose aspirin therapy for the prevention of preeclampsia. *Semin Perinatol, 14,* 152.

250. Wang, Y., et al. (1992). Placenta lipid peroxidases and thromboxane are increased and prostacyclin is decreased in women with preeclampsia. *Am J Obstet Gynecol, 167,* 946.

251. Watson, M.J. (1991). Fetal responses to maternal swimming and cycling exercise during pregnancy. *Obstet Gynecol, 77,* 382.

252. Wenstrom, K.D. & Gall, S.A. (1988). Incidence, morbidity and mortality, and diagnosis of twin gestations. *Clin Perinatol, 15,* 1.

253. Wilson, M., et al. (1980). Blood pressure, the renin-aldosterone system, and sex steroids throughout normal pregnancy. *Am J Med, 68,* 97.

254. Winberg, P. (1998). In search of the keys to the neonatal pulmonary vascular bed. *Acta Paediatr, 87,* 357.

255. Wolfson, R.N., et al. (1982). Autonomic Control of Fetal Cardiac Activity. In U. Elkayam & N. Gleicher (Eds.). *Cardiac problems in pregnancy: diagnosis and management of maternal and fetal disease.* New York: Alan R. Liss.

256. Yeh, T.F., et al. (1984). Increased O_2 consumption and energy loss in premature infants following medical care procedures. *Biol Neonate, 46,* 157.

257. Zahka, K.G. (2002). Principles of neonatal cardiovascular hemodynamics. In A.A. Fanaroff & R.J. Martin (Eds.). *Neonatal and perinatal medicine, diseases of the fetus and infant* (7th ed.). St. Louis: Mosby.

258. Zahka, K.G. & Lane, J.R. (2002). Approach to the neonate with cardiovascular disease. In A.A. Fanaroff & R.J. Martin (Eds.). *Neonatal and perinatal medicine, diseases of the fetus and infant* (7th ed.). St. Louis: Mosby.

259. Zahka, K.G., et al. (2002). Congenital heart defects. In A.A. Fanaroff & R.J. Martin (Eds.). *Neonatal and perinatal medicine, diseases of the fetus and infant* (7th ed.). St. Louis: Mosby.

260. Zahka, K.G. (2002). Causes and associations. In A.A. Fanaroff & R.J. Martin (Eds.). *Neonatal and perinatal medicine, diseases of the fetus and infant* (7th ed.). St. Louis: Mosby.

261. Ziegler, J.W., et al. (1995). The role of nitric oxide, endothelin, and prostaglandins in the transition of the pulmonary circulation. *Clin Perinatol, 22,* 387.

CHAPTER 9

Respiratory System

Respiration is the totality of those processes that ultimately result in energy being supplied to the cells. In pregnancy the respiratory system undergoes significant changes. The increased metabolic needs of the pregnant woman, fetus, and placenta require increased maternal respiratory efficiency to ensure adequate oxygenation. The placenta functions as the respiratory system for the fetus, providing nutrients and oxygen and removing carbon dioxide. This makes the relationship between the mother and fetus not only intimate but also interdependent. At birth, tremendous energy is expended by the neonate to generate sufficient negative pressure to convert to an air-liquid interface in the alveoli and maintain functional residual capacity (FRC). Transitional events continue over the first week of life as the neonate adjusts to the new environment, more alveoli are recruited, and the surfactant system stabilizes. This chapter examines alterations in the respiratory system and acid-base homeostasis during the perinatal period and their implications for the mother, fetus, and neonate.

MATERNAL PHYSIOLOGIC ADAPTATIONS

Changes in the respiratory system during pregnancy are mediated by hormonal and biochemical changes as well as by the enlarging uterus. As the muscles and cartilage in the thoracic region relax, the chest broadens and tidal volume (V_T) is improved with a conversion from abdominal to thoracic breathing. This leads to a 50% increase in air volume per minute. These changes result in a mild respiratory alkalosis. For the fetus, this mild alkalosis is essential for the exchange of gases across the placenta.[256]

Antepartum Period

Pregnancy is associated with major changes in the respiratory system in lung volumes and ventilation. Both biochemical and mechanical factors interact to increase the delivery of oxygen and the removal of carbon dioxide.

Factors Influencing Respiratory Function

Mechanical factors. The gradual enlargement of the uterus leads to changes in abdominal size and shape, shifting the resting position of the diaphragm up to 4 cm above its usual position. The transverse diameter of the chest increases about 2 cm in response to the increased intraabdominal pressure, and a flaring of the lower ribs occurs. The subcostal angle progressively increases from 68 to 103 degrees in late gestation. Not all of these changes can be attributed to intraabdominal pressure, since the increase in the subcostal angle occurs before the increasing mechanical pressure.[14,48,63,249,257] Relaxation of the ligamentous rib attachments increases rib cage elasticity. This change is similar to those seen in the pelvis and mediated by similar factors, especially relaxin (see Chapter 14).[214]

Although the aforementioned changes suggest that diaphragmatic motion decreases, the reverse is actually true. Several studies indicate that diaphragmatic movement actually increases during pregnancy, with the major work of breathing being accomplished by the diaphragm rather than by the costal muscles.[24,256] These changes in thoracic structures modify the abdominal space. This modification may be in preparation for the increase in uterine size. The changes in thoracic configuration have a major impact on lung volumes, however, to which the increasing intraabdominal pressure contributes.

Biochemical factors. Hormones and other biochemical factors are important in stimulating changes in the respiratory system in pregnancy. These substances can act centrally via stimulation of the respiratory center or directly on smooth muscle and other tissues of the lung. The most important influences are mediated by progesterone and prostaglandins (PGs).

Serum progesterone levels increase progressively throughout pregnancy and are thought to be a major factor in the changes seen in ventilation.[257] Progesterone is a respiratory stimulant. The administration of progesterone to normal subjects increases minute ventilation and enhances

310

responses to hypercapnia.[249] This suggests that there is an increased sensitivity to carbon dioxide by the respiratory center and that progesterone lowers the carbon dioxide threshold of the respiratory center.[171,257] This increased sensitivity most likely contributes to the sensation of dyspnea that is experienced by a large percentage of pregnant women and may also lead to some of the hyperventilation that occurs during the second stage of labor after pushing efforts (as carbon dioxide levels increase during breath holding).[249] Conversely, postmenopausal women and women with amenorrhea have lower resting ventilation.[63] Progesterone may also exert a local effect on the lung, causing water retention in the lung that results in decreased diffusion capacity. Therefore hyperventilation is an attempt to maintain normal PO_2 levels.[63,87,103,114,155]

Progesterone may also play a role in decreasing airway resistance (up to 50%), thereby reducing the work of breathing and facilitating a greater airflow in pregnancy. Relaxation of bronchiole smooth muscle has been attributed to progesterone. This counteracts the expected increase in airway resistance that would be the result of lungs that are less distended.[88]

PGs may also play a role in ventilatory changes by affecting the smooth muscle tissue of the bronchial airways. $PGF_{2\alpha}$ is a bronchial smooth muscle constrictor, whereas PGE_1 and PGE_2 have bronchodilatory effects.[102,114] PGs may balance or counteract some of the results of the structural changes in the respiratory system during pregnancy (e.g., decreased lung distention as a result of elevated diaphragm) and modify respiration to meet fetal requirements (maternal respiratory alkalosis promotes carbon dioxide transfer from the fetus).

Lung Volume

Changes in lung volumes begin in the middle of the second trimester and are progressive to term (Figure 9-1).[260] The most significant change is a 25% to 40% increase in V_T, with a progressive decrease in expiratory reserve volume (ERV), residual volume (RV), and FRC. Along with the change in V_T, there is a concomitant increase in inspiratory capacity (IC), thereby allowing the total lung capacity (TLC) to remain relatively stable. Vital capacity (VC) and inspiratory reserve volume (IRV) are essentially unaltered, although some literature notes a small change in IRV.[48,63,194,249,257] Figure 9-2 summarizes static lung volumes during normal pregnancy and the postpartum period.

The decreased RV, in conjunction with an elevated metabolic rate, increases the risk of hypoxia if respiratory depression occurs.[257] On the other hand, forced expiratory volume in 1 second (FEV_1) does not change nor does the FEV_1/VC ratio.[3,249,257] These assessments are

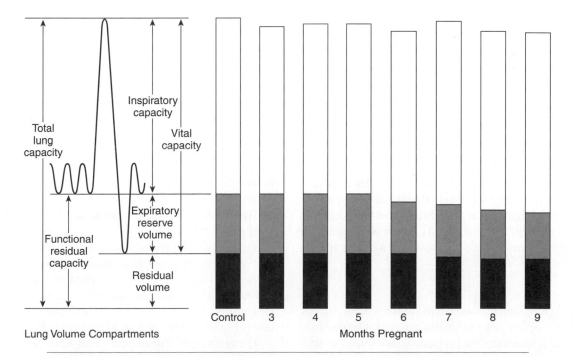

FIGURE **9-1** Changes in lung volumes with pregnancy. (From Bonica, J.J. [1967]. *Principles and practice of obstetric analgesia and anesthesia*. Philadelphia: F.A. Davis.)

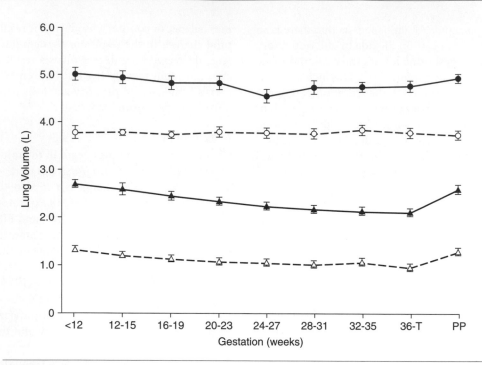

FIGURE **9-2** Serial values of static lung volume during normal pregnancy and postpartum *(PP)*. Values are mean ± SEM. *Solid circles,* Total lung capacity; *open circles,* vital capacity; *solid triangles,* functional residual capacity; *open triangles,* residual volume. (From Milne, J. [1979]. The respiratory response to pregnancy. *Postgrad Med J, 55,* 316.)

used in individuals with asthma, and therefore can still be used reliably in pregnant women.[249,257]

Changes in lung volumes result from the elevation of the diaphragm and the changes in the configuration of the chest. The alteration in RV is also the result of a 35% to 40% decrease in chest wall compliance; lung compliance is unchanged.[43,249] The decreased chest wall compliance is caused by hormonal influences as well as changes in abdominal pressure.[40] This reduction in compliance allows for more inward movement of the chest wall and reduces the amount of trapped air (residual trapped volume) that contributes to the RV. Therefore the RV decreases 200 to 300 ml. This, along with an approximately 200 ml decrease in ERV, brings the total deficit in the FRC to 500 ml (see Figure 9-1). There is a progressive drop in FRC from 20 weeks' gestation for a change of 10% to 24% by term.[249,257]

Lung Function

Changes in lung function are related to three major factors: ventilation, airflow, and diffusing capacity. Oxygen consumption increases during pregnancy; however, the arterial oxygen pressure (PaO_2), though it increases, does not change significantly, even though the arteriovenous oxygen

difference decreases. This indicates that there must be a change in ventilation.[63]

Ventilation. Minute ventilation ($V_T \times$ respiratory rate [RR]) increases 30% to 50% during pregnancy. Changes begin early in pregnancy and result in an increase in minute volume, from 6.5 to 7.5 L/min in early pregnancy to 10 to 10.5 L/min at term (Figure 9-3). The elevated resting ventilation exceeds the demands in oxygen consumption (which increases by approximately 20% to 30%), indicating that women hyperventilate during pregnancy.[43,63,201,249,257] The greater increase in resting ventilation is thought to be due to the stimulatory effects of progesterone.[83,249]

The increase in minute ventilation is probably due primarily to a 40% increase in V_T, rather than changes in respiratory rate.[63] It is much more efficient to increase alveolar ventilation through an increase in V_T than with a proportionately equal increase in respiratory rate.[241] The increased metabolic rate and carbon dioxide production also influence V_T changes.[257] Maximal inspiratory and expiratory pressures are not altered in pregnancy.[40]

The reduced RV further enhances alveolar ventilation. This change in RV decreases the amount of gas mixing that occurs with each tidal exchange in the alveolus,

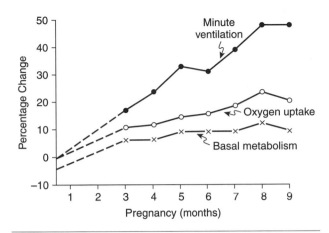

FIGURE **9-3** Time course of percentage changes in minute ventilation, oxygen uptake, and basal metabolism during pregnancy. (From Prowse, C.M. & Gaensler, E.A. [1965]. Respiratory and acid-base changes during pregnancy. *Anesthesiology, 26,* 381.)

thereby improving gas exchange at the alveolar level. Alveolar ventilation increases by 5% to 70% during pregnancy.[13,42,63,201,221]

Airflow. Airflow is dependent upon resistance encountered in the bronchial tree. Two of the important determining factors for resistance are smooth muscle tone in the bronchi and the degree of congestion encountered in bronchial wall capillaries. Despite the changes in minute ventilation and the concomitant increase in alveolar ventilation, the work of breathing (airway resistance and lung compliance) remains unchanged. In the larger airways, congestion has very little to do with resistance. Although study results conflict, airway resistance probably does not change during pregnancy because of a balance between bronchoconstricting ($PGF_{2\alpha}$, decreased RV, and decreased $PaCO_2$) and bronchodilating (PGE_2 and progesterone) forces.[73,114,249]

Assessment of small airway function is most often determined by the evaluation of closing volume (CV) and closing capacity (CC). CV is the point at which the small airways close (collapse and cease to ventilate) in the lowest part of the lung. Small airway (<1 mm) patency is believed to be the result of transpulmonary pressure, compliance of the airway walls, and the presence of sufficient surfactant. Closure in the lung bases normally occurs somewhere between the RV and FRC. CV is usually expressed as a percentage of vital capacity (CV/VC). CC is the term applied to the sum of the CV and RV (CC = CV + RV) and is expressed as a percentage of total lung capacity (CC/TLC).[102,249,257]

Under normal circumstances, closure does not occur during tidal breathing. When closure occurs at a higher than normal volume, however, gas exchange may be affected because ventilation to the lung bases is decreased. In pregnancy, airway closure above the FRC has been reported and is attributed to the 20% decrease in ERV. This alteration changes gas distribution and results in a fall in PaO_2.[50,63,249,257]

Whether closing volumes are normally altered in pregnancy is unclear; however, small airway dysfunction is not a feature of normal pregnancy pulmonary dynamics. If airway closure is at or above FRC, there is the possibility of altering PaO_2 due to ventilation-perfusion ($\dot{V}/\dot{Q}$) differences in the bases. If these differences are significant, compensatory maternal physiologic responses such as an increase in respiratory rate may result.

Diffusing capacity. Diffusing capacity refers to the ease with which gas is transferred across the pulmonary membrane. Diffusion capacity of carbon dioxide may show an increase or no change in early pregnancy, followed by a decrease reaching a plateau in the second half of pregnancy. These changes are not thought to be clinically significant.[30,249] Carbon dioxide production increases by 30% due to changes in cholesterol and fat metabolism.[257] Oxygen consumption increases by 37 ml/min. This change is accounted for by the needs of the fetus (12 ml/min) and placenta (4), and by increased maternal cardiac output (7), ventilation (2), renal function (7), and extra tissue in the breasts and uterus (5).[62] The increase in carbon dioxide production exceeds the changes in oxygen consumption, leading to an increase in the respiratory quotient from 0.70 to 0.83 by term.[63]

Acid-Base Changes

The normal pregnant woman is in a state of compensated respiratory alkalosis, which is thought to be the result of the effects of progesterone on the respiratory system and lung volume changes, especially the increased minute volume.[257] The result is a reduction in arterial and alveolar carbon dioxide and a slight increase in PaO_2. The fall in carbon dioxide begins early in pregnancy.[28] It is unclear whether the change in carbon dioxide is progressive or maintained at low levels throughout pregnancy.[249]

The purpose of the respiratory alkalosis seems to be facilitation of carbon dioxide transfer from the fetus to the mother by increasing the arterial carbon dioxide pressure ($PaCO_2$) gradient. Hyperventilation leads to average $PaCO_2$ values of 27 to 32 mmHg and a concomitant decrease in serum bicarbonate levels between 18 and 21 mEq/L with a base deficit of −3 to −4 mEq/L. The latter is a consequence

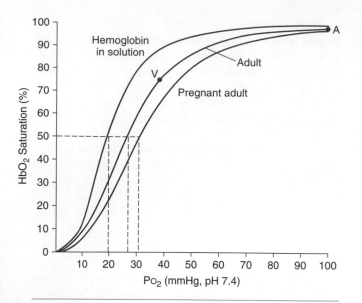

FIGURE **9-4** Oxyhemoglobin dissociation curve under standard conditions for normal blood of pregnant and nonpregnant adults. Also shown is the dissociation curve for hemoglobin in solution. (From Delivoria-Papadopoulos, M. & McGowen, J.E. [1998]. In R.A. Polin & W.W. Fox [Eds.]. *Fetal and neonatal physiology* [2nd ed.]. Philadelphia: W.B. Saunders.)

of increased renal excretion of bicarbonate, reflecting a metabolic compensation for the low $PaCO_2$. The pH therefore increases to the high end of normal (7.40 to 7.45). The reduction in blood buffer reduces the mother's ability to compensate for the metabolic acidosis that could develop during prolonged labor or other states in which tissue perfusion may be reduced. These changes are stable throughout pregnancy until the onset of labor.[30,50,107,249,247]

In contrast, PaO_2 levels increase from those of prepregnancy (95 to 100 mmHg) due to the increase in alveolar ventilation. During the first trimester, PaO_2 levels range from 106 to 108 mmHg, dropping to 101 to 104 mmHg by the third trimester. Even though the PaO_2 level remains elevated, the alveolar-arterial PO_2 gradient ($AaDO_2$) may not increase until near term due to an attempt to offset hyperventilation. Whether there is clinical significance to these changes is unclear. However, supine positioning versus sitting in late pregnancy does decrease PaO_2 levels and increase the $AaDO_2$ gradient.[63,249,237]

The oxygen-hemoglobin dissociation curve (Figure 9-4 and the box on p. 313) demonstrates that once the plateau of the curve is achieved it takes large changes in oxygen concentration in order to make small changes in PaO_2. The P_{50} increases from 26 to 30 mmHg by term (Figure 9-4), thus decreasing the affinity of hemoglobin and enhancing transfer of oxygen from mother to fetus.[63,257] It is unclear whether

the small changes seen in PaO_2 levels during pregnancy are significant to the maternal-fetal oxygen gradient and therefore to the fetus. Considering that fetal PaO_2 levels are between 25 and 35 mmHg, this seems unlikely. However, this increase may reflect increased maternal pulmonary circulation, with a greater volume of blood contained within the pulmonary vasculature at any given point in time. This may be very significant at higher altitudes. SaO_2 does not change significantly during pregnancy, although saturations below 96% may be seen in women who smoke.[245]

With increasing altitude, decreases in PaO_2 can be seen as compensatory in nature. The change in altitude has a significant effect on oxygen saturation, with a change in the oxygen-hemoglobin dissociation curve seen. The hyperventilation of pregnancy is also accentuated, and maternal dyspnea may be more prominent; therefore patients need to be given assurance that it is normal. All these factors are an attempt by the maternal system to maintain higher PaO_2 levels under relatively hypoxic conditions.[63,105,162,249] Pregnancy at high altitude is also associated with morphologic differences in placental villi with increased capillary diameter.[75]

Commercial aircraft are usually pressurized to 5000 to 8000 feet above sea level, so flying results in a transient exposure to altitude. Pregnant women who travel by airplane may also experience an increase in dyspnea and respiratory rate as their bodies attempt to compensate for the increased altitude. Fetal hemoglobin (HbF) and the fetal circulation protect the fetus from desaturation during commercial flights.[209] Flying in commercial aircraft is generally not a risk in women with uncomplicated pregnancies. However, pregnant women are at greater risk of thromboembolism during air travel due to changes in hemostasis (see Chapter 7) and should be sure to stretch, perform isometric exercises, and walk around the cabin at regular intervals.[16,209] The women should also maintain hydration with frequent intake of nonalcoholic beverages, because hydration is important for placental blood flow.[209]

Intrapartum Period

The major effect of labor upon the respiratory system is related to the increased muscular work, metabolic rate, and oxygen consumption. Consequently, alterations in ventilation and acid-base status can be anticipated.

With the onset of labor there is an increased demand for oxygen, and oxygen consumption increases with uterine muscle activity. If there is insufficient time for uterine relaxation and restabilization after a contraction, oxygen content is lower and myometrial hypoxia as well as metabolic acidosis may occur with the next contraction. Over time this can lead to inadequate oxygenation, which increases

Oxygen-Hemoglobin Dissociation Curve

The oxygen-hemoglobin dissociation curve demonstrates the equilibrium between oxygen and hemoglobin (see Figure 9-4). The curve relates the partial pressure of oxygen to the percentage of hemoglobin that is saturated. There are two aspects of the curve that must be considered: its shape and its position. The shape of the curve is sigmoid, indicating that at higher levels (>50 mmHg) the curve flattens and an increase in PO_2 produces little increase in saturation. This upper region is the PO_2 range in which oxygen binds to hemoglobin in the lungs. At low PO_2 levels the curve is steep and small changes in PO_2 result in large changes in hemoglobin saturation. In this range oxygen is released from hemoglobin and cellular activities occur. A small drop in PO_2 here allows a large amount of oxygen to be unloaded to the tissues.

The position of the curve, whether it is shifted to the right or the left, depends on the oxygen affinity for the hemoglobin molecule. The affinity of hemoglobin for oxygen must be sufficient to oxygenate the blood during its movement through the pulmonary circulation. However, it must be weak enough to allow release of oxygen to the tissues. This affinity is expressed as the P_{50}, the oxygen tension at which hemoglobin is half saturated. The higher the affinity the lower the P_{50} and vice versa, indicating an inverse relationship. The P_{50} for adult blood at a pH of 7.40 and a temperature of 37° C is normally 26 mmHg. Numerous factors, both genetic and environmental, can influence the affinity of hemoglobin and shift the oxygen-hemoglobin dissociation curve.

A shift to the right implies a lowered affinity; a shift to the left indicates that oxygen is more tightly bound to hemoglobin. The structure of the hemoglobin molecule regulates the affinity and can be affected by pH, PCO_2, and temperature. Increasing amounts of carbon dioxide reduce hemoglobin affinity for oxygen. This is termed the Bohr effect. Because of the Bohr effect the reciprocal exchange of oxygen for carbon dioxide is facilitated. Elevations in temperature also shift the curve to the right such that saturation is decreased at any given PO_2. The pH increases with release of CO_2, and the curve shifts to the left. The shift indicates an increased affinity for oxygen and favors the uptake of oxygen by hemoglobin.

Because of the sigmoid shape of the curve, a shift in position has little effect on the saturation when the PO_2 is within the normal arterial range (95 to 100 mmHg). However, in the venous system, in which the PO_2 range is around 40 mmHg, there is a right shift in the curve, leading to an increased unloading of oxygen to the tissues and improving tissue oxygenation.

---

the severity of the pain experienced. Most studies have evaluated respiratory system changes during active and painful labor. There are few studies evaluating the labor process with the use of sporadic analgesia and psychoprophylaxis. The pain experienced during labor is the result of the interaction of a number of factors (see Chapter 14). The subjective component includes the discomfort that is perceived by the mother. Objective factors are related to changes in the functioning of the cardiorespiratory system, alterations in the autonomic nervous system, and physical changes that occur during labor and delivery.

Ventilatory alterations related to pain vary significantly from patient to patient; therefore each laboring woman must be evaluated independently. Changes seen during the intrapartum period include an increase in respiratory rate and a change in V_T, with a tendency toward further hyperventilation. Hyperventilation is a natural response to pain and becomes evident as the pain and apprehension of labor increase. Hyperventilation is greatly diminished when pain is alleviated by methods such as lumbar epidural anesthesia.[111] With strong expulsive efforts, maximal inspiratory pressure decreases, possibly as a result of development of transient diaphragmatic fatigue.[183]

Although pain seems to be the major cause of this hyperventilatory response, anxiety, drugs, and oxygen mask application, as well as voluntary use of psychoprophylactic breathing exercises, can contribute to the elevated respiratory rate. V_T may be further increased during the second stage of labor as hyperventilation following breath holding with expulsive efforts is encountered. Risks of the Valsalva maneuver, which is not recommended, are discussed in Chapter 4.

Increases in oxygen uptake and minute ventilation are seen during labor, with a significant increase noted between early latent and active phases. Oxygen intake further increases (up to twofold) with contractions.[30] The increase in ventilation can lead to a progressive and substantial decline in $PaCO_2$. Once again, there are wide variations in values between patients; however, a $PaCO_2$ level around 25 mmHg is representative of what might be encountered during the first stage of labor. It has been suggested that there is a transient decline in $PaCO_2$ with each contraction until cervical dilatation is complete, at which time the decline in $PaCO_2$ can be seen even between contractions. Arterial carbon dioxide levels as low as 17 mmHg have been recorded in some women experiencing painful contractions. The changes in $PaCO_2$ are markedly reduced or eliminated when continuous lumbar epidural anesthesia is used during labor. Variables affecting $PaCO_2$ levels that need to be considered include breath holding (which elevates $PaCO_2$ levels), compensatory hyperventilation following breath holding, length of contractions, and frequency of contractions. The timing of analgesia administration as well as the frequency and efficacy of the analgesia may also alter $PaCO_2$ values.[50,38]

The respiratory alkalosis that ensues from hyperventilation is normally associated with a drop in base excess and possibly a decrease in arterial pH, according to some researchers. Other investigators have documented a rise in pH. In either case, the degree of change indicates that labor and hyperventilation are highly significant events that may lead to dramatic alterations in physiologic parameters.[18,38,41]

Labor studies demonstrate that maternal acidosis is not uncommon and can be attributed to isometric muscular contractions that reduce the blood flow to working muscles, leading to tissue hypoxia and anaerobic metabolism in the face of a normal PaO_2. The degree of maternal acidosis is dependent upon the extent of maternal anxiety and tension, intensity of muscular workload, degree of isometric contractions, and duration of labor. Studies have shown that changes in pH may also be minimized through the use of epidural anesthesia throughout labor.[38,208]

In the first stage of labor, the maternal and fetal $PaCO_2$ levels parallel each other. This may reflect the respiratory nature of these changes. As labor progresses, this paralleling of values is lost, which may be an indication of the difficulty that charged ions have in crossing the placental membrane.[208]

Fetal $PaCO_2$ levels rise when maternal acidosis occurs, reflecting not only fetal base deficit alterations but also the hypoxia within the uterine muscle. Contractions not only decrease the blood flow within the intervillous space but also reduce the oxygen supply to the uterus. The longer and stronger the contractions, the more pronounced the effects are. The local buildup of $PaCO_2$ decreases the fetal elimination of carbon dioxide, which may lead to a drop in fetal pH.[208]

During the second stage of labor, maternal $PaCO_2$ levels may rise during pushing efforts. During this stage, a further increase in blood lactate levels due to voluntary muscle activity during bearing down is seen. This is reflected in a substantial decline in blood pH and a fall in blood buffering capability (base excess).

Changes in acid-base status due to hyperventilation and increased oxygen consumption are potentially hazardous to both the mother and fetus.[41] Extremely low $PaCO_2$ levels result in cerebral vasoconstriction and possibly reduce intervillous perfusion and blood flow. The alkalemia that results shifts the oxygen-hemoglobin dissociation curve to the left. This shift impairs the release of oxygen from maternal blood to fetal blood, thereby decreasing the availability of oxygen to the fetus during a time when oxygenation may already be impaired due to uterine contractions.[14,41]

Hyperventilation may lead to dizziness and tingling in the mother due to low $PaCO_2$ levels. Interventions can include counting respirations out loud to help the mother slow her respiratory rate, letting her know when the contraction is ending so that she can begin to relax, avoiding the Valsalva maneuver, and promoting deep breathing between contractions to cleanse the system and promote oxygenation and restabilization.

The acid-base changes encountered in the first and second stages of labor quickly reverse in the third stage and postpartum period with compensatory respiratory efforts. These efforts are largely due to a decrease in respiratory rate. Acid-base levels return to pregnancy values within 24 hours of delivery and to nonpregnant levels by several weeks after delivery. Table 9-1 summarizes the changes in arterial blood gases during the intrapartum period.

Although it may appear that the use of epidural anesthesia is being advocated here, it is not. Research on the effects of labor on acid-base status has been conducted in conjunction with the delivery of epidural analgesia. Psychoprophylaxis (psychoanalgesia) has been shown to reduce the need for medication, to reduce tension and pain by self-report, and to engender a positive attitude toward the labor and delivery experience. Lamaze psychoprophylaxis is based on the hypothesis that childbirth is a natural physiologic process and that pain can be minimized through education and specified exercises. Education and antenatal preparation are designed to reduce anxiety through knowledge of the processes of labor. Relaxation techniques are designed to reduce skeletal muscle spasm and tension that may contribute to pain. Reduction of pain sensations and perception is achieved through distraction by utilizing conditional responses such as breathing patterns.[57,65,213]

Postpartum Period

The respiratory tract rapidly returns to its prepregnant state after delivery. This is a direct result of the separation of the placenta and consequential loss of progesterone production, as well as the immediate reduction in intraabdominal pressure with delivery of the neonate that allows increased excursion of the diaphragm.

Chest wall compliance changes immediately after delivery due to a decrease in pressure on the diaphragm and reduction in pulmonary blood volume. A 20% to 25% increase in static compliance has been reported following delivery[37,160] Changes in rib cage elasticity may persist for months after delivery.[257] V_T and RV return to normal soon after delivery, whereas ERV may remain in an abnormal state for several

TABLE **9-1**   **Maternal Blood Gas Alterations during the Intrapartum Period**

STAGE OF LABOR	PARAMETER	RANGE VALUE	ACID-BASE STATUS
Early	PaCO$_2$	21-26 mmHg	Respiratory alkalosis
	Plasma base deficit	−0.9 to −6.9 mEq/L	
	Blood pH	7.43-7.49	
End of first stage	PaCO$_2$	21-35 mmHg	Mild metabolic acidosis compensated by respiratory alkalosis
	Plasma base deficit	−1.2 to −9.2 mEq/L	Mild respiratory acidosis during bearing down
	Blood pH	7.41-7.54	
End of second stage (delivery)	PaCO$_2$	16-24 mmHg	Metabolic acidosis uncompensated by respiratory alkalosis
	Plasma base deficit	−2.3 to −12.3 mEq/l	
	Blood pH	7.37-7.45	

From Burgess, A. (1979). *The nurse's guide to fluid and electrolyte balance.* New York: McGraw-Hill.

months. As progesterone levels fall in the first 2 days after delivery, a rise in PaCO$_2$ levels can be seen during the first 2 days after delivery. Diffusing capacity, which at term is slightly below postpartum levels, increases during the post partum period. Overall, anatomic changes and ventilation return to normal 1 to 3 weeks after delivery.[37,166,173]

CLINICAL IMPLICATIONS FOR THE PREGNANT WOMAN AND HER FETUS

The respiratory changes that occur with pregnancy can be annoying as well as limiting in some circumstances. Common complaints and experiences include, among others, dyspnea and capillary engorgement of the upper respiratory tract. As a result, modifications in activity levels as well as in the activities themselves may need to be considered. Discussions with women regarding their usual activities can help provide sufficient information for determining when change is needed. In addition, changes in the maternal respiratory system can influence the course of disease processes (e.g., asthma), affecting not only the mother but also the fetus. Specific areas addressed in this section include dyspnea of pregnancy, upper respiratory capillary engorgement, respiratory infections, asthma, smoking, and anesthesia. Exercise is discussed briefly; further information can be found in Chapter 8.

Dyspnea

The sensation of dyspnea is reported by 60% to 70% of pregnant women, beginning in the first or second trimester (Figure 9-5) and with a maximal incidence between 28 and 31 weeks.[63,257] Because abdominal girth has not increased

significantly at the time of dyspnea onset, intraabdominal pressure cannot be ascribed as the cause.[77,87]

Dyspnea during pregnancy is a physiologic dyspnea; that is, it occurs at rest or with mild exertion.[257] The actual cause remains unclear, but it is thought to be due to the increased respiratory drive and load, changes in oxygenation, or a combination of these events.[87,257] Increased sensitivity to carbon dioxide and hypoxia may be important contributing factors.[87]

Dyspnea of pregnancy has been explained in relation to the hyperventilation of pregnancy. Decreased PaCO$_2$ levels and an increased awareness of the V$_T$ changes that occur in normal pregnancy have been implicated in these theories. As early as 1953, it was suggested that the heightened awareness of the normal hyperventilation of pregnancy might result in the sensation of dyspnea. The frequent improvement in symptoms with increasing gestation suggests an adjustment to this normal process.[49]

Dyspnea has also been correlated with altered PaCO$_2$ levels, suggesting a physiologic basis for this sensation. The women most likely to experience dyspnea had relatively high PaCO$_2$ levels before pregnancy, and the researchers felt that the marked change in PaCO$_2$ (from nonpregnant to pregnant levels) might account for the dyspnea. Women who experienced dyspnea have been reported to have an increased ventilatory response to carbon dioxide that led to a heightened awareness of the hyperventilation associated with pregnancy.[90]

For whatever reasons dyspnea occurs, it can be quite uncomfortable and anxiety provoking for some women. The hyperventilation and dyspnea may decrease the ability of some pregnant women to maintain their usual activity levels.

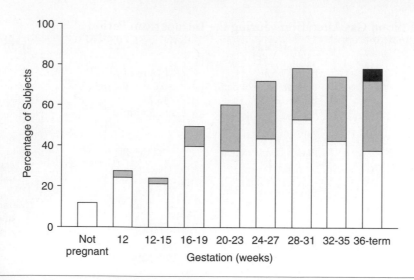

FIGURE **9-5** Incidence, time course, and severity of dyspnea during normal pregnancy. *Solid white areas*, dyspnea present climbing hills or more than one flight of stairs; *solid gray areas*, present on climbing one flight of stairs, walking at an even pace on level ground, during routine performance of housework; *solid black area*, dyspnea present on slightest exertion or at rest. (From Milne, J. [1979]. The respiratory response to pregnancy. *Postgrad Med J, 55*, 318.)

Early descriptions of dyspnea to the patient are appropriate and encouraged. Pathologic dyspnea—which may occur with disorders such as pulmonary emboli (a complication sometimes seen in pregnancy)—must be differentiated from physiologic dyspnea during pregnancy. Pathologic dyspnea is characterized by respiratory rates greater than 20, PCO_2 below 30 or greater than 35, or abnormal FEV_1.[77,257]

Upper Respiratory Capillary Engorgement

Hormonal changes (especially the increase in estrogens) result in capillary engorgement throughout the respiratory tract. Progesterone may contribute to engorgement by inducing vascular smooth muscle relaxation and nasal vascular pooling. Increased circulating blood volume may also play a role in this pooling. The results of these changes can be uncomfortable to some women and in certain situations can be hazardous.[116]

The nasopharynx, larynx, trachea, and bronchi may become swollen and reddened. For some individuals this may be uncomfortable, but it usually does not pose any unusual difficulties. These symptoms can be markedly aggravated with minor upper respiratory infections and preeclampsia. The swelling can lead to inflammation (noninfective in nature) that causes changes in the voice (e.g., hoarseness), make nose breathing difficult, and increase the incidence of nosebleeds. The swelling can also increase the hazard of intubation. Abrasions and lacerations of the mucosa may occur, and bleeding may ensue.[41]

Respiratory Infection and Injury

The altered cell-mediated immunity in the pregnant woman may place her at risk for upper respiratory infections (see Chapter 12). These changes, along with hypererythema and edema, not only make having an upper respiratory infection more uncomfortable but can also potentiate movement of the infection into the lungs. Infections associated with lung involvement could potentially increase airway resistance, thereby increasing the work of breathing, and lead to decreased V_T and RV. This may lead to decreased maternal and subsequently fetal PaO_2 levels. Although difficult to accomplish for some women, avoidance of those situations in which infections might be contracted and avoidance of individuals carrying infections is a good practice. Most upper respiratory infections are only annoyances and do not lead to significant consequences for the mother or fetus.

The prevalence of bacterial pneumonia is minimally changed in pregnancy.[115,198] However, there is some evidence that viral pneumonia may progress more rapidly during pregnancy and that pregnant women are more susceptible to viral pneumonia.[30] For example, varicella pneumonia is associated with a 20% mortality in nonpregnant women versus a 45% mortality during pregnancy.[17] Pneumonia increases the risk of preterm labor and perinatal mortality.[30] Although chronic infections such as tuberculosis have often been reported to reactivate and worsen with pregnancy, recent evidence suggests that there is no increased risk of relapse or adverse effects in women who have received adequate therapy.[249]

Adult respiratory distress syndrome (ARDS) is an acute lung injury involving diffuse interstitial infiltrates, decreased lung compliance, and hypoxia.[30] ARDS is usually triggered by sepsis but may also be triggered by other factors, including disseminated intravascular coagulation (see Chapter 7), preeclampsia, amniotic fluid embolism, abruptio placenta, or fetal demise.[63,249] Physiologic changes during pregnancy, especially changes in colloid osmotic pressure, may increase the risk of ARDS following lung injury.[30]

Exercise

The effect of exercise on the respiratory system is related to alveolar ventilation and is dependent upon the age, body weight, body composition, and physical condition of the individual. Cardiovascular function, uterine blood flow, respiratory function, blood gases, aerobic capacity, metabolism, temperature, and psychological state are all affected by exercise. Maternal respiratory function, aerobic capacity, oxygen consumption, and blood gases are considered here, along with fetal blood gases, activity, and breathing movements.[247] Cardiovascular changes with exercise during pregnancy are discussed in Chapter 8.

Maternal Respiration and Blood Gases

Studies of respiratory rates with exercise in pregnant and nonpregnant women demonstrate that respiratory rates in pregnant women are higher than those in nonpregnant women during mild exercise, but this difference disappears during moderate exercise. V_T and minute volume remain higher in pregnant subjects during all levels of exercise.[10,139] Ventilation increases 38% and oxygen consumption is 15% greater during exercise in pregnant versus nonpregnant women.[221,249] The efficiency of gas exchange does not seem to be impaired in the pregnant woman during exercise. During prolonged exercise, however, PaO_2 increases and $PaCO_2$ decreases. This decrease in $PaCO_2$ is most likely due to the effects of progesterone on the respiratory center.[150]

Oxygen Consumption

Oxygen consumption (VO_2) increases during exercise. In pregnancy, oxygen consumption also increases with advancing gestational age. Part of this increase is due to the increased work of carrying the extra weight associated with pregnancy.[7,243] Exercise-induced changes in acid-base balance are similar in pregnant and nonpregnant women.[186,252]

Non–weight-bearing exercise seems to result in little or no increased energy cost (difference between resting and exercising VO_2) during pregnancy, with a slight increase occurring during late gestation. These same findings hold

true in weight-bearing exercise, with some investigators finding no change in oxygen consumption during treadmill exercise and others reporting an increase. A decrease in oxygen consumption has been reported during strenuous exercise, possibly because of decreased fuel availability or a protective mechanism on the mother's part to prevent hypoxia.[10,139,243]

Aerobic Capacity

Aerobic capacity (the measure of an individual's ability to perform exercise) is dependent upon the intake, circulation, and utilization of oxygen. Aerobic capacity is also known as maximum oxygen consumption (VO_2max) and is the maximum oxygen volume that can be extracted from the air during exercise. Aerobic capacity is influenced by age, sex, heredity, hemoglobin content, inactivity (or, conversely, exercise), and disease.[7] Aerobic capacity can be increased by as much as 33% with exercise conditioning.[7,247]

Studies have demonstrated an increase in work rate with a concomitant decrease in VO_2max when exercise was instituted during pregnancy; for nonexercising women work rate and VO_2max decreased. This suggests that overall fitness was maintained during pregnancy with exercise, whereas not exercising led to a decline in fitness levels.[33] Others have reported a progressive decline in aerobic capacity during pregnancy—even though the fit group maintained a higher VO_2max in the first and second trimesters—as well as postpartally.[247]

Fetal Blood Gases

In the fetus, PaO_2 and $PaCO_2$ tensions decrease with the intensity and duration of exercise. However, these are not significantly different from control groups, unless exercise is prolonged and exhaustive. Although fetal PaO_2 does provide information about fetal status, it is not a good indicator of fetal oxygen consumption or of whether tissue requirements are being met. In this light, changes in PaO_2 without further indications of hypoxia may be indicative of adjustments in the oxygen-hemoglobin dissociation curve.[150]

Asthma

Asthma is an obstructive disease characterized by increased airway resistance, decreased expiratory flow rates, hyperinflation with premature airway closure, and some loss of lung compliance. These factors lead to an increase in the work of breathing. Along with this, hyperinflation and exaggerated negative pleural pressures can lead to increased demands on the right ventricle. This can be seen as a rise in pulmonary arterial pressure. These factors decrease left stroke volume, arterial systolic pressure, and pulse pressure.[249]

The restrictive processes in asthma are usually reversible and are due to an increased responsiveness of the airways to a variety of stimuli. When stimulated, the characteristic responses include contraction of the bronchial smooth muscle, mucous hypersecretion, and mucosal edema. The mechanism for this responsiveness is unclear and may be different from patient to patient.[17,97,249]

Several mechanisms have been implicated in the etiology of the disease. These include an immunologic response, blocked β-adrenergic function, β-adrenergic amine deficiency, cholinergic dominance, intrinsic smooth muscle defect, and some combination of two or more of these. Other possibilities include an imbalance in cyclic nucleotides. Cyclic adenosine monophosphate (cAMP) and cyclic guanosine monophosphate (cGMP) are involved in the modulation of airway tone, with the former contributing to bronchodilation and the latter to bronchoconstriction.[47,97] A major pathogenic characteristic is airway inflammation with release of inflammatory mediators (e.g., leukotrienes, histamine, eosinophil chemotactic factor of anaphylaxis, platelet-activating factor) and disruption of the mucosal epithelial barrier.[249]

Asthma is the most common pulmonary problem seen during pregnancy, occurring in 0.4% to 1.3% of pregnant women.[17,63,180] Asthma may improve (28% to 29%), worsen (22% to 35%), or remain unchanged (22% to 49%) during pregnancy.[212,241] Trying to predict an individual's course during pregnancy is extremely difficult. Women with more severe asthma before pregnancy are more likely to have severe asthma during pregnancy, although this is not always the case.[241,249]

Retrospective studies have suggested that women with asthma were at significant risk for serious adverse effects during pregnancy, including preterm labor and low–birth-weight infants. However, recent studies have demonstrated no change in perinatal mortality when asthma was methodically managed, although preeclampsia and neonatal hypoglycemia occurred more frequently.[97,249] Close monitoring, good education, and consistent therapy (including inhaled and oral corticosteroids) have improved outcome.[97,210,249]

Asthma may lead to maternal hypoxia or hyperventilation with resultant hypocapnia and alkalosis, potentially affecting fetal well-being.[42] Transient hypoxia is therefore not generally as great a concern as chronic hypoxia, in which prematurity, being small for gestational age (SGA), and mortality rates are all increased.[42,211] Acute hypocapnia and alkalosis, however, can contribute to fetal depression by reducing umbilical and uterine blood flow secondary to vasoconstriction. Alkalosis also increases maternal hemoglobin affinity for oxygen, thereby reducing availability to the fetus.

The normal alterations of the respiratory system during pregnancy may influence asthma in both positive and negative ways. The increase in circulating cortisol levels may augment cAMP functioning as well as reduce inflammation through steroid action. Progesterone levels decrease bronchomotor tone—relaxing smooth muscle tissue—and thereby decrease airway resistance. Elevated serum cAMP levels may also promote bronchodilation (Table 9-2). Thus improvement of asthma during pregnancy may be secondary to increased free cortisol, decreased plasma histamine, decreased bronchial smooth muscle tone due to progesterone, and decreased airway resistance due to decreased tone.[63,249] Conversely worsening may be due to increased progesterone and mineral steroids that compete for glucocorticoid receptors, increased viral respiratory infections and thus bronchial inflammation, increased $PGF_{2\alpha}$, and hyperventilation.[53,249] Therefore the effect of pregnancy on the course of asthma in an individual woman depends on the balance of these factors in her system.

Pharmacologic treatment and the selection of an appropriate agent are based on the risk-to-benefit ratio of bronchodilator effect and hypoxia avoidance versus possible adverse consequences. General management in-

TABLE 9-2   Factors Affecting Asthma in Pregnancy

IMPROVEMENT

Increased progesterone-mediated bronchodilation
β-adrenergic-stimulated bronchodilation
Decreased plasma histamine levels
Increased free cortisol levels
Increased glucocorticoid-mediated β-adrenergic responsiveness
Increased PGE-mediated bronchodilation
PGI_2-mediated bronchial stabilization
Increased half-life of bronchodilators
Decreased protein-binding of bronchodilators

WORSENING

Pulmonary refractoriness to cortisol effects
Increased $PGF_{2\alpha}$-mediated bronchoconstriction
Decreased functional residual capacity, causing airway closure and altered ventilation-perfusion ratios
Increased major basic protein in lung
Increased incidence of viral or bacterial respiratory infection
Increased gastroesophageal reflux
Increased stress

Data from Schatz, M. & Hoffman, C. (1987). Interrelationships between asthma and pregnancy: Clinical and mechanistic considerations. *Clin Rev Allergy, 5,* 301.

cludes careful history taking and evaluation, patient education, avoidance of known precipitants, and medical therapy. Education about the medical regimen and recognition of early symptoms so that treatment may be initiated early and hypoxia prevented are essential. Women need to be counseled to use only those medications prescribed and to avoid over-the-counter medications. Prescribed medications should be taken only as directed; maternal and fetal side effects need to be explained clearly and concisely.[97,249]

Cystic Fibrosis

Cystic fibrosis (CF) is an autosomal recessive disorder seen in 1 out of 2500 Caucasians. CF is due to an abnormal gene on chromosome 7. This gene codes for a protein needed for regulating chloride transport across cell membranes. With decreasing mortality, more women with CF are surviving to childbearing age. Kent and Farquaharson reviewed 217 pregnancies in 192 women with CF and found no increase in spontaneous abortion, but did find an increase in preterm delivery and perinatal mortality.[136] The rate of preterm delivery is about 25%.[136,141] Assuming the partner of a woman with CF is not a carrier, all of their children will be carriers. If the partner is a carrier, there is a 50% risk with each pregnancy of having a child with CF; all non-affected offspring will be carriers.

Prepregnancy pulmonary function is a predictor of pregnancy outcome. Women with mild CF generally do well during pregnancy.[17,63,136,249] However, women with moderate to severe CF— especially those with hypoxemia, cor pulmonale, and poor nutritional status—often do not do well.[63,141,249] Particularly ominous is preexisting pulmonary hypertension. In these women the usual pregnancy increase in cardiac output cannot be accommodated within the pulmonary vasculature. This leads to further desaturation, myocardial hypoxia, decreased cardiac output, and increased hypoxia.[63] Weight loss or poor weight gain during pregnancy is associated with a poor outcome.[71,81] Mortality is similar to that of nonpregnant women with CF when matched for age.[83,136,249]

Smoking

Smoking may interfere with a woman's ability to conceive, which may need to be addressed if fertility problems are present. Additional risks for the mother include a spontaneous abortion rate two times greater than in the nonsmoking population, an increased risk of abruption, placenta previa, early or late bleeding, premature rupture of membranes and prolonged rupture of membranes, and preterm labor. These are relatively significant conse-

quences, and mothers who smoke need to be informed of the possibilities and that the effects of cigarette smoking are also dose related. The risk of preeclampsia to the mother is reportedly decreased with cigarette smoking; however, if it does occur, the risk of perinatal mortality is greatly increased.[1,249]

Fetal and neonatal risks of maternal smoking include low birth weight, preterm delivery, intrauterine growth restriction, placenta previa, abruptio placentae, and premature rupture of membranes.[1,8,108,157,249] There is a twofold increase in deaths related to sudden infant death syndrome, and the incidence of respiratory disorders is higher due to an impairment of the immunologic system.[19,154] An increased risk of malformations has been reported, though the reports have been controversial. The most frequently reported defects are urinary tract anomalies, cleft lip and palate, and absence of the distal portion of the limbs.[146,261]

There is a dose-related effect of the number of cigarettes per day and the decrease in birth weight.[72,249] Generally by 6 months' postnatal age, there is not significant difference in weight of offspring of smokers versus nonsmokers, although long-term effects are unknown.[72] Fetal and infant mortality has also been reported to be related to dose in primiparas (25% increase with 1 pack or less per day; 56% increase with more than 1 pack), but not in multiparas (30% increase regardless of the number of packs per day).[137]

Children of smokers may be at risk for later problems as well, including behavioral difficulties and attention-deficit disorders.[1,168] Alterations in lung function have been reported with in utero exposure to smoking, with no effect of postnatal exposure.[51,225,231] An increased risk of asthma, pneumonia, and bronchitis has been reported in children of smokers.[23,225,249,250] Offspring of smokers also are reported to have a higher incidence of non-Hodgkin lymphoma, acute lymphoblastic leukemia, and Wilms tumor, with a dose-response relationship.[225]

Placentas of smokers are proportionately greater in weight (as related to fetal weight) than placentas of nonsmokers. This is thought to be evidence that smoking results in hypoxia and that compensatory hypertrophy occurs. To maintain the efficiency of oxygen transfer that is needed for the well-being of the fetus, the diffusing distance (distance between maternal and fetal blood) in the placenta is decreased, whereas the surface area and vascularity increase. In this way the fetus is assured of an adequate oxygen supply. Women who experience chronic anemia or live at high altitudes have similar compensatory mechanisms because of the chronic intrauterine hypoxia.[31] The placentas of smokers have more areas of calcification;

an increased incidence of fibrin deposits; an increased frequency of necrosis, inflammation in the margin, and placental lesions; and evidence of deoxyribonucleic acid (DNA) changes.[249] In addition, an increased risk of placental lesions has also been identified. These findings suggest that smoking causes some direct damage to the blood vessels of the placenta that may lead to placental underperfusion.[1,8,31]

If the alterations seen in the placenta are due to a decrease in uterine blood flow, the fetal consequences may be acidosis and hypoxemia. Because diffusion of oxygen to the fetus is dependent on blood flow, a decrease in flow could lead to hypoxia; therefore heavy smoking may subject the fetus to frequent periods of hypoxia that may have a cumulative effect on development.[1] This decrease in uterine blood flow may be mediated through the release of catecholamines from the adrenals when exposed to nicotine. Nicotine readily crosses the placenta, and fetal levels are generally 90% of maternal levels.[66] Nicotine may compete with nutrients for placental nutrient carriers, thus reducing nutrient transfer and thus fetal growth. An increased maternal heart rate and an elevation of blood pressure are clinical indications of catecholamine release with smoking. The catecholamines trigger peripheral vasoconstriction, which leads to a decrease in perfusion of the uteroplacental vasculature (underperfusion). Chronic underperfusion leads to fibrin deposition in arteries, inflammation and necrosis of tissue, and the development of lesions and calcifications. The perimeter of the placenta would be affected first, because perfusion is lower in these regions. The reduction of blood flow brought about by these defects could affect the placenta such that it would not be able to sustain itself, leading to an increased incidence of abruption. The overall impact of these changes would be a reduction in placental blood flow, leading to a decrease in available oxygen to the fetus and hypoxia.[1,8,222]

The risk of hypoxia is further increased by carbon monoxide, a by-product of smoking. Because carbon monoxide has a higher affinity for hemoglobin than does oxygen, the oxygen-carrying capacity of the blood in smokers is reduced. These effects have been demonstrated by highly elevated levels of carboxyhemoglobin in the fetus at birth.[8] Along with this, carbon monoxide greatly increases the affinity of oxygen for hemoglobin. With increased affinity, oxygen is less readily unloaded to the fetal tissues.[1] This, in turn, reduces fetal oxygenation further.

Fetal behavior changes that have been associated with cigarette smoking are changes in fetal heart rate (FHR) and fetal movements.[1] Fetal tachycardia has long been believed to occur with maternal smoking. More recent studies have indicated that FHR does not change during or after smoke inhalation; however, beat-to-beat variability is reduced, as is the number of accelerations.[96] A reduction in fetal movements and an increase in the number of epochs without fetal movement have also been reported.

After delivery, the neonate may continue to be exposed to the effects of nicotine through breast milk. Smoking is reported to decrease the volume of breast milk.[246] Once again, concentrations are related to cigarette consumption but can be detected in breast milk up to 8 hours after smoking.[1]

Inhalation Anesthesia

The use of inhalation anesthesia on pregnant women usually occurs only during an emergency situation. The effect on the maternal respiratory system is related to maternal cardiorespiratory status before induction and the type and adequacy of ventilation following induction. Because of the reduced functional residual capacity and increased closing volumes during pregnancy, as well as the higher metabolic requirements, the pregnant woman is less tolerant of apnea or a difficult or failed intubation.[9,150] Oxygen partial pressure levels drop rapidly in these situations, leading to hypoxia, hypoxemia, and acidosis. These events not only place the mother at risk, but also jeopardize the status of the fetus. Light to moderate anesthesia with adequate oxygen mixing should provide no difficulties to the well-hydrated, stable pregnant woman.[41]

Use of anesthesia can place the fetus at risk for depression and asphyxia. Fetal metabolic acidosis may be encountered following the administration of certain intravenous agents used for induction. If depression does occur, it is an indication of impaired placental blood flow, possibly due to decreased maternal cardiac output.[41,50,111] Most of the time, no serious depression occurs.

Inhalation agents are dose- and time-dependent compounds affecting the fetus directly through transplacental crossing of drugs or indirectly by altering maternal homeostasis or changing uteroplacental blood flow.[41] Uteroplacental blood flow may be altered through several mechanisms: (1) change in perfusion pressure, (2) modification of vascular resistance, (3) alterations in uterine contractions and basal tone, and (4) interference in fetal cardiovascular function (umbilical circulation). Uterine blood flow varies directly with perfusion pressure across the uterine vascular bed (uterine arterial pressure minus uterine venous pressure) and inversely with uterine vascular resistance. The balance between perfusion pressure and vascular

TABLE **9-3**   Clinical Implications for the Respiratory System in the Pregnant Woman and Fetus

Understand the normal respiratory changes that occur during pregnancy (pp. 310-314). Explain to the pregnant woman the changes that can occur in the respiratory system early in pregnancy and how they can affect daily activities and exercise tolerance (pp. 310-314, 317-318). Encourage prelabor preparation to reduce discomfort, hyperventilation, and anxiety during labor (pp. 314-316). Reduce hyperventilation during labor by counting respirations slowly, discouraging breath holding, and encouraging deep breathing between contractions (pp. 314-316). Discuss upper airway changes that may lead to nasal congestion (p. 318).	Counsel women regarding respiratory infections during pregnancy (pp. 318-319). Discuss usual exercise routines and changes that may be necessary owing to reduced tolerance and increased dyspnea (p. 319 and Chapter 8). Counsel asthmatic women who are pregnant to follow their medical regimen as directed, to avoid known precipitating factors, and seek medical intervention when symptoms persist (pp. 319-321). Encourage and support pregnant women in reducing or eliminating cigarette consumption both during and after pregnancy (pp. 321-322).

resistance is the primary basis for acute changes in uterine blood flow.[41]

Adverse responses or heavy anesthesia can precipitate a hazardous sequence of events. Maternal cardiac output may fall, precipitating a fall in blood pressure and an increased likelihood of maternal acidosis and decreased uterine blood flow. The result is a decreased uteroplacental blood flow with decreased nutrient supply to the fetus. Fetal heart rate and blood pressure may fall due to direct fetal cardiovascular depression (drug response) or the indirect effect of decreased uteroplacental perfusion. The decreased cardiac output and low blood pressure culminate in fetal hypoxia and acidosis, as reflected in low oxygen saturations, elevated PCO_2 levels, and falling base excess. Fetal status before induction affects the severity of the response.[41,111] This same sequence of events may occur with severe maternal hyperventilation. Marked reductions in maternal PCO_2 reduce uteroplacental blood flow and maternal cardiac output and can lead to fetal hypoxemia and acidosis.

Induction time, in conjunction with time to placental separation, may influence fetal outcome and neonatal response. Prolonged induction to delivery time allows accumulation of the anesthetic agent within the fetus. This may result in progressive depression, culminating in asphyxia. Caval occlusion may also contribute to these events (see Chapter 8).[18] A left lateral tilt surgical table can reduce the possibility of caval occlusion.

SUMMARY

The maternal respiratory alterations that occur during pregnancy ensure an adequate supply of oxygen to the developing fetus and its supporting structures. These demands are increased with activity and labor and are usu-

ally compensated for without difficulty. However, subjective interpretation of labor and the pain experienced can trigger maternal hyperventilation and place the fetus in jeopardy. Adequate education of the mother about the normal physiologic changes and the labor experience is essential to maternal-fetal well-being. Psychoprophylaxis, analgesia, and anesthesia can moderate the experience and can be used safely during the intrapartum period. Careful monitoring with all these methods is important to safeguard the fetus from deleterious effects. Clinical implications for the pregnant woman and her fetus are summarized in Table 9-3.

DEVELOPMENT OF THE RESPIRATORY SYSTEM IN THE FETUS

Embryonic development of the lung and the role of lung fluid and fetal breathing movements in development, as well as surfactant synthesis and secretion, sets the stage for understanding the changes that occur with transition to extrauterine life.

Anatomic Development

Lung growth occurs in five stages: embryonic (conception to 7 weeks' gestation), pseudoglandular (7 to 16 weeks' gestation), canalicular (16 to 25 or 26 weeks' gestation), saccular (26 to 35 weeks' gestation) and alveolar (25 weeks' gestation to postterm). These stages are summarized in Figure 9-6. Lung growth and development is mediated by growth factors (GFs) such as fibroblast GF, keratocyte GF, insulin-like GF, platelet-derived GF, epidermal GF, vascular epithelial GF, and transforming GF–α and GF–β.[140]

The embryonic stage of lung development lasts from conception to 7 weeks' gestation. Around day 24, a ventral

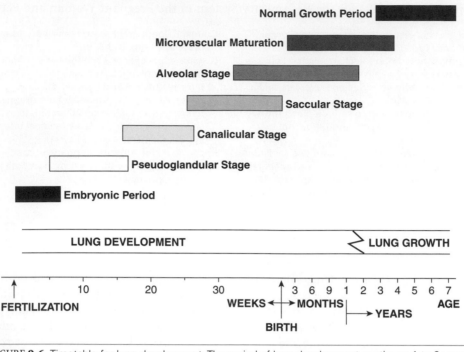

FIGURE **9-6** Timetable for lung development. The period of lung development continues 1 to 2 years, followed by continued lung growth into childhood. The timing of the saccular and alveolar stages and the period of microvascular maturation overlap with indeterminate initiation and end points. (Modified from Zeltner, T.B., et al. [1987]. The postnatal development and growth of the human lung. II: Morphology and end points. *Respir Physiol, 67,* 269.)

diverticulum (outpouching) can be seen developing from the foregut. This groove extends downward and is gradually separated from the future esophagus by a septum (see Chapter 11). Between 2 and 4 days later, the first dichotomous branches can be seen (Figure 9-7). At the end of this stage, three main divisions are evident on the right and two on the left, with 10 rudimentary bronchopulmonary segments on the right and nine on the left.[112,175]

Between 7 and 16 weeks' gestation, a tree of narrow tubules forms. New airway branches arise through a combination of cell multiplication and necrosis. These tubules have thick epithelial walls made of columnar or cuboidal cells. This morphologic structure, along with the loose mesenchymal tissue surrounding the tree, gives the lungs a glandular appearance (hence the term *pseudoglandular stage*).[112,175] By 16 weeks, branching of the conducting portion of the tracheobronchial tree is established. These preacinar airways can from this point forward increase only in length and diameter, not in number. The most peripheral structures by this time are the terminal brochioles.[112]

The mesenchymal tissue surrounding the airways has an inductive influence on the branching that occurs. Removal of this tissue interrupts epithelial branching until regeneration occurs.[230] This mesenchyme is of two types. The cellular type surrounds the endodermal tree and contributes to the nonepithelial elements of the tree. The other type fills the remainder of the space and develop into the pleura, subpleural connective tissue, intralobular septa, and cartilage of the bronchi.[230] Toward the end of the pseudoglandular period, rudimentary forms of cartilage, connective tissue, muscle, blood vessels, and lymphatics can be identified.[117] Ciliated cells appear by 13 weeks, and mucus-producing glands by 16 weeks.[112]

The epithelial cells of the distal air spaces (future alveolar lining) begin to flatten (becoming more cuboidal), signaling the beginning of the canalicular stage.[200] This change is called canalicular because of the vascular capillaries (rudimentary capillaries) that approximate the potential air spaces.[112] A rich vascular supply begins to proliferate, and with the changes in mesenchymal tissue the capillaries are brought closer to the airway epithelium.

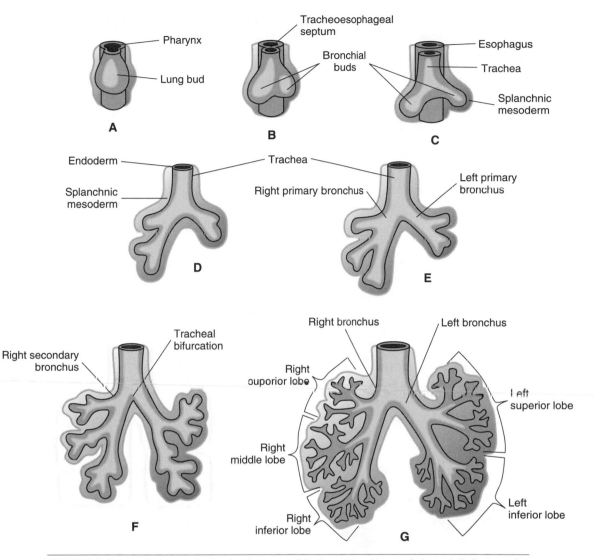

FIGURE **9-7** Successive stages in the development of the bronchi and lungs. **A** through **C,** Four weeks. **D** and **E,** Five weeks. **F,** Six weeks. **G,** Eight weeks. (From Moore, K.L. & Persaud, T.V.N. [1993]. *The developing human: Clinically oriented embryology* [5th ed.]. Philadelphia: W.B. Saunders.)

Primitive respiratory bronchioles begin to form during this stage, delineating the acinus (gas-exchanging section of the lung) from the conducting portion of the lung (Figure 9-8, *A*).

The canalicular stage continues until 25 to 26 weeks' gestation. At that time, terminal air sacs appear as outpouchings of the terminal bronchioles, marking the beginning of the saccule stage (Figure 9-8, *B*). During this stage the number of terminal sacs increases, forming multiple pouches off a common chamber (the alveolar duct). Around 30

weeks' gestation, lung surface area and volume increase sharply.[112,125] The surface epithelium thins considerably as vascular proliferation increases. As the vessels develop, they stretch and thin the epithelium that covers them even more, bringing the capillaries into proximity with the developing airways (Figure 9-8, *B* and *C*).[112,175] Eventually this leads to fusion of the basement membrane between the endothelium and the epithelium, thus creating the future blood-gas barrier. The alveolar stage begins around 35 weeks' gestation. Shallow indentations in the saccule walls can be detected (see

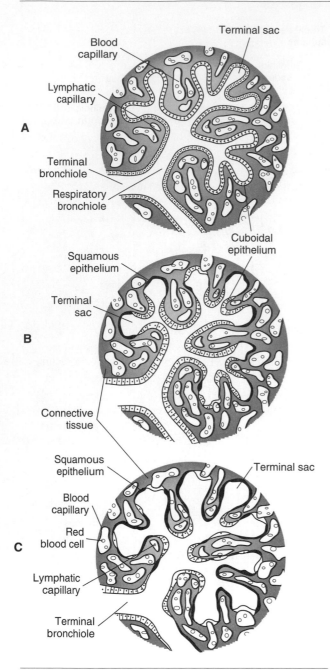

FIGURE **9-8** Diagrammatic sketches of histological sections illustrating progressive stages of lung development. **A,** Late canalicular stage (approximately 24 weeks' gestation). **B,** Early saccular stage (approximately 26 weeks' gestation). **C,** Newborn infant (early alveolar stage). Note that the alveolar capillary membrane is thin and some of the capillaries have begun to bulge into the terminal air sacs (future alveoli). (From Moore, K.L. & Persaud, T.V.N. [1993]. *The developing human: Clinically oriented embryology* [5th ed.]. Philadelphia: W.B. Saunders.)

Figure 9-8, *C*). These are primitive alveoli and will deepen and multiply postnatally.[112]

Lung structures and cells are differentiated to the point that extrauterine life can usually be supported at between 24 and 26 weeks' gestation. Although the normal number of air spaces has not developed, the epithelium has thinned enough and the vascular bed has proliferated to the point that oxygen exchange can occur. The 24- to 26-week lung, however, is markedly different than that of the term neonate, just as the term infant's lung is different from that of the child or adult.

The respiratory portion of the lung has a continuous epithelial lining composed mainly of two cell types: type I and type II pneumocytes. These cell types begin to differentiate by 20 to 22 weeks.[112] Type I cells attenuate or flatten. These pneumocytes cover approximately 95% of the alveolar surface with its long cytoplasmic extensions.[112] The thinnest area of the alveolus is composed of these extensions, and it is here that gas exchange occurs most rapidly.

The type II pneumocytes, although more numerous than type I, occupy less than 5% of the alveolar surface.[112,200] These cells retain their cuboidal shape and contain more organelles than do type I cells. Mitochondria are larger, and the Golgi apparatus, rough endoplasmic reticulum, ribosomes, and multivesicular bodies are more extensive.[207] Lamellar bodies and glycogen lakes appear within the cytoplasm.[112] Surfactant is produced and secreted by the lamellar bodies. With development, numbers and size of lamellar bodies increase with storage of surfactant lipids. As the density of lamellar bodies increases, cytoplasmic glycogen decreases.[112]

The first type II cells are seen between 20 and 24 weeks' gestation. Once they appear, the number of cells increases, with a concomitant increase in the number of lamellar bodies within the cells. The organelles migrate toward the luminal plasma membrane (alveolar duct surface), which forms prominent microvilli extending into the alveolar duct toward the end of gestation. Surfactant secretion occurs along this border.

Surfactant secretion is detectable between 25 and 30 weeks' gestation, although the potential for alveolar stability does not occur until between 33 and 36 weeks.[112,200] Surfactant proteins (SPs) also begin forming. SP-A expression begins at 75% of gestation; SP-B and SP-C begin by mid-gestation.[112] Along with surfactant production and secretion, type II pneumocytes appear to be the chief cells involved in the repair of the alveolar epithelium. This suggests that type I cells are more susceptible to injury and differentiate from type II pneumocytes.

Pulmonary Vasculature

Pulmonary vessel development occurs in conjunction with the branching of the bronchial tree.[109,222] The arteries have more branches than the airways; the veins develop more tributaries. The preacinar region has an arterial branch that runs along each conducting airway (termed *conventional artery*); supernumerary arteries feed the adjacent alveoli. All the preacinar arteries are present by 16 weeks' gestation. If for any reason there is a decrease in the number of airways, there is a concomitant decrease in conventional and supernumerary arteries.[109,222] From 16 weeks on, the preacinar vessels increase in length and diameter only.[112,117,200]

With movement into the canalicular and saccular stages, intraacinar arteries appear and continue their development into the postnatal period.[109] The conventional arteries continue their development for the first 18 months of life, and the supernumerary arteries continue to be laid down for the first 8 years.[202,222] These latter vessels are smaller and more numerous, servicing the alveoli directly.[117] If blood flow is reduced or blocked through the conventional arteries, the supernumerary arteries may serve as collateral circulation, thereby maintaining lung function during periods of ischemia or increased pulmonary vascular resistance.[237] Postnatally, the intraacinar vessels multiply rapidly as alveoli appear.[68]

The pulmonary veins develop more slowly. By 20 weeks, however, preacinar veins are present.[109] The development of the veins parallels that of the arteries and conducting airways, although supernumerary veins outnumber supernumerary arteries. Both types of veins (supernumerary and conventional) appear simultaneously.[117] Formation of additional veins as well as lengthening of existing veins continues postnatally.

Further development of the pulmonary circulation is related to the changes in muscle wall thickness and extension of muscle into arterial walls. Because of the low intrauterine oxygen tension, the pulmonary artery wall is very thick. The wall thins as oxygen tension rises after birth. With thinning, the medial layer elastic fibrils become less organized. The pulmonary vein, in contrast, is found to be deficient in elastic fibers at birth and progressively incorporates muscle and elastic tissue over the first 2 years of life.[10,109]

The intrapulmonary arteries have thick walls as well. The smaller arteries have increased muscularity and dilate actively with the postnatal increase in oxygen tension. There is a concomitant fall in pulmonary vascular resistance.[117] Between 3 and 28 days postnatally, these vessels achieve their adult wall thickness–to–external diameter ratio; the larger arteries take longer to achieve adult levels (4 to 18 months).[68,109]

The arteries of the fetus are more muscular than those of the adult or child. Muscle thickness–to–external diameter ratio decreases postnatally based on postnatal age and the size of the vessel.[117] After delivery, muscle distribution changes, and this process continues over the first 19 years of life. Prenatally, muscle development can be seen in the arteries of the terminal bronchioles; by 4 months' postnatal age the arteries of the respiratory bronchioles have incorporated muscle tissue.

Congenital Anomalies of the Lungs

Pulmonary agenesis in the embryonic period probably occurs secondary to failure of initial (lung agenesis) or later (lobarbronchial agenesis) branching. Agenesis is rare, but when it occurs is often associated with tracheal stenosis or esophageal atresia.[112] Pulmonary hypoplasia may arise due to intrinsic abnormalities in lung development, but it is often due to external compression from congenital diaphragmatic hernia, with lung compression by the herniated portions of the gastrointestinal system, or oligohydramnios, as occurs with renal agenesis (and thus inadequate amniotic fluid production [see Chapter 3]) in Potter syndrome. The mechanisms for pulmonary hypoplasia with oligohydramnios is not well understood but may be due to mechanical restriction of the chest wall (lack of space to grow due to lack of amniotic fluid in the amniotic sac), interference with fetal breathing movements, or failure to produce adequate fetal lung fluid.[112,143]

Bronchiogenic cysts—usually single lesions ranging in size from small cysts to those covering an entire lobe—develop early in gestation. These cysts may arise due to atresia of the bronchial or distal airway with development of a fluid-filled mass.[112]

Functional Development

The functional development of the lung revolves around the biochemistry of surfactant. However, the lung does secrete other substances and has its own macrophage function. Macrophages are found in groups of three or four cells lying free within the alveolar space. Ingested foreign bodies are seen as osmiophilic inclusions within the cell. These cells are spherical in shape and are derived from hematopoietic tissue.[164] Larger particles (e.g., bacteria) not swept away by ciliary action are removed and destroyed by pulmonary macrophages. Foreign material, once identified, is engulfed and destroyed by the macrophage. These cells are critical for maintaining the sterility of the lung environment and removing surfactant from the alveolar surface.

Surfactant

Surfactant is of major importance to the adequate functioning of the lung and has many roles (Table 9-4). Pulmonary surfactant is a lipoprotein, with 90% of its dry weight composed of lipid (Figure 9-9).[254] The majority of the lipid is saturated phosphatidylcholine (PC), of which dipalmitoyl phosphatidylcholine (DPPC) is the most abundant. The latter is the component responsible for decreasing the surface tension to almost zero when compressed at the surface during inspiration. Phosphatidyl-glycerol (PG) accounts for another 8% of the phospholipids present in surfactant, a substantial quantity. PG is unique to lung cells, bronchoalveolar fluid, and amniotic fluid. This makes PG a good marker for surfactant. The other components are involved in intracellular transport, storage, exocytosis, adsorption, spreading of the monolayer, clearance at the alveolar lining, and immunoprotection (see the box below).[22,254]

Four SPs have been identified (SP-A, SP-B, SP-C, and SP-D), and these make up 8% of the molecule. SP-A is the

TABLE **9-4** Classic and "Nonsurfactant" Functions of Pulmonary Surfactant

CLASSIC FUNCTIONS	"NONSURFACTANT" FUNCTIONS
Lung mechanics	Nonspecific host defenses
Reduction of surface tension in relation to surface area	Maintaining the surfactant film stability as a pathogen barrier
Stabilizing lung volume at low transpulmonary pressures	Facilitating microcilliary transport
	Antioxidant activity
	Antibacterial-antiviral activity
Prevention of lung collapse and atelectasis	Specific host defenses role: SP-A and SP-D are "collectins" with a pathogen-recognizing function
Gas exchange: Maintaining the gas exchange area of the lung	SP-A and Sp-D serve as opsonins, modulating chemotaxis and phagocytosis
Reduction of pulmonary shunt flow	SP-A interacts with alveolar macrophages through a specific receptor
	Alteration of cytokine/inflammatory mediator release

From Frerking, I., et al. (2001). Pulmonary surfactant: Functions, abnormalities and therapeutic options. *Intensive Care Med, 27,* 1700. *SP,* Surfactant protein.

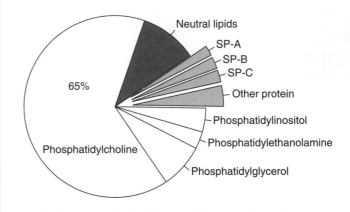

FIGURE **9-9** Composition of pulmonary surfactant. (From Jobe, A.H. [1999]. Fetal lung development, tests for maturation, induction of maturation, and treatment. In R.K. Creasy & R. Resnik [Eds.]. *Maternal-fetal medicine* [4th ed.]. Philadelphia: W.B. Saunders.)

Surfactant Biosynthesis

Surfactant is synthesized in the type II alveolar cells. Phospholipids are synthesized in the endoplasmic reticulum from glucose, phosphate and fatty acids. The surfactant components then move from the endoplasmic reticulum to the Golgi apparatus and lamellar bodies (see Figure 9-10). The lamellar bodies contain surfactant lipids, surfactant protein B (SP-B), and SP-C, but minimal SP-A. The lamellar bodies are secreted by exocytosis into the alveolar hyperphase. Here the lamellar body unravels to form tubular myelin. This process requires the interaction of SP-A, SP-B and calcium. Tubular myelin is a long, rectangular tubule that forms a lattice-like structure with SP-A at the corners. This structural change enhances spreadability and adsorption. Tubular myelin spreads over the alveolar surface in a monolayer.[123,128,192]

Surfactant reduces surface tension within the alveoli. Surface tension is the attraction between molecules at the gas liquid interface within the alveoli. Surface tension is constricting force causing alveoli to constrict and collapse. Surfactant acts to prevent this attractive force. Phospholipids contain hydrophilic (polar) and hydrophobic (nonpolar) groups. The surface film is oriented so that the polar groups interact with the moist alveolar lining and the nonpolar with the air molecules. During expiration the molecules of this surface film are compressed preventing interaction of gas and liquid molecules in the alveoli and thus reducing surface tension (see Figure 9-11).[128,254]

With repeated expansion and compression of the surface layer during breathing, the layer gradually breaks down. Compression squeezes out unsaturated lipid and some protein that form vesicles. The surfactant components are taken back up into the type II cell for degradation and recycling. New surfactant is constantly entering the surface layer as "used" surfactant leaves.[123,181]

most abundant and is needed for surfactant turnover, formation of tubular myelin (Figure 9-10 and the box on p. 328), and nonimmune host defenses within the lungs. SP-A maintains the surfactant monolayer at the air-liquid interface.[52] Deficiency of SP-A increases the risk of pulmonary infection. SP-B acts with SP-A to form tubular myelin.[24,36,53,125,130,254]

SP-B maintains the surface tension–lowering effects of surfactant, enhances spreading of the monolayer, and stimulates lipid adhesion and surface film formation.[164,214] SP-B is an essential component of surfactant.[52] Complete lack of SP-B results in severe respiratory distress syndrome (RDS) that does not respond to surfactant replacement therapy. These infants need a lung transplant to survive. Infants with partial or transient SP-B defects have a better outcome.[24,47,125,238] SP-C facilitates spreading, surface absorption, and lipid uptake; SP-D is thought to have a role in host defenses.[24,125]

The biosynthesis of surfactant entails a series of events including glycerophospholipid production, apoprotein synthesis, glycosylation and surfactant apoprotein processing, integration of surfactant component parts, and transport of components from synthesis sites to integration sites. This process is summarized in the box on p. 328 and Figure 9-10.

PC and PG are composed of a three-carbon glycerol backbone with fatty acids esterified to the hydroxyl groups.

The asymmetric arrangement of these molecules results in a hydrocarbon-rich fatty acid tail, which is nonpolar, and a phosphodiester region, which is polar. This allows for a monolayer film to be established at the air-liquid interface within the alveoli (Figure 9-11).[128,199]

There are two pathways for phosphatidylcholine (also called *lecithin*) synthesis. Key precursors for PC synthesis include glycerol, fatty acids, choline, glucose, and ethanolamine. The major pathway is the cytidine diphosphate (CDP) choline system, which is critical for mature alveolar structural integrity and stability. The other pathway leads to phosphatidylethanolamine (PE) formation and is termed the *methyltransferase system*. This has minor significance in the adult lung and seems to play a relatively insignificant role in fetal lung development. This may be because choline is incorporated more effectively into PC than is methionine. However, the ability of the human fetus to synthesize PC by N-methylation of PE early in gestation may contribute to survival with premature delivery.

The biosynthesis of phosphatidylcholine, phosphatidylinositol, and phosphatidylglycerol depends on the biosynthesis of phosphatidic acid. The increased production of phospholipids seen in late gestation is dependent upon the increased synthesis of this acid. The majority of phospholipid produced is PC.[22] The choline pathway and the diglyceride synthesis mechanisms that yield increased PC synthesis in late gestation interact. Although this inter-

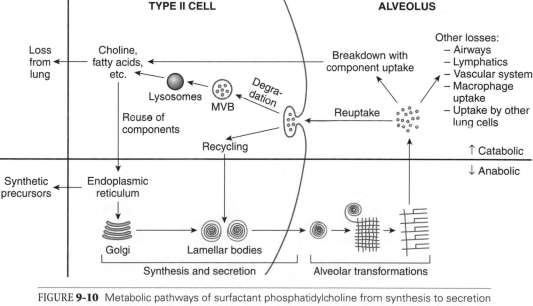

FIGURE **9-10** Metabolic pathways of surfactant phosphatidylcholine from synthesis to secretion by type II cells to alveolar transformation and reuptake by the type II cell. *MVB*, Multivesicular body. (From Jobe, A.H. [1999]. Fetal lung development, tests for maturation, induction of maturation, and treatment. In R.K. Creasy & R. Resnik [Eds.]. *Maternal-fetal medicine* [4th ed.]. Philadelphia: W.B. Saunders.)

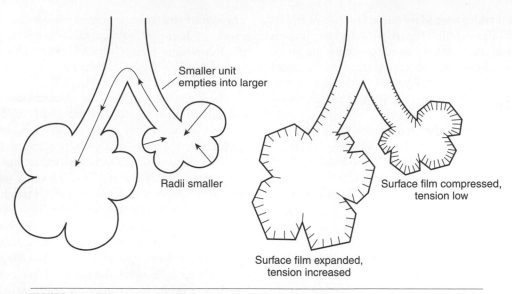

Smaller unit empties into larger

Radii smaller

Surface film compressed, tension low

Surface film expanded, tension increased

FIGURE **9-11** Effect of surfactant on lung stability as illustrated by a two-alveolus model. The surfactant-sufficient lung has stable alveoli of different sizes because of the variable effect of surfactant on surface tension. In the absence of surfactant, the wall tension on the small alveoli (as calculated by the LaPlace equation) exceeds that on the large airway. (Modified from Netter, H.H. [1977]. *CIBA collection of medical illustrations.* Copyright by CIBA Pharmaceutical Co., Division of CIBA-Geigy Corporation. Note: Modification in Jobe, A.A. [2002]. Lung development and maturation. In A.A. Fanaroff & & R.J. Martin [Eds.]. *Neonatal and perinatal medicine: Diseases of the fetus and infant* [7th ed.]. St. Louis: Mosby.)

action yields increased quantities of PC, it is not the highly saturated version identified in the final surfactant compound. The remodeling of PC that occurs in the phosphatidylcholine-lysophosphatidylcholine cycle provides the DPPC required for surfactant.[125,199]

As gestation advances, phospholipid content and saturation increase. This is accompanied by an increase in lamellar bodies within the type II pneumocytes. Choline incorporation, which is low in early gestation, increases abruptly in late gestation. This suggests that pathway regulatory mechanisms are enhanced in order to meet postnatal needs. Increases in surfactant before birth are due to increased synthesis; increases after birth are due to increased secretion.[199] Table 9-5 summarizes differences in surfactant components in mature versus immature lungs. Markers of lung maturation include loss of glycogen lakes in type II cells, increased fatty acid synthesis, increased β-receptors, and increased production of PC via the choline incorporation pathway.[125]

Enzymatic changes in the phospholipid synthesis pathway correlate to the surge in saturated PC and increase in PG with concomitant decrease in PI.[125,199] Whether this surge is due to a change in enzyme or substrate concentra-

tion, an adjustment in catalytic efficiency, a change in substrate affinity, or the activation of latent enzymes is not clear.

Influences on Fetal Lung Maturation

A complex interaction of several hormones and factors controls surfactant synthesis. Normal lung function is dependent upon the presence of surfactant, which permits a decrease in surface tension at end-expiration (to prevent atelectasis) and an increase in surface tension during lung expansion (to facilitate elastic recoil on inspiration). Surfactant provides the lung with the stability required for maintenance of homeostatic blood gas pressures while decreasing the work of breathing.[94]

Hormones that stimulate or accelerate lung maturity include glucocorticoids, thyroid hormones, prolactin, thyrotropin-releasing hormone, catecholamines, TGF-α, estrogens, bombesin, and epidermal growth factor. Androgens and insulin (or perhaps hyperglycemia) delay lung maturation.[101] Factors such as chronic maternal hypertension, preeclampsia, maternal cardiovascular disease, intrauterine growth restriction, prolonged rupture of membranes, and other maternal-fetal events that lead to stress and increased

TABLE **9-5** Changes in Surfactant with Development

VARIABLES	IMMATURE LUNG	MATURE LUNG
Type II cells:		
Glycogen lakes	High	Gone
Lamellar bodies	Few	Many
Microvilli	Few	Many
Surfactant composition:		
Sat PC/total PC	0.6	0.7
Phosphatidylglycerol (%)	<1	10
Phosphatidylinositol (%)	10	2
SP-A (%)	Low	5
Surfactant function	Decreased	Normal

From Jobe, A.H. (2002). Lung development and maturation. In A.A. Fanaroff & R.J. Martin (Eds.). *Neonatal and perinatal medicine: Diseases of the fetus and infant* (7th ed.). St. Louis: Mosby.
PC, Phosphatidylcholine; *SP,* surfactant protein.

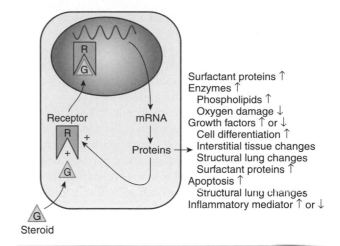

FIGURE **9-12** Synopsis of proposed glucocorticoid effects on fetal pulmonary development. *G,* Glucocorticoids; *R,* glucocorticoid receptor; ↑, increase; ↓, decrease. (From Bolt, R.J., et al. [2001]. Glucocorticoids and lung development in the fetus and preterm infant. *Pediatr Pulmonol, 32,* 79.)

fetal catecholamine and corticosteroid levels have been associated with accelerated lung maturity and a decreased risk of RDS.[125] However, stressed infants do not consistently have a lower incidence of RDS.[86,104,207,242] Lung maturation is delayed in infants of diabetic mothers and infants with RH isoimmunization with hydrops.[125] Some infants seem to have spontaneous early lung maturation.[207]

Glucocorticoids. Glucocorticoids such as betamethasone and dexamethasone are probably the best known of the hormones that accelerate the normal pattern of surfactant synthesis and fetal lung maturation.[45,101] These glucocorticoids increase the rate of glycogen depletion and glycerophospholipid biosynthesis. The depletion in glycogen leads to direct anatomic changes in alveolar structures by thinning the interalveolar septa and increasing the size of the alveoli. Morphologic changes include an increase in the number of type II pneumocytes and an increase in the number of lamellar bodies within those cells. These changes occur in conjunction with functional maturation, leading to an accelerated synthesis of surfactant phospholipid.[22,24,76,101,125,142] Actions of glucocorticoids on the type II cell are summarized in Figure 9-12. Glucocorticoids may also play a role in early lung development.[24] Pneumocyte glucocorticoid action centers on surfactant synthesis rather than secretion, and it affects more than just synthesis. Glucocorticoids act directly on lung tissue, increasing the number of β-adrenergic receptors and enhancing elastin and collagen production, thus improving lung compliance.[76,125,199]

Current recommendations for antenatal steroids are for use of a single course for women between 24 and 34 weeks' gestation who are at risk for preterm delivery within 7 days.[181,182] Either betamethasone or dexamethasone may be used, with no clear proof of efficacy of one drug over the other, although there is some suggestion that betamethasone may be safer and more protective.[181,253] Concerns have been raised about the effects of corticosteroids on the developing brain with repeated courses of antenatal steroids.[132,253] Therefore, until the results of further clinical trials are available (several are currently in progress), recommendations are for a single course.[182] Antenatal corticosteroid treatment reduces the incidence of RDS by about 50% in infants younger than 31 weeks' gestational age, decrease neonatal mortality by 30%, and decrease the incidence of intraventricular hemorrhage and necrotizing enterocolitis.[45,126]

Thyroid hormones. Thyroxine (T_4) and triiodothyronine (T_3) have also been shown to increase the rate of phospholipid synthesis.[22,95,199] Thyroid hormones, like glucocorticoids, enhance production of phosphatidylcholine through choline incorporation. They do not, however, increase phosphatidylglycerol synthesis or stimulate the production of surfactant-specific proteins.[12,142] Whereas glucocorticoids increase fatty acid synthetase activity, thyroid hormone seems to decrease its activity. These differences suggest different sites of action for these hormones as well as the need for action in conjunction with other hormones.[142] However, trials of thyrotropin-releasing hormone for preterm birth have demonstrated a lack of efficacy and an increase in complications.[47]

Catecholamines. Whereas glucocorticoids and thyroid hormones play a role in enhancing the synthesis of phospholipids, catecholamines stimulate the secretion of surfactant into the alveolar space. This appears to be a direct action of adrenergic compounds on type II cells.[64] The response is prompt, occurring in less than an hour. Further research has shown that there is an increase in surfactant and saturated phosphatidylcholine in lung fluid and improved lung stability. This is demonstrated in an increased lecithin-to-sphingomyelin (L/S) ratio. An added benefit is the inhibition of fetal lung fluid secretion and possible reabsorption of the fluid within the alveoli at the time of delivery. These two effects (the increase in surfactant and decrease in lung fluid) work together in preparing for respiratory conversion at birth.[64]

Factors inhibiting lung maturation. Delayed maturation of surfactant synthesis is observed in infants of diabetic mothers (IDMs) whose disease is not well controlled. It is unclear whether the causative factor is the hyperglycemia, the hyperinsulinemia, or both; research continues to provide conflicting results.[199] Maturation of surfactant synthesis occurs at the same time that glycogen is depleted from the lungs and liver. Insulin inhibits glycogen breakdown, thereby decreasing the substrate available for PC synthesis as well as altering the natural anatomic changes that occur with glycogen depletion.[22,142] The effect of cortisol on choline incorporation may be altered by insulin, although some have found

either no effect or a synergistic effect. In vivo studies suggest that hyperglycemia may be the cause of altered lung maturation in an IDM, rather than hyperinsulinemia.[199]

Androgens also delay lung maturation. At any stage of gestation, the female fetal lung is about 1 week more mature. This may be why male preterm infants are more prone to RDS than female infants of similar gestations.[199]

Assessment of Fetal Lung Maturity

To manage preterm birth, it is important to accurately assess fetal lung maturity. This is especially true when the date of the last menstrual period is not known or if preeclampsia, placenta previa, multiple pregnancy, Rh isoimmunization, diabetic pregnancy, or intrauterine growth restriction is present. The presence of surfactant phospholipids in the amniotic fluid allows determination of lung maturity because their concentrations change as the surfactant system matures. Gluck et al initially demonstrated that the ratio of lecithin (L) to sphingomyelin (S) (the L/S ratio) is a reliable index and a good predictor of whether RDS will develop if the infant is born within the 48 hours following amniocentesis. This is still one of the most widely used assessment tools in obstetrics.[125]

Sphingomyelin is a general membrane phospholipid not related to lung maturation. Levels remain constant throughout gestation. Lecithin levels rise sharply at around 34 to 35 weeks' gestation, thereby providing the basis for achieving a ratio between the two (Figure 9-13). If the L/S

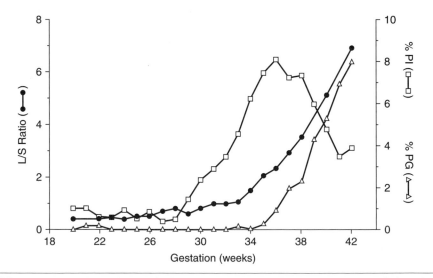

FIGURE **9-13** Lecithin (phosphatidylcholine)-sphingomyelin *(L/S)* ratio, percentage of phosphatidylglycerol *(PG)*, and percentage of phosphatidylinositol *(PI)* in amniotic fluid in normal pregnancies as a function of gestational age. Each measurement has as distinct profile relative to gestational age. (Redrawn and modified from Gluck, L., et al. [1974]. The interpretation and significance of the lecithin-sphingomyelin ratio in amniotic fluid. *Am J Obstet Gynecol, 120,* 142. Note: Modification in Jobe, A.A. [2002]. Lung development and maturation. In A.A. Fanaroff & R.J. Martin [Eds.]. *Neonatal and perinatal medicine: Diseases of the fetus and infant* [7th ed.]. St. Louis: Mosby.)

ratio is greater than or equal to 2, it indicates lung maturity and a negligible risk for RDS. A ratio less than 1.5 indicates lung immaturity.[125] A higher incidence of inaccurate readings is found in complicated pregnancies.

Factors that influence phospholipid concentrations in the amniotic fluid include volume of amniotic fluid (varies inversely) and contamination of the sample with blood, meconium, or antiseptics. PC levels are falsely high with blood contamination (fetal or maternal). PG is only slightly affected, however, because blood does not contain PG in significant amounts. The presence of PG is an indication that the major synthesis pathway for surfactant is present and functioning. Therefore, when PG is present in the amniotic fluid, there is little risk for RDS regardless of the L/S ratio value.[125] Other techniques for assessing fetal lung maturity include the complete lung profile, a modified profile (L/S ratio and PG only), and techniques such as the fluorescent polarization (FP) assay. The lung profile consists of the L/S ratio, percentages of PG and PI, and the ratio of cold-acetone precipitable PC to total PC. The FP assay measures the effects of phospholipids in amniotic fluid on a fluorescent probe. Results are comparable to the L/S ratio in predictive value.[125]

A low L/S ratio is not an absolute indication that RDS will develop and may in fact predict RDS in only 50% of cases.[125] The presence of PG, however, makes it less likely that the infant will develop RDS, even when diabetes or perinatal asphyxia is present.[190] PG has been seen in infants of less than 30 weeks' gestational age who have spontaneous or stress-induced early lung maturation.[106] Regardless, the use of fetal lung maturity tests has decreased the incidence of RDS.

Oxygen Antioxidants

The other biochemical system that develops prenatally and is needed for successful adaptation to extrauterine life is the antioxidant system (AOS). The AOS is designed to scavenge or detoxify the highly reactive oxygen metabolites produced during aerobic respiration. The potentially cytotoxic oxygen metabolites (e.g., superoxide radical, hydrogen peroxide, hydroxyl radical, singlet oxygen, peroxide radical) are produced intracellularly in excess amounts under hyperoxic conditions. The detoxifying antioxidant enzymes include superoxide dismutase, catalase, and glutathione peroxidase.

The transition to the extrauterine environment is a move from a relatively hypoxic state to a hyperoxic one. In utero, the fetal lung is exposed to low PaO_2 levels, with even lower oxygen tensions existing in the fetal lung fluid that fills the alveolar spaces and bronchiole tubes. At delivery the alveolar and airway cells are abruptly exposed to hy-

peroxic tensions. Therefore it is important to have an AOS in place that can reduce damage by oxygen radicals.[82]

The development of the antioxidant enzymes occurs late in gestation.[82] Antioxidant levels appear to be strongly correlated to the degree of protection that can be expected from oxygen radical–induced lung injury. When enzyme levels are increased (as with exogenous treatment), there is increased tolerance to hyperoxia. Although there are other protective mechanisms in place, it does not appear that increased amounts of these will result in an increased level of protection. However, deficiencies within these other pathways will result in an increased susceptibility to cellular damage. This suggests that the other antioxidants play a secondary role in providing protection. Antioxidant enzymes provide primary protection by direct detoxification of reactive oxygen radicals. This prevents damage to cell proteins and DNA structure. The other systems terminate reactions already initiated by oxygen radical attack.

Lung Fluid

Lung fluid is secreted beginning in the canalicular stage. This fluid is derived from alveolar epithelium secretions and is not an ultrafiltrate or mixture of plasma or amniotic fluid.[181] Active transport is required to attain the final ion concentrations found in the fluid; this is probably achieved by the active transport of chloride, with sodium following passively. The water flux can be attributed to the osmotic force of sodium chloride (NaCl).[21,158] Osmolarity and sodium and chloride levels are lower in amniotic fluid than in tracheal fluid, whereas pH and glucose and protein levels are higher.[21]

Estimated lung fluid production in term infants is 250 to 300 ml per day or about 10 to 30 ml per kg body weight.[75] Of the fluid produced, some is swallowed and some (~15 ml/hr) moves into the amniotic fluid via periodic opening of the larynx. Movement of lung fluid into amniotic fluid increases with fetal breathing movements.[112] The amount of lung fluid contributed to the amniotic pool is relatively insignificant when compared to that contributed by micturition. The volume of fluid in the lungs is equal to the functional residual capacity (FRC).[21,117,125,158]

Although the functional importance of lung fluid is not entirely known, it does play an important part in cell maturation and development as well as in determining the formation, size, and shape of the developing air space. Alterations in fluid dynamics affect pulmonary cell proliferation and differentiation. In fetal lambs whose tracheas were ligated, the lungs were relatively large but were immature when type II cells were assessed.[7] For those fetal lambs whose lungs were drained, the alveolar walls were thick and lung size was decreased, with fewer alveoli and

TABLE 9-6 Normal Fetal pH and Blood Gas Data

	UMBILICAL VEIN	DESCENDING AORTA	ASCENDING AORTA
pH	7.40-7.43	7.36-7.39	7.37-7.40
PO$_2$ (torr)	28-32	20-23	21-25
PCO$_2$ (torr)	38-42	43-48	41-45

From Clyman, R.I & Heymann, M.A. (1999). Fetal cardiovascular physiology. In R.K. Creasy & R. Resnik (Eds.). *Maternal-fetal medicine* (4th ed.). Philadelphia: W.B. Saunders.

type II cells.[4] Therefore, if production of lung fluid is decreased or leakage of amniotic fluid is experienced, there is risk of lung hypoplasia. In comparison, tracheal obstruction of a chronic nature leads to hyperplasia, with an increase in the number of alveoli, although functionally immature.[112,237]

Lung fluid production slows in late pregnancy, with a decrease in volume to 65% of previous values. Absorption of lung fluid begins in early labor so that after birth only about 35% of the original lung fluid volume needs to be cleared (see Transitional Events).[125,200,228]

Fetal Blood Gases

Usual fetal blood gases are listed in Table 9-6. Factors that affect maternal-to-fetal diffusion of oxygen include maternal and fetal PO$_2$ relationships, maternal and fetal oxygen-hemoglobin dissociation curves (see the box on p. 315), maternal and HbF concentrations, and the Bohr effect. Carbon dioxide transfer is affected by hydrogen ion concentration and the Haldane effect.

Fetal acid-base status can be evaluated during the antepartum period by percutaneous umbilical blood sampling, and during the intrapartum period by scalp blood sampling, or at birth by umbilical cord blood sampling. More recently, techniques for fetal pulse oximetry and lactate measurements using small aliquots of blood have become available.[32,170,186] Studies evaluating fetal pulse oximetry to refine the technique and interpretation of findings are ongoing.

Oxygen transfer. The placenta is separated into cotyledons, which are subdivided into lobules. The lobules are fed by uteroplacental arteries that direct blood toward the apex of the intervillous space. Depending on where blood is located in the cavity, the maternal-fetal oxygen gradient varies. The PaO$_2$ of the blood within the maternal arteries is at the most 100 mmHg. By the time blood reaches the apex of the lobule, the PaO$_2$ is 17 mmHg and the maternal-fetal

gradients are the greatest. At the rim of the cavity, the maternal PaO$_2$ is approximately 35 mmHg and fetal PaO$_2$ is around 28 mmHg. This gradient facilitates the transfer of oxygen from the mother to the fetus.[165,166]

As noted earlier, the fetal oxygen-hemoglobin dissociation curve is placed to the left of the adult curve, indicating that HbF has a higher affinity for oxygen. This can be seen in the larger quantity of oxygen that each gram of HbF carries. Besides the higher affinity, the fetus has an increased number of red blood cells and therefore increased hemoglobin content. This leads to a higher oxygen-carrying capacity when compared with the mother.[30]

When the maternal blood releases oxygen to the fetus, it accepts fetal metabolites in return, leading to a fall in maternal pH. This shifts the maternal oxygen-hemoglobin dissociation curve to the right (the Bohr effect), which increases the movement of oxygen from the mother to the fetus. As the fetus gives up carbon dioxide, the pH rises, shifting the fetal dissociation curve to the left. This allows the fetus to accept more oxygen as the affinity increases. This movement of hydrogen ions results in a displacement of both dissociation curves, moving them further apart (double Bohr effect). As the distance between the two curves increases, oxygen transfers at a faster rate from maternal blood to fetal blood. This process is unique to the placenta.

Maternal oxygen therapy during the intrapartum period is useful in treating fetal hypoxia, even though, because of differences in the oxygen-hemoglobin dissociation curve between the fetus and mother, fetal PO$_2$ does not increase as dramatically as that of the mother. Administration of oxygen to the mother increases maternal arterial PO$_2$, increasing the gradient between maternal and fetal values in the placenta. This increases oxygen transfer to the fetus, increasing fetal oxygen content and fetal cerebral oxygenation.[5,30] Fetal cerebral oxygenation has been reported to also be enhanced by maternal left lateral versus supine positioning.[30]

Maternal hypoxia (especially below 60 mmHg) can have significant consequences for the fetus. In this situation the maternal oxygen-hemoglobin dissociation curve shifts to the left (toward the fetal curve), decreasing oxygen availability to the fetus.[42] Maternal hyperventilation with decreased PCO$_2$ can also lead to decreased fetal oxygenation by decreasing uterine blood flow and shifting the maternal oxygen-hemoglobin dissociation curve to the left.[3]

Carbon dioxide transfer. The carbon dioxide combining power of blood is dependent upon the amount of hemoglobin that is not combined with oxygen. This uncombined hemoglobin is free to buffer the hydrogen ions formed by the dissociation of carbonic acid. This means

TABLE **9-7**   Factors Affecting Fetal Breathing Movements

FACTOR	EFFECT
Glucose concentrations; glucose infusions	Increased FBM in patients who have fasted
Cigarette smoking	Increased frequency of FBM, although incidence remains unchanged
Caffeine	Increased FBM with chronic exposure; no effect with acute exposure
Ethanol	Dramatic decrease in FBM
Methadone	Decreased FBM with chronic exposure
Tocolytics	Dramatic increase in FBMs

Adapted from Richardson, B.S. & Gagnon, R. (1999). Fetal breathing and body movements. In R.K. Creasy & R. Resnik (Eds.). *Maternal-fetal medicine* (4th ed.). Philadelphia: W.B. Saunders.
FBM, Fetal breathing movement.

that as maternal blood gives up oxygen it is able to accept increased amounts of carbon dioxide (the Haldane effect). The fetus gives up carbon dioxide as oxygen is accepted, without altering the local $PaCO_2$ levels. This double Haldane effect is unique to the placenta and is probably responsible for half the transplacental carbon dioxide transfer.

Fetal Breathing Movements

Fetal breathing movements (FBM) can be seen on ultrasound as early as 10 weeks' gestation, and they occur 6% of the time by 19 weeks.[56,159] FBM are rapid and irregular, occurring intermittently early in gestation. As gestation progresses, the strength and frequency of FBMs increase, and they occur approximately 30% to 40% of the time in the last 10 weeks, with a rate of 30 to 70 breaths per minute.[55,159,174,204] Large movements (gasping) occur 5% of the total breathing time, one to four times per minute.[159]

The rapid and irregular respiratory activity may contribute to lung fluid regulation, thereby influencing lung growth. The diaphragm seems to be the major structure involved, with minimal chest wall excursion encountered (4- to 8-mm change in transverse diameter). Movement of the diaphragm is necessary for chest wall muscle and diaphragm training and development, building adequate strength for the initial breath.[55,56] The movement of the diaphragm also influences the course of lung cell differentiation and proliferation. Bilateral phrenectomy in animal models results in altered lung morphology with an increase in type II over type I cells. Presumably the innervated diaphragm increases the size of the thorax and thereby increases tissue stress, affecting morphology. In addition, however, hypoplastic lungs are found when fetal breathing movements do not occur.[230]

With increasing gestational age, FBMs become more organized and vigorous.[174] Even with these gestational changes, tracheal fluid shifts are negligible—the pressure generated being no more than 25 mmHg.[230] Fetal matura-tion leads to the appearance of FBM cycles, with an increase in breathing movements during daytime hours.[159] Although the patterns of FBMs vary according to rate, amplitude, and character, they seem to be correlated mostly with fetal behavioral states and occur the most often during active sleep.[55,159,203,204]

The mechanism for the initiation of FBMs is unknown, although they seem to be stimulated by maternal inhalation of carbon dioxide, adrenergic and cholinergic compounds, and PG synthesis inhibitors. Other factors affecting FBMs include maternal glycemia, nicotine and alcohol ingestion, and labor.[164,203] These are summarized in Table 9-7.

Abnormal breathing patterns can be seen during periods of fetal hypoxia. Mild hypoxemia decreases the incidence of FBMs, while severe hypoxemia may lead to cessation of FBMs for several hours. The onset of asphyxia leads to gasping.[204] Interestingly, the onset of mild hypoxemia (as with umbilical artery occlusion of short duration) may lead to quiet sleep, which decreases activity expenditure and oxygen consumption in the fetus.[159] Although paradoxical in nature, this conservation mechanism may protect the fetus while cardiac output is redistributed toward the placenta.

NEONATAL PHYSIOLOGY

The neonatal respiratory system is still immature at birth and undergoes significant changes during transition to extrauterine life and in early postnatal life. As described in Development of the Respiratory System of the Fetus, the final stage of lung development begins around 35 weeks' gestation and continues well into the postnatal period. Changes in the lungs with growth are summarized in Table 9-8.

Transitional Events

Transitional events are all those activities that must occur within organ systems to achieve appropriate functioning

TABLE **9-8** Changes in Lung Size with Growth

Parameter	30 Weeks' Gestation	Full Term	Adult	Fold Increase after Birth
Lung volume	25 ml	150-200 ml	5 L	23
Lung weight	20-25 g	50 g	800 g	16
Alveolar number		50 m	300 m	6
Surface area	0.3 m^2	3-4 m^2	75-100 m^2	23
Surface area/kg		0.4 m^2	1 m^2	2.5
Alveolar diameter	32 μ	150 μ	300 μ	22
Number of airways	24	23-24	22-24	0
Tracheal length		26 mm	184 m	7
Main bronchi length		26 mm	254 m	10

From Hodson. W.A. (1998). Normal and abnormal structural development of the lung. In R.A. Polin & W.W. Fox (Eds.). *Fetal and neonatal physiology* (2nd ed.). Philadelphia: W.B. Saunders.

in the extrauterine environment. The most critical of these is the establishment of an air-liquid interface at the alveolar level and the acquisition of sustained rhythmic respiration by the neonate. This must occur within seconds of placental separation, or pulmonary and cardiovascular changes will not occur and resuscitation will be necessary. Respiratory changes at birth are linked with the cardiovascular changes discussed in Chapter 8.

Establishment of Extrauterine Respiration

Before discussing first breath events, a brief review of intrauterine status immediately before birth is warranted. At term, the acinar portion of the lung is well established, although "true" alveoli are only now beginning to develop. The pulmonary blood vessels are narrow; less than 10% to 12% of the cardiac output perfuses the lungs to meet cellular nutrition needs. This low volume circulation is in part due to the high pulmonary vascular resistance created by constricted arterioles.

Before term the lung holds approximately 10 to 30 ml per kg of lung fluid. Lung aeration is complete when this liquid is replaced with an equal volume of air and the FRC is established. A substantial amount of air is retained from the early breaths, and within an hour of birth 80% to 90% of the FRC is created. The retention of air is due to surfactant and a decrease in surface tension. Surfactant decreases the tendency toward atelectasis; promotes capillary circulation by increasing alveolar size, which indirectly dilates precapillary vessels; improves alveolar fluid clearance; and protects the airway.[169] The blood gas levels that are encountered in the fetal state would result in significant hyperventilation if encountered postnatally. This indicates a diminished responsiveness of the respiratory centers to chemical stimuli in the blood in the prenatal period. Postnatal breathing is responsive to stimuli from arterial

and central chemoreceptors (via oxygen and carbon dioxide tension in the blood); stimuli from the chest wall and lungs, musculoskeletal system, and skin; and emotions and behavioral stimuli. The change that takes place at birth and the increase in aerobic metabolism are not only rapid but irreversible. Within a few hours of birth, the full-term neonate is responsive to hypoxia and hypercapnia in much the same manner as an adult.[327] Changes in blood gases with transition are summarized in Figure 9-14.

The actual mechanics of respiratory conversion begins with the passage of the fetus through the birth canal. The thorax is markedly depressed during this passage, and external pressures of 160 to 200 cmH$_2$O and intrathoracic pressures of 89 cmH$_2$O or greater are generated.[131,184] As the face or nares are exposed to atmospheric pressure, a small amount of lung fluid is expelled.[23] Recoil of the chest to predelivery proportions allows for passive inspiration of air. This initial step helps to reduce viscous forces that must be overcome in order to establish an air-liquid interface in the alveoli.[284]

The forces that must be overcome in the first breaths include the viscosity of the lung fluid column, the tissue resistive forces (compliance), and surface tension forces at the air-liquid interfaces. The viscosity of lung fluid provides resistance to movement of fluid in the airways. The maximal resistance takes place at the beginning of the first breath, and the greatest displacement occurs in the trachea.[184] The dissipation of tracheal fluid during the vaginal squeeze reduces the amount of pressure that must be generated to move the liquid column down the conducting airways.

As the column progresses down the conducting branches, the total surface area of the air-liquid interface increases as the bronchiole diameter is progressively reduced. The surface tension, however, increases.[174] The sur-

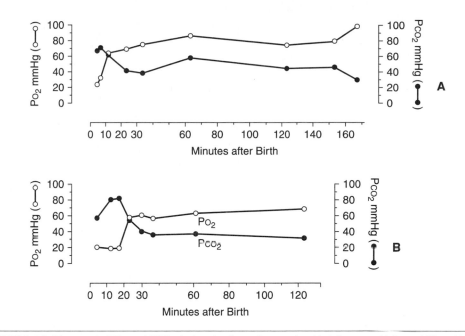

FIGURE **9-14** Changes in PO$_2$ and PCO$_2$ during the first minutes after birth in normal infants **(A)** and in asphyxiated infants **(B)** with delayed onset of respiration. (Courtesy of R.Turnell, M.D. From Carlo, W.A. & DiFiore, J.M. [2002]. Assessment of pulmonary function. In A.A. Fanaroff & R.J. Martin [Eds.]. *Neonatal and perinatal medicine: Diseases of the fetus and infant* [7th ed.]. St. Louis: Mosby.)

face tension forces are the most difficult forces to overcome during the first breath events. The maximal forces are encountered where the radial curvature of the airways is smallest (terminal bronchioles); here the viscous forces are at their nadir.[174,184,251] In this locality the intraluminal pressure must be at its peak in order to prevent closure by tension in the intraluminal walls (Laplace relationship).[251] If these smaller airways were fluid-filled only (no air-liquid interface), the pressures needed would be considerably less; however, this would make alveolar expansion more difficult. Surface tension forces drop again once air enters the terminal air sacs.[174,251] As the air-liquid interface is established, tubular myelin is formed and spreads over the lining layer.[200] During labor and immediately after birth, alveolar surfactant production increases with secretion of lamellar bodies and formation of tubular myelin.[123]

Tissue resistive forces at birth are unknown. However, the fluid within the terminal air sacs enhances air introduction, possibly by modifying the configuration of the smaller units of the lung. The fluid enlarges the radius of the alveolar ducts and terminal air sac, thereby facilitating expansion (Laplace relationship). The lung fluid also reduces the possibility of obstruction of the small ducts by cellular debris.

At birth the lungs must move from secretion to absorption of lung fluid or the infant would rapidly succumb, drowning in his or her own secretions. Because lung fluid production slows in late pregnancy and absorption of lung fluid begins in early labor, after birth only about 35% of the original lung fluid volume needs to be cleared.[125,200,228] Ventilation of the lungs leads to liquid dispersion across the pulmonary epithelium (Figure 9-15). The pulmonary epithelium undergoes a reversible increase in solute permeability, leading to a rapid transfer of lung fluid solutes. The interstitial spaces and lymphatics become distended during the first 5 to 6 hours of life and an increase in pulmonary lymph flow can be seen.[248] Removal of lung fluid is mediated by differences in protein in the interstitial space and blood versus lung fluid. This creates an osmotic gradient that pulls liquid from the lungs into the interstitial space and then into the capillaries.[21,164] Approximately 10% to 20% of lung fluid is reabsorbed by the lymphatics.[21]

The drop in pulmonary vascular resistance with aeration and the rise in oxygen tension increase the number of alveolar capillaries perfused, resulting in an increase in blood flow and fluid removal capacity. With the increased lymphatic flow and the dramatic change in the pulmonary blood flow, lung fluid is dispersed within the first few hours after delivery.

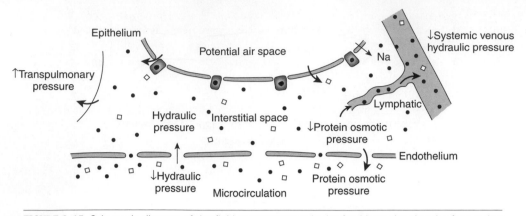

FIGURE **9-15** Schematic diagram of the fluid compartments in the fetal lung showing the forces that affect fluid clearance near birth. *Circles,* albumin molecules; *squares,* globulin. (From Bland, R.D. [1987]. Pathogenesis of pulmonary edema after preterm birth. *Adv Pediatr, 34,* 175.)

During the interval between recoil and the generation of first breath pressures, the infant may generate a positive pressure within the mouth by glossopharyngeal breathing. This "frog breathing" may build enough pressure to facilitate lung expansion and reduce the pressure needed during the first inspiration. This is probably not a significant source of pressure in most infants.[174,183]

Another contributor to lung expansion is the increase in pulmonary blood flow with birth. The increased flow is due to compression of the placenta during labor and delivery with transfer of blood to the fetus and neonate.[164] Jaykka proposed that this flow leads to capillary erection (expansion) as pulmonary capillaries uncoil and may increase transpulmonary pressure and lung stability.[120,121] Because alveoli are attached to their surrounding capillary network by elastic fibers in the extracellular matrix, expansion of the capillaries would pull open the alveoli to allow air entry.[69,164] Mercer and Skovgaard recently proposed that neonatal transition was dependent on the presence of adequate blood volume (to mediate capillary erection and alveolar opening in the lungs) and red blood cell volume for oxygen delivery to stimulate respiration and maintenance of oxygenation.[164] Thus placental transfusion may have an important role in respiratory transition.[164]

The first diaphragmatic inspiration has been noted to begin within 9 seconds of delivery and generates very large positive intrathoracic pressures (mean, 70 cmH$_2$O). Air enters as soon as the intrathoracic pressure begins to drop, with mean inspiratory pressures of 30 to 35 cmH$_2$O pressure.[174] The large transpulmonary pressure generated by the diaphragm lasts only 0.5 to 1 second, pulling in 10 to 70 ml of air. The alveolar lining layer becomes es-

tablished after the first breath, allowing the molecules of surfactant to reduce the surface tension during expiration.[184] The first expiration is also active, establishing a residual volume of air. The magnitude of the expiratory pressure contributes to FRC formation, even distribution of air, and elimination of lung fluid.[174] The second and third breaths are similar to the first but require less pressure in that the small airways are open and surface active forces are diminished.[184] Lung expansion augments surfactant secretion, providing alveolar stability and FRC formation.

By 10 minutes of age, the FRC is equal to 17 ml/kg, and at 30 minutes it is equal to 25 to 35 ml/kg.[106] The return of muscle tone after the first breath helps to maintain FRC by providing chest wall stability.[174]

Lung compliance is four times greater by day 1 and continues to increase gradually over the first week. Flow resistance decreases by one half to one fourth during this time, and the distribution of ventilation is as even after day 1 as it is on day 3.[174] The total work of the first breath is equivalent to the cry of an infant who is several days old.

Structural and functional changes in the pulmonary circulation occur after birth, with extensive remodeling of the pulmonary arteries during the first weeks after birth. Changes in the pulmonary vasculature and pulmonary vascular resistance after birth are discussed further in Chapter 8. In conjunction with the local vascular changes in the pulmonary bed, there are major organizational changes within the cardiovascular system. The first breath events and cardiovascular events (see Chapter 8) are interdependent and must occur together for transition to be successful.

Control of Respiration

The goal of respiration is to meet the oxygen and carbon dioxide metabolic demands of the organism through extraction of oxygen from the atmosphere and removal of carbon dioxide produced by the organism. The brain's respiratory center is responsible for matching the level of ventilation to the metabolic demand. The assessment of metabolic needs and alteration of ventilation is accomplished by the chemoreceptors.

Chemoreceptors

The peripheral chemoreceptors (carotid and aortic bodies) sense PaO_2 and $PaCO_2$, and the central chemoreceptors (medullary) are sensitive to PCO_2^- [H^+] in the extracellular fluid of the brain. When the PaO_2 falls below the acceptable range, the chemoreceptors increase the efferent neural activity to the respiratory center (brain), resulting in an increase in ventilation. At birth, the fetal PaO_2 of approximately 25 mmHg (sufficient for intrauterine growth) increases to 50 mmHg with the first few breaths and then to 70 mmHg in the first hours. This increase in oxygen tension exceeds the fetal demands for oxygen, yielding a relative neonatal hyperoxia at birth. This change in oxygen tension causes the chemoreceptors to become less responsive to stimuli during the first few days of life.[20] This implies that fluctuations in oxygen tension levels may not lead to a chemoreceptor response during these early days of neonatal life.[55] After this lag time, however, the chemoreceptors reset and become oxygen-sensitive and a major controller of respiration.[55,204]

Sustained hyperventilatory efforts during hypoxia cannot be maintained by the neonate. Studies in human and animal newborns have demonstrated that an initial hyperventilatory response is achieved but is followed by a subsequent fall in ventilation and oxygen tensions.[3,28] The reason for this lack of sustained response is unknown but may be due to feeble chemoreceptor output, a central inhibitory effect of hypoxia on ventilation, or changes in pulmonary mechanics.[55]

The neonate's response to carbon dioxide is also limited in the early neonatal period. Although this is more mature than the response to hypoxia, the neonate can only increase ventilation by 3 to 4 times baseline ventilation in comparison to the tenfold to twentyfold increase that can be achieved by adults.[54] Along with this, the threshold of tolerance is initially higher, progressively declining over the first month of life.[95,257] This too may be due to the increased $PaCO_2$ levels found in the fetal state (45 to 50 mmHg) and the need to reset chemoreceptors.[55,204]

Modification of ventilatory patterns is dependent upon inspiratory muscle strength, rib cage rigidity and compliance, airway resistance, and lung compliance. The status of these parameters at any given time, as well as their integrative functioning, affects the performance of the respiratory pump and is mediated by specific reflex arcs.[55]

Chest Wall Reflexes

Most of the reflexes for the respiratory pump arise from the chest wall via the muscle spindles through local spinal reflex arcs and centrally mediated reflexes. The diaphragm is scantily innervated; however, the intercostal muscles have abundant fibers from which this information is obtained. These stretch-sensitive mechanoreceptors detect chest wall and workload forces.[79]

Excessive stretch is modulated by alpha motoneuron activity altering respiratory muscle activity or recruiting more muscles. Further sensory information is obtained by proprioreceptors that sense changes in rib position and tension applied across the joint space. Cutaneous stimulation of the thoracic wall causes a generalized increase in sensory and motoneuron stimulation of the respiratory muscles, augmenting muscle contractions and ventilation.[44]

Chest wall distortion during inspiration stimulates muscle spindles that trigger central reflex arcs, leading to reflex inhibition of intercostal, phrenic, and laryngeal neurons. This is possibly a protective mechanism in the neonate. Termination of distorted inefficient breathing may lead to energy conservation and reduce the possibility of muscle fatigue.[78]

Lung Reflexes

The mechanoreceptors of the large lung airways include stretch receptors, irritant receptors, and C receptors. The sensory feedback mechanisms for these receptors are along the vagus nerve to the central respiratory center.

The stretch receptors sense lung inflation and deflation, with neural output proportional to lung volume or tension.[55] Lung inflation initiates inhibitory impulses that terminate inspiration and prolong expiratory time. This is termed the *Hering-Breuer reflex.* Once triggered, respiratory frequency slows. Although not found in adults, this reflex is active in the neonate for reasons that are not well understood. It may be a protective mechanism for the neonate, because inspiratory occlusion results in an increase in inspiratory effort and inspiratory time in the term neonate. Responses in term infants vary.[135,233]

The irritant receptors of the mucosal lining in the airways are extremely sensitive to mechanical stimulation and are responsible for the cough reflex seen clinically. In infants over 35 weeks' gestation, there is the typical adult response to stimulation: increased breathing, coughing, arousal, and gross body movement. For infants less than

35 weeks, however, these responses are not usually elicited. These infants may have either no response or a brief cough followed by apnea, slowing of respiration, or immediate respiration.[80] The reason for this difference is unknown but may be due to a functional immaturity or the possibility that unmyelinated irritant receptors may be inhibitory in nature.[80,233]

Chemoreceptors provide information about the metabolic needs of the infant, and the mechanoreceptors provide information about the status of the respiratory pump. The central respiratory center integrates this information and establishes the ventilatory pattern that efficiently meets the infant's needs. Each respiratory cycle during a stable state (e.g., quiet sleep) is uniform for amplitude, duration, and waveform. Behavioral influences as well as active sleep states (rapid eye movement [REM] sleep) alter the regularity of breathing. The information received from the various receptors helps to determine the inspiratory time, the expiratory time, the lung volume at which the breath should occur (FRC), the rate of inspiration, and the braking of the expiration. The recruitment and adjustment of the various respiratory muscle groups result in the predetermined lung volume being achieved.[55,251]

The information just described is received by the respiratory controller in the brainstem, which is responsible for initiating automatic respiration and adjustments.[251] This respiratory control center is divided into three areas: the apneustic center, the pneumotaxic center, and the medullary center. The pneumotaxic center may be responsible for switching inspiration to expiration. The apneustic center seems to be responsible for cutting off inspiration. Both centers are located in the pons and neither seems to be necessary for rhythmic expiration. However, destruction of the medullary center results in apnea and is therefore thought to be responsible for respiratory rhythm.[155]

These centers are connected to the cerebral cortex via the spinal cord, thereby allowing voluntary control of respiration. The spinal cord is responsible for the integration and relay of commands to the muscles of the respiratory pump via the phrenic and intercostal nerves.

Upper Airway

The nares are oriented more vertically in infants with a shorter anteroposterior diameter. Nasal resistance is about one third the total pulmonary resistance (versus 45% in adults).[67] Neonates tend to be nasal breathers, although many term infants will breath orally with nasal occlusion.[169,208] The nasal route is the primary route due to the high position of the epiglottis and the position of the soft palate.[67]

The epiglottis and hyoid, thyroid, and cricoid cartilage are stabilized in the term infant by fatty superficial fascia. This fascia is absent in preterm infants, leading to flexibility and increasing the risk of airway obstruction.[67] The pharyngeal airway is shorter and wider in neonates, with the cricoid cartilage at the level of the fourth cervical vertebrae (versus the seventh in adults). The pharyngeal airway is also prone to collapse in preterm infants, leading to obstruction and apnea.[67]

Newborns are able to adduct their vocal cords during expiration to increase their FRC. This can lead to grunting as expired air is released across the partially closed glottis. This mechanism is often seen in more mature preterm infants or term infants with respiratory distress, but it is also noted in healthy infants during the first few days after birth. In these infants use of this mechanism is thought to assist in maintaining lung volumes during transition.[67]

Respiratory Pump

The movement of gas in and out of the lungs is based on the functioning of the respiratory pump, which is composed of the rib cage and respiratory muscles. The pump must move sufficient oxygen and carbon dioxide into and out of the lungs to replace the oxygen consumed and wash out the carbon dioxide that accumulates in the alveoli. Ventilatory efforts in the neonate are dependent upon the strength and endurance of the diaphragm. When the diaphragm is unable to generate the necessary energy to sustain ventilatory efforts, ventilatory assistance is required.[55]

Diaphragm

The diaphragm inserts on the lower six ribs, the sternum, and first three lumbar vertebrae. It is innervated bilaterally by the phrenic nerves and expends its work on the lung, the rib cage, and the abdomen. In order to maximize diaphragmatic work, the intercostal muscles must stabilize the rib cage and the abdominal muscles should stabilize the abdomen.[55,178] In the full-term infant the coordination of these efforts is almost nonexistent; the preterm infant is even less effective at coordinating these events. During REM sleep (the most predominant sleep state in the neonate), the intercostal and abdominal muscles are less efficient, contributing to respiratory instability.

The diaphragm works most efficiently when the dome is high in the thorax (relaxed position, optimal fiber length), increasing the thoracic volume while compressing the abdominal contents and moving the abdominal wall.[178] The neonatal diaphragm is situated differently than that of the adult. In its relaxed state it is located higher in the thorax, favoring more efficient generation of inspiratory pressures. In the adult the diaphragm is flatter and generally lower, making it more inefficient mechanically. This difference is made up for by the stability of the chest wall in the adult.

The composition of the muscle fibers in the neonate is also different. In adults, 60% of the fibers are fast-oxidative, fatigue-resistant type I fibers; 30% are type IIa fast-oxidative fatigue-sensitive fibers; and the rest are type IIb slow-oxidative, fatigue-resistant fibers.[133] In contrast, the neonatal diaphragm and intercostal muscles have a lower proportion of fatigue-resistant muscle fibers (20% type I fibers) and more type IIa fibers.[55,133] Type I fibers increase in number from 24 weeks' gestation on. At 24 weeks, they comprise 10% of the total fiber content, reaching the adult proportion at 8 months' postnatal age.[55,133]

Contraction and relaxation times, as well as the latent period, are longer in premature babies when compared with adults. A lack of sarcoplasmic reticulum in the diaphragmatic muscle may result in a slower initiation as well as termination of contractions. Therefore, when high respiratory rates occur, there may be ischemia of the muscle with fatigue related to inadequate substrate availability.[79,161] Because of these developmental patterns and other limitations (Table 9-9), the infant is particularly vulnerable to diaphragmatic muscle fatigue, especially when the work of breathing is increased. This vulnerability increases with lower gestational age.[221]

The diaphragm is attached to a chest wall that is more pliable than that of the adult. This can lead to distortion of the lower portion of the chest wall during contraction, especially if it is forceful. The decreased efficiency of the contraction and reduced V_T can make ventilation less effective, requiring adjustments in the respiratory pattern.[55]

Rib Cage and Chest Wall Muscles

The muscles of the rib cage include the external intercostal muscles (inspiration); the internal intercostal muscles (expiration); and the accessory muscles, including the sterno-cleidomastoid, pectoral, and scalene muscles. The major role of these muscles is to fixate the chest wall by tonic contraction during diaphragmatic excursion. If they are unable to accomplish this goal, collapse and distortion of the chest wall is likely to occur during inspiratory efforts. If the needed stability is provided, the contraction of the inspiratory muscles of the rib cage can contribute to the thoracic volume by elevating the anterior end of each rib. During sighing, the increase in V_T is largely due to this increased chest wall excursion.

The rib cage of the newborn is more boxlike, with nearly equal anteroposterior and transverse diameters (versus the elliptical shape of the adult) (Figure 9-16). The ribs are articulated to the rib cage more horizontally, in a position similar to that of the adult at full inspiration. This reduces the mechanical efficiency of chest wall excursions in the newborn.[153]

Rib Cage Compliance

The chest wall in the infant is cartilaginous, soft, and pliable. This design allows for compression during passage through the birth canal without rib fractures and for further growth and development. Nelson has described the rib cage as a loosely fitting glove surrounding the neonatal lung.[184] The high compliance dictates that for any given change in volume there is almost no change in pressure.[105] This increased compliance is highest in the preterm infant but is significant in the full-term infant as well. As a result, there is a tendency of the chest wall to collapse and the infant to retract as he or she tries to generate the negative pressure needed for lung expansion.[178]

Elastic recoil is that property of a body that causes it to return to its resting position after having been stretched or deformed.[185] In the older child and adult, once the chest wall has reached the FRC it tends to recoil outward; however, the tendency of the lung to collapse toward the RV provides a counterbalance.[185,251] In other words, at resting

TABLE **9-9** **Potentially Important Predisposing Factors for Diaphragmatic Fatigue in Newborns**

Problem	Predisposing Factors
Decreased efficiency	Thoracic shape/rib orientation
	Soft rib cage (magnified by prematurity)
	Rapid eye movement sleep–induced intercostal muscle activity depression
	Normally flat diaphragm with decreased zone of apposition
Decreased oxygen and/or substrate supply	Hypoxemia acidosis and/or hypotension
	Poor compensatory increase in diaphragmatic blood flow
	Insufficient nutritional intake and/or decreased substrate stores
Decreased maximal force potential	Small muscle fiber diameter
	Increased lung volume at end expiration

From Murphy, T. & Woodrum D. (1998). Functional development of respiratory muscles. In R.A. Polin & W.W. Fox (Eds,). *Fetal and neonatal physiology* (2nd ed.). Philadelphia: W.B. Saunders.

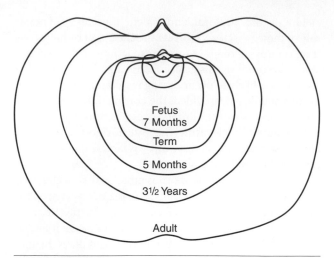

FIGURE **9-16** Superimposed outlines of thoracic skeletal contours at various ages. Outlines are aligned relative to the vertebral body. (From Fenn, W.O. & Rahn, H. [1964]. *Handbook of physiology.* Bethesda, MD: American Physiological Society.)

lung volumes (FRC) the elastic recoil of the chest wall is equal and opposite to that of the lungs.

At V_T, the chest wall of the neonate is nearly infinitely compliant. The lack of opposition by the thorax to the recoil of the lung causes the newborn's respiratory system to come to equilibrium at a resting volume very close to the collapse volume (Figure 9-17).[184] The activity of the intercostal muscles during normal breathing is a major determinant of the elastic characteristics of the chest wall and therefore the functional residual capacity. Therefore, during tidal breathing, some of the dependent airways fall into their closing volume range and the bronchioles collapse and are not in communication with the main stem bronchus. Bronchiole compliance contributes to these dynamics.

Elastic recoil of the chest wall increases during the 2 weeks after birth, although it remains considerably less than that of the adult for a long period of time. The continued change in recoil pressures is presumed to be the result of progressive ossification, improvement in intercostal muscle tone, and development of a negative pressure on the abdominal side of the diaphragm.[185]

For the infant (with a small abdomen) lying in the supine position, the outward recoil of the chest is presumably inhibited. Once the infant learns to stand and the abdomen has grown, the contents of the abdominal cavity shift away from the upper abdomen, thereby creating an increase in negative subdiaphragmatic pressure. This change in pressure favors outward recoil of the chest wall.[185]

The clinical implications of this highly compliant chest are related to the ease at which lung collapse is possible in the neonate. The low elastic recoil pressure of the neonatal lung and the high compliance of the thorax result in the majority of tidal breathing in the infant occurring near the closing capacity of the lung. This contributes to the possibility of collapse and affects gas distribution.

The mechanical liabilities of a highly compliant chest wall after delivery include a compromised ability to produce a large V_T, requiring the generation of greater pressures. This requires the infant to perform more work to move the same amount of V_T.[185] This is especially true in preterm infants with lung diseases associated with decreased lung compliance (e.g., RDS). Lung disease causes the respiratory drive (response to stimulus) to increase in an attempt to generate stronger contractions with high inspiratory pressures in order to expand stiff, noncompliant lungs.

Increased diaphragmatic force and the pliable chest wall lead to chest distortion.[55,184] Therefore a portion of the energy and force of the contraction is wasted. Retractions are the clinical signs of these distortions and are indications of the degree of inward rib cage collapse during forceful diaphragmatic contractions.[185] This increase in work of breathing can lead to fatigue and eventually apnea.

The compliance of the chest wall—combined with the compliance of the lungs—affects the closing volume, closing capacity, expiratory reserve volume, and functional residual capacity. For the neonate, this means that a high closing volume and high closing capacity combine with a low expiratory reserve volume and FRC, culminating in a propensity toward lung collapse.[184]

Mechanical Properties of the Respiratory System

The work of breathing is the cumulative product of the pressure and volume of air moved at each instant. The work is done by the muscles as energy is expended to overcome the elastic and resistive forces (compliance and resistance) of the lung and thorax as well as the frictional resistance to air movement. The respiratory muscles expend about half their energy on inspiration. The rest is stored within the tissues (which have been stretched) as potential energy. As the potential energy is released, expiration occurs passively.

There are two major sources of resistance that the respiratory muscles must overcome during each breath. These are: (1) tissue elastic resistance that is created by displacement of the lung and chest wall from their resting positions (compliance), and (2) resistance presented by gas molecules flowing through the airways.

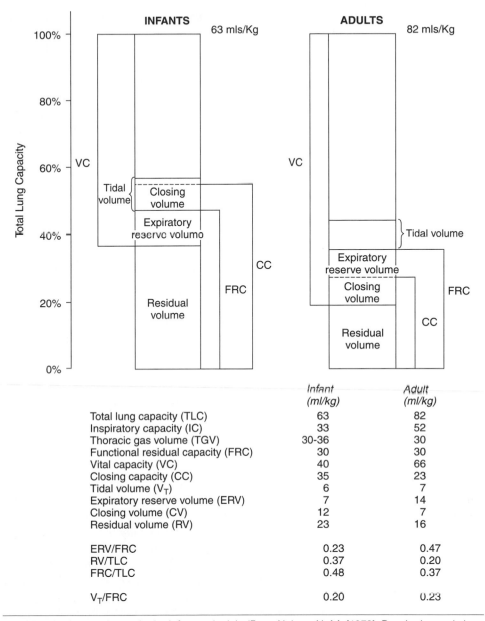

	Infant (ml/kg)	Adult (ml/kg)
Total lung capacity (TLC)	63	82
Inspiratory capacity (IC)	33	52
Thoracic gas volume (TGV)	30-36	30
Functional residual capacity (FRC)	30	30
Vital capacity (VC)	40	66
Closing capacity (CC)	35	23
Tidal volume (V_T)	6	7
Expiratory reserve volume (ERV)	7	14
Closing volume (CV)	12	7
Residual volume (RV)	23	16
ERV/FRC	0.23	0.47
RV/TLC	0.37	0.20
FRC/TLC	0.48	0.37
V_T/FRC	0.20	0.23

FIGURE **9-17** Lung volumes in the infant and adult. (From Nelson, N. M. [1976]. Respiration and circulation after birth. In C. A. Smith & N. M. Nelson [Eds.]. *The physiology of the newborn infant*. Springfield, IL: Charles C Thomas.)

The system is most efficient when the respiratory rate and V_T are set to require the minimum expenditure of work. This can be assessed by evaluating the amount of oxygen used in performing the work. Under normal circumstances the oxygen consumed is only a small fraction of the total metabolic requirement. The newborn infant expends the least amount of energy when breathing 30 to 40 breaths per minute.

Lung Compliance

The pressure gradient necessary to overcome the elastic recoil force encountered in the lung depends on V_T and lung compliance. Compliance is the measurement of the elastic properties opposing a change in volume (ml) per unit of change in pressure (cm H_2O) (Hooke law). This can be demonstrated in a pressure-volume curve (Figure 9-18) that relates a change in lung volume to the change in the

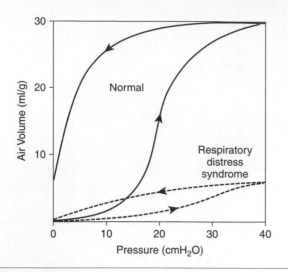

FIGURE **9-18** Air-pressure-volume curves of neonatal and abnormal lung. Volume is expressed as milliliters of air per gram of lung. The lung of an infant with respiratory distress syndrome accepts a smaller volume at all pressures. Note also that the deflation pressure-volume curve follows very closely the inflation curve for the affected lung. (From Klaus, M.H. & Fanaroff, A.A. [2001]. *Care of the high risk neonate* [5th ed.]. Philadelphia: W.B. Saunders.)

alveolar-to-intrapleural pressure gradient (i.e., transpulmonary pressure). The slope of the curve indicates the compliance. The flatter the curve, the stiffer the lung is.[176,184]

Lung compliance depends on the tissue elastic characteristics of the parenchyma, connective tissue, and blood vessels, as well as the surface tension in the alveoli and the initial lung volume before inflation. When the lung must be inflated from a very low lung volume, the required pressure gradient is greater.

For the healthy, more mature preterm infant, lung compliance is similar to that of the full-term infant. The change in lung compliance is sensed by lung stretch receptors. These receptors, along with muscle spindle fibers from the respiratory muscles, transmit information to the respiratory center in order to modify the drive necessary to maintain ventilation. Lung disease usually leads to a decrease in lung compliance, which translates to a smaller volume change for pressure change.

The most significant determinant of elastic properties is the alveolar air-liquid interface. When molecules are aligned at an air-liquid interface, they lack opposing molecules on one side; this means that the intermolecular attractive forces are unbalanced and there is a tendency for the molecules to move away from the interface. This reduces the internal surface area of the lung and therefore augments elastic recoil.

Surfactant varies surface tension, allowing for high surface tensions at large lung volumes and low tensions at low volumes. Surfactant forms an insoluble folded surface film upon compression and thereby lowers surface tension. This tends to stabilize air spaces of unequal size and prevents their collapse. Without surfactant, smaller alveoli tend to empty into larger ones, resulting in microatelectasis alternating with hyperaeration (see Figure 9-11 and the box on p. 328).

Alveolar collapse occurs in a number of diseases; probably the most notable is RDS (see Respiratory Distress Syndrome). In RDS, surfactant deficiency is directly related to gestational age and developmental immaturity of the lungs. Surfactant synthesis, however, is also dependent on normal pH and pulmonary perfusion. Therefore any disease or event that interferes with these processes may lead to surfactant deficiencies (e.g., asphyxia, hemorrhagic shock, pulmonary edema).[176]

Airway Resistance

Lung resistance is dependent upon the size and geometric arrangements of the airways, viscous resistance of the lung tissue, and the proportion of laminar to turbulent airflow. Resistance varies inversely with lung volume—meaning that the greater the lung volume, the less resistance is encountered, and vice versa. This is because the diameter of the airways increases with the expansion of the parenchyma.

Gas flows through a tube from a point of higher pressure to a point of lower pressure. Two patterns of flow have been identified based on the magnitude of the pressure drop and its relationship to the rate of gas flow. These patterns are termed *laminar* and *turbulent*. In laminar flow, resistance is determined by the radius and length of the tube during the flow. Laminar flow can become turbulent if the flow rate rises excessively or when the angle or diameter of the tube changes abruptly (e.g., at branch points).

In adults, the upper airways (especially the nose) account for the major portion of total airway resistance.[184] In neonates and children under 5 years of age, it is the peripheral airways that contribute the most to airway resistance.[174] The decreased diameter of airways (especially in the periphery) is the reason for this increased resistance. The distal airway growth in diameter and length lags behind proximal growth during the first 5 years of life. Therefore a small decrement in the caliber of airways can lead to a very large increase in peripheral airway resistance.[185]

Cartilage provides the support for stability of the conducting airways. With ongoing development, there is an increase in number of cartilage rings during the first

2 months of life and an increase in total area of support over the remainder of childhood. The lack of support in the neonate can lead to dynamic compression of the trachea during situations associated with high expiratory flow rates and increased airway resistance (e.g., crying).

In disease states, resistance is increased either by a decrease in the intraluminal size of the airway or through compression or contraction of the walls of the airway.[185] Peripheral airways are tethered open by the elastic mesh of the pulmonary parenchyma and the transmural pressure gradient (intraluminal airway pressure greater than the intrapleural pressure). During forced expiration, intrapleural pressure rises significantly; this is transmitted to the alveoli and increased even further by the pulmonary parenchyma elastic recoil pressure. Initially this maintains a favorable pressure gradient. However, a pressure drop must occur from alveolus to mouth during active expiration, and there will be a point in the airway at which intraluminal pressure will equal intrapleural pressure (equal pressure point). As the gas continues to move toward the mouth, the forces maintaining airway patency are overwhelmed and the airway will collapse.[185] If the elastic parenchyma meshwork is destroyed, as with bronchopulmonary dysplasia (BPD), airway collapse is even more likely.

Resistance increases with decreasing gestational age and with specific lung diseases (e.g., RDS, BPD) that are more prominent in preterm infants. The increased resistance is sensed by respiratory muscles, leading to an increase in ventilatory drive. Changes in the radius of the larynx or trachea because of edema (e.g., with repeated intubation for meconium aspiration) or as a result of intubation also increase resistance. This effect may be quite pronounced because the resistance is generated in the large airways, where resistance should be at its lowest.

Time Constants

Time constants reflect the combined effect of resistance and compliance on the lung (Figure 9-19). The time needed for a given lung unit to fill to 63% of its final capacity is the product of resistance and compliance. Nichols and Rogers noted that if the resistance and compliance are equal in two adjacent lung units (alveoli), the time constant will be the same and there will be no redistribution of gases between the alveoli.[185] If the time constant of one unit is longer, but the compliances remain equal, the two alveoli will eventually reach the same volume. However, the longer the time constant, the slower the filling will be due to the increased resistance. In this instance, the intraluminal pressure in the alveolus with the least resistance will be higher and lead to redistribution of its gases into the adjacent, slower-filling alveolus.

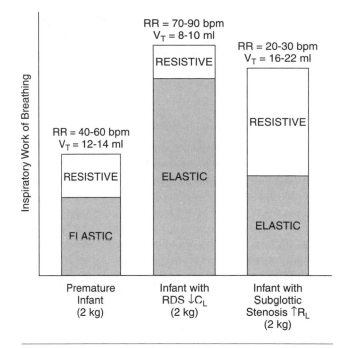

FIGURE **9-19** Relative contributions of the elastic and resistive compartments of the work of breathing in infants with normal pulmonary function, decreased compliance (C_L), and increased resistance (R_L). (From Carlo, W.A., & DiFiore, J.M. [2002]. Assessment of pulmonary function. In A.A. Fanaroff & R.J. Martin [Eds.]. *Neonatal and perinatal medicine, diseases of the fetus and infant* [7th ed.]. St. Louis: Mosby.)

The time constant can also be lengthened when compliance is increased, but resistance remains the same. In this circumstance the less compliant alveolus will fill faster than its adjacent, more compliant neighbor. This is due to the decreased volume that the less compliant alveoli can hold. Redistribution of gases will occur if inflation is interrupted prematurely due to the increased pressure in the less compliant alveolus as compared to the adjacent lung unit.[185] This redistribution of gases in the lung is not a major factor in the normal lung, in that the alveoli are relatively stable and do not change much in size.[185] This is a result of the effect of surfactant upon the lung.

Ventilation

Once air enters the lungs, it must come in contact with the blood in order to effect gas exchange. The drop in negative pressure causes air to move by bulk flow down the air passages to the level of the bronchioles. From this point forward, the movement of air into the acinar portion of the lungs is due to the random movement of the molecules from a higher area of concentration to a lower area of concentration (diffusion). Any factor that impedes the flow of gas to the acinus reduces gas exchange and influences the partial pressure of gas within the blood. Therefore the effective interface of ventilation with blood flow is responsible for the adequacy of oxygen uptake and carbon dioxide removal. In this section, the factors that affect ventilation at the alveolar level are discussed.

Dead Space Ventilation

A variable portion of each breath is not involved in gas exchange and is therefore wasted; this is considered dead space ventilation. There are two types of dead space: anatomic dead space and alveolar dead space. Anatomic dead space is that volume of gas within the conducting airways that cannot engage in gas exchange. Alveolar dead space is the volume of inspired gas that reaches the alveolus but does not participate in gas exchange because of inadequate perfusion of that alveolus. The total dead space (anatomic and alveolar) is termed physiologic dead space. Physiologic dead space is usually expressed as a fraction of the V_T and is approximately 0.3 in infants and adults.[185] Patients experiencing respiratory failure have elevated dead space–to–V_T ratios, which results in hypoxia and hypercarbia unless counteracted by an increase in the amount of air expired per minute.[185]

Pleural Pressure

The differences in pleural pressure within the lung play a significant role in determining the distribution of gases. During spontaneous breathing, a greater proportion of gas is distributed to the dependent regions of the lung. It is assumed that the difference in subatmospheric (negative) intrapleural pressure at the base and at the apex is the reason for this distribution pattern. Interestingly, alveolar pressure remains constant in all regions of the lung. Subsequently, the transpulmonary distending pressure in the dependent regions is decreased, leading to a reduced lung volume in these areas. The smaller alveoli in the dependent lung regions lie on the steeper slope of the transpulmonary pressure–to–lung volume curve, resulting in a greater portion of the V_T being directed to the dependent alveoli during normal breathing.[185] A greater portion of the pulmonary perfusion goes to the dependent regions as well, thereby matching ventilation and perfusion more closely.

Lung Volumes

Lung volumes in the newborn are illustrated in Figure 9-17.

Functional Residual Capacity

The FRC is established during the first breaths, forming the alveolar reservoir at end-expiration and allowing for continuous gas exchange between respiratory efforts and sta-

bilization of PaO_2. Normally the FRC comprises 30% to 40% of the total capacity of the lung and may change volume from breath to breath. Immediately following birth the FRC is low, increasing rapidly with successive breaths. In preterm infants with lung disease, the FRC stays low until the lung disease resolves. The goal is to keep the FRC above the passive resting volume of the lung, which may be difficult for neonates due to their pliable chest wall. The role of the FRC is crucial in the energy expenditure of the respiratory musculature. FRC minimizes the work of breathing while optimizing the compliance of the system and maintaining a gas reservoir during expiration.[55]

Closing Capacity

As noted earlier, in the neonate (especially the preterm infant) it is possible for lung volumes to be reduced below the FRC during quiet breathing, with dependent regions of the lung being closed to the main bronchi (closing capacity). When the closing capacity exceeds the FRC, the ventilation-perfusion ratio drops and hypoxia and hypercarbia occur. If total atelectasis exists, then the closing capacity exceeds not only the FRC but also the V_T, and these portions of the lung are closed during expiration and inspiration. The use of end-expiratory pressure is designed to raise the FRC above closing capacity.[185] Continuous distending pressure is used in the neonatal population when chest wall compliance leads to marked distortion and altered lung volumes, as well as during disease states associated with alveolar collapse (e.g., RDS).

The greater closing capacity seen in children under 6 years and in adults over 40 years is probably due to decreased elastic recoil in the lung.[177,179] Elastic recoil is that property of the lung that allows it to retract away from the chest wall, creating a subatmospheric pressure in the intrapleural space. The decrease in elastic recoil results in the subatmospheric pressure in the intrapleural space being raised, leading to increased airway closure in dependent regions.[185]

Perfusion

Alveolar ventilation is dependent not only on the functioning of the airways, but also on the functioning of the pulmonary vasculature. Pulmonary vascular muscle thickness is a function of gestational age, with the preterm infant having less well-developed smooth muscle. This incomplete development results in a drop in pulmonary vascular resistance much sooner after delivery, predisposing the infant to a faster onset of congestive heart failure and left-to-right shunting.[185]

Normal Pulmonary Blood Flow

The majority of pulmonary blood flow is distributed to the dependent regions of the lungs due to gravitational forces.

Ventilation-Perfusion Ratios

Ventilation-perfusion ($\dot{V}/\dot{Q}$) ratios are based on the distribution of gases, the distribution of the pulmonary circulation, and the interrelationship between these two factors. This interrelationship is affected by the rate of airflow into the lungs (which is a function of depth of inspiration, rate of inspiration, airway resistance, and lung compliance) and pulmonary circulation (which is influenced by cardiac output and pulmonary vascular resistance). The ideal ratio occurs when ventilation and perfusion are matched such that the sites available on the hemoglobin molecules are equal to the concentration of oxygen molecules in the alveoli and there is sufficient time for the diffusion of oxygen across the membranes and attachment of hemoglobin. The "ideal" lung is depicted in Figure 9-20. In this instance neither ventilation (oxygen) nor blood flow is wasted. Interestingly, the usual distribution of gases and blood is neither equal nor ideal.

Maldistribution of pulmonary blood flow is the most frequent cause of reduced oxygenation of arterial blood. The degree of nonuniformity of distribution is probably greater for pulmonary circulation than it is for gas distribution. The uneven distribution not only occurs between the two lungs but also between lobes and alveolar segments. This is usually manifested by a reduction in the PaO_2.

Distribution can range from the unventilated to the unperfused alveoli, with all degrees of variation in between. Ventilated alveoli that are not perfused compose the alveolar dead space and have PaO_2 and $PaCO_2$ values that are essentially equivalent to those of inspired air. This is because there is no alveolar gas exchange with the blood to modify the gas concentrations in the alveoli. On the other hand, alveoli that are perfused but not ventilated result in intrapulmonary shunts in which PaO_2 and $PaCO_2$ values are the same as those in mixed venous blood. In this situation, the air trapped within the alveoli equilibrates with the venous blood traversing the capillaries of the alveoli (see Figure 9-21). Some degree of gas exchange occurs in all other situations.

When there is a low ventilation-perfusion ratio (<1) the alveoli are underventilated with respect to perfusion or overperfused with respect to ventilation. In circumstances in which the alveoli are overventilated for the perfusion available, there is a high ventilation-perfusion ratio (>1). In these abnormal or disease states the ventilation-perfusion inequalities may increase in magnitude, involving greater and greater numbers of alveoli. The net result is a significant impact on gas exchange and blood gases.

In zone 1 (apex of the lung), the alveolar pressure is greater than the pulmonary artery and venous pressures. As a result, the pulmonary vessels collapse, with concomitant loss of gas exchange and wasted ventilation.[185] In zone 2, pulmonary artery pressure exceeds alveolar pressure, and blood flow resumes. The perfusion pressure increases as blood flows downward; this results in a linear increase in blood flow. Slowing of blood occurs when the pulmonary venous pressure and alveolar pressure are equal.[185] Pulmonary venous pressure and pulmonary artery pressure increase, exceeding alveolar pressure in zone 3, the base of the lungs. In the more dependent regions of this zone, the transmural pressure increases, with resultant dilation of the vessels, and blood flow increases.[185]

Posture differences between the upright adult and supine lying infant probably also affect pulmonary blood distribution. The general principles still apply, but maybe to a lesser extent. Wasted ventilation in the apices due to lack of perfusion is probably much less likely in the supine position, helping to balance some of the limitations encountered in the neonatal lung.

Abnormal Distribution of Pulmonary Blood Flow
There are numerous factors that may influence the distribution of pulmonary blood flow in the lung. One of the most significant to the neonate is hypoxia. Vasoconstriction occurs when alveolar hypoxia is encountered. If diffuse, hypoxia may result in an increase in intravascular pulmonary artery pressure, which is more intense in infants than in adults.[251]

Ventilation-Perfusion Relationships
Mismatching of ventilation and perfusion is the most common reason for hypoxia and is a frequent result of the neonatal respiratory system's liabilities. Efficient gas exchange in the lungs requires matching of pulmonary ventilation and perfusion. The relationship between ventilation and perfusion is expressed as a ratio and reflects the correlation between alveolar ventilation and capillary perfusion for the lung as a whole. $\dot{V}/\dot{Q}$ relationships are summarized in the box above.

The ventilation of the air space should be adequate to remove the carbon dioxide delivered to it from the blood, and the perfusion of the air space should be no greater than that which allows oxygenation and complete saturation of the blood on its brief passage through the alveolar capillaries. Ideal efficiency would occur if ventilation were perfectly matched to perfusion, yielding a ratio of 1 (Figure 9-20).

In healthy adults, capillary blood spends 0.75 second in the alveolus, and the oxygen/carbon dioxide exchange occurs across the 0.5-μm alveolar-capillary membrane. As the blood leaves the alveolus, the blood gas tensions are identical with those of the alveolar gas. The gas tensions achieved

Ventilation-Perfusion Relationships
($\dot{V}_A = \dot{Q}$)

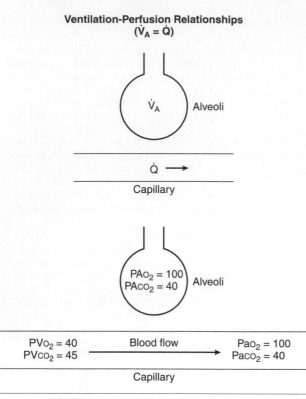

FIGURE **9-20** Ideal lung ventilation-perfusion.

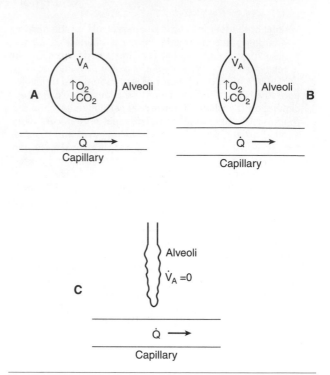

FIGURE **9-21** Ventilation-perfusion mismatching. **A,** High ventilation-perfusion. **B,** Low ventilation-perfusion. **C,** Shunt.

at equilibrium are dependent upon rate of ventilation, membrane thickness, membrane area, capillary blood flow, venous gas tensions, and inspired gas tensions.[239,261] In order for equilibrium to be achieved rapidly, the area for exchange must be large enough to allow the blood to be spread thinly over the vessel wall and blood and gas must actively mix together.[251]

Matching of ventilation to perfusion is dependent upon gravity to a large extent. Both ventilation and perfusion increase as air and blood move down the lung, with perfusion increasing more than ventilation. Right ventricular pressure is inadequate to fully perfuse the apices of the lung. On the other hand, lung weight leads to a relatively greater negative intrapleural pressure at the apex than at the base, resulting in the apical alveoli being better expanded but receiving a smaller portion of each V_T than the bases. Along with this, there is reduced perfusion in the apices creating a high $\dot{V}/\dot{Q}$ ratio.[184,239,251]

$\dot{V}/\dot{Q}$ ratios of zero are characteristic of shunts. In this situation, no ventilation takes place during the passage of blood through the lungs. The pulmonary capillary blood arrives in the left atrium with the same gas tensions it had when it was mixed venous blood. Examples of shunts include the normal bronchial and thebesian circulations, perfusion of an atelectatic area, venoarterial shunts, and cyanotic congenital heart disease with blood flow directly from the right to the left side of the heart.

High $\dot{V}/\dot{Q}$ ratios (Figure 9-21, *A*) are the result of increased dead space and may occur if the blood is spread in an extremely thin film over a very large surface area or if blood is vigorously mixed with large volumes of air. Rapid equilibration occurs, but a large amount of ventilation is required.[251] Here there is wasted ventilation, either in anatomic conducting airways or in poorly perfused alveoli (alveolar dead space). Thus a large amount of ventilation is wasted on a relatively small amount of blood without significantly changing the oxygen content. This inefficient gas exchange will eventually result in carbon dioxide retention.[185]

On the other hand, alveolar underventilation results in low $\dot{V}/\dot{Q}$ ratios (Figure 9-21, *B*). In this situation, ventilation is low in relation to perfusion but not entirely absent. This is the normal state for the lung bases in an erect position. It is also found in disease in which airway obstruction reduces ventilation to alveolar units (e.g., asthma, CF).

The blood perfusing the underventilated alveoli is incompletely oxygenated and a lower amount of carbon dioxide is removed. Partial venoarterial shunts contribute incomplete arterialized blood to the arterial stream; this is termed *venous admixture*. This is reflected in an elevated partial pressure of carbon dioxide upon blood gas evaluation.

Abnormalities of $\dot{V}/\dot{Q}$ ratios may be secondary to either too much or too little ventilation to an area with normal blood flow, too much or too little blood flow with normal ventilation, or some combination of the two. Whichever occurs, the lung's regulatory mechanisms work to achieve and maintain the ideal. In areas where the $\dot{V}/\dot{Q}$ ratio is high and carbon dioxide levels are low, local airway constriction occurs in order to reduce the amount of ventilation going to the area. When the opposite occurs, the airways dilate in an attempt to increase ventilation to the area and improve the carbon dioxide exchange. When oxygenation is also affected and low alveolar oxygen concentrations are found, the lung reduces blood flow to the region. These mechanisms are finite, however.

In newborns, most of the ventilated areas are well perfused and there is little dead space. However, in newborn infants significant amounts of perfusion are wasted on unexpanded air spaces (intrapulmonary shunts) as transitional events progress. The lower PaO_2 in the newborn demonstrates the widened alveolar-to-arterial PO_2 gradient, reflecting the increased venous admixture. Although perfusion of unexpanded air spaces may play a significant role in this, the continued right-to-left shunting through transitional circulatory circuits is another contributory factor. The premature infant is at even greater risk for shunting and venous admixture due to developmental immaturity.[139]

Intrapulmonary shunting (Figure 9-21, *C*) and wasted ventilation are normal features of the newborn lung. The latter results from transition from fluid-filled to air-filled lungs, in which alveoli are underventilated but normally perfused. These effects begin to dissipate after 1 to 2 hours of air breathing. During the first few days of life, the neonatal lung—compared to that of the adult—has a greater shunt component and a larger proportion of low $\dot{V}/\dot{Q}$ areas. However, V_T, alveolar volume, and dead space volume per breath are similar (when expressed in ml/kg). These arterial-alveolar differences in both oxygen and carbon dioxide persist in the full-term infant for about a week due to the venoarterial shunting. These gradually dissipate and adult values are achieved.[184,239]

Effect of $\dot{V}/\dot{Q}$ Mismatching on Oxygen

As inspired gas moves to the level of the arterial circulation, there is a stepwise decrease in oxygen tension. This results in reduced oxygen content in the alveoli; however, alveolar oxygen levels remain higher than those in the arterial blood. This maintains a concentration gradient that supports oxygen diffusion. If the ideal were maintained, at the end of equilibration the alveolar and arterial oxygen concentrations would be the same. This, however, is not the case. There remains a difference between the two ($AaDO_2$), which is reflective of the imperfect matching of ventilation to perfusion (see Figure 9-21).

Under normal circumstances this difference is relatively small and is secondary to the anatomic shunts through the thebesian and bronchial circulations. The hypoxemic patient, however, may have additional shunts (congenital heart disease) or increased $\dot{V}/\dot{Q}$ mismatching. Both situations result in an increased venous admixture.

$\dot{V}/\dot{Q}$ mismatching affects oxygenation by lowering the arterial PO_2 and widening the $AaDO_2$. This occurs for two reasons, the first being an increased blood flow through low $\dot{V}/\dot{Q}$ segments rather than high $\dot{V}/\dot{Q}$ segments. This results in an increased volume of desaturated blood. The second reason is the sigmoid shape of the oxygen-hemoglobin dissociation curve. This implies that the alveolar PO_2 is not proportional to oxygen content or saturation.

On the oxygen-hemoglobin dissociation curve, low $\dot{V}/\dot{Q}$ segments, with lower alveolar PO_2 values, will have a proportionately greater drop in oxygen content. This is because of their position on the steep portion of the curve. The high $\dot{V}/\dot{Q}$ segments will have higher alveolar PO_2 values but will not exhibit the expected increase in oxygen content because they lie on the flat portion of the curve. In this area of the curve, changes in PO_2 have very little effect on oxygen content or saturation. The net effect is one of low $\dot{V}/\dot{Q}$ segments negating high ones. Although the oxygen content is higher in the latter, it is not high enough to compensate for the markedly lower oxygen content found in the low $\dot{V}/\dot{Q}$ segments. Therefore arterial desaturation occurs.

Measurement of $\dot{V}/\dot{Q}$ mismatching as it relates to desaturation is difficult. Venous admixture is a convenient way to describe the amount of mixed venous blood it would take to obtain the observed arterial oxygen content. Venous admixture can be expressed as the ratio of shunted blood to total pulmonary blood flow, reflecting the efficiency of the lung in oxygenating the blood. The magnitude of this ratio determines in part what effect an increase in fractional inspired oxygen (FIO_2) will have on PaO_2. If the ratio is equal to zero, there will be a linear increase in PaO_2 with increasing inspired oxygen. Once the ratio is 0.5 or greater, increasing the FIO_2 will have no effect on PaO_2.[185]

Effect of $\dot{V}/\dot{Q}$ Mismatching on Carbon Dioxide

$PaCO_2$ is determined mainly by the degree of alveolar ventilation in relation to the carbon dioxide produced by the cells. When alveolar ventilation is reduced secondary to an increase in alveolar dead space (alveoli are ventilated but not perfused or underperfused), carbon dioxide levels in the blood begin to rise. This is reflected in the widened gradient between end-expiratory PCO_2 and alveolar PCO_2, with end-expiratory PCO_2 being lower due to the addition of alveolar dead space gas, which does not contain carbon dioxide.[185]

The difference between alveolar and capillary PCO_2 is usually low due to the diffusibility of carbon dioxide. This means that even with a large venous admixture load there would be only a slight increase in arterial PCO_2. The small change occurs because the carbon dioxide dissociation curve is linear and relatively steep (within the normal range), meaning that large changes in carbon dioxide content produce small changes in carbon dioxide tension.

Developmental Differences in V̇/Q̇ Matching

In full-term infants, markedly lower PaO_2 levels are found. This is indicative of a widened alveolar-to-arterial PO_2 gradient and an increase in venous admixture being added to the arterial blood. The persistent right-to-left shunting through fetal vascular channels—along with atelectatic areas of the lung being perfused—is the source of the admixture. In adults the major component of venous admixture is the maldistribution of ventilation.[185]

This alteration stabilizes as transition progresses, lasting a week or so in the full-term infant. The preterm infant, however, is at greater risk for desaturation because of increased chest wall deformation and increased ductal shunting. For the preterm infant it may be several weeks before complete transition and stabilization occur.[184]

Hypoxemia and thermal stress may result in ductal opening and shunting during the early transitional period for both full-term and preterm infants. It is not until late infancy and early childhood that venous admixture falls to adult levels. Beyond 7 years of age, the PaO_2 does not vary much, stabilizing between 95 and 100 mmHg.[185]

Alveolar-Capillary Membrane

The alveolar-capillary membrane is the physical barrier separating the alveolar gases from the pulmonary capillary blood. The barrier also helps prevent liquid movement from the circulation to the alveolus, thereby avoiding alveolar flooding and collapse. Transudation of fluid resulting in pulmonary edema is a major cause of respiratory failure in all age groups.

Diffusion is the movement of gases from an area of high concentration to an area of lower concentration until equi-

librium is achieved. This is the mechanism by which gas exchange occurs at the alveolar-capillary membrane. The rate of diffusion is directly proportional to the surface area available, and the solubility of the gases and is inversely proportional to the diffusion distance. The diffusion capacity for oxygen is greatly affected by the time it takes for the oxygen to combine with hemoglobin. The surface area in the normal lung is determined by the amount of ventilated and perfused tissue available, increasing with age, height, and body surface area.

Oxygen-Hemoglobin Dissociation Curve

Because of the low-oxygen environment in which the fetus lives, the need for an increased affinity for oxygen is essential to survival. HbF (see Chapter 7) alters this affinity, and 2,3-diphosphoglycerate (2,3-DPG) regulates it.[59] When 2,3-DPG binds with fetal gamma chains, it does not lower oxygen affinity as it does with adult hemoglobin beta chains. The fetal oxygen-hemoglobin dissociation curve therefore lies to the left of the adult curve (Figure 9-22). This means that in the fetus and neonate the affinity of oxygen for hemoglobin is greater and the release of oxygen to the tissues is somewhat less than in the adult at any given PO_2. The oxygen-hemoglobin dissociation curve is reviewed in the box on p. 315.

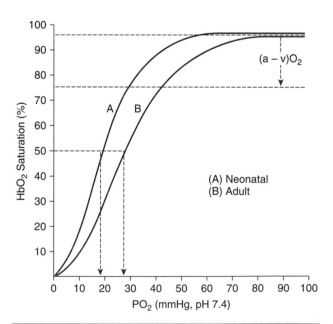

FIGURE **9-22** Oxyhemoglobin curves of blood from term infants at birth and from adults. (From Delivoria-Papadopoulos, M. & McGowen, J.E. [1998]. In R.A. Polin & W.W. Fox [Eds.]. *Fetal and neonatal physiology* [2nd ed.]. Philadelphia: W.B. Saunders.)

Oxygen Consumption

Oxygen consumption in the newly born infant is twice that of the adult in relation to weight. One of the major factors affecting oxygen consumption in the neonate is temperature (see Chapter 19). The neutral thermal environment is that environmental temperature at which oxygen consumption is minimal. Small changes in environmental temperature can result in dramatic increases in oxygen consumption. A decrease of 2° C in environmental temperature can double oxygen requirements. If the infant is unable to increase delivery to meet these needs, tissue oxygenation falls and may become insufficient. When oxygen consumption is no longer possible, the cell switches to anaerobic metabolism to meet energy and work needs.

Tissue Respiration

The ultimate purpose of oxygenation of arterial blood is for consumption by the cells during aerobic metabolism. Aerobic metabolism is desirable because 20 times more energy is made available when substrates are metabolized aerobically versus anaerobically.[185] Molecular oxygen is used in oxidation-reduction reactions in cells, in which oxidation is the loss of electrons from an atom or molecule and reduction is the gain of electrons.[177]

When one substance is oxidized, another is reduced. Reducing agents give up electrons; electron acceptors are oxidizing agents. Oxygen is an oxidizing agent. Food molecules (substrate), such as glucose, are reducing agents. Within the cells of the body, oxygen serves as final acceptor in the process of cell respiration. Energy is derived from this process and is used to form adenosine triphosphate (ATP) from adenosine diphosphate (ADP) and inorganic phosphate. When energy is later released, ATP is hydrolyzed to ADP. It is the hydrolysis reaction and cellular work activities that allow ATP to provide the energy to accomplish cellular functions. Hypoxia and hyperoxia are discussed in Clinical Implications for Neonatal Care.

CLINICAL IMPLICATIONS FOR NEONATAL CARE

Although there are many liabilities within the neonatal respiratory system, the healthy term infant achieves transition to the extrauterine environment without any difficulties. However, the developmental stage of the system does increase the possibility of respiratory distress and failure above that seen in older individuals. Both anatomic and functional development are required to achieve adult functioning; therefore both contribute to respiratory vulnerability and the risk of distress. Implications of neonatal respiratory system characteristics are summarized in Table 9-10.

Anatomic risk factors include the incomplete development of the bone and cartilage that make up the thoracic cavity and are a part of the respiratory pump. The increased compliance of the thorax makes it extremely important that the intercostal muscles be able to contract and fixate the chest so that adequate pressure can be generated and inspiration occurs. Although full-term infants appear to compensate well, the intercostal muscles and accessory muscles are still not completely developed. This contributes to diaphragmatic breathing and chest wall instability, which can lead to higher closing volumes and a decreased FRC. In disease states in which decreased resistance occurs, the inspiratory pressures necessary to fill the lungs may result in deformation of the chest wall.

The ability to stabilize the chest wall is directly related to increasing gestational age. Therefore, premature infants are highly susceptible to chest wall deformation and atelectasis during tidal breathing. This may result in hypoxemia, hypercarbia, and apnea, necessitating supplemental oxygen or ventilatory support.

Airway resistance is increased due to the smaller nares, shorter airways with multiple bifurcations, and peripheral airway diameter. Therefore upper airway congestion and minor small airway infections may create tremendous resistance and place the infant at risk for respiratory distress, muscle fatigue, and respiratory failure. Edema secondary to trauma or infection of upper airway passages can easily result in obstruction with a marked increase in resistance to airflow. This distress can be seen in nasal flaring, retractions, and tachypnea.

Until the age of 5 years, the small peripheral airways contribute 50% of the airway resistance that must be overcome. This is compared with 20% in the adult, who has a much larger cross-sectional area for flow. Bronchi constrict in response to numerous factors, including inhaled irritants, hypoxemia, hypercarbia, and cold. This constriction significantly increases airway resistance and the work of breathing.

The surface area of the lung is also decreased because of the characteristic structure of the chest. The ribs are rounder, giving the typical barrel chest configuration seen in the full-term infant. However, this results in thoracic crowding due to the relative size of the abdominal organs. The surface area of the lung is consequently decreased and lung expansion is reduced.

The lung is smaller and because of this the compliance is decreased. If compounded by disease states that reduce elasticity (e.g., pulmonary congestion, pulmonary fibrosis), the compliance drops even further and the work of breathing must increase in order to compensate.

TABLE **9-10**   Implications of Alterations in Respiratory Function in Neonates

ALTERATION	IMPLICATION
Immature alveoli; decreased size and number of alveoli	Risk of respiratory insufficiency and pulmonary problems
Thicker alveolar wall; decreased alveolar surface area	Less efficient gas transport and exchange
Continued development of alveoli until childhood	Possibly opportunity to reduce effects of discrete lung injury
Decreased lung elastic tissue and recoil	Decreased lung compliance requiring higher pressures and more work to expand
	Increased risk of atelectasis
Fewer pores and channels for collateral ventilation	Greater distress with airway obstruction
	Increased risk of air leak and pulmonary edema
	Increased risk of atelectasis
Compliant boxlike rib cage with almost horizontal insertion of ribs and immature musculature	Difficulty in taking deep breaths
	Less effective movement of thoracic cage
	Less effective in generating intrathoracic pressures needed for lung expansion
	Greater reliance on diaphragmatic and abdominal musculature for respiration
	Retractions
	Difficulty maintaining functional residual capacity and increasing tidal volume
	Risk of atelectasis
	Increased work of breathing
Reduced diaphragm movement and maximal force potential, with more horizontal position and smaller muscle fiber diameter	Less effective respiratory movement
	Difficulty generating negative intrathoracic pressures
	Risk of atelectasis
	Possible increased risk of muscle fatigue with respiratory insufficiency and failure
Tendency to nose breathe; altered position of larynx and epiglottis	Enhanced ability to synchronize swallowing and breathing
	Risk of airway obstruction
	Possibly more difficult to intubate
Small compliant airway passages with higher airway resistance and immature reflexes	Risk of airway obstruction and apnea
Increased pulmonary vascular resistance with sensitive pulmonary arterioles	Risk of ductal shunting and hypoxemia with events such as hypoxia, acidosis, hypothermia, hypoglycemia, and hypercarbia
	Possible protection against the development of congestive heart failure in first few weeks in infants with defects (e.g., a large ventricular septal defect)
Increased oxygen consumption	Increased respiratory rate and work of breathing
	Risk of hypoxia
Increased intrapulmonary right-left shunting	Increased risk of atelectasis with wasted ventilation
	Lower $PaCO_2$
Immature development of lung capillary basement membrane	More vulnerable to collapse of terminal bronchioles and alveoli
Decreased functional residual capacity	Less oxygen reserves with increased risk of atelectasis and hypoxia
	Increased work of breathing
Closing volume nearer tidal volume	Areas of airway collapse and atelectasis
	Risk of hypoxia and hypercarbia
	Increased work of breathing
Immaturity of pulmonary surfactant system in immature infants	Increased risk of atelectasis and respiratory distress syndrome
	Increased work of breathing
Immature respiratory control	Irregular respiration with periodic breathing
	Altered respiratory threshold
	Instability of respiratory drive
	Risk of apnea
	Inability to rapidly alter depth of respiration
	Difficulty in compensating for hypoxemia and hypercarbia

Adapted from Blackburn, S. (1992). Alterations in the respiratory system in the neonate: Implications for practice. *J Perinat Neonat Nurs, 6*(2), 46.

Cartilaginous support is essential for the stability of the conducting airways. This too is a function of gestational age and development. Cartilage rings continue to increase in number for up to 2 months in age. Weakness secondary to lack of support can result in dynamic compression of the trachea in situations associated with high expiratory flow rates and increased airway resistance. Although bronchiolitis and asthma are common disease entities that cause this, it can also occur during episodes of crying, resulting in reduced saturations.

The gas-exchanging portion of the lung in the full-term infant is made up of terminal air sacs and alveoli. Terminal air sacs lack the cupped shape of alveoli and are longer and narrower. They require higher pressures in order to maintain expansion, and once collapsed, increased pressures must be generated in order to open them. The alveoli that are present are smaller and predisposed to collapse.

The surface area available for diffusion is reduced in the neonate. During disease states, this may be reduced even further, requiring an increase in minute ventilation. Much of neonatal disease may be related to an alteration in functional residual capacity, closing capacity, or both. When the closing capacity is high, the pleural pressure exceeds the intraluminal pressure resulting in early closure of bronchi, making them unavailable for gas exchange. A reduction in FRC can lead to unstable blood gases between respiratory efforts.

Without collateral ventilation the neonate cannot divert ventilation to distal airways when obstruction occurs. Currently no anatomic pathways have been found on histologic sectioning of neonatal lungs. However, radiologic evidence suggests that these alternative pathways may exist. Without channels for collateral ventilation, there is an increased risk for atelectasis or emphysematous change and ventilation-perfusion mismatching.[185]

Biochemical immaturity of the surfactant system can result in progressive atelectasis. Primary surfactant deficiency is found in premature infants, resulting in RDS. However, surfactant production may be interrupted by numerous causes, including cytogenic oxygen toxicity, ischemia of the pulmonary bed, pulmonary edema, and hemorrhagic shock. Synthesis of surface-active material is dependent upon a normal pH and adequate pulmonary perfusion.

Prematurity may also result in increased susceptibility to oxygen-induced cytotoxicity. This AOS parallels the maturation of the surfactant system, both occurring late in gestation. Without the ability to detoxify reactive oxygen metabolites, the metabolites are released into the immediate environment, where they can injure normal cells.[50] This may lead to cell death and cause pulmonary edema, surfactant synthesis disruption, and scarring of lung tissues.

Physiologic Basis for Clinical Findings

The presence of increased work of breathing indicates a primary pulmonary disorder. The signs of increased work of breathing are chest wall retractions (subcostal, intercostal, suprasternal) and the use of accessory muscles (alar flare). Patients with respiratory failure have elevated ratios of dead space volume to V_T; such a condition results in hypoxia and hypercarbia unless counteracted by an increase in expired minute ventilation.[283] Respiratory patterns change with increased respiratory work.

In mild to moderate disease there is tachypnea, slight substernal and intercostal retractions, slight increase in anterior-to-posterior diameter, and intermittent expiratory grunting without cyanosis. Retractions occur because of the increased compliance of the chest wall, the immaturity of the intercostal muscles, and the increased inspiratory pressure generated. As the severity of the disease increases, the retractions become more marked. Deformation of the chest leads to paradoxical breathing (asynchrony of chest and abdominal movements), which is the result of diaphragm fatigue, inability of the intercostal muscles to fixate the chest wall, and increased inspiratory pressures.

Expiratory grunting elevates the end-expiratory pressure and slows the expiratory flow rate. This is accomplished by laryngeal braking through partial closure of the glottis. These maneuvers help maintain expansion and preserve oxygenation between respirations. The severity of lung disease can be determined by the frequency and loudness of the grunting. Nasal flaring results from increased inspiratory pressure.

Tachypnea may be the only sign of abnormalities in lung functioning. It is the most efficient way for neonates to increase ventilation and compensate for hypoxia and hypercarbia. Respiratory rates drop as fatigue sets in.

Periodic Breathing and Apnea of Prematurity

Breathing in newborn, especially preterm infants, tends to be irregular, with marked breath-to-breath variability and episodes of periodic breathing.[204] Periodic breathing is defined as "pauses in respiratory movements that last for up to 20 seconds alternating with breathing."[204] Periodic breathing is common in preterm infants and is also seen in term infants, and even adults, at altitude. Periodic breathing is thought to be benign.[204] Mechanisms for periodic breathing and apnea are unclear but probably due to alterations in or instability of the respiratory control center. These patterns are more common during REM sleep, possibly due to decreased intercostal muscle tone, diaphragmatic activity, and upper airway adductor muscles during REM sleep.[171,204]

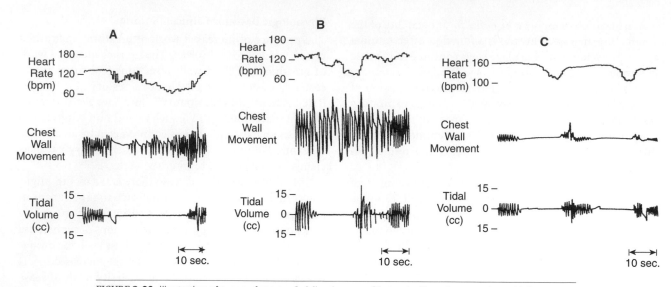

FIGURE **9-23** Illustration of types of apnea. **A,** Mixed apnea. Obstructed breaths precede and follow a central respiratory pause. **B,** Obstructive apnea. Breathing efforts continue, although no nasal airflow occurs. **C,** Central apnea. Both nasal airflow and breathing effort ceases simultaneously. (From Miller, M. [1986]. Diagnostic methods and clinical disorders in children. In N. Edelman & T. Santiago [Eds.]. *Breathing disorders of sleep.* New York: Churchill Livingstone.)

Apnea involves longer pauses and changes in heart rate, often to less than 80 beats per minute. Three types of apnea have been described in preterm infants: central (10% to 25% of the episodes), obstructive (10% to 20%) and mixed (50% to 75%).[170,204] Central apnea is characterized by no air flow or breathing effort and obstructive apnea by no air flow with breathing efforts. Mixed apnea begins as central apnea and ends as obstructive.[171,204] These patterns are illustrate in Figure 9-23.

Apnea is common in preterm infants, and more frequent in infants with chronic lung disease or other respiratory problems. Physiologic immaturity and depression of the respiratory drive, sleep state, less well-developed ventilatory responses to carbon dioxide and perhaps oxygen, altered responses to sensory input by the upper airway and a predisposition to pharyngeal collapse may all contribute to apnea of prematurity.[171,204] Factors related to apnea in the preterm infant are summarized in Table 9-11. Methylxanthines (e.g., caffeine, theophylline) are used in management of the preterm infant with apnea. These agents have a central stimulatory effect on brainstem respiratory structures.[171]

Hypoxia and Hyperoxia
Hypoxia

Hypoxia is a decreased oxygen level of the tissues, while hypoxemia is a decreased oxygen content of the blood. When hypoxia occurs, aerobic metabolism is impaired and there is a subsequent depletion in the supply of ATP available.

Therefore those processes that require energy will not occur. If the hypoxic event is not too severe or too long, cellular activities may be disrupted only for a period of time, and any damage is reversible.

Cell death occurs when the loss of ATP leads to failure of the sodium pump. Once pump failure develops, sodium is free to flow into the cell, bringing water with it. The cell and intracellular structures swell with this increased fluid volume. Along with this, anaerobic metabolism is activated, leading to a fall in cellular pH. The lowered pH interferes with enzyme activities and alters the permeability of the cell membrane. Increased permeability allows calcium to diffuse into the cell, resulting in oxidative phosphorylation uncoupling and a further reduction in ATP formation. As the fluid influx increases, the ribosomes located on the endoplasmic reticulum are shed, and protein synthesis is disrupted.[177,185]

Cell rupture and death may occur if enzymes leak from the intracellular lysosomes. Once released into the intracellular fluid, the enzymes are activated by the low pH, and cell disintegration is inevitable. Enzyme levels (e.g., creatinine phosphokinase) can be measured once cellular disintegration occurs and the enzymes are released into the extracellular fluid.

Abnormal functioning of the organ systems is due to the energy-dependent cellular activities. In the brain, aerobic metabolism is necessary for maintaining the sodium-potassium pump, which allows for nerve impulse transmission and synthesis of the synaptic chemi-

TABLE **9-11**   **Factors Related to Apnea in Immature Infants**

OBSERVATION	EXPLANATION
Hypoxemia causes respiratory depression and results in hypoventilation in the neonate instead of sustain hyperventilation as in the adult.	Hypoxemic depression in the young infant is centrally mediated and not overridden by stimulation from peripheral chemoreceptors.
Hypercapnea causes hyperventilation as in the adult, with diminished response in apneic versus nonapneic infants.	Decreased hypercapnic ventilatory response in apneic infants may be secondary to central neural mechanisms or respiratory muscle fatigues.
Obstructed inspiratory efforts may occur during apnea and may be misdiagnosed as primary bradycardia when breathing movements persist.	Pharyngeal hypotonia and failure of upper airway respiratory muscles (e.g., genioglossus, alae nasi) to contract during inspiration may compromise upper airway patency.
Apnea is common during active sleep.	During active sleep, respiration is irregular, the rib cage collapses, lung volume drops, and arterial oxygen pressure falls.
Infants with apnea exhibit delayed auditory evoked responses.	There may be fewer dendritic synaptic connections in the brainstem, associated with instability of respiratory control.

Modified from Klaus, M.II. & Fanaroff, A.A. (2001). *Care of the high risk neonate* (5th ed.). Philadelphia: W.B. Saunders.

cals. Decreased mental activity, impaired judgment, and neuromuscular incoordination may occur when cellular hypoxia is present.

Muscle weakness and fatigue are signs of muscle cell hypoxia. Skeletal muscles have increased compensatory mechanisms and are therefore less susceptible to hypoxic damage than other organ systems.

Respiratory responses include an increase in frequency and depth of respiration. This is an attempt to provide an increased oxygen supply to the blood. Acidosis may occur, contributing to the respiratory compensation. Heart rate and cardiac output also increase as the cardiovascular system attempts to deliver more oxygenated blood to the tissues.

Hematologic responses include stimulation of erythropoietin by low circulating oxygen levels through the kidneys. This results in stimulation of the bone marrow with formation and maturation of red blood cells, which are then released into vascular circulation. In acute hypoxia, immature red blood cells are released. If a chronic hypoxic state exists, the marrow produces more cells and the volume of mature cells increases. This response is an attempt to increase the oxygen-carrying capacity of the blood, thereby improving the oxygen availability to the tissues.

There are several factors that affect the availability of oxygen to the cells. Hypoxia can be categorized depending on which of these factors is responsible for the alterations in tissue oxygenation into hypoxic, anemic, circulatory, and histologic hypoxia.

Hypoxic hypoxia occurs when tissue oxygenation is inadequate because the PaO_2 is reduced and hemoglobin is only partially saturated. This situation may be the result of decreased inspired oxygen (altitude), impaired pulmonary diffusion (pulmonary edema), altered perfusion of the lung (persistent pulmonary hypertension), or some combination of these events.[177]

Anemic hypoxia indicates that the hemoglobin available to transport oxygen is reduced although completely saturated. PaO_2 levels are usually normal in this situation. Anemia may be the result of excessive loss or destruction of red blood cells or impaired production of hemoglobin or red blood cells. Physiologic compensation for anemia includes an increased heart rate and cardiac output. Hypoxia results in vasodilatation and decreased blood viscosity, thereby increasing blood flow in an attempt to maintain normal tissue oxygenation.[177,185]

When tissue oxygenation is decreased due to inadequate blood flow (as with hyperviscosity syndrome), the infant is at risk for circulatory hypoxia. The oxygen content of the blood may be normal, but the blood flow to the tissues is reduced; consequently oxygen availability is also reduced.

Histotoxic hypoxia is reduced oxygen uptake capacity of cells or the reduced oxygen utilization of the cells. Blood flow and oxygen tensions are usually not disturbed. Some toxins (e.g., cyanide, arsenic, and some barbiturates) may interfere with oxidative phosphorylation. Deficiencies in thyroid hormone or niacin also can impair cellular energy production and oxygen use, thereby potentiating cellular hypoxia and altered cellular activity levels.[177]

Hyperoxia

Oxygen can be a toxic agent when too much is available. Prolonged exposure in high concentrations (as in ventilatory support) or increased oxygen pressure (e.g., deep sea diving) can lead to oxygen toxicity. In either situation, time is a critical factor. Toxic responses require prolonged exposure to hyperoxia.

For the premature infant, hyperoxia is a relative term and must be evaluated in light of the PaO_2 levels that are normally encountered in utero. Therefore, small increases in PO_2 may represent a hyperoxic state and place the infant at risk for oxygen injury. Currently, the pulmonary system, central nervous system, and retina have been identified as being susceptible to oxygen injury. In the neonate the organ systems that are affected are the pulmonary system and the retina.

Hyperoxia results in excessive production of highly reactive metabolites of oxygen called free radicals. These metabolites are normally produced during oxidation-reduction reactions within the cells and are detoxified by the antioxidant system. In hyperoxic states this system is overwhelmed and unable to keep up with the generation of free radicals. This can result in cellular damage through irritation (lungs, see section on BPD) or vasoconstriction (retina).

In the eye, high concentrations of PaO_2 cause reversible vasoconstriction. In premature infants this constriction of blood vessels leads to obliteration of the immature vessels and retinal hypoxia (retinopathy of prematurity). Capillary development is stimulated but is abnormal. There is a lack of organization, and the blood vessels may actually extend beyond the retinal surface into the vitreous body. Once the hyperoxia is resolved, there can be resolution with normal retinal development. However, in severe cases, retinal hemorrhages can occur and fibrous scar tissue forms, causing buckling of the retina, leading to detachment and blindness. Similar changes have been reported in severely hypoxic term infants. Transfusion of preterm infants with adult blood rapidly increases the amount of adult hemoglobin, altering the oxygen-carrying capacity, and may transiently increase the risk of retinopathy of prematurity.

Asphyxia

Asphyxia is defined as "a condition of impaired gas exchange leading, if it persists, to progressive hypoxemia and hypercapnia with a metabolic acidosis."[152] There are two categories of asphyxia most frequently encountered in the fetus and neonate; these are perinatal asphyxia and in-

trauterine asphyxia. Intrauterine (fetal) asphyxia is the reduction or cessation of placental gas exchange that occurs either before or during delivery. This type of event places the infant at greater risk for perinatal asphyxia secondary to central nervous system depression, respiratory depression, and cardiac compromise. Perinatal asphyxia is failure of the newly born infant to establish adequate alveolar ventilation at birth with subsequent hypoxemia and respiratory and metabolic acidosis.

Intrauterine asphyxia is the most frequent cause of acidosis encountered in the neonate. The obstetric risk factors that can result in asphyxia are subdivided into three general categories: altered placental gas exchange, altered maternal perfusion of the placenta, and maternal hypoxemia. Specific risk factors are listed in Table 9-12.

The maintenance of a normal fetal acid-base balance in utero requires the maternal and fetal systems to balance the production and elimination of carbon dioxide. Certain factors favor the release of carbon dioxide from the fetus to the mother; these include the increased affinity of HbF for oxygen. This means that as hemoglobin becomes oxygenated at the placental barrier, the affinity for carbon dioxide is driven lower, increasing the release of carbon dioxide to the mother. At the same time, as maternal blood releases oxygen to the fetus, affinity for carbon dioxide is enhanced.[88,200]

The driving force behind carbon dioxide diffusion from fetal to maternal blood is the difference between maternal and fetal $PaCO_2$ levels. Fetal $PaCO_2$ values are higher than those in the maternal system. The hyperventilation of pregnancy creates a mild maternal alkalosis, which helps maintain a gradient that facilitates carbon dioxide transfer to the maternal system by driving maternal $PaCO_2$ levels lower. This gradient is estimated to be between 14 and 17 mmHg.[200]

When fetal hypoxemia occurs due to disturbances in base excess production (anaerobic metabolism) or circumstances in which carbon dioxide concentrations are altered (uterine contractions, placental infarcts, placental abruption), alterations in fetal heart rate minute volume and redistribution of fetal circulation occur. Increased fetal cardiac minute volume, seen clinically as fetal tachycardia, increases the delivery of carbon dioxide to the placenta in much the same way as hyperventilation increases the delivery of carbon dioxide to the alveoli. Fetal tachycardia is frequently encountered after the hypoxic episodes of labor. Uterine contractions are repetitive stress events that impede intervillous blood flow by shutting off venous outflow and compromising the exchange of carbon dioxide between maternal and fetal systems. $PaCO_2$ levels subsequently rise, and hypoxemia and metabolic acidosis may result.

TABLE **9-12**   Risk Factors for Fetal Asphyxia

PRENATAL AND MATERNAL RISK FACTORS	FETAL RISK FACTORS
Preeclampsia	Premature delivery
Hypertension	Postmaturity ($\geq$43 weeks' gestation)
Diabetes mellitus	Intrauterine growth restriction
Older (>35 years) or younger (<15 years) primigravida	Multiple birth
	Polyhydramnios
Chronic renal disease	Meconium stained amniotic fluid
Maternal malnutrition or severe obesity	**INTRAPARTUM RISK FACTORS**
Sickle cell disease	
Anemia (<9 g Hgb)	Breech or other abnormal presentations
Rh or ABO incompatibility	Forceps delivery (other than low)
Heart disease	Cesarean section
Pulmonary disease	Prolapsed umbilical cord
Third trimester bleeding	Nuchal cord
Drug or ethanol abuse	Prolonged general anesthesia
Maternal infection	Excessive sedation or analgesia
Uterine or pelvic anatomic abnormalities	Anesthetic complications (hypotension or hypoxia)
Prolonged rupture of membranes	Prolonged or precipitous labor
Previous fetal or neonatal deaths	Uterine hypertonus
	Abnormal heart rate or rhythm

Conversely, a decrease in cardiac minute volume (fetal bradycardia) secondary to hypoxia or anoxia also results in impaired gas exchange and an increase in fetal carbon dioxide levels. The fetus can tolerate these episodes only for brief periods if protracted hypoxic metabolic acidosis ensues.[200]

During asphyxial episodes, fetal blood flow is redistributed in order to spare the brain, heart, and adrenals as much as possible. The sequelae of intrauterine asphyxia are cardiovascular deterioration with hypotension, bradycardia, and central nervous system depression. The latter may affect the infant's ability to establish spontaneous respirations following delivery. A characteristic pattern of fetal response to asphyxia has been extrapolated by Dawes from his primate work and has been translated to neonates.[56]

Once an asphyxial event occurs (in utero, during delivery, or immediately after delivery), there is an initial period of rapid gasping, with a concomitant rise in heart rate and flailing movements of arms and legs. Blood pressure begins to slowly rise. These events last approximately a minute and are followed by a cessation of respirations (primary apnea), a falling heart rate, and a gradual decrease in blood pressure. During this period, spontaneous respirations can usually be induced by tactile stimulation.

If the asphyxial episode continues for another 2 to 4 minutes, gasping begins again. Initially the gasping is deep and sporadic. Gasping efforts increase briefly and then begin to slow. The heart rate falls to below 100 beats per minutes, and blood pressure rapidly declines. Respiratory efforts completely cease in another 7 to 8 minutes. This is secondary apnea. The heart rate continues to fall, and bradycardia becomes pronounced. At this time, sensory stimulation will not lead to recovery. Brain damage begins after 8 minutes of total asphyxia and is maximal after 12 to 13 minutes. Death usually ensues.[195] Because dysphageal episodes can begin in utero, it may be difficult to determine exactly where in this pattern the infant is at birth. Therefore resuscitative efforts need to be initiated quickly with any depressed infant at birth.

The oxygen content of the blood falls rapidly during the first 2 minutes of asphyxia. Anaerobic metabolism leads to lactic acid buildup and metabolic acidosis. At the same time, carbon dioxide accumulates and respiratory acidosis sets in. The respiratory system experiences ischemia during asphyxial events because blood flow is shunted away from the lungs. This ischemia results in cellular damage to the alveoli with cell membrane disruption and concomitant leakage of fluid into the alveolar space. Death of the type II alveolar cells destroys the surfactant-producing ability of the lung, leading to RDS. Supplemental oxygen and possible ventilatory support may be necessary in order to prevent hypoxia.

Pulmonary hypoxia can also lead to pulmonary vasoconstriction and the persistence of high pulmonary vascular resistance. This reduces blood flow to the pulmonary vascular bed and compounds the local hypoxia. The hypoperfusion, hypoexpansion, and hypoxia can delay the normal closure of fetal shunts, causing right-to-left shunting to persist.

Not only does asphyxia place neonates at risk for RDS and persistent pulmonary hypertension, but intrauterine stress events can result in the passage of meconium into the amniotic fluid (fetuses of more than 35 weeks' gestation), with subsequent aspiration during gasping efforts or with spontaneous respirations. This increases the risk of pneumonitis and pneumonia during the early neonatal period and may necessitate respiratory support.

Transient Tachypnea of the Newborn

The population that is most likely to experience transient tachypnea is full-term infants born by cesarean section or having suffered some sort of perinatal hypoxic stress event. The exact cause of transient tachypnea is unknown. Possible explanations include alteration in permeability of the pulmonary capillary vessels, aspiration of amniotic fluid during gasping efforts in utero, and lack of or decreased vaginal thoracic squeeze. The first two explanations would result in an increased protein concentration in the lung fluid, preventing transfer of fluid into the pulmonary circulation (see Figure 9-15). The vaginal thoracic squeeze during a vertex delivery was once thought to be an important mechanism of lung fluid removal. However, because much of the lung fluid is removed before birth, this mechanism probably has only a minor effect on fluid clearance.[23] The net result of transient tachypnea is a delay in physiologic adjustment and respiratory transition, with an increase in diffusion distance, a decrease in V_T, and an increased risk of $\dot{V}/\dot{Q}$ mismatching.

The most common clinical sign is tachypnea with respiratory rates in the range of 80 to 100 breaths per minute. Mild to moderate retractions and grunting may be exhibited. Cyanosis is not a prominent finding; if oxygen supplementation is necessary, it rarely needs to be greater than 40%. Air exchange is good; breath sounds may initially be moist but clear quickly.

Radiographic findings demonstrate vascular engorgement with increased pulmonary vascular markings. Central markings are ill defined, but there is branching outward toward the periphery. Moderate cardiomegaly may be evident, and occasional air bronchograms can be identified. The overall lung volume is increased, indicating hyperaeration. The diaphragm is depressed, and the anterior-to-posterior diameter is increased. Symptoms and findings clear within 1 to 5 days. Treatment modalities are supportive in nature and based on symptomatology exhibited. Sepsis must be ruled out.

Respiratory Distress Syndrome

RDS is a developmental deficiency in surfactant synthesis accompanied by lung hypoperfusion. The incidence of RDS is inversely related to gestational age. RDS is the most common cause of respiratory failure in the preterm infant and is exacerbated by asphyxia. The pathophysiology of RDS is summarized in Figure 9-24.

RDS is characterized by alterations in surface tension, in which increased pressure is required to keep the alveoli open. Pressures in adjacent alveoli are unequal, therefore time constants are changed, with some alveoli taking longer to fill and others filling normally. This leads to overdistention of the normal alveoli. As the alveoli reach their elastic limit, the infant must generate greater transpulmonary pressure in order to inspire the same amount of volume. The loss of elasticity and the progressive collapse of smaller alveoli reduce lung compliance. This results in uneven $\dot{V}/\dot{Q}$ ratios, with concomitant hypoventilation, decreased functional residual capacity, and increased closing capacity.

When the closing capacity exceeds the functional residual capacity, some segments of the lung are closed during a portion of tidal breathing. As a result, the $\dot{V}/\dot{Q}$ ratio falls and hypoxemia and hypercarbia ensue. The hypoxemia and carbon dioxide retention are usually progressive, culminating in metabolic and respiratory acidosis, which further affect the ability of the type II cells to produce surfactant.[123,206,210,211,249]

If the closing capacity exceeds both the functional residual capacity and V_T, lung segments are closed during inspiration and expiration. This represents complete atelectasis and is characterized as a "white-out" on chest roentgenogram. The use of continuous positive airway pressure (CPAP) and positive end-expiratory pressure (PEEP) prevents alveolar collapse during expiration and increases FRC above closing capacity.

Atelectatic areas of the lung contribute to the dead space within the entire lung. This changes the dead space–to–V_T ratio and leads to hypoxia and hypercarbia unless there is a concomitant increase in expired minute ventilation. An increase in respiratory rate reflects the infant's attempt to compensate. If dead space has increased to the point that alveolar ventilation is compromised, respiratory failure may be the result. Dead space may increase up to 70% in severe RDS.[185]

As hypoxemia and hypercarbia become more severe, pulmonary artery vasoconstriction occurs. Pulmonary perfusion is compromised, and right-to-left shunting occurs through the foramen ovale and ductus arteriosus. Hypoperfusion and hypoxemia compound local ischemia, leading to continued alveolar and capillary epithelial damage.[206]

The increased subatmospheric intrapleural pressure created by the infant in an attempt to maintain adequate airflow, along with the low serum protein that is common in

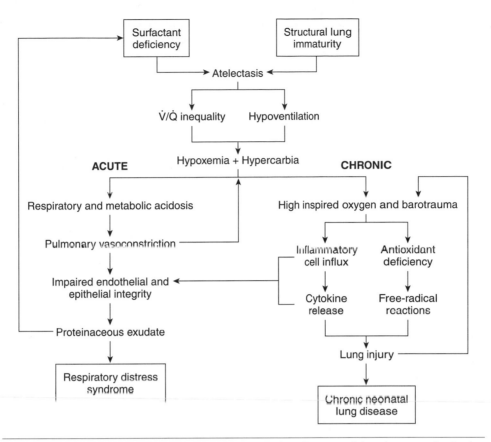

FIGURE **9-24** Schematic representation of the complex series of acute and chronic events that lead to neonatal respiratory distress syndrome and chronic neonatal lung disease. (From Rodriguez, R.J., et al. [2002]. Respiratory distress syndrome and its management. In A.A. Fanaroff & R.J. Martin [Eds.], *Neonatal and perinatal medicine, diseases of the fetus and infant* [7th ed.]. St. Louis: Mosby.)

preterm infants, causes the shift of alveolar and interstitial fluid toward the alveolar space. Combined with the increased alveolar surface tension, pulmonary edema and alveolar flooding ensue. Fibrinogen in the exudate is converted to fibrin. Fibrin lines the alveoli; it binds blood products and cellular debris found in the alveoli, resulting in formation of hyaline membranes.

The excess alveolar fluid and membrane formation result in an increased diffusion distance and reduced lung surface area. Gas exchange is hampered, and ventilation-perfusion mismatching is compounded. Further hypoxemia and hypercarbia are the end result. This becomes a vicious circle that may increase in severity over the first days of life. Recovery is characterized by regeneration of alveolar tissue and concomitant increase in surfactant activity.

RDS is characterized by impaired or delayed surfactant synthesis (see Figure 9-24). The preterm infant has a decreased number of type II pneumocytes secondary to gestational age. Surfactant must not only be present at the time of delivery, but also must be regenerated at a rate consonant with its use. This implies that type II cells must be present, viable, and intact in order to maintain normal surface tension. Inadequate amounts of surfactant at birth may be due to a variety of problems. These include extreme immaturity of the alveolar lining cells, diminished or impaired production rates resulting from transient fetal or neonatal stress, impaired release mechanisms from within the cell, and death of type II cells. The extreme immaturity and impaired release mechanisms probably explain the inability of the very early fetus to survive.

Surfactant is also altered in immature infants. Surfactant produced by these infants has a decreased SP–to–lipid ratio, is more rapidly converted to immature forms, is less effective in improving lung compliance, and is more susceptible to inactivation by proteinaceous pulmonary edema.[123]

Lung hypoperfusion is another component of RDS pathogenesis. An ischemic injury that occurs either in utero or at the time of delivery results in hypoperfusion of the lung. The more immature the lung and smaller the capillary bed, the greater the ease with which the nutritional blood supply to the developing lung can be compromised. At 35 weeks the type II cells are presumably differentiated to the point that the pathway for PC synthesis is more resistant to fetal stress and the nutritional blood supply is more abundant and therefore more difficult to compromise.

Oxidative stress may also have a role. Preterm infants are more vulnerable to this stress as a result of decreased levels of antioxidant enzymes (e.g., catalase, glutathione peroxidase) and endogenous free-radical scavengers (e.g., α-tocopherol) and decreased binding proteins (e.g., transferrin, ceruloplasmin).[91]

Clinical Manifestations

Clinically the infant attempts to compensate for the progressive respiratory and metabolic acidosis by increasing both inspiratory pressures and respiratory rate. Grunting occurs in an attempt to slow expiratory flow rates and maintain a higher FRC. All of the clinical signs appear early and usually increase in severity over the first 72 hours. The infant may also present with pitting edema, cyanosis, and diminished breath sounds.

Cyanosis is a result of an excessive concentration of deoxygenated hemoglobin in the capillaries, although hypoxia can occur without cyanosis. Factors contributing to cyanosis include the alveolar hypoventilation, impaired diffusion across the alveolar-capillary membrane, and right-to-left shunting through fetal channels or through completely atelectatic lungs. Hypoxia and cyanosis are usually progressive, requiring increasing concentrations of oxygen.

Grunting is forced expiration against a partially closed glottis so that end-expiratory pressure is increased and expiratory flow is retarded. This maintains the lung at a slightly higher volume for a longer period of time, thereby increasing gas exchange time. There is usually a very short expiratory phase; this reduces the time in which the lung can become airless before the next inspiratory effort. The tachypnea and grunting help to maintain a more normal FRC.

Retractions are indicative of the increased inspiratory pressure, decreased lung compliance, and increased chest wall compliance. They can be quite marked in RDS, with substernal retractions pulling to the backbone. This dysfunctional respiratory effort results in cephalocaudal expansion only (paradoxical breathing), with increased negative pressures being generated in the bases. Therefore hyperinflation occurs in the bases and atelectasis in the apices. Marked abnormalities in $\dot{V}/\dot{Q}$ ratios are the result.

Treatment

Interventions are supportive as well as active in nature. Adequate, effective resuscitation with maintenance of body temperature is essential for reducing the incidence and severity of the disease. Therapy is aimed at maintaining oxygenation, adequate ventilation, normal pH, and adequate perfusion and tissue oxygenation. Hydration is important, but overhydration increases the risk of congestive heart failure. A systolic murmur, bounding pulses, active precordium, tachycardia, tachypnea, apnea, and carbon dioxide retention, as well as worsening ventilatory requirements, are indications of patent ductus arteriosus (see Chapter 8) and congestive heart failure. Active interventions include administration of exogenous surfactant and the use of continuous distending pressure or continuous negative pressure in an attempt to keep FRC above closing capacity. Ventilatory support may be needed if the infant is unable to compensate for hypoxemia, hypercarbia, and acidosis by generating sufficient negative pressure and increasing minute ventilation.

Surfactant replacement therapy. Exogenous surfactant replacement therapy (SRT) stabilizes the lung until postnatal surfactant synthesis matures. SRT became generally available in 1990 after a series of successful clinical trials. "Surfactant therapy has been the single most important factor in reducing overall neonatal mortality rates."[52] Use of SRT has been associated with a 30% reduction in mortality and a decrease in pneumothorax, oxygen requirements, and ventilator requirements.[91,124] Effects on bronchopulmonary dysplasia have been inconsistent.[91] The combined use of antenatal corticosteroids and SRT have additional beneficial effects.[131]

Both synthetic and natural surfactant preparations are used. Surfactant phospholipids and proteins are recycled with little catabolism. Exogenous surfactant mixes with the infant's own surfactant. This mixture appears to enhance the function of endogenous surfactant, making it less sensitive to inactivation.[123]

Timing of the initial dose and type of surfactant are still unclear. Both natural and synthetic surfactants are effective in reducing RDS.[216-219] Natural surfactant use has a greater reduction in air leak and possibly an improved survival rate.[52,216] Exogenous surfactant has been given shortly after birth in at-risk infants (prophylactic) or once the infants begins to show signs of RDS (treatment). Currently SRT requires that the infant be intubated, although other modes of delivery are being investigated. Prophylactic therapy (generally within 15 minutes of birth) has usually been used in infants weighing less than 1000 grams. A meta-analysis of prophylactic versus treatment use demonstrated decreased mortality, pulmonary interstitial emphysema, and pneumothrorax.[219] It is unclear which babies benefit most from prophylactic use, although general practice is to reserve prophylactic use for the most immature babies.[52] Surfactant therapy is currently being investigated or used for other disorders, including ARDS, bronchiolitis, and meconium aspiration.[52,223,258]

Chronic Neonatal Lung Disease

In 1967, Northway and colleagues originally described a sequence of radiographic changes in infants with RDS that came to be known as bronchopulmonary dysplasia (BPD).[187] This sequence of events is rarely seen in current clinical practice, particularly in infants above 1200 grams or older than 30 weeks' gestational age.[129] Instead, there is a slower subtler onset, with the gradual development of lung abnormalities that persist after 20 to 30 days of life.[13,24] Up to 30% of very-low–birth-weight (VLBW) preterm infants still require oxygen at 36 weeks' postconceptional age.[129] Currently, VLBW preterm infants are more likely to develop what has been termed chronic lung disease (CLD) or the "new" BPD, characterized by oxygen requirements after 28 days of age or at 36 weeks' postconceptional age, but without the characteristic sequence of BPD radiographic changes.[24] Infants with this disorder have decreased alveolarization, including alveolar hypoplasia and variable saccule wall fibrosis but with minimal airway disease.[34]

Participants in a recent workshop organized by the National Institute of Child Health and Human Development; National Heart, Lung, and Blood Institute; and the Office of Rare Diseases reviewed the definition of BPD and CLD.[129] This group recommended that the name BPD be retained rather than CLD as the term for chronic neonatal lung disease. They proposed a revised definition with new diagnostic criteria based on gestational age and severity as evidenced by need for oxygen and/or positive pressure ventilation.[129] These criteria—which do not include specific radiographic criteria due to inconsistent interpretation of findings—await clinical validation.

Chronic neonatal lung disease is due to lung injury, probably mediated by an inflammatory reaction with cytokine release and oxidative damage (see Figure 9-24). These responses can be caused by many factors, including structural lung immaturity, oxidant injury, infection, inflammation, volutrauma/barotrauma, edema, and undernutrition.[13,24,34] Mechanisms increasing the risk from lung injury in immature infants and potential preventive strategies are summarized in Table 9-13.

Treatment for BPD has been multifaceted. Some modalities are centered on primary prevention, and others are employed after the disease process is diagnosed. Primary prevention includes reducing the incidence of premature births through patient education and recognition of early labor, the use of drugs to inhibit premature labor, using glucocorticoids to mature surfactant synthesis pathways, provision of effective resuscitation, and providing exogenous surfactant. Secondary treatment modalities include ventilatory support (either negative or positive pressure); adequate nutrition for growth and healing, facilitating closure of the ductus arteriosus through pharmacologic or surgical treatment; diuretic therapy to mobilize fluids and reduce pulmonary edema; bronchodilators and antiinflammatory agents to decrease resistance to airflow and improve distribution of ventilation; and various ventilatory techniques (e.g., high-frequency ventilation). Corticosteroid

TABLE **9-13**   **Mechanisms of Increased Risk for Lung Injury in the Immature Lung and Prevention Strategies**

MECHANISM	REASONS FOR SUSCEPTIBILITY TO LUNG INJURY	POTENTIAL PREVENTION STRATEGIES
Volutrauma	Poorly compliant alveoli but highly compliant airways	Small tidal volume
Oxidant injury	Immature antioxidant defense systems	Superoxide dismutase
Infection	Immature macrophages and leukocytes; altered airway clearance	Prevention of infection
Inflammation	Poorly developed antioxidant, antiproteolytic and antielastolytic systems	Corticosteroids
Edema	Increased permeability of alveolar-capillary membrane	Lung injury prevention
Undernutriton	Impaired repair, growth and development	Vitamin A

From Carlo, W.A., et al. (2002). Assisted ventilation and complications of respiratory distress. In A.A. Fanaroff & & R.J. Martin (Eds.). *Neonatal and perinatal medicine: Diseases of the fetus and infant* (7th ed.). St. Louis: Mosby.

therapy has been used to reduce inflammation and facilitate weaning from the ventilator. Steroid use is currently controversial as a result of adverse neurologic and other outcomes reported in infants on prolonged therapy.[13] Further studies are needed on the safety and efficacy of these drugs, as well as on the optimal dose and dosing schedule. Research has also focused on enhancing or modifying lung maturation through the antioxidant and surfactant pathways to improve adaptation to extrauterine life.

Meconium Aspiration Syndrome

Meconium aspiration syndrome (MAS) is a cause of respiratory failure in term and postmature infants. Elimination of meconium into amniotic fluid is associated with some degree of fetal distress, but it may occur in normal or breech delivery without evidence of asphyxia.[106] Meconium may be passed in utero due to hypoxic stress. The hypoxia and acidosis are probably responsible for the gasping activity that leads to aspiration of meconium before delivery.

Approximately 12% to 14% of all babies delivered release meconium into the amniotic fluid.[134,171] These infants are usually SGA, postterm, or with cord compression or alterations in uteroplacental circulation. Of infants with meconium-stained fluid, only about 4% to 11% develop MAS.[24,171]

Postnatal aspiration into the pulmonary tree can be prevented most of the time with oropharyngeal suction before the first breath. This suctioning decreases development of mild to moderate MAS, but not severe MAS.[24,233] Thus the basis for mild/moderate and severe MAS are likely different.[24] It is currently believed that antepartum or intrapartum aspiration of meconium—along with alteration in meconium clearance from the lungs—leads to severe MAS.[24,122,148] Endotracheal suctioning (ETS) after birth is indicated for infants with cardiorespiratory depression or need for positive pressure ventilation after birth. ETS is not indicated if the infant with meconium-stained fluid is vigorous at birth, oropharyngeal suctioning has been performed, and the meconium is thin.[171] Implications of thick versus thin meconium for management is unclear.

Meconium can damage type II cells and inhibit surfactant action.[24,98] Thus SRT has been used with additional trials in progress.[98] Free fatty acids in meconium inactivate surfactant; the cholesterol tends to fluidize the surface film and interfere with the ability of surfactant to lower surface tension during compression.[53,98] In addition, meconium has a high adhesive tension that may "glue" unstable airways closed.[98] Surfactant inactivation, along with the chemical pneumonitis, leads to atelectasis and intrapulmonary shunting (Figure 9-25). These infants develop hy-

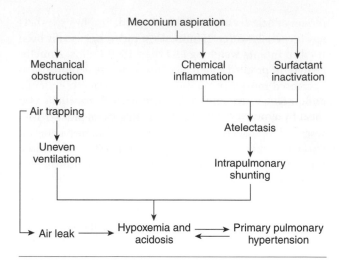

FIGURE **9-25** Pathophysiology of meconium aspiration syndrome. (From Miller, M.J., et al. [2002]. Respiratory disorders in preterm and term infants. In A.A. Fanaroff & R.J. Martin [Eds.]. *Neonatal and perinatal medicine: Diseases of the fetus and infant* [7th ed.]. St. Louis: Mosby.)

poxemia and acidosis and are at risk for persistent pulmonary hypertension (see Chapter 8).

The lower airways become partially obstructed, resulting in air trapping and overinflation distal to the obstruction (see Figure 9-25). Small airway obstruction produces an alteration in $\dot{V}/\dot{Q}$ ratios and reduced lung compliance. The alveolar hypoventilation leads to carbon dioxide retention, hypoxemia, and acidosis. When the obstruction is complete, the distal alveoli collapse, increasing the intrapulmonary shunt and compounding arterial hypoxemia. Obstruction may also be potentiated by epithelial inflammation in the bronchi and alveoli. This results in a chemical pneumonitis with increased airway resistance and decreased diffusing capacity. Each of these events contributes to the hypoxemia seen clinically. The pneumonitis may also explain the decreased lung compliance, because elasticity is lost with inflammation.

Minute ventilation is increased in order to compensate for the $\dot{V}/\dot{Q}$ alterations. The increase is usually due to an increase in respiratory rate; however, carbon dioxide retention continues because the V_T is reduced, thereby increasing dead space and reducing alveolar ventilation. The chest radiograph demonstrates patchy areas that have reduced aeration. There are sometimes confluent areas alternating with hyperlucent ones. The diaphragm may be depressed. Blood gas levels show a metabolic acidosis and hypoxemia that are dependent upon the degree of pulmonary bed involved. These findings are more pronounced if persistent pulmonary hypertension is present. The infant may be able to compensate initially; therefore $PaCO_2$ levels may be normal. However, this usually does not last.

If the process continues, respiratory failure is likely. Pneumothorax or pneumomediastinum may also occur because of the alveolar distention that occurs with air trapping. Right-to-left shunting is common, especially if persistent pulmonary hypertension is present. Secondary bacterial infections frequently occur but may be difficult to diagnose by chest roentgenogram, especially during the acute phase of the syndrome.

Assisted ventilation may be necessary in these infants in order to ensure adequate oxygenation, drive the $PaCO_2$ level toward normal, and facilitate transitional events. Cord gases and arterial gas should be assessed in order to evaluate the asphyxial insult and determine adequate recovery. Chest percussion, postural drainage, and suctioning are used to continue the removal of meconium from lung passages. Extracorporeal membrane oxygenation (ECMO) may be used to treat critically ill infants who do not respond to conventional therapy.

MATURATIONAL CHANGES DURING INFANCY AND CHILDHOOD

The functional and anatomic maturation of the respiratory system continues through childhood until the bony thorax stops growing. Functional development is essentially secondary to anatomic development and is tied to the continued growth of the airways and multiplication of the alveoli (see Table 9-8).

At the time of birth there are up to 20 to 50 million air spaces—a combination of terminal air sacs and alveoli.[112] From then on, alveoli beget alveoli, gradually replacing all of the terminal air sacs. The greatest change is in the first 1 to 2 years. By 8 years of age (range, 5 to 13 years), the alveolar number has increased to approximately 300 million.[68] It is unclear whether alveolar multiplication continues after this time, or whether further lung growth is related only to alveoli enlarging in size.[237]

Alveolar diameter doubles in size during maturation. At 2 months of age, alveoli measure 150 to 180 μm; by adulthood, they are 250 to 300 μm.[68,112] This indicates that there is a steady increase in surface area during childhood. Alveolar surface area increases from 3 to 4 m^2 at birth to 32 m^2 at 8 years, reaching 75 to 100 m^2 by adulthood.[68,112] This improves the oxygen-diffusing capacity of the organ system.

Oxygen affinity continues to increase over the first 6 months of life with conversion from fetal to adult hemoglobin (see Chapter 7). At that time, over 90% of the hemoglobin is the adult type. This improves the diffusion of oxygen to the tissues, meeting the increased metabolic needs of the cells. From 10 months to 11 years, the pulmonary arteries grow and enlarge; the small arteries are mostly nonmuscular or minimally muscular during this time. At the end of this growth period, the muscular arteries have reached the level of the alveolar duct where the vessels are 130 μm in diameter. Between 11 years and maturation, which occurs around 19 years of age, muscle extension continues, reaching the alveolus where vessels are 75 μm in diameter.[68,108] Intrapulmonary veins, on the other hand, are thinner than their counterparts, and muscle extension does not spread as far peripherally. Once this is achieved, the system is considered mature.

Lung compliance increases rapidly during the first year and then more slowly.[96] Lung elastic tissue continues to develop until early adulthood. Collateral ventilation also develops during childhood, thereby providing protection against obstruction of small airways and atelectasis. The pores of Kohn appear sometime between the first and second years of life. Lambert channels begin to be evident by 6 years of age. Interbronchiolar channels are not found in normal lungs but may develop in disease situations.[156]

By 8 months the muscle fiber content of the diaphragm reaches adult proportions. Rib cage compliance remains altered during infancy. The peripheral airways contribute the most to airway resistance until 5 years, when the upper airways predominate (as in adults).[153] Cartilage support for the conducting airways increases rapidly in the first 2 months and then more slowly throughout childhood. Closing capacity decreases after 6 years.[177] Venous admixture does not reach adult values until early childhood.[185]

Changes in the shape of the thorax to adulthood are illustrated in Figure 9-16. Infants are predominately nose breathers for the first 3 to 4 months. Until 8 years the cricoid cartilage is the narrowest portion of the larynx (versus the vocal cords in older individuals). Density of mucus glands decreases to adulthood, from 10 to 20 per mm^2 to 1 per mm^2.

SUMMARY

Although the respiratory system is not fully developed at birth, the infant does demonstrate capabilities and strategies necessary to achieve sustained respirations, blood gas tension, and acid-base homeostasis and compensatory mechanisms to maintain that balance even in disease states. Transition must be seen as a process that takes several days, with initial responses relating to the fetal state. Knowledge of these differences and the progression toward extrauterine stability can guide therapeutic interventions and determine clinical assessment.

TABLE **9-14** Clinical Implications for the Respiratory System in Neonates

Understand the normal anatomic and functional development of the respiratory system (pp. 323-335 and Tables 9-8 and 9-10). Know what factors stimulate fetal lung development, what factors inhibit functional development, and what therapies are utilized with potential preterm delivery (pp. 330-333). Discuss the various tests utilized to assess fetal lung maturity (pp. 332-333). Describe the expected changes in fetal blood gases during the intrapartum and transitional periods (pp. 334-335). Identify various steps in respiratory conversion at birth (pp. 335-338). Identify infants at risk for asphyxia (pp. 356-357 and Table 9-12) Understand the consequences of hypoxia, hyperoxia, asphyxia (pp. 354-358). Acquire and maintain neonatal resuscitation skills (pp. 356-358).	Monitor head and neck positioning in preterm infants to maintain airway patency (p. 340). Assess respiratory function on a regular basis (pp. 351-353). Evaluate preterm infants for periodic breathing and apnea (pp. 353-354 and Table 9-11). Identify and evaluate infants at risk for transient tachypnea (p. 358). Identify and evaluate risk factors and clinical symptomatology associated with respiratory distress syndrome (pp. 358-361). Identify and evaluate infants at risk for developing chronic neonatal lung disease (pp. 361-362 and Table 9-13). Monitor blood gases and ventilatory parameters in infants with chronic neonatal lung disease (pp. 361-362). Identify and monitor infants who either are at risk for or who have meconium aspiration (pp. 362-364).

The infant has prepared throughout gestation for this transition. The respiratory muscles have exercised and trained to take over the function of the respiratory pump itself, although fatigue may be encountered quite quickly. Intercostal muscles can stabilize the chest wall, so that effective ventilation can be achieved. The difficulties come when disease or immaturity is encountered. There is little reserve to increase ventilatory efforts or sustain increased respiratory activity. The ability to recruit accessory muscles, the use of laryngeal braking (grunting), and the recruitment of new alveoli help to improve gas exchange and increase the pulmonary surface area. Each infant responds uniquely to the process of transition and to pathology. The development of refined clinical skills and further research may give us more clues as to when and how the respiratory system prepares and achieves its sustained activity. Clinical implications for the neonate are summarized in Table 9-14.

REFERENCES

1. Abel, E.L. (1983). *Marijuana, tobacco, alcohol, and reproduction.* Boca Raton, FL: CRC Press.
2. Adamson, S.L. (1991). Regulation of breathing at birth. *J Dev Physiol, 15,* 45.
3. Albersheim, S., et al. (1976) Effect of CO_2 on the immediate response to O_2 in preterm infants. *J Appl Physiol, 41,* 609.
4. Alcorn, D., et al. (1977). Morphological effects of chronic tracheal ligation and drainage in fetal lamb lung. *J Anat, 123,* 649.
5. Aldritch, C.J., et al. (1994). The effect of maternal oxygen administration on human fetal cerebral oxygenation measured during labor by near infrared spectroscopy. *Br J Obstet Gynaecol, 101,* 509.
6. Aldritch, C.J., et al. (1995). The effect of maternal position on fetal cerebral oxygenation during labor. *Br J Obstet Gynaecol, 102,* 14.
7. Alexander, S. (1984). Physiologic and biochemical effects of exercise. *Clin Biochem, 17,* 126.
8. Andres, R.L. (1999). Social and illicit drug use in pregnancy. In R.K. Creasy & R. Resnik (Eds.). *Maternal-fetal medicine* (4th ed.). Philadelphia: W.B. Saunders.
9. Archer, G.W. & Marx, G.F. (1974). Arterial oxygen tension during apnoea in parturient women. *Br J Anaesth, 46,* 358.
10. Artal, R., et al. (1986). Pulmonary responses to exercise in pregnancy. *Am J Obstet Gynecol, 154,* 378.
11. Baier, R.J., et al. (1990). Effects of various concentrations of O_2 and umbilical cord occlusion on fetal breathing and behaviors. *J Appl Physiol, 68,* 1597.
12. Ballard, P.L., et al. (1986). Human pulmonary surfactant apoprotein: effects of development, culture and hormones on the protein and its mRNA. *Pediatr Res, 20,* 422A.
13. Bancalari, E. (2002). Neonatal chronic lung disease. In A.A. Fanaroff & R.J. Martin (Eds.). *Neonatal and perinatal medicine: Diseases of the fetus and infant* (7th ed.). St. Louis: Mosby.
14. Bassell, G.M. & Marx, G.F. (1984). Physiologic changes of normal pregnancy and parturition. In E.V. Cosmi (Ed.). *Obstetric anesthesia and perinatology.* New York: Appleton-Century-Crofts.
15. Bergeson, P.S. & Shaw, J.C. (2001). Are infants really obligatory nasal breathers? *Clin Pediatr (Phila), 40,* 567.
16. Bettes, T.M. & McKenas, D.K. (1999). Medical advice for commercial air travelers. *Am Fam Physician, 60,* 801.
17. Bhatia, P. & Bhatia, K. (2000). Pregnancy and the lungs. *Postgrad Med J, 76,* 683.

18. Birnbach, D.J., et al. (2000). *Textbook of obstetric anesthesia.* New York: Churchill Livingstone.

19. Blair, P.S., et al. (1996). Smoking and sudden infant death syndrome: results from 1993-5 case control study for confidential inquiry into stillbirths and deaths in infancy. *BMJ, 313,* 195.

20. Blanco, C.E., et al. (1985). Studies in utero of the mechanisms of chemoreceptor resetting. In C.T. Jones & P.W. Nathaniel (Eds.). *The physiologic development of the fetus and the newborn.* London: Academic Press.

21. Bland, R.D. (1998). Formation of fetal lung fluid and its removal near birth. In R.A. Polin & W.W. Fox (Eds.). *Fetal and neonatal physiology* (2nd ed.). Philadelphia: W.B. Saunders.

22. Bleasdale, J.E. & Johnston, J.M. (1985). Developmental biochemistry of lung surfactant. In G.H. Nelson (Ed.). *Pulmonary development: transition from intrauterine to extrauterine life.* New York: Marcel Dekker.

23. Bloom, R.S. (2002). Delivery room resuscitation of the newborn. In A.A. Fanaroff & R.J. Martin (Eds.). *Neonatal and perinatal medicine, diseases of the fetus and infant* (7th ed.). St. Louis: Mosby.

24. Bolt, R.J., et al. (2001). Glucocorticoids and lung development in the fetus and preterm infant. *Pediatr Pulmonol, 32,* 76.

25. Boyton, B.R. (1988). The epidemiology of bronchopulmonary dysplasia. In T.A. Merritt, W.H. Northway, & B.R. Boyton (Eds.). *Contemporary issues in fetal and neonatal medicine: Bronchopulmonary dysplasia.* Boston: Blackwell Scientific Publications.

26. Brancazio, L.R., et al. (1997). Peak expiratory flow rate in normal pregnancy. *Obstet Gynecol, 89,* 383.

27. Brouillette, R.T., et al. (1997). Evaluation of the newborn's blood gas status. National Academy of Clinical Biochemistry. *Clin Chem, 43,* 215.

28. Bureau, M.A., et al. (1985). The ventilatory response to hypoxia in the newborn lamb after carotid body deneravation. *Respir Physiol, 60,* 109.

29. Campbell, L.A. & Klocke, R.A. (2001). Implications for the pregnant patient. *Am J Respir Crit Care Med, 163,* 1051.

30. Catanzarite, V. & Cousins, L. (2000). Respiratory failure in pregnancy. *Immunol Allergy Clin N Am, 20,* 775.

31. Christenson, R. (1979). Gross differences observed in the placentas of smokers and nonsmokers. *Am J Epidemiol, 110,* 178.

32. Chua, S., et al. (1997). Fetal oxygen saturation during labour. *Br J Obstet Gynaecol, 104,* 1080.

33. Clapp, J.F. (1985). Fetal heart rate response to running in midpregnancy and late pregnancy. *Am J Obstet Gynecol, 153,* 251.

34. Clark, R.H., et al. (2001). Lung injury in neonates: causes, strategies for prevention and long-term consequences. *J Pediatr, 139,* 478.

35. Cleary, G.M. & Wiswell, T.E. (1996). Meconium-stained amniotic fluid and the meconium aspiration syndrome: An update. *Pediatr Clin North Am, 45,* 511.

36. Clements, J.A. & Avery, M.E. (1998). Lung surfactant and neonatal respiratory distress syndrome. *Am J Respir Crit Care Med, 157,* S59.

37. Cohen, S. & Mazze, R. (1985). Physiology of pregnancy. In J. M. Baden & J.B. Brodsky (Eds.). *The pregnant surgical patient.* New York: Futura.

38. Cole, P.V. & Nainby-Luxmoore, R.C. (1962). Respiratory volumes in labour. *Br Med J, 1,* 1118.

39. Conter, V., et al. (1995). Weight growth in infants born to mothers who smoked during pregnancy. *BMJ, 310,* 768.

40. Contreras, G., et al. (1991). Ventilatory drive and respiratory muscle function in pregnancy. *Am Rev Respir Dis, 144,* 837.

41. Cosmi, EV. (1984). *Obstetric anesthesia and perinatology.* New York: Appleton-Century-Crofts.

42. Cousins, L. (1999). Fetal oxygenation, assessment of fetal well-being, and obstetric management of the pregnant patient with asthma. *J Allergy Clin Immunol, 103,* S34.

43. Crapo, R.O. (1996). Normal cardiopulmonary physiology during pregnancy. *Clin Obstet Gynecol, 39,* 3.

44. Crewels, L.A., et al. (1997). The pulmonary surfactant system: biochemical and clinical aspects. *Lung, 175,* 1.

45. Crowley, P. (1995). Antenatal corticosteroid therapy: A meta-analysis of the randomized trials, 1972 to 1974. *Am J Obstet Gynecol, 173,* 322.

46. Crowley, P. (2000). Prophylactic corticosteroids for preterm birth. *Cochrane Database Syst Rev 2000, 2,* CD000065.

47. Crowther, C.A., et al. (2000). Prenatal thyrotropin-releasing hormone for preterm birth. *Cochrane Database Syst Rev 2000, 2,* CD000019.

48. Cruikshank, D. & Hays, P. (1986). Maternal physiology in pregnancy. In S. Gabbe et al. (Eds.), *Obstetrics: normal and problem pregnancies.* New York: Churchill Livingstone.

49. Cugell, D.W., et al. (1953). Pulmonary function in pregnancy: serial observations in normal women. *Am Rev Tuberc, 67,* 568.

50. Cunningham, F.G & Whitridge, W.J. (1997). *Williams obstetrics* (20th ed.). Stamford, CT: Appleton & Lange.

51. Cunningham, J., et al. (1994). Maternal smoking during pregnancy as a predictor of lung function in children. *Am J Epidemiol, 139,* 1139.

52. Curley, A.E. & Halliday, H.L. (2001). The present status of exogenous surfactant for the newborn. *Early Hum Dev, 61,* 67.

53. Dargaville, P.A., et al. (2001). Surfactant and surfactant inhibitors in meconium aspiration syndrome. *J Pediatr, 128,* 113.

54. Davis, G.M., Hobbs, S. & Bureau, M.A. (1986). Limitation of the ventilatory response to CO_2 in newborn lambs. *Am Rev Respir Dis, 133*(suppl), A136.

55. Davis, G.M. & Bureau, M.A. (1987). Pulmonary and chest wall mechanics in the control of respiration in the newborn. *Clin Perinatol, 14,* 551.

56. Dawes, G.S. (1968). *Foetal and neonatal physiology.* Chicago: Year Book Medical.

57. Delke, I., et al. (1985). Effect of Lamaze childbirth preparation on maternal plasma beta-endorphin immuno-reactivity in active labor. *Am J Perinatol, 2,* 317.

58. De Dooy, J.J., et al. (2001). The role of inflammation in the development of chronic lung disease in neonates. *Eur J Pediatr, 160,* 457.

59. Delivoria-Papadopoulos, M. & McGowen, J.E. (1998). In R.A. Polin & W.W. Fox (Eds,). *Fetal and neonatal physiology* (2nd ed.). Philadelphia: W.B. Saunders.

60. DeMello, D.E. & Lin, Z. (2001). Pulmonary alveolar proteinosis: a review. *Pediatr Pathol Mol Med, 20,* 413.

61. Dennehy, K.C. & Pian-Smith, M.C. (2000). Airway management of the parturient. *Int Anesthesiol Clin, 38,* 147.

62. DeSwiet, M. (1991). The respiratory system. In F. Hytten & G. Chamberlain (Eds.). *Clinical physiology in obstetrics* (3rd ed.). Oxford: Blackwell Scientific.

63. DeSwiet, M. (1999). Pulmonary disorders. In R.K. Creasy & R. Resnik (Eds.). *Maternal-fetal medicine* (4th ed.). Philadelphia: W.B. Saunders.

64. Dobbs, L.G. & Mason, R.J. (1979). Pulmonary alveolar type II cells isolated from rats. Release of phosphatidylcholine in response to beta-adrenergic stimulation. *J Clin Invest, 63,* 378.

65. Doering, S.G. & Entwisle, D.R. (1975). Preparation during pregnancy and ability to cope with labor and delivery. *Am J Orthopsychiatry, 45,* 825.

66. Donnenfield, A.F., et al (1993). Simultaneous fetal and maternal nicotine levels in pregnant women smokers. *Am J Obstet Gynecol, 168,* 781.

67. Duara, S. (1998). Structure and function of the upper airway in neonates. In R.A. Polin & W.W. Fox (Eds.). *Fetal and neonatal physiology* (2nd ed.). Philadelphia: W.B. Saunders.

68. Dunnill, M.S. (1962). Postnatal growth of the lung. *Thorax, 17,* 329.

69. Dunsmore, S.E. & Rannels, D.E. (1996). Extracellular matrix biology in the lung. *Am J Physiol, 270,* L3.

70. Ecker, J.L. & Parer, J.T. (1999). Obstetric evaluation of fetal acid-base balance. *Crit Rev Clin Lab Sci, 36,* 407.

71. Edenborough, F.P., et al. (1995). Outcome of pregnancy in women with cystic fibrosis. *Thorax, 50,* 170.

72. Ellard, G.A., et al. (1996). Smoking during pregnancy: the dose dependence of birth weight deficits. *Br J Obstet Gynaecol, 103,* 806.

73. Ellegard, E.K. & Karlsson, N.G. (2000). Nasal mucociliary transport in pregnancy. *Am J Rhinol, 14,* 375.

74. Erik, J., et al. (2000). Treatment with exogenous surfactant stimulates endogenous surfactant synthesis in premature infants with respiratory distress syndrome. *Crit Care Med, 28,* 3383.

75. Espinoza, J., et al. (2001). Placental villus morphology in relation to maternal hypoxia at high altitude. *Placenta, 22,* 606.

76. Fiascone, J., et al. (1986). Differential effect of betamethasone on alveolar surfactant and lung tissue of fetal rabbits. *Pediatr Res, 20,* 428A.

77. Field, S.K., et al. (1991). Relationship between inspiratory effort and breathlessness in pregnancy. *J Appl Physiol, 71,* 1897.

78. Fishburne, J., et al. (1972). Bronchospasm complicating intravenous prostaglandin $F_{2\alpha}$ for therapeutic abortion. *Obstet Gynecol, 39,* 892.

79. Fisher, J.T., et al. (1998). Regulation of lower airway function. In R.A. Polin & W.W. Fox (Eds,). *Fetal and neonatal physiology* (2nd ed.). Philadelphia: W.B. Saunders.

80. Flemming, P., et al. (1978). Functional immaturity of pulmonary irritant receptors and apnea in newborn preterm infants. *Pediatrics, 61,* 515.

81. Frangolias, D.D., et al. (1997). Pregnancy and cystic fibrosis: a case-controlled study. *Chest, 111,* 963.

82. Frank, L. & Sosenko, I.R.S. (1987). Development of lung antioxidant enzyme system in late gestation: possible implications for the prematurely born infant. *J Pediatr, 110,* 9.

83. Frank, L. & Sosenko, I.R.S. (1987). Prenatal development of lung antioxidant enzymes in four species. *J Pediatr, 110,* 106.

84. Frederiksen, M.C. (2001). Physiologic changes in pregnancy and their effect on drug disposition. *Semin Perinatol, 25,* 120.

85. Frerking, I., et al. (2001) Pulmonary surfactant: functions, abnormalities and therapeutic options. *Intensive Care Med, 27,* 1699.

86. Friedman, S.A., et al. (1995). Neonatal outcome after preterm delivery for preeclampsia. *Am J Obstet Gynecol, 172,* 1785.

87. Garcia-Rio, F., et al. (1996). Regulation of breathing and perception of dyspnea in healthy pregnant women. *Chest, 110,* 446.

88. Gee, J.B.L., et al. (1967). Pulmonary mechanics during pregnancy. *J Clin Invest, 46,* 945.

89. Ghidini, A. & Spong, C.Y. (2001). Severe meconium aspiration syndrome is not caused by aspiration of meconium. *Am J Obstet Gynecol, 185,* 931.

90. Gilbert, R., et al. (1962). Dyspnea of pregnancy: a syndrome of altered respiratory control. *JAMA, 182,* 1073.

91. Gitto, E., et al. (2001). Respiratory distress syndrome in the newborn: the role of oxidative stress. *Intensive Care Med, 27,* 1116.

92. Gleicher, N. (1998). *Principles and practice of medical therapy in pregnancy* (3rd ed.). Stamford, CT: Appleton & Lange.

93. Gnanaratnem, J. & Finer NN. Neonatal acute respiratory failure. *Curr Opin Pediatr, 12,* 227.

94. Goldsmith, J.P. & Karotkin, E.H. (1996). *Assisted ventilation of the neonate* (3rd ed.). Philadelphia: W.B. Saunders.

95. Gonzales, L.W., et al. (1986). Glucocorticoids and thyroid hormone stimulate biochemical and morphological differentiation of human fetal lung in organ culture. *J Clin Endocrinol Metab, 62,* 678.

96. Goodman, J.D.S., Visser, F.G.A. & Dawes, G.S. (1984). Effects of maternal cigarette smoking on fetal trunk movements, fetal breathing movements, and the fetal heart rate. *Br J Obstet Gynecol, 91,* 657.

97. Greenberger, P.A. (1992). Asthma in pregnancy. *Clin Chest Med, 13,* 597.

98. Greenough, A. (2000). Expanded use of surfactant replacement therapy. *Eur J Pediatr, 159,* 635.

99. Greenough, A. (2001). Respiratory support techniques for prematurely born infants: new advances and perspectives. *Acta Paediatr Taiwan, 42,* 201.

100. Gregory, G.A., et al. (1974). Meconium aspiration in infants—a prospective study. *J Pediatr, 85,* 848.

101. Gross, I. & Ballard, P.L. (1998). In R.A. Polin & W.W. Fox (Eds.). *Fetal and neonatal physiology* (2nd ed.). Philadelphia: W.B. Saunders.

102. Guyton, A.C. & Hall, J.E. (1996). *Textbook of medical physiology* (9th ed.). Philadelphia: W.B. Saunders.

103. Halbower, A.C. & Jones, M.D. Jr. (1999). Physiologic reflexes and their impact on resuscitation of the newborn. *Clin Perinatol, 26,* 621.

104. Hallak, M., et al. (1993). Accelerated pulmonary maturation from preterm premature rupture of membranes: a myth. *Am J Obstet Gynecol, 169,* 1905.

105. Hankins, G.D., et al. (1996). Third-trimester arterial blood gas and acid base values in normal pregnancy at moderate altitude. *Obstet Gynecol, 88,* 347.

106. Haworth, S.G. & Hislop, A.A. (1981). Normal structural and functional adaptation to extrauterine life. *J Pediatr, 98,* 915.

107. Heenan, A.P. & Wolfe, L.A. (2000). Plasma acid-base regulation above and below ventilatory threshold in late gestation. *J Appl Physiol, 88,* 149.

108. Heffner, I.J., et al. (1993). Clinical and environmental predictors of preterm birth. *Obstet Gynecol, 81,* 750.

109. Hislop, A. & Reid, L.M. (1977). Formation of the pulmonary vasculature. In W.A. Hodson (Ed.). *Development of the lung.* New York: Marcel Dekker.

110. Ho, J.J., et al. (2000). Continuous distending pressure for respiratory distress syndrome in preterm infants. *Cochrane Database Syst Rev 2000, 4,* CD002271.

111. Hodgkinson, R. & Marx, G.F. (1984). Effects of analgesia-anesthesia on the fetus and neonate. In C.V. Cosmi (Ed.). *Obstetric anesthesia and perinatology.* New York: Appleton-Century-Crofts.

112. Hodson, W.A. (1998). Normal and abnormal structural development of the lung. In R.A. Polin & W.W. Fox (Eds.). *Fetal and neonatal physiology* (2nd ed.). Philadelphia: W.B. Saunders.

113. Huch, R. (1986). Maternal hyperventilation and the fetus. *J Perinat Med, 14,* 3.

114. Hyman, A., et al. (1978). Prostaglandins and the lung: state of the art. *Am Rev Respir Dis, 117,* 111.

115. Ie, S., et al. (2002). Respiratory complications of pregnancy. *Obstet Gynecol Surv, 57,* 39.

116. Incaudo, G.A. (1987). Diagnosis and treatment of rhinitis during pregnancy and lactation. *Clin Rev Allergy, 5,* 325.

117. Inselman L.S. & Mellins R.B. (1981). Growth and development of the lung. *J Pediatr, 98,* 1.

118. Jain, L. (1999). Alveolar fluid clearance in developing lungs and its role in neonatal transition. *Clin Perinatol, 26,* 585.

119. James, A.W. (2001). Asthma. *Obstet Gynecol Clin North Am, 28,* 305.

120. Jaykka, S. (1954). A new theory concerning the mechanism of the initiation of respiration in the newborn. *Acta Paediatr Scand, 43,* 399.

121. Jaykka, S. (1958). Capillary erection and the structural appearance of fetal and neonatal lungs. *Acta Paediatr Scand, 47,* 484.

122. Jeffrey, P.K. (1998). The development of large and small airways. *Am J Respir Crit Care Med, 157,* 174.

123. Jobe, A.H. (1998). Pathophysiology of respiratory distress syndrome and surfactant metabolism. In R.A. Polin & W.W. Fox (Eds.). *Fetal and neonatal physiology* (2nd ed.). Philadelphia: W.B. Saunders.

124. Jobe, A.H. (1998). Surfactant treatment. In R.A. Polin & W.W. Fox (Eds.). *Fetal and neonatal physiology* (2nd ed.). Philadelphia: W.B. Saunders.

125. Jobe, A.H. (1999). Fetal lung development, tests for maturation, induction of maturation, and treatment. In R.K. Creasy & R. Resnik (Eds.), *Maternal-fetal medicine* (4th ed.). Philadelphia: W.B. Saunders.

126. Jobe, A.H. & Ikegami, M. (2000). Lung development and function in preterm infants in the surfactant treatment era. *Annu Rev Physiol, 62,* 825.

127. Jobe, A.H. & Bancalari, E. (2001). NICHD/NHLBI/ORD workshop summary: Bronchopulmonary dysplasia. *Am J Respir Crit Care Med, 163,* 1723.

128. Jobe, A.H. & Ikegami, M. (2001). Biology of surfactant. *Clin Perinatol, 28,* 655.

129. Jobe, A.H. & Ikegami, M. (2001). Prevention of bronchopulmonary dysplasia. *Curr Opin Pediatr, 13,* 124.

130. Johansson, J., et al. (1994). The proteins of the surfactant system. *Eur Respir J, 7,* 372.

131. Kari, M.A., et al. (1994). Prenatal dexamethasone treatment in conjunction with rescue therapy of human surfactant: a randomized placebo-controlled multicenter study. *Pediatrics, 93,* 730.

132. Kay, H.H., et al. (2000). Antenatal steroid treatment and adverse fetal effects: what is the evidence? *J Soc Gynecol Investig, 7,* 269.

133. Keens, D.H. & Ianuzzo, C.D. (1979). Development of fatigue-resistant muscle fibers in human ventilatory musculature. *Am Rev Respir Dis, 119*(suppl), 139.

134. Keijzer, R., et al. (2000). Hormonal modulation of fetal pulmonary development: Relevance for the fetus with diaphragmatic hernia. *Eur J Obstet Gynecol Reprod Biol, 92,* 127.

135. Kemp, J.G., et al. (1997). Acid-base regulation after maximal exercise testing in late gestation. *J Appl Physiol, 83,* 644.

136. Kent, N.E. & Farquharson, D.F. (1993). Cystic fibrosis in pregnancy. *Can Med Assoc J, 140,* 809.

137. Kleinman, J.C., et al. (1988). The effects of maternal smoking on fetal and infant mortality. *Am J Epidemiol, 127,* 274.

138. Knill, R. & Bryan, A.C. (1976). An intercostal-phrenic inhibitory reflex in the human newborn infant. *J Appl Physiol, 40,* 352.

139. Knuttgen, H.G. & Emerson, K. (1974). Physiological response to pregnancy at rest and during exercise. *J Appl Physiol, 36,* 549.

140. Kotecha, S. (2000). Lung growth: Implications for the newborn infant. *Arch Dis Child Fetal Neonatal Ed, 82,* F69.

141. Kotloff, R.M., et al. (1992). Fertility and pregnancy in patients with cystic fibrosis. *Clin Chest Med, 13,* 623.

142. Kresch, M.J. & Gross, I. (1987). The biochemistry of fetal lung development. *Clin Perinatol, 14,* 481.

143. Laudy, J.A. & Wladimiroff, J.W. (2000). The fetal lung. 2: Pulmonary hypoplasia. *Ultrasound Obstet Gynecol, 16,* 482.

144. Lehmann, V. (1975). Dyspnea in pregnancy. *J Perinat Med, 3,* 154.

145. Levinson, G., et al. (1974). Effect of maternal hyperventilation on uterine blood flow and fetal oxygenation and acid-base status. *Anesthesiology, 40,* 340.

146. Li, D.K., et al. (1996). Maternal smoking during pregnancy and the risk of congenital urinary tract anomalies. *Am J Public Health, 86,* 249.

147. Liggins, G.C. & Howie, R.N. (1972). A controlled trial of antepartum glucocorticoid treatment for prevention of the respiratory distress syndrome in premature infants. *Pediatrics, 50,* 515.

148. Liggins, G.C. (1994). The role of cortisol in preparing the fetus for birth. *Reprod Fertil Dev, 6,* 141.

149. Lim, W.S., et al. (2001). Pneumonia and pregnancy. *Thorax, 56,* 398.

150. Lotgering, F., et al. (1985). Maternal and fetal responses to exercise during pregnancy. *Physiol Rev, 65,* 1.

151. Lotgering, F.K., et al. (1998). Respiratory and metabolic responses to endurance cycle exercise in pregnant and postpartum women. *Int J Sports Med, 19,* 193.

152. Low, J.A. (1997). Intrapartum fetal asphyxia: definition, diagnosis, and classification. *Am J Obstet Gynecol, 176,* 957.

153. Lowrey, G.H. (1986). *Growth and development of children.* Chicago: Year Book.

154. MacDorman, M.F., et al. (1997). Sudden infant death syndrome and smoking in the United States and Sweden. *Am J Epidemiol, 1436,* 249.

155. Machida, H. (1981). Influence of progesterone on arterial blood and CSF acid-base balance in women. *J Appl Physiol, 51,* 1433.

156. Macklem, P.T. (1971). Airway obstruction and collateral ventilation. *Physiol Rev, 51,* 368.

157. Malloy, M.H., et al. (1992). Sudden infant death syndrome and maternal smoking. *Am J Public Health, 82,* 1380.

158. Maloney, J.E. (1987). Lung liquid dynamics in the perinatal period. In J. Lipshitz et al. (Eds.). *Perinatal development of the heart & lung.* New York: Perinatology Press.

159. Marchal, F. (1987). Neonatal apnea. In L. Stern & P. Vert (Eds.). *Neonatal medicine.* New York: Masson.

160. Marx, G.F., et al. (1970). Static compliance before and after vaginal delivery. *Br J Anaesthiol, 42,* 1100.

161. Maxwell, L.C., et al. (1983). Development of the histochemical and functional properties of baboon respiratory muscles. *J Appl Physiol, 54,* 551.

162. McAuliffe, F., et al. (2001). Blood gases in pregnancy at sea level and at high altitude. *BJOG, 108,* 980.

163. McMurray, R.G., et al. (1993). Recent advances in understanding maternal and fetal responses to exercise. *Med Sci Exerc, 25,* 1305.

164. Mercer, J. & Skovgaard. (2002). Neonatal transitional physiology: A new paradigm. *J Perinat Neonat Nurs, 15,* 56.

165. Meschia, G. (1999). Placental respiratory gas exchange and fetal oxygenation. In R.K. Creasy & R. Resnik (Eds.). *Maternal-fetal medicine* (4th ed.). Philadelphia: W.B. Saunders.

166. Metcalfe, J., Stock, M. & Banon, P. (1988). Maternal physiology during gestation. In E. Knobil et al. (Eds.). *The physiology of reproduction.* New York: Raven.

167. Meyrick, B. & Reid, L.M. (1977). Ultrastructure of alveolar lining and its development. In W.A. Hodson (Ed.). *Development of the lung.* New York: Marcel Dekker.

168. Milberger, S., et al. (1996). Is maternal smoking during pregnancy a risk factor for attention deficit hyperactivity disorder in children? *Am J Psychiatry, 153,* 1138.

169. Miller, M.G., et al. (1987). Oral breathing in newborn infants. *J Pediatr, 107,* 465.

170. Miller, M.J. (1998). Pathophysiology of apnea of prematurity. In R.A. Polin & W.W. Fox (Eds.). *Fetal and neonatal physiology* (2nd ed.). Philadelphia: W.B. Saunders.

171. Miller, M.J., et al. (2002). Respiratory disorders in preterm and term infants. In A.A. Fanaroff & & R.J. Martin (Eds.). *Neonatal and perinatal medicine: Diseases of the fetus and infant* (7th ed.). St. Louis: Mosby.

172. Milne, J., et al. (1977). Maternal gas exchange and acid-base status during normal pregnancy. *Scott Med J, 22,* 108.

173. Milne, J.A., et al. (1977). The effect of human pregnancy on the pulmonary transfer factor for carbon monoxide as measured by the single-breath method. *Clin Sci Mol Med, 53,* 271.

174. Milner, A.D. & Vyas, H. (1982). Lung expansion at birth. *J Pediatr, 101,* 879.

175. Moore, K.L. & Persaud, T.V.N. (1998). *The developing human: clinically oriented embryology* (6th ed.). Philadelphia: W.B. Saunders.

176. Mortola, J.P. (1998). Mechanics of breathing. In R.A. Polin & W.W. Fox (Eds.). *Fetal and neonatal physiology* (2nd ed.). Philadelphia: W.B. Saunders.

177. Muir, B.L. (1988). *Pathophysiology* (2nd ed.). New York: John Wiley.

178. Murphy, T. & Woodrum D. (1998). Functional development of respiratory muscles. In R.A. Polin & W.W. Fox (Eds.). *Fetal and neonatal physiology* (2nd ed.). Philadelphia: W.B. Saunders.

179. Naeye, R.L. (1980). Abruptio placentae and placenta previa: frequency, perinatal mortality and cigarette smoking. *Obstet Gynecol, 55,* 701.

180. National Asthma Education Program, Report of the Working Group on Asthma and Pregnancy. (1993). *Management of asthma during pregnancy* (NIH publication no. 93-3279). Bethesda, MD: National Institutes of Health.

181. National Institutes of Health Consensus. (1995). Consensus Developmental Conference on the Effects of Corticosteroids for Fetal Maturation on Perinatal Outcomes. *JAMA, 273,* 413.

182. National Institutes of Health. (2000). Antenatal corticosteroids revisited: Repeated courses. *NIH Consensus Statement, 17*(2), 1.

183. Nava S., et al. (1992). Evidence of acute diaphragmatic fatigue in a "natural condition": the diaphragm during labor. *Am Rev Respir Dis, 146,* 1226.

184. Nelson, N.M. (1976). Respiration and circulation after birth. In C.A. Smith & N.M. Nelson (Eds.). *The physiology of the newborn infant.* Springfield, IL: Charles C Thomas.

185. Nichols, D.G. & Rogers, M.C. (1987). Developmental physiology of the respiratory system. In M.C. Rogers (Ed.). *Textbook of pediatric intensive care* (vol. 1). Baltimore: Williams & Wilkins.

186. Nordstrom, L. (2001). Lactate measurements in scalp and cord arterial blood. *Curr Opin Obstet Gynecol, 13,* 141.

187. Northway, W.H., et al. (1967). Pulmonary disease following respiratory therapy of hyaline membrane disease: Bronchopulmonary dysplasia. *N Engl J Med, 276,* 357.

188. O'Day, M.P. (1997). Cardio-respiratory physiological adaptation of pregnancy. *Semin Perinatol, 21,* 268.

189. Ohtake, P.J. & Wolfe, L.A. (1998). Physical conditioning attenuates respiratory responses to steady-state exercise in late gestation. *Med Sci Sports Exerc, 30,* 17.

190. Painter, P.C. (1980). Simultaneous measurement of lecithin, sphingomyelin, phosphatidylglycerol, phosphatidylinositol, phosphatidylethanolamine and phosphatidylserine in amniotic fluid. *Clin Chem, 26,* 1147.

191. Poets, C.F. (1998). When do infants need additional inspired oxygen? A review of the current literature. *Pediatr Pulmonol, 26,* 424.

192. Possemayer, F. (1998). Physiochemical aspects of pulmonary surfactant. In R.A. Polin & W.W. Fox (Eds.). *Fetal and neonatal physiology* (2nd ed.). Philadelphia: W.B. Saunders.

193. Prowse, C.M. & Gaensler, E.A. (1965). Respiratory and acid-base changes during pregnancy. *Anesthesiology, 26,* 381.

194. Purinak, B.M., et al. (1994). Longitudinal study of pulmonary function tests during pregnancy. *J Physiol Pharmacol, 38,* 129.

195. Quirk, J.G. & Bleasdale, J.E. (1986). Fetal lung maturation in the pregnancy complicated by diabetes mellitus. In G.C. Di Renzo & D.F. Hawkins (Eds.). *Perinatal medicine: Problems and controversies.* New York: Raven Press.

196. Rabbette, P.S., et al. (1994). Hering-Breuer reflex and respiratory system compliance in the first year of life: a longitudinal study. *J Appl Physiol, 76,* 650.

197. Rajadurai, V.S., et al. (1992). Effect of fetal haemoglobin on the accuracy of pulse oximetry in preterm infants. *J Paediatr Child Health, 28,* 43.

198. Ramsey, P.S. & Ramin, K.D. (2001). Pneumonia in pregnancy. *Obstet Gynecol Clin North Am, 28,* 553.

199. Ramsey, S.A. (1998). Regulation of surfactant-associated phospholipid synthesis and secretion. In R.A. Polin & W.W. Fox (Eds.). *Fetal and neonatal physiology* (2nd ed.). Philadelphia: W.B. Saunders.

200. Randell, S.H. & Young, S.L. (1998). Structure of alveolar epithelial cells and the surface layer during development. In R.A. Polin & W.W. Fox (Eds.). *Fetal and neonatal physiology* (2nd ed.). Philadelphia: W.B. Saunders.

201. Rees, C.B., et al. (1990). Longitudinal study of respiratory changes in normal human pregnancy with cross-sectional data on subjects with pregnancy induced hypertension. *Am J Obstet Gynecol, 162,* 826.

202. Reid L.M. (1984). Structural development of the lung and pulmonary circulation. In K. Raivio, et al. (Eds.). *Respiratory distress syndrome.* London: Academic Press.

203. Richarson, B.S. & Gagnon, R. (1999). Fetal breathing and body movements. In R.K. Creasy & R. Resnik (Eds.). *Maternal-fetal medicine* (4th ed.). Philadelphia: W.B. Saunders

204. Rigatto, H. (1998). Control of breathing in fetal life and onset and control of breathing in the newborn. In R.A. Polin & W.W. Fox (Eds.). *Fetal and neonatal physiology* (2nd ed.). Philadelphia: W.B. Saunders.

205. Rodenstein, D.O., et al. (1985). Infants are not obligatory nasal breathers. *Am Rev Respir Dis, 131,* 343.

206. Rodriquez, R.J., et al. (2002). Respiratory distress syndrome and its management. In A.A. Fanaroff & R.J. Martin (Eds.). *Neonatal and perinatal medicine: Diseases of the fetus and infant* (7th ed.). St. Louis: Mosby.

207. Rojas, M.A. (1995). Changing trends in the epidemiology and pathogenesis of neonatal chronic lung disease. *J Pediatr, 126,* 605.

208. Rooth, G. (1980). Fetal homeostasis. In S. Aladjem, A.K. Brown & C. Surreau (Eds.). *Clinical perinatology.* St. Louis: Mosby.

209. Samuel, B.U. & Barry, M. (1998). The pregnant traveler. *Inf Dis Clin N Am, 12,* 325.

210. Schatz, M., et al. (1985). Distinguishing clinical and biochemical characteristics associated with improvement or deterioration of asthma during pregnancy. *J Allergy Clin Immunol, 75,* 133.

211. Schatz, M. & Hoffman, C. (1987). Interrelationships between asthma and pregnancy: Clinical and mechanistic considerations. *Clin Rev Allergy, 5,* 301

212. Schatz, M., et al. (1988). The course of asthma during pregnancy, postpartum, and with successive pregnancies: A prospective analysis. *J Allergy Clin Immunol, 81,* 509.

213. Scott, J.R. & Rose, N.B. (1976). Effects of psychoprophylaxis (Lamaze preparation) on labor and delivery in primiparas. *N Engl J Med, 294,* 1205.

214. Sherwood, O.D., et al. (1993). The physiological effect of relaxin during pregnancy: Studies in rats and pigs. *Oxf Rev Reprod Biol, 15*, 143.

215. Soll, R.F. (1998). Surfactant treatment of the very preterm infant. *Biol Neonate, 74*(suppl 1), 35

216. Soll, R.F. (2000). Synthetic surfactant for respiratory distress syndrome in preterm infants. *Cochrane Database Syst Rev 2000, 2,* CD001149

217. Soll, R.F. (2000). Prophylactic synthetic surfactant for preventing morbidity and mortality in preterm infants. *Cochrane Database Syst Rev 2000, 2,* CD001079.

218. Soll, R.F. (2000). Natural surfactant extract for preventing morbidity and mortality in preterm infants. *Cochrane Database Syst Rev 2000, 2,* CD000511.

219. Soll, R.F & Morley, C.J. (2000). Prophylactic versus selective use of surfactant for preventing morbidity and mortality in preterm infants. *Cochrane Database Syst Rev 2000, 2,* CD000510

220. Spaeth, J.P., et al. (1998). Anesthesia for the micropremie. *Semin Perinatol, 22*, 390.

221. Sparling, I., et al. (1992). The variability of cardiopulmonary adaptation to pregnancy at rest and during exercise. *Br J Obstet Gynecol, 99*(suppl 8), 1.

222. Spira, A., et al. (1977). Smoking during pregnancy and placental pathology. *Biomedicine, 27*, 266.

223. Spragg, R. (2000). Surfactant replacement therapy. *Clin Chest Med, 21*, 531.

224. Stick, S. (2000). Pediatric origins of adult lung disease. 1: The contribution of airway development to paediatric and adult lung disease. *Thorax, 55*, 587.

225. Stick, S.M., et al. (1996). Effects of maternal smoking during pregnancy and a family history of asthma on respiratory function in newborn infants. *Lancet, 348*, 1050.

226. Stjernfeldt, M., et al. (1986). Maternal smoking during pregnancy and risk for childhood cancer. *Lancet, 1*, 1350.

227. Strang, L.B. (1978). Pulmonary circulation at birth. In L.B. Strang (Ed.). *Neonatal respiration: Physiological and clinical studies.* Philadelphia: J.B. Lippincott.

228. Strang, L.B. (1991). Fetal lung liquid: secretion and reabsorption. *Physiol Rev, 71*, 991.

229. Sykes, M.K. (1975). Arterial oxygen tension in parturient women. *Br J Anaesth, 47*, 530.

230. Taeusch, H.W., et al. (1981). *Schaffer and Avery's diseases of the new born* (6th ed.). Philadelphia: W.B. Saunders.

231. Tager, I.B., et al. (1995). Maternal smoking during pregnancy: effects on lung function during the first 18 months of life. *Am J Respir Crit Care Med, 152*, 977.

232. Tan, K.S. & Thomson, N.C. (2000). Asthma in pregnancy. *Am J Med, 109*, 727.

233. Thach, B.T. (2001). Maturation and transformation of reflexes that protect the laryngeal airway from liquid aspiration from fetal to adult life. *Am J Med, 111*(suppl 8A), 69S.

234. Thompson, M.W. (2001). Surfactant protein B deficiency: Insights into surfactant function through clinical surfactant protein deficiency. *Am J Med Sci, 321*, 26.

235. Thorp, J.A. & Rushing, R.S. (1999). Umbilical cord blood gas analysis. *Obstet Gynecol Clin North Am, 26*, 695.

236. Thurlbeck, W.M. & Angus, G.E. (1975). Growth and aging of the normal human lung. *Chest, 67* (suppl), 3S.

237. Thurlbeck, W.M. (1975). Postnatal growth and development of the lung. *Am Rev Respir Dis, 111*, 803.

238. Tredano, M., et al. (2001). Clinical biological and genetic heterogeneity of the inborn errors of pulmonary surfactant metabolism. *Clin Chem Lab Med, 39*, 90.

239. Truog, W.E. (1998). Pulmonary gas exchange in the developing lung. In R.A. Polin & W.W. Fox (Eds.). *Fetal and neonatal physiology* (2nd ed.). Philadelphia: W.B. Saunders.

240. Turnbull, G.L., et al. (1996). Managing pregnancy-related nocturnal nasal congestion: the external nasal dilator. *J Reprod Med, 41*, 897.

241. Turner, E.S., et al. (1980). Management of the pregnant asthmatic patient. *Ann Intern Med, 6*, 905.

242. Tyson, J.F., et al. (1995). The small for gestational age infants: accelerated or delayed pulmonary maturation? Increased or decreased survival? *Pediatrics, 95*, 534.

243. Ueland, K., et al. (1973). Cardiorespiratory responses to pregnancy and exercise in normal women and patients with heart disease. *Am J Obstet Gynecol, 115*, 4.

244. Vander, A., Sherman, J. & Luciano, D. (2000). *Human physiology: The mechanism of body function* (8th ed.). New York: McGraw-Hill.

245. Van Hook, J.W., et al. (1996). Effect of pregnancy on maternal oxygen saturation values: Use of reflectance pulse oximetry during pregnancy. *South Med J, 89*, 1188.

246. Vio, F., et al. (1991). Smoking during pregnancy and lactation and its effects on breastmilk volume. *Am J Clin Nutr, 54*, 1011.

247. Wallace, A.M. & Engstrom, J.L. (1987). The effects of aerobic exercise on the pregnant woman, fetus, and pregnancy outcome: A review. *J Nurse Midwifery, 32*, 277.

248. Weibel, E.R. & Gil, J. (1977). Structure-function relationships at the alveolar level. In J.B. West (Ed.). *Bioengineering aspects of the lung.* New York: Marcel Dekker.

249. Weinberger, S.E. & Weiss, S.T. (1999). Pulmonary diseases. In G.N. Burrow & T.P. Duffy (Eds.). *Medical complications during pregnancy* (5th ed.). Philadelphia: W.B. Saunders.

250. Weltzman, M., et al. (1990). Maternal smoking and childhood cancer. *Pediatrics, 85*, 505.

251. West, J.B. (1988). Pulmonary pathophysiology—the essentials (5th ed.). Baltimore: Williams & Wilkins.

252. Westgren, M., et al. (1999). Role of lactate measurements during labor. *Obstet Gynecol Surv, 54*, 43.

253. Whitelaw, A. & Thoresen, M. (2000). Antenatal steroids and the developing brain. *Arch Dis Child Fetal Neonatal Ed, 83*, F154.

254. Whitsett, J.A. (1998). Composition of pulmonary surfactant lipids and proteins. In R.A. Polin & W.W. Fox (Eds.). *Fetal and neonatal physiology* (2nd ed.). Philadelphia: W.B. Saunders.

255. Whitsett, J.A. & Stahlman, M.T. (1998). Impact of advances in physiology, biology, and molecular biology on pulmonary disease in neonates. *Am J Respir Crit Care Med, 1157*, 567.

256. Wilkening, R. & Meschia, G. (1983). Fetal oxygen uptake, oxygenation, and acid-base balance as a function of uterine blood flow. *Am J Physiol, 244*, 749.

257. Wise, R.A. & Polito, A.J. (2000). Respiratory physiologic changes in pregnancy. *Immunol Allergy Clin N Am, 20*, 663.

258. Wiswell, T.E. (2001). Expanded uses of surfactant therapy. *Clin Perinatol, 28*, 695.

259. Witlin, A.G. (1997). Asthma in pregnancy. *Semin Perinatol, 21*, 284.

260. Wolfe, L.A., et al. (1998). Acid-base regulation and control of ventilation in human pregnancy. *Can J Physiol Pharmacol, 76*, 815.

261. Wyszynski, D.F., et al. (1997). Maternal cigarette smoking and oral clefts: a meta-analysis. *Cleft Palate Craniofac J, 34*, 206.

262. Zeldis, S.M. (1992). Dyspnea during pregnancy: distinguishing cardiac from pulmonary causes. *Clin Chest Med, 13*, 567.

CHAPTER 10

Renal System and Fluid and Electrolyte Homeostasis

The kidneys are critical organs in maintaining body homeostasis by regulation of water and electrolyte balance, excretion of metabolic waste products and foreign substances, regulation of vitamin D activity and erythrocyte production (via erythropoietin), and gluconeogenesis.[182] The kidneys also have an important role in control of arterial blood pressure through the renin-angiotensin system and regulation of sodium balance. This chapter examines the alterations in basic renal processes and regulation of fluids and electrolytes observed in the pregnant woman, fetus, and neonate, and discusses the implications of these changes in clinical practice. Basic renal processes are summarized in Figure 10-1 and in the box on p. 371.

MATERNAL PHYSIOLOGIC ADAPTATIONS

The renal system undergoes a variety of structural and functional changes during pregnancy, with many of the structural changes persisting well into the postpartum period. Pregnancy is characterized by sodium retention and increased extracellular volume, both of which are mediated by alterations in renal function. Many parameters normally used to evaluate renal function and fluid and electrolyte homeostasis are altered in pregnancy, and subclinical renal problems may not be recognized.

Antepartum Period

The renal system must handle the effects of increased maternal intravascular and extracellular volume and metabolic waste products as well as serve as the primary excretory organ for fetal wastes. Changes in the renal system are related to hormonal effects (particularly the influence of progesterone on smooth muscle), pressure from the enlarging uterus, effects of position and activity, and alterations in the cardiovascular system and vasoactive substances. Cardiovascular system changes that interact with alterations in renal hemodynamics include increased cardiac output, increased blood and plasma volume, and alterations in the venous system and plasma proteins (see Chapters 7 and 8). The predominant structural change in the renal system during pregnancy is dilatation of the renal pelvis and ureters; functional changes include alterations in hemodynamics, glomerular filtration, and tubular handling of certain substances. Changes in fluid and electrolyte homeostasis result from changes in renal handling of water and sodium and alterations in the renin-angiotensin system. Table 10-1 summarizes changes in the renal system during pregnancy and their clinical implications. Even with these changes, renal reserve is maintained during pregnancy, so that the pregnant woman has the capacity for further vasodilatation and dilatation above baseline if needed.[63,172]

Structural and Urodynamic Changes

Pregnancy is characterized by physiologic hydroureter and hydronephrosis with significant dilatation of the renal calyces, pelvis, and ureters beginning as early as the seventh week. The mean kidney length increases by approximately 1 cm due to the increased renal blood flow and vascular volume and the renal hypertrophy.[135] Renal volume increases by 30%.[31] Hydronephrosis is generally reported to occur in more than 80% of pregnant women.[15,61,125,148] Recent ultrasound studies have demonstrated dilatation of the urinary tract in 50% of women in the second and third trimesters.[58] The diameter of the ureteral lumen increases with hypertonicity and hypomotility of the ureteral musculature.[148] Ureteral hypomotility and reduced peristaltic movements may be mediated by prostaglandin E_2 (PGE_2).[15,21,61,142]

The ureters elongate and become more tortuous during the last half of pregnancy as they are laterally displaced by the growing uterus.[15] These changes are seen in the renal pelvis and the upper portion of the ureters to the pelvic brim. The portion of the ureters below the pelvic brim (linea terminalis) is usually not enlarged. The ureters may contain as much as 300 ml of urine.[61] This reservoir of urine can interfere with accuracy of 24-hour urine collections and increases the risk of urinary tract infection (UTI).

The etiology of physiologic hydroureter is unclear. Dilatation begins before the uterus reaches the pelvic brim, so initial changes are probably hormonally mediated.[58] Hormonal influences, particularly progesterone, may induce hypertrophy of the longitudinal smooth muscles surrounding distal portions of the ureters and hyperplasia of periurethral connective tissue.[15,61] This may lead to a temporary stenosis and mild dilatation of the upper portion of the ureters. These findings are similar to those seen in women on oral contraceptives and in postmenopausal women given estrogen and progesterone.[61] The major contributing factor to hydronephrosis in later pregnancy is probably external compression of the ureters at the pelvic brim by the uterus, iliac arteries, and enlarging ovarian vein complexes.[58] As pregnancy progresses, the ureters are compressed at the pelvic brim by blood vessels in the area and by the growing uterus, leading to further, marked dilatation and urinary stasis. Dilatation is more prominent in the primipara, whose firmer abdominal wall may increase resistance and pressure on the ureters.[15] Increased urine flow in pregnancy results in some ureteral dilatation even without any obstruction to flow.[123]

In most women the right ureter is dilated to a greater extent than the left.[50,64] These differences become more prominent after 21 weeks.[58] The right ureter makes a right-angle turn as it crosses the iliac and ovarian veins at the pelvic brim; the turn of the left ureter is less acute, and it

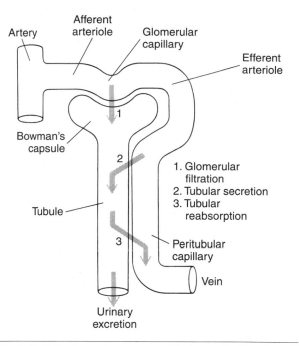

FIGURE **10-1** Basic renal processes: (1) glomerular filtration, (2) tubular reabsorption, and (3) tubular secretion. Substances are processed by a combination of filtration, secretion, and reabsorption. (See the box below for descriptions of these processes.) (From Vander, A.J., et al. [1985]. *Human physiology: Mechanisms of body function* [3rd ed.]. New York:

Basic Renal Processes

Glomerular filtration—Plasma is filtered from blood moving through the glomerulus into the Bowman capsule. The glomerulus is freely permeable to water and small molecules but impermeable to colloids and larger molecules, including most protein-bound substances. Filtration is influenced by hydrostatic and colloid osmotic pressure.

Tubular reabsorption—Water and other substances appear in the urine in smaller quantities than were originally filtered due to reabsorption in the tubules. Tubular reabsorption of substances from the tubular lumen back into the blood in the peritubular capillaries occurs through simple diffusion, facilitated diffusion, and active transport. These mechanisms can only transport limited amounts (transport maximum [Tm]) of certain substances, such as glucose, due to saturation of the carriers. Any amount filtered in excess of this quantity cannot be reabsorbed and appears in the urine. The proximal tubule is the major site for reabsorption of glucose, amino acids, sodium, protein, and other organic nutrients. The movement of water, sodium, and chloride

through the kidneys is interrelated and affected by concentration gradients within various segments of the nephron and the surrounding interstitial spaces. These substances are freely filtered and 99% of the amount filtered is reabsorbed, 65% to 80% in the proximal tubule, 20% to 25% in the ascending limb of the loop of Henle, and the remainder in the distal and collecting tubes. The processes through which sodium is reabsorbed vary in different portions of the tubule. Reabsorption of sodium in the proximal tubule is an active, carrier-mediated process. In the ascending limb of the loop of Henle, chloride is actively reabsorbed and sodium follows passively. Sodium reabsorption is mediated by aldosterone in the distal tubule and collecting duct, where sodium is exchanged for potassium and hydrogen ions. Water reabsorption by passive diffusion or osmosis is sodium dependent but also depends on permeability of the tubular membrane (which is altered by arginine vasopressin).

Tubular secretion—This involves the movement of substances from the peritubular capillaries into the lumen of the tubules.

Adapted from Vander, A., Sherman, J., & Luciano, D. (2000). *Human physiology: The mechanism of body function* (8th ed.). New York: McGraw-Hill.

TABLE **10-1**   Changes in the Renal System during Pregnancy

PARAMETER	ALTERATION	SIGNIFICANCE
Renal calyces, pelvis, and ureters	Dilatation (more prominent on right)	Increased risk of urinary tract infection in pregnancy and postpartum
	Elongation, decreased motility, and hypertonicity of ureters	Altered accuracy of 24-hour urine collections
	May last up to 3 months postpartum	
Bladder	Decreased tone, increased capacity	Risk of infection
		Urinary frequency and incontinence
		Alteration in accuracy of 24-hour urine collections
	Displaced in late pregnancy	Urinary frequency
	Mucosa edematous and hyperemic	Risk of trauma and infection
	Incompetence of vesicoureteral valve	Risk of reflux and infection
		Alteration in accuracy of 24-hour urine collections
Renal blood flow	Increases 35%-60%	Increased glomerular filtration rate
		Increased solutes delivered to kidney
Glomerular filtration rate	Increases 40%-50%	Increased filtration and excretion of water and solutes
		Increased urine flow and volume
		Decreased serum blood urea nitrogen, creatinine, uric acid
		Altered renal excretion of drugs with risk of subtherapeutic blood and tissue levels
Renal tubular function	Increased reabsorption of solutes (may not always match increase in filtered load)	Maintenance of homeostasis
		Avoid pathologic solute or fluid loss
	Increased renal excretion of glucose, protein, amino acids, urea, uric acid, water-soluble vitamins, calcium, hydrogen ions, phosphorus	Tendency for glycosuria, proteinuria
		Compensation for respiratory alkalosis
		Increased nutritional needs (i.e., calcium, water-soluble vitamins)
	Net retention of sodium and water	Accumulation of sodium and water to meet maternal and fetal needs
Renin-angiotensin-aldosterone system	Increase in all components	Maintain homeostasis with expanded extracellular volume
	Resistance to pressor effects of angiotensin II	Retention of water and sodium
		Balance forces favoring sodium excretion
		Maintain normal blood pressure
Arginine vasopressin and regulation of osmolarity	Retention of water	Expansion of plasma volume and other extracellular volume
	Osmostat reset	Maintenance of volume homeostasis in spite of reduction in plasma osmolarity

parallels rather than crosses the left ovarian vein. The iliac vessels are more rigid on the right than on the left, thus further compressing the ureters. Compression is maximal by around 30 weeks' gestation, with no further significant changes to term.[30] The sigmoid colon, which lies between the left ureter and the pelvis, probably does not have a cushioning effect, as had previously been proposed.[61] The sigmoid colon does contribute to dextroversion of the uterus and may increase ureteral compression on the con-tralateral side during the last trimester.[15,61] The position of the fetus does not seem to influence ureteral dilatation. The site of placental attachment may increase venous flow on that side with subsequent compression of the ureters by the dilated vessels.[61]

Bladder tone decreases as a result of the effects of progesterone on smooth muscle. Bladder capacity doubles by term. The bladder becomes displaced anteriorly and superiorly by the end of the second trimester. Under the influence of estrogen, the trigone undergoes hyperplasia with hypertrophy of the bladder musculature. The bladder mucosa becomes hyperemic with increased size and tortuosity of the blood vessels. The mucosa becomes more edematous and vulnerable to trauma or infection after engagement of the presenting part.[61]

The baseline intravesical pressure doubles due to the enlarged uterus.[123] The decreased bladder tone and flaccidity may lead to incompetence of the vesicoureteral valve and reflux of urine. Vesicourethral reflux is seen in up to 3.5% of pregnant women, especially in the third trimester.[123] Predisposing factors for this reflux include hypertrophy and hyperplasia of the urethral wall, increased elasticity of the ureters, increased bladder pressure, and decreased peristalsis in the distal ureter.[123,135] Alterations in bladder placement by the growing uterus stretch the trigone and displace the intravesical portion of the ureters laterally. This shortens the terminal ureter, decreasing intravesical pressure. If intravesical pressure subsequently increases with micturition, urine regurgitates into the ureters.[61]

Changes in Urodynamics

Urine output increases from a mean of 1475 to 1919 ml per 24 hours primarily because of changes in sodium excretion.[123] Mean flow rate decreases in the second and third trimesters with an increase in flow time and time to maximal flow throughout pregnancy.[123] The number of voids per day and mean daily urine output increase throughout gestation.[177] Studies of changes in bladder capacity during pregnancy have reported variable findings. Increased bladder capacity due to the decreased tone has been reported, especially in primiparas.[5] Others have found a mean bladder capacity similar to that of the nonpregnant state in the first two trimesters, but decreased capacity in the third trimester due to elevation of the trigone and the size of the presenting part.[163] A recent study reported that the pregnant woman's bladder has a larger capacity with a lower pressure per volume.[153] In nonpregnant women the first urge to void was at a bladder capacity of 150 to 200 ml and maximum at 450 to 550 ml with an intravesicular pressure of 20 cmH$_2$O; in pregnant women the first urge to void was at a bladder capacity of 250 to 400 ml (intravesical pressure of 4 to 8 cmH$_2$O) and often did not reach maximum until 1000 to 1200 ml (intravesicular pressure of 12 to 15 cmH$_2$O).[153]

Changes in Renal Hemodynamics

Significant hemodynamic changes occur within the kidneys beginning early in pregnancy in conjunction with systemic vasodilatation (see Chapter 8). Renal blood flow (RBF) increases 35% to 60% by the end of the first

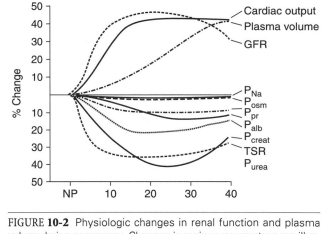

FIGURE **10-2** Physiologic changes in renal function and plasma values during pregnancy. Changes in various parameters are illustrated by percentage of increase or decrease from nonpregnant baseline. *GFR,* Glomerular filtration rate; *NP,* nonpregnant; P_{Na}, plasma sodium; P_{osm}, plasma osmolality; P_{pr}, plasma protein; P_{alb}, plasma albumin; P_{creat}, plasma creatinine; P_{urea}, plasma urea; *TSR,* total systemic resistance; *10-40,* weeks of pregnancy. (From Davison, J.M. [1997]. Edema in pregnancy. *Kidney Int Suppl, 59,* S93.)

trimester then decreases from the second trimester to term.[21,45,63,148] This change is accompanied by increased glomerular filtration rate (GFR), decreased renal vascular resistance (RVR), and activation of the renin-angiotensin-aldosterone system.[29] Renal hemodynamic changes begin before significant expansion of plasma volume and are thought to be primarily related to the decrease in systemic vascular resistance (SVR), which may stimulate sodium retention.[98] These changes may be mediated by nitric oxide (NO), prostacyclin (PGI$_2$), and atrial natriuretic factor (ANF), possibly via effects on GFR. Increased flow is enhanced by vasodilatation of preglomerular and postglomerular capillaries. Another measure of renal hemodynamics is the effective renal plasma flow (ERPF), which increases 80% by midpregnancy.[44,91,125,159,167,178] ERPF then gradually decreases by 25% during the third trimester to values 50% greater than nonpregnant values.[63,109,125,135,171]

Changes in Glomerular Filtration

The GFR increases 40% to 50% during pregnancy.[12,44,45,53,178] The rise begins soon after conception and precedes plasma volume expansion.[13] Changes in GFR are detectable 3 to 4 weeks after conception, peak at 9 to 16 weeks, then remain relatively stable to around 36 weeks. (Figure 10-2).[13,45,53,187] A decrease of up to 15% to 20% may occur in the last few weeks of pregnancy.[13,54,63,154] Values for GFR in pregnancy average 110 to 180 ml/min. Differences in reported values for RBF and GFR during pregnancy relate to the method of measurement. The increased GFR is related to increased glomerular blood flow (and glomerular capillary hydrostatic pressure) and decreased colloid osmotic (plasma oncotic) pressure due to a reduction in the concentration of plasma proteins. Failure of the GFR to increase early in pregnancy has been associated with pregnancy loss.[187]

The increases in renal plasma flow (RPF) and GFR parallel each other, although RPF changes are slightly greater than those of the GFR. This alters the filtration fraction (GFR/RPF), the portion of the renal blood flow that is filtered.[13,109,125,137,148] As a result, renal excretion of amino acids, glucose, protein, electrolytes, and vitamins increases, whereas serum urea, creatinine, blood urea nitrogen (BUN), and uric acid levels decrease (Table 10-2). The causes of the increased RPF and GFR during pregnancy are unknown. Current interest is focused in the role of NO as a mediator.[13,29,48,154] NO is a potent renal vasodilator. NO and its second messenger, guanosine 3′,5′-monophosphate (cGMP), increase in pregnancy.[154] In animal studies, inhibition of the usual NO increase during pregnancy reverses renal vasodilatation.[154] Other factors that may play a role in renal hemodynamic changes are prostacyclin, ANF, human placental lactogen, and human chorionic gonadotropin.[13,29,48,130,154]

During pregnancy, 24-hour urine volumes are higher. The degree to which renal handling of substances is altered during pregnancy depends on the renal process involved (see Figure 10-1). For example, since urea and creatinine are processed only by glomerular filtration, the increased GFR leads to a significant decrease in serum urea and creatinine levels.[137] The increased GFR also alters renal excretion of drugs (see Chapter 6).

Alterations in Tubular Function

The elevated GFR increases the concentration of solutes and volume of fluid within the tubular lumen by 50% to 100%. Tubular reabsorption increases in order to prevent rapid depletion from the body of sodium, chloride, glucose, potassium, and water. There is actually a net retention of most of these substances during pregnancy. Conversely, tubular reabsorption rates cannot always accommodate the increased filtered load and lead to excretion of substances such as glucose or amino acids. Changes in tubular function are summarized in Figure 10-3.

TABLE 10-2   Changes in Laboratory Values Associated with Renal Function during Pregnancy

VARIABLE	NONPREGNANT VALUES	VALUES DURING PREGNANCY	CRITICAL VALUES
Creatinine clearance	85-120 ml/min	110-180 ml/min	
Plasma creatinine	0.65 ± 0.14 mg/dl	0.46 ± 0.13 mg/dl	>0.80 mg/dl
Blood urea nitrogen	13 ± 3 mg/dl	8.7 ± 1.5 mg/dl	>14 mg/dl
Urinary protein	<150 mg/24 hours	<250-300 mg/24 hours	>300 mg/24 hours
Urinary glucose	20-100 mg/24 hours	>100 mg/24 hours (up to 10 g/24 hours)	
Plasma urate	4-6 mg/dl	2.5-4 mg/dl	>5.8 mg/dl
Urinary amino acids		Up to 2 g/24 hours	>2 g/24 hours

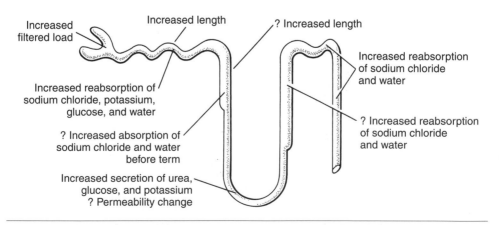

FIGURE 10-3 Tubular changes during pregnancy. (From Green, R. & Hatton, T.M. [1987]. Renal tubular function in gestation. *Am J Kid Dis, 9,* 265.)

Alterations in GFR and tubular function result in altered plasma values of many substances during pregnancy (see Figure 10-2).

Renal glucose excretion increases soon after conception and remains high to term. Urinary glucose values may be 10- to 100-fold greater than nonpregnant values (20 to 100 mg per 24 hours).[45,125] Glycosuria is more common during pregnancy and can vary from day to day and within any 24-hour period. Glycosuria is discussed in Clinical Implications for the Pregnant Woman and Her Fetus.

Excretion of amino acids, urea, and protein increases in pregnancy. Protein excretion rises from less than 150 mg per 24 hours to up to 250 to 300 mg per 24 hours, with marked day-to-day variation.[45] Increased urea clearance leads to decreased plasma urea nitrogen levels by 8 to 10 weeks.[45] Plasma urea levels may be only 63% of nonpregnant values by the third trimester.[112]

Proteinuria occurs more frequently during pregnancy. The filtered load of amino acids during pregnancy may exceed tubular reabsorptive capacity with small amounts of protein lost in the urine. Values of 1+ protein on dipsticks are common and do not necessarily indicate the presence of glomerular pathology or preeclampsia.[148] Urinary protein excretion during pregnancy is not considered abnormal until values exceed 300 mg per 24 hours.[171] Protein excretion does not correlate with the severity of renal disease, and increased protein excretion in a pregnant woman with known renal disease does not necessarily indicate progression of the disease.[44,45] However, proteinuria associated with hypertension in the pregnant woman is associated with a greater risk of an adverse pregnancy outcome.[83]

Uric acid is normally handled by filtration, secretion, and reabsorption (see Figure 10-1), so less than 10% of the filtered load appears in urine. During pregnancy, filtration of uric acid increases up to 30% in the first 16 weeks, and net reabsorption is decreased and secretion enhanced.[42,187] As a result, serum uric acid levels decrease up to 25% as early as 8 weeks. Levels gradually increase toward nonpregnant values after that point as tubular reabsorption of uric acid increases. This increase may possibly be a result of the rise in RPF that alters the filtration fraction at this stage of gestation.[45,62,125,154,148,171]

Potassium excretion is decreased, with retention of an additional 300 to 350 mEq due to increased proximal tubular reabsorption.[107,154] Serum potassium levels do not rise, since the additional potassium is used for maternal tissues and by the fetus. The mechanisms for increased potassium reabsorption in pregnancy are not well documented. These changes occur in spite of the increase in aldosterone that normally would increase urinary potassium loss. Therefore the altered potassium excretion may be due to

antagonistic action of progesterone on renal tubular actions of aldosterone.[107,154]

Renal acid-base balance is altered to compensate for the respiratory alkalosis that develops secondary to an increased loss of carbon dioxide from hyperventilation (see Chapter 9). The respiratory alkalosis is compensated for by increased renal loss of bicarbonate. This is accomplished by renal retention of H^+ ions and a decrease in serum bicarbonate. As a result, serum bicarbonate levels fall 4 to 5 mEq/L to 18 to 22 mEq/L.[42,135,137]

Urinary calcium excretion is increased, possibly due to the increased GFR, and serum calcium and phosphorus levels decrease. This is balanced by increased intestinal absorption of calcium, so serum ionic calcium levels remain stable (see Chapter 16).[125] To maintain homeostasis and meet fetal demands, women need 1200 mg of calcium per day in their diet.[137] Excretion of water-soluble vitamins also increases, so maternal diet must be evaluated to ensure adequate supplies of vitamins B_1, B_2, B_6, and C; folate; and niacin (see Chapter 11 and Table 11-5).

Fluid and Electrolyte Homeostasis

The pregnant woman must retain additional fluid and electrolytes to meet her needs and those of her growing fetus. In order to do this, renal excretory responses are modified and a new balance achieved. Since fluid and electrolyte balance is mediated predominantly by sodium and water homeostasis, pregnancy changes primarily involve alterations in these substances. The hormonal systems involved in regulation of sodium and water homeostasis, arginine vasopressin (AVP) (antidiuretic hormone), and the renin-angiotensin-aldosterone system must also be altered in order to react appropriately to the new equilibrium.

Sodium Homeostasis

The filtered load of sodium increases up to 50% as a result of the increased GFR. The nonpregnant woman filters approximately 20,000 mEq of sodium per day; the pregnant woman filters 30,000.[48,62] In order to prevent excessive urinary sodium loss, tubular reabsorption of sodium also increases (Figure 10-3). Not only does tubular sodium reabsorption increase so that 99% of the filtered sodium is reabsorbed, but there is a net retention of approximately 950 mg (2 to 6 mEq/day) of sodium during pregnancy.[44,48,54,154,173] Sodium retention occurs gradually with an increase in late pregnancy.[48] Much of the sodium is used by the fetus and placenta; the rest is distributed in maternal blood and extracellular fluid (ECF) (Table 10-3).[148,187]

Despite these alterations the pregnant woman remains in sodium balance and responds normally to changes in

TABLE **10-3**   Storage of Sodium during Pregnancy

Storage Site	Sodium (mEq)
Fetus	290
Edema fluid	240
Plasma	140
Amniotic fluid	100
Uterus	80
Placenta	57
Breasts	35
Red cells	5
Total	947

From Sullivan, C.A. & Martin, J.N. (1994). Sodium and pregnancy. *Clin Obstet Gynecol, 37,* 560.

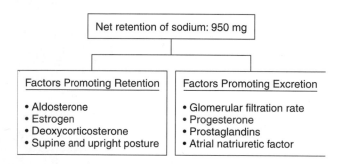

FIGURE **10-4** Factors influencing the regulation of sodium excretion in pregnancy. (From Monga, M. [1999]. Maternal cardiovascular and renal adaptation to pregnancy. In R.K. Creasy & R. Resnik [Eds.]. *Maternal-fetal medicine* [4th ed.]. Philadelphia: W.B. Saunders.)

both sodium and water balance.[64] The specific mechanisms for sodium retention during pregnancy are unclear. The maintenance of sodium balance during pregnancy is multifactorial and related to a balance (Figure 10-4) between natriuretic factors favoring sodium excretion (increased GFR, decreased RVR, decreased plasma oncotic pressure, decreased serum albumin, vasodilating prostaglandins, increased ANF, and the diuretic-like and aldosterone-antagonistic actions of progesterone) and antinatriuretic factors favoring sodium conservation (increased renin, aldosterone, deoxycorticosterone, and human placental lactogen and estrogen).[21,54,109,125,135,173,182,187] ANF is released by the atrial endothelial lining and increases early in pregnancy. ANF opposes the action of progesterone and inhibits the renin-angiotensin-aldosterone system, thus stimulating sodium loss.[54,98,168] As a result of these changes, sodium retention in pregnancy is proportional to water accumulation and the woman remains in homeostatic balance.

Renin-Angiotensin-Aldosterone System

The renin-angiotensin-aldosterone system is important in fluid and electrolyte homeostasis and maintaining arterial blood pressure (Figure 10-5 and the box on p. 378.) Pregnancy is characterized by increases in components of the renin-angiotensin-aldosterone system and decreased sensitivity to the pressor effects of angiotensin II (ATII). These changes are mediated by estrogens, progesterone, prostaglandins, and alterations in renal processing of sodium.[29,87,148,156]

During pregnancy, major sites for renin production include the uterus, placenta, and fetus as well as the kidneys.[25,80,119] Renin peaks at levels two to three times higher than normal during the first trimester and remains elevated, with a tendency to reach a plateau by about 32 weeks. The increase in renin is due primarily to increases in inactive renin; however, both active renin and plasma renin activity (PRA) (a measure of the capacity of plasma to generate angiotensin I) also increase.[175] PRA increases 4 to 10 times during the first trimester, peaking at 12 weeks, then remaining high to term with a possible decrease in the third trimester noted by some investigators.[157,175]

Renin release is stimulated by estrogens (which also increase concentrations of angiotensinogen), decreased blood pressure, increased levels of plasma and urinary PGE, and aldosterone-antagonizing effects of progesterone.[148,157,175] Increases in plasma renin are also seen during the later part of the secretory phase of the menstrual cycle, peaking at twice normal levels with the luteinizing hormone surge and persisting until midway into the luteal phase. These changes coincide with progesterone release.

Angiotensinogen (plasma renin substrate) levels double by 8 to 10 weeks, increase twofold to threefold by 20 weeks, and peak at 30 to 32 weeks.[25] This increase is due to the effects of estrogen on the liver, which synthesizes this α-globulin.[156,157] Low angiotensinogen levels are associated with spontaneous abortion and may reflect reduced placental estrogen production.

Angiotensin-converting enzyme (ACE) levels may be similar or slightly lower than nonpregnant values, although increases after 30 weeks have been reported.[25,157] ATII increases early in pregnancy and peaks at two to three times nonpregnant levels by 30 weeks.[25,157] ATII levels may fall in the third trimester but are still above nonpregnant values.[148]

Plasma aldosterone levels and turnover begin to increase as early as two weeks after and plateau by 24 weeks at levels two to five times (or more) those in nonpregnant women.[48,137,175] Aldosterone increases again later in gestation, peaking at about 36 weeks at levels eight to ten times higher than nonpregnant values.[64] The increased aldosterone

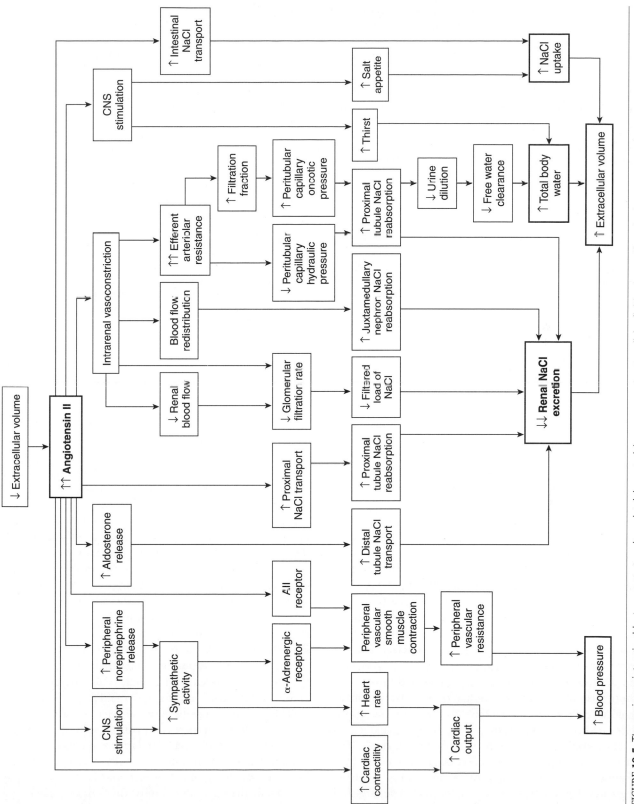

FIGURE **10-5** The renin-angiotensin-aldosterone system in maintaining arterial pressure and extracellular fluid volume. (See the box on p. 378 for a description of the renin-angiotensin-aldosterone system.) (From Ballerman, B.J., et al. [1996]. Vasoactive peptides and the kidney. In B.M. Brenner [Eds.]. *The kidney* [5th ed.]. Philadelphia: W.B. Saunders.)

Renin-Angiotensin-Aldosterone System

Angiotensinogen (plasma renin substrate) is produced in the liver and is always present in the blood. Renin is a proteolytic enzyme found in blood in active and inactive forms. Renin is secreted and stored primarily in the juxtaglomerular cells surrounding afferent arterioles of cortical nephron glomeruli. Renin is also synthesized in extrarenal sites such as the brain, vascular smooth muscle, the genital tract, and the fetoplacental unit. Stretch receptors in the juxtaglomerular cells sense changes in renal perfusion and afferent arteriole pressures and increase renin release.

Renin release is also influenced by the sympathetic nervous system and concentrations of circulating potassium, angiotensin II (ATII), and possibly sodium. Renin acts on angiotensinogen to form angiotensin I, whose actions include stimulating catecholamine release, facilitating norepinephrine release from peripheral sympathetic veins, and reducing renal blood flow in the cortex and the medulla. A measure of the capacity of plasma renin to generate angiotensin I (ATI) is plasma renin activity (PRA). Angiotensin I is broken down by angiotensin-converting enzyme (ACE) to ATII in the pulmonary circulation. ATII is a potent vaso-constrictor that stimulates adrenal production and release of aldosterone and constriction of the renal vasculature to reduce glomerular filtration rate (GFR) and the effective renal plasma flow (ERPF). ATII helps to maintain the arterial blood pressure and peripheral perfusion. Atrial natriuretic factor (ANF) also influences blood pressure and stimulates urinary sodium excretion.

Aldosterone is a mineralocorticoid secreted by the outer zona glomerulosa cells of the adrenal cortex. The two major activities of aldosterone are regulation of extracellular fluid (ECF) balance by altering sodium retention and excretion and regulation of potassium balance. Aldosterone regulates fluid volume via a direct effect on renal distal tubular transport of sodium to increase sodium reabsorption and decrease potassium reabsorption. As sodium is reabsorbed, potassium and hydrogen ions are secreted into the tubular lumen. Increased reabsorption of sodium results in increased water retention, since water is passively reabsorbed along with the sodium, thus increasing body ECF volume. Aldosterone is regulated via feedback mechanisms involving potassium and ECF volume.[10,73,78,175,182]

opposes the sodium-losing effects of progesterone and allows a progressive accumulation of sodium in maternal and fetal tissues.

Despite these changes the pregnant woman remains responsive to both sodium depletion and loading, suggesting that a new equilibrium has been established.[48,137,175] The expanded intravascular and ECF compartments are sensed as "normal" by the woman's vascular and renal volume-regulating mechanisms. The elevated levels of aldosterone may be necessary to maintain the expanded extracellular volume. This new equilibrium is protected against further increases or depletion in a manner similar to that in nonpregnant individuals.[148]

ATII is also a potent vasopressor. Yet despite markedly elevated levels during pregnancy, the blood pressure does not rise and in fact actually decreases along with the peripheral vascular resistance (see Chapter 8). The basis for resistance of the pregnant woman to the pressor effects of ATII and other vasoactive substances is unclear. This refractoriness may be due to decreased vascular smooth muscle responsiveness to ATII, perhaps mediated by local action of vasodilating prostaglandins or to activation of the renal kallikrein-kinin system.[66,176,189] Other mechanisms include downregulation of angiotensin receptors and the effects of endothelial-derived relaxing factors such as NO.[176] The result is an estimated 60% decrease in sensitivity of the systemic vasculature to the pressor effects of ATII during pregnancy. Preeclampsia is associated with a suppression of the renin-angiotensin-aldosterone system (see Chapter 8).[25,87] Diurnal variations in PRA, ATII, aldosterone, and angiotensin sensitivity during pregnancy have been reported.[51]

Volume Homeostasis and Regulation of Osmolarity

Because ECF volume is determined by sodium, the accumulation of sodium in pregnancy is accompanied by accumulation of water.[24] Both extracellular and intravascular volumes expand during pregnancy. The largest portion of this expansion is in the vascular component, favoring placental perfusion.[24,98] The amount of water filtered by the kidneys increases 50% or more during pregnancy due to the increased GFR. Pregnant women accumulate 6 to 8 L of water (Table 10-4) to meet their needs and those of the fetoplacental unit.[21,48,91,125] About 70% to 75% of maternal weight gain is due to increased body water in the extracellular spaces. Interstitial fluid volume increases 2 to 3 L beginning at 6 weeks and peaks at 24 to 30 weeks, with the greatest accumulation during the second half of pregnancy.[48,187] Accumulation of greater than 1.5 L of interstitial fluid is associated with edema.[21] Alterations in blood volume are discussed in Chapters 7 and 8.

The exact mechanisms for water retention in pregnancy are still unclear. The increase in plasma volume occurs despite decreases in plasma osmolarity and colloid osmotic pressure, changes that would normally stimulate decreases in intravascular volume. Estrogen and progesterone may play a role through dilatation of the venous capacitance vessels so that they can accommodate additional volume

TABLE **10-4**   Estimates (in ml) of Accumulated Extracellular and Intracellular Water at the End of Pregnancy

	TOTAL WATER	EXTRA-CELLULAR	INTRA-CELLULAR
Fetus[a]	2414	1400	1014
Placenta[b]	540	260	280
Amniotic fluid[c]	792	792	0
Uterus[d]	800	528	272
Mammary gland[e]	304	148	156
Plasma	920	920	0
Red cells	163	0	163
Total	5933	4048	1885

From Davison, J.M. (1997). Edema in pregnancy. *Kidney Int Suppl, 59,* S91. For the purposes of the above estimates, the following assumptions have been made: [a]extracellular space = 41.2% of body weight; [b]48% of extracellular water as liver; [c]99% water, [d]66% of water to be extracellular; and [e]49% of water to be as in 'viscera'.

without stimulation of atrial baroreceptors to alter AVP and aldosterone release.[44]

Plasma osmolarity decreases from conception, reaching 8 to10 mOsm/kg below nonpregnant values by 10 weeks' gestation (and possibly earlier) and remaining low (273 ± 3 mOsm/kg) to term.[48,54,106,110,125,176] This change is associated with changes in sodium, urea, and other ions and may arise from the decrease in PCO_2 and subsequent compensatory adjustments in renal ion excretion (Figure 10-2).[46,54,91,98,106,186] A decrease in plasma osmolarity of this magnitude in a nonpregnant person would significantly reduce the osmotic threshold for thirst, suppress AVP release, and lead to a massive water diuresis (as occurs in diabetes insipidus). However, the pregnant woman senses this change in osmolarity as normal. At this new baseline, she responds to water loading and deprivation and concentrates and dilutes urine in a manner similar to that in nonpregnant individuals.[91,106,110,125]

Arginine Vasopressin

AVP (previously called antidiuretic hormone) secretion and its effect on renal reabsorption of water are similar in pregnant and nonpregnant women, as is AVP secretion in response to changes in baseline plasma osmolarity.[187] During pregnancy the osmostat for AVP is reset, so the threshold at which the osmoreceptors signal the need for increased release is reduced from 280 to 270 mOsm/kg.[48,148] The pregnant woman concentrates her urine at levels below nonpregnant values.[53]

AVP metabolites increase in pregnancy, probably due to placental metabolism, but maternal circulating AVP levels do not change significantly.[54] The threefold to fourfold increase in plasma AVP clearance is secondary to placental vasopressinases.[108,126,176] These changes in osmoregulation parallel the progressive increase in vasopressin metabolism and placental vasopressinases.[47] Nonosmotic factors regulating AVP secretion in pregnancy are poorly understood. In nonpregnant individuals a decrease in arterial blood pressure stimulates AVP secretion. In pregnancy the fall in plasma osmolarity occurs weeks before the fall in blood pressure, and the lowered osmolarity is still sensed as normal at term when the blood pressure has returned to nonpregnant values. AVP release is also influenced by plasma volume (decreased plasma volume increases AVP release and increased plasma volume decreases AVP release). During pregnancy the threshold for the release of AVP is reset to accommodate the increase in extracellular volume at a lower baseline plasma osmolarity.[44,106] Human chorionic gonadotropin may also have a role in resetting the thirst and osmostat receptors during pregncnay.[135,154]

Intrapartum Period

The renin-angiotensin systems of both the fetus and the mother are altered during labor and delivery. At delivery, maternal renin, PRA, and angiotensinogen, as well as fetal renin and angiotensinogen levels, are elevated.[108,109] These changes may be important in control of uteroplacental blood flow during the intrapartum and early postpartum periods.

Since the changes in renal function may also affect handling and excretion of drugs, drug doses and responses must be carefully monitored (see Chapter 6). General anesthesia decreases GFR, RPF, and sodium excretion and is associated with renal vasoconstriction, which may be magnified by the effects of stress with catecholamine release.[140] Thus monitoring of fluid and electrolyte status is especially important following use of general anesthesia for cesarean birth or with nonobstetric surgery during pregnancy.

The pregnant woman is also at risk for iatrogenic water intoxication during late pregnancy and the intrapartum period. This risk may result from the loss of electrolytes by use of saluretics; forcing fluids in a woman with preeclampsia and compromised renal function; or oxytocin infusion during labor, since the antidiuretic action of oxytocin reduces water excretion.[21]

Some bladder and urethral trauma probably occurs in most women during the intrapartum period.[123] With contractions, intravesicular pressure increases by about 5 cmH$_2$O; however, bearing down increases pressure by up to 50 cmH$_2$O. Therefore prolonged straining during the second stage of labor may be more important in causing injury to the bladder than are contractions.[123]

Postpartum Period

Renal plasma flow, GFR, plasma creatinine, and BUN return to nonpregnant levels by 2 to 3 months postpartum.[5,99,101,109] Urinary excretion of calcium, phosphate, vitamins, and other solutes generally returns to normal by the end of the first week, but hyperfiltration may be maintained for up to 4 weeks due to decreased glomerular oncotic pressure.[31,100,175] Immediately after delivery, the creatinine clearance increases but by 6 days is similar to nonpregnant levels.[44,45] PRA and ATII concentrations fall to nonpregnant values immediately after delivery, then rise again and remain elevated for up to 14 days.[175] These changes may reflect the loss of renin from the fetoplacental unit, with subsequent "overshooting" by the maternal system.[175] Urinary glucose excretion returns to nonpregnant patterns by 1 week postpartum, and pregnancy-associated proteinuria is resolved by 6 weeks.[15,45,148] Plasma osmolality returns to nonpregnant levels by 2 weeks.[110,176]

The postpartum period is characterized by a rapid and sustained natriuresis and diuresis, especially prominent on days 2 to 5, as the sodium and water retention of pregnancy is reversed.[44] Fluid and electrolyte balance is generally restored to nonpregnant homeostasis by 21 days postpartum and often earlier.[88] Persistence of more than a trace of edema after this time is indicative of sodium retention or a protein-losing state.

The decrease in oxytocin contributes to diuresis since oxytocin acts similarly to AVP in promoting reabsorption of free water. As oxytocin levels decrease, the diuresis becomes more pronounced, with up to 3000 ml of urine excreted per 24 hours on the second through fifth days after delivery.[43,121,135] A normal voiding for the postpartum woman may be 500 to 1000 ml, several times greater than a nonpostpartum individual. Water may also be lost via night sweats.

Women with preeclampsia may become hypervolemic during the postpartum period as water accumulated in the interstitial space returns to the vascular compartment. If the woman's renal function remains impaired, the normal diuresis may be delayed. She may be unable to rapidly excrete this increased fluid volume and may develop congestive heart failure or pulmonary edema.

The alterations in tone of the ureters and bladder during pregnancy do not permanently impair function of these structures unless infection has incurred.[15,123] Morphologic changes in the urinary tract may last 3 to 4 months or longer.[109,135] In many women the dilatation of the bladder, ureters, and renal pelvis has decreased significantly by the end of the first week, although the potential for distensi-bility of these structures may persist for several months. In most women these structures return to their nonpregnant state by 6 to 8 weeks; in some women these changes may persist for 12 to 16 weeks or longer.[38,44,135] In some women, mild residual dilatation, especially on the right side, may persist for years with no pathologic significance.

The decreased tone, edema, and mucosal hyperemia of the bladder can be aggravated immediately postpartum by prolonged labor, forceps delivery, analgesia, or anesthesia.[15] These events may also lead to submucosal hemorrhages. Pressure of the fetal head on the bladder during labor can result in trauma and transient loss of bladder sensation in the first few days or weeks postpartum. This can lead to overdistention of the bladder, with incomplete emptying and an inability to void. Stress incontinence is also seen postpartum, although most develops prior to delivery.[52,79,151,177,185] Altered sphincter tone may increase the frequency of incontinence with events such as coughing.

Decreased urine flow rates are seen after vaginal delivery, with an increased voided volume, total flow time, and time to peak flow on the first day postpartum, returning to nonpregnant levels by 2 to 3 days.[141] Urinary retention is reported in 1.7% to 17.9% of women and is more common after the first vaginal delivery, epidural anesthesia, and catheterization prior to delivery.[153] Retention is a result of the continuing bladder hypotonia after delivery without the weight of the pregnant uterus to limit its capacity.[153]

CLINICAL IMPLICATIONS FOR THE PREGNANT WOMAN AND HER FETUS

Changes in the renal system and fluid and electrolyte homeostasis during pregnancy are associated with events such as urinary frequency, nocturia, dependent edema, and an inability to void postpartum that are experienced by many pregnant women. These events are usually not pathologic but can be annoying and are often amenable to nursing interventions. However, renal changes are also associated with an increased risk of pathologic events such as UTI and pyelonephritis and can interfere with the recognition and evaluation of renal disease during pregnancy. In addition, renal system changes interact with or are aggravated by preeclampsia and other renal and hypertensive disorders.

Urinary Frequency, Incontinence, and Nocturia

Urinary frequency (more than 7 daytime voidings) occurs in about 60% of women.[123] Most textbooks state that urinary frequency is most common during the first and third trimesters due to compression of the bladder by the uterus, and less common during the second trimester because the bladder is displaced upward and over the pelvis. However, Thorp notes there is little research to support this belief and that urinary frequency is progressive and maximum at term.[177] Frequency begins in the first trimester before the uterus is large enough to put significant pressure on the bladder.[177] Throughout most of pregnancy, urinary frequency is primarily due to the effects of hormonal changes, hypervolemia, and the increased RBF and GFR.[26,177] Pressure of the pregnant uterus probably influences urinary frequency only in the last weeks of pregnacy.[19] Alterations in bladder sensation postpartum can lead to overdistention with incomplete emptying and overflow incontinence.[15]

During pregnancy, 30% to 50% of women (versus about 8% of nonpregnant women) experience incontinence.[123] Urinary incontinence can begin in any trimester, but once it begins, an increase in severity until delivery is noted.[123,163,177] True stress incontinence is seen in about one third of pregnant women, urge incontinence in 13% to 26%.[41,123] Urinary incontinence regresses after delivery in the majority of women, but often returns in subsequent pregnancies.[79,123]

Nocturia results from increased sodium excretion, with an obligatory, concomitant loss of water. It has been thought that, during the day, water and sodium are trapped in the lower extremities because of venous stasis and pressure of the uterus on the iliac vein and inferior vena cava. At night, when the pregnant woman lies down, pressure on the iliac and inferior vena cava is reduced, promoting increased venous return, cardiac output, renal blood flow, and glomerular filtration with subsequent increase in urine output. However, since pregnant women excrete large amounts of sodium at night, diurnal differences in sodium, and therefore water, excretion may be the primary cause of nocturia.[123] Nursing interventions for women experiencing urinary frequency and nocturia are summarized in Table 10-5.

TABLE **10-5**   Nursing Interventions for Common Problems during Pregnancy Related to the Renal System

PROBLEM	NURSING INTERVENTIONS
Urinary frequency	Restrict fluids in evening.
	Ensure adequate intake over 24-hour period.
	Encourage to void when there is sensation to reduce accumulation of urine.
	Limit intake of natural diuretics (e.g., coffee, tea, cola with caffeine).
	Teach the mother the signs of urinary tract infection.
Nocturia	Use the left lateral recumbent position in the evening to promote diuresis.
	Reduce fluid intake in evening.
	Ensure adequate fluid intake over 24-hour period.
	Avoid coffee, tea, and cola with caffeine in the evening.
Dependent edema	Avoid the supine position.
	Avoid the upright position for extended periods.
	Rest in the left lateral recumbent position with legs slightly elevated.
	Elevate the legs and feet at regular intervals and when sitting.
	Use water immersion.
	Use support hose or elastic stockings.
	Avoid tight clothing on lower extremities (e.g., tight pants, socks, girdles, garter belts, knee-high stockings).
	Engage in regular exercise.
	Restrict the intake of high-salt foods and beverages.
	Assess for signs of preeclampsia (e.g., increased blood pressure, proteinuria, generalized edema).
Inability to void postpartum	Assess for bladder distention and urine retention.
	Promote adequate hydration.
	Promote early ambulation.
	Provide privacy.
	Administer analgesic before voiding attempt.
	Place ice on perineum to reduce swelling and pain.
	Pour warm water over perineum.
	Turn on the water in the bathroom.
	Provide fluid during the voiding attempt.
Risk of urinary tract infection	Screen urine culture on initial prenatal visit.
	Encourage use of the left lateral position to maximize renal output and urine flow.
	Teach perineal hygiene.
	Encourage adequate fluid intake.

Dependent Edema

Dependent edema is seen in up to 70% of pregnant women and is more common as pregnancy progresses.[48,148] Edema is more common in obese women and is associated with larger babies.[48] The forces resulting in the movement of fluid out of the vascular space include capillary hydrostatic pressure and colloid osmotic (plasma oncotic) pressure, which is generated primarily by albumin.[48] Compression of the iliac vein and inferior vena cava by the growing uterus increases capillary hydrostatic pressure below the uterus, with filtration of fluid into the interstitial spaces of the lower extremities. The net reduction in plasma albumin during pregnancy reduces plasma colloid osmotic pressure, interfering with return of fluid to the vascular compartment. However, Theunissen et al suggest that the increased interstitial fluid is not due to the decreased plasma oncotic pressure, since interstitial oncotic pressures is reduced to an even greater degree by increased flow of protein into the lymphatic system to maintain the transcapillary osmotic gradient.[176] They suggest the basis of the edema is alterations in capillary permeability and changes in interstitial ground substance. These changes reduce the margin of safety against edema, but increase the margin of safety for vascular engorgement and provide a transcapillary pool of fluid that can be mobilized with delivery.[176]

Dependent edema is more likely to develop in women who are in supine or upright positions for prolonged periods. The development of edema in pregnancy is associated with the amount of water accumulation. Women with no visible edema have an accumulation of approximately 1.5 L. Pedal edema is associated with an accumulation of 2 or more liters; women with generalized edema have accumulated 4 to 5 or more L of water. Edema in the lower legs increases the risk of varicosities and thromboembolic complications (see Chapter 7). Nursing interventions are summarized in Table 10-5 and include leg elevation, increased fluids, activity changes, and water immersion.[48,91,95,100] Leg elevation uses gravity to decrease capillary hydrostatic pressure and thus reabsorption of interstitial fluid into the vascular space.[48,91] Water immersion also changes hydrostatic pressure to help move water back into the vascular space.[6] Increased urine flow and diuresis are noted after immersion.[100]

Effects of Position on Renal Function

Position can markedly alter renal function during pregnancy, especially during the third trimester (Table 10-6). These postural effects are magnified in women with preeclampsia.[106] As pregnancy progresses, there is pooling of blood in the pelvis and lower extremities while sitting, lying supine, or standing. The pooling of blood leads to a relative hypovolemia and decreased cardiac output. In order to compensate and maintain adequate perfusion of vital organs such as the heart and brain, blood vessels supplying less vital organs such as the kidneys are constricted.[8,21] Renal plasma flow is maximal in the left lateral (versus supine) sitting or standing positions.[125]

During the second half of pregnancy, the supine and upright positions are associated with a reduction in GFR and in urine output.[21,137] As a result, pregnant women excrete water poorly and have a reduced urine volume when lying supine and, to a lesser extent, when upright.[104] For example, renal excretion of a water load while in the supine position may be decreased by 40% in late pregnancy.[21] Water excretion is enhanced by the lateral recumbent position. However, this position interferes with the ability of the woman to concentrate urine, possibly because of mobilization of fluid from the lower extremities with increased intravascular volume and subsequent suppression of AVP.[104]

Renal handling of sodium is also affected by postural changes. Moving from a lateral recumbent to a supine or

TABLE **10-6**   Physiologic and Pathophysiologic Changes in Glomerular Filtration Rate, Renal Plasma Flow, and Sodium Excretion

Function	Normal Pregnancy*	Postural Effect	Preeclampsia	Essential Hypertension
GFR	50%	17%	33%	30%
RPF	35%	20%	20%	26%
Sodium excretion	50%	60%	50%	30%

From Brinkman, C.R. & Meldrum, D. (1979). Physiology and pathophysiology of maternal adjustments to pregnancy. In S. Aladjem, A.K. Brown, & C. Surreau (Eds.). *Clinical perinatology* (2nd ed.). St. Louis: Mosby.
*The standard for the percent changes in normal pregnancy is normal nonpregnant values; other percentages represent changes from the normal pregnant values.
GFR, Glomerular filtration rate; *RPF,* renal plasma flow.

sitting position is associated with sodium retention and, in some cases, with an increase in plasma renin and aldosterone levels.[187] Sodium excretion may be decreased in the supine and upright positions.[104] This sodium retention is associated with weight gain and occasional ankle swelling that comes and goes rapidly depending on the woman's activity patterns and position and does not necessarily indicate pathology. Therefore, in evaluating sudden weight gain and edema in the extremities during pregnancy, data regarding recent activity patterns are essential.

Inability to Void Postpartum

Immediately after delivery, the woman has a hypertonic bladder with an increased capacity and decreased sensation, leading to incomplete emptying. Women should void within 6 to 8 hours of delivery. Inability to void after delivery is related to the following factors: (1) trauma to the bladder from pressure of the presenting part during labor, with transient loss of bladder sensation; (2) edema of the urethra, vulva, and meatus and spasm of the sphincter from the forces of delivery; (3) decreased intraabdominal pressure immediately postpartum due to continuing distention of the abdominal wall; (4) decreased sensation of the bladder due to regional anesthesia and catheter use; and (5) hematomas of the genital tract.[121] Nursing interventions are summarized in Table 10-5.

Risk of Urinary Tract Infection

UTI occurs with increased frequency during pregnancy and is related to anatomic changes in the renal system. Asymptomatic bacteriuria (ASB) occurs in 5% to 10% of pregnant women, which is similar to rates in sexually active nonpregnant women.[112,123] However, during pregnancy, 30% to 40% of women with untreated ASB develop a UTI.[33,49,112,136,169] This a threefold to fourfold increase over rates in nonpregnant women.[49,69] The rate of ASB is stable throughout gestation.[123]

Dilatation of the urinary tract, along with partial obstruction of the ureters from ureteral compression at the pelvic brim, results in urinary stasis. Large volumes of urine may be sequestered in the ureters and hypotonic bladder during pregnancy. These static pools increase the risk of ASB, especially because the urine may contain glucose, protein, and amino acids, which provide additional substrates for bacterial growth. Edema and hyperemia of the bladder mucosa also increase susceptibility to infection. The static column of urine in the hypoactive ureters also facilitates ascending bacterial migration, increasing the risk of pyelonephritis.[33,108,123,169] UTI is associated with preterm labor (see Chapters 4 and 12).[40,49]

UTIs are also more common during the postpartum period. Factors that increase the risk of UTIs postpartum include pregnancy-induced changes in the bladder (hypotonia, edema, and mucosal hyperemia) that may be aggravated by the trauma of labor and delivery. Decreased bladder sensation from pressure of the fetal head during labor leads to incomplete emptying and urinary stasis, further predisposing to UTI for the first few postpartum weeks.[26] Recommendations to reduce the risk of UTI during pregnancy and the postpartum period are summarized in Table 10-5.

Fluid Needs in Labor

Fluid needs of women in labor are controversial; the routine use of intravenous (IV) infusions has been questioned and even discontinued in some practices.[89,96,118,128,129,164,165,180,186] Prior to the use of general anesthesia for delivery, food and fluid intake was maintained during labor. With introduction of general anesthesia, food and fluid were prohibited and IV administration of fluids and glucose became routine to provide fluid and calories to prevent dehydration and ketosis.[118,180] Routine IV use has continued in many settings even with the decline in use of general anesthesia. There is little documentation supporting either the benefits of this therapy or the risk of oral intake for most women.[56,133,180] Complications such as infection, phlebitis, hyponatremia, and fluid overload can occur with IV therapy.[128] For example, Cotton et al. found that the amount of IV fluid given during the intrapartum period was often double that ordered.[38] In addition, it may be harder for the woman to change her position during IV therapy, leading to increased use of the supine position. IV therapy is also linked to increased use of medications since there is an accessible line.[96]

Acute hydration can lead to hypervolemia, with a greater risk in pregnant women who already have expanded body water and plasma volume.[28] The use of hypertonic glucose infusions can lead to elevations in maternal blood glucose, which can in turn result in fetal hyperglycemia and hyperinsulinemia and eventually neonatal hypoglycemia.[27,96,118,128,129,180,186] Lower cord blood sodium values and increased neonatal weight loss in the first 48 hours have been reported following the administration of 5% dextrose solutions to laboring women.[43] Conditions associated with IV fluid administration during labor are summarized in Table 10-7.

Oxytocin infusions have been associated with water intoxication and maternal and fetal hyponatremia.[21,186] The risk of water intoxication is increased when oxytocin is administered with large volumes of hypertonic dextrose solution. The hypertonic solution pulls fluid into the vascular compartment from the interstitial space, resulting in hemodilution.

TABLE **10-7**   Conditions Associated with Intravenous Fluid Administration during Labor

Use of Intravenous Dextrose (Glucose or Sorbitol)	Use of Intravenous Lactated Ringer's Solution
Maternal and fetal hyperglycemia Maternal hyponatremia Fetal hyperinsulinism Neonatal hypoglycemia Neonatal hyponatremia associated with transient tachypnea Neonatal jaundice associated with maternal hyperglycemia Fluid shift from mother to baby with greater weight loss in the neonate in the first 48 hours	Fewer problems than with dextrose, glucose, or sorbitol When combined with dextrose, problems with maternal and fetal hyperglycemia, fetal hyperinsulinism, neonatal hypoglycemia, and jaundice Possible fluid shifts from mother when large amounts of intravenous fluids are given

From Keppler, A.B. (1988). The use of intravenous fluids during labor. *Birth, 15*(2), 75.

However, the additional fluid cannot be readily excreted due to the antidiuretic effects of oxytocin. Water intoxication results in electrolyte imbalances such as hyponatremia, which can affect both mother and fetus and in severe cases can lead to seizures and hypoxia.[21] Thus, not only must oxytocin infusions be carefully monitored, but maternal electrolyte and fluid status and urine output must also be carefully evaluated for any woman receiving this type of infusion.

IV infusions may be needed for anesthesia or medication administration and must be carefully monitored where used. However, there is little evidence to support routine use of IV infusions in otherwise healthy women not receiving these agents. O'Sullivan notes the following: "Intravenous therapy is seldom necessary during the first 12 hours of labor, irrespective of the finding of ketonuria; when it is prescribed, the indication for its use should be clearly documented and fluid balance charts should be meticulously maintained. In fact, the judicious use of oral fluids should mitigate the need for intravenous fluids in many patients."[134,p.39]

Maternal-Fetal Fluid and Electrolyte Homeostasis

Fetal fluid and electrolyte balance is dependent on maternal homeostasis and placental function. Since serum osmolarity is similar in the fetus and the mother, changes in maternal or fetal osmolarity will lead to transfer of water from the opposite compartment to achieve homeostasis. Water is continuously exchanged between mother and fetus, with a net flux in favor of the fetus, placenta, and amniotic fluid. Factors that influence the rate and direction of water exchange between the mother and the fetus include maternal and fetal blood flow to and from the placenta, osmotic and hydrostatic pressure gradients across the placenta, and availability of cellular transport mechanisms.[105]

Fetal balance is affected by any maternal or fetal conditions that alter the supply, demand, and transfer of water. Maternal events such as altered nutrition, electrolyte imbalance, diabetes, hypertension, or the excessive use of diuretics are associated with alterations in fetal fluid and electrolyte status, amniotic fluid volume, and fetal growth.[18] For example, fetal urine flow can be increased by volume loading of maternal blood or administration of diuretics, since acute changes in maternal plasma osmolarity induce parallel changes in the fetus due to transplacental movement of fluid with decreased urine flow and increased AVP.[18] In addition, since fetal free water is derived from the mother, net movement of water to the fetus is decreased when maternal osmolarity increases; this leads to decreased fetal urine flow and increased tubular reabsorption of water.[97]

The fluid and electrolyte status of the infant reflects maternal balance during labor.[176] A reduction in fetal plasma volume with increased fetal osmolarity occurs in most infants during labor. These changes are more pronounced following prolonged labor, with administration of hyperosmolar glucose solutions to the mother, or during fetal hypoxia because fluid is redistributed from the extracellular to intracellular fluid (ICF) compartments.[21] Maternal electrolyte imbalances result in similar alterations in the fetus. For example, infants of mothers who receive large volumes of fluid during the 6 hours preceding birth have increased ECF and a higher incidence of hyponatremia.[20] In addition, mothers receiving IV fluids are more likely to have hyponatremic newborns than women who receive only oral fluids.[57] Administration of hypotonic fluid to the mother can, by increasing the maternal ECF volume, lead to decreases in fetal osmotic pressure and serum sodium and has resulted in maternal and neonatal hyponatremia and an increased risk of neonatal complications.[57] If this therapy is used, the fluid and electrolyte status of both mother and infant must be carefully monitored.

Measurement of Renal Function during Pregnancy

The marked increase in GFR during pregnancy significantly reduces serum BUN, plasma urea, uric acid, and creatinine by the end of the first trimester.[112] As a result, values that are normal for nonpregnant individuals may actually be elevations for the pregnant woman and reflect pathologic alterations in renal function. Thus it is critical for health care providers to know the normal values for these parameters during pregnancy (see Table 10-2) so that early signs of renal impairment are not missed. In a pregnant woman, plasma creatinine levels greater than 0.80 mg per 100 ml, plasma urea nitrogen levels greater than 13 to 14 mg per 100 ml, or plasma BUN and creatinine levels that do not decrease to expected values by mid-gestation may indicate a significant reduction in renal function and require further investigation.[45,91,154,171,187]

GFR is usually measured by either inulin or endogenous creatinine clearance (C_{cr}). The 24-hour C_{cr} is generally a good index of GFR in both pregnant and non pregnant women but is less valid in women with severe renal impairment or diminished urine production. In the latter case the amount of creatinine secreted by the proximal tubule can markedly alter urinary creatinine values.[45] The C_{cr} rises approximately 45% by 6 to 8 weeks and remains elevated to or near term, when it may begin to fall.[45] C_{cr} can be approximated by several formulas:

$$C_{cr} = 70 \times \frac{\text{24-Hour urinary creatinine (mg)}}{}$$

Or, if only the serum creatinine is known:

$$C_{cr} = \frac{140 - \text{age} \times 0.88 \text{ (for females)}}{}$$

Dilatation of the urinary tract with stasis and retention of large volumes of urine can lead to collection errors. Accuracy of clearance measures in pregnancy can be improved by using 24-hour collections to avoid "washout" from diurnal changes in urine flow, ensuring that the woman is well hydrated to ensure a high urine flow rate, discarding the first morning specimen, and having the woman assume a lateral recumbent position for 1 hour before the start and 1 hour prior to the end of the collection. Dietary intake has to be evaluated in the timing of blood samples during a clearance period since recent ingestion of cooked meat can increase plasma creatinine levels up to 0.18 mg per 100 ml. Plasma creatinine levels, used to estimate GFR, are influenced by age, height, weight, and gender. In the pregnant woman, body size and weight may not accurately reflect kidney size.[44,45]

Interpretation of diagnostic studies such as ultrasound or IV pyelography in the pregnant women must be done in light of the normal structural changes.[91] Since structural changes in the urinary system may persist for several months after delivery, these alterations also need to be considered when evaluating postpartum renal function. Evaluation of renal function is considered if the GFR during the postpartum period decreases more than 25% to 30% from predelivery values or if the serum creatinine rises above nonpregnant levels.[14]

Glycosuria

Chemically detectable glycosuria is found in the majority of pregnant women.[148,187] Glucose excretion may be up to 10 times greater than the nonpregnant levels of 20 to 100 mg per 24 hours.[125] About 70% of pregnant women excrete more than 100 mg of glucose per 24 hours; in up to 50%, glucose excretion is greater than 150 mg per 24 hours.[14,44,187] Large day to day variation in glucose excretion is reported, with little correlation between excretion rate, plasma glucose levels, and the stage of pregnancy.[44,187] Few women with glycosuria have abnormal glucose tolerance test results. Thus glycosuria in pregnancy does not reflect alterations in carbohydrate metabolism but rather alterations in renal function.[125,187]

The basis for glycosuria in pregnancy is not well understood. For many years it was thought that glycosuria developed from a decrease in the transport maximum (T_m) for glucose in the proximal tubules. Recent evidence demonstrates that this is not the case. The T_m for glucose is not a constant value but varies with changes in extracellular volume and GFR and with hyperglycemia.[44] As the GFR increases during pregnancy, renal reabsorptive capacity for glucose also increases but not to the same extent. As the filtered load of glucose increases, more glucose is excreted, leading to glycosuria at normal plasma glucose levels.[148,187] When increased glucose excretion occurs, alterations in reabsorption seem to occur primarily in that portion of the glucose load that escapes reabsorption in the proximal tubules (usually 5% of the filtered glucose) and is normally reabsorbed in the loops of Henle and collecting duct.[44,125]

Glycosuria during pregnancy has not been associated with alterations in perinatal mortality or morbidity or with subsequent development of diabetes or renal disorders.[1148] However, Davison suggests that women with greater than the usual degree of glycosuria during pregnancy may have sustained renal tubular damage from earlier untreated UTIs.[44,45] How this alters renal handling of glucose is unclear. Infection is known to cause a temporary impairment of distal tubular function. In some women, sites for glucose reabsorption may not be completely healed and thus are unable to deal with the stresses imposed by the increased filtered load of glucose during pregnancy.

Because of the high incidence of glycosuria in normal pregnant women, random testing of urine samples is not useful in the diagnosis and control of diabetes during pregnancy. In addition, urinary glucose may not be a reliable indicator of plasma glucose control in pregnant diabetics, thus decreasing the usefulness of urinary glucose concentrations for monitoring these women.[44,148] In the pregnant diabetic, any elevation of blood glucose results in a greater urinary loss of glucose than in the nonpregnant state. Because water and electrolytes are normally lost along with glucose, volume depletion and polydipsia occur sooner in the pregnant than in the nonpregnant diabetic woman (see Chapter 15).[148]

Hypertension and the Renal System

The kidneys play a critical role in the regulation of blood pressure (Figure 10-5); therefore alterations in renal function often lead to hypertension. During the perinatal period, renal disorders associated with hypertension often have a poorer outcome for both mother and infant. Preeclampsia involves specific lesions and functional alterations in the renal system (see Table 8-5). The renal lesion usually seen in preeclampsia is glomerular capillary endotheliosis, which decreases the diameter of the glomerular capillary lumina, resulting in decreased GFR and RPF.[21] In addition, in women with preeclampsia, GFR and RPF are decreased from values seen in healthy pregnant women (see Table 10-6).[21] The renin-angiotensin-aldosterone system is altered in preeclampsia. A impaired response to infusion of ATII, which antedates the onset of clinically detectable hypertension, has also been noted in women with preeclampsia.[65,175] Sodium excretion is reduced in these women (see Table 10-6) due to the decreased GFR, increased vascular resistance, decreased RPF (with decreased perfusion of the peritubular capillaries), alterations in plasma and blood volume, and possibly inadequate tubular reabsorptive mechanisms.[21,64] Further discussion of vascular changes associated with pregnancy, preeclampsia, and the impact of preeclampsia and chronic hypertension can be found in Chapter 8.

Renal Disease and Pregnancy

As the severity of renal disease and reduction in renal function increase, the ability to conceive and sustain a pregnancy also decreases.[45] In general, women with mild renal disease prior to pregnancy have few problems, whereas those with moderate to severe disease have a greater risk of worsening renal function, hypertension, or other pregnancy complications.[49,90,91] A normal pregnancy is rare if,

before conception, the woman has a plasma creatinine greater than 3 mg/dl or a urea nitrogen above 30 mg/dl—values representing a 50% to 75% decrease in renal function. Table 10-8 summarizes the effects of pregnancy on chronic renal problems. Management of women with chronic renal problems includes careful monitoring of maternal functional status and signs of increasing severity of the disease and fetal assessment.

Pregnancy Following Renal Transplant

Many women have conceived following renal transplant. Approximately 40% of these have miscarried or chosen to terminate the pregnancy.[125] Of those women who carried the pregnancy beyond the first trimester, 90% to 92% have had a successful pregnancy outcome, although there is an increased frequency of preeclampsia (30%), preterm birth (45% to 60%), and intrauterine growth restriction (20% to 30%).[125,146] The transplanted kidney undergoes the usual renal changes seen in pregnancy. Renal hemodynamics often improve with pregnancy, but 15% to 18% have permanent impairment of renal function.[135,145,170] Pregnancy is generally not recommended for at least 2 years following transplant to ensure that the transplant is successful and able to function under the increased demands of pregnancy. The frequency of rejection is not altered by pregnancy.[135,145,170] Concerns regarding teratogenicity of immunosuppressive drugs, which must be continued during pregnancy, have not been realized to date, although long-term follow-up data are still sparse.[39,46,62] Cyclosporine is associated with lower birth weights and an increase in very-low–birth-weight (VLBW) infants.[7]

SUMMARY

The renal system is critical to maintenance of fluid and electrolyte homeostasis within the body. Relatively small changes in renal function can significantly alter this homeostasis, leading to a variety of volume and electrolyte disorders. Renal function and many related laboratory parameters are altered significantly during pregnancy to levels that would be considered pathologic in a nonpregnant individual. In most cases the pregnant woman readily adapts to these changes and establishes a new equilibrium for volume and electrolyte homeostasis. At this new equilibrium, she responds to alterations in fluid and electrolyte intake in a manner similar to that of a nonpregnant individual. Pathophysiologic conditions that alter renal function or volume homeostasis affect the health of both the pregnant woman and her infant. Monitoring and health counseling related to fluid and electrolyte status are essential during pregnancy. Clinical recommendations for nurses working

TABLE **10-8**   Chronic Renal Disease and Pregnancy

RENAL DISEASE	EFFECTS
Chronic pyelonephritis (infectious tubulointerstitial disease)	Bacteriuria in pregnancy and may lead to exacerbation.
Chronic glomerulonephritis and focal glomerular sclerosis	Increased incidence of high blood pressure late in gestation but usually no adverse effect if renal function is preserved and hypertension is absent before gestation. Some disagree, believing coagulation changes in pregnancy exacerbate disease, especially immunoglobulin A nephropathy, membranous glomerulonephritis, and focal glomerular sclerosis.
Immunoglobulin A nephropathy	Some cite risks of sudden escalating or uncontrolled hypertension and renal deterioration. Most note good outcome when renal function is preserved.
Systemic lupus erythematosus	Prognosis is most favorable if disease is in remission 6 or more months prior to conception. Some authorities increase steroid dosage in immediate postpartum period.
Periarteritis nodosa	Fetal prognosis is poor. Associated with maternal death. Therapeutic abortion should be considered.
Scleroderma	If onset during pregnancy, there can be rapid, overall deterioration. Reactivation of quiescent scleroderma can occur during pregnancy and postpartum.
Diabetic nephropathy	No adverse effects on the renal lesion. Increased incidence of infection, edema, and preeclampsia.
Polycystic kidney disease	Functional impairment and hypertension usually minimal in childbearing years.
Reflux nephropathy	In the past, some emphasized risks of sudden escalating hypertension and worsening of renal function. Consensus now is that results are satisfactory when preconception function is only mildly affected and hypertension is absent. Vigilant screening for urinary tract infection is necessary.
Urolithiasis	Ureteral dilatation and stasis do not seem to affect natural history, but infections can be more frequent. Stents have been successfully placed and sonographically controlled ureterostomy has been performed during gestation.
Previous urologic surgery	Depending on original reason for surgery, there may be other malformations of urogenital tract. Urinary tract infection is common during pregnancy and renal function may undergo reversible decrease. No significant obstructive problem but cesarean section may be necessary for abnormal presentation or to avoid disruption of the continence mechanisms if artificial sphincters or neourethras are present.
After nephrectomy, solitary and pelvic kidneys	Pregnancy is well tolerated. May be associated with other malformations of the urogenital tract. Dystocia rarely occurs with a pelvic kidney.

From Davison, J.M. & Lindheimer, M.D. (1999). Renal disorders. In R.K. Creasy & R. Resnik (Eds.). *Maternal-fetal medicine* (4th ed.). Philadelphia: W.B. Saunders.

with pregnant women based on alterations in the renal system and fluid and electrolyte balance are summarized in Table 10-9.

DEVELOPMENT OF THE RENAL SYSTEM IN THE FETUS

Although functionally different, the renal and genital systems (see Chapter 1) are closely linked embryonically and anatomically. Both develop from a common ridge of mesodermal tissue and end in the cloaca. Anatomic development of the kidneys begins early in gestation, with formation of the adult number of nephrons by 32 to 36 weeks. Urine formation begins by 9 to 10 weeks; during the second half of gestation, urine production by the fetus is a major component of amniotic fluid. Renal function does not reach levels comparable to adults until about 2 years of age.

Anatomic Development
Development of the Kidneys

The kidneys arise from a ridge of mesodermal tissue (called the nephrogenic cord) that runs along the posterior wall of the abdominal cavity on either side of the primitive aorta. The kidney develops through three successive, overlapping

TABLE **10-9**   Recommendations for Clinical Practice Related to Changes in the Renal System and Fluid and Electrolyte Homeostasis in Pregnant Women

Recognize the usual values for renal function tests and patterns of change during pregnancy and postpartum (pp. 370-379 and Tables 10-1 and 10-2).

Recognize that individual laboratory values must be evaluated in light of clinical findings and previous values (pp. 385-386 and Table 10-2).

Teach women to recognize and reduce the risk of urinary tract infection during pregnancy and postpartum (p. 383 and Table 10-5).

Monitor and teach women with pyelonephritis to recognize signs of initiation of preterm labor (p. 383).

Recognize the effects of altered renal function on pharmacokinetics of drug eliminated by glomerular filtration (pp. 374, 379, and Chapter 6).

Monitor and evaluate maternal responses to drugs for evidence of subtherapeutic doses (pp. 374, 379 and Chapter 6).

Assess maternal nutritional status in relation to calcium and water-soluble vitamins and provide nutritional counseling (p. 374-375 and Chapters 11 and 16).

Know the influences of position on renal function (pp. 382-383 and Table 10-6).

Counsel women regarding appropriate positions and activity patterns (pp. 380-384 and Table 10-6).

Assess activity patterns and position in evaluating changes in weight gain and edema (p. 382).

Monitor fluid and electrolyte status and renal function following use of general anesthetics (pp. 383-384).

Monitor oxytocin and intravenous infusions during labor and delivery to avoid overload (pp. 383-384 and Table 10-7).

Use fluids, ice chips, and other alternatives to use of intravenous (IV) infusions with women with uncomplicated labors (pp. 383-384).

Know the benefits and risks for the mother, fetus, and neonate of different types of IV fluids (pp. 383-384 and Table 10-7).

Avoid use of hypertonic solutions during labor (pp. 383-384).

Monitor maternal fluid and electrolyte status and urine output (especially in women receiving an oxytocin infusion or with preeclampsia or compromised renal function) during labor and delivery for development of water intoxication (pp. 383-384).

Teach women the common experiences associated with changes in renal system (urinary frequency, dependent edema, nocturia) and implement appropriate interventions (pp. 380-382 and Table 10-5).

Monitor women with dependent edema for varicosities and thromboembolism (p. 382).

Teach women involved in 24-hour urine collections strategies to enhance the accuracy of the collection (pp. 370, 385).

Know usual values and monitor for glycosuria and proteinuria in the pregnant woman (pp. 374-375; 383-385).

Monitor the fluid and electrolyte status of women with preeclampsia, chronic hypertension, and diabetes, recognizing that alterations may occur more rapidly than in other pregnant women (pp. 383-384).

Counsel women with renal disorders regarding the impact of their disorder on pregnancy and of pregnancy on their disorder (p. 386 and Table 10-8).

Monitor women with chronic renal problems for signs of initiation of preterm labor, intrauterine fetal growth retardation, hypertension, and alterations in maternal renal function (p. 386 and Table 10-8).

Evaluate bladder function and voiding postpartum (pp. 380, 383, and Table 10-5).

Implement interventions to encourage postpartum voiding (p. 383 and Table 10-7).

Observe for signs of pulmonary edema and congestive heart failure post birth in women with preeclampsia and impaired renal function (p. 380).

Recognize that structural changes in the urinary system may persist for 6 months or more following birth (p. 381).

---

stages. The initial steps involve formation of transient nonfunctional structures (called the pronephros and mesonephros) on either side of midline, from which the metanephros, or permanent kidney, develops (Figure 10-6, *A*). The pronephros arises in the cervical region in the third week, extends in a cranial-to-caudal direction, then degenerates beginning in the fourth week. Each pronephros consists of seven to ten solid cell groups. The pronephric ducts are incorporated into the mesonephric kidneys.

The mesonephros appears late in the fourth week, forming a large ovoid organ on either side of midline next to the developing gonads in the thoracic and lumbar regions (see Figure 10-6, *A*). The mesonephros and gonad form the urogenital ridge. The mesonephros consists of S-shaped tubules with glomeruli and collecting ducts that enter a common large duct. This mesonephric duct persists in the male as the wolffian duct and gives rise to the male genital ducts (see Chapter 1). The rest of the mesonephros regresses by 8 to 10 weeks as the metanephros begins to function.[127,190]

The permanent kidneys (metanephros) arise during the fifth week from the ureteric bud at the caudal end of the mesonephric duct (see Figure 10-6, *A*). Formation of the permanent kidney involves two separate, interrelated processes. These processes are under the control of genes that are differentially expressed to form proteins that encode for extracellular matrix, cell adhesion, growth factors, and cell receptor proteins.[77] Factors influencing nephrogen-

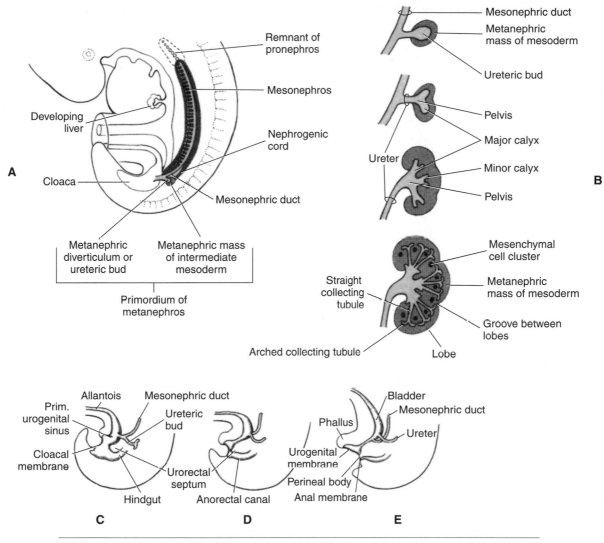

FIGURE **10-6** Embryology of the kidney. **A,** formation of the ureteric bud (fifth week); **B,** formation of nephrons (fifth to eighth weeks); partitioning of the cloaca into the urogenital sinus and anorectal canal with formation of the bladder at end of the 5th week (**C**), 7 weeks (**D**), and 8 weeks (**E**). (A and B, From Moore, K.L. [1998]. *The developing human* [6th ed.]. Philadelphia: W.B. Saunders. C to E, From Sadler, T.W. [2000]. *Langman's medical embryology* [8th ed.]. Baltimore: Williams & Wilkins.)

esis include platelet-derived growth factor, protein phosphatases, and the renin-angiotensin system.[76] The ureteric bud grows out into the surrounding mesoderm (metanephric blastema), dilates, and subdivides to form the ureters, renal pelvis, and collecting ducts (Figure 10-6, *B*). The growth of the ureteric bud into the surrounding mesoderm induces formation of small vesicles that elongate to form primitive renal tubules. The proximal ends of these tubules form the Bowman capsule. The distal end comes into contact with the blind ends of the collecting ducts and fuses.[127,149,190] Nephron formation begins at

about 8 weeks in the juxtamedullary area and progresses toward the cortex. By 20 weeks, branching of the collecting ducts is complete and one third of the nephrons have been formed.[81] Nephrons develop until 35 to 36 weeks (or a weight of 2100 to 2500 g and length of 46 to 49 cm), when adult numbers of nephrons are reached (Figure 10-7).[22] Nephron development continues in the preterm infant born before 35 weeks' gestation until the infant reaches 34 to 35 weeks' postconceptional age. Maturation and hypertrophy of the nephrons continue into infancy with growth of glomeruli and tubules.[127] Renal vascularization

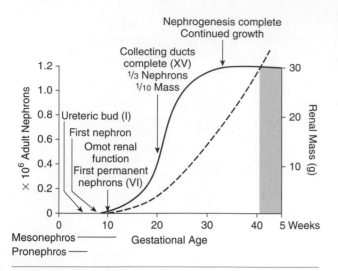

FIGURE **10-7** Schematic illustration of fetal renal development. Note that by 20 weeks of gestation branching of the collecting system (15 generations) is complete and one third of nephrons have been formed. (From Harrison, M.R., et al. [1982]. Management of the fetus with congenital hydronephrosis, *J Pediatr Surg, 17*, 728.)

parallels nephrogenesis.[78] A timeline for development of the permanent kidney is illustrated in Figure 10-7.

Initially the kidneys are in the pelvic area. With straightening of the embryo and growth of the sacral and lumbar areas, the kidneys undergo a series of positional changes and migrate upward. During this process the kidneys rotate 90 degrees so that the renal pelvises face midline.[190] Failure of the kidneys to ascend leads to pelvic kidneys. Abnormal ascent and rotation can result in configurations such as horseshoe-shaped kidneys (in which the kidneys are pushed together and fuse).

Urinary System

The urinary system develops following division of the cloaca. The cloaca is the dilated end of the hindgut and is involved in the development of the terminal portions of the genital (see Chapter 1), urinary, and gastrointestinal (see Chapter 11) systems. Downward growth of the urorectal septum at 5 to 6 weeks divides the cloaca into the posterior anorectal canal and anterior primitive urogenital sinus (Figure 10-6, *C* and *D*). The upper and largest part of the urogenital sinus becomes the bladder and is initially continuous with the allantois (Figure 10-6, *E*). The allantois eventually becomes a thick fibrous cord (the urachus, or median umbilical ligament). The ureters are incorporated into the bladder wall. The urethra develops from the lower urogenital sinus along with portions of the external genitalia.[127,190]

Developmental Basis for Common Anomalies

Factors that alter renal development include maternal hyperglycemia, alterations in the renin-angiotensin system, reduction in vitamin A to the fetus, and pharmacologic agents.[102,122] Major malformations of the renal system and urinary tract can be divided into three broad categories: agenesis-dysplasia of the renal system, polycystic kidneys, and malformations of the lower urinary tract.[67] Several events are critical for the normal development of the kidneys. If the ureteric bud does not arise from the end of the mesonephric duct or if the ureteric bud does not induce formation of the renal cortex and nephrons, unilateral or bilateral renal agenesis, aplasia, or hypoplasia results. If the ureteric bud splits early or if two buds arise on one side, there may be duplication of the kidneys or ureters. Renal agenesis and hypoplasia are often associated with oligohydramnios. The marked decrease in amniotic fluid with bilateral renal agenesis is thought to result in adverse effects on extrarenal fetal development (see Chapter 3).[57]

Polycystic kidneys are a heterogeneous group of disorders that arise from environmental and genetic causes. The specific embryological basis for these defects is unknown. Theories that have been proposed include: (1) failure of the collecting ducts to develop, with subsequent cystic degeneration; (2) failure of the developing nephrons to unite with the collecting tubules; and (3) persistence of remnants of early rudimentary nephrons, which normally degenerate but instead remain and form cysts.[67,127] The last theory has been proposed as a possible cause of adult-onset polycystic kidneys.

Malformations of the lower urinary tract include obstructive uropathy and exstrophy. Obstructive uropathy arises from obstructions at the uteropelvic junction due to adhesions, aberrant blood vessels, or strictures, or in the urethra from posterior urethral valves. Severe forms result in fetal renal damage from hydronephrosis. Anomalies of other systems may occur secondary to oligohydramnios (see Chapter 3). Fetal surgery has been utilized to promote drainage of the urinary tract and prevent irreversible renal damage before birth. Exstrophy of the bladder arises from incomplete midline closure of the inferior part of the anterior abdominal wall, with concurrent abnormalities in the mesoderm of the bladder wall.[127] Timing for development of renal and urinary system anomalies is summarized in Table 10-10.

Functional Development

Urine production and glomerular filtration in the fetus begin at 9 to 10 weeks; loop of Henle function and tubular reabsorption begin by 12 to 14 weeks.[77,144] Renal blood flow

TABLE **10-10**   **Stages of Developmental Abnormalities of the Kidneys and Urinary Tract**

STRUCTURE FORMED	TIME (WEEKS)	MORPHOLOGIC ABNORMALITIES
Pronephros and mesonephros	3-4	Renal agenesis, unilateral and bilateral (Potter syndrome)
Ureteric bud and initiation of metanephros	5	Renal agenesis or hypoplasia
Urogenital sinus	6	Urorectal abnormalities
Cephalad migration of kidney	7-9	Renal ectopia, horseshoe kidney
Major calyces, pelvis, ureter, urinary bladder, fetal urine formed	8-11	Ureteral abnormalities, posterior urethral valves, abnormal pelvis and calyces, multicystic dysplasia
Minor calyces, collecting tubules, papillary duct	13-14	Medullary cystic disease, medullary sponge kidney
Number of lobes in mature kidney (14-16) established	16	
Demarcation of cortex and medulla, growth of nephron, one third of nephrons formed	20-22	Renal hypoplasia, polycystic and medullary cystic kidney disease
Nephron induction ceases ($\approx$ million nephrons per kidney)	32-36	

From Yared, A., Barakat, A.Y., & Ichikawa, I. (1990). Fetal nephrology. In R.D. Eden & F.H. Boehm (Eds.). *Assessment and care of the fetus.* Norwalk, CT: Appleton & Lange.

(RBF) and the glomerular filtration rate (GFR) are low throughout gestation, due to the high RVR and low systemic blood pressure, but increase between 20 and 35 weeks, then level off to birth.[82,179] This increase is concurrent with increases in numbers and growth of nephrons. In adults, 20% to 25% of the cardiac output goes to the kidneys. In the fetus, 40% to 50% of the combined ventricular output goes to the placenta and only 2% to 3% to the kidneys.[22] Fetal fluid and electrolyte balance is maintained primarily by the placenta and influenced by maternal balance.

Although fetal RBF and GFR are low, this does not lead to low fetal urine output.[57] Fetal urine is an important component for amniotic fluid production, and the primary component of amniotic fluid after 18 weeks.[144] Fetal urine output and amniotic fluid production both increase with gestation. The fetal bladder fills and empties every 20 to 30 minutes.[144] Mean hourly flow rates of urine are about 2 ml at 20 weeks, 10 ml at 30 weeks, 17 ml at 35 weeks, and 27 ml at 40 weeks.[57] Urine flow rates are decreased in infants with intrauterine growth restriction.[14] Alterations in urine production or excretion can significantly alter both amniotic fluid volume and development of other systems (see Chapter 3).

Fetal ability to concentrate urine and conserve sodium is limited, with a concentrating ability about 20% to 30% of adult values.[146] Fetal urine is hypotonic (100 to 250 mOsm/kg) due to greater tubular reabsorption of solute than water.[77] Fetal urine becomes less hy-

potonic with increasing gestation.[22] The major solute in fetal urine is sodium, decreasing from 120 mEq/L at 16 weeks to 50 mEq/L from 24 to 40 weeks.[166] The fetus is not dependent on the kidneys for sodium conservation since sodium is readily transported across the placenta. The expanded ECF compartment of the fetus may also stimulate decreased tubular reabsorption of sodium and water.[53] During the third trimester, fetal urine may become isotonic with plasma during severe stress.[18] The fetal kidney is less sensitive to AVP, which is present by 11 weeks, possibly as a result of immaturity of AVP receptors or presence of antagonists such as prostaglandins.[22,147,190] Osmoreceptors and volume receptors in the fetus stimulate prolonged secretion of AVP from about 26 weeks.[72]

The renin-angiotensin system (see Figure 10-5 and the box on p. 378) is active in the fetus, with increased renal and extrarenal production of all components. An intact RAS is necessary for normal development.[78,85] ATII acts as a growth modulator and renal growth factor.[2] In animal models, $ATII_2$ receptors are more dense early in development; later in gestation, both $ATII_2$ and $ATII_1$ receptors increase in the fetus. After birth the density of $ATII_2$ (but not $ATII_1$) receptors decreases.[2,85] Therefore it is thought that $ATII_2$ receptors regulate morphogenesis, whereas $ATII_1$ may be important in later neurovascular development.[2,85,173] Blocking of ATII receptors in developing animals leads to congenital anomalies of the kidneys and urinary track.[60,83,89] Exposure to angiotensin-converting

TABLE 10-11 Implications of Alterations in Renal Function in Neonates

ALTERATION	IMPLICATIONS
Decreased glomerular filtration rate	Difficulty excreting water loads with risk of overhydration and water intoxication
	Narrow margin of safety for fluid management
	Tendency for water retention and edema (especially pulmonary edema
	Increased half-lives of drugs such as antibiotics, barbiturates, and diuretics
	Altered drug doses and dosing intervals
	Risk of hyperglycemia in very-low–birth-weight (VLBW) infants
Altered tubular function: sodium	Increased sodium loss in urine, especially in VLBW infants
	Alterations in other electrolytes with risk of acidosis, hyperkalemia, hypocalcemia, and hypoglycemia
	Limited ability to excrete excess sodium
Altered tubular function: glucose	Unable to handle an exogenous glucose
	Risk of glycosuria
	Load with risk of hyperglycemia
	Risk of hyponatremia and dehydration
Altered tubular function: bicarbonate	Less able to compensate for acid-base abnormalities with risk of acidosis, especially in VLBW infants
Decreased concentrating ability	Risk of dehydration

From Blackburn, S. (1994). Renal function in the neonate. *J Perinat Neonat Nurs, 8*(1), 37.

enzyme (ACE) inhibitors is associated with altered renal hemodynamics and anomalies.[78]

Angiotensinogen is produced in the yolk sac and found in the immature tubule by 30 days.[161] Renin is found by 4 to 6 weeks in the mesonephros and by 8 weeks in the metanephros.[85] Renin concentration and activity are both elevated in the fetus, decreasing to term but still higher than adult levels.[131] The juxtamedullary cells produce increasing amounts of renin from the third month of gestation.[69] Renal responsiveness to aldosterone is decreased in the fetus, which may lead to increased sodium loss. Endothelial cells lining the villous capillaries and the cells of the trophoblast are rich in ACE; the fetal membranes and amniotic fluid contain large amounts of renin. ACE is found by 30 days, primarily in the proximal tubules.[161] The chorion also produces renin and angiotensinogen.[175] Placental circulation is a major site for conversion of angiotensin I to ATII (similar to processes in the pulmonary circulation after birth), which is involved in control of placental blood flow in the fetus. The increased ATII appears important in modulating fetal blood pressure and renal hemodynamics, especially at birth.[147]

During the last 20 weeks of gestation, the weight of the kidney increases in a linear relationship to gestational age, body weight, and body surface area.[72] Before 5 months, renal growth occurs primarily in the inner medullary area, which contains mostly collecting ducts. From 5 to 9 months, major growth is in the cortex and outer medullary areas. After birth, nephron growth occurs primarily in the tubules and the loop of Henle. At birth, approximately 20% of the infant's loops of Henle are too short to reach into the medulla, which can lead to problems in concentrating urine.[92] The rate of tubular growth after birth is reflected in changes in glomerular-to-tubular surface area. This ratio is 27:1 at birth, 8:1 by 6 months, and 3:1 in adults.[60]

NEONATAL PHYSIOLOGY

The newborn's kidney differs from that of the older child and adult in glomerular and tubular function. The adult number of nephrons is achieved by 34 to 35 weeks, but the nephrons are shorter and less functionally mature. Alterations in renal function and fluid and electrolyte balance are heightened in preterm infants who have not yet achieved their full complement of nephrons. When evaluating postnatal renal function, both gestational age and postbirth age must be considered, since postnatal renal maturation is more a function of postbirth than gestational age; that is, a preterm infant who is several weeks old may have more mature renal function than a newborn term infant. Basic renal processes are summarized in Figure 10-1 and the box on p. 371. Alterations in neonatal renal function and their implications are summarized in Table 10-11.

Transitional Events

During intrauterine life the placenta is the major organ of excretion, handling many functions that are normally performed by the lungs and kidney. With birth the kidneys must rapidly take over control of fluid and electrolyte bal-

TABLE **10-12**   Changes in Body Water and Electrolyte Composition during Intrauterine and Early Postnatal Life

Component	24 Weeks	28 Weeks	32 Weeks	36 Weeks	40 Weeks	1-4 Weeks After Term Birth
Total body water (%)	86	84	82	80	78	74
Extracellular water (%)	59	56	52	48	44	41
Intracellular water (%)	27	28	30	32	34	33
Sodium (mEq/kg)	99	91	85	80	77	73
Potassium (mEq/kg)	40	41	40	41	41	42
Chloride (mEq/kg)	70	67	62	56	51	48

From Bell, E.F. & Oh, W. (1999). Fluid and electrolyte management. In G.B. Avery, M.A. Fletcher, & M.G. MacDonald (Eds.). *Neonatology, pathophysiology and management of the newborn* (5th ed.). Philadelphia: J.B. Lippincott.

ance, excretion of metabolic wastes, and other renal functions. Activity of AVP and the renin-angiotensin system increases with birth, perhaps stimulated by catecholamines, prostaglandins, hypercarbia, and the renin-angiotensin and kinin-kallikrein systems. As a result, blood pressure increases, with peripheral vasoconstriction and redistribution of blood flow to the vital organs (see Chapter 8).[139] Tubular sodium reabsorption decreases during the intrapartum period, so the first urine has a higher fractional sodium excretion.[22] RBF may not increase immediately at birth, but does increase significantly by 24 hours as RVR falls.[93] Activity of the renin-angiotensin system increases further during the first few days after birth. Transient increases in GFR may occur during the first 2 hours after birth. These changes are variable, decreasing to previous levels by 4 hours.[14,167]

Body Composition

Body composition changes with gestational age and is influenced by maternal fluid and electrolyte balance. Newborns have higher total body and extracellular water and less intracellular water than older individuals. With advancing gestation, total body water content and extracellular water decrease, whereas intracellular water increases as cells proliferate and organs mature.[17,19] Body water and electrolyte composition at different gestations is summarized in Table 10-12. The fetus is 82% water at 32 weeks' gestation and 78% at term. ECF decreases from 59% at 24 weeks' gestation to 44% at term, and intracellular water increases from 27% to 34% (Table 10-12 and Figure 10-8).[124,14,25,132] The relative interstitial volume of the newborn is three times greater than that of the adult.[133]

Electrolyte composition also changes with gestational age. Since the electrolyte composition of extracellular water is primarily Na^+ and Cl^-, the preterm infant (with more extracellular water) has more Na^+ and Cl^- and fewer intracellular ions (K^+, Mg^{2+}, PO_4) per unit weight. Protein, fat,

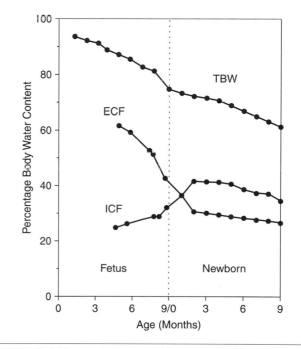

FIGURE **10-8** Total body water *(TBW)* content and fluid distribution between intracellular fluid *(ICF)* and extracellular fluid *(ECF)* compartments in humans during the fetal and neonatal periods and during the first 9 months after birth. (From Brace, R.A. [1998]. Fluid distribution in the fetus and neonate. In R.A. Polin & W.W. Fox [Eds.]. *Fetal and neonatal physiology* [2nd ed.]. Philadelphia: W.B. Saunders.)

and carbohydrate composition of the body also increases with age. Infants that are small for gestational age (SGA) have more water and less fat, whereas infants that are large for gestational age (LGA) have more fat and less water.

Shortly after birth, ECF increases, possibly related to withdrawal of maternal hormones. This increase in ECF volume is followed by a diuresis as fluid in the interstitial space is mobilized and eliminated and the extracellular space contracts.[37,132] The postbirth fluid decrease in ECF volume may be related to decreases in ANF, which is elevated in the fetus and for the first week after birth.[16,179] The fluid shifts are greater in the extremely low–birth-weight (ELBW) infant.[12,114] In the first 72 hours the ELBW infant may have a water loss of 5 to 7 mL/kg due to immature renal function, high transepidermal insensible water loss (IWL), and changes in the extracellular space.[11] Loss of fluid from the interstitial space may lead to hypernatremia, hyperglycemia, and hyperkalemia.[12] Changes in water and sodium homeostasis after birth are summarized in Table 10-13.

Loss of 5% to 10% of birth weight (up to 10% to 15% in preterm infants) is usually seen during the first week following birth due to these changes in body water compartments.[19,37] Contraction of the extracellular space increases with decreasing gestational age at birth.[115] Losses are higher in preterm infants because they produce a more dilute urine and have greater urine sodium (and therefore additional obligatory water) loss.[35] Fluid therapy during the first week must account for these changes, otherwise fluid overload—which is associated with a risk of congestive heart failure, necrotizing enterocolitis, and symptomatic patent ductus arteriosus (PDA)—may occur.[132]

Urine Output

Urine output varies with fluid and solute intake, renal concentrating ability, perinatal events, and gestational age. Generally, term infants excrete 15 to 60 ml/kg of urine per day and preterm infants 1 to 3 ml/kg/hour (24 to 48 ml/kg/day) during the first few days. Urine output less than 0.5 ml/kg/hour after 48 hours is considered oliguria.[22] Output increases over the first month to 250 to 400 ml/day.[73] In the first 2 days after birth, frequency of micturition is 2 to 6 times per hour; subsequently, micturition occurs one or more times with each feeding.[22] Preterm infants of less than 32 weeks' gestational age tend to void once per hour, have more interrupted voids (2 to 3 small voids within 10 minutes), and have smaller voids with residuals.[162] These differences may be due to immaturity of the detrusor sphincter complex. Bladder capacity is about 13 ml at 32 weeks and 20 ml by 36 weeks.[162]

The initial voiding after birth usually occurs within 24 hours but may be delayed. Approximately 13% to 21% of newborns void in the delivery room, over 95% by 24 hours, and all (unless there are problems) by 48 hours.[30,32] If infants urinate for the first time in the delivery room, this event may be missed or not recorded. The force and direction of the urine stream are as important in assessing the urinary system as is the time of first voiding. A delay in spontaneous voiding, in the absence of renal anomalies, is usually due to inadequate perfusion with contraction of the intravascular compartment and temporary expansion of interstitial fluid volume. Delayed voiding may occur in infants whose mothers received magnesium sulfate prior to delivery. Side effects of magnesium sulfate in the newborn include neuromuscular blockade with hypotonia and urine retention.

Renal Blood Flow and Glomerular Filtration

Renal blood flow is reduced in both term and preterm infants at birth, primarily because the RVR is high. RVR is inverse to gestational age and falls after birth, but is still higher than in adults.[93] RVR is high in the fetus, since renal function is primarily needed in utero only for amniotic fluid production. Therefore only a small percentage of the fetal cardiac output perfuses the kidney. During the first 12 hours after birth, 4% to 6% of the cardiac output perfuses the kidneys, increasing to 8% to 10% (versus 25% in adults) over the next few days.[14] RVR falls as RBF and GFR increase at birth.[78] A similar pattern is seen in preterm infants greater than 34 to 35 weeks of gestational age, but the decrease in RVR is more gradual, with a slower increase in GFR.[69] The higher RVR and low blood flow to the outer cortex of the kidney in preterm infants may be due to the predominance of sympathetic tone in these infants.[69]

TABLE 10-13   Postnatal Phases of Water and Sodium Homeostasis

Parameters	Phase I	Phase II	Phase III
Age	Birth-36 hours	12-96 hours	After 2-4 days
Glomerular filtration rate	Low	Increases rapidly	Decreases slightly, then continues to slowly increase with maturation
Water and sodium excretion	Minimal regardless of intake-ability to excrete water and sodium very limited	Diuresis and natriuresis occur independent of intake	Excretion of water and sodium varies appropriately with intakes
Water and sodium balance	Zero water and sodium balance on restricted intake	Negative water and sodium balance regardless of intake	Water and sodium balance stabilize and then become positive with growth

From Jose, P.A., et al. (1994). Neonatal renal function and physiology. *Curr Opin Pediatr, 6,* 175.

Effective renal blood flow (ERBF) increases with postconceptional age. ERBF is 20 mL/min per 1.73 m² at 30 weeks, increasing to 45 at 35 weeks and 83 at term, versus about 300 mL/min per 1.73 m² at 3 months and 650 in the adult (1.73 m² is a correction factor for differences in surface area that allows comparison of values between persons of different sizes).[82] Changes in RBF after birth are due to formation of new glomeruli; vascular remodeling; and vasoactive sub-

stances such as adenosine, endothelin, ANF, NO, and the renin-angiotensin and kallikrein-kinin systems.[94] Since the newborn has a higher RVR and sensitivity to vasoconstrictors than older individuals, the increase in RBF in early infancy is related to decreases in vasoconstrictor influences.[94] In newborns the juxtamedullary nephrons are more mature than the outer cortical nephrons and a greater proportion of the blood perfuses the inner cortical and medullary nephrons versus the outer cortical nephrons. After birth, perfusion of the outer cortex increases rapidly, perhaps in response to catecholamines and redistribution of placental blood flow.[93,167]

A major difference in renal function between the newborn and the adult is the lower GFR in the newborn, which is even lower when the infant's smaller size and surface area are considered. The GFR is approximately 20 to 25 ml/min per 1.73 m² at term or after 35 weeks, 10 to 13 ml/min per 1.73 m² in infants less than 28 weeks' gestational age, and as low as 2 ml/min per 1.73 m² at 25 weeks.[23,93] The GFR (Figure 10-9) and RBF increase rapidly after birth, doubling by 2 weeks of age. The pattern of maturation is similar in preterm infants over 34 to 35 weeks' gestation and term infants, although these preterm infants may exhibit a slower increase, especially during the first week. The GFR is lower in preterm infants less than 34 to 35 weeks' gestational age and remains low until their full complement of nephrons has developed at about 35 weeks' gestational age. After this point, maturation of RBF and GFR increases rapidly (up to fivefold) and is similar to that of term infants (Figure 10-10).[4,23,71]

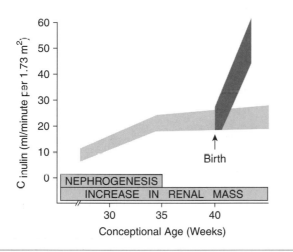

FIGURE **10-9** Maturation of glomerular filtration rate in relation to conceptional age (From Guignard, J.P. [1981]. The neonatal stressed kidney. In A.B. Gruskin & M.E. Norman [Eds.]. *Pediatric nephrology.* The Hague: Martinus Nijhoff.)

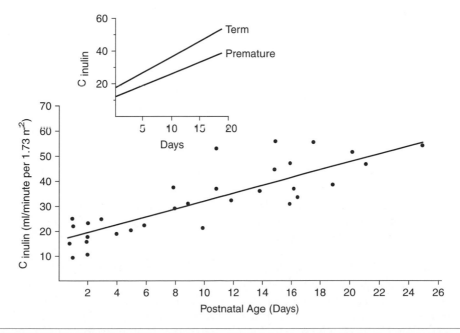

FIGURE **10-10** Postnatal maturation of glomerular filtration rate in term and preterm neonates. (From Guignard, J.P. [1981]. The neonatal stressed kidney. In A.B. Gruskin & M.E. Norman [Eds.]. *Pediatric nephrology.* The Hague: Martinus Nijhoff.)

The increase in GFR after birth (see Figure 10-9) is due to redistribution of placental blood flow with increased RBF and perfusion pressure, decreased RVR, and increased systemic blood pressure, which increases glomerular capillary hydrostatic pressure, along with increasing glomerular surface area (initially glomerular surface area is about 10% of adult) and increased permeability of the glomerular membrane.[4,72,167] Increased ATII may help maintain the GFR in the face of a low mean arterial pressure.[179] The pattern of postnatal changes in GFR is summarized in Table 10-13. GFR correlates with gestational age in infants prior to 35 weeks.[72] After 35 weeks, GFR is more closely related to weight, length, and age. Maturation of GFR and other aspects of renal function may occur at varying rates in preterm infants, so infants must be evaluated individually in determining dosages of many pharmacologic agents (see Chapter 6).[158]

Tubular Function

Tubular function is also altered in the neonate. The decreased RBF and GFR reduce the volume of solutes per unit time that the tubules must handle. Tubular thresholds for reabsorption of many solutes are also reduced and neonates are more likely to lose sodium, glucose, and other solutes in urine. Although tubular function is quite adequate for the healthy infant, immature infants or infants with health problems are at high risk for fluid and electrolyte problems.[103]

Sodium

Rapidly growing infants are in positive sodium balance (sodium intake greater than output). Excretion of sodium is reduced in comparison to adults, possibly because of increased PRA and aldosterone levels as well as incorporation of sodium into the new tissue.[57] Renal tubular handling of sodium undergoes rapid changes after birth as the reabsorptive capacity for sodium and other solutes increases.

Term newborns readily conserve sodium.[22] The pattern for renal reabsorption of sodium is different in the infant as compared with an older child or adult primarily because of the altered distribution of blood flow and changes in reabsorption in the proximal versus distal tubules. In infants a greater portion of RBF is to juxtamedullary nephrons, whereas in the adult the majority of RBF is to the cortical area and only about 10% goes to the medullary area. Since the juxtamedullary nephrons tend to be more involved in conservation than excretion of sodium, an infant's ability to excrete a sodium load is limited. This limitation increases the tendency toward sodium retention, with increased ECF volume and edema formation if excess sodium is given.[14,23]

In addition, proximal tubule reabsorption of sodium in infants is decreased; distal tubule reabsorption is relatively increased, perhaps as a compensatory mechanism to reduce renal sodium loss.[22,69] The increased distal tubule reabsorption is enhanced by elevated levels of aldosterone. Tubular reabsorption of sodium is greater in term infants than in preterm infants, who have increased urinary sodium losses and lower plasma sodium levels. Factors that influence natriuresis are summarized in Table 10-14.

Sodium balance in preterm infants. Preterm infants are more likely to be in negative sodium balance (sodium intake less than output) during the first few weeks after birth.[93,167] Negative sodium balance has been observed in 100% of infants less than 30 weeks' gestation, 70% at 30 to 32 weeks, and 40% between 33 and 35 weeks.[2,4] Factors leading to the negative sodium balance in these infants include immature NA^+/K^+-ATPase, high ECF volume, tubular aldosterone insensitivity, and other factors listed in Table 10-14.[22] Even though the GFR is lower in the preterm infant (so the kidneys have less sodium to handle), the altered tubular reabsorption with decreased proximal tubular reabsorption and increased distal tubule load results in increased fractional sodium excretion. Decreased proximal tubule reabsorption of sodium in preterm infants may be due to the shorter length of the tubules and immature transport mechanisms.[93] As a result, greater amounts of fluid and electrolytes such as Na^+ remain in the lumen and are sent to the distal tubule. The distal tubule is unable to increase its reabsorptive capacity to handle the additional sodium load despite elevated PRA and aldosterone levels, so more sodium is lost in the urine. The ability of the distal tubule to respond to aldosterone may be reduced or the distal tubule may already be under maximal aldosterone stimulation and thus may be unable to further increase its reabsorptive capacity.[22,167]

The fractional sodium excretion (FE_{Na}) is the amount of urinary sodium excretion as a percent of the filtered sodium.[59] There is an inverse relationship between (FE_{Na}) and gestational age. In the larger preterm infant FE_{Na} is 1% to 5% versus 5% to 15% in VLBW infants and 0.5% in term infants.[72] FE_{Na} is highest in the first 10 days after birth and by one month is less than 0.4% to 1%.[93] FE_{Na} is a measure of tubular function (as GFR is a measure of glomerular function) and calculated as follows:

$$FE_{Na} = \frac{Urine\ sodium}{Serum\ sodium} \times \frac{Serum\ creatinine}{Urine\ creatinine} \times 100$$

Tubular reabsorption of sodium (T_{Na}) can be estimated by the formula $T_{Na} = 100\% - FE_{Na}$. The greater the FE_{Na}, the more sodium is lost in the urine. To determine if FE_{Na} is excessive, sodium and fluid intake must be considered.[57,167]

TABLE **10-14** Factors Affecting Natriuresis and Urine Output in Fetuses and Newborn Infants

FACTOR	EFFECT ON NATRIURESIS	EFFECT ON URINE OUTPUT
Low renal blood flow (e.g., PDA)	↓	↓
Indomethacin for PDA	Variable	↓
Limited GFR:		
Prerenal failure	↓	↓
Intrinsic or postrenal failure	↑	↑ or ↓
Tubular function: low tubular Na$^+$/K$^+$-ATPase	↑	
Prenatal glucocorticoids administration (upregulates transcription)	↓	
High cord levels of EDLS (inhibit Na$^+$/K$^+$-ATPase)	↑	
Dysfunction: aminoglycosides, amphotericin	↑	↑
Dopamine (note that the receptor is probably not present in ELBW infants)	↑	↑
Renin-angiotensin-aldosterone system: high PRA and angiotensin activity:		
Aldosterone (low level at birth later stimulated by sodium depletion)	↓	
Progesterone (limits tubule sensitivity to aldosterone)	↑	
High circulating level of atrial natriuretic factors	↑	
High concentration of AVP	May ↑	↓
Prostaglandins (limit effect of AVP)		↑
Osmotic diuresis caused by hyperglycemia	↑	↑
Diuretics	↑	↑

From Brion, L.P., Bernstein, J. & Spitzer, A. (1997). Kidney and urinary tract. In A.A. Fanaroff & R.J. Martin (Eds.). *Neonatal-perinatal medicine, diseases of the fetus and infant* (6th ed.). St. Louis: Mosby.
*Increased natriuresis caused by extracellular fluid expansion mediated by ADH; decreased natriuresis if sodium depletion.
AVP, arginine vasopressin; *EDLA*, circulating endogenous digoxin-like immunoreactive substances; *ELBW*, extremely low–birth-weight; *GFR*, glomerular filtration rate; *Na$^+$/K$^+$-ATPase*, sodium potassium adenosine triphosphatase; *PDA*, patent ductus arteriosus; *PRA*, plasma renin activity.

By several weeks of age, most preterm infants are in positive sodium balance as tubular function matures. Maturation takes longer in VLBW infants, who are at risk for fluid and electrolyte disturbances for a longer period.[4,22,93]

Glucose

The ability of the tubules to reabsorb glucose and the transport maximum (T_m) for glucose are decreased in the preterm infant and increase to term.[22,69] The lower T_m is due to low levels of sodium-glucose transporters in the proximal tubule.[22] Even at term, the renal threshold for glucose (corrected for surface area) is lower in the infant. However, even with this lower threshold, most normoglycemic infants (unless very immature) are not glycosuric.[4] This is probably because the glucose T_m-to-GFR ratio is high.[22] Although the glomerulotubular balance for glucose filtration and reabsorption can be demonstrated as early as 25 weeks' gestation, low renal thresholds for glucose (<100 to 150 mg/dl) and increased fractional excretion of glucose are seen in some VLBW infants.[23,72] Urinary glucose levels are increased in preterm infants, with higher fractional glucose excretion, less reabsorption of glucose, and a tendency toward glycosuria.[14] VLBW infants are also at risk for hyperglycemia, since they are unable to readily excrete a glucose load. Since renal handling of glucose is interrelated with that of water, Na$^+$, K$^+$, and other solutes, attempts to excrete a glucose load may lead to hyponatremia, dehydration, and other abnormalities. Therefore VLBW infants with glucose IV must be monitored for hyperglycemia, glycosuria, and fluid and electrolyte status. Glucose metabolism is discussed in Chapter 15.

Renal Handling of Other Solutes

In general, renal excretion of solutes increases with gestation and postnatal age. Potassium excretion is low during gestation, and the newborn is less able to excrete a potassium load. With the lower GFR, less sodium is delivered to and reabsorbed by the tubules. Since K$^+$ is exchanged for Na$^+$ in the distal tubule, less K$^+$ is secreted and subsequently excreted.[14] Healthy term and growing preterm infants are in positive potassium balance; stressed or ill infants may have a negative balance. Transient hyperkalemia (up to 5.5 to 6 mEq/L) occurs in some VLBW infants (especially those less than 27 to 28 weeks of gestational age), probably due to their low GFR, decreased tubular response to aldosterone, and decreased renal adenosine triphosphatase (ATPase) activity.[70,115,58] The turnover of potassium is related to that of energy needs and nitrogen. Stressed infants have greater energy needs. After other energy sources (i.e., carbohydrate and fat stores) have been used, protein will be catabolized for energy, with release of nitrogen. This leads to a negative nitrogen balance and increase in K^+ secretion and excretion. A negative potassium balance is also associated with the use of diuretics and parenteral fluid therapy.[179]

Uric acid levels are higher in preterm than term infants (averaging 7.7 versus 5.2 ml/dl) and decrease with gestation. Serum levels are higher in infants due to increased production of uric acid as a by-product of nucleotide breakdown.[190] Serum uric acid levels may also be elevated in hypoxic infants or following asphyxia.[72] Uric acid crystals may occasionally be seen as reddish staining of the diaper in normal newborns and can be misinterpreted as blood. Urea excretion is usually decreased in the neonate since they are using nitrogen for growth. Urinary protein excretion is greater at birth, gradually decreasing over the first few weeks. Transient proteinuria may occur during the first 5 days.[4,22,173]

Renal excretion of phosphorus, calcium, and magnesium is interrelated with sodium reabsorption and excretion. During the first week, calcium excretion varies inversely with gestational age and directly with urine flow and sodium excretion, thus increasing the risk for hypocalcemia in the VLBW infant.[14] Alterations in sodium intake and excretion alter renal handling of these solutes in ill infants, so liberal sodium supplementation may lead to development or exacerbation of hypocalcemia.[72] Phosphorus excretion is higher during the first weeks after birth and is related to gestational age and type of oral feeding. Calcium and phosphorus metabolism are discussed in Chapter 16.

Acid-Base Homeostasis

Serum bicarbonate levels and plasma pH are lower in neonates due to a lower renal threshold for and reduced capacity to reabsorb bicarbonate. The lower threshold (serum level at which bicarbonaturia occurs) might be the result of altered transport capacity for bicarbonate or may be related to expansion of ECF volume.[14,190] The more immature the infant, the lower the bicarbonate levels are. Serum bicarbonate levels may be as low as 12 to 16 mEq/L in VLBW, 18 to 20 in LBW, and 20 to 22 in term infants (versus 24 to 28 in adults).[73,167,190] Serum bicarbonate levels in preterm infants increase to values greater than 20 mEq/L within the first 1 to 2 weeks. Urinary pH is 6 to 7 initially, with minimum values (4.5 to 5.3) reached by 1 to 2 weeks.[73] The occurrence of alkaline urine along with a metabolic acidosis suggests renal tubular acidosis.[73]

Term and preterm infants are able to excrete an acid load, although the ability of the kidneys to respond to an acid load increases with gestational and postnatal age.[22] The decreased response to an acid load in the VLBW infant may result from immaturity of the hydrogen ion–secreting mechanism, decreased excretion of urinary buffers, or unresponsiveness of the distal tubule to aldosterone.[23,72] Normally most newborns are probably secreting near to their maximal ability, with little reserve to cope with any disorders that produce acidosis. Thus any event that increases the potential for acidosis, such as cold stress, hypoxemia or starvation, is more likely to produce alterations in acid-base status in the newborn.

Water Balance

Regulation of water balance by the newborn is similar to that of adults but occurs within a narrower range. The ability of newborns to dilute urine is similar to that of adults, while their ability to concentrate urine is limited. The ability to dilute is defined as the minimum amount of solute (electrolytes, protein) that can be excreted in a volume of urine; that is, there is an obligatory amount of solute that the body must lose in order to excrete water in urine. Since diluting segments of the distal tubule and ascending loop of Henle develop early, term newborns and preterm infants of more than 35 weeks' gestation can dilute their urine to osmolarities of 50 mOsm/L (similar to adult values) or lower; preterm infants of less than 35 weeks' gestation can dilute to 70 mOsm/L.[111] However, neither term nor preterm infants can handle large or rapidly administered water loads due to the low GFR.[23,35,111] Therefore the neonate is at risk for overhydration, water retention, and overload. The decreased ability to excrete a water load is related primarily to a lower GFR and perhaps decreased sensitivity of the tubules to AVP. The ability to excrete water load increases after 3 to 4 days in term infants and preterm infants born at 35 or more weeks' gestation.[190]

The ability to concentrate urine relates to the maximum amount of solute that can be excreted within a volume of urine (i.e., the ability to excrete a solute load without becoming dehydrated). To excrete more solute, the body would have to increase the amount of urine water. The ability to concentrate urine is mediated by vasopressin and occurs via aquaporins (water channel proteins).[111] The concentration of solutes in urine depends on a complex interaction of events called the *countercurrent multiplier system* (Figure 10-11 and the box on p. 399). The newborn

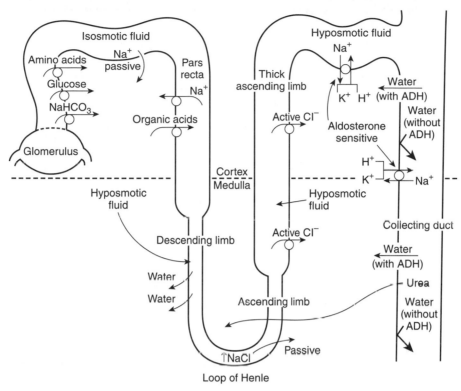

FIGURE **10-11** The countercurrent mechanism (see the box below). (From Ramanathan, S. & Turndorf, H. [1988]. Renal disease. In F.M. James, A.S. Wheeler, & D.M. Dewan [Eds.]. *Obstetric anesthesia: The complicated patient* [2nd ed.]. Philadelphia: F.A. Davis. Modified by the authors from Petersdorf, R.G., et al. [1983]. *Harrison's principles of internal medicine* [10th ed.]. New York: McGraw-Hill.)

Countercurrent Multiplier System

The ability to concentrate urine is the maximum amount of solute that can be excreted within a volume of urine. Adults concentrate to a maximum of 1200 to 1400 mOsm/L; term newborns to 600 to 700 mOsm/L. To excrete more solute, the amount of urine water would have to be increased. Concentration of solutes in urine depends on the countercurrent system, which involves movement of Na$^+$ water, and other solutes between the tubular lumen, collecting ducts, and the surrounding interstitial fluid.

This system can be summarized as follows. Fluid entering the descending limb of the loop of Henle is hyposmotic due to movement of solutes out of the proximal tubule. Since water but not Na$^+$ is reabsorbed in the descending limb, the fluid in the loop of Henle becomes hyperosmotic. As the filtrate moves through the ascending limb, Na$^+$ and Cl$^-$ (but not water) move out of the lumen, so that the filtrate again becomes hyposmotic and the surrounding interstitial fluid becomes hyperosmotic. The longer the loops of Henle, the more concentrated the urine. As the filtrate passes through the distal tubule and collecting duct, Na$^+$ reabsorption is mediated by aldosterone and Na$^+$ is exchanged for secreted H$^+$ and K$^+$. There is little water movement in the distal tubule. In the collecting duct, arginine vasopressin (AVP) controls water reabsorption. When AVP is present, water reabsorption increases, resulting in a hypertonic urine.

From Ramanathan, S. & Turndorf, H. (1988). Renal disease. In F.M. James, A.S. Wheeler, & D.M. Dewan (Eds.). *Obstetric anesthesia: The complicated patient* (2nd ed.). Philadelphia: FA Davis.

can maximally concentrate urine to approximately half of adult levels (600 to 800 mOsm/L versus 1200 to 1400 mOsm/L). This ability is further decreased in preterm infants, with maximum urinary concentration of 245 to 450 mOsm/kg/L in 1300- to 1500-g infants at 1 to 3 weeks of age and even lower levels in more immature infants.[72] By 4 to 6 weeks after birth, preterm infants can concentrate similarly to term infants.[22] The limitation in concentrating ability is due to several factors:

1. Decreased medullary osmotic gradient related to decreased accumulation of urea and other solutes and increased medullary blood flow.
2. Lower concentrations of blood urea. Urea is a solute that sets up the concentration gradient. Since urea is an end product of nitrogen metabolism, growing infants—who use nitrogen to make protein and new tissue—metabolize less nitrogen and produce less urea.
3. Decreased solute levels for the concentration gradients in the interstitial space due to decreased reabsorption and increased excretion of Na^+, Cl^-, glucose, and urea, possibly mediated by increased prostaglandin production.
4. Decreased length of loops of Henle and collecting ducts and immature tubular function.
5. Decreased response to circulating AVP.
6. Interference of prostaglandins with the hyposmotic action of AVP.[22,23,35,69,72,174,190]

Hormonal Regulation
Renin-Angiotensin-Aldosterone System

Renin-angiotensin-aldosterone system (see Figure 10-5 and the box on p. 378) activity is inversely related to gestational age.[162] Values in the newborn are higher than in adults and decrease gradually over the first months.[23,69,73,131,162,181] Angiotensinogen and PRA are particularly high (Figure 10-12).[23,131,181] PRA remains high for the first 2 to 3 weeks in all newborns, then decreases.[181] Circulating ATII is also high at birth, and the decrease parallels the decrease in PRA.[131] The high ATII levels may be mediated by decreased potency in the newborn.[131] Hyperfunction of this system may be due to the low systemic blood pressure and RBF, sodium wasting, and the normal decrease in ECF volume after birth.[190] The increased renin and aldosterone concentrations may be mediated by prostaglandins, which are also elevated at birth.[14] By increasing sodium reabsorption by the distal tubules, or by influencing vasoconstriction, aldosterone modulates changes in GFR to protect the renal tubules from overload with loss of electrolytes and other solutes in the urine.

In the VLBW infant, adrenal production of aldosterone is decreased, as is distal tubule response to aldosterone.[22,69] These changes increase the risk of hyponatremia and dehydration. Hypertension in the newborn is usually related to factors (e.g., renal vein thrombosis, coarctation of the aorta, bronchopulmonary dysplasia, and glucocorticoids admin-

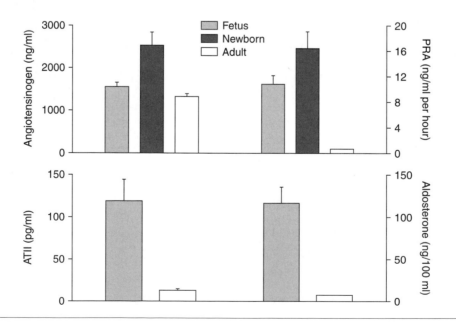

FIGURE **10-12** Circulating levels of angiotensinogen, plasma renin activity *(PRA)*, angiotensin II *(ATII)*, and plasma aldosterone in fetal cord blood, newborn infants, and normal adults. (From Tufro-McReddie, A. & Gomez, R.A. [1993]. Ontogency of the renin-angiotensin-aldosterone system. *Semin Nephrol, 13*, 519.)

istration) that activate the renin-angiotensin system to stimulate ATII production.[131] The basis for the decreased response to aldosterone is uncertain but may relate to lack of receptors, the presence of an undetermined antagonist, or the deficiency of intracellular transport system enzymes.[4]

Arginine Vasopressin

Both the distal tubule and the collecting ducts of the infant respond to AVP. AVP increases at birth, especially in infants born vaginally (possibly stimulated by head compression). Sensitivity of volume receptors and osmoreceptors in neonates is similar to that in adults. However, tubular response to circulating AVP is decreased, especially in preterm infants.[22,23] Plasma and urinary AVP are increased following perinatal asphyxia (possibly mediated by catecholamines) and in infants with intracranial hemorrhage, RDS, meconium aspiration syndrome, and pneumothorax. These findings may be due to decreased osmolarity in the medullary interstitium (from decreased tubular function and decreased reabsorption of solutes) or inhibition of AVP by increased levels of PGE_2.[57,174] The increase in AVP at birth may enhance extrauterine adaptation by increasing blood pressure and peripheral vasoconstriction and enhancing postnatal fluid homeostasis.

Factors regulating AVP secretion in neonates are not fully understood. Increased AVP and water retention may be important in the etiology of later hyponatremia in VLBW infants.[22,174] Chronically increased sodium excretion with contraction of the ECF compartment may stimulate the renin-angiotensin-aldosterone system and AVP secretion. AVP increases renal water reabsorption to restore ECF volume but may also decrease plasma sodium.

Other Regulating Factors

Renal function and hemodynamics are influenced by other substances in addition to the renin-angiotensin-aldosterone system and AVP. The kallikrein-kinin system modulates renal blood flow and handling of sodium and water.[68] The kidneys produce dopamine (precursor to norepinephrine and epinephrine) in the proximal tubules of superficial nephrons[9] Dopamine inhibits renal sodium absorption (thus increasing sodium excretion), increases water excretion by inhibiting AVP release from the pituitary, and alters water transport in the collecting ducts.[84] Prostaglandins also mediate renal blood flow and may be important in regulating renal blood flow during stress; they may also balance the increased renin activity.[9]

Bladder

The neonate's bladder is almost entirely in the abdominal cavity and is cigar shaped (as opposed to the pyramidal shape in adults); therefore the ureters are short. As a result, distention of the bladder compresses the abdomen and increases pressure on the diaphragm. As the pelvic cavity increases in size during infancy and early childhood, the bladder gradually sinks into the pelvis and the ureters lengthen.[117]

CLINICAL IMPLICATIONS FOR NEONATAL CARE

The newborn infant is able to regulate sodium and water balance, but within a much narrower range than the older child or adult. As a result, the neonate is much more likely to develop fluid and electrolyte disturbances within a shorter period of time, with a small margin between homeostasis and overload or underload. Careful calculation and monitoring of needs are essential to maintain homeostasis. Immaturity of renal function limits the ability of the infant, especially if preterm or ill, to cope with additional stress and increases the risk of renal dysfunction following pathophysiologic events such as perinatal asphyxia or with RDS. In addition, alterations in renal function affect excretion of drugs and influence serum levels and drug half-life values, increasing the risks of side effects and toxicity.

Management of Fluid and Electrolyte Balance

Birth represents a major change in the infant's fluid and electrolyte status, which in fetal life is maintained by the placenta and mother. Lorenz notes that, in light of these changes after birth, "the goal is not to maintain fluid and electrolyte status after birth but rather to allow these changes to occur approproately."[115,p.205] Calculation of fluid needs for any infant involves consideration of maintenance needs, replacement of losses, and provision of allowances for growth. Maintenance needs include consideration of endogenous water produced by oxidative metabolism plus IWL and loss of water in urine and stool. Usual values for these parameters are known and can be used to calculate fluid needs. In healthy term or large preterm infants, individual variations from these values, unless major, are probably not crucial, since the infant's kidneys will adjust to ensure fluid and electrolyte homeostasis.[132] However, ill or VLBW infants may not be able to adjust, since their renal function is inefficient or compromised by illness. In addition, these infants are more likely to be in environments (e.g., an incubator, a radiant warmer, phototherapy) that markedly alter IWL.[55,132]

Stool water loss is estimated at 5 to 10 ml/kg/day under basal conditions but can increase markedly with diarrhea. Stool water losses are considered to be minimal during the first few days after birth and thus are not included in calculation of initial fluid needs. Approximately 5 to 10 ml/kg/day of endogenous water is produced by oxidation. This water is often ignored in calculation of fluid requirements.[14] Water for growth varies with body water composition. For example, if an infant is assumed to have a water content of 70%, water needed for growth would be 0.70 ml per g of weight gain. Since body water composition is not static, water for growth is generally estimated at 10 to 20 ml/kg/day, with the higher values used for more immature infants who have a larger proportion of body water.[132] In the first week after birth, during the period of physiologic weight loss, calculation of maintenance fluid needs does not include replacement of water for growth but is based primarily on calculation of IWL and urine water loss.

Insensible Water Loss

IWL is water loss from the skin (70%) and respiratory tract (30%). IWL generally consists of about 32% of the total water requirement, unless IWL is markedly increased.[14] Basal levels of IWL in the neonate are 20 ml/kg/day or 0.7 to 1.6 g/kg/hour.[14] IWL is markedly increased in the preterm infant. In ELBW infants with thin, gelatinous skin, these losses are particularly high.[12] Skin water loss is proportional to surface area, and these infants have greater ratios of surface area to weight. Preterm infants also have greater IWL because of increased permeability of their epidermis to water, greater percentage of body water, and increased skin blood flow in relation to metabolic rate.[14,132] IWL can be significantly altered by conditions that increase the basal metabolic rate and by therapeutic modalities such as phototherapy, radiant warmers, heat shields, humidity, semipermeable dressings, and incubators.[12,14,97,130,184] Factors that increase or decrease IWL in neonates are summarized in Table 10-15.

Urine Water Loss

Urine water loss generally accounts for about 56% of total body water requirements (generally about 50 to 100 ml/kg/

day).[14] The amount of water the infant must excrete in urine, maximum urine concentrating ability (urine osmolarity), and renal solute load are all interrelated (Figure 10-13) and can be calculated using the following formula:

$$\text{Urine volume (ml/kg)} = \frac{\text{Solute load (mOsm/kg)}}{\text{Urine osmolarity (mOsm/L)}} \times 1000$$

Variations in renal solute load can markedly alter obligatory urinary water losses. For example, a nongrowing infant who could concentrate to a maximum of 300 mOsm/L would have to excrete about 25 ml/urine/kg to get rid of a solute load of 7.5 mOsm/kg; the same infant would be obligated to lose 50 ml/urine/kg if receiving a solute load of 15 mOsm/kg (7.5/300 × 1000 = 25 ml/kg urine versus 15/300 × 1000 = 50 ml/kg urine) and would be at greater risk for dehydration.

The renal solute load is the amount of solutes from metabolic end products (especially nitrogenous compounds and electrolytes) and exogenous sources that must be excreted by the kidneys. Endogenous solutes are produced from catabolism of tissues when caloric and protein intake is inadequate. Exogenous solutes are derived from parenteral solutions and enteral intake.[174] The solute load from exogenous sources can be calculated from the following formula:

$$\text{Solute load (mOsm/L)} = 4 \text{ (g protein per dl)} + 1 \\ (\text{mEq } Na^+ + K^+ + Cl^-)$$

Renal solute load varies with the type of oral intake and whether or not the infant is receiving an intravenous solution with additional electrolytes and other solutes.

Daily solute excretion in most infants ranges from 7.5 to 30 mOsm/dl or more.[50] Renal solute load is lowest for growing infants fed human milk and highest for infants

---

TABLE **10-15**   Factors Influencing Insensible Water Loss in Neonates

INCREASE INSENSIBLE WATER LOSS	DECREASE INSENSIBLE WATER LOSS
Immaturity (50%-300%)	Plastic heat shields (30%-50%)
Radiant warmer (50%-200%)	Double-wall incubator or heat shield (30%-50%)
Forced convection incubator (30%-50%)	Plastic blanket under radiant warmer (30%-50%)
Phototherapy (40%-100%)	High humidity (50%-100%)
Respiratory distress	Transport thermal blanket (70%)
Elevated body or ambient temperature*	Assisted ventilation with warmed and humidified air (20%-30%)
Skin breakdown or injury	Increasing postnatal age
Congenital defects (omphalocele, gastroschisis, neural tube defect)	Semipermeable dressing or topical agents (50%)
Motor activity, crying (up to 70%)	
Other factors that increase metabolic rate	

Compiled from references 12, 14, 35, 60, 97, 184, and 188.
*A 1° increase in body temperature is equal to a 30% increase in insensible water loss.

who are starved or receiving high osmolar parenteral fluids or a high-protein formula. Renal solute loads for commercial formulas can be found in the manufacturer's formula handbook. Renal solute loads for parenteral fluids average 10 to 20 mOsm of solute per 100 kcal expended (in infants <10 kg, ml/kcal = cc/kg). For example, an intravenous line with a 10% glucose solution would average 10 mOsm/kg/day, and a maintenance IV with 3 mEq NaCl and 2 mEq KCl would yield an additional 10 mOsm/L of solute from these electrolytes.[14]

Various factors can modify renal solute load and urine water excretion. In the growing preterm infant who is incorporating protein and other solutes into new tissue, each gram of weight gain decreases the renal solute load by about 1 mOsm. The decrease in solute load is reflected in decreased obligatory urine water loss. Urine water volume and thus fluid needs may be increased with glycosuria or furosemide therapy and decreased in infants on positive-pressure ventilation or with inappropriate ADH secretion or acute renal tubular necrosis.[14]

Estimating Fluid and Electrolyte Needs

During the first few days following birth, maintenance fluid requirements are based on IWL and urine water loss. With increasing postbirth age, fluid requirements increase due to increased stool water losses and growth. There are many variations in specific recommendations for fluid and elec-

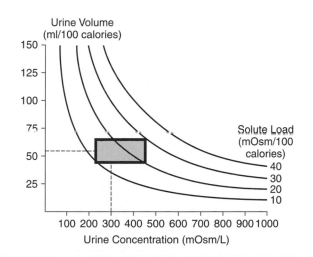

FIGURE **10-13** Interrelationships of urine volumes, concentrations, and renal solute loads in the neonate. Urine volume as a function of urine concentration for various solute loads, varying from high (40 mOsm/100 cal) to low (10 mOsm/100 cal). If urine volume were 55 ml/100 cal expended, both high- and low-solute loads could be excreted without taxing the minimum (about 50 mOsm/L) or maximum (about 1400 mOsm/L) concentrating power of the normal mature kidney. (From Winters, R.W. [1973]. *The body fluids in pediatrics.* Boston: Little, Brown.)

trolyte needs. Fluid needs for the first few days are generally calculated to account for the normal physiologic weight loss of 5% to 10% (10% to 15% in VLBW) of birth weight. If IWL is increased (see Table 10-15), fluid needs are also increased. On the other hand, fluid needs are reduced in infants with acute renal failure or congestive heart failure. Fluid needs are higher in infants less than 1000 g due to markedly increased IWL and decreased renal concentrating ability (which increases obligatory urine water loss). These infants may need up to 200 to 300 ml/kg/day.[14]

Sodium Requirements of Preterm Infants

There are conflicting viewpoints on the management of fluid and electrolyte status in preterm infants. Sodium intake is usually calculated at 1 to 3 mEq/kg/day. Preterm infants, particularly those less than 30 to 32 weeks' gestation, may be unable to maintain sodium balance on the standard sodium intake due to increased urinary Na loss, and may require sodium intakes up to 4 to 8 mEq/kg/day.[3,4] Others feel that these infants can be maintained on lower sodium intakes and that increasing fluid leads to increased sodium loss.[113] However, most agree that sodium supplementation is necessary in VLBW infants after the initial decrease in extracellular volume.[22]

VLBW infants are also at risk for hyperkalemia because of alterations in renal function and changes in fluid dynamics after birth. As a result, potassium needs must be carefully monitored and routine replacement may need to be decreased in the first few days.[12,35,115] Some infants less than 26 to 27 weeks of age have signs of dehydration at 24 to 48 hours, with elevated sodium, potassium, and glucose without oliguria, acidosis, or shock. This may result from excessive evaporative losses (up to 100 to 200 ml/kg/day) due to the immature skin and greater surface area–to–body mass ratio, aldosterone insensitivity, and immaturity of renal Na^+/K^+-ATPase activity or a shift in potassium from the intracellular to extracellular space.[1,115,116,152] These infants have an initial weight loss of up to 20% and high urine output.[35] Management may require insulin and glucose infusions.[12]

Various protocols have been recommended for management of fluids and electrolytes in VLBW infants. The more immature the infants, the less able they are to adapt to a low sodium intake.[22] Lorenz et al. noted that preterm infants given increased fluid and sodium in the first week actually had lower serum sodium values than infants who received less fluid.[113] Restriction of sodium intake in the first five days decreased the incidence of hypernatremia, while fluid restriction led to hyponatremia.[36,159] Engle found that conservative fluid management during the first few weeks was associated with a positive sodium balance and fewer complications.[57] Modi notes that, if given liberal fluid intake with sodium supplementation, infants will not have the usual initial postbirth weight loss. However, eventually most infants will experience the typical postbirth changes in fluid compartments.[124] "The well recognized diuresis that accompanies improving respiratory function in babies with RDS is in fact a natriuresis and is an example of delayed postnatal maturation."[124] All infants have a reduction in ECF volume in the first few days, which is associated with increased excretion of fluid and sodium excretion. This in part accounts for the increased sodium losses in the first week. Thus correcting the high sodium excretion by increasing sodium intake in the first week may impede the normal postbirth adjustments in body fluid compartment values.[22,124] However, after these adjustments have occurred, sodium balance in the VLBW infant must be carefully evaluated and monitored. Some artificial formulas as well as human milk may not contain adequate sodium for the VLBW infant with immature renal function. These infants may require sodium supplementation until sodium balance is positive.

Risk of Overhydration and Dehydration

Although the infant can dilute urine to osmolarities of 50 to 70 mOsm/L, the usual diuretic response to a water load often diminishes before the entire load can be excreted.[37,73] This decreased ability to excrete a water load makes the infant more susceptible to fluid overload. Term and larger preterm infants are more vulnerable to overhydration in the first 5 days following birth, since maximal dilution is not achieved until after that time.[132] GFR remains low in preterm infants until a gestational age greater than 34 to 35 weeks is reached; thus these infants are at risk for volume overload for a longer period.[35] Fluid overload in preterm infants has been associated with an increased risk of PDA and possibly necrotizing enterocolitis (NEC).[1] The expanded extracellular volume secondary to fluid overload may stimulate production of PGE_2, which maintains a patent ductus. In infants with PDA and a large shunt, blood flow to the intestines is reduced, which may result in hypoperfusion, ischemia, and NEC.

Because of decreased concentrating ability, neonates (especially preterm infants) are at risk for dehydration, particularly if fluid intake is inadequate or extrarenal losses are elevated, as with transepidermal loss in VLBW infants.[158] In evaluating dehydration in the first week, the usual postbirth weight loss must be considered so that infants do not become overhydrated.[132]

Electrolyte Imbalances

Limitations in renal function in preterm and ill neonates increase the risk of electrolyte disturbances from iatrogenic causes. Electrolyte imbalances can also arise from pathophysiologic problems, but these are not considered here.

Hyponatremia. Hyponatremia in preterm or sick infants can occur secondary to alterations in fluid (dilutional hyponatremia) or in sodium balance. Dilutional hyponatremia can arise from excess transfer of free water across the placenta because of rapid or excessive administration of fluids to the woman in labor. Excessive administration of a hypotonic solution overwhelms the limited fetal or neonatal renal capacity to deal with a water overload. This may occur if maintenance fluid requirements for the first week after birth do not allow for the physiologic weight loss, especially in VLBW infants. These events lead to rapid expansion of extracellular volume and reduced serum sodium and are associated with an increased incidence of PDA, congestive heart failure, NEC, intracranial hemorrhage, and bronchopulmonary dysplasia.[72]

Dilutional hyponatremia can also occur subsequent to water retention associated with the syndrome of inappropriate secretion of antidiuretic hormone (SIADH).[72] (ADH is the former term for AVP). This syndrome is seen with a variety of pathophysiologic problems such as asphyxia, respiratory distress, sepsis, and central nervous system problems, and following PDA ligation and other stressful situations. SIADH involves excessive secretion of AVP with normal fluid intake, serum hyponatremia and hyposmolality, increased urine osmolality and renal sodium excretion, absence of volume depletion and dehydration, and normal renal and adrenal function.[72]

Hyponatremia can also arise from negative sodium balance and excessive loss of sodium by immature kidneys of VLBW infants. In these infants the greater sodium loss increases water loss (renal excretion of sodium must be accompanied by excretion of water), leading to decreased ECF volume and hyponatremia.[72,167] Urinary sodium loss and subsequent hyponatremia in VLBW infants interfere with renal concentrating ability by changing the osmotic gradient and impairing AVP response. This further reduces water reabsorption and increases sodium loss and risk of hyponatremia.[59,174] Dilutional hyponatremia is an ever-present risk for VLBW infants in the early postnatal period. This risk may be reduced by increasing sodium intake in VLBW infants during the first few weeks and careful monitoring intake, output, electrolytes, weight, and fluid status.[14]

Hypernatremia. Hypernatremia related to immaturity of renal function may arise from dehydration caused by excessive sodium intake or increased IWL. The dehydration may be aggravated by limited concentrating ability of the immature kidney.[72,111] Hypernatremia can also follow intravenous administration of sodium bicarbonate, since the infant may not be able to rapidly excrete this sodium load.

Hypernatremia in VLBW infants is usually secondary to high transepidermal water losses in the first week.[59]

Late metabolic acidosis. Late metabolic acidosis can also occur due to limitations in renal function, especially in VLBW infants. This disorder usually occurs at 2 to 3 weeks of age and is characterized by a mild metabolic acidosis accompanied by an alkaline urine. Late metabolic acidosis may also be related to the amount of protein in the infant's diet, the amino acid composition of the protein, and the lower renal threshold for bicarbonate; the disorder often corrects with maturation of renal function.[73] In VLBW infants, this may be secondary to sodium depletion.[22]

Measurement of Renal Function and Hydration Status

Parameters used to assess hydration status in the neonate include weight, fluid intake, urine specific gravity (1.002 to 1.010) and osmolarity (60 to 300 mOsm), urine output (minimum 1 to 3 ml/kg/hour) and electrolytes, and serum electrolytes and osmolarity. Findings indicative of adequate renal function in the newborn include urine volume greater than 1 to 3 ml/hour, FE_{Na} less than 3%, and urine specific gravity of 1.008 to 1.012.[132,138] Changes in urine specific gravity are often an early response to alterations in hydration. Urine for this measurement can be obtained reliably from either collecting bags or aspirating several drops from the diaper.[120,143] Urine output can be assessed by weighing diaper before and after use and noting the difference (1 g = 1 ml urine). Since urine rapidly evaporates from diapers of infants under radiant warmers, this assessment must be done soon after the infant voids.[34]

Serum osmolarity can be estimated by doubling the serum sodium value (since sodium and its anions are the major components of ECF), or more precisely by the following formula:[86]

$$\text{Serum osmolality (mOsm/L)} = 2Na + \frac{\text{BUN (mg/dl)}}{2.8} + \frac{\text{Blood glucose (mg/dl)}}{18}$$

2.8 and 18 represent molecular weights divided by 10. Measurement of renal function also involves assessment of GFR.

Plasma creatinine levels at birth reflect maternal values and increase shortly after birth (possibly because of a shift in ECF), followed by a decrease and stabilization at about 0.35 to 0.40 mg/dl (range, 0.14 to 0.70) by 1 to 2 weeks in term infants and up to 3 weeks in preterm infants.[72,75,155] The elevated creatinine levels may be due to immature tubular function with "leaky" tubular membranes.[75] Plasma creatinine levels are higher at birth in VLBW infants and inversely related to gestational age. Because GFR increases more slowly after birth in these infants, the decrease in

plasma creatinine is slower, taking up to 5 or more days. Therefore, plasma creatinine levels are a poor predictor of renal function in ELBW infants.[115,150] This measure is also limited in infants and children in general due to the progressive changes in GFR and muscle mass.[155]

Creatinine clearance generally approximates GFR in term infants (as in adults) but is considerably more variable in preterm infants. At lower GFR values, creatinine clearance tends to overestimate GFR.[74,155] Creatinine clearance correlates with birth weight, length, and gestational age.[72] Plasma creatinine and creatinine clearance are useful measurements in stable infants but are less accurate in infants with renal failure or preterm infants whose renal function is rapidly changing with maturation.[155] The formula GFR (ml/min per 1.73 m^2) = KL/P_{cr} (L − length in cm; P_{cr} = plasma creatinine; K = estimate of muscle mass) is a better estimate of GFR than plasma creatinine alone, since it accounts for percentage of muscle mass. In this formula, K = 0.27 for VLBW, 0.33 for preterm infants with weight appropriate for gestational age (AGA), 0.31 for SGA preterm infants, 0.45 for AGA term infants, and 0.33 for SGA term infants less than 1 year.[155] This formula can be used after the first week in term infants, and until 1 year of age for preterm infants greater than 34 to 35 weeks' gestational age. The accuracy of this formula has been questioned, especially because variations in hydration status and various pathophysiologic states can alter the results.[59,74]

Renal Function during Neonatal Illness

Immaturity in renal function in infants, especially preterm infants, limits their ability to cope with additional stresses and can lead to significant alterations of renal function in association with specific pathologic problems such as RDS, perinatal asphyxia, congestive heart failure, bronchopulmonary dysplasia, and PDA. These disorders can also interfere with maturation of renal hemodynamics and tubular function (Figure 10-14).[179]

During perinatal asphyxia, severe RDS, or other hypoxemic events, vascular resistance is increased, GFR decreased, and the renin-angiotensin-aldosterone system activated, further magnifying alterations that normally occur in normal newborns. In addition, cardiac output is redistributed, with increased blood flow to vital organs (heart, brain, and adrenal glands) and reduced flow to less essential areas such as the renal and gastrointestinal systems. The percentage of decrease in flow to these nonessential systems is greater in immature animals and perhaps in human preterm infants as well.[132] The decreased blood flow increases the risk of renal and intestinal ischemia and disorders such as NEC and acute tubular necrosis. Following asphyxia episodes, infants are at risk for SIADH, reduced urine output, impaired electrolyte

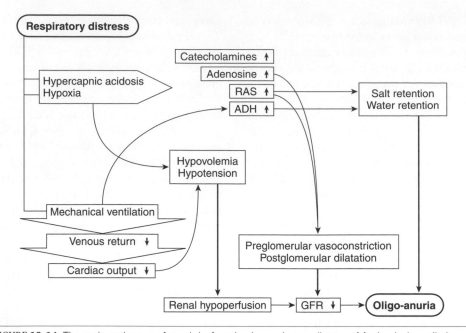

FIGURE **10-14** The main pathways of renal dysfunction in respiratory distress. Mechanical ventilation as well as the hypoxemia-induced activation of vasoactive factors contribute to the development of systemic hypotension and hypovolemia. (From Toth-Heyn, P., et al. [2000]. The stressed neonatal kidney: From pathophysiology to clinical management of neonatal vasomotor neuropathy. *Pediatr Nephrol, 14,* 230.)

reabsorption, hyperkalemia, and hyponatremia.[22] These infants require careful calculation and titration of fluid intake. Oliguria or anuria is most likely to develop within the first 24 hours. Initial fluid intake is limited to replacement of insensible and urinary water losses.

Infants with RDS and hypoxemia have marked changes in renal function with impairment of renal perfusion and reduced urine output by hypoxemia. Oliguria is associated with renal tubular necrosis, decreased renal perfusion, and impaired diluting ability. These impairments can lead to a decreased ability to excrete water, water retention, and edema. The reduction in perfusion is due to vasoconstriction with increased RVR possibly mediated by elevated activity of the renin-angiotensin system.[73] The decreased urine output is due to increased AVP and altered renal hemodynamics with a decreased GFR.[72] In hypoxemic infants an increase in urine output may occur prior to improvement in the alveolar-arterial oxygen gradient, suggesting that the improvement in respiratory function may be secondary to renal excretion of fluid sequestered in the lungs.[35,72] Renal tubular function is also altered in these infants, with increased renal loss of protein, glucose, and sodium, decreased concentrating ability, and impairment of the ability to excrete acid (increasing the risk of renal tubular acidosis).

Positive-pressure ventilation further alters renal function by decreasing cardiac output and renal perfusion, redistributing blood flow, and increasing intrathoracic and inferior vena caval pressure. Positive-pressure ventilation and constant positive airway pressure alter renal function by decreasing GFR.[35,72] Adequate hydration and careful monitoring of fluid and electrolyte status are especially critical for infants with respiratory problems and those on assisted ventilation.

MATURATIONAL CHANGES DURING INFANCY AND CHILDHOOD

Renal function undergoes rapid maturation during the first 2 years, increasing the risk of fluid and electrolyte problems in infants. Function comparable to that of adults is achieved by around 2 years. ERPF increases rapidly from birth to 3 months, then more slowly reaching adult values by 12 to 24 months.[94] GFR also increases rapidly during the first 3 months, then increases more slowly to reach adult values by 1 to 2 years.[92,93] Values may remain lower in preterm infants, with a lag in reaching values seen in term infants.[93] For example, by 9 months of age, GFR in preterm infants was only two thirds that of term infants.[183] Creatinine output per unit of body weight increases throughout childhood as muscle mass increases.[72] Plasma creatinine values are stable at values averaging 0.35 to 0.40 mg/dl until 2 years of age, when they increase further until adolescence.[155]

By 2 months the infant is able to maximally excrete a water loss; concentrating ability does not reach adult levels until around 18 months or later.[78] The ability to concentrate urine is probably related to increasing protein content in the

TABLE **10-16**   Recommendations for Clinical Practice Related to Changes in the Renal System and Fluid and Electrolyte Homeostasis in Neonates

Monitor fluid and electrolyte status of infants of mothers who received large volumes or rapidly administered intravenous fluids during labor or hypertonic intravenous (IV) solutions (p. 384 and Table 10-7).

Know normal values for parameters used to assess renal function and fluid and electrolyte status and recognize abnormalities (pp. 396-398, 401-404).

Know expected patterns of weight loss following birth and monitor status (pp. 393-394).

Carefully calculate fluid and electrolyte requirements (pp. 394, 401-404).

Record fluid intake and output and maintain within calculated limits (pp. 401-404).

Use an infusion device to administer IV fluids, calculate intake hourly, and adjust as needed (pp. 398, 401-404).

Assess hydration status of infants using weight, intake and output, urine specific gravity and osmolality, serum osmolality and electrolytes) (pp. 401-404).

Observe for signs of overhydration, water retention, vascular overload, and dehydration (pp. 404-405).

Know and monitor complications associated with excess fluid (pp. 404-405).

Record the time and character of the first voiding (p. 394).

Monitor voiding and fluid and electrolyte status in infants born with perinatal asphyxia or after maternal magnesium sulfate administration (pp. 394, 405-406).

Monitor infants on glucose IVs (especially very-low–birth-weight [VLBW] infants) for glycosuria, hyperglycemia, and fluid and electrolyte status (p. 397 and Chapter 15).

Monitor potassium levels in infants with increased energy needs or who are stressed, or on diuretics or volume expanders (pp. 397-398).

Monitor calcium and magnesium levels in VLBW infants or those on sodium supplementation or with increased sodium excretion (pp. 397-398 and Chapter 16).

Monitor blood and urine pH values in low–birth-weight (LBW) or ill infants (pp. 398, 405).

Know the risk factors for acidosis and observe for acid-base alterations in infants with cold stress, starvation, and fluid and electrolyte alterations (pp. 398, 405).

Observe for renal sodium loss and hyponatremia, especially in VLBW infants (pp. 396-397, 403-404).

Know the effects of illness on renal function and monitor ill or stressed infants for problems such as hyponatremia and dehydration (pp. 403-404).

Recognize and monitor for drug side effects related to immature renal function (p. 396 and Chapter 6).

Know the components (e.g., maintenance, replacement of loss, provision for growth) of usual fluid and electrolyte needs for infants and how these needs vary at different gestational ages (pp. 401-404).

Calculate infant fluid and electrolyte needs and renal solute load (pp. 398-404).

Avoid use of high solute load formulas, especially in LBW infants (pp. 402-403).

Recognize the factors influencing insensible water loss and act to minimize the effects of these losses (p. 402 and Table 10-15).

Recognize and monitor for effects of neonatal pathophysiologic problems on renal function (pp. 405-406).

Recognize the factors placing the infant at risk for overhydration, dehydration, and electrolyte imbalances and monitor infants for these problems (pp. 398-400, 404-405).

Recognize the parameters associated with syndrome of inappropriate secretion of antidiuretic hormone (SIADH) and late metabolic acidosis (pp. 404-405).

diet, which increases urea levels in serum and tubular filtrate. This increase is important in creating the necessary gradient essential for maximizing renal concentrating mechanisms.[167]

PRA decreases significantly from 1 to 6 weeks, then more slowly. Adult values for PRA and aldosterone levels are reached by 6 to 9 years, possibly earlier.[68,93,131] The decrease in ATII parallels the decrease in PRA.[131]

Further maturation and growth of nephrons continues to about 2 years of age.[6,131] Anatomically the lobulation seen in the newborn kidney disappears and the glomerulus and tubules approach adult relationships by about 6 months.[14] The cuboidal epithelium of the newborn's glomerulus is gradually replaced by thin epithelium by 1 year of age.[138] Total body water decreases to 70% by 3 months and 60% to 65% by 12 months.[117] ECF volume decreases to 30% by 3 to 6 months, then gradually to adult values of 10%.[82] Urine output increases to 500 to 600 ml per 24 hours by 1 year of age.[73] The bladder remains a cigar-shaped abdominal organ until early childhood, with achievement of the adult pelvic position and pyramidal shape by about 6 years.[117]

SUMMARY

The neonate is vulnerable to significant alterations in volume homeostasis and electrolyte balance due to immaturity of renal function. This vulnerability is especially marked in the preterm infant, in whom there is very little margin for errors in management of fluid and electrolyte status. These infants can rapidly become overhydrated or dehydrated or develop hyponatremia, hypernatremia, and other electrolyte disorders. By careful assessment and observation, the nurse can prevent or minimize the effects of many of these disorders. Recommendations for clinical practices related to alterations in the renal system and fluid and electrolyte balance are summarized in Table 10-16. By providing care to minimize these alterations, neonatal health can be enhanced, with a reduction in the risks associated with pathophysiologic complications.

REFERENCES

1. Adamkin, D.H. (1998). Issues in the nutritional support of the ventilated baby. *Clin Perinatol, 25,* 79.
2. Alcorn, D., et al. (1996). Angiotensin receptors and development of the kidney. *Clin Exp Pharmacol Physiol Suppl, 3,* S88.
3. Al-Dahhan, J., et al. (1984). Sodium homeostasis in term and preterm infants. III: The effects of salt supplementation. *Arch Dis Child, 59,* 945.
4. Al-Dahhan, J., et al. (1983). Sodium homeostasis in term and preterm infants. I: Renal aspects. *Arch Dis Child, 58,* 335.
5. Andriole, V.T. & Patterson, T.F. (1991). Epidemiology, natural history, and management of urinary tract infections in pregnancy. *Med Clin North Am, 75,* 359.
6. Arant, B.S. (1987). Postnatal development of renal function during the first year of life. *Pediatr Nephrol, 1,* 308.
7. Armenti, V.T., et al. (1994). National Transplantation Pregnancy Registry: outcomes of 154 pregnancies in cyclosporine treated female kidney transplant recipients. *Transplantation, 57,* 502.
8. Assali, N.S., Digman, W.J. & Dasgupta, K. (1979). Renal function in human pregnancy. II. Effects of venous pooling on renal hemodynamics and water, electrolyte, and aldosterone excretion during normal gestation. *J Lab Clin Med, 54,* 394.
9. Bailie, M.D. (1992). Development of the endocrine function of the kidney, *Clin Perinatol, 18,* 59.
10. Ballerman, B.J., et al. (1991). Vasoactive peptides and the kidney. In B.M. Brenner & F.C. Rector (Eds.). *The kidney.* Philadelphia: W.B. Saunders.
11. Baumgardt, S. (1990). Water metabolism. In R.M. Cowett, & W.W. Hay (Eds.). *The micropremie: The next frontier* (report of the 99th Ross Conference on Pediatric Research. Columbus). OH: Ross Laboratories.
12. Baumgardt, S. & Costarino, A.T. (2000). Water and electrolyte metabolism of the micropremie. *Clin Perinatol, 27,* 131.
13. Baylis, C. (1999). Glomerular filtration rate in normal and abnormal pregnancies. *Semin Nephrol, 19,* 133.
14. Bell, E.F. & Oh, W. (1999). Fluid and electrolyte management. In G.B. Avery, M.A. Fletcher & M.G. MacDonald (Eds.). *Neonatology, pathophysiology and management of the newborn* (5th ed.). Philadelphia: J.B. Lippincott.
15. Beydoun, S.N. (1985). Morphologic changes in the renal tract in pregnancy. *Clin Obstet Gynecol, 28,* 249.
16. Bierd, T.M., et al. (1990). Interrelationships of atrial natriuretic peptide, atrial volume, and renal function in premature infants. *J Pediatr, 116,* 753.
17. Boineau, F.G. & Lewy, J.E. (1990). Estimation of parenteral fluid requirements. *Pediatr Clin North Am, 37,* 257.
18. Brace, R.A. (1986). Amniotic fluid volume and its relationship to fetal fluid balance: Review of experimental data. *Semin Perinatol, 10,* 103.
19. Brace, R.A. (1998). Fluid distribution in the fetus and neonate. In R.A. Polin & W.W. Fox (Eds.). *Fetal and neonatal physiology* (2nd ed.). Philadelphia: W.B. Saunders
20. Brans, Y. (1986). Fluid compartments in neonates weighing 1000 grams or less. *Clin Perinatol, 13,* 403.
21. Brinkman, C.R. & Meldrum, D. (1979). Physiology and pathophysiology of maternal adjustments to pregnancy. In S. Aldjem, A.K. Brown, & C. Surreau (Eds.). *Clinical perinatology* (2nd ed.). St. Louis: Mosby.
22. Brion, L.P., Bernstein, J., & Spitzer, A. (1997). Kidney and urinary tract. In A.A. Fanaroff & R.J. Martin (Eds.). *Neonatal-perinatal medicine, diseases of the fetus and infant* (6th ed.). St. Louis: Mosby.
23. Brion, L.P., et al. (1999). Renal disease. In G.B. Avery, M.A. Fletcher, & M.G. MacDonald (Eds.). *Neonatology, pathophysiology and management of the newborn* (5th ed.). Philadelphia: J.B. Lippincott.
24. Brown, M.A. & Gallery, E.D. (1994). Volume homeostasis in normal pregnancy and pre-eclampsia: physiology and clinical implications. *Baillieres Clin Obstet Gynecol, 8,* 287.
25. Brown, M.A., et al. (1997). The renin-angiotensin-aldosterone system in pre-eclampsia. *Clin Exp Hypertens, 19,* 713.
26. Cardozo, L. & Cuter, A. (1997). Lower urinary tract symptoms in pregnancy. *Br J Urol, 80,* 14.
27. Carmen, S. (1986). Neonatal hypoglycemia in response to maternal glucose infusion before delivery. *J Obstet Gynecol Neonatal Nurs, 15,* 319.
28. Carvalho, J.C. & Mathias, R.S. (1994). Intravenous hydration in obstetrics, *Int Anesthesiol Clin, 32,* 103.
29. Chapman, A.B., et al. (1998). Temporal relationships between hormonal and hemodynamic changes in early human pregnancy. *Kidney Int, 54,* 2056.
30. Chih, T.W., et al. (1991). Times of the first urine and the first stool in Chinese newborns. *Acta Paediatr Sin, 32,* 17.
31. Christensen, T., et al. (1989). Changes in renal volume during normal pregnancy. *Acta Obstet Gynecol Scand, 68,* 541.
32. Clark, D.A. (1977). Time of first void and first stool in 500 newborns. *Pediatrics, 60,* 457.
33. Connolly, A. & Thorp, J.M. (1999). Urinary tract infections during pregnancy. *Urol Clin North Am, 26,* 779.
34. Cooke, B.J., Werkman, S. & Watson, D. (1989). Urine output measurement in premature infants. *Pediatrics, 83,* 116.
35. Costarino, A.T. & Baumgart, S. (1988). Controversies in fluid and electrolyte management for the preterm infant. *Clin Perinatol, 15,* 863.
36. Costarino, A.T., et al. (1992). Sodium restriction versus daily maintenance replacement in low birth weight premature infants: A randomized, blind therapeutic trial. *J Pediatr, 120,* 999.
37. Costarino, A.T. & Brans, Y. (1998). Fetal and neonatal body and fluid composition with relevance to growth and development. In R.A. Polin & W.W. Fox (Eds.). *Fetal and neonatal physiology* (2nd ed.). Philadelphia: W.B. Saunders
38. Cotton, D.B., et al. (1984). Intrapartum to postpartum changes in colloid osmotic pressure. *Am J Obstet Gynecol, 149,* 174.
39. Crowe, A.V., et al. (1999). Pregnancy does not adversely affect renal transplant function. *QJM, 92,* 631.
40. Culpepper, L. & Jack, B. (1990). Prevention of urinary tract infection complications during pregnancy. In I.R. Merkatz & J.E. Thompson (Eds.). *New perspectives on prenatal care.* New York: Elsevier.
41. Cutner, A., et al. (1992). Assessment of urinary symptoms in the second half of pregnancy. *Int Urogynecol J, 3,* 30.
42. Dafnis, E. & Sabatini, S. (1992). The effects of pregnancy on renal function: Physiology and pathophysiology. *Am J Med Sci, 303,* 184.
43. Dahlenburg, G.W., Burnell, R.H., & Braybrook, R. (1980). The relation between cord serum sodium levels in newborn infants and maternal intravenous therapy during labour. *Br J Obstet Gynaecol, 87,* 519.
44. Davison, J.M. (1985). The physiology of the renal tract in pregnancy. *Clin Obstet Gynecol, 28,* 257.
45. Davison, J.M. (1987). Overview: Kidney function in pregnant women. *Am J Kidney Dis, 9,* 248.

46. Davison, J.M. (1991). Dialysis, transplantation, and pregnancy. *Am J Kidney Dis, 17,* 127.

47. Davison, J.M., et al. (1992). Metabolic clearance of vasopressin and an analogue resistant to vasopressinase in human pregnancy, *Am J Physiol, 264,* F348.

48. Davison, J.M. (1997). Edema in pregnancy, *Kidney Int Suppl, 59,* S90.

49. Davison, J.M. & Lindheimer, M.D. (1999). Renal disorders. In R.K. Creasy & R. Resnik (Eds.). *Maternal-fetal medicine* (4th ed.). Philadelphia: W.B. Saunders.

50. De Curtis, M., Senterre, J. & Rigo, J. (1990). Renal solute load in preterm infants. *Arch Dis Child, 65,* 357.

51. Delemarre, F. (1996). Diurnal variation in angiotensin sensitivity in pregnancy, *Am J Obstet Gynecol, 174,* 259.

52. Dimpfl, T., et al. (1992). Incidence and cause of postpartum urinary stress incontinence. *Eur J Obstet Gynecol Reprod Biol, 43,* 29.

53. Duvekot, J.J., et al. (1993). Early pregnancy changes in hemodynamics and volume homeostasis are consecutive adjustments triggered by a primary fall in systemic vascular tone. *Am J Obstet Gynecol, 169,* 1382.

54. Duvekot, J.J. & Peeters, L.L. (1994). Renal hemodynamics and volume homeostasis in pregnancy. *Obstet Gynecol Surv, 49,* 830.

55. El-Dahr, S.S. & Chevalier, R.L. (1990). Special needs of the newborn infant in fluid therapy. *Pediatr Clin North Am, 37,* 323.

56. Elkington, K.W. (1991). At the water's edge: where obstetrics and anesthesia meet. *Obstet Gynecol, 77,* 304.

57. Engle, W.D. (1986). Development of fetal and neonatal renal function. *Semin Perinatol, 10,* 113.

58. Faundes, A., et al. (1998). Dilatation of the urinary tract during pregnancy: Proposal of a curve of maximal caliceal diameter by gestational age. *Am J Obstet Gynecol, 178,* 1082.

59. Feld, L.G. & Waz, W.R. (1998). Renal transport of sodium during early development. In R.A. Polin & W.W. Fox (Eds.). *Fetal and neonatal physiology* (2nd ed.). Philadelphia: W.B. Saunders

60. Fetterman, G.H., et al. (1965). The growth and maturation of human glomeruli and proximal convolutions from term to adulthood. *Pediatrics, 35,* 601.

61. Freed, S.Z. (1981). Hydronephrosis of pregnancy. In S.Z. Freed & N. Herzig (Eds.). *Urology in pregnancy.* Baltimore: Williams & Wilkins.

62. Gabert, H.A. & Miller, J.M. (1985). Renal disease in pregnancy. *Obstet Gynecol Surv, 40,* 449.

63. Gaboury, C.L. & Woods, L.L. (1995). Renal reserve in pregnancy. *Semin Nephrol, 15,* 449.

64. Gallery, E.D.M. & Brown, M.A. (1987). Control of sodium excretion in human pregnancy. *Am J Kidney Dis, 9,* 290.

65. Gant, N.F., et al. (1973). A study of angiotensin II pressor response throughout primigravid pregnancy. *J Clin Invest, 52,* 2682.

66. Gant, N.F., et al. (1987). Control of vascular reactivity in pregnancy. *Am J Kidney Dis, 9,* 303.

67. Gillerot, Y. & Koulischer, L. (1988). Major malformations of the urinary tract. *Biol Neonate, 53,* 186.

68. Gomez, R.A. & Norwood, V.F. (1995). Developmental consequences of the renin-angiotensin system. *Am J Kidney Dis, 26,* 409.

69. Green, T.P. (1987). The pharmacologic basis of diuretic therapy in the newborn. *Clin Perinatol, 14,* 951.

70. Gruskay, J.A., et al. (1988). Non-oliguric hyperkalemia in the premature infant <1000 gms. *J Pediatr, 113,* 381.

71. Guignard, J.P. (1981). The neonatal stressed kidney. In A.B. Gruskin & M.E. Norman (Eds.). *Pediatric nephrology.* The Hague: Martinus Nijhoff.

72. Guignard, J.P. & John, E.G. (1986). Renal function in the tiny, premature infant. *Clin Perinatol, 13,* 377.

73. Guignard, J.P. & Torrado, A. (1987). Neonatal renal function and disease. In L. Stern & P. Vert (Eds.). *Neonatal medicine.* New York: Masson.

74. Guignard, J.P. (1998). Measurement of glomerular filtration rate in neonates. In R.A. Polin & W.W. Fox (Eds.). *Fetal and neonatal physiology* (2nd ed.). Philadelphia: W.B. Saunders.

75. Guignard, J.P. & Drukker, A. (1999). Why do newborn infants have a high plasma creatinine? *Pediatrics, 103,* e49.

76. Guillery, E.N. (1997). Fetal and neonatal nephrology. *Curr Opin Pediatr, 9,* 148

77. Guillery, E.N., et al. (1998). Functional development of the kidney in utero. In R.A. Polin & W.W. Fox (Eds.). *Fetal and neonatal physiology* (2nd ed.). Philadelphia: W.B. Saunders.

78. Guron, G. & Friberg, P. (2000). An intact renin-angiotensin system is a prerequisite for normal renal development. *J Hyperten, 18,* 123.

79. Haadem, K. (1994). The effects of parturition on female pelvic floor anatomy and function. *Curr Opin Obstet Gynecol, 6,* 326.

80. Hagemann, A., et al. (1994). The uteroplacental renin-angiotensin system: A review. *Exp Clin Endocrinol, 102,* 252.

81. Harrison, M.R., et al. (1982). Management of the fetus with congenital hydronephrosis, *J Pediatr Surg, 17,* 728.

82. Heisler, D. (1993). Pediatric renal function. *Int Anesthesiol Clin, 31,* 103.

83. Henderson, P. & Little, G.A. (1990). The detection of pregnancy-induced hypertension. In I.R. Merkatz & J.E. Thompson (Eds.). *New perspectives on prenatal care.* New York: Elsevier.

84. Hertzberg, B.S., et al. (1993). Doppler USS assessment of maternal kidneys. Analysis of intrarenal reactivity indexes in normal, pregnancy and physiologic pelvicaliectasis. *Radiology, 186,* 689.

85. Hilgers, K.F. (1997). Angiotensin's role in renal development. *Semin Nephrol, 17,* 492.

86. Hill, L.L. (1990). Body composition, normal electrolyte concentrations, and the maintenance of normal volume, tonicity, and acid-base metabolism. *Pediatr Clin North Am, 37,* 241.

87. Israel, A. & Pecano, A. (2000). Renin-angiotensin aldosterone system in pregnancy-induced hypertension. *J Hum Hypertens, 14*(suppl 1), S36.

88. Jaffe, D.J. (1985). Postpartum evaluation of renal function. *Clin Obstet Gynecol, 28,* 298.

89. Johnson, C., et al. (1989). Nutrition and hydration in labour. In I. Chalmers, M. Enkin, & M.J.N.C. Keirse (Eds.). *Effective care in pregnancy and childbirth.* Oxford, England: Oxford University Press.

90. Jones, D.C. & Hayslett, J.P. (1996). Outcome of pregnancy in women with moderate or severe renal insufficiency. *N Engl J Med, 335,* 226.

91. Jones, D.C. (1997). Pregnancy complicated by chronic renal disease. *Clin Perinatol, 24,* 483.

92. Jose, P.A. & Fildes, R.D. (1990). Postnatal development of renal function. In *The tiny baby* (Mead-Johnson Symposium on Perinatal and Developmental Medicine, no. 33). Evansville, IN: Mead Johnson.

93. Jose, P.A., et al. (1994). Neonatal renal function and physiology, *Curr Opin Pediatr, 6,* 172.

94. Jose, P.A. (1998). Postnatal maturation of renal blood flow. In R.A. Polin & W.W. Fox (Eds.). *Fetal and neonatal physiology* (2nd ed.). Philadelphia: W.B. Saunders.

95. Katz, V.L., et al. (1992). Effect of daily immersion on the edema of pregnancy. *Am J Perinatol, 9,* 225.

96. Keppler, A.B. (1988). The use of intravenous fluids during labor. *Birth, 15*(2), 75.

97. Knauth, A., et al. (1989) A semipermeable polyurethane dressing as an artificial skin in premature neonates. *Pediatrics, 83,* 943.

98. Kolkot, F. (1997). Starvation in the midst of plenty-the problems of volemia in pregnancy and pre-eclampsia. *Nephrol Dial Transplant, 12,* 388.

99. Krutzen, E., et al. (1992). Glomerular filtration in pregnancy: a study in normal subjects and in patients with hypertension, pre-eclampsia and diabetes. *Scan J Clin Lab Invest, 53,* 387.

100. Kwee, A., et al. (2000). The effect of immersion on haemodynamics and fetal measures in uncomplicated pregnancies of nulliparous women. *Br J Obstet Gynaecol, 107,* 663.

101. Lafayette, R.A., et al. (1999). The dynamics of glomerular filtration after cesarean section. *J Am Soc Nephrol, 10,* 1561.

102. Lelievre-Pegorier, M. & Merlet-Benichou, C. (2000). The number of nephrons in the mammalian kidney: environmental influences play a determining role. *Exp Nephrol, 8,* 63.

103. Linday, L.A. (1994). Developmental changes in renal tubular function. *J Adolesc Health, 15,* 648.

104. Lindheimer, M.D. & Ehrlich, E.N. (1979). Postural effects on renal function and volume homeostasis during pregnancy. *J Reprod Med, 23,* 135.

105. Lindheimer, M.D. & Katz, A.D. (1986). The kidney in pregnancy. In B.M. Brenner & F.C. Rector (Eds.). *The Kidney* (3rd ed.). Philadelphia: Ardmore Medical Books.

106. Lindheimer, M.D., et al. (1987). Water homeostasis and vasopressin release during rodent and human gestation. *Am J Kidney Dis, 9,* 270.

107. Lindheimer, M.D., et al. (1987). Potassium homeostasis in pregnancy. *J Reprod Med, 32,* 517.

108. Lindheimer, M.D., et al. (1991). Osmotic and volume control of vasopressin release in pregnancy. *Am J Kidney Dis, 17,* 105.

109. Lindheimer, M.D. & Katz, A.I. (1992). Renal physiology and disease in pregnancy. In D.W. Seldin & G. Giebisch (Eds.). *The kidney: physiology and pathophysiology* (2nd ed.). NY: Raven.

110. Lindheimer, M.D. & Davison, J.M. (1995). Osmoregulation, the secretion of arginine vasopressin, and its metabolism during pregnancy. *Eur J Endocrinol, 132,* 133.

111. Lindshaw, M.A. (1998). Concentration of the urine. In R.A. Polin & W.W. Fox (Eds.). *Fetal and neonatal physiology* (2nd ed.). Philadelphia: W.B. Saunders

112. Lockitch, G. (1997). Clinical biochemistry of pregnancy. *Crit Rev Clin Lab Sci, 34,* 67.

113. Lorenz, J.M., et al. (1982). Water balance in very low-birth-weight infants: Relationship to water and sodium intake and effect on outcome. *J Pediatr, 101,* 423.

114. Lorenz, J.M., et al. (1995). Phases of fluid and electrolyte homeostasis in the extremely low birth weight infant. *Pediatrics, 96,* 484.

115. Lorenz, J.M. (1997). Assessing fluid and electrolyte status in the newborn. National Academy of Clinical Biochemistry. *Clin Chem, 43,* 205.

116. Lorenz, J.M., et al. (1997). Potassium metabolism in extremely low birth weight infants in the first week of life. *J Pediatr, 131,* 81.

117. Lowrey, G.H. (1986). *Growth and development of children.* Chicago: YearBook Medical.

118. Ludka, L.M. & Riberst, C.C. (1993). Eating and drinking in labor. A literature review. *J Nurse Midwifery, 38,* 199.

119. Lumbers, E.R. (1995). Functions of the renin-angiotensin system during development. *Clin Exp Pharmacol Physiol, 22,* 499.

120. Lybrand, M., Medoff-Cooper, B. & Munro, B.H. (1990). Periodic comparisons of urinary specific gravity using urine from a diaper and collecting bag. *MCN, 15,* 238.

121. Malinowski, J. (1978). Bladder assessment in the postpartum patient. *JOGN Nursing, 7,* 14.

122. Merlet-Benichou, C. (1999). Influences of fetal environment on kidney development. *Int J Dev Biol, 43,* 453.

123. Mikhail, M.S. & Anyaegbunam, A. (1995). Lower urinary tract dysfunction in pregnancy: a review. *Obstet Gynecol Surv, 50,* 675.

124. Modi, N. (1999). Renal function, fluid and electrolyte balance and neonatal renal disease. In J.M. Rennie & N.R.C. Robertson (Eds.). *Textbook of neonatology* (3rd ed.). Edinburgh: Churchill Livingstone.

125. Monga, M. (1999). Maternal cardiovascular and renal adaptation to pregnancy. In R.K. Creasy & R. Resnik (Eds.). *Maternal-fetal medicine* (4th ed.). Philadelphia: W.B. Saunders.

126. Monson, J.P. & Williams, D.J. (1992). Osmoregulatory adaptation in pregnancy and its disorders. *J Endocrinol, 132,* 7.

127. Moore, K., Persaud, T.V.N. & Schmitt, W. (1998). *The developing human: Clinically oriented embryology* (6th ed.). Philadelphia: W.B. Saunders.

128. Newton, N., Newton, M., & Broach, J. (1988). Psychologic, physical, nutritional and technologic aspects of intravenous infusion during labor. *Birth, 15*(2), 67.

129. Nordstrom, L., et al. (1995). Continuous maternal glucose infusion during labor: effects of maternal and fetal glucose and lactate levels. *Am J Perinatol, 12,* 357.

130. Norris, M., et al. (1996). The role of vasoactive molecules of endothelial origin in the pathophysiology of normal pregnancy and pregnancy induced hypertension. *Curr Opin Nephrol Hypertension, 5,* 347.

131. Norwood, V.F., et al. (1998). Development of the renin-angiotensin system. In R.A. Polin & W.W. Fox (Eds.). *Fetal and neonatal physiology* (2nd ed.). Philadelphia: W.B. Saunders.

132. Oh, W. (1997). Fluid, electrolyte and acid-base homeostasis. In A.A. Fanaroff & R.J. Martin (Eds.). *Neonatal-perinatal medicine, diseases of the fetus and infant* (6th ed.). St. Louis: Mosby.

133. O'Reilly, S.A., et al. (1993). Low risk mothers: oral intake and emesis in labor. *J Nurse Midwifery, 38,* 228.

134. O'Sullivan, G. (1994). The stomach-fact and fantasy: eating and drinking during labor. *Int Anesthesiol Clin, 32,* 31.

135. Paller, M.S. (1999). Renal diseases. In G.N. Burrow & T.P. Duffy. *Medical complications during pregnancy* (5th ed.). Philadelphia: W.B. Saunders.

136. Patterson, T.F. & Andriole, V.T. (1997). Detection, significance, and therapy of bacteriuria in pregnancy. *Infect Dis Clin North Am, 11,* 593.

137. Pauerstein, C.J. (1987). *Clinical obstetrics.* New York: John Wiley & Sons.

138. Pereira, G.H. (1995). Nutritional care of the extremely premature infant. *Clin Perinatol, 22,* 61.

139. Pohjavuori, M. (1983). Obstetric determinants of plasma vasopressin concentrations and renin activity at birth. *J Pediatr, 103,* 966.

140. Ramanathan, S. & Turndorf, H. (1988). Renal disease. In F.M. James, A.S. Wheeler, & D.M. Dewan (Eds.). *Obstetric anesthesia: The complicated patient.* Philadelphia: F.A. Davis.

141. Ramsay, I.N., et al. (1993). Uroflowmetry in the puerperium. *Neurol Urodyn, 12,* 33.

142. Rasmussen, P.E. & Nielsen, F.R. (1988). Hydronephrosis during pregnancy: A literature survey. *Eur J Obstet Gynecol Reprod Biol, 27,* 249.

143. Reams, P.K. & Deane, D.M. (1988). Bagged versus diaper urine specimens and lab values. *Neonatal Network, 6*(6), 17.

144. Reznik, V.M. & Budorick, N.E. (1995). Prenatal detection of congenital renal disease. *Urol Clin North Am, 22,* 21.

145. Rizzoni, G., et al. (1992). Successful pregnancies in women on renal replacement therapy: Report from the EDTA registry. *Nephrol Dial Transplant, 7,* 279.

146. Robillard, J.E., Nakamura, K.T., & Ayres, N.A. (1985). Control of fluid and electrolyte balance during fetal life. In C.T. Jones & P.W. Nathanielsz (Eds.). *The physiological development of the fetus and newborn.* New York: Academic Press.

147. Robillard, J.E. & Nakamura, K.T. (1988). Hormonal regulation of renal function during development. *Biol Neonate, 53,* 201.

148. Rowe, J.W., Brown, R.S., & Epstein, F.H. (1981). Physiology of the kidney in pregnancy. In S.Z. Freed & N. Herzig (Eds.). *Urology in pregnancy.* Baltimore: Williams & Wilkins.

149. Sadler, T.W. (2000). *Langman's medical embryology* (8th ed.). Philadelphia: Lippincott, Williams & Wilkins.

150. Sahgal, N., et al. (1990). Plasma creatinine concentration is a poor predictor of glomerular filtration in extremely low birth weight infants. *Clin Res, 38,* 789A.

151. Sampselle, C.M. (1990). Changes in pelvic muscle strength and stress urinary incontinence associated with childbirth. *J Obstet Gynecol Neonatal Nurs, 19,* 371.

152. Sato, K., et al. (1995). Internal potassium shift in premature infants: cause of nonoliguric hyperkalemia. *J Pediatr, 126,* 109.

153. Saultz, J.W., et al. (1991). Postpartum urinary retention. *J Am Board Fam Pract, 4,* 341.

154. Schobel, H.P. (1998). Pregnancy-induced alterations in renal function. *Kidney Blood Press Res, 21,* 274.

155. Schwartz, G.J., Brion, L.P. & Spitzer, A. (1987). The use of plasma creatinine for estimating glomerular filtration rate in infants, children and adolescents. *Pediatr Clin North Am, 34,* 571.

156. Sealey, J.E., et al. (1994). Estradiol- and progesterone-related increases in renin-aldosterone system: studies during ovarian stimulation and early pregnancy. *J Clin Endo Metab, 79,* 258.

157. Seely, E.W. & Moore, T.J. (1994). The renin-angiotensin aldosterone system and vasopressin. In D. Tulchinsky & A.B. Little (Eds.). *Maternal-fetal endocrinology* (2nd ed.). Philadelphia: W.B. Saunders.

158. Shaffer, S.E. & Norman, M.E. (1989). Renal function and renal failure in the newborn. *Clin Perinatol, 16,* 199.

159. Shaffer, S.G. & Meade, V.M. (1989). Sodium balance and extracellular volume regulation in very low birth weight infants. *J Pediatr, 115,* 285.

160. Shaffer, S.G. & Weismann, D.N. (1992). Fluid requirements in the preterm infant. *Clin Perinatol, 19,* 233.

161. Shutz, S. & Le Mollec, J.M. (1996). Early expression of the components of the renin-angiotensin system in human development. *Am J Pathol, 149,* 2067.

162. Sillen, U., et al. (2000). The voiding patterns of healthy preterm neonates. *J Urol, 163,* 278.

163. Simeonova, A. & Bengtsson, C. (1992). Prevalence of urinary incontinence among women in a Swedish primary health care centre. *Scan J Prim Health Care, 8,* 203.

164. Singhi, S., et al. (1985). Iatrogenic neonatal and maternal hyponatremia following oxytocin and aqueous glucose infusion during labour. *Br J Obstet Gynaecol, 92,* 356.

165. Sleutel, M. & Golden, S.S. (1999). Fasting in labor: relic or requirement. *J Obstet Gynecol Neonatal Nurs, 28,* 507.

166. Spitzer, A. (1996). The current approach to the assessment of fetal renal function: fact or fiction? *Pediatr Nephrol, 10,* 230.

167. Stewart, C.L. & Jose, P.A. (1985). Transitional nephrology. *Urol Clin North Am, 12,* 143.

168. Stjernquist, M., et al. (1995). Vasoactive peptides and uterine vessels. *Gynecol Endocrinol, 9,* 165.

169. Stray-Pederson, B. (1990). Screening and treatment of bacteriuria in pregnancy and the postpartum period. *Int Urogynecol J, 1,* 100.

170. Sturgis, N.N. & Davison, J.M. (1992). Effect of pregnancy on long-term function of renal allograft. *Am J Kidney Dis, 19,* 167.

171. Sturgiss, S.N., et al. (1994). Renal haemodynamics and tubular function in human pregnancy. *Baillieres Clin Obstet Gynaecol, 8,* 209.

172. Sturgiss, S.N., et al. (1996). Renal reserve during pregnancy. *Am J Physiol, 271,* F16.

173. Sullivan, C.A. & Martin, J.N. (1994). Sodium and pregnancy. *Clin Obstet Gynecol, 37,* 558.

174. Sulyok, E. (1988). Renal response to vasopressin in premature infants: What is new? *Biol Neonate, 53,* 212.

175. Symonds, E.M. (1988). Renin and reproduction. *Am J Obstet Gynecol, 158,* 754.

176. Theunissen, I.M. & Parer, J.T. (1994). Fluid and electrolytes in pregnancy. *Clin Obstet Gynecol, 37,* 3.

177. Thorp, J.M., et al. (1999). Urinary incontinence in pregnancy and the puerperium: A prospective study. *Am J Obstet Gynecol, 181,* 266.

178. Thornburg, K.L., et al. (2000). Hemodynamic changes in pregnancy. *Semin Perinatol, 24,* 11.

179. Toth-Heyn, P., et al. (2000). The stressed neonatal kidney: From pathophysiology to clinical management of neonatal vasomotor neuropathy. *Pediatr Nephrol, 14,* 227.

180. Tourangeau, A., et al. (1999). Intravenous therapy for women in labor: implementation of a practice change. *Birth, 26,* 1.

181. Tufro-McReddie, A. & Gomez, R.A. (1993). Ontogeny of the renin-angiotensin-aldosterone system. *Semin Nephrol, 13,* 519.

182. Vander, A., Sherman, J. & Luciano, D. (2000). *Human physiology: The mechanism of body function* (8th ed.). New York: McGraw-Hill.

183. Vanpee, M., et al. (1992). Renal function in very low birth weight infants: normal maturity reach during early childhood. *J Pediatr, 121,* 784.

184. Vernon, H.J., et al. (1990). Semipermeable dressing and transepidermal water loss in premature infants. *Pediatrics, 86,* 357.

185. Viktup, L., et al. (1992). The symptom of stress incontinence caused by pregnancy or delivery in primiparas. *Obstet Gynecol, 79,* 945.

186. Wasserstrum, N. (1992). Issues in fluid management during labor: general considerations. *Clin Obstet Gynecol, 35,* 505.

187. Winston, J. & Levitt, M.F. (1985). Renal function, renal disease and pregnancy. In S.H. Cherry, R.L. Berkowitz & N.G. Kase (Eds.). *Rovinsky and Guttmacher's medical, surgical and gynecologic complications of pregnancy.* Baltimore: Williams & Wilkins.

188. Winters, R.W. (1973). *The body fluids in pediatrics.* Boston: Little, Brown.

189. Worley, R.J., et al. (1979). Vascular responsiveness to pressor agents during human pregnancy. *J Reprod Med, 3,* 115.

190. Yared, A., Barakat, A.Y., & Ichikawa, I. (1990). Fetal nephrology. In R.D. Eden & F.H. Boehm (Eds.). *Assessment and care of the fetus.* Norwalk, CT: Appleton & Lange.

CHAPTER 11

Gastrointestinal and Hepatic Systems and Perinatal Nutrition

The gastrointestinal (GI) system consists of processes involved in intake, digestion, and absorption of nutrients and elimination of byproducts in bile and stool.[273] Utilization of nutrients for production of energy and other vital functions is discussed in Chapters 15 and 16. This chapter focuses on the processes involved in preparing food substances for absorption of nutrients across the intestinal villi. These processes are summarized in Figure 11-1; GI enzymes are summarized in Table 11-1.

Maternal nutrition is one of the most important factors affecting pregnancy outcome. The maternal GI tract must digest and absorb nutrients needed for fetal and placental growth and development and to meet the altered demands of maternal metabolism as well as eliminate unneeded byproducts and waste materials from both the woman and the fetus. Structural and physiologic immaturity of the neonate's GI tract can result in alterations in neonatal nutritional status and increase the risk of malabsorption and dehydration. This chapter reviews GI and hepatic function in the pregnant woman, fetus, and neonate and implications for clinical practice.

MATERNAL PHYSIOLOGIC ADAPTATIONS

The GI and hepatic systems during pregnancy are characterized by marked anatomic and physiologic alterations that are essential in supporting maternal and fetal nutrition. These changes are related to mechanical forces such as the pressure of the growing uterus and hormonal influences such as effects of progesterone on GI smooth muscle and effects of estrogen on liver metabolism.

Antepartum Period

The antepartum period is characterized by anatomic and physiologic changes in all the organs of the GI system. These changes and their implications are summarized in Table 11-2. Pregnancy is associated with increased appetite; increased consumption of food; and alterations in the types of food desired, including cravings, avoidance of certain foods, and pica (craving for nonnutrient substances).

Specific changes in food consumption and the types of foods craved or avoided are strongly influenced by cultural and economic factors. Food consumption has been reported to increase 15% to 20% beginning in early pregnancy, peak at mid-gestation, and decrease near term.[220] Changes in maternal caloric intake do not parallel changes in basal metabolism or fetal growth (Figure 11-2).

The basis for changes in patterns of food intake is unclear but may be a response to the drain of glucose and other nutrients by the fetus, alterations in taste threshold and acuity, and hormonal changes. Estrogen acts as an appetite suppressant and progesterone as an appetite stimulant. Influences of estrogen and progesterone on patterns of food intake are supported by similar changes during the menstrual cycle. Decreased appetite and food intake have been reported during the follicular phase of the menstrual cycle (when estrogen peaks), with increased appetite during the luteal phase (when progesterone peaks).[61,272] During pregnancy, alterations in insulin and glucagon combine with estrogen and progesterone to influence food intake.[273] Leptin (see Chapter 15) may also mediate maternal appetite changes.

Mouth and Pharynx

Contrary to the old wives' tale regarding the loss of a tooth per baby, pregnancy does not result in demineralization of the woman's teeth. Fetal calcium needs are drawn from maternal body stores, not from the teeth (see Chapter 16). The major component of tooth enamel (hydroxyapatite crystals) is not reduced by the biochemical or hormonal changes of pregnancy.[186,233] As a result of gingival alterations, however, the pregnant woman may become more aware of preexisting or newly developed dental caries. In addition there may be a transient increase in tooth mobility.[233] Calculus and debris deposits increase during pregnancy and are associated with gingivitis.[55,233]

Gingivitis occurs in 30% to 100% of pregnant women, generally beginning around the second month and peaking in the middle of the third trimester.[55,186,225,233] Estrogen

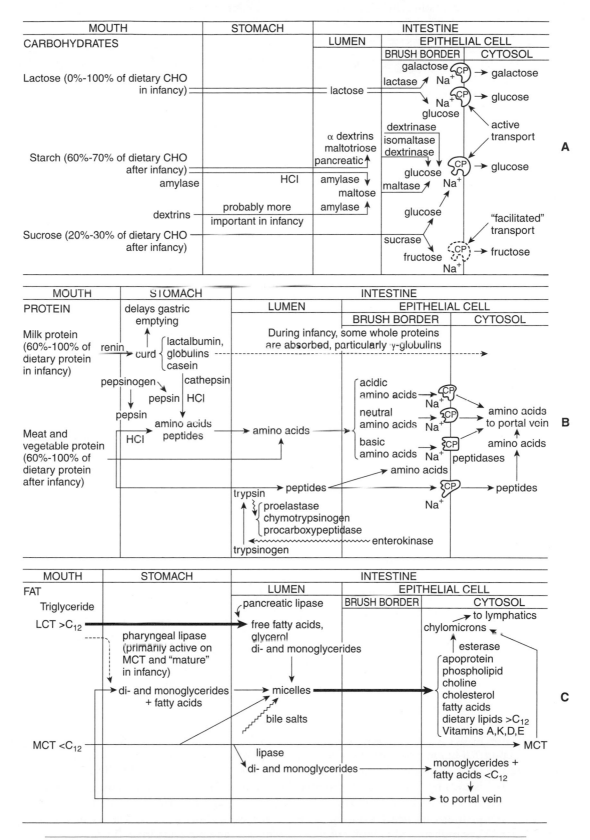

FIGURE **11-1** Summary of digestion and absorption. **A,** Carbohydrate digestion. **B,** Protein digestion.
C, Lipid digestion. (From Johnson, T.R., Moore, W.M. & Jeffries, J.E. [1978]. *Children are different*.
Columbus, OH: Ross Laboratories.)

TABLE **11-1** Gastrointestinal Enzymes

ENZYME	SOURCE	SUBSTRATE	SITE
INVOLVED IN FAT DIGESTION			
Human milk lipase	Human milk	Triglyceride, lipovitamins	Small intestine
Lingual lipase	Oral glands (Ebner)	Triglyceride	Stomach
Gastric lipase	Gastric mucosa	Triglyceride	Stomach
Pancreatic lipase-colipase	Pancreas	Triglyceride	Small intestine
Phospholipase A_2	Pancreas	Phospholipid	Small intestine
Cholesterol esterase, nonspecific lipase	Pancreas	Cholesterol esterase, monoglyceride, lipovitamins	Small intestine
Intestinal lipase	Intestinal mucosa	Triglyceride	Small intestine
Alkaline lipases and phospholipases	Microbes	Triglyceride, other (?)	Colon, feces
INVOLVED IN PROTEIN DIGESTION			
Gelatinase	Gastric mucosa	Gelatin	Stomach
Pepsins	Gastric mucosa	Protein	Stomach
Enterokinase	Duodenal mucosa	Activates trypsinogen to trypsin	Duodenum
Trypsin	Pancreas	Peptides and basic amino acids (lysine, arginine)	Small intestine
Chymotrypsin	Pancreas	Peptides and aromatic amino acids (phenylalanine, leucine, tyrosine, tryptophan, methionine, glutamine)	Small intestine
Elastase	Pancreas	Peptides and aliphatic amino acids (valine, leucine, alanine, serine)	Small intestine
Carboxypeptidase A	Pancreas	Peptides, aliphatic and aromatic amino acids	Small intestine
Carboxypeptidase B	Pancreas	Peptides and basic amino acids	Small intestine
Intestinal peptidases	Small intestine	Dipeptides and tripeptides	Small intestine
Oligopeptidases	Intestinal brush border	Larger peptides	Small intestine
INVOLVED IN CARBOHYDRATE DIGESTION			
Salivary amylase	Salivary glands	Starch	Mouth, stomach
Pancreatic amylase	Pancreas	Starch	Small intestine
Maltases	Small intestine brush border	Maltose, sucrose, dextrins	Small intestine
Lactase	Small intestine brush border	Lactose	Small intestine
Sucrase-isomaltase	Small intestine brush border	Sucrose, dextrins	Small intestine
Glucoamylase	Small intestine brush border	Glucose polymers	Small intestine
Mammary amylase	Human milk	Glucose polymers	Small intestine

Adapted from Watkins J.B. (1985). Lipid digestion and absorption. *Pediatrics, 75*(suppl.), 151, as modified from Patton, J.S. (1983). Gastrointestinal lipid digestion. In Johnson, L.R. (Ed.). *Physiology of the gastrointestinal tract.* New York: Raven; and Sunshine, P. (1977). Digestion and absorption of carbohydrates. In *Selected aspects of perinatal gastroenterology* (Mead Johnson Symposium on Perinatal and Developmental Medicine, no. 11). Evansville, IN: Mead Johnson.

increases blood flow to the oral cavity and accelerates turnover of gum epithelial lining cells. The gums become highly vascularized (with proliferation of small blood vessels and connective tissue), hyperplastic, and edematous.[64,186,294] Development of gingivitis may also be related to alterations in the inflammatory process during pregnancy (see Chapter 12), with increased intensity of localized irritation. These changes, along with the decreased thickness of the gingival epithelial surface, result in friable gum tissues that may bleed easily or cause discomfort with chewing. Bleeding with brushing occurs more frequently during pregnancy. The incidence of gingivitis is higher with increasing maternal age and parity, preexisting periodontal disease, and poor dentition.[186,225]

TABLE **11-2**   **Alterations in the Gastrointestinal System during Pregnancy**

ORGAN	ALTERATION	SIGNIFICANCE
Mouth and pharynx	Gingivitis	Friable gum tissue with bleeding and discomfort with chewing
		Increased periodontal disease
	Epulis formation	Bleeding and interference with chewing
	Increased saliva production	Annoyance
Esophagus	Decreased lower esophageal sphincter pressure and tone	Increased risk of heartburn
	Widening of hiatus with decreased tone	Increased risk of hiatal hernia
Stomach	Decreased tone and mobility with delayed gastric emptying time	Increased risk of gastroesophageal reflux and vomiting
		Increased risk of vomiting and aspiration with use of sedatives or anesthetics
	Incompetence of pyloric sphincter	Reflux of alkaline biliary material into stomach
	Decreased gastric acidity and histamine output	Improvement of peptic ulcer symptoms
Small and large intestines	Decreased intestinal tone and motility with prolonged transit time	Facilitated absorption of nutrients such as iron and calcium
		Increased water absorption in large intestine with tendency toward constipation
		Increased flatulence
	Increased height of duodenal villi	Increased absorption of calcium, amino acids, other substances
	Altered enzymatic transport across villi	Increased absorption of specific vitamins and other nutrients
	Displacement of cecum and appendix by uterus	Complicate diagnosis of appendicitis
Gallbladder	Decreased tone and motility	Alteration in measures of gallbladder function
		Increased risk of gallstones
Liver	Altered position	Mask mild to moderate hepatomegaly
	Altered production of liver enzymes, plasma proteins, bilirubin, and serum lipids	Some liver function tests less useful in evaluating liver disorders
		Early signs of liver dysfunction may be missed
	Presence of spider angiomata and palmar erythema	Altered early recognition of liver dysfunction
		Discomfort because of itching

In 3% to 5% of pregnant women, a specific angiogranuloma known as an *epulis* or pregnancy tumor develops.[233,273] Epulis formation generally occurs between the third and ninth month and may gradually increase in size. With epulis formation, the gingivitis is advanced and severe, with a hyperplastic outgrowth that is generally found along the maxillary gingiva on the palatal side. This mass is very friable, bleeding easily and often interfering with chewing. Epulis usually regresses spontaneously after delivery. Occasionally these growths may need excising during pregnancy due to bleeding, interference with chewing, or increasing periodontal disease.[186,233]

Saliva becomes more acidic during pregnancy with alterations in electrolyte content but generally does not increase in volume. Some women may experience a sense of increased saliva production due to difficulty in swallowing saliva during the period of nausea and vomiting in early pregnancy.[186] A few women do experience excessive salivation (ptyalism). This uncommon disorder begins as early as 2 to 3 weeks and ceases with delivery. The excessive salivation seems to occur primarily during the day.[64] The pathogenesis of ptyalism is unknown, but it is thought to be due to increased saliva, the inability to swallow due to nausea, or activation of the esophagosalivary reflex during gastroesophageal reflux (GER).[173,233]

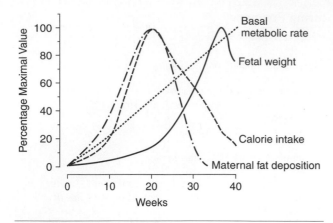

FIGURE **11-2** Changes in maternal caloric intake, maternal fat deposition, fetal weight, and basal metabolic rate during pregnancy. (Values are expressed as a percentage of marginal change). (From Rosso, P. [1987]. Regulation of food intake during pregnancy and lactation. *Ann NY Acad Sci, 499,* 191.)

Esophagus

Lower esophageal sphincter (LES) tone decreases primarily because of the smooth muscle relaxant activity of progesterone. The LES is a pressure barrier between the stomach and the esophagus, acting as a protective mechanism to prevent or minimize GER. LES pressure decreases during pregnancy, with the magnitude of pressure change positively correlated with gestational length.[64,154] At the beginning of the second trimester, basal LES tone is unchanged, although a marked decrease in the normal rise in LES pressure in response to stimulation with a protein meal has been reported.[25,64,85] This suggests an inhibitory effect and may signal the loss of an important protective response—that is, the ability to modify LES pressure in response to increased intragastric pressure so that reflux is prevented.[64]

Changes in the LES in pregnancy are similar to changes seen during the ovarian or menstrual cycle and in women on oral contraceptives, supporting the theory of a hormonal cause for this alteration. An increased incidence of acid reflux with heartburn, which is associated with decreased LES pressure, is seen in nonpregnant women during the luteal phase of the ovarian cycle, when progesterone levels are highest.[75,273] Women on sequential oral contraceptives (as opposed to agents that contain only an estrogen component) demonstrate similar decreases in LES pressure during the progesterone phase of the cycle. After delivery or discontinuance of oral contraceptives, LES function returns to normal.[25,64,77,85,115,273] Alterations in LES tone and pressure are major etiologic factors in the development of heartburn during pregnancy.

Other changes in the esophagus during pregnancy include an increase in secondary peristalsis and nonpropulsive peristalsis and increased incidence of hiatal hernia. Flattening of the hemidiaphragm causes a loss of the normal acute esophageal-gastric angle, which may also lead to reflux.[64]

Stomach

The stomach of the pregnant woman tends to be hypotonic with decreased motility due to actions of progesterone. GI motility is decreased, with prolonged small intestinal transit time. Incompetence of the pyloric sphincter may result in alkaline reflux of duodenal contents into the stomach.[64]

The effects of pregnancy on gastric emptying time (particularly during early pregnancy) are unclear, with contradictory findings due in part to use of different measurement techniques and study methodologies.[77,154,202,215,233,250,296] As gestation advances, decreased smooth muscle tone and motility secondary to progesterone production tend to delay emptying time, with a tendency toward reverse peristalsis. Gastric emptying time is especially prolonged following ingestion of solid foods. In this situation, reduction in acid production and pepsin secretion due to progesterone action may slow digestion even further.[77]

The effect of pregnancy on gastric acid secretion is also unclear. In several studies, gastric volume was not increased nor was gastric pH decreased during early pregnancy.[154,202,296] Others have reported a decrease in acidity during the first and second trimesters along with normal gastrin levels, with an increase in acidity to greater than nonpregnant values during the third trimester, accompanied by an increase in gastrin.[233] In general there seems to be a tendency for decreased gastric acidity in pregnancy, especially during the first and second trimesters, with an increase in the third along with a small but statistically significant decreases in both basal and histamine-stimulated acid output.[64] Thus production of hydrochloric acid is reduced during the first 6 months of pregnancy, with a gradual return to nonpregnant levels or above during the third trimester.[64]

Secretion of pepsin parallels changes in gastric acid output.[64] Decreased gastric acidity is thought to result from hormonal influences (particularly estrogen) and increased levels of placental histaminase.[64,225] Placental histaminase is thought to mediate acid and pepsin secretion by reducing parietal cell responsiveness to endogenous histamine.[64] Gastrin levels are normal during most of pregnancy, with marked increases late in the third trimester, at delivery, and immediately after delivery. The additional gastrin is probably of placental origin.[59]

Small and Large Intestines

The action of progesterone on smooth muscles also decreases intestinal tone and motility. The decreased motility observed in pregnancy may not necessarily be a direct effect of progesterone but rather due to inhibition by plasma motilin.[250] Decreased GI tone leads to prolonged intestinal transit time, especially during the second and third trimesters.[154] Alterations in transit time increase with advancing gestation, paralleling the increase in progesterone.

Intestinal transit times during stages of pregnancy have been compared with phases of the ovarian cycle in nonpregnant women.[154] Intestinal motility is altered and transit time prolonged during late pregnancy and the luteal phase of the ovarian cycle when progesterone secretion is elevated. The prolonged transit time in late pregnancy was due to an increase in small bowel transit secondary to inhibition of smooth muscle contraction and not to delayed gastric emptying time.[154,236] The woman may experience a sense of "bloating" and abdominal distension secondary to the delayed intestinal transit toimes.[233]

The height of the duodenal villi increases (hypertrophies), which in turn increases absorptive capacity.[239] This change—along with the influences of progesterone on intestinal transit time—increases the absorptive capacity for substances such as calcium, lysine, valine, glycine, proline, glucose, sodium, chloride, and water during pregnancy.[273] Progesterone also increases lactase and maltase activity. Absorption of other nutrients (including niacin, riboflavin, and vitamin B_6) is reduced, perhaps due to the influence of progesterone on enzymatic transport mechanisms.[233,239,273] Duodenal absorption of iron increases nearly twofold by late pregnancy, probably in response to depletion of maternal circulating iron stores by the placenta and fetus.[233] As a result of the decreased intestinal motility, nutrients and fluids tend to remain in the intestinal lumen for longer periods of time. This may facilitate absorption of nutrients such as iron and calcium.[70] The amount and efficiency of intestinal calcium absorption increases, mediated primarily by increased 1,25-dihydroxyvitamin D (see Chapter 16).

Progesterone also enhances colonic absorption of calcium, sodium, and water and increases net secretion of potassium.[233,273] The reduced motility and prolonged transit time in the large intestine increase water absorption in the colon. Stools are smaller with lower water content, which contributes to development of constipation during pregnancy. Increased flatulence may also occur due to decreased motility along with compression of the bowel by the growing uterus. The appendix and cecum are displaced superiorly by the growing uterus, so that by term the ap-

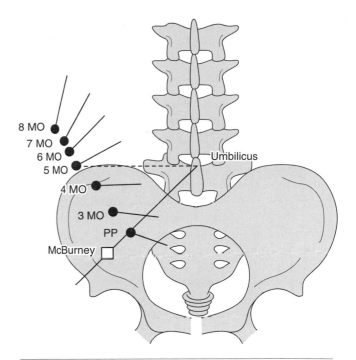

FIGURE **11-3**   Rise of the appendix during pregnancy. Changes in position and direction of the appendix during pregnancy: After the fifth month, the appendix lies at the crest level and rises above this levels during the third trimester. The postpartum position *(PP)* of the appendix corresponds to its position in the nonpregnant state. On x-ray, the base of the appendix is usually found medial to McBurney's point. The average position of the umbilicus corresponds to the point at which a line extended horizontally form the iliac crest crosses the spine. (From Baer, J.L., et al. [1932]. Appendicitis in pregnancy with changes in position and axis of the normal appendix during pregnancy. *JAMA, 98,* 1359.)

pendix tends to be located along the right costal margin (Figure 11-3).

Pancreas

The pancreas contains estrogen receptors, which in the rich estrogen environment of pregnancy may increase the risk of pancreatitis.[22,273] Serum amylase and lipase decrease during the first trimester. The significance of this change is unclear. Changes in the islet cells associated with increased production and secretion of insulin are discussed in Chapter 15.

Gallbladder

Muscle tone and motility of the gallbladder decrease during pregnancy, probably due to the effects of progesterone on smooth musculature. As a result, gallbladder volume is increased and emptying rate decreased, especially in the second and third timesters.[76,154,233] Most measures of gallbladder function are altered during pregnancy, especially after 14 weeks. Recent studies have demonstrated that fasting and residual volumes increase to about 20 weeks' gestation, then remain high to term, paralleling the increase in progesterone.[77] The residual gallbladder volume after fasting and emptying is nearly twice as large in the pregnant woman as in nonpregnant women who are not taking oral contraceptives.[264] The increased fasting volume may also be due to decreased water absorption by the mucosa of the gallbladder. This change results from reduced activity of the sodium pump in the mucosal epithelium secondary to estrogens.[24] As a result, bile is more dilute, with a decreased ability to solubilize cholesterol. The sequestered cholesterol may precipitate to form crystals and stones, increasing the tendency to form cholesterol-based gallstones in the second and third trimesters.[24,77] In the third trimester, bile is supersaturated with lithogenic cholesterol, which, in conjunction with biliary stasis and sludging, increases the risk of gall stones.[75,77] Alterations in gallbladder tone also lead to a tendency to retain bile salts, which can lead to pruritus.

Liver

During pregnancy the enlarging uterus displaces the liver superiorly, posteriorly, and anteriorly. The liver edge may be palpable by late in the third trimester.[233] Hepatic blood flow per se is not significantly altered in spite of marked changes in total blood volume and cardiac output. This is because much of the increased cardiac output is sent to the uteroplacental circulation. As a result the proportion of cardiac output delivered to the liver is decreased by one third.[143,215,233] Histologically only minor nonspecific changes such as increased fat and glycogen storage and variations in cell size have been reported. The size of the liver does not increase.

Liver production of plasma proteins, bilirubin, serum enzymes, and serum lipids is altered. These changes arise primarily from estrogen and in some cases from hemodilution. Changes in liver products during pregnancy and their significance are summarized in Table 11-3. Although liver function is not impaired during pregnancy, most of the changes in liver function tests are in the same direction as seen in individuals with liver disorders. Some liver function tests are less useful in evaluating liver disorders during pregnancy; other tests such as aspartate aminotransferase (AST, or serum glutamic-oxaloacetic transaminase [SGOT]), alanine aminotransferase (ALT, or serum glutamic-pyruvic transaminase [SGPT]), and bilirubin are still reliable. Changes in hepatic metabolism of drugs during pregnancy are discussed in Chapter 6.

Spider angiomata (also called *spider nevi*) and palmar erythema (common findings in many liver disorders) thought to be caused by estrogens are seen in many pregnant women (see Chapter 13). These findings tend to develop between the second and fifth months and disappear or diminish following delivery. Increases in the size of previously existing spider angiomata may also be noted.

Weight Gain during Pregnancy

Weight gain during pregnancy reflects increased maternal stores as well as those of the developing fetus and placenta. Approximately 62% of the gain is water, 30% fat, and 8% protein. About 25% of the total gain is attributable to the fetus, 11% to the placenta and amniotic fluid, and the remainder to the mother.[117] Optimal weight gain during pregnancy varies with maternal prepregnancy weight; greater weight gain is most important in women who are underweight, and a lower total weight gain is preferable for women who are obese. Results from the Collaborative Perinatal Project suggest that weight gains associated with lowest perinatal mortality rates were 30 lb in underweight women, 20 lb in normal weight women, and 16 lb in overweight women (Figure 11-4).[105]

The usual recommendation for weight gain in pregnancy in healthy women has been a gain of 24 to 28 lb (11 to 13 kg). The Institute of Medicine's (IOM) guidelines for weight gain and the pattern of gain based on prepregnancy weight for height are in Table 11-4.[118] According to these guidelines the recommended gain for normal weight women is 25 to 35 lb (11.5 to 16 kg), with less for overweight women and more for underweight women, especially during the second and third trimesters. The recommended pattern for normal weight women is approximately 8 lb during the first trimester, followed by about 1 lb (0.4 kg) per week for the remainder of gestation, with higher gains (0.5 kg/wk) in underweight and less (0.3 kg) in overweight women.[105,118]

This pattern results in the addition of approximately 8 lb of fat stores, acquired primarily during the first half of pregnancy. Weight gained during the second half of pregnancy goes toward growth of the fetus and maternal supportive tissues. Marked or persistent deviations from these patterns—including gains of less than 1 lb (0.5 kg) per month in an obese woman or less than 2 lb (1 kg) per month in a woman of normal weight—necessitate evaluation and counseling.[118] Women whose weight gain significantly exceeds these limits or deviates from the expected pattern also require similar interventions. For example, if a woman gains 30 lb in the first 20 weeks of pregnancy, she

TABLE 11-3   Liver Function Tests in Normal Pregnancy and Postpartum

Substance	Pregnancy Effect	Trimester of Maximum Change	Return to Nonpregnant Level	Basis and Implication
Albumin	↓ 20%	2	?	Result of hemodilution and increased catabolism; leads to decreased protein for binding and increased concentrations of free substances
γ-Globulin	N to sl ↓	3	?	Transfer of immunoglobulin G (IgG) to fetus in third trimester for protection of fetus from infection
α-Globulin	↑	3	?	Facilitation of transport of lipids and carbohydrates to the placenta, as well as transport of increased maternal thyroid hormones
β-Globulin	↑	3	?	Facilitatation of transport of lipids, carbohydrates, and iron to placenta, as well as transport of hormones
Total protein	↓ 20%	2	?	Primarily related to a fall in albumin; decreases protein-bound substances and increases concentrations of free protein for transport across the placenta
Fibrinogen	↑ 50%	2	2 weeks	Protection against excessive blood loss at delivery by facilitation clotting
Ceruloplasmin	↑	3	?	Involved in the transport of most of the body copper needed by mother, fetus, and placenta
Transferrin	↑	3	?	Involved in the binding and transport of iron to meet increased maternal and fetal needs
Bilirubin	N to sl ↑	3	?	May be a slight increase in bilirubin clearance due to maternal clearance of bilirubin from fetus
BSP	N to sl ↑	3	Soon after delivery	Increased removal associated with decreased albumin; alterations may reflect the mild cholestasis seen in pregnancy
AST (SGOT) and ALT (SGPT) in pregnancy	N	—	—	Do not change during pregnancy, so these enzymes can be used as indicators of liver or other organ damage during pregnancy; increase during labor and delivery, perhaps reflecting the effects of the mechanical forces of labor
AST (SGOT) and ALT (SGPT) in labor	↑	In labor	By 2-3 weeks	
GGTP	↑	3	?	Important in synthesis of amino acids for maternal and fetal use
Alkaline phosphatase	2-4 fold ↑	3	Usually by 3 weeks	Much of increase is probably a result of increased production by the placenta rather than the maternal liver
Lactic dehydrogenase in pregnancy	sl ↑	3	?	Enzyme associated with tissue injury that catalyzes lactic acid to pyruvic acid; increases further during labor, perhaps reflecting the effects of the mechanical forces of labor
Lactic dehydrogenase in labor	↑	In labor	By 2-3 weeks	
Cholesterol	1½-2 fold ↑	2-3	Significant decrease within 24 hours	Essential precursor for many lipid substances; needed for alterations in lipid metabolism and increased demands for lipids during pregnancy including production of estrogens and progesterone by the placenta

Modified from Monheit, A.G., Cousins, L., & Resnik, R. (1980). The puerperium: Anatomic and physiologic adjustments. *Clin Obstet Gynecol, 23, 973.*
ALT (SGPT), Serum alanine aminotransferase; *AST (SGOT)*, serum aspartate aminotransferase; *BSP*, sulfobromophthalein; *GGTP*, serum γ-glutamyl transpeptidase; *N*, normal; *sl*, slight.

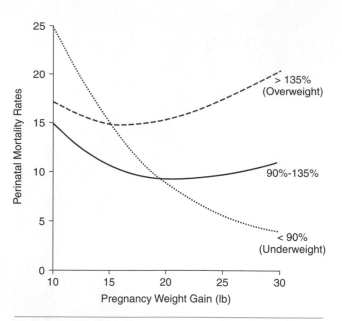

FIGURE **11-4** The relationship between weight gain in pregnancy and perinatal mortality. (From Naeye, R.L. [1979]. Weight gain and the outcome in pregnancy. *Am J Obstet Gynecol, 135,* 3.)

TABLE **11-4**   Recommended Total Weight Gain Ranges for Pregnant Women by Prepregnant Body Mass Index

WEIGHT-FOR-HEIGHT CATEGORY	RECOMMENDED TOTAL WEIGHT GAIN*	
	kg	lb
Low (BMI† <19.8)	12.5-18	28-40
Normal (BMI = 19.8—26.0)	11.5-16	25-35
High (BMI 26.0—29.0)	7.0-11.5	15-25
Obese (BMI [>] 29)	At least 6	At least 15

From Institute of Medicine. (1990). *Nutrition during pregnancy.* Washington, DC: National Academy Press.
*Young adolescents and African-American women should strive for gains at the upper end of the recommended range. Short women (<157 cm or 62 in) should strive for gains at the lower end of the range.
†BMI is calculated using metric units (BMI = kg/m² × 100).

has added approximately 25 lb of fat to her stores (and additional fat is often difficult to lose postpartum). This woman will still need to gain approximately 20 lb during the second half of pregnancy to ensure adequate growth of the fetus and her own tissues.[225]

Greater gains are needed in women with multifetal pregnancies. Recommended weight gain is 35 to 45 lb (16 to 20.5 kg) for twins and 50 pounds for triplets with a gain of approximately 1.5 lb per week in the second and

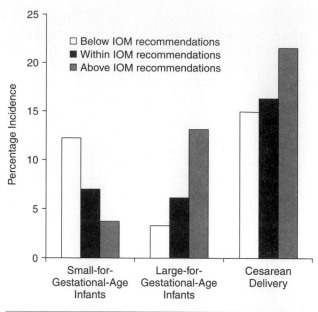

FIGURE **11-5** Incidence of small-for-gestational age, large-for gestational-age, and cesarean delivery for women from San Francisco with pregnancy weight gains within, below, and above the Institute of Medicine recommendations (see Table 11-4). (Adapted from Parker, J. & Abrams, B. [1992]. Prenatal weight gain advice: an examination of the recent prenatal weight gain recommendations of the Institute of Medicine. *Obstet Gynecol, 79,* 664.)

third trimesters.[45,118] These women also have increased nutritional needs, including higher energy, vitamin D, linolenic and linoleic acid, calcium, and other minerals.[45]

The IOM guidelines have generated controversy and concern that using them would increase the numbers of large-for-gestational-age (LGA) infants and maternal and fetal complications.[83,126] Abrams et al reviewed pregnancy outcomes from studies using the IOM guidelines and found that weight gain within these recommendations was associated with the best maternal and fetal outcome (Figure 11-5).[3] However, they also noted that in most women, weight gain was not within the IOM guidelines.[3] Maternal weight gain per se lacks sensitivity and specificity as a predictor of pregnancy outcome, since many women with good pregnancy outcomes have weight gains outside the recommended range.[52,65,126,255] However, higher or lower than usual weight gains do increase the risk of maternal and fetal complications (see Figure 11-5).[2,3]

Intrapartum Period

Gastric motility is further decreased during labor. This decrease is probably influenced by anxiety and pain as well as effects of opioid administration.[59] The reduced competency of the LES—along with decreased gastric motility and increased gastric acidity—delay gastric emptying time and increase the risk of aspiration with sedatives or anesthesia.

Labor is accompanied by delays in gastric emptying times that differ (although perhaps not to the extent that was reported in earlier studies) from both third-trimester and nonpregnant values.[72,202] The combination of gastric volumes greater than 25 ml and pH less than 2.5 is thought to increase the risk of chemical aspiration pneumonitis.[40] Opioids also delay gastric emptying and increase the risk of aspiration if used in conjunction with general anesthesia. Opioids may be the main factor in delayed gastric emptying during labor. Reduced use of general anesthesia for delivery has reduced the numbers of women at risk for intrapartum aspiration. However, any use of general anesthesia with a pregnant woman, whether for delivery or nonobstetric surgery, requires careful monitoring and use of interventions to prevent vomiting and aspiration. Pharmacologic interventions include prophylactic use of antacids or H_2-receptor agonists.[40]

During labor, alkaline phosphatase levels, which double during pregnancy, increase further. Serum aminotransferases (AST and ALT), which do not change in pregnancy, and lactic dehydrogenase increase up to twice normal values.[292] These enzymes are associated with tissue injury and may reflect the stresses of labor on the mother and placenta.

Postpartum Period

During the postpartum period the anatomic and physiologic changes within the GI and hepatic systems gradually return to their prepregnant state. Delivery results in an average weight loss of 4.5 to 5.8 kg (10 to 13 lb).[62] Findings regarding postpartum weight loss are inconsistent.[62,146,198,208] Some women have further weight loss during the first week; others have no change or gain weight. The increased adrenocortical hormone and arginine vasopressin activity associated with the stress of labor tends to lead to water and sodium retention that may prevent weight loss or lead to a gain. In general, after 4 days, most women begin to show some additional loss, averaging another 2.3 to 3.6 kg (5 to 8 lb) due to diuresis and 0.9 to 1.4 kg (2 to 3 lb) from involution and lochia by the end of the first week.[62] Drugs used to suppress lactation plus alterations in energy utilization may alter losses in nonlactating women.[37]

Most women lose weight steadily over the first 3 to 6 months, with the greatest loss in the first 3 months. Weight loss occurs sooner and to a greater degree in women of lower parity, age, and prepregnant weight.[37,62,208] Lactation may facilitate postpartum weight and body fat loss as maternal tissue stores are catabolized to use as energy for milk production.[37] Most women do not lose all of the pregnancy weight gain, with an average retention of 1 kg (2.2 lb) with each pregnancy; 10% retain more than 15 lb.[62] Women who are overweight or normal weight before pregnancy are more likely to retain weight following pregnancy than women who were underweight.[62] Abrams et al. found no evidence that weight gain during pregnancy within the IOM recommendations increased the risk of weight retention following birth.[3]

Gingivitis often disappears after delivery but may last for up to 6 months postpartum.[233] Epulis regresses and also usually disappears postpartum, but a scarred area may remain.[233] LES pressure and tone return to normal levels by 6 to 8 weeks postpartum.[233] Gallbladder volume returns to normal by 2 weeks postpartum.[77] Gallbladder contractility is enhanced postpartum, enabling the previously atonic gallbladder to empty a larger proportion of its volume and expel microgallstones that developed during pregnancy.[273] Expulsion of these stones can lead to a gallstone pancreatitis.

Most of the liver enzymes return to nonpregnant levels within 3 weeks of delivery.[214] Fatty acids, cholesterol, triglycerides, and lipoproteins tend to reach normal levels by about 10 days.[214] AST, ALT, and lactic dehydrogenase, which rose during the intrapartum period, reach nonpregnant levels by 2 to 3 weeks. Alkaline phosphatase decreases after delivery and usually returns to nonpregnant levels by 20 days, but may remain elevated for up to 6 weeks.[214,292]

The appendix returns to its usual position by 10 days postpartum.[250] GI muscle tone and motility are decreased during the intrapartum and early postpartum periods. Decreased gastric motility along with relaxation of the abdominal musculature can result in gaseous distention 2 to 3 days postpartum. Decreased intestinal motility can lead to postpartum ileus and constipation. Bowel movements usually resume 2 to 3 days after birth, with resumption of normal bowel patterns by 8 to 14 days.

CLINICAL IMPLICATIONS FOR THE PREGNANT WOMAN AND HER FETUS

The normal alterations in GI function and structure in the pregnant woman are responsible for some of the more common discomforts of pregnancy, including heartburn and constipation. Alterations in the anatomic position of structures such as the appendix and liver and in concentrations of liver enzymes and other substances, as well as concerns about potential hazards with the use of radiographic contrast studies on the fetus, can lead to difficulty in assessing and diagnosing pathologic processes that arise. This section examines the basis for development of these problems and reviews the effect of pregnancy on selected chronic disorders such as peptic ulcer disease (PUD) and cholelithiasis.

Nutritional Requirements of Pregnancy

The physical and physiologic demands of pregnancy on the mother, along with fetal needs for nutrients, significantly increase nutritional requirements during pregnancy (Table 11-5). Nutrient needs are also altered postpartum and during lactation (see Chapter 5). During pregnancy an additional 300 calories per day are needed in the second and third trimesters to meet energy and growth demands of the mother and fetus and to conserve protein for cell growth. Energy needs vary considerably from woman to woman with adaptations in individual metabolism to spare energy for fetal growth (see Chapter 15 and Figure 15-3).[52,139,255] Protein re-

quirements increase 15 to 60 g to provide nitrogen for maternal, fetal, and placental tissue synthesis and growth.[87] Sources of protein should contain all the essential amino acids.

Maternal plasma levels of most vitamins and minerals gradually decline during gestation. This decline is probably due primarily to the effects of hemodilution rather than to greater fetal and maternal demands.[222] With the exception of vitamin D (see Chapter 16) and iron (see Chapter 7), little is known about the effects of pregnancy on metabolism of most vitamins and minerals. Recommended dietary allowances (RDAs) for childbearing-age, pregnant, and lactating women are available from the Food and Nutrition Board of the National Academy of Science.[87]

During pregnancy, daily dietary allowances for many vitamins are increased by 20% to 100%, including vita-

TABLE **11-5**   Basis for Increased Nutrient Needs in Pregnancy

NUTRIENT	REASON FOR INCREASED NEED IN PREGNANCY
Protein	Rapid fetal tissue growth
	Placental growth and development
	Maternal tissue growth (e.g., uterus, breasts)
	Increased blood volume (increased hemoglobin, plasma proteins)
	Maternal storage reserves (for labor, delivery, and lactation)
Calories	Increased basal metabolic rate (BMR), energy needs, and protein sparing
Calcium	Fetal skeleton and tooth bud formation
	Increased maternal calcium metabolism
Phosphorus	Fetal skeleton and tooth bud formation
	Increased maternal phosphorus metabolism
Iron	Increased maternal circulating blood volume and increased hemoglobin
	Fetal liver iron storage; iron cost of pregnancy
Iodine	Increased BMR and thyroxine production
Magnesium	Coenzyme in energy and protein metabolism; enzyme activator
	Tissue growth; cell metabolism; muscle action
Vitamin A	Essential for cell development and thus for tissue growth
	Fetal tooth bud formation (development of enamel forming cells in gum tissue)
	Bone growth
Vitamin D	Absorption of calcium and phosphorus
	Mineralization of fetal bone tissue and tooth buds
Vitamin E	Tissue growth
	Cell wall integrity and red blood cell integrity
Vitamin C	Tissue formation and integrity
	Increased iron absorption
	Integrity of connective and vascular tissues
Folic acid	Increased metabolic demands of pregnancy and increased heme production
	Production of cell nucleus materials
Niacin	Coenzyme in energy and protein metabolism
Riboflavin	Coenzyme in energy and protein metabolism
Thiamin	Coenzyme for energy metabolism
Vitamin B_6	Coenzyme in protein metabolism
	Increased fetal growth requirement
Vitamin B_{12}	Coenzyme in protein metabolism, especially proteins in nucleic acid
	Formation of red blood cells

Adapted from Worthington-Roberts, B.S. & Williams, S.R. (1996). *Nutrition in pregnancy and lactation.* New York: McGraw-Hill.

min E (10 mg), vitamin C (70 mg), thiamin (1.5 mg), riboflavin (1.6 mg), niacin (17 mg), vitamin B_6 (2.2 mg), and vitamin B_{12} (2.2 μg).[2,87,118,168] Vitamin E is essential during pregnancy for tissue growth and integrity of cell and red blood cell membranes. Vitamin C increases iron absorption and is needed for collagen formation and tissue formation and integrity. Thiamin, niacin, riboflavin, and vitamins B_6 and B_{12} serve as coenzymes for protein and energy metabolism, which are increased in the pregnant woman.[288] Zinc supplementation has been reported to increase birth weight in undernourished women with low serum zinc levels and decrease the risk of intrauterine growth restriction (IUGR).[101,140] Requirements for minerals and other vitamins are discussed in Chapters 7 (iron and folate), 16 (calcium, phosphorus, magnesium, and vitamin D), and 18 (iodine). Excessive intake or marked deficiency of specific vitamins and minerals has been reported to be associated with adverse pregnancy outcome, although the number of observations is limited. For example, excess (>15,000 IU/day) vitamin A (retinol) is associated with an increase in birth defects.[123,189] The reader is referred to texts on nutrition during pregnancy for further discussion of nutritional assessment and requirements.[118,222,288]

The practice of routine multivitamin supplementation is controversial.[130,141] The Institute of Medicine recommends that pregnant women with balanced diets do not need routine multivitamin/mineral supplementation, except for iron (see Chapter 7).[118] Folic acid supplementation is recommended for all women of childbearing age to reduce the incidence of neural tube defects (see Chapter 14). Folic acid in late pregnancy may also reduce the risk of preterm delivery and low birth weight.[208] Additional multivitamin/mineral supplementation or supplementation of specific nutrients may be needed by women whose diet is inadequate (and this may apply to women above the poverty level) or who have a multiple pregnancy, smoke, or are alcohol or drug abusers.[130] Scholl et al. reported that supplementation of low-risk pregnant adolescents reduced the risk of preterm labor and low birth weight.[235] Other studies suggest that maternal vitamin supplementation may reduce the incidence of some birth defects.[2,48,243]

Fetal Nutritional Needs

The fetus is dependent on the mother and placenta for transfer of nutrients essential for normal fetal growth and development. (Fetal growth and alterations are discussed in Development of the Gastrointestinal and Hepatic Systems in the Fetus.) Nutritional needs of the fetus are met by three mechanisms depending on the stage of development. Prior to implantation, the blastocyst absorbs nutrients from its surrounding tissues and from fluids within the fallopian tube and uterus. Between implantation and placental development, nutrients are absorbed via a sinusoidal space between maternal and fetal tissues. With formation of the placenta, nutrients are transferred across this structure from mother to fetus via a variety of mechanisms (see Chapter 3). The energy needs of the fetus near term are met through carbohydrates (80%) and amino acids (20%).[222] Fat is not used as an energy source by the fetus due to immaturity of fat metabolism. The major fetal energy source is glucose from the mother; free fatty acids are an alternative source as well as substrate for lipid formation (see Chapter 15).

Amino acids are actively transported from mother to fetus, and imbalances in maternal plasma amino acid concentrations can result in excessive fetal concentrations and subsequent damage. For example, women with phenylketonuria (PKU) have, in the past, often discontinued their low phenylalanine diet by adolescence. As a result, these women have elevated levels of phenylalanine in their blood. If they become pregnant, phenylalanine crosses the placenta and can damage the fetus. Infants born to mothers with elevated phenylalanine levels (regardless of whether the infant has PKU or not) are at high risk for IUGR, mental retardation, microcephaly, and congenital heart disease.[58,168,240] The risk increases with increasing maternal phenylalanine levels, which should be maintained at 2 to 8 mg/dl.[168] Elevated levels in the first 9 weeks are associated with increased birth defects; increased levels later are associated with altered brain and fetal growth.[224] Since fetal damage often occurs before the woman is aware that she is pregnant, women with PKU are advised to return to a low phenylalanine diet prior to conception and remain on the diet during pregnancy (to keep maternal blood levels of phenylalanine below 600 μmol/L).[116] Current recommendations are for individuals with PKU to remain on a low phenylalanine diet for life to enhance neurological functioning.

Fetal needs for most vitamins and minerals can be met if maternal intakes follow recommended dietary allowances.[87,118] Lipid-soluble vitamins (A, D, E, and K) cross the placenta more readily than water-soluble vitamins and with increasing ease with advancing gestation.[129] The vitamins most often associated with deficiencies during pregnancy are folate and B_6 (see Chapter 7).

Calcium and phosphorus are actively transported across the placenta, which allows accumulation of calcium and calcification of the fetal skeleton (see Chapter 16). The fetus needs trace elements such as zinc, copper, chromium, iodine, magnesium, and manganese. Maternal dietary intake of these elements is usually sufficient. Iron supplementation is recommended to enhance maternal iron stores (see Chapter 7).

Heartburn and Gastroesophageal Reflux

Heartburn (reflux esophagitis with retrosternal burning) arises from reflux of gastric acids into the lower esophagus. Heartburn has been reported in 30% to 70% of women at some time during pregnancy and in 50% to 90% in the third trimester.[21,173,233,239] Heartburn usually begins during the second trimester, although about 25% experience heartburn in the first trimester,[25] Heartburn intensifies with advancing gestation and disappears following delivery. Interventions are summarized in Table 11-6.

TABLE **11-6**   Recommendations for Common Problems during Pregnancy Related to the Gastrointestinal System

Problem	Nursing Recommendations
Heartburn	Eat small, frequent meals.
	Eat bland foods.
	Avoid fatty or spicy foods and citric juices.
	Avoid late night or large meals.
	Avoid foods that reduce lower esophageal sphincter pressure (e.g., alcohol, chocolate, caffeine).
	Avoid lying down for 1 hour following meals.
	Chew gum.
	Sleep with torso elevated.
	Avoid lying flat or bending.
	Use antacids (aluminum and magnesium hydroxide combination is best because aluminum tends to cause diarrhea and magnesium constipation) after meals and at bedtime.
	Avoid the use of antacids containing phosphorus (alter calcium-phosphorus balance, leading to leg cramps) or sodium (increase water retention).
	Monitor for side effects of chronic antacid use (alteration in muscle tone and deep tendon reflexes, electrolyte imbalance).
	Recognize potential effects of chronic antacid use on malabsorption of K, P, Ca, and drugs such as anticoagulants, salicylates, vitamin E.[79]
Constipation	Drink fluids.
	Drink hot or cold liquids (especially on an empty stomach).
	Eat high-fiber/bulk laxative foods such as fruits and raw vegetables.
	Eat high fiber bran and wheat foods.
	Encourage regular light exercise during pregnancy.
	Early ambulation postpartum.
	Use stool softeners.
	Use bulk-forming fiber containing agents (which are not absorbed and are therefore the safest).
	Avoid use of mineral oil in pregnancy (absorbs fat-soluble vitamins including vitamin K).
	Monitor for side effects if laxatives are prescribed (fluid accumulation, sodium retention and edema, cramping).
	Monitor for drug interactions if laxatives are prescribed (decreased serum K with diuretics, decreased effectiveness of anticoagulants and salicylates).[79]
Hemorrhoids	Use sitz bath.
	Eat bulk foods.
	Use astringents such as witch hazel (Tucks), lemon juice, or vinegar.
	Prevent constipation and straining (see above).
Nausea and vomiting	Small, frequent high-carbohydrate, low fat meals and snacks (others suggest high-protein meals).
	Avoid strong odors, fatty or spicy foods, and cold liquids.
	Consume dry crackers or toast before arising.
	Consume ginger (e.g., soda, tea, cookies, supplement).
	Suck on hard candy.
	Try elastic wrist bands (SeaBands)
	Lie down when first experiencing symptoms.
	Teach relaxation techniques.
	Avoid factors and situations that precipitate symptoms.
	Monitor for side effects of pharmacologic agents (see text).

The pathogenesis of heartburn during pregnancy is multifactorial. The major etiologic factor is relaxation of the LES along with alterations in pressure gradients across the sphincter. In nonpregnant women, LES tone increases in response to elevations in intragastric pressure as a protective mechanism to prevent or minimize reflux. Alterations in LES tone during pregnancy eliminate or significantly reduce this protective mechanism.[25,59] Pregnant women without heartburn tend to have LES pressures sufficient to maintain the normal pressure gradient across the gastroesophageal junction, whereas women with heartburn do not demonstrate this compensatory mechanism.[225,250] Pregnant women (regardless of whether or not they experience heartburn) have increased nonpropulsive esophageal motor activity with decreased wave amplitude and slower spread of peristaltic waves, with a 50% reduction in secondary peristalsis.[225,269] These findings are suggestive of reflux and are more prominent in women who experience symptoms of heartburn during pregnancy.[269]

Pressure from the growing uterus increases intragastric pressure and along with flattening of the hemidiaphragm causes anatomic distortion of the stomach and decreases the acuteness of the angle at the gastroesophageal junction.[59,64] Elevations in intragastric and intraabdominal pressure are intensified by multiple pregnancy, hydramnios, obesity, lithotomy position, bending over, or application of fundal pressure.[59,250] The tendency toward reflux is increased by the decreased GI tone and relaxation of the cardiac sphincter.[64] As a result of gastric stasis and pyloric incompetence, the refluxed material may be alkaline or acidic. Prolonged reflux of normal pH or alkaline duodenal material can lead to esophagitis.[64]

The frequency of hiatal hernia is also increased, occurring in 15% to 20% of pregnant women primarily after 7 to 8 months' gestation. This disorder arises from alterations in muscle tone and pressure with widening of the hiatus. Interventions are similar to those for heartburn (Table 11-6).

Constipation

Constipation occurs in 10% to 30% of women and tends to be worse in the first and third trimesters.[36,233,250] Constipation probably arises primarily from alterations in water transport and reabsorption in the large intestine. The smooth muscle relaxant effects of progesterone decrease intestinal motility and prolong transit time, which increases electrolyte and subsequently water absorption in the large intestine. Other predisposing factors are compression of the rectosigmoid area by the enlarging uterus and changes in dietary habits and activity and exercise patterns. Interventions for women with constipation are summarized in Table 11-6.

Hemorrhoids

Hemorrhoids arise more frequently during pregnancy and are aggravated by constipation. Factors that contribute to hemorrhoid formation during pregnancy include poor support for hemorrhoidal veins in the anorectal area; lack of valves in these vessels, leading to reversal in the direction of blood flow and stasis; gravity; pressure of the expanding uterus; increased venous pressure in the pelvic veins; venous congestion and engorgement; and enlargement of the hemorrhoidal veins. Interventions for women with hemorrhoids are summarized in Table 11-6.

Nausea and Vomiting

Nausea with or without vomiting is a self-limiting event experienced by approximately two thirds of pregnant women in Western cultures.[86,176,225] Vomiting occurs in 30% to 45% of these women.[233] Nausea and vomiting in pregnancy (NVP) generally begins at between 4 and 6 weeks, but may occur as early as 2 to 3 weeks after the last menstrual period, and peaks at 8 to 12 weeks.[250] NVP usually resolves by 3 to 4 months, although a few women (~10%) may experience symptoms to term.[49,250] The most frequent food aversions are to meat, fish, poultry, and eggs.[86] NVP is often reported to occur most prominently prior to rising in the morning and ingestion of food (hence the term "morning sickness"), but women often experience symptoms in the afternoon, evening, or throughout the day.[297] NVP usually disappears by 10 to 12 weeks but persists to 14 weeks in 40% of women, 16 weeks in less than 20%, and 20 weeks in less than 10%.[225,233]

The exact cause and function of nausea and vomiting is unknown. Many theories have been proposed, focusing on mechanical, endocrinologic, allergic, metabolic, genetic, and psychosomatic etiologies, but none have substantial research support.[42,67,71,100,116,225,233,250] The major schools of thought are that this phenomenon is physiologic-hormonal or psychogenic in origin, although recently several researchers have postulated adaptive and protective mechanisms.[86,116]

The most common hormonal theories are related to rapidly increasing and high levels of estrogen, human chorionic gonadotropin (hCG), and possibly thyroxine. Support for a hormonal theory comes from studies documenting nausea in women on estrogen medications or combined oral contraceptive pills, the high correlation between women who experience nausea with both oral contraceptive use and pregnancy, and parallels between hCG patterns and the timing of symptom appearance and disappearance in NVP.[116,176] However, studies examining the correlation of hCG levels with symptom appearance and intensity in individual women have produced inconsistent results. Increased NVP is seen in women with multiple and molar pregnancies, both of which are characterized by increased hCG. Perhaps a combination of endocrine factors leads to NVP, and individual women may have different sensitivities to these substances. NVP has been associated with favorable pregnancy outcomes such as decreased miscarriage rates, low birth weight, and perinatal mortality, although some researchers have found no differences in perinatal mortality and low birth weight.[86,116,122,251,280,281]

Support for a psychologic (although not necessarily pathologic) component to NVP comes from placebo studies in which over half of women with NVP experienced dramatic improvement in their symptoms when given a placebo.[176] Some proponents of the psychogenic origin suggest that it may be related to emotional factors with ambivalence or unconscious rejection of the pregnancy. Few studies have been done to document this theory, and many available reports are case studies of women in psychotherapy. Studies that have been done on more representative populations present conflicting findings. Several investigators reported that women without NVP were more prone to psychologic difficulties during pregnancy and postpartum, felt less close to their mothers, and were less likely to breastfeed.[286] Conversely, NVP has also been associated with greater identification with the maternal role.[286]

Another hypothesis is that NVP may have an adaptive function to protect the embryo for potentially toxic substances in foods, such as animal products that might contain parasites and other pathogens if not handled correctly, caffeinated beverages, and alcohol.[116] A study of 20 societies in which women experience NVP and 7 in which NVP is rare found that the societies in which NVP was rare were more likely to have plants (corn) as the primary staple rather than animal products.[86] Decreased energy intake in early pregnancy is correlated with increased placental weight in animal and human studies.[86] Huxley suggests that hCG activates the thyroid, and thus increases thyroxine secretion, which stimulates placental growth. As noted above, hCG (and thyroxine) levels correlate with severity and onset of NVP in some but not all studies. Huxley postulates that NVP reduces maternal energy intake. Maternal levels of anabolic hormones, insulin, and insulin-like growth factor I (IGF-I) are lowered as is maternal tissue synthesis, favoring early placental growth and development, and later fetal growth.[116] Underweight women tend to experience less severe NVP than women with normal preconceptional body mass index (BMI).[116]

Interventions for women experiencing NVP are summarized in Table 11-6. Pharmacologic treatment may occasionally be required due to severity of symptoms or interference with the woman's responsibilities. Use of pharmacologic agents is fraught with potential problems, since

NVP and thus the administration of any drugs occur during the period of embryonic organogenesis. Until the early 1980s, Bendectin (which combined an antihistamine and pyridoxine) was commonly used to treat NVP. Litigation over the relationship of Bendectin and congenital defects resulted in removal of this drug from the market, although a causal relationship has never been documented.[176,274] Since Bendectin was removed from the market, there has been an increase in hospital admissions for hyperemesis in North America.[194] Medications currently used include antihistamines and phenothiazines.[176] As with any drug during pregnancy, these agents must be used with caution (see Chapter 6). Alternative therapies have been investigated.[124,177,274,295] Ginger has been reported to be effective in reducing nausea.[274] However, studies on the use of acupuncture for NVP have had equivocal findings.[124,144,177,194]

Hyperemesis gravidarum, an uncommon disorder seen in up to 2% of pregnant women, is intractable vomiting associated with alterations in nutritional status, dehydration, electrolyte imbalance, significant weight loss (>5%), ketosis, and acetonuria.[181,176,248,250] These women often require hospitalization. Hyperemesis has been linked to alterations in thyroid hormones (see Chapter 18).

Food and Fluid Intake in Labor

Food and fluid intake during labor is controversial. For many years most hospitals in the United States have not allowed women in active labor to eat or consume beverages other than ice chips or clear liquids. These prohibitions developed during the period when general anesthesia was commonly utilized during the second stage of labor; accordingly, there were concerns regarding the risk of aspiration should the anesthetized woman vomit. These constraints are currently being questioned, with many practitioners advocating more liberal food and fluid policies during labor.[38,39,72] There is little documentation supporting either the benefits of this therapy or the risk of oral intake for most women (see Chapter 10).[167,200]

Individuals opposed to a more liberal food and fluid policy in labor argue that, although rare, aspiration has devastating consequences and can still occur with an endotracheal tube in place or use of regional anesthesia. Pregnant women are at particular risk for pulmonary aspiration because of delayed gastric emptying time, increased levels of gastrin (resulting in increased gastric volume and lowered gastric pH), and decreased LES tone (which allows stomach contents in an unconscious woman to passively move into the pharynx and into the lungs).[72] Antacids have been used to increase gastric pH and reduce the risk of damage to lung tissue should aspiration occur.[39,40]

Those advocating relaxation of restrictions note that: (1) general anesthesia has been replaced by regional anesthesia; (2) the incidence of maternal mortality from aspiration of stomach contents in normal labor is rare; (3) gastric emptying may not be significantly altered in normal women who have not received narcotics; (4) use of intravenous fluid administration is increased; and (5) prolonged fasting during labor has physiologic and psychologic effects.[38,39,167,200] General anesthesia, if used, is safer than in the past as the result of changes in anesthetic agents and administrative techniques, such as the use of endotracheal tubes, which prevent aspiration of vomitus. Potential physiologic effects of fasting include increased ketones and fatty acids with decreased alanine, glucose, and insulin. Psychologic effects include increased anxiety and stress.[39] Use of intravenous fluids has been associated with maternal and infant fluid and electrolyte problems (see Chapter 10). Low-risk women who deliver at home or in alternative settings and women in other cultures often consume food and beverages during labor with few complications.

Effects of Altered Maternal Nutrition

Weight gain during pregnancy is associated with improved infant growth and development. Most studies demonstrate a correlation between maternal weight gain and birth weight even when other variables that influence birth weight (gestational age, maternal height, and birth order)

are held constant. The relationship between weight gain during pregnancy and perinatal mortality varies with maternal prepregnancy weight and pregnancy weight gain (see Figure 11-4). Specific effects of altered maternal nutrition are listed in Table 11-7. Effects of maternal nutrition on the fetus are discussed further in "Fetal Growth."

Undernutrition and Pregnancy

Women who are underweight have a higher incidence of pregnancy loss and small-for-gestational-age (SGA) infants. These women may fail to gain adequate weight during pregnancy, further increasing the risk of fetal growth restriction and maternal nutritional anemia and malnutrition. Kristal and Rush reviewed studies examining the effects of maternal undernutrition on fetal growth and concluded the following: (1) limitations in the overall amount of maternal food intake from either starvation or iatrogenic limitations lead to a consistent depression in birth weight (up to 550 g); (2) relief of acute undernutrition up to the beginning of the third trimester is associated with return of birth weight to previous levels; (3) results of supplementation studies with pregnant women at risk nutritionally (in developed and developing countries) are consistent, with increases in birth weight of 40 to 60 g; (4) there seems to be a limit in the amount of supplementation a given individual can tolerate and to the effect of these supplements; and (5) a consistent depression in birth weight is

TABLE **11-7**   Expected Consequences of Inadequate Nutrition in Women during a Reproductive Cycle

| | DEFICIENCY NUTRITION | |
PREPREGNANCY	PREGNANCY	POSTPREGNANCY
Low stature Low body weight Low adiposity Low lean body mass Delayed menarche Low nutrient reserves (Ca, Fe, I, Zn, vitamin A, and so on) Low discretionary activity	Small placenta Reduced duration of pregnancy Risk of low birth weight and intrauterine growth restriction Inadequate weight gain Low deposition of fat Inadequate volume expansion Inadequate hormonal response Nutrient deficiencies (Fe, I, Zn, vitamin A, folate, vitamin D, and so on) Perinatal complications Lower discretionary activity	Body weight deficient Poor lactation performance Prolonged amenorrhea Longer birth interval Nutrient deficiencies (Fe, Ca, Zn, vitamin A, and so on) Low discretionary activity Poorer prepregnancy nutrition
	RELATIVE EXCESS OF ENERGY (OBESITY)	
Poor health (higher prevalence of hypertension, diabetes) Low discretionary activity	Increased adiposity Risk of macrosomic baby Perinatal complications Risk of preeclampsia Risk of diabetes	Worsening of diabetes and health consequences Low discretionary activity

Adapted from Viteri, F.E., Schumacher, L., & Silliman, K. (1989). Maternal malnutrition and the fetus. *Semin Perinatol, 13*, 236.

seen with use of high-density protein supplements in which more than 20% of calories supplied are protein.[147] High-density protein diets have also been associated with an increased incidence of prematurity and neonatal morbidity in some populations.[105,287] Both caloric and protein deprivation affect the fetus, although it is controversial as to which is most detrimental to fetal growth and development. Human and animal studies suggest that restrictions in caloric intake have the most marked effects on fetal growth, whereas protein deprivation leads to alterations in later development.[105]

Maternal Obesity and Pregnancy

Maternal obesity is associated with an increased incidence of macrosomia, LGA infants, delivery complications, and perinatal mortality.[66,93,162,125] These LGA infants are usually larger than expected in weight but not length due to increased deposition of adipose tissue.[105] The woman's excess adipose tissue reserves may be supplying some of the fuel needed for fetal growth. Cord blood triglyceride levels are elevated, reflecting enhanced fat synthesis by fetal liver and adipose tissue.[105,287] Since obese women tend to have LGA infants even when pregnancy weight gain is inadequate, it is difficult to determine if their infants are growth restricted.

Many of the metabolic changes seen in pregnancy (such as increased circulating insulin, insulin resistance) are similar to those seen in obese women.[105] Obese women tend to have more problems during delivery due to increased fetal growth and macrosomia. The incidence of preeclampsia and chronic hypertension, thrombophlebitis, varicose veins, and diabetes mellitus is increased in obese woman.[293,105,145,191] These women may gain excess weight during pregnancy, which can be difficult to lose later. Maternal obesity also has been reported to be a risk factor for neural tube defects.[66,93,191]

Caloric restriction during pregnancy is generally not recommended because of potential adverse effects on the fetus. Severe caloric restriction can significantly reduce the availability of glucose (the major fetal energy substrate) and increase maternal serum amino acid and ketone levels. Maternal ketosis has been associated with poor neurologic development in offspring, although some studies have not confirmed this finding.[105] However, caloric restriction may be indicated in the obese pregnant woman to maintain a weight gain that has been associated with an improved pregnancy outcome.

Pregnancy and Gastrointestinal Disorders

The physiologic and anatomic changes of the GI tract during pregnancy have varying effects on disorders of this system. The course of some disorders is minimally affected by pregnancy. For example, one of the more common GI disorders occurring in the childbearing population—inflammatory bowel disease (IBD), which includes ulcerative colitis and Crohn disease—is not adversely affected by pregnancy. If these disorders are quiescent at the time of pregnancy, outcome for both mother and fetus is usually good. If the disorder is active at the time of conception, there is a higher rate of spontaneous abortion and preterm delviery.[250] The risk of exacerbation of ulcerative colitis during pregnancy is similar to the risk in nonpregnant women. Risk of exacerbation is highest during the first trimester and postpartum. Maternal immune tolerance or increases in corticosteroids during the second and third trimesters may have a protective effect.[12,250] Appendicitis and cholelithiasis are the most common reasons for nonobstetric surgery during pregnancy.[241,247]

Pregnancy and Acute Appendicitis

Appendicitis is not more common during pregnancy, but may be more severe due to delayed diagnosis.[75] Diagnosis of appendicitis during pregnancy is complicated by anatomic and physiologic changes of pregnancy. Since the appendix is displaced upward and laterally to the right, the point of maximal tenderness may be as high as the right costal margin. By the second trimester, the appendix lies above the iliac crest (see Figure 11-3). As a result, radiated pain associated with suppuration or perforation tends to be felt at the point where the appendix abuts the peritoneum, which becomes higher and more lateral as gestation progresses.[12,242,247,251]

Guarding and rebound tenderness are often milder and less well localized, since the uterus is between the appendix and the parietal peritoneum.[250] Nausea is common in the first trimester, and changes in white blood cell (WBC) counts associated with appendicitis are similar to changes in pregnancy. Suidan and Young suggest that one way to differentiate uterine from appendiceal pain is to turn the woman onto her left side while pressing the point of maximal tenderness. If the pain decreases or ceases, the pain is probably uterine in origin; if not, appendicitis should be suspected.[251] Appendicitis increases the risk of spontaneous abortion and preterm labor, especially if accompanied by peritonitis.[250] The risk of perforation is greatest in the third trimester.[250]

Pregnancy in Women with Peptic Ulcer Disease

PUD in women is seen more often after menopause and is uncommon during the childbearing years.[90] The risk of PUD is greatest with use of nonsteroidal antiinflammatory agents and colonization with *Helicobacter pylori.*[250] In women of childbearing age, estrogen may protect the gastric lining from ulcer formation, perhaps by increasing gastric and duodenal mucus secretion.[90,273] Pregnancy has a further protective effect on the development and progression of PUD.[50,225] Up to 80% of women with PUD improve during pregnancy, although 50% experience recurrence of symptoms by 3 months postpartum and almost all by 2 years after delivery.[64,225] Women with persistent symptoms during pregnancy usually have other problems such as hyperemesis gravidarum and albuminuria.[225]

The basis for improvement during pregnancy is still conjectural but is thought to lie in the normal changes in gastric acidity that accompany pregnancy. Production of hydrochloric acid (both basal and in response to histamine) decreases in pregnancy, with a tendency to return to normal or increased levels of acidity in the third trimester.[50] Decreased gastric acidity, delayed gastric emptying, increased plasma histaminase (thought to mediate acid and pepsin secretion by reducing parietal cell responsiveness to endogenous histamine), increased prostaglandins (protective of gastric mucosa), and increased mucin secretion (which protects the gastric mucosa from the effects of acid) may all contribute to improvement in peptic ulcer symptoms.[47,50,64,184,233]

Gastrin levels are normal during most of pregnancy, with marked increases late in the third trimester, at delivery, and immediately after delivery. Thus, by late pregnancy, gastric pH and pepsin output have returned to nonpregnant levels. It is at this time that peptic ulcer symptoms tend to recur.[64,225]

Cholelithiasis and Pregnancy

The incidence of cholelithiasis, which is more common in women, is increased further during pregnancy and in women taking oral contraceptive agents.[24,77,178] Cholelithiasis is the second most common nonobstetric surgical problem (acute appendicitis being the most common) during pregnancy.[264] A hormonal basis for the risk of gallstones in women has been suggested, since the increased risk is seen primarily between menarche and menopause. Elevated estrogen and progesterone levels during pregnancy may further aggravate the tendency toward cholelithiasis, as does the increased bile stasis and sludging during pregnancy.[75]

There are three forms of gallstones: cholesterol, pigment, and mixed (composed primarily of calcium bilirubinate). The increased incidence of gallstones associated with females and pregnancy is seen primarily with cholesterol gallstones. The process of gallstone development involves (1) production of bile supersaturated with choles-

terol; (2) nucleation and crystallization of cholesterol, which initiates stone formation; and (3) growth of the stone.[215] Supersaturation of bile with cholesterol occurs when cholesterol secretion is high or bile acid secretion is low (concentrated bile is more likely to hold cholesterol in solution). Cholesterol production increases during pregnancy. In addition, estrogens and progesterone increase biliary cholesterol saturation and estrogen decreases the proportion of chenodeoxycholic acid. This acid is a component of the bile acid pool that dissolves gallstones by decreasing biliary cholesterol secretion. Altered gallbladder tone during pregnancy, with incomplete emptying and increased fasting and residual volumes, may also increase the risk of gallstone formation by sequestering cholesterol crystals.[24,77,215]

Cholecystitis and pancreatitis. Acute cholecystitis is rare during pregnancy.[170] Severe abdominal pain is more likely due to appendicitis, which occurs four to five times more often during pregnancy than does cholecystitis.[24] The incidence of pancreatitis, although rare, increases in pregnancy and postpartum. Pancreatitis in pregnancy is usually associated with gallstone formation and develops when gallstones traveling down the common bile duct collide with and traumatize the ampulla.[12,193,215,225,250]

Pregnancy and Liver Disease

Liver disease in pregnancy can be divided into two categories: (1) disorders seen only in pregnancy and associated with jaundice and abnormal liver tests (intrahepatic cholestasis, pregnancy-induced hypertension, and fatty liver of pregnancy); and (2) liver diseases that may occur during and are affected by pregnancy.[51] The most common liver disease seen in pregnant woman is viral hepatitis. Major effects of pregnancy on liver disorders are potential difficulties with diagnosis; increased fetal risk; and, especially with hepatitis B, transmission to the fetus. Alterations in some liver function tests during pregnancy can make diagnosis of liver disorders more difficult, although jaundice is always abnormal. Jaundice during pregnancy is discussed in Chapter 17.

Severe pruritus and jaundice characterize intrahepatic cholestasis. The risk of postpartum hemorrhage, gallstones, fetal distress, stillbirth, and prematurity is increased. The basis for this disorder is unclear, although it may have a genetic basis or hormonal cause, since a similar syndrome occurs with oral contraceptive use.[215] Fatty liver of pregnancy is a rare disorder of unknown cause that usually appears during the third trimester, often in association with pregnancy-induced hypertension (PIH), with high fetal and maternal mortality rates. Delivery of the infant results in rapid improvement.[215]

TABLE **11-8** Recommendations for Clinical Practice Related to Changes in the Gastrointestinal System in Pregnant Women

Counsel women regarding changes in appetite, food preferences, and intake during pregnancy (p. 412).

Counsel women regarding gingival changes during pregnancy and the need for dental hygiene (pp. 412-415).

Counsel women regarding common problems (heartburn, nausea and vomiting, constipation, hemorrhoids) associated with the gastrointestinal (GI) system (pp. 424-426 and Table 11-2).

Implement interventions to reduce or relieve heartburn, nausea and vomiting, constipation, and hemorrhoids (pp. 424-426 and Table 11-6).

Counsel women regarding the presence of spider angiomata and palmar erythema (p. 418 and Chapter 13).

Recognize the usual parameters for liver function tests and patterns of change during pregnancy and the postpartum period (p. 418 and Table 11-3).

Know the expected parameters for weight gain during pregnancy and monitor maternal patterns (pp. 418-420 and Table 11-4).

Know the recommended nutritional requirements during pregnancy (pp. 422-423 and Table 11-5).

Assess maternal nutritional status and provide nutritional counseling (pp. 422-423 and Table 11-5).

Recognize potential maternal and fetal/neonatal complications associated with undernutrition and obesity during pregnancy (pp. 427-428 and Table 11-7).

Counsel women regarding the risk of caloric restriction during pregnancy (p. 428).

Monitor fluid, food, and caloric intake during labor and the early postpartum period (pp. 426-427).

Counsel women regarding weight loss patterns following delivery (p. 421).

Recommend postpartum exercises to enhance weight loss and return of abdominal and perineal tone (p. 421).

Evaluate GI function postpartum (p. 421).

Recognize factors that increase the risk of gallstone formation and recognize signs of cholelithiasis (p. 429).

Counsel women with GI and liver problems regarding the effect of their disorder on pregnancy and of pregnancy on the disorder (pp. 428-430).

Recognize signs of appendicitis during pregnancy (p. 428).

Recognize signs of liver disorders that are unique to pregnancy (p. 429 and Chapter 17).

Counsel women with phenylketonuria and other metabolic disorders regarding risks to their infant and need for dietary restrictions (p. 423).

Provide support for women who must use special diets during pregnancy (p. 423).

Know fetal nutritional requirements and counsel women regarding fetal needs and growth patterns (pp. 423-424, 439-440).

Know factors that can alter fetal growth and monitor fetal growth patterns (pp. 439-440 and Figure 11-2 and Table 11-7).

Counsel women regarding changes in GI function with use of oral contraceptive agents (pp. 416, 425, 429).

Liver function and histologic changes are associated with preeclampsia (see Table 8-5), with alterations in liver function tests (AST, ALT, GGT, and bilirubin) reported in about half.[99] The degree of liver abnormality tends to parallel the severity of preeclampsia. Some women with preeclampsia develop an additional group of findings, the HELLP syndrome, that includes hemolysis (H); elevated serum levels of liver enzymes, especially SGOT and SGPT (EL); and low platelets (LP) (see Chapter 8).[79,215]

SUMMARY

The pregnant woman experiences changes in GI and hepatic function that enhance absorption of nutrients for herself and her fetus. These changes are associated with common experiences and discomforts of pregnancy such as heartburn, constipation, nausea, and vomiting. A major component of interconceptional and prenatal care is nutritional assessment and counseling. Maternal nutrition before and during pregnancy is critical for optimal growth and development of the fetus and prevention of maternal, fetal, and neonatal disorders. Table 11-8 summarizes recommendations for clinical practice related to the GI system and perinatal nutrition.

DEVELOPMENT OF THE GASTROINTESTINAL AND HEPATIC SYSTEMS IN THE FETUS

The development of the GI system can be divided into three phases. During early gestation, anatomic development gives rise to the organs and other structures of the system. During middle to late gestation, functional components such as hormones, enzymes, and reflexes develop (Figure 11-6). Finally, after birth, coordinated function develops with interaction of hormones and enzymes in the digestion of food substances along with maturation of suck-swallow coordination. Characteristics and timing

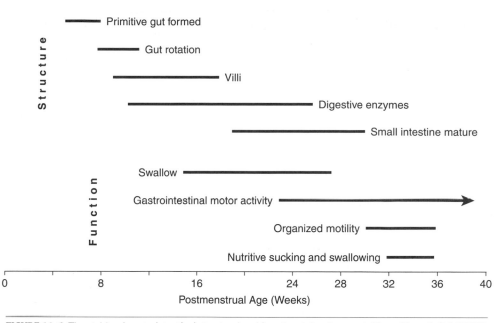

FIGURE **11-6** Timetable of gastrointestinal structural and functional development. (From Newell, S.J. [1996]. Gastrointestinal function and its ontogeny: How should we feed the preterm infants? *Semin Neonatol, 1,* 60.)

of common GI anomalies are listed in Table 11-9. GI anomalies account for about 5% to 7% of all anomalies identified by prenatal ultrasound.[246]

Anatomic Development

Anatomic development of the GI system begins during the fourth week with partitioning of the yolk sac into intra- and extraembryonic portions. Initially the cranial portion of the GI system develops concurrently with the respiratory system (see Chapter 9). The epithelium of the trachea, the bronchi, and the lungs and digestive tract arise from the primitive gut, a derivation of the yolk sac. The GI system develops in a cranial-to-caudal direction. The yolk sac arises at 8 days and by the fourth week has divided into two parts. The extraembryonic or secondary yolk sac provides for nutrition of the embryo, prior to development of the mature placenta, then is assimilated into the umbilical cord by 3 to 4 months. The intraembryonic portion is incorporated into the embryo as the primitive gut (Figure 11-7).

The primitive gut is initially closed at both ends by membranes. The cranial (buccopharyngeal) membrane is reabsorbed during the third week, and the caudal (cloacal) membrane during the ninth week. The midgut remains temporarily connected to the yolk sac by the vitelline duct. Development of the primitive gut and its derivatives can be divided into four sections: pharyngeal gut, foregut, midgut, and hindgut.[189]

Development of the Pharyngeal Gut

The pharyngeal gut extends from the buccopharyngeal membrane to the tracheobronchial diverticulum, forming the pharynx and its derivative, lower respiratory tract, and upper esophagus (Figure 11-8). The pharyngeal area develops from bands of mesenchymal tissue (branchial or pharyngeal arches) separated by deep clefts (branchial or pharyngeal clefts) on the exterior of the embryo. A series of indentations (pharyngeal pouches) appear on the lateral walls of the pharyngeal gut and penetrate into the surrounding mesenchyme but do not communicate with the external clefts.[227] The pharyngeal arches form the muscular and skeletal components of the pharyngeal area, aortic arch, and nerve networks; mandible; dorsal portion of the maxillary process; hyoid bone; thyroid bone; laryngeal cartilage; and their associated vascular and nerve supplies. The pharyngeal pouches form the eustachian tube, tonsils, thymus, parathyroid, and part of the thyroid.[189,227]

Development of the Foregut and Common Anomalies

The foregut extends from the tracheobronchial diverticulum to the upper part of the duodenum. Structures formed from the foregut (lower esophagus, stomach, liver, upper portion of the duodenum to the entry of the common bile duct, liver, biliary tree, and pancreas) are all supplied by the celiac artery.[189]

TABLE **11-9**   Incidence, Time of Occurrence, and Associated Defects of Various Gastrointestinal Anomalies

ANOMALY	INCIDENCE (PER LIVE BIRTHS)	FETAL AGE AT WHICH DEFECT OCCURS	PRESENCE OF HYDRAMNIOS	ASSOCIATED DEFECTS
Diaphragmatic hernia	1:4000	Eighth-tenth week of fetal life	>75%	Lung hypoplasia, malrotation of bowel, patent ductus arteriosus (PDA), coarctation of aorta, and neurologic malformations
Tracheoesophageal fistula and esophageal atresias	1:3000 1:4000	Fourth-fifth week of fetal life	>60%	Encourage in more than 50% of patients and include gastrointestinal (GI), skeletal, and cardiac defects
Duodenal atresia	1:10,000-1:40,000	Eighth-tenth week of fetal life	Approx. 50%	Down syndrome, GI malformations, and congenital heart disease
Jejunoileal atresia	1:330-1:1500	During fetal life after embryogenesis (after twelfth week of gestation)	35% jejunal 10%-15% ileal	Infrequent, but may be associated with volvulus, malrotation, and meconium peritonitis
Colonic atresia	1:5000-1:20,000	Vascular accidents in gestation	Rare	Occur in 30%-40% and are associated with abdominal wall defects, vesicointestinal fistulae, and jejunal atresias
Anorectal anomalies	1:5000-1:15,000	Fifth-eighth week of fetal life	Rare	May be familial-associated anomalies in 30%-70% and include cardiac, GI, and vertebral anomalies
Omphalocele	1:3000-1:10,000	Eighth-eleventh week of fetal life	Common, but incidence unknown	Occur in 60%; cardiac defects 15%-20%; tetralogy of Fallot; associated with specific syndromes: Beckwith and trisomy D, E, and 21
Gastroschisis	1:6000	? Ninth-eleventh week of fetal life	Incidence unknown	Foreshortened gut and intestinal atresias 15%; cardiac defects <10%
Duplications of GI tract	1:100-1:4000	Fourth-sixth week of fetal life	Unknown	Most common in ileum and esophagus
Meckel's diverticulum	1:50-1:100	Fifth-seventh week of fetal life	Rare	Usually occurs as isolated defect

From Sunshine, P. (1990). Fetal gastrointestinal physiology. In R.D. Eden & F.H. Boehm (Eds.). *Assessment and care of the fetus.* Norwalk, CT: Appleton & Lange.

Esophagus. During the fourth week the tracheobronchial diverticulum appears along the ventral wall of the foregut, dividing the foregut into the ventral respiratory primordium and dorsal esophagus (Figure 11-9, *A*). The esophagus is initially short, but quickly elongates with ascent of the pharynx and cranial growth. The rapidly growing endothelium temporarily obliterates the esophageal lumen, with recanalization of the lumen by 8 weeks.

Incomplete division of the foregut into respiratory and digestive portions at 4 to 5 weeks leads to tracheoesophageal fistula with or without esophageal atresia (Figure 11-9, *B*; also see Table 11-9). This malformation probably arises from posterior deviation or unequal development of the septum developing between the primitive trachea and esophagus. Failure of the lumen to recanalize during the eighth week leads to esophageal stenosis or atresia.

Stomach, duodenum, and pancreas. The stomach arises during the fourth week as a spindle-shaped dilation in the caudal area of the foregut (see Figure 11-8), and its structure is well established by 6 weeks. The stomach dilates and enlarges, rotating around a longitudinal and an anteroposterior axis. During the longitudinal rotation the stomach rotates 90 degrees clockwise, ending with the left side facing anteriorly and the right posteriorly. The subsequent greater growth of the posterior wall in comparison with the ante-

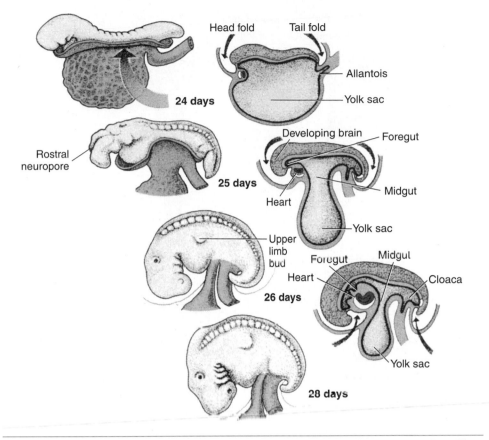

FIGURE **11-7** Development of the primitive gut and folding of the embryo from 24 to 28 days. (From Moore, K.L. [1988]. *Essentials of human embryology.* Philadelphia: B.C. Decker.)

rior wall leads to the lesser and greater curvatures of the stomach. Initially the cephalic and caudal ends of the stomach are in midline. During the second or anteroposterior rotation of the stomach, the caudal (pyloric) portion moves right and upward, and the cephalic (cardiac) portion moves left and slightly downward.[189,227] Embryonic anomalies of the stomach are rare, probably because stomach development is relatively simple. The most common stomach anomaly is pyloric stenosis, which is thought to be genetic in origin.

The duodenum arises from both the foregut and midgut. As the stomach rotates, the duodenum takes on a C-shaped form and rotates to the right. The lumen of the duodenum becomes obliterated by rapidly growing epithelium, with later recanalization. Failure to recanalize leads to duodenal atresia or stenosis.

The pancreas appears at about 5 weeks as dorsal and ventral buds in the duodenal area. As the duodenum rotates to the right and becomes C-shaped, the ventral pancreatic bud migrates toward the lower end of the common bile duct. The two pancreatic buds meet and fuse to form

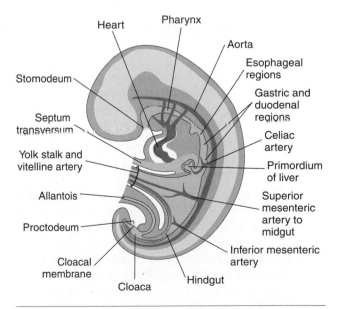

FIGURE **11-8** Early development of the digestive system and its blood supply. (From Moore, K.L. & Persaud, T.V.N. [1998]. *The developing human: Clinically oriented embryology* [6th ed.]. Philadelphia: W.B. Saunders.)

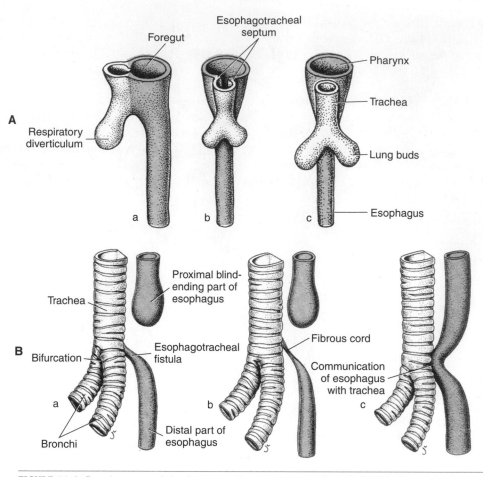

FIGURE **11-9** Development of the foregut and common anomalies. **A,** Partitioning of the foregut to form the respiratory diverticulum and esophagus during the third (a) and fourth (b and c) weeks of development. **B,** Abnormalities of the esophagus: (a) esophageal atresia and esophagotracheal fistula; (b) esophageal atresia with a connection between the distal part of the esophagus and trachea with a fibrous cord; and (c) connection of the proximal and distal parts of the esophagus to the trachea by a narrow canal. (From Sadler, T.W. [1985]. *Langman's medical embryology* [5th ed.]. Baltimore: Williams & Wilkins.)

the final pancreas by 7 weeks.[153] In individuals with an annular pancreas, the ventral bud encircles the duodenum and may cause obstruction.[227] All cell types are seen by 9 to 10 weeks.[238]

Liver and gallbladder. The liver appears during the third week as a ventral thickening (liver bud or hepatic diverticulum) consisting of rapidly proliferating strands of cells at the distal end of the foregut (see Figure 11-8). The hepatic diverticulum divides into a large cranial portion, which forms the hepatic parenchyma and main bile duct, and a smaller caudal portion, from which the gallbladder arises.[227] The liver initially grows into the septum transversum, a thick mesodermal plate separating the yolk sac and the thoracic cavity. The liver grows rapidly, eventually

bulging into the caudal part of the abdominal cavity and stretching the mesoderm of the septum transversum until it becomes a thin membrane. The ventral portion of this membrane forms the falciform ligament; the dorsal portion forms the lesser omentum. The cranial portion of the septum transversum forms part of the diaphragm. Further growth of the liver promotes closure of the pleuroperitoneal canals (two large openings on either side of the foregut).

The lumina of the gallbladder and the intrahepatic and extrahepatic bile ducts are initially open, becoming temporarily obliterated by proliferating epithelium and later recanalizing. Biliary atresia can arise from failure of recanalization. With complete failure, the ducts are narrow nonfunctional fibrous cords. Failure of part of a bile duct to recanalize results in partial obstruction or atresia of that duct, with distention of the gallbladder and hepatic duct proximal to the atretic area.[189,227]

Development of the Midgut and Common Anomalies

Development of the midgut is characterized by rapid elongation of the gut and associated mesentery.[189] The midgut begins caudal to the liver and gives rise to the small intestine (except for the upper duodenum), cecum, appendix, ascending colon, and proximal portion of the transverse colon. These structures are supplied by the superior mesenteric artery.[189]

Initially midgut growth parallels the neural tube; however, the rapid growth of the midgut quickly exceeds that of the rest of the body, including the abdominal cavity. This occurs at a time when the liver and kidneys are relatively large, occupying much of the available space in the abdominal cavity. As a result, the midgut herniates into the extraembryonic coelom of the proximal umbilical cord. This physiologic herniation begins in the sixth week, with return of the midgut to the abdominal cavity during the tenth week.

Development of the midgut involves four steps: herniation, rotation, retraction, and fixation (Figure 11-10).[189,227] The midgut initially elongates and forms a U-shaped loop, which projects (herniates) into the proximal umbilical cord. The cranial limb of this loop grows rapidly, forming coils characteristic of the small intestine with little change in the caudal portion except for appearance of the cecal bud.

The midgut rotates a total of 270 degrees in a counterclockwise direction around an axis formed by the superior mesenteric artery. Midgut rotation occurs in two stages. The initial 90-degree rotation occurs while the midgut is in the umbilical cord (see Figure 11-10, *A-B*); the second rotation (180 degrees) takes place as the gut returns to the abdomen at 10 weeks (see Figure 11-10, *C-D*). The initial 90-degree rotation is in a counterclockwise direction. As a result, the cranial limb moves to the right and down and the caudal limb moves to the left and up (see Figure 11-10). The lumen of the intestines becomes temporarily obliterated by rapid epithelial growth, with later recanalization.

Retraction or return of the midgut to the abdominal cavity occurs rapidly during the tenth week. The stimulus for this return is unknown, but it occurs as the rate of liver growth slows, the relative size of the kidney decreases, and the abdominal cavity enlarges. As the midgut reenters the abdominal cavity, the gut rotates 180 degrees counterclockwise. The jejunum returns first and the area of the cecal bud last; the cecum and appendix end up near the liver in the right upper quadrant (see Figure 11-10, *D*).[227]

The final step in development of the midgut is fixation (see Figure 11-10, *E*). The cecum and appendix descend into the lower right quadrant. The proximal colon lengthens, becoming the ascending colon. The mesenteries are pressed against the posterior abdominal wall and fuse with the wall. In some regions of the midgut, the mesenteries also fuse with the parietal peritoneum so that the ascending colon is rectoperitoneal.

Congenital anomalies of the midgut. Congenital anomalies of the midgut include omphalocele, gastroschisis, umbilical hernia, intestinal stenosis and atresia, and malrotation (see Table 11-9). Omphalocele arises at 8 to 11 weeks' gestation from a developmental arrest at the stage of herniation of the midgut into the umbilical cord with failure of all or part of the gut to return to the abdominal cavity (bowel-containing omphalocele). There is often an associated defect in development of the abdominal musculature at the junction of the umbilical cord (liver-containing omphalocele).[249] This results from a primary failure in the formation of the lateral folds, which along with the cephalic and caudal folds form the abdominal wall.[189] The size of this defect influences the size of the omphalocele, which can range from a single loop of intestine to a mass containing most of the intestines and parts of the liver, bladder, and other organs. The omphalocele is covered by a thin, avascular membrane (derived from amnion) that may be ruptured. The umbilical cord generally inserts into the apex of the omphalocele sac. Omphalocele is associated with Beckwith-Wiedemann syndrome, congenital heart disease, trisomy 13, trisomy 18, and urinary tract problems.[80]

In gastroschisis the extrusion of the intestines results from a defect in the anterior abdominal wall that probably arises between 9 and 11 weeks but may occur as early as 5 to 6 weeks.[164] This defect is usually to the right of, and not necessarily continuous with, the umbilical ring. Since there is usually no hernial sac present, the intestines extrude into the amniotic cavity and are embedded in a gelatinous mass. Gastroschisis arises secondary to a paraumbilical abdominal wall defect that may be a result of: (1) failure of differentiation of the lateral fold somatopleure after the bowel has returned to the peritoneal cavity and the umbilical ring has formed; (2) failure in formation of the umbilical coelom with rupture of the amniotic membrane at the base of the umbilical cord; (3) intrauterine rupture of an incarcerated hernia into the cord; or (4) weakness in the abdominal wall arising from alterations in the normal involution of the second umbilical vein or ischemic damage.[13,106,164,249]

An umbilical hernia is associated with an enlarged umbilical ring and failure of the rectus muscles to come

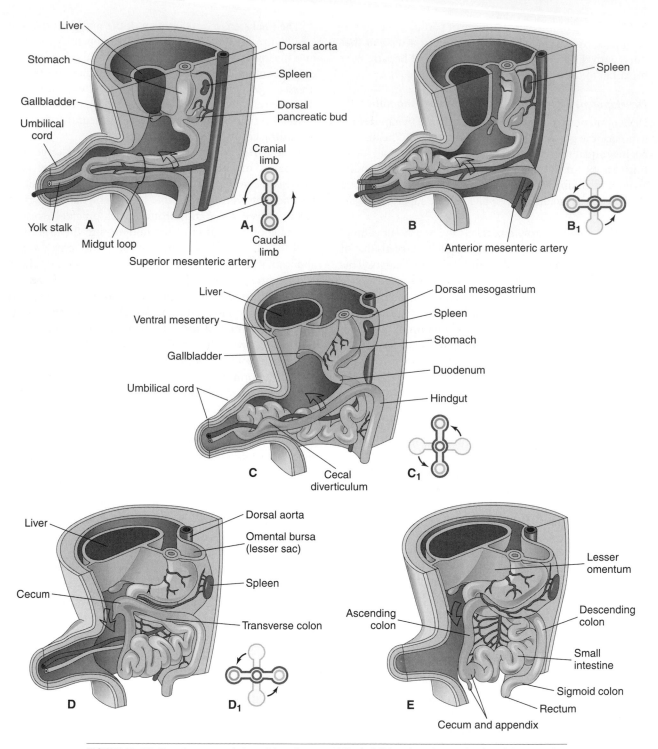

FIGURE **11-10** Development of the midgut (see p. 435). **A,** Midgut loop in proximal umbilical cord at 6 weeks. **A₁,** Transverse section through midgut, showing initial relationships of limbs of midgut loop to artery. **B,** Beginning midgut rotation. **B₁,** 90-Degree counterclockwise rotation. **C,** Return of intestines to abdomen at 10 weeks. **C₁,** Additional 90-degree rotation. **D,** After return to abdomen. **D₁,** Final 90-degree rotation (for a total of 270 degrees). **E,** Late fetal period, with cecum rotated to normal position. (From Moore, K.L. & Persaud, T.V.N. [1998]. *Before we are born: Essentials of human embryology and birth defects* [5th ed.]. Philadelphia: W.B. Saunders.)

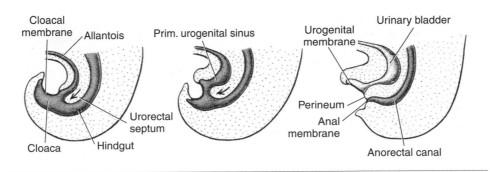

FIGURE **11-11** Development of the hindgut. (From Sadler, T.W. [1985]. *Langman's medical embryology* [5th ed.]. Baltimore: Williams & Wilkins.)

together in midline. The protruding viscera are covered with normal skin.

Intestinal stenoses and atresias can arise as primary or secondary defects. Primary stenosis or atresia arises at 8 to 11 weeks, and perhaps as early as 6 to 7 weeks, as a result of partial or complete failure of the intestinal lumen to recanalize. Secondary stenosis or atresia is a result of: (1) fetal vascular accidents or infarction (with interruption of blood supply to part of the intestines), or (2) secondary to twisting or inflammatory changes. Vascular accidents and infarction are common causes of jejunal and ileal atresias and probably occur after 12 weeks (see Table 11-9).

Alterations in midgut development can also lead to malrotation. Three of the more common forms are nonrotation, mixed malrotation, and reverse rotation. With nonrotation the midgut rotates 90 degrees instead of 270 degrees, without the 180-degree rotation that normally occurs upon reentry of the gut into the abdominal cavity. As a result, the colon enters the abdomen first instead of last so that the colon ends up on the left and the small intestine on the right. This form of malrotation is sometimes referred to as left-sided colon. In mixed malrotation the midgut rotates only 180 degrees, so that the terminal ileum reenters first. The cecum is subpyloric and fixed to the abdominal wall, which may compress the duodenum. In reverse rotation the initial 90-degree rotation is clockwise instead of counterclockwise, resulting in placement of the transverse colon behind the duodenum. Malrotation increases the risk of volvulus, with twisting of the intestinal loops and abnormal fixation of the mesenteries resulting in excessive mobility of the bowel. This can lead to kinking of the bowel and blood vessels and necrosis.[189,227]

Development of the Hindgut and Common Anomalies

Development of the hindgut and urogenital system is interrelated. The cloaca is the expanded terminal end of the gut; the hindgut ends at the cloacal membrane (Figure 11-11). The hindgut gives rise to the distal transverse colon, descending and sigmoid colons, rectum, upper anal canal, bladder, and urethra, which are supplied by the inferior mesenteric artery.[189]

At 5 to 7 weeks, the cloaca is divided into two parts by the urorectal septum, a wedge of downward-growing mesenchymal tissue. During weeks 6 to 7, the urorectal septum reaches and fuses with the cloacal membrane, forming the perineum. The area of fusion is the perineal body. The cloacal membrane has now been divided into two parts. The ventral urogenital membrane will be incorporated in the terminal portion of the urogenital system (see Chapters 1 and 10); the dorsal part becomes the anal membrane. A pit that develops in the anal membrane ruptures at 8 to 9 weeks, resulting in an open communication between the rectum and the body exterior. The lower portion of the anal canal develops around the site of the anal pit from ectodermal tissues.[227]

Imperforate anus and associated malformations arise from abnormal development of the urorectal septum. In the simplest form of imperforate anus, the anal membrane fails to rupture and the anal canal ends at the membrane. In more complex forms there may be a layer of connective tissue between the end of the rectum and the body surface. Failure of the anal pit to develop or atresia of the end of the rectum can cause these forms. If the descent of the urorectal septum is arrested, the cloaca may remain, with abnormalities of the urogenital and lower GI systems.

Functional Development

Anatomically the fetal GI tract develops to the stage seen in the newborn by about 20 weeks.[157,279] Functional development begins during fetal life with development of digestive and liver enzyme systems and the absorptive surfaces of the intestine (Table 11-10; see also Figure 11-6) and continues into the postbirth period. Most of the processes needed for enteral nutrition are in place by 33 to 34 weeks' gestation.[279] Although the placenta takes care of the nutrient needs of the fetus, function of the fetal GI tract is important in amniotic fluid homeostasis (see Chapter 3). Amniotic fluid in turn contains nutrients, hormones, and growth factors that stimulate secretion of hormones and regulatory peptides and enhance growth and maturation of the gut.[31,185,271]

The major gut-regulating polypeptides, including gastrin, motilin, and somatostatin, are all present by the end of the first trimester and act as local inducing agents regulating growth and development of the gut.[15,33,197,271] Initially, cells that produce these substances are more widely distributed than in the adult, but they reach adult distribution by 24 weeks.[131,132,197] Gastric epidermal growth factor (EGF) receptors appear by 18 weeks.[133] EGF enhances growth and development of the gut and may protect the stomach from hydrochloric acid.[132] Transport of amino acids begin by 14 weeks, glucose transport by 18 weeks, and fatty acids by 24 weeks (see Table 11-10).[160]

The intestinal villi begin to develop around 7 weeks and are present in the entire small intestine by 14 weeks, with well-developed villi and crypts seen by 19 weeks.[47] Intestinal motility and peristalsis develop gradually and mature during the third trimester.[47] Meconium begins to form at about 16 weeks.

Swallowing begins at 10 to 14 weeks, and by 16 weeks the fetus swallows 2 to 6 ml of amniotic fluid per day, increasing to 200 to 600 ml/day (average, 450 ml/day) by term. Failure of the fetus to swallow amniotic fluid is associated with GI obstruction and polyhydramnios (see Chapter 3).

Most of the metabolic functions of the fetal liver are handled by the maternal liver. The fetal liver is primarily a hematopoietic organ until the latter part of gestation, when bone marrow erythropoiesis and liver metabolic activity increase. Many liver enzyme systems are still immature at birth.

Enzymes involved in protein digestion and absorption develop early in gestation and may be important in fetal life to prevent bowel obstruction by cellular debris.[97] Glucose from the mother is the major source of fetal energy (see Chapter 15). Disaccharidase enzymes are present by 9 to 10 weeks, increase rapidly after 20 weeks, and become very active after 27 to 28 weeks (except for lactase, which does not reach mature levels until 36 to 40 weeks).[127,138,158,252] Bile acids can be detected in the liver and gallbladder by 14 to 16 weeks and in the intestines by 22 weeks; however, the bile acid pool remains low even at term. The fetal jejunum and liver have decreased capacity for reabsorbing bile acids and poorer enterohepatic recirculation of taurine-conjugated bile acids, the major bile acid at birth.[106,237]

Fetal Growth

Fetal growth is dependent on factors such as genetic determinants, general maternal health and nutrition, availability

TABLE **11-10**   Development of the Gastrointestinal Tract in the Fetus

Development	Gestation (Weeks)
ANATOMIC DEVELOPMENT	
Esophagus	
Superficial glands develop	20
Squamous cells appear	28
Stomach	
Gastric glands form	14
Pylorus and fundus defined	14
Pancreas	
Differentiation of endocrine and exocrine tissue	14
Liver	
Lobules form	11
Small Intestine	
Crypt-villi develop	14
Lymph nodes appear	14
Colon	
Diameter increases	20
FUNCTIONAL DEVELOPMENT	
Sucking and Swallowing	
Swllowing begins	10-14
Only mouthing	28
Immature suck-swallow	33-36
Stomach	
Gastric motility and secretion	20
Pancreas	
Zymogen granules	20
Liver	
Bile metabolism	11
Bile secretion	22
Small Intestine	
Active transport of amino acids	14
Glucose transport	18
Fatty acid absorption	24
Enzymes	
α-Glucosidases	10
Dipeptidases	10
Lactase	10
Enterokinase	26

From Lebenthal, A. & Lebenthal, E. (1999). The ontology of the small intestinal epithelium. *J Parenter Enteral Nutr, 23,* S5.

of growth substrates, presence of fetal growth–promoting hormones, and vascular support via changes in plasma volume during pregnancy and the maternal blood supply to the placenta. Availability of growth substrates depends on perfusion of the intervillous spaces and availability of glucose, amino acids, and fats in maternal blood (see Chapter 15). Fetal growth does not seem to be greatly dependent on hormones such as growth hormone, thyroid hormones, glucocorticoids, and sex steroids that are critical for postnatal growth. Hormones and peptide growth factors believed to be necessary for fetal growth include insulin, human placental lactogen (hPL), insulin-like growth factors I and II (IGF-I and IGF-II), epidermal growth factor, platelet-derived growth factor, leptin, and transforming growth factor–α.[96] Insulin probably has a permissive rather than a direct effect on fetal growth by stimulating nutrient uptake and utilization. Growth factors appear early in gestation, beginning at the 4- to 8-cell stage.[96]

Early in gestation, placental and embryonic growth are regulated primarily by IGF-II. IGF-II is unaffected by nutrient availability. Thus embryo and placental growth are maintained even if maternal energy intake is decreased, as often occurs with NVP.[116] During the second and third trimesters, fetal growth becomes dependent on IGF-I. IGF-I is sensitive to nutrient status.[100,116,188] Another factor that is thought to have a role in fetal growth is placental leptin. Leptin secretion peaks around 8 weeks. Leptin is thought to act on hypothalamus to regulate food intake and satiety. During pregnancy, placental leptin may signal satiety to the maternal hypothalamus, thus resulting in reduced food intake and energy intake, which stimulates placental growth.[100,116] These factors are discussed further in Chapter 15.

Initial growth is slow during the first 2 months (period of organ formation), then accelerates rapidly. Maximum growth rate is achieved from the fourth to eighth months, when the fetus grows at the rate of 5% to 9% per week. Growth velocity slows after 32 weeks, with a mean increase of 12 to 15 g/day until term.[190] At the cellular level, growth occurs through hypertrophy (increased cell size) or hyperplasia (increased cell numbers). The human fetus undergoes primarily hyperplastic growth in early gestation (similar increases in deoxyribonucleic acid [DNA] and organ protein content), followed by a period of simultaneous hyperplasia and hypertrophy. From 34 to 35 weeks on, growth is predominantly hypertrophic.[104]

Maternal nutrition influences fetal growth. The effects of maternal nutrient restriction depend on the stage of pregnancy, length of restriction, and type of restriction. For example, if maternal nutrients are restricted throughout pregnancy, fetal growth restriction develops. If the restriction is only during the first trimester, infant birth weights tend to be within normal limits, with increased placental weight. Increased food intake in early gestation tends to be associated with infants with lower birth and placental weights. High carbohydrate intake in early pregnancy is associated with lower placental and birth weights. Restricted protein intake (and thus restricted intake of essential amino acids) in early pregnancy has a detrimental effect on both fetal and placental development.[116,169] Epidemiologic data suggest that averse in utero nutrition may have long-term effects on the infants, with a predisposition to chronic disease in adult life.[289]

Intrauterine Growth Restriction

Fetal growth restriction is "the failure of a fetus to achieve its growth potential,"[120] which in practice is stated as measures of absolute (i.e., low birth weight [LBW]) and relative (i.e., SGA) size. Measures of relative size often vary (e.g., less than the third or less than the tenth percentile, or more than 2 standard deviations below mean), making comparisons between different centers difficult.[120] Fetal growth restriction is evaluated by serial ultrasonographic measurements.

Factors that cause alterations in growth, such as malnutrition during the period of hyperplasia, can decrease the rate of cell division and result in organs or a fetus that is smaller in size with fewer cells. This form of growth alteration is not reversible after the time when hyperplastic cell growth would normally have ceased. Malnutrition during the period of hypertrophy results in organs or a fetus that is smaller in size (due to reduction in cell size) but has a normal number of cells. Hypertrophic growth alterations may be reversible with adequate nutrition. Since fetal tissues are undergoing hyperplastic growth throughout gestation, the fetus is especially vulnerable to irreversible changes at the cellular level.[273]

Factors altering fetal growth can be intrinsic or extrinsic (Figure 11-12).[70,100,217] Intrinsic factors are those within the fetus arising from chromosomal or genetic abnormalities or infectious agents that alter the normal process of cell division. Extrinsic factors include placental insufficiency and fetal malnutrition. Placental insufficiency due to maternal, fetal, or placental factors often results in caloric restriction to the fetus (inadequate glucose transported to meet fetal growth needs) and tends to occur later in gestation. Caloric restriction usually leads to an asymmetric growth failure in which brain growth is spared. Fetal malnutrition due to maternal protein restriction (arising from maternal malnutrition or significantly protein-reduced diets) results in symmetric fetal growth failure in which the brain is not spared.[273]

Management of fetal growth restriction varies with the underlying cause. Strategies range from prepregnancy counseling and preventative interventions such as cessation

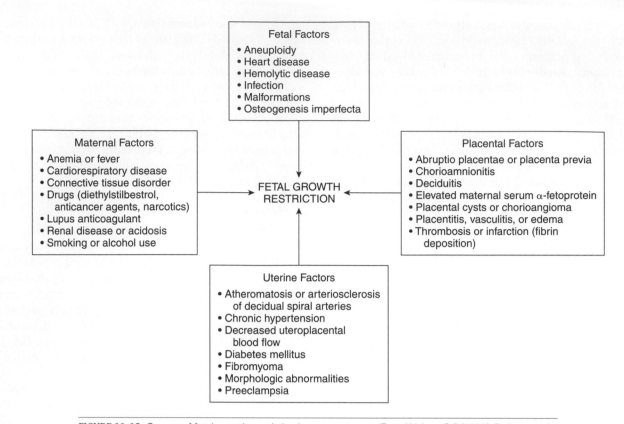

FIGURE **11-12** Causes of fetal growth restriction by compartment. (From Weiner, C.P. [1989]. Pathogenesis, evaluation and potential treatments from severe, early onset growth retardation. *Semin Perinatal, 13*, 321.)

of smoking and alcohol use, promotion of adequate nutrition, and early identification of and interventions for pathologic problems such as preeclampsia to fetal therapies. Fetal therapies that have been proposed or implemented include providing nutrient supplements (glucose and amino acids) to the fetus via infusions into the maternal circulation, the amniotic fluid, or directly into the fetus (by intraperitoneal catheter or cordocentesis) and improving uteroplacental blood flow (through maternal oxygen therapy, bed rest, and low-dose aspirin to reduce vasospasm).[104,120] The growth-restricted fetus and neonate are at risk for perinatal asphyxia, meconium aspiration, hypoglycemia, and other problems (Table 11-11).

NEONATAL PHYSIOLOGY

GI function in the neonate is characterized by functional, anatomic, and physiologic limitations, which are increased in the preterm infant. Provision of adequate nutritional support for growth and development is an ongoing challenge for nurses and other health care providers. As a result of the limitations in GI function, infants are at risk for dehydration, reflux, malabsorption, and electrolyte imbalance.

Transitional Events

Although the fetal GI system is involved with removal of amniotic fluid, digestive and absorptive functions are performed by the placenta. With birth the infant's GI system, although still functionally immature, must assume responsibility for supplying the infant's energy, nutrient, and fluid needs. The intestinal mucosal barrier (glycocalyx) remains immature for 4 to 6 months. During this period, antigens and other macromolecules can be transported across the intestinal epithelium into the systemic circulation, increasing the risk for both infection and the development of allergies.[14,268] With maturation of the epithelium (gut closure), uptake of macromolecules decreases. Gut closure and the development of intestinal flora are discussed further in Chapter 12.

Maturation of Gastrointestinal Function

Postnatal development of GI function is influenced by the infant's genetic endowment, intrinsic timing mechanisms,

TABLE **11-11**   Perinatal Adaptive Problems of Small for Gestational Age Infants

PROBLEM	PATHOGENESIS	PREVENTION
Perinatal asphyxia	↓ Placental reserve (insufficiency) ↓ Cardiac glycogen stores	Antepartum and intrapartum fetal heart rate monitoring
Meconium aspiration	Hypoxia/stress phenomenon	Oral-pharyngeal-tracheal suction
Fasting hypoglycemia	↓ Hepatic glycogen ↓ Gluconeogenesis	Early alimentation
Alimented hyperglycemia	"Starvation diabetes"	Avoid excessive carbohydrate loads
Polycythemia-hyperviscosity	Fetal hypoxia, ↑erythropoietin Placental transfusion	Neonatal partial exchange transfusion
Temperature instability	↓ Adipose tissue ↑ Heat loss	Ensure neutral thermal environment
Pulmonary hemorrhage (rare)	Hypothermia, ↓ oxygen, disseminated intravascular coagulation	Avoid cold stress and hypoxia
Immunodeficiency	"Malnutrition" effect	Unknown

Adapted from Kliegman, R.M. & Hulman, S.E. (1987). Intrauterine growth retardation: Determinants of aberrant fetal growth. In A.A. Fanaroff & R.J. Martin (Eds.), *Neonatal-perinatal medicine: Diseases of the fetus and infant*. St. Louis: Mosby.

TABLE **11-12**   Gastrointestinal Trophic Factors

GENERAL TROPHIC FACTORS FOR THE GI TRACT	FACTORS AFFECTING GI SECRETION	FACTORS AFFECTING GI MOTILITY
Nutrients, especially iron, zinc, vitamin B$_{12}$, vitamin A, folate, arginine, and glutamine	Secretin	Motilin
Hormones and peptides:	Gastrin	Enteroglucagon
Epidermal growth factor	Gastric inhibitory peptide	Vasoactive intestinal peptide
Transforming growth factor	Pancreatic polypeptide	Neurotensin
Insulin-like growth factor	Vasoactive intestinal peptide	Cholecystokinin
Insulin	Neurotensin	
Growth hormone		
Glucocorticoids		
Somatostatin		
Bombesin		
Intestinal peptide Y		
Others:		
Polyamines		
Nucleotides		

From Carver, J.D. & Barness, L.A. (1996). Trophic factors for the gastrointestinal tract. *Clin Perinatol*, 23, 266.

initiation of feeding, composition of the diet, hormonal regulatory mechanisms, and gut trophic factors (Table 11-12).[15,47,53,160] Hormonal regulatory mechanisms have a critical role in mediating development of the gut after birth. Postnatal gut maturation is stimulated by increases in specific GI hormones and enteric neuropeptides, including enteroglucagon (growth of the intestinal mucosa), gastrin (growth of gastric mucosa and exocrine pancreas), motilin and neurotensin (development of gut motor activity), and gastric inhibitory peptide (initiation of enteroinsular axis and subsequent glucose tolerance).[160,164,192,217,271] A major stimulus for increases in these hormones is initiation of enteral feeding, which induces surges in plasma concentrations of the hormones listed above in both term and preterm infants. The response is delayed in preterm infants and in infants on parenteral-only nutrition. Human milk is rich in many GI trophic factors and thus enhances postbirth GI adaptation and maturation.[53] Term infants with fetal distress have increased concentration of GI hormones, especially motilin, which may account for meconium passage. Increases in other hormones may cause redistribution of visceral blood flow in these infants.[15]

Term infants demonstrate marked changes in intermediary metabolites and secretions from the gut, pancreas, and pituitary within hours after birth (Table 11-13). Marked differences are seen in hormonal secretion with human milk versus formula by 6 days, with a greater insulin response in formula-fed infants that lasts to at least 9 months. This suggests that early feeding practices may have prolonged and subtle effects on programming hormonal responses to feeding.[271] Similar changes in interme-

diary metabolites and secretions are not seen in infants who are being given nothing by mouth (NPO) or are on only parenteral or intravenous feedings.[15,271] These responses are delayed for several days in preterm infants on enteral feeding, reflecting immaturity of gut responses.[15]

These surges seem to be triggered by small amounts of enteral feeding and are absent in unfed neonates.[15,29,164] This finding has implications for gut maturation in infants fed from birth by total parenteral nutrition (TPN) and has led to the use of minimal enteral feeding.[164] Small amounts of enteral feeding may be important to induce surges in gut hormones and maturation of the gut (see Minimal Enteral

TABLE 11-13   Changes in Gastrointestinal Hormones and Enteric Neuropeptides in Neonates

Substance	Site: Role	Postnatal Changes*	Implications
Gastrin	Stomach: Regulates gastric secretions; trophic effect on gastric mucosa.	Cord blood levels 4-5 fold higher than adult and remain higher for several weeks. Increase further with first feeding. Basal levels decline after 3 to 4 weeks and surge with feeding.	Gastric acid low in spite of high gastrin levels; may be a result of a lack of receptors or inhibitory effects of peptide YY and neurotensin, which allow gastrin to stimulate gastric mucosal maturation without excess acid secretion
Secretin	Duodenum: Neutralizes acidic chyme entering duodenum	Higher basal levels with a more marked increase with feeding in first 3 weeks.	May protect mucosa during maturation. Occurs even in absence of feeding.
Cholecystokinin (CCK)	Upper small intestine: Stimulates pancreatic enzyme secretion and gall bladder contraction	Postnatal surge	May enhance pancreatic growth.
Motilin	Small intestine: Increases gastric emptying and stimulates intestinal motility (interdigestive myoelectric complexes) between feedings.	Cord blood levels are low with marked postnatal surge peaking at 2 weeks. Peak is enhanced but delayed in preterm infants.	Increased motor activity in the neonatal gut
Glucose-dependent insulinotrophic peptide (GIP)	Jejunum: Increases insulin after meals	Low at birth, increasing gradually in first month	Increases associated with development of glucose responses
Neurotensin	Ileum: Inhibits gastric secretion and motility	Increases after feeding Response develops in first month	Decreases entry of chyme, enhancing early nutrient absorption
Peptide YY	Distal intestine: Inhibits gastric emptying and slows small bowel transit.	Elevated in cord blood, increasing further to 2 weeks at 50 times higher than adult levels	Prevents hyperacidity with increased gastrin in neonate
Enteroglucagon and glucagon-like peptides I and II	Small and large intestine: Secreted in parallel; enhance insulin secretion after feeding	Marked postnatal surge peaking in first week	Enhance gut maturation

Based on material from Vanderhoof, J.A., et al. (1999). Gastrointestinal disease. In G.B. Avery, M.A. Fletcher & M.G. MacDonald (Eds.). *Neonatology, pathophysiology and management of the newborn* (5th ed. Philadelphia: J.B. Lippincott.
*Surges seen only in infants who are fed enterally. All except secretin are low in infants on parenteral-only feedings.

Feedings). Maturation of gut functions and enzymes is described in the next section and summarized in Tables 11-13 and 11-14.

Initiation of Enteral Feeding

At birth the GI system must adapt to enteral nutrition. This process begins in fetal life and is still immature in the preterm infant (see Table 11-13). In addition to stimulating release of hormones critical for maturation of gut function, enteral feedings are also important as a source of energy and fluid for the infant. Human milk is the preferred feeding for both term and preterm infants. A healthy infant can be breastfed immediately after delivery. Colostrum is rich in antibodies, nonirritating, easily swallowed, and enhances meconium passage (see Chapter 5). Bottle-fed infants are usually fed within 6 to 8 hours, but can certainly be fed sooner, especially if at risk for hypoglycemia. Animal studies suggest that 5% dextrose water (D5W) is as damaging to the lungs if aspirated as formula. 10% Dextrose water (D10W) may be more damaging due to its lower pH and higher glucose content.[199] Aspiration of regurgitated sterile water mixed with gastric acid can also be irritating to lung tissue. Early feeding and adequate fluid intake are associated with decreased bilirubin levels (see Chapter 17). Initiation of feeding in ill or preterm infants depends on infant health status, maturity, and ability to tolerate feeding.

Minimal enteral feedings. Minimal enteral feeding, also called gut or GI priming, is early (within the first week after birth) introduction of small amounts of enteral feeding to induce surges in gut hormones and maturation of the gut rather than to meet the infant's nutritional needs, which are supplied by parenteral nutrition.[164,231] As noted above, providing even small amounts of enteral feeding in the first weeks following birth is important to stimulate gut hormones and subsequent maturation of the intestine.[29,164,197,231,245] There is no postbirth rise in gut hormones in preterm infants on total TPN, whereas infants fed orally demonstrate a marked increase in these hormones over the first week.[47] Surges of gut hormones still occur after up to 10 days (and perhaps longer) without oral feeding.[15] As little as 0.5 to 1.0 ml/kg/hour of enteral feeding appears to be beneficial.[197] These small volumes help build up mucosal bulk and stimulate development of brush border enzymes and pancreatic function; enhance maturation of GI hormones; and reduce the distention, vomiting, and malabsorption that often occur with resumption of enteral feeding. Early minimal feedings have also been reported to improve maturation of gut motor patterns, decrease feeding intolerance; improve weight gain; enhance transition to oral feedings; and decrease physiologic jaundice, cholestasis, osteopenia, glucose intolerance, and sepsis.[27,28,127,197,245] Early feeding with human milk may also stimulate maturation of lactase activity in the preterm infants.[230] Minimal

TABLE 11-14 Adaptation of the Gastrointestinal System to Enteral Nutrition*

INTRAUTERINE	TRANSITIONAL	EXTRAUTERINE
BARRIER FUNCTION		
"Immature" MVM	Maturing MVM, mucus, glycocalyx	"Mature" apical cellular barrier
SIgA in gut wall	SIgA in meconium and amniotic fluid	Low serum IgA; human milk rich in IgA
Cellular immunity	Inability of GALT to mount immune response	Capacity to make immunoglobulins with milk proteins
IELs, M cells, Peyer's patches		
MOTILITY		
Contrast moves down gut	Disorganized random contractions ("fetal complexes")	Coordinated MMCs
DIGESTION		
Uptake and intracellular sorting of macromolecules	End of intracellular MM processing, development of extracellular proteases	Near- to full-term exocrine pancreatic function
WEEKS OF GESTATION		
20	25-30	35-40

From Weaver, L.T. (1997). Digestive system development and failure. *Semin Neonatol, 2,* 228.
*Features of the human gastrointestinal tract during development that may determine success of adaptation to enteral nutrition. The transitional period is the time during which the tract changes from one adapted primarily to fetal life to one adapted to neonatal life.
GALT, Gut-associated lymphoid system; *IEL,* intraepithelial lymphocyte; *MMC,* migrating motor complex; *MM,* macromolecular; *MVM,* microvillous membrane; *SIgA,* secretory immunoglobulin A.

enteral feedings do not increase the risk of necrotizing enterocolitis (NEC) and may reduce the risk.[165,228]

Human milk is the preferred substance for minimal enteral feeding.[28,127] Use of sterile water does not provide the same enhancement of gut maturation as provision of feeding with nutrients.[28] Berseth and Nordyke compared small-volume nutrient feedings with sterile water feeding during the first 2 weeks in preterm infants. Infants fed sterile water had delayed maturation of motor activity and establishment of full enteral nutrition.[28] Other studies have also demonstrated enhancement of GI motility with full strength (versus dilute or water) feedings.[18,28] Although minimal enteral feeding is usually provided via continuous infusion, Schandler et al recently reported that bolus feeding may lead to greater feeding tolerance and weight gain.[231]

Passage of Meconium

Passage of meconium is an essential step in initiation of intestinal function. Meconium consists of vernix caseosa, lanugo, squamous epithelial cells, occult blood, and bile and other intestinal secretions. Initially meconium is sterile, with bacteria appearing by 24 hours of age. Most term infants pass meconium by 12 (69%) to 24 (94%) hours and almost all (99.8%) by 48 hours of age.[244] Meconium passage is delayed in preterm infants, probably due to immaturity of gut motility patterns. Only 37% of preterm infants pass meconium by 24 hours, 69% by 48 hours and 99% by 9 days.[278] Although failure to pass meconium is a frequent sign of intestinal obstruction, infants with a high-level complete obstruction such as a duodenal atresia may occasionally pass meconium stool. Delayed passage of meconium is associated with elevated bilirubin levels, probably due to continued action of the intestinal deconjugating enzyme, β-glucuronidase, with reabsorption of the unconjugated bilirubin and recirculation to the liver via the enterohepatic circulation (see Chapter 17).

Functional and Anatomic Limitations

GI function is still maturing at birth, especially in preterm infants, which increases the risk of malabsorption and malnutrition. Functional and anatomic maturation includes suck-swallow reflexes, esophageal motility, function of the LES, gastric emptying, intestinal motility, and development of absorptive surface area.

Sucking and Swallowing

Reflexes needed for food intake mature in the fetus during the third trimester (Figure 11-6). The swallow reflex is well developed by 28 to 30 weeks but easily exhausted. This reflex is complete by about 34 weeks. In newborns, air enters the stomach via the nasal passages with swallowing. Since air can compete with milk for space in the infant's stomach and lead to regurgitation, burping is used to release this air. The gag reflex may be present by 18 weeks but is not complete until around 34 weeks.

Infants demonstrate nutritive and nonnutritive sucking (NNS). Nutritive sucking brings milk into the oral cavity by compression of the nipple and generation of negative pressure. NNS occurs either with or without stimulation by a nipple, is more rapid than nutritive sucking, and has a regular burst-pause pattern.[108,157] Fetuses by 13 to 15 weeks respond to oral stimulation with tongue protrusion, rooting, and sucking. Older fetuses have been noted on ultrasound to suck reflexively on their fingers.[12,107] NNS is present in preterm infants by at least 24 weeks, and possibly earlier, but does not develop a rhythmic pattern until about 33 weeks and is not mature until 37 weeks.[31,107,210] The sucking reflex usually is not well enough developed for nutritive sucking until 32 to 34 weeks. Sucking is thought to stimulate secretion of GI regulatory peptides and thus enhance gastric emptying.[271] Sucking can be affected by maternal medications and perinatal complications.

Although all components of sucking and swallowing are present by 28 weeks, the infant is unable to coordinate these activities. Some suck-swallow synchrony is seen by 32 to 34 weeks; synchrony is complete by 36 to 38 weeks. Suck-swallow coordination has been demonstrated earlier for breastfeeding than for bottle feeding.[182]

Gryboski and Walker described three stages in the development of suck-swallow patterns: (1) mouthing with no effective sucking; (2) an immature sucking pattern with short bursts of sucking not synchronized with swallowing; and (3) a mature pattern with long bursts of sucking accompanied by swallowing and associated with propulsive peristaltic waves in the esophagus.[106] Sucking is observed in term infants from birth; however, the mature suck-swallow pattern does not appear for several days. A transient immature suck-swallow pattern seen with the first few feedings is characterized by short bursts of three to five sucks followed by swallowing.[106] Within 24 to 48 hours, a mature pattern emerges, characterized by a prolonged burst of 30 or more sucks, with approximately 1 to 2 sucks per second and swallowing every 5 to 6 sucks.[157,159]

In contrast, preterm infants tend to have short bursts of sucking, followed by swallowing, often accompanied by a rest period (for breathing) before sucking resumes. Preterm infants are limited in their ability to suck by their weaker flexor control (important for firm lip and jaw closure) and immature musculature. Organization of sucking into a burst-pause pattern seems to occur earlier with breast-feeding than with bottle feeding. Meier reported that by 32 weeks, breastfed infants have an organized sucking pattern with bursts of two to three sucks followed by a pause.[182] Assessment of an infant's suck, swallow, and gag capabilities is important before initiation of enteral feeding.

Infants must also be able to coordinate breathing with sucking and swallowing. From 38 weeks to 6 months, infants can easily coordinate these activities. After 6 months this ability is gradually lost. Until about 3 months of age, solids placed in the infant's mouth will be forced up against the palate by the tongue and then either swallowed or flow out the mouth.[60] By 3 to 4 months of age, the infant begins to be able to selectively transfer semisolid food to the back of the mouth for swallowing.

Esophageal Motility and Lower Esophageal Sphincter Function

Esophageal motility is decreased in the newborn, especially during the first 12 hours after birth. Esophageal peristalsis is increased and accompanied by simultaneous nonperistaltic contractions, with poor coordination of esophageal motility and swallowing. (GI motility refers to oscillating contractions in small segments that mix food versus the large peristaltic waves that propel food along the tract.) Basal tone and length of the LES are reduced in infants. The LES, which forms a pressure barrier between the esophagus and stomach, is divided into three sections. In children and adults, the upper section is above the diaphragm (under the influence of intrathoracic pressure), the middle section is at the level of the LES, and the lower is below the diaphragm (under the influence of abdominal pressure). This anatomy protects against reflux. In the neonate the LES is primarily above the diaphragm and reflux more likley.[34,114] LES pressure increases from 4 mm Hg at 27 to 28 weeks to 18 mm Hg at term.[197] Although LES pressures increase with gestation, even the very-low–birth-weight (VLBW) infant is able to generate effective LES pressures.[185]

The infant has transient periods of LES relaxation that increase the risk of reflux.[44] The LES may also relax transiently from pressure on the fundus of the stomach from overdistention, as may occur with delayed gastric emptying.[34] In addition infants have a shorter esophagus and the angle formed by the fundus of the stomach and esophagus is less acute, also increasing the risk of reflux.[34] Alterations in the LES are related to incomplete development and possibly decreased responsiveness to gastrin (which enhances LES pressure) due to delayed maturation of hormonal receptors. LES tone develops rapidly during the first week; however, the sphincter may remain immature for up to 6 to 12 months.

Gastric Emptying

Gastric motility and muscle tone are decreased and emptying time is delayed in the newborn. The delay in gastric emptying may have a hormonal basis with delayed maturation of feedback control mechanisms. The elevated gastrin level in the newborn also delays emptying.[159] Antroduodenal activity (coordination of contractions between the antral portion of stomach and the duodenum) is five times lower in preterm as compared to term infants, markedly delaying gastric emptying.[119] Gastric emptying may take 2 to 6 hours or longer in these infants.[97]

Gastric emptying is influenced by other factors such as muscle tone, mucus, pyloric sphincter tone, presence of amniotic fluid, hormones, and type of food. Carbohydrate increases emptying time, and fat decreases emptying time. Medium-chain triglycerides empty faster than long-chain ones.[31,197] Human milk empties more rapidly than formula or dextrose water, and D5W empties faster than D10W.[78,230] Formulas with higher caloric density are retained in the stomach for longer periods (although these formulas are associated with emptying of more calories over comparative periods).[197]

Mucus delays gastric emptying, especially during the first 24 hours after birth. Upright or semiupright positions decrease the likelihood of air passing from the stomach to the duodenum. The gastric capacity of an infant is approximately 6 ml per kilogram of body weight. In preterm infants, large residual gastric volumes may develop, leading to gastric distention, compromised respiratory function, and interference with delivery of adequate nutrients.[197]

Intestinal Motility

Mature intestinal interdigestive motility patterns involve three phases, which recycle over a 60- to 90-minute period. Phase I is quiescence, phase II is characterized by irregular contractions, and phase III by regular phasic contractions. Contractions during phase II and III migrate down the intestine and are called *migratory motor complexes* (MMCs).[30,31,44] Intestinal motility patterns and gastric emptying begin to mature after 30 to 32 weeks but are still somewhat disorganized to near term age.[192] Between 29 and 32 weeks, infants begin to develop periods of gut quiescence interspersed with short bursts of activity called *clusters*. Between 32 and 36 weeks, motor activity becomes more organized, with cycling between quiescence and activity clusters.[31] Frequency of cluster decreases with increasing gestational age (from 12 to 14 per min at 27 to 28 weeks to 6 to 8 per min by term).[33] As cluster frequency decreases, MMCs appear.[33] MMCs are first seen by 32 to 34 weeks' gestation and are mediated by motilin.[30] Motilin receptors are not functional until 32 weeks' gestation, with an absence of cyclic motilin release in the preterm infants.[30] MMCs are rare during fasting in infants who instead have periods of quiescence alternating with nonmigratory phasic activity. With increasing gestational age, the length of the activity clusters increases and their frequency decreases.[30]

In adults given milk, motor activity increases (mature fed response). Most (85%) term infants have a mature gut fed response.[30,69] Preterm infants may have a mature fed response but are more likely to have an immature response (motor activity decreases with feeding) or interdeterminate response (motor activity does not change with feeding).[30] For example, two thirds of preterm infants less than 35 weeks of age have an immature response, 10% an interdeterminate response, and 25% a mature response.[11] By term only 15% have an immature response. Thus most term infants have increased intestinal motility with feeding, whereas in most preterm infants contractions cease, possibly due to vagal immaturity.[7] The cessation of contractions with feeding in the preterm infants lasts for 15 to 20 minutes and then gradually resumes. Alterations in motility in the preterm infants may limit the ability of these infants to tolerate enteral feedings due to less efficient propulsion of food, delayed gastric emptying, and slower intestinal transit time.[30,197] Antenatal corticosteroids may enhance maturation of GI motor activity.[19]

Intestinal movement tends to be more disorganized and slower in newborns due to immaturity of the intestinal musculature, poor coordination of peristaltic waves, and a tendency for segmentation of peristalsis.[97] Disorganized motility results in a decreased ability to clear the upper gut, with impaired absorptive function, prolonged transit time in the upper intestine, and more rapid emptying of the ileum and colon. Intestinal transit time averages 4 to 12 hours in adults versus 8 to 96 hours in the preterm infant.[30] Prolonged transit time in the small intestine may also be an advantage by increasing chances for absorption of specific nutrients. However, faster emptying of the colon reduces the time for water and electrolyte absorption, increasing stool water content and the risk of dehydration and electrolyte imbalance. The gastrocolonic reflex is active in the neonate: entry of food into the beginning of the small intestine or colon causes reflexive propulsion of food toward the rectum.

The preterm infant experiences even more irregular and less predictable peristaltic waves along with antiperistaltic waves. These limitations further increase transit time and impair absorption. GI peristalsis develops gradually in the fetus from 33 to 40 weeks' gestation. Immaturity of peristalsis in the preterm infant is one reason that fetal passage of meconium is rarely seen before 34 weeks' gestation.

Intestinal Surface Area

The immature surface of the small intestine decreases absorptive area, especially in preterm infants. Numbers of intestinal villi and epithelial cells increase with gestation. In the mature intestine, epithelial cells in the crypts are undifferentiated and develop the ability to hydrolyze and transport nutrients as they migrate toward the top of the villus, replacing older cells. Turnover of intestinal epithelial cells is decreased in the newborn, impairing absorptive efficiency.

Alterations in the normal crypt-to-villous cell turnover rate lead to inadequate functional surface area along the brush border and glycocalyx and alter digestion, absorption, and host defense mechanisms. The surface area of the small intestine can be altered by anoxia and infection, further impeding absorption of nutrients. Enteric intake after birth induces epithelial hyperplasia, increasing cell turnover and stimulating production of microvillous enzymes such as pancreatic lipase, amylase, and trypsin.[29,164] Gut regulatory peptides and hormones increase at birth and have a trophic effect on the intestine (Tables 11-12 and 11-13).[26,160,195] Colostrum and human milk contain factors that stimulate epithelial cell turnover and maturation.[25,195] The gut mucosal immune system is still immature at term, increasing the risk of infection and other disoders.[25,174,276] Human milk contains substances that not only protect the infants from infection but also enhance maturation of this system ("gut closure").[25] Gut closure is discussed further in Chapter 12.

Physiologic Limitations

Newborns are limited in their ability to digest and absorb certain nutrients due to decreased activity of specific enzymes and other substances as well as functional and anatomic limitations. However, newborns, especially if fed human milk, have mechanisms available that partially compensate for these alterations, resulting in relatively proficient digestion in term and many preterm infants.

A prominent difference in digestive processes between the neonate and adult is immaturity of exocrine pancreatic function, which forces the infant to use compensatory mechanisms that rely on nonpancreatic enzymes found in the lingual area and salivary secretions, intestinal brush border, enterocyte, and human milk. Slow development of pancreatic exocrine function may be a protective mechanism to prevent degradation and loss of intestinal epithelial cells and brush border enzymes by the pancreatic proteolytic enzymes.[109] Limitations of the newborn related to digestion and absorption of protein, carbohydrate, and fat and compensatory mechanisms are summarized in Table 11-15. Digestion and absorption are summarized in Figure 11-1.

TABLE **11-15**   Physiologic Limitations in Digestion and Absorption of Protein, Carbohydrate, and Fat in the Neonate

FACTOR	LIMITATION IN NEONATE	IMPLICATION	COMPENSATORY MECHANISMS
DIGESTION AND ABSORPTION OF PROTEIN			
Gastric acid	50% of adult values	Increased gastric pH Decreased pepsin activity Decreased gastric proteolysis	
Pepsinogen	50% of adult values	Decreased pepsin Decreased gastric proteolysis	
Trypsin	Near adult levels (but activity reduced)	Decreased proteolysis	
Enterokinase	10% of adult activity	Decreased activation of trypsin and other pancreatic peptidases	
Chymotrypsin	10%-60% of adult activity	Decreased proteolysis	
Carboxypeptidases	10%-60% of adult activity	Decreased proteolysis	
Intestinal mucosal dipeptidases	Adequate	Promote protein digestion	
Amino acid absorption	Adequate	Adequate absorption of amino acids and some intact proteins	
DIGESTION AND ABSORPTION OF CARBOHYDRATE			
Salivary amylase	⅓ of adult levels	Decreased starch digestion (infants ingest little starch)	Increased gastric pH helps retain activity in stomach Used to digest glucose polymers
Pancreatic amylase	0.2%-5% of adult levels	Decreased starch digestion	Mammary amylase
Sucrase, maltases, isomaltase	Adequate digestion of sucrose, maltose, isomaltose		
Adequate			
Glucoamylase	50%-100% of adult levels	Enhances digestion of glucose polymers	
Lactase	Term is two to four times greater than older children; preterm is 30% of term by 28-30 weeks	Term infant able to digest lactose well; preterm infant has limited lactose digestion	Colonic salvage
Glucose absorption	Term is 50%-60% of adult; lower in preterm	Adequate absorption at low levels; more problems in handling glucose load	
DIGESTION AND ABSORPTION OF FAT			
Pancreatic lipase	10%-20% of adult levels	Decreased fat digestion	Lingual and gastric lipase Human milk bile salt–stimulated lipase
Bile acids	Synthesis and bile acid pool Term is ½ adult values; preterm is ⅙ adult values Decreased reabsorption through the enterohepatic circulation	Decreased fat digestion and absorption Steatorrhea in preterm infants	Human milk bile salt–stimulated lipase

Digestion and Absorption of Proteins

In spite of limitations in amounts and function of proteolytic enzymes, term and many preterm infants digest and absorb proteins relatively well.[157,253] The newborn's initial gastric pH is neutral or slightly alkaline.[156] Decreased secretion of gastric acid and prolonged buffering by the stomach contents due to delayed gastric emptying in newborns increase gastric pH. Amniotic fluid in the stomach further elevates gastric pH during the initial 24 hours. Acid secretion is further decreased and gastric pH increased in preterm infants. However, even the extremely LBW infant can achieve a gastric pH lower than 4.[197]

Gastric acid secretion increases within 24 hours of birth, then falls and remains low for at least 3 weeks, with varying findings in different studies.[102,282] Werchil notes that most studies agree that the highest acid concentration is found within the first 10 days and the lowest between 10 to 30 days.[282] Pepsinogen production is low (corrected for weight) for the first few months and is even lower in preterm infants.[24,157] The elevated pH reduces pepsin activity and gastric peptic hydrolysis in both term and preterm infants.[47,111,156] Although circulating levels of gastrin (which normally stimulates secretion of gastric acid and pepsin) are elevated, receptors for this hormone may be immature.[157,160] The decreased gastric acidity and pepsinogen levels may enhance development of gut host defense mechanisms by promoting activity of immunoglobulins and antigen recognition by the GI tract.[157,291]

Term and preterm infants have near adult levels of trypsin, but activity of trypsin and the other pancreatic proteolytic hormones is reduced. Chymotrypsin and carboxypeptidase B activity are 10% to 60% and enterokinase activity is 10% of adult values. Since enterokinase activates trypsin, which in turn activates the other pancreatic proteolytic enzymes, the level of enterokinase is the rate-limiting step for intestinal protein digestion.[111,157,232,253] This limitation does not seem to have a major impact on infants over 26 to 28 weeks' gestation, who are usually able to digest and absorb 85% of the dietary protein in human milk and most formulas.[47] Preterm infants cannot handle excessive protein loads (>5 g/kg/day). Intestinal mucosal dipeptidase activity, along with the ability to transport and absorb amino acids, develops early in gestation. The newborn's intestine absorbs more intact proteins and macromolecules, which may increase the risk for development of allergies (see Chapter 12) and NEC in infants fed formula.[14,156] In breastfed infants, absorption of macromolecules from breast milk enhances passive immunity.[195]

Digestion and Absorption of Carbohydrates

Carbohydrate digestion in adults is dependent on salivary and pancreatic amylase and disaccharidases (see Figure 11-1, A). Salivary amylase activity at birth is one third that of adults. Levels increase after 3 to 6 months of age and may be related to the addition of starch (solid foods) to the infant's diet.[102,158,187,232,171] Salivary amylase, although inactivated by gastric acid, retains some activity in the infant's stomach and is effective in digestion of glucose polymers.[271]

Pancreatic amylase activity is decreased in term and preterm infants to 0.2% to 5% of adult values. Adequate levels are achieved after 4 to 6 months.[109,127] Cholecystokinin and secretin have little effect on pancreatic amylase secretion prior to 1 month. Amylase activity increases significantly after this time.

Mammary amylase in human milk compensates for the decreased pancreatic amylase. Mammary amylase is highest in colostrum, gradually decreasing after 6 weeks.[56,109] Buffers in human milk and the higher gastric pH in the neonate help maintain mammary amylase activity.[53,158]

The term newborn has adequate levels of α-glucosidases such as sucrase, maltases, isomaltase, and glucoamylase. Sucrase and maltases attain maximal activity by 32 to 34 weeks' gestation or earlier. Glucoamylase is an intestinal brush border enzyme that digests glucose polymers found in many formulas.[47,158] Levels of glucoamylase are 50% to 100% of adult values and increase rapidly after birth.[157,271] Glucoamylase is less susceptible than disaccharidases to intestinal mucosal injury. This enzyme is evenly distributed along the small intestine, which along with the prolonged transit time seen in infants contributes to more efficient hydrolysis and mucosal uptake.[158,160] Digestion of glucose polymers depends on salivary amylase, glucoamylase, and human milk amylase. Neonates can effectively hydrolyze and absorb glucose polymers, especially those of short- to medium-chain length.

The major carbohydrate in human and cow's milk is lactose. Lactase activity increases rapidly in late gestation and is adequate after 36 weeks. At term, lactase levels are two to four times higher than in older infants.[136,187] Lactase activity at 28 to 34 weeks is only 30% of term values, but increases after birth with exposure to lactose.[127,156] In spite of low lactase activity, most preterm infants digest lactose adequately, especially lactose in human milk.[127,136,195] Lactose that is not absorbed in the small intestines is conserved by colonic salvage.

Colonic salvage involves bacterial fermentation of carbohydrate to hydrogen gas and short-chain fatty acids, which are absorbed by the colon, minimizing carbohydrate loss in stools (Figure 11-13).[31,127,136,138,187] These fatty acids are a source of calories, enhance fluid and electrolyte ab-

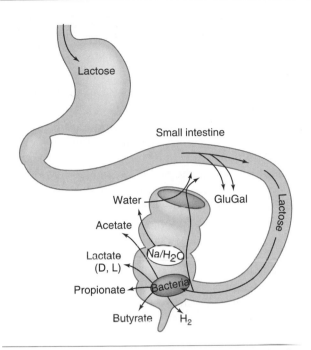

FIGURE **11-13** The two major fates of dietary lactose: (1) digestion in the small intestine with absorption of glucose *(Glu)* and galactose *(Gal)*, or (2) fermentation in the colon to various gases such as H₂; lactate; and short-chain fatty acids including acetate, propionate, and butyrate. The absorption of short-chain fatty acids simulates sodium and water absorption in the colon. Unfermented lactose may exert and osmotic stimulus causing fecal excretion of water. (From Kien, C.L. [1996]. Digestion, absorption, and fermentation of carbohydrates in the newborn. *Clin Perinatol, 23,* 213.)

sorption by the colon, and promote cell replication in the gut.[127] In preterm infants, two thirds of the ingested lactose may reach the colon. Changes in colonic bacterial flora following antibiotic use or surgery may alter the infant's ability to conserve energy via colonic salvage.[47] Lactase deficiency generally resolves when the preterm infant reaches a postconceptional age of 36 to 40 weeks.[156] These infants need some lactose intake since lactose enhances calcium absorption.

Mechanisms for glucose, galactose, and fructose absorption develop early in gestation and are relatively mature. The capacity for mucosal glucose uptake at term is 50% to 60% of adult values.[157] Absorption of glucose is slower in preterm infants, with further reductions in SGA infants suggesting that IUGR may delay maturation of these processes. Infants seem to absorb glucose as well as adults at low glucose concentrations but have a maximal absorptive capacity about 20% that of the adult.[252] Glucose transport increases by 2 to 3 weeks of age.[158] Hypoxia and ischemia decrease intestinal perfusion, altering the ultra-

structure of intestinal cells, which decreases active transport and uptake of glucose.[252]

Digestion and Absorption of Fats

Fat digestion in the adult relies on pancreatic lipase to break down triglycerides and bile acids to emulsify fat droplets prior to and during lipolysis (see Figure 11-1, *C*). These processes are decreased in term and especially in preterm and SGA infants.[156] Lipase activity at term is 10% to 20% of that seen in older children, partly due to minimal responsiveness by pancreatic acinar cells to secretin and cholecystokinin during the first month. Term infants fail to absorb 10% to 15% and preterm infants 30% or more of ingested fat.[31,97] Thus steatorrhea is more common in preterm infants.[97]

Bile acid synthesis and pool size are one half of adult values in term infants, and one sixth of adult and one third of term infant values in preterm infants.[156,271] Since hepatic conjugation of bile acids in infants is taurine dependent (versus glycine dependent in the adult), adequate intake of taurine is essential in infancy.[157] The decreased bile acid pools are due to reduced hepatic synthesis and poorer recirculation and conservation of bile salts through enterohepatic shunting as a result of immaturity of liver and intestinal active transport processes.[47,157,236,277] Antenatal corticosteroids may enhance maturity of bile salt pools in preterm infants.[97]

In preterm infants, concentrations of bile acids in the duodenal lumen may be below critical levels necessary for micelle formation (water-soluble aggregates of lipids and lipid-soluble substances).[47,272] Decreased micelle formation results in poor absorption of long-chain triglycerides, which are dependent on micelle formation for solubilization and subsequent hydrolysis (see Figure 11-1C). Infants are better able to absorb medium- and short-chain triglycerides, which are not dependent on micelle formation.

Alternative pathways to compensate for the decreased levels of pancreatic lipase and bile acids include human milk bile salt stimulated lipase (also called *mammary lipase* or *milk digestive lipase*), lingual lipase, and gastric lipase. Both gastric and lingual lipase have high activity at birth.[31,111] Gastric lipase activity is high by at least 25 weeks' gestation and remains high until 34 weeks, when it increases about 40%, then falls slightly to term.[194] Lingual and gastric lipases hydrolyze 50% and mammary lipase 20% to 40% of dietary fat in infants.[97,109] Intragastric lipolysis by these extrapancreatic lipases breaks down triglycerides in the milk fat globule. As a result, the fat globule is a better substrate for the available pancreatic lipase and enhances action of bile salts. Extensive hydrolysis of fat in the stomach can be documented in preterm infants as young as 26 to 32 weeks' gestation.[109,111]

Sucking is a stimulus for secretion of lingual lipase. Since lingual lipase is decreased in some preterm infants, NNS with gavage feedings may stimulate secretion of this enzyme with subsequent improvement of fat digestion and absorption. This has been suggested, although not well documented, as a basis for the improved weight gain reported with NNS.[41]

Mammary lipase is present in the milk of term and preterm mothers. This enzyme is stable at low pH (and not inactivated in the stomach) and hydrolyzes triglycerides at low concentrations of bile salts.[109,110] Mammary lipase works in the duodenum, and its activity is stimulated by bile salts at concentrations below those required for micelle formation such as are found in many preterm infants.[277] Temperatures above 55° C inactivate this enzyme; freezing (to −80° C) does not seem to affect its activity.[109,110] This lipase also produces monolauryl, a substance with antibacterial, antiviral, and antifungal activity.

Absorption of Other Substances

Alterations in fat absorption affect absorption of fat-soluble vitamins, especially in preterm infants who may need supplementation with water-soluble analogues. Absorptive capacity for folate is also lower. Lower gastric secretion of intrinsic factor may interfere with absorption of vitamin B_{12}.[156] Neonates are less able to adapt to changes in osmotic load in the large intestine, increasing the risk of diarrhea and electrolyte imbalance.

Mechanisms for absorption of iron are relatively well developed in term and preterm infants, with a high rate of iron absorption for the first 10 weeks.[156] Iron in human milk is absorbed better than iron in formula, with absorption of up to 50% of the iron in human milk, even in preterm infants.[157,271] For the first few months, preterm infants may not absorb large quantities of iron due to saturation of transferrin with iron from turnover of red blood cells (see Chapter 7).

Calcium absorption is influenced by vitamin D, calcium, and phosphorus concentrations; fatty acids; and lactose (see Chapter 16). The complex relationship between calcium and lipid intake makes determining calcium concentrations for formulas difficult. A high calcium intake alters absorption and retention of fatty acids; a high lipid intake can decrease calcium absorption.[156] Calcium absorption is lower in infants than in adults when calcium concentrations are low, but more efficient at higher levels.[157] Zinc and copper are well absorbed in term infants but not in preterm infants, who may be in negative zinc or copper balance for several months.[157,283,296] Mechanisms for

absorption of many nutrients have not been well studied in human neonates.

Liver Function in the Neonate

Portal blood flow is lower in the fetus, with shunting of blood flow away from the portal sinuses and liver parenchyma into the inferior vena cava via the ductus venosus. Many excretory and detoxification functions of the fetal liver are assumed by the placenta and maternal liver. With removal of the placenta, blood flow through the ductus venosus ceases, with anatomic closure by proliferation of connective tissue by approximately 2 weeks in most term infants (see Chapter 8).

The newborn liver accounts for about 5% of the infant's weight. This physiologic enlargement is a result of: (1) increased labile connective tissue (possibly in response to hypoxic stress with the abrupt shift in the oxygenation of blood supplying the liver at birth [i.e., from well-oxygenated blood from the placenta to systemic venous blood]); (2) active liver hematopoiesis, which decreases in a few weeks as liver metabolic functions increase; (3) increased liver glycogen; and (4) hepatic congestion due to changes in blood flow with removal of the placenta.[106]

Infants have a unique pathologic response to liver dysfunction, with active fibroblastic proliferation and early bile stasis that can alter the presentation of liver disorders. Decreased bile flow (cholestasis)—often in association with a direct (conjugated) hyperbilirubinemia—is seen with many liver disorders in infants. The cholestasis is due to disruption of the canalicular membrane, poor development of bile acid secretory mechanisms, and immaturity of bile acid synthesis.[106,237]

Liver enzyme systems necessary for metabolism of some drugs are depressed in the newborn. In the mature liver, oxidation and conjugation result in water-soluble drugs that are more readily excreted into bile. In the fetus, depression of these processes is an advantage, since lipid-soluble metabolites are more readily transferred across the placenta, where they can be handled by the maternal system. The liver smooth endoplastic reticulum (SER) is the location of many hepatic microsomal enzymes. The neonatal liver has little SER, and activities of microsomal enzymes are reduced or undetectable at birth, interfering with drug metabolism.[106] Hepatic metabolism of drugs is discussed in Chapter 6.

CLINICAL IMPLICATIONS FOR NEONATAL CARE

Food and warmth are "two of the most important controllable factors in determining survival and normal development."[206,p.645] Limitations of GI function in term and preterm neonates have major implications for the infant's nutritional needs and the composition and method of feedings. The feeding of sick and preterm infants is associated with many controversies, including when, what, and how to feed. Decisions regarding feeding can lead to other problems such as an increased risk of NEC and metabolic or nutritional alterations. This section reviews nutritional requirements of infants and implications of GI limitations for the selection of method and composition of feedings. Problems related to neonatal physiologic limitations such as reflux, dehydration, diarrhea, and NEC are also examined.

Infant Growth

Growth rates during the neonatal period are more rapid than at any other time. The method for growth assessment of term infants generally involves use of standardized charts from the National Center for Health and Statistics.[205] These charts have been recently revised to include a broader population base as well as more breastfed infants. Expected patterns and assessment of growth for preterm infants in the immediate postbirth period are controversial, especially regarding whether these infants should be expected to follow intrauterine or extrauterine patterns. Both intrauterine and extrauterine growth standards are available.

Generally recommendations have been that postnatal growth of preterm infants follow the pattern for intrauterine growth of a fetus of the same gestation, although it is unclear whether intrauterine rates are appropriate or realistic for these infants.[205] A variety of intrauterine growth charts are available, all of which have limitations in that they were developed from measurements of preterm infants at various gestations who may not represent a normal fetal population.[205] The growth chart used should be one that is most appropriate for the location and patient population (ethnic, socioeconomic, and demographic characteristics). General parameters for daily weight gain are in Table 11-16. New postnatal growth grids for LBW and VLBW infants for the first 3 years (using gestation-adjusted ages) have been developed recently for postdischarge care.[94,95]

Nutritional Requirements of Full and Preterm Infants

Nutritional requirements of infants vary with gestational age and health status. Requirements for healthy term infants are assumed to be those found in human milk. Recommended dietary allowances for term infants are in Table 11-17. For infants who are not breastfed, commercial formulas are alternatives for meeting nutritional needs. Whole cow's milk and evaporated milk do not meet cur-

TABLE **11-16**   Approximate Daily Weight Gain for Infants

Age	Weight
GESTATIONAL AGE	
24-28 weeks	15-20 g/kg/day
29-32 weeks	17-21 g/kg/day
33-36 weeks	14-15 g/kg/day
37-40 weeks	7-9 g/kg/day
CORRECTED AGE	
40 weeks-3 months	30 g/day
3-6 months	12 g/day
6-9 months	15 g/day
9-2 months	10 g/day
12-24 months	6 g/day

From Kalhan, S.C. & Price, P.T. (1999). Nutrition and selected disorders of the gastrointestinal tract. I: Nutrition for the high risk infant. In M.H. Klaus & A.A. Fanaroff (Eds.). *Care of the high risk neonate* (5th ed.). Philadelphia: W.B. Saunders.

rent standards for infant nutrition.[193] Nutritional requirements for preterm infants are less clear. One problem is lack of knowledge and agreement on what is the optimal growth rate for the preterm infants and how closely this rate should parallel that of the fetus. Nutritional requirements for preterm infants are often estimated by assaying the body composition of fetuses at different gestational ages and examining fetal accretion of different nutrients. Water, energy, and caloric requirements are higher for preterm infants because of greater insensible water loss (see Chapter 10), increased exposure to stressors, and increased expectations for growth.

Energy needs vary depending on the infant's age, thermal environment, activity, maturation, growth rate, and health status.[127] Maintenance caloric requirements are calculated based on resting energy expenditure, activity, cold stress, and fecal losses (Table 11-18). Growth requires additional calories (approximately 45 kcal for each 1 g weight gain).[127] The caloric (energy) maintenance and growth requirement for breastfed term newborns averages 85 to 100 kcal/kg/day, with 100 to 110 kcal/kg/day for formula-fed newborns.[97]

Preterm infants have maintenance requirements of approximately 50 to 60 kcal/kg/day, although this may be higher for some infants, depending on the infant's basal metabolic rate (increased with health problems), activity level (decreased in infants on morphine or fentanyl), cold stress (increases metabolic rate), specific dynamic action (efficiency of nutrient absorption), and fecal losses. For growth these infants need an additional 45 to 70 kcal/kg/day.[127] Increasing the growth allowance above this level will

TABLE **11-17** Recommended Dietary Allowances for Full-Term Infants

COMPONENT, UNITS/DAY	0-6 MONTHS	6-12 MONTHS
Estimated body weight, kg	6	9
Energy, kcal	650	850
Protein, g	13	14
Calcium, mg	400	600
Phosphorus, mg	300	500
Magnesium, mg	40	60
Sodium, mg	120	200
Potassium, mg	500	700
Chloride, mg	180	300
Zinc, μg	5000	5000
Copper, μg	400-600	600-700
Chromium, μg	10-40	20-60
Manganese, μg	300-600	600-1000
Selenium, μg	10	15
Vitamin A, IU	1250	1250
Vitamin D, IU	300	400
Vitamin E, IU	3	4
Vitamin K, μg	5*	10
Thiamine (vitamin B_1), μg	300	400
Riboflavin (vitamin B_2), μg	400	500
Pyridoxine (vitamin B_6), μg	300	600
Niacin, mg	5	6
Biotin, μg	10	15
Pantothenic acid, mg	2	3
Folic acid, μg	25	35
Vitamin B_{12}, μg	0.3	0.5
Ascorbic acid, mg	30	35

Data from National Academy of Science (1989). *Recommended dietary allowances* (10th ed.). Washington, DC: National Academy of Science; table from Schandler, R.J., et al. (1998). Parenteral and enteral nutrition. In H.W. Taeusch & R.A. Ballard (Eds.). *Avery's diseases of the newborn* (7th ed.). Philadelphia: W.B. Saunders.
*Vitamin K, 0.5 mg also administered at birth.

TABLE **11-18** Estimated Energy Expenditure in a Growing Preterm Infant

EXPENDITURE	kcal/kg/DAY
Resting energy expenditure	47
Minimal activity*	4
Occasional cold stress*	10
Fecal loss of energy (1% to 16% of intake)	15
Growth† (includes dietary induced thermogenesis)	45
Total	121

From Kalhan, S.C. & Price, P.T. (1999). Nutrition and selected disorders of the gastrointestinal tract. I: Nutrition for the high risk infant. In M.H. Klaus & A.A. Fanaroff (Eds.). *Care of the high risk neonate* (5th ed.). Philadelphia: W.B. Saunders.
*As infant matures, energy expanded in activities, such as crying and nursing, increases; at the same time, energy expended as a result of cold stress decreases.
†Calculated assuming 3.0 to 4.5 kcal/g weight gain at a rate of gain of 10 to 14 g/kg/d

day of a whey-predominant feeding.[296] Inadequate protein leads to alterations in cardiorespiratory, liver, and renal function; decreased immunocompetence; altered brain growth; and poor weight gain and somatic growth. Excessive intake (>5 g/kg/day) results in a metabolic overload with irritability, and can lead to late metabolic acidosis, azotemia, edema, fever, lethargy, diarrhea, elevated blood urea nitrogen (BUN), and poorer developmental outcome.[23,92,106]

A major energy source in human milk and most formulas is fat, which accounts for 30% to 55% of the total calories (3.3 to 6 g per 100 kcal).[8] Specific requirements include those for linoleic acid and possibly linolenic acid, essential fatty acids needed as precursors for synthesis of other fatty acids. Approximately 2.7% to 3% (300 mg linoleic acids per 100 kcal) of the infant's energy intake should be essential fatty acids.[8,23] Inadequate fats or lack of essential fatty acids can lead to metabolic problems, skin disorders, and poor growth; excessive fats can lead to ketosis.

Carbohydrates make up 30% to 50% (usually 41% to 44%) of the caloric content.[127] Inadequate carbohydrate can lead to hypoglycemia; excessive carbohydrate, to diarrhea. Infants, especially preterm infants who have poor stores and a higher growth rate, have increased needs for calcium, phosphorus, and vitamins to support growth and bone mineralization. Nutrient requirements for enteral and parental nutrition are summarized in Table 11-19.

increase weight gain, but not exponentially because the energy cost of weight gain also increases.[127] Most stable preterm infants achieve satisfactory growth on approximately 120 kcal/kg/day.[283,296] Caloric requirements for infants on parenteral feedings tend to be lower, averaging 80 to 110 kcal/kg/day, since activity level and fecal losses are lower.[31,97,127]

Fetal protein accretion is 3 to 4 g/kg/day. The type of dietary protein affects daily protein requirements. For example, infants can achieve adequate growth with 2 to 2.5 g/kg/

TABLE **11-19** Comparison of Suggested Parenteral and Enteral Fluid (Energy and Nutrient Intakes for Low–Birth Weight Infants)

COMPONENT, UNIT	PARENTERAL INTAKE (UNIT/kg/DAY)	ENTERAL INTAKE (UNIT/kg/DAY)
Water, mL	150	150
Energy, kcal	80-100	120-130
Protein, g	3.0-3.5	3.5
Fat, g	1.0-4.0	5-7
Carbohydrate, g	16	12-14
Calcium, mg	80-120	200-220
Phosphorus, mg	60-90	100-110
Magnesium, mg	9-10	7-10
Sodium, mEq	2.0-4.0	2-8
Potassium, mEq	2.0-3.0	2-3
Chloride, mEq	2.0-3.0	2-3
Zinc, μg	350-450	1000 2000
Copper, μg	65	65-300
Chromium, μg	0.4	0.1-0.4
Manganese, μg	10	7.5
Selenium, μg	2.0	1-2
Vitamin A, IU	500	700-2000
Vitamin D, IU	160	400
Vitamin E, IU	2.8	5-25
Vitamin K, μg	80	7-9*
Thiamine (vitamin B_1), μg	350	20-40
Riboflavin (vitamin B_2), μg	150	60
Pyridoxine (vitamin B_6), μg	180	35-60
Niacin, mg	6.8	0.8
Folic acid, μg	56	50
Vitamin B_{12}, μg	0.3	0.1-0.5
Ascorbic acid, mg	32	35

Adapted from American Academy of Pediatrics Committee on Nutrition (1985). Nutritional needs of low–birth-weight infants. *Pediatrics, 75,* 976; and Greene, H.L., et al. (1988). Guidelines for the use of vitamins, trace elements, calcium, magnesium, and phosphorus in infants and children receiving parenteral nutrition: Report of the Subcommittee on Pediatric Parenteral Nutrient Requirements for the Committee on Clinical Practice Issues of the American Society of Clinical Nutrition. *Am J Clin Nutr, 48,* 1324; adapted by Schandler, R.J., et al. (1998). Parenteral and enteral nutrition. In H.W. Taeusch & R.A. Ballard (Eds.).
Avery's diseases of the newborn (7th ed.). Philadelphia: W.B. Saunders.
*Vitamin K, 0.5-1 mg at birth.

Composition of Feedings

To maximize growth and reduce stress, the limitations of the neonate's GI, renal, and metabolic systems must be considered in selecting substances for feeding. This can be accomplished through analysis of the composition of human milk and commercial formulas and consideration of

TABLE **11-20** Nutrient Composition of Preterm and Mature Human Milk

COMPONENT	PRETERM HUMAN MILK (1 WEEK)	MATURE HUMAN MILK (1 MONTH)
Volume (ml)	100	100
Energy (kcal)	67	70
Protein (g)	2.4	1.8
% Whey/casein	70/30	70/30
Fat (g)	3.8	4
% MCTs/LCTs	2/98	2/98
Carbohydrate (g)	6.1	7.0
% Lactose	100	100
Calcium (mg)	25	22
Phosphorus (mg)	14	14
Magnesium (mg)	3.1	2.5
Sodium (mg)	50	30
Potassium (mg)	70	60
Chloride (mg)	90	60
Zinc (μg)	500	320
Copper (μg)	80	60
Vitamin A (IU)	560	400
Vitamin D (IU)	4	4
Vitamin E (mg)	1	0.3
Vitamin C (mg)	5.4	5.6

Adapted from Schandler, R.J., et al. (1998) Parenteral and enteral nutrition. In H.W. Taeusch & R.A. Ballard (Eds). *Avery's diseases of the newborn* (7th ed.). Philadelphia: W.B. Saunders.
LCT, Long-chain triglyceride; *MCT,* medium-chain triglyceride.

the advantages and disadvantages of each for that individual infant. This section discusses considerations in selecting feedings for term and preterm infants. Composition of human milk is summarized in Table 11-20. Table 11-21 compares the composition of premature, standard, and soy formulas.

Protein

Milk protein consists of casein and whey proteins. Whey forms soft, flocculent curds. Casein forms tougher, more rubbery curds; it requires a greater energy expenditure to digest and is more likely to be incompletely digested. Human milk has a whey-to-casein ratio around 70:30 (versus 20:80 in cow's milk). Whey is easier to digest in the presence of low levels of trypsin and pepsin and is associated with fewer imbalances in plasma amino acids in preterm infants.[230] Whey protein contains a different mixture of amino acids than does casein, with increased levels of cystine and decreased methionine. Human milk contains less protein than cow's milk but has higher levels of nonprotein nitrogen with an amino acid composition that is easy for the infant to use.[213,229] The major whey protein in human milk is α-lactalbumin, which is high in amino acids that are essential

TABLE **11-21** Comparison of Premature, Standard, and Soy Formulas

	PREMATURE	STANDARD	SOY
Energy	24 kcal/oz	20 kcal/oz	20 kcal/oz
Protein	Whey-to-casein (60:40)	Whey-to-casein (60:40 or 18:82)	Spy protein isolate
Fat	MCTs and LCTs	LCTs	LCTs
Carbohydrate	Glucose polymers Lactose polymers	Lactose	Sucrose and/or glucose
Ca and P	Fortified to meet needs of preterm infants; Ca-to-P ratio 1.8-2:1	Not fortified to meet needs of preterm infant; Ca-to-P ratio 1.3-1.5:1	Ca-to-P ratio 1.3-1.4:1
Iron	Available with or without iron fortification	Available with or without iron fortification	Available with iron fortification only

Adapted from Kalhan, S.C. & Price, P.T. (1999). Nutrition and selected disorders of the gastrointestinal tract. I: Nutrition for the high risk infant. In M.H. Klaus & A.A. Fanaroff (Eds.). *Care of the high risk neonate* (5th ed.). Philadelphia: W.B. Saunders.
Ca, Calcium; *LCT,* long-chain triglyceride; *MCT,* medium-chain triglyceride; *P,* phosphorus.

for the infant. Other human milk proteins include lactoferrin, lysozyme, and secretory immunoglobulin A.

The use of whey-dominant feedings reduces the risk of lactobezoar formation. Lactobezoars are milk curd balls that develop within the stomach and were seen predominantly in preterm infants on whey-dominant, high-caloric-density formulas. This disorder, now rare, usually resolved spontaneously in asymptomatic infants. Symptomatic infants (abdominal distention, gastric residuals, and vomiting) often responded to discontinuation of feeding and gastric gavage, although about 11% to 14% developed gastric perforation.[106]

The amino acid composition of feedings is critical for optimal neonatal growth and development. Some amino acids are essential in the neonate that are not essential for adults due to the decreased ability of the infant to synthesize these amino acids.[127] For example, taurine is essential for central nervous system (CNS) growth, maintaining optimal retinal integrity and function, and bile acid synthesis. Intermediary metabolic pathways for synthesis of some amino acids are immature. The last enzyme in transsulfuration is absent in the fetus and develops slowly in preterm infants. These infants cannot synthesize cystine and have limited tolerance for methionine (which is normally converted to cystine). Similar deficiencies exist in the ability of the infant to oxidize tyrosine and phenylalanine. Transamination pathways are also not well developed, so histidine is an essential amino acid in the neonate but not in the adult.[157] Thus infants need a feeding that contains lower levels of methionine, phenylalanine, and tyrosine and adequate cystine, taurine, and histidine.[41,127,293] Glutamine may have an important role in gut maturation, fat metabolism, and gut immune function in addition to producing glutamate, a neurotransmitter needed for CNS development (see Chapter 14).

Phenylalanine and tyrosine can significantly increase net acid loads, which along with high-protein feedings contributes to development of late metabolic acidosis. This disorder is seen in preterm infants usually at 2 to 3 weeks of age. Late metabolic acidosis is associated with the amount of protein in the diet, the amino acid composition of the diet, and the decreased ability of the immature kidney to conserve bicarbonate (see Chapter 10).

Carbohydrate

Immaturity of lactase activity in preterm infants may interfere with their ability to optimally use lactose-based formulas, although many infants have little difficulty digesting lactose. Preterm infants can absorb up to 90% of the lactose in human milk.[229,230] Carbohydrates other than lactose are often included in feedings if greater carbohydrate absorption is needed or if lactose is poorly tolerated.[157] Use of low-lactose feedings reduces the risk of overwhelming the infant's available lactase. Infants do require some lactose for calcium absorption.

Glucose polymers are often used as an alternative carbohydrate substrate in formulas. Preterm infants hydrolyze and absorb glucose polymers in a manner similar to that with lactose in term infants.[157] Glucose polymers have several advantages: (1) ready availability from natural sources, including corn syrup solids; (2) high caloric density without significantly increasing the renal solute load (see Chapter 10); (3) incorporation into feedings without significantly increasing the osmotic load and risk of increased water loss and diarrhea; (4) more rapid emptying from the stomach of young infants than lactose or glucose; (5) independence from lactase and amylase; and (6) digestion by glucoamylase, which is present in adequate quantities in preterm infants and whose secretion is less likely to be altered by mucosal injury.[109,157,158] Oligosaccharides are glucose polymers that prevent bacterial attachment to the intestinal mucosa, thus providing protection against infection. Oligosaccharides are present in human milk.[230]

Fat

Fats are the primary source of energy in human milk and many formulas. Fats provide a higher caloric density without significantly increasing osmotic load. Limitations in neonatal fat digestion and absorption can reduce the usefulness of this energy source. High-caloric-density formulas tend to be retained in the stomach for longer periods, thus delaying gastric emptying.

Infants need both saturated and unsaturated fatty acids in their diet. Human milk and vegetable oils (corn, coconut, and soy) are absorbed better than saturated fat (cow's milk or butter fat).[41] Human milk fat is contained in fat globules that consist of fatty acids such as linoleic, linolenic, oleic, palmitic, arachidonic, and docosahexaenoic acids. These latter two acids are precursors for prostaglandins and phospholipids and may be important in cognition, vision, and growth.[229,230] Milk fat globules are more easily absorbed in the presence of a reduced bile acid pool.[230] Human milk contains long-chain polyunsaturates that are well absorbed and may enhance nervous system devlopment.[127]

In formulas, unsaturated fats in vegetable oils are a source of the essential fatty acid linoleic acid. Short- and medium-chain triglycerides (MCTs) can be absorbed intact across the gastric and intestinal mucosa. These triglycerides are not dependent on the reduced bile acid pools for emulsification and do not require carnitine, often low in preterm infants, for transfer into the mitochondria.[56,127] MCTs are associated with more rapid gastric emptying and enhanced calcium, magnesium, and fat absorption.[229] MCTs may also increase the level of plasma ketones, which can be used as an alternative substrate to glucose for brain metabolism. About 10% to 50% of the fat in preterm formulas is in the form of MCTs to enhance fat absorption. Infants need some long-chain fatty acids for integrity of cell membranes and brain development.[100,267]

Vitamins, Minerals, and Trace Elements

Infants need adequate amounts of essential vitamins, minerals, and trace elements in their diet to support normal growth and development. Immature infants have decreased stores of most of these substances since stores accumulate late in gestation, and dietary supplementation may be needed. Specific requirements for many vitamins and trace elements in preterm infants are unknown. Increased quantities of fat-soluble vitamins (A, D, E, K) and their water-

soluble analogues compensate for the inadequate bile acid pools and poorer absorption of fat, especially in preterm infants. Requirements for B vitamins (coenzymes for metabolic processes and energy production) and folic acid (a cofactor for DNA synthesis) may also be increased because of the infant's greater growth rate and decreased intestinal absorption. Vitamin K is discussed in Chapter 7.

Vitamin A. Vitamin A enhances light perception and tissue integrity along with repair and growth of epithelial tissue. Higher levels are needed in preterm infants due to poor absorption and stores. Decreased vitamin A has been reported in infants with chronic lung disease (CLD).[97] This may be due to lowered intake or consumption of vitamin A in the repair of damaged lung epithelial tissue. Administration of vitamin A to prevent CLD has been only marginally effective.[97,103,265] Vitamin A levels should be monitored in infants on parenteral alimentation. Vitamin A in parenteral solutions decreases markedly over 24 hours as a result of adherence of the vitamin to IV tubing and photodegradation.

Vitamin C. Vitamin C is water soluble, readily absorbed, and not stored in significant amounts. It is important in amino acid metabolism (needed for growth) and intestinal iron absorption. Deficiencies are associated with scurvy (rare) and transient hypertyrosinemia.[296]

Vitamin D. Vitamin D facilitates intestinal calcium and phosphorus absorption, bone mineralization, and calcium reabsorption from bone (see Chapter 16). Preterm infants have lower serum concentrations of vitamin D and increased needs due to more rapid growth and immaturity of enzymes involved in metabolism of dietary vitamin D to active substrates. These infants are at greater risk of osteopenia and rickets (see Chapter 16).[296]

Vitamin E. An important consideration related to both the fat and vitamin composition of feeding is the ratio of polyunsaturated fatty acid (especially linoleic acid) to vitamin E. The fat content of the red blood cell membrane is determined by dietary fat. Diets that contain high levels of polyunsaturated fatty acid (PUFA) or iron necessitate increased levels of vitamin E to protect red blood cells from oxidative injury and hemolysis. Recommended concentrations of vitamin E (α-tocopherol) to PUFA are 0.9 IU vitamin E per g of linoleic acid.[8,23]

Preterm infants have lower vitamin E stores, poor absorption, and increased needs to protect cell membranes from peroxidative damage and prevent hemolytic anemia. Elevated serum vitamin E levels have been associated with NEC and cerebral hemorrhage, so high doses must be avoided. Vitamin E supplementation has not been effective in preventing retinopathy of prematurity or bronchopulmonary dysplasia, with conflicting results from studies.[23,127,293] Vitamin E may have a role in prevention of intraventricular hemorrhage in extremely LBW infants, but additional research is needed.[23,127,293]

Folate. Folate deficiency, which can lead to anemia, poor growth, and delayed CNS maturation, is seen more often in preterm infants. Folate needs are increased in VLBW infants, who have decreased stores and absorption and more rapid growth.[31,283] Supplementation with 50 to 70 μg/dl/day has been recommended for preterm infants during the first 2 to 3 months, when intake is limited.[127,296]

Calcium, phosphorus, and magnesium. Calcium, phosphorus, and magnesium are essential in the neonate for bone mineralization and growth. The newborn with lower levels of parathyroid hormone (PTH) is less able to remove calcium from the bone, increasing the risk of hypocalcemia (see Chapter 16). Calcium levels in feedings may be increased to allow for calcium storage and support bone mineralization and growth. If calcium levels are altered, phosphorus intake also needs to be adjusted to maintain a homeostatic calcium-phosphorus balance. Vitamin D and magnesium are also needed for adequate bone mineralization and to prevent rickets.

Iron. Term and preterm infants develop a physiologic anemia during the first few months after birth because of postnatal suppression of erythropoiesis (see Chapter 7). During this period, iron from destroyed red blood cells is stored for use when erythropoiesis resumes. Once the stored iron is used up, the infant's hemoglobin will again fall if adequate iron is not available from dietary sources or supplementation. Iron supplementation is usually started before the point of depletion to maintain and build up stores. Supplementation is started earlier in preterm infants, since their iron stores are lower at birth and often further depleted by iatrogenic blood losses. Recommendations regarding iron supplementation are discussed in Chapter 7.

Trace elements and other substances. Stores of trace elements such as zinc, copper, iodine, chromium, selenium, and molybdenum are accumulated late in gestation. Requirements for trace elements are often also increased in preterm infants due to poor stores and increased growth rates. Specific requirements and absorptive mechanisms for many of these elements are unknown. Concentrations in human milk are generally adequate, and commercial formulas are supplemented. Parenteral alimentation solutions must be supplemented with these elements or infants will rapidly become deficient. Other substances found in human milk are inositol, choline, and nucleotides and many antiinfective substances (see Chapter 12). Inositol is a lipotrophic growth factor that may enhance surfactant function and reduce cell damage by free radicals.[112]

Nucleotides enhance growth and development, GI function, and host defenses. Choline, a component of phospholipids and acetylcholine precursor, may enhance neural development and function.[112]

Zinc. Zinc is an essential cofactor for over 70 enzymes needed for protein and nucleic acid synthesis. Zinc deficiencies inhibit uptake of fat-soluble vitamins and protein synthesis and can lead to growth restriction. Deficiencies have been reported in preterm infants fed human milk and infants on parenteral nutrition with inadequate supplementation. Excessive losses may occur in infants with ostomies or chronic diarrhea.[6,206,219,283]

Copper. Copper is also an enzyme component and essential for hemoglobin synthesis, myelinization, and formation of antioxidant enzymes and collagen. Copper deficiency (failure to thrive, iron-resistant anemia, pallor, edema, seborrheic dermatitis, and hypotonia) has been reported in preterm infants fed formulas with low levels of copper and in infants with ostomies or chronic diarrhea.[6,267]

Electrolytes. Levels of potassium and sodium may be increased in preterm formulas to compensate for increased intestinal potassium and renal sodium losses and to support growth (sodium is co-precipitated in the bone during periods of active bone growth). Concentrations of specific electrolytes are also determined by fluid composition and levels of other electrolytes. Electrolytes are discussed in Chapter 10.

Calories and Renal Solute Load

The caloric level of the feeding should reflect the infant's energy needs, but at an osmolality that the infant's kidneys and other systems can handle (see Chapter 10). Caloric content of human milk is generally 20 kcal/oz but may vary considerably. Preterm human milk has a slightly higher caloric density (see Table 11-20), but it also varies. Standard formulas contain 20 kcal/oz and preterm formulas 24 kcal/oz. Higher calorie formulas may be used, but problems with osmotic and solute load often offset the advantages of extra calories. Osmolalities should be similar to those of physiologic fluids (250 to 300 mOsm per kg water).

Caloric supplements such as Polycose (Ross Laboratories) and MCT Oil (Mead Johnson) may be used to increase the caloric density of feedings without significantly altering mineral content and solute load. These supplements may reduce the percentage of calories as protein (which may limit growth) and increase the percentage of calories as fat and carbohydrate (increasing the potential for ketosis and loose stools).[296] There is a risk of a lipoid pneumonia if MCT Oil is aspirated.

Use of Human Milk with Preterm Infants

Human milk is an ideal, nutritionally adequate feeding for term and most preterm infants that meets the infant's unique nutritional needs and provides over 45 other enzymes, growth factors, and bioactive substances to enhance growth and development, protect the infant from infection, and enhance gut maturation.[9,50] Human milk also contains substances such as human milk bile salt stimulated (mammary) lipase and mammary amylase, and has a low renal solute load (see Chapter 10), an amino acid composition ideal for the newborn, and lipids in a form that can be easily digested and absorbed. These and other characteristics of human milk compensate for the neonate's physiologic limitations. Preterm infants fed human milk have a lower incidence of NEC and infection, enhanced fat absorption, and more rapid gastric emptying.[165,197,293] Composition of human milk is described further in Chapter 5 and Table 11-20. The nutrient content of human milk can vary due to methods of expression and storage, portion of the milk used (i.e., foremilk versus hindmilk), and use of feeding tubes.[230]

Milk from mothers of preterm infants is different from that of term mothers and more closely approximates what are thought to be the nutritional needs of these infants (see Table 11-20).[13,102,197] However, the composition of this milk changes gradually over the first month after birth and by 1 month is similar to term milk. Preterm human milk is low (in terms of the preterm infant's nutrient requirements) in protein, calcium, phosphorus, iron, vitamins, and sodium, even though nutrients such as protein, iron, and calcium are in forms that are more readily absorbed by the infant. For example, it has been estimated that preterm infants fed human milk retain calcium and phosphorus equivalent to 15% to 20% of the calcium and 30% to 35% of the phosphorus accumulated by the fetus in utero.[283] Most preterm infants fed their own mother's milk gain at rates similar to intrauterine rates or those of infants fed whey formulas.[13,127,205] VLBW infants fed human milk may need supplementation to promote growth and prevent deficiencies. Human milk fortifiers that contain protein, glucose polymers, calcium, phosphorus, fat-soluble vitamins, and sodium may be used.[229,230] Use of these fortifiers results in short-term increases in weight gain, length and head circumference.[148,149] Fortifiers may however, alter percentages of other nutrients. The effect of fortification on antiinfective and other nonnutrient milk components is unclear.[230]

Parenteral Nutrition Solutions

TPN is the intravenous administration of a hypertonic solution containing amino acids, carbohydrates, fats, electrolytes, vitamins, minerals, and trace elements in order to maintain positive nitrogen balance. Partial parenteral nutrition involves infusion of amino acids and carbohydrates with or without fats to supplement enteral feedings.[296] Infants generally cannot tolerate glucose loads over 6 to 8 mg/kg/min in the first 1 to 2 weeks; the usual range in solutions is 3 to 8 mg/kg/minute. Parenteral alimentation has been associated with nitrogen retention and weight gain in LBW infants.[127] Nutritional requirements of infants on parenteral feedings differ from those of infants on enteral feedings since these solutions are infused directly into the blood rather than the immature gut. Nutrient requirements for preterm infants on parenteral nutrition are summarized in Table 11-19.

Problematic components of parenteral nutrition solutions have been amino acid mixtures and lipid emulsions. Abnormal plasma amino acid profiles have been reported in infants on parenteral nutrition.[97] These profiles have generally occurred with the use of adult solutions that were not constituted for neonates with immature liver function and intermediary metabolic pathways for synthesis of some amino acids. Use of pediatric/neonatal mixtures with addition of specific amino acids are now used. These solutions, which contain higher levels of taurine, cytosine, and tyrosine and branched-chain amino acids, with reduced methionine and phenylalanine, improve nitrogen retention and normalize plasma values and approximate the amino acid pattern of human milk.[97,127] Early parenteral amino acid administration (within the first 1 to 2 days) seems to be well tolerated by most infants and is associated with greater nitrogen retention and a positive nitrogen balance.[97,128,216,256,257,258,272,297]

Lipid emulsions are isotonic with a high caloric density and can be used to provide adequate caloric intake through a peripheral infusion. These emulsions are started within the first few days and gradually increased as tolerated. Lipid emulsions can lead to hyperlipidemia and hyperglycemia (reasons for alteration in glucose metabolism are unclear), especially with rates greater than 0.2 to 0.25 g/kg/hour (equivalent to 6g/kg/day) or with use in VLBW and SGA infants with little adipose tissue.[23,97,207,257,258] Generally 20% emulsions are preferred over 10% emulsions, since 10% emulsions have a higher phospholipid content, which slows triglyceride clearance.[97,207,258] These 20% solutions also provide more calories without increasing fluid. Excess free fatty acids may compete with and displace bilirubin from albumin, thus levels may need to be kept lower until hyperbilirubinemia resolves (see Chapter 17).[97] Fats have been associated with decreased oxygenation and increased pulmonary vascular tone.[258] Effects on oxygenation may be minimized by prolonging the infusion period and using rates less than 0.2 g/kg/hour.[127,258]

Feeding Infants with Various Health Problems

Immature infants generally tolerate feeding with preterm formulas or preterm breast milk better than standard formulas. Considerations discussed below for selecting feedings for preterm infants are also important in planning nutritional support for infants with specific health problems. These infants have individualized nutritional needs that may require use of specialized formulas or feeding methods. For example, critically ill infants may need to be fed via total or partial parenteral nutrition because of their inability to digest and absorb enteral feedings or the risk of complications. Nutrient needs of preterm and term infants with specific problems are summarized in Table 11-22.

Very-Low–Birth-Weight Infants

The considerations in selecting the feedings described above are even more critical in planning for nutritional support of VLBW infants, whose body systems are even more immature. Unique nutritional problems of these infants include the following:

1. Limited protein and energy reserves (e.g., a 1000-g preterm has only 10 g of stored fat versus 400 g in a term neonate). Energy needs may be increased by intermittent cold stress, infection, or stresses of the neonatal intensive care unit environment.
2. High ratio of surface area to body weight.
3. Small gastric capacity, which limits intake.
4. High water requirements due to increased insensible water losses and immature renal function. These factors limit the ability of the infant to tolerate high-caloric-density formulas due to risks associated with hyperosmolar solutions.

5. Immature digestive and absorptive capacities for fats, carbohydrates, vitamins, and trace elements.
6. Immature brain and liver, which are vulnerable to damage from elevated plasma concentrations of amino acids such as tyrosine, methionine, and phenylalanine.[5,41,92]

Infants with Respiratory Problems

Infants with respiratory distress, including infants with bronchopulmonary dysplasia (BPD), may be unable to feed by bottle or breast due to rapid respiratory rates, fatigue, and inability to coordinate sucking, swallowing, and breathing. These infants need to be fed by other enteral (intragastric) or parenteral methods. Fluid and caloric requirements are often increased because of the increased metabolic demands, respiratory workload, oxygen consumption, and insensible water losses. Energy needs may increase up to 20% to 40% above baseline in infants with BPD. Oxygen consumption, energy expenditure, and work load are higher for infants with respiratory problems who are breathing spontaneously than those on assisted ventilation. Intestinal disaccharidases may be diminished in infants following shock or ischemia, with a temporary carbohydrate intolerance.[106] Infants recovering from respiratory distress syndrome have been reported to have decreased functional residual capacity, with increases in respiratory rate and minute ventilation during nasogastric feedings.[106] Feeding these infants in a prone position may improve their oxygenation during feeding.[106]

Infants with Cardiac Problems

Infants with cardiac problems often grow poorly due to increased metabolic demands and difficulty with feed-

TABLE **11-22** Effect of Disease on Selected Nutrient Requirements in Preterm and Term Infants

Nutrient	Preterm Infants			Term Infants			Both
	RDS	CLD	NEC/SBS	Cyanotic CHD	CHF	Sepsis	IUGR
Free water	↓	↓	↑	↔	↓	↔	↑
Energy	↑	↑↑	↑↑	↑	↑↑	↑	↑
Fat	↔	↑	↑[a]↑	↑	↑	↔	↑
Carbohydrate	↑	↓	↑	↑	↑	↑	↑
Protein	↔	↑	↑	↑	↑	↑↑	↑
Calcium	↔	↑[b,c]	↑[a]	↑[d]	↑[c,d]	↔	↑
Iron	↔	↑[b]	↑	↑	↔	↓	↑

From Townsend, S.F., et al. (1998) Enteral nutrition. In G.B. Merenstein & S.L. Gardner (Eds.). *Handbook of neonatal intensive care* (4th ed.). St. Louis: Mosby.
[a]Particularly with loss of terminal ileum.
[b]In preterm infants less than 1500 g.
[c]Particularly with calciuric diuretics such as furosemide.
[d]Particularly if postoperative.
CHD, Congenital heart disease; *CHF,* congestive heart failure; *CLD,* chronic lung disease; *IUGR,* intrauterine growth restriction; *NEC,* necrotizing enterocolitis; *RDS,* respiratory distress syndrome; *SBS,* short bowel syndrome.

ing. Caloric requirements are increased because of hypermetabolism (higher metabolic rate and oxygen consumption secondary to increased cardiac and respiratory workload), tissue hypoxia, protein loss, increased frequency of infection, and poorer nutrient absorption due to decreased splanchnic blood flow.[98] Infants with cardiac problems may be fluid and sodium restricted. Feeding problems may limit intake since the infant may become fatigued, tachypneic, and stressed with feeding. Intervention strategies include use of higher-caloric-density and low-sodium formulas, frequent smaller feedings, feeding on demand and in an upright position, avoidance of feeding immediately after prolonged crying or when the infant is exhausted, and administration of oxygen with feeding as needed. Infants with cardiac or renal problems may need to be on low-sodium or solute-load formulas.

Infants with Short-Bowel Syndrome

Infants with reduction in the length of their small intestine, which usually results from surgical resection because of a congenital anomaly or NEC, are at very high risk for nutritional and growth problems due to reduction in intestinal absorptive surface area. In addition, the remaining sections of bowel may have been ischemic with villous atrophy. Loss of intestinal surface area results in loss of brush border enzymes such as the disaccharidases, resulting in carbohydrate intolerance and a pool of unabsorbed sugars that act as a rich substrate for bacterial growth. Infants who have less than 25 cm of residual small intestine (normal small intestinal length is 250 to 270 cm at term) if the ileocecal valve is intact or more than 40 cm without this valve are likely to eventually be able to tolerate enteral only feedings.[271] During resection, particular efforts are made to preserve the ileum (because of its critical role in bile acid and vitamin B_{12} absorption) and cecal valve.[106] Ileocecal resection is associated with gastric hypersecretion and hypersecretion of regulatory peptides (including motilin, enteroglucagon, and peptide YY) for several weeks.[271] Other problems in digestion and absorption of nutrients resulting from small-bowel resection include disaccharide intolerance; decreased pancreatic and biliary secretions; impaired vitamin (especially folate and vitamin B_{12}), calcium, iron, zinc, and magnesium absorption; protein malabsorption; and bile salt depletion.[106]

With adequate enteral nutrition, the remaining bowel usually undergoes villous hyperplasia with increased cell proliferation and migration.[96,270,98] This response is similar to maturational responses seen in the newborn following initiation of enteral feedings and is related to exposure of the gut to enteral feedings and to the trophic effect of GI

hormones. Most infants receive parenteral nutrition immediately after surgery, but initiation of minimal enteral feedings—using an elemental lactose free feeding as soon as the bowel has recovered—is important in enhancing villous hyperplasia.[156,198] Vitamin, mineral, and trace element supplementation is needed due to increased intestinal loss.[96]

Considerations Related to Feeding Method

The healthy term infant is fed by breast or bottle depending on the parent's choice. The choice of feeding method for preterm or ill infants also depends on the choice of breast milk or formula, as well as maturity, health status, growth pattern, and individual responses to specific methods. These infants can be fed by enteral or parenteral methods, each of which have specific advantages and disadvantages (Table 11-23). Clinically stable preterm infants can be breastfed. Infants as young as 32 weeks (1200 g) have been reported to have an organized sucking pattern at the breast, with two to three sucks per burst followed by a pause and stable transcutaneous oxygen pressures.[182]

Infants who have not developed suck-swallow coordination, who fatigue easily, or for whom oral feeding is contraindicated due to health status require an alternative feeding method. With preterm infants this method is usually gavage (intragastric), given either as a bolus or in a continuous drip and using either breast milk or formula.

Intragastric gavage permits normal digestive processes and hormonal responses to occur. Tube insertion is generally easy since most infants who require gavage do not have a well-developed gag reflex. Infants who are fed intragastrically are generally able to tolerate higher osmotic loads than those fed transpylorically, with less distention, vomiting, and diarrhea. Risks of intragastric gavage such as regurgitation, aspiration, and gastric distention—which may compromise respiratory function—are reduced with transpyloric feedings. Transpyloric feeding tubes are harder to insert, and this feeding method is associated with complications such as impaired fat absorption, intestinal perforation, and ileus (see Table 11-23). Routine use of transpyloric feedings is not recommended due to the increased mortality risk.[197,293]

The enteral feeding–induced surge of gut hormones following birth may be enhanced by bolus methods, although others have reported that continuous feeding may enhance intestinal motility.[15,18,28,68] Bolus feedings stimulate cyclic responses in the secretion of gut hormones, insulin, and glucagon that are not seen in infants fed by continuous drip, although which response is best at this age is unknown.[15] Use of syringe pump infusion systems to deliver human milk by continuous infusion has been associated with loss of milk fat, decreased fat

TABLE **11-23**   **Advantages and Risk of Various Feeding Methods**

METHOD	ADVANTAGES	DISADVANTAGES
Peripheral venous nutrition	Not dependent on GI function No danger of aspiration Low infection risk	Repeated infants thermal and physiologic stress Personnel effort to start and maintain Risk of tissue injury with extravasation Lack of nutrients into gut to promote intestinal growth and maturation
Central venous nutrition: surgical line	Higher concentration of glucose can be given Possible when other methods fail Not dependent on GI function No danger of aspiration Low risk of necrotizing enterocolitis Once catheter inserted, less handling and cold stress	General anesthesia Vena cava thrombosis Infection Lack of nutrients into gut to promote intestinal growth and maturation
Central venous nutrition: Percutaneous line	Same as above No need for general anesthesia Less risk of thrombosis	Infection Lack of nutrients into gut to promote intestinal growth and maturation
Intermittent intragastric feeding	Promotes intestinal growth, gut hormone secretion, and bile flow Avoids risk associated with parenteral nutrition	Bypasses salivary and lingual enzymes
Continuous intergastric feeding	Larger volumes may be tolerated without respiratory compromise Slightly lower energy expenditure	Bypasses salivary and lingual enzymes
Transpyloric feeding	Does not rely on gastric emptying	Difficult tube placement Loss of gastric emptying as guide to feeding intolerance Possible increased mortality

Adapted from Bell, E.F. (1996). Nutritional support. In J.P. Goldsmith & E.H. Karotkin (Eds.). *Assisted ventilation of the neonate* (3rd ed.). Philadelphia: W.B. Saunders.
GI, Gastrointestinal.

concentrations (especially at low infusion rates), and terminal delivery of a large fat load if fat in the tubing is recovered using an air infusion. Similar findings were not demonstrated with intermittent gavage or bolus feedings.[171] The method and type of feeding influence gastric emptying. Increasing caloric density inhibits gastric emptying, supporting the practice of using diluted formula for the initial feedings.

Parenteral solutions may be given via central or peripheral lines, which have advantages and risks (see Table 11-23). Infants on parenteral nutrition require careful monitoring since they are at greater risk for metabolic derangements, electrolyte imbalances, sepsis, anemia, and thromboembolytic complications.

Monitoring Nutritional Status

Nutritional needs are affected by age, weight, maturity, growth rate, and health status. Monitoring nutritional status includes assessment of physical status, tolerance of enteral or parenteral feeding, and growth. McLaren divides nutritional assessment into three areas: status (balance between intake and expenditures), process (how infant's growth has progressed over time and factors affecting this growth), and nonnutritional factors (genetics, psychosocial environment, stress).[180]

An indicator of health and nutritional status is growth. There is general consensus regarding growth rates for term infants. Although preterm infants are often expected to grow initially at a relatively faster rate than term infants, there is a lack of agreement on optimal growth rates and how closely this rate should approximate that of fetuses of similar gestations.

Growth is monitored by daily weight gain and loss and by weekly monitoring of other anthropometric parameters (length, head circumference, mean arm circumference, and triceps skin fold thickness).[97,163] There are problems with these measurements. Length is often measured inaccurately, and both length and head circumference are spared relative to weight in malnutrition. Mean arm circumference reflects muscle and fat deposition, and although sensitive to current protein and energy intake, few standards are available for preterm infants.[163] Triceps skin fold thickness estimates fat stores, but values are difficult to interpret and standards are not available for preterm infants.[163]

The use of weight to monitor growth is particularly problematic in VLBW infants. The need for daily weights should be considered against the stress (and increased energy and caloric consumption) of this procedure. Weight gain may be due to water retention and not new tissue, or may be influenced by the type of equipment attached to the infant.[163] As noted earlier, different early growth charts for preterm infants exist, each reflecting the characteristics of the population from which the chart was developed.[205] These curves were not developed using many subjects fed human milk or human milk–like preterm formulas, as is current practice. An awareness of the limitations of different charts and use of a chart based on a population with characteristics similar to those of the infant being assessed are important for their optimal use.

Nutritional status is also monitored by calculating daily caloric, fluid, and nutrient intake; physical assessment of the infant; biochemical monitoring; and assessment for signs of nutritional deficiencies. Biochemical monitoring to assess the adequacy of protein intake may involve evaluation of serum proteins with short half-lives such as prealbumin and retinol-binding protein. Assessment and monitoring of nutritional tolerance for infants on enteral feedings involve testing of stools for reducing substances and blood, measuring feeding residuals and abdominal girth, and observing for vomiting.[97,163]

Regurgitation and Reflux

Newborns are more prone to regurgitation, vomiting, and GER due to anatomic and functional immaturity of their GI system. Regurgitation peaks at 3 months of age; 40% to 50% of infants regurgitate more than once a day.[175] Regurgitation is common in infants as a result of immaturity of the LES, decreased LES basal tone, alterations in esophageal and gastric motility, delayed gastric emptying, entry of air into the stomach with swallowing, less acute esophageal-stomach angle, increased esophageal peristalsis, and a tendency toward reverse peristalsis.[34] These limitations and the frequency of regurgitation are more marked in preterm infants.

Interventions to reduce regurgitation include frequent burping; feeding slowly in a semiupright position to reduce air swallowing and passage of swallowed air into the duodenum; using small, frequent feedings; and placing the infant in a prone or right lateral position after feeding to enhance gastric emptying.

Regurgitation does not mean that an infant has gastroesophageal reflux disease (GERD), although GERD is also seen more frequently in infants, particularly in preterm and ill neonates. GERD is the retrograde flow of gastric contents into the esophagus often accompanied by regurgitation, but may occur in the absence of regurgitation.[46,82,106] Although this is a temporary phenomenon that generally resolves by 8 to 12 months, probably due to maturation of the GI system and introduction of solid food, GER can be severe enough to result in failure to thrive, aspiration, esophagitis, and dysphagia.[34,175] Infants with reflux may present with choking, gagging, apnea, or other respiratory symptoms.

Reflux in preterm infants is related to immaturity: decreased LES tone, pressure, and size; intrathoracic LES position; delayed gastric emptying; and impaired intestinal motility, with abdominal distention and higher pressure. Altered esophageal motility and peristalsis lead to poor clearance of refluxed material and increased risk of aspiration.[47,114,177] Most infants with reflux respond to interventions such as positioning; small, frequent, or thickened feedings; or drugs that enhance gastric emptying or reduce acid secretion. Some infants may require surgical correction.

Necrotizing Enterocolitis

NEC is a disorder seen primarily in preterm infants. Although the entire gut can be involved, NEC is most prominent in the jejunum, ileum, and colon. Clinical manifestations range from signs of feeding intolerance (abdominal distention, residuals, gross or occult blood in the stools, vomiting) or general systemic signs (lethargy, apnea, respiratory distress, thermal instability) to sepsis, shock, and peritonitis, with intestinal perforation in about 30% of these infants.[80,97]

The cause of NEC is unclear, with no single etiologic factor found in all infants. NEC is associated with prematurity, infection, hypertonic feedings, hypovolemia, perinatal asphyxia, and hypothermia. An immature GI tract with immature immune function, barrier function, and luminal stasis also plays a role in the pathogenesis of NEC (Figure 11-14).[196] Although 90% to 95% of infants have had enteral feedings prior to the development of symptoms, significant mortality from NEC has been reported in VLBW infants before the first feeding.[23,161]

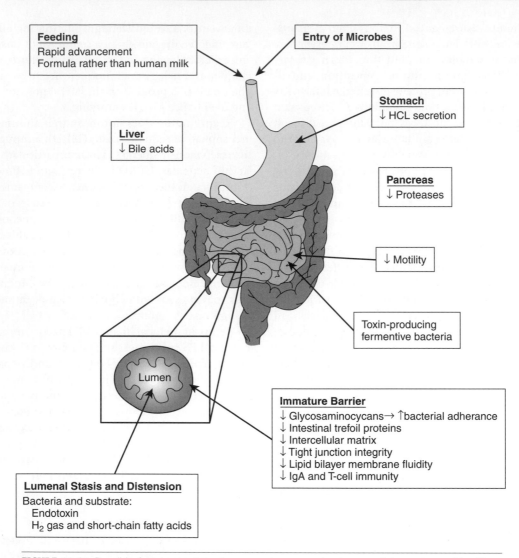

Feeding
Rapid advancement
Formula rather than human milk

Entry of Microbes

Stomach
↓ HCL secretion

Liver
↓ Bile acids

Pancreas
↓ Proteases

↓ Motility

Toxin-producing
fermentive bacteria

Lumen

Immature Barrier
↓ Glycosaminocycans→ ↑bacterial adherance
↓ Intestinal trefoil proteins
↓ Intercellular matrix
↓ Tight junction integrity
↓ Lipid bilayer membrane fluidity
↓ IgA and T-cell immunity

Lumenal Stasis and Distension
Bacteria and substrate:
   Endotoxin
   H_2 gas and short-chain fatty acids

FIGURE **11-14** Possible factors predisposing premature neonates to necrotizing enterocolitis. (From Neu, J. & Weiss, M.D. [1999]. Necrotizing enterocolitis: Pathophysiology and prevention. *J Parenter Enteral Nutr, 23,* S15.)

In addition early feeding does not necessarily predispose to an increased incidence of NEC.[27,74,141,181] Small enteral feedings of human milk (along with parenteral feedings) may protect the bowel from NEC by stimulating gut maturation, promoting mucosal integrity, providing substrate for intestinal enzymes, reducing ileus, and increasing perfusion.[151,165,181,196]

Ischemia, feeding, and infection have been proposed as major etiologic events. With asphyxia, blood is redistributed to the brain and heart. The bowel may become ischemic, with mucosal damage, ileus, and stasis. Initial gut colonization is followed by bacterial overgrowth and invasion of the injured mucosa. With initiation of enteral intake, feedings remain in the intestinal lumen for extended periods (due to mucosal damage and limitations in absorptive function in immature infants) and serve as a substrate for further bacterial growth and intramural gas formation. The source of this gas is uncertain, but it may arise from bacterial fermentation of carbohydrates.[80,97]

The specific relationships between feeding and NEC are unclear. Excessive volume or rapid increases in feeding may be the critical factors rather than early feeding per se.[136,141] Rapid advances in feeding (especially >20 cal/kg/day) along with impaired absorptive function secondary to immaturity or ischemia may result in intraluminal accumulation of fermentation products and bacteria-derived peptides that lead to mucosal inflammation.[11,135,136,179,266,290] A large volume might further stress the mucosa (already injured from ischemia) and further impede blood flow by distention. This may lead to a local hypoxemia, vascular insufficiency, and accumulation of fermentation products due to impaired absorption.[141,271] Finally, hyperosmolar feedings may overwhelm the immature or damaged mucosa.[268]

MATURATIONAL CHANGES DURING INFANCY AND CHILDHOOD

Digestive and absorptive capabilities gradually mature over the first 6 months to 2 years following birth. An important aspect of intestinal maturation is gut closure, which provides protection against the transport of macromolecules across the intestinal mucosa, reducing the risk of infection and allergy development (see Chapter 12). The LES lengthens from 1 cm at birth to 2.5 cm by 6 months, with most of the increased length in the portion of the esophagus below the diaphragm.[106] LES basal tone increases after 6 months and is associated with resolution of reflux in most infants.[47] The esophagus, which is 10 cm (range, 7 to 14 cm) in length at term, grows about 0.65 cm per year, reaching an adult length of 25 cm in childhood.[16,279]

Gastric acid and pepsinogen levels reach adult levels by 3 months. Gastric acid production and pepsin activity do not reach adult levels until 2 years, limiting gastric proteolysis in infants.[58,253] Levels of trypsin reach adult levels by 1 month.[157]

Pancreatic enzymes are minimal for the first 4 to 6 months; thus the infant is dependent on salivary and mammary amylase for initial digestion of carbohydrate. Pancreatic amylase activity increases after 4 to 6 months at about the time that starch (cereal) is introduced into the diet. Cereal is not efficiently digested before this time. Since hydrolysis of amylopectin (starch) is incomplete up to about 6 months, neonates given formula thickened with cereal may develop diarrhea.[56,155]

Activity of maltase, isomaltase, and sucrase remains high into adulthood, with some decrease seen in the elderly.[252] Retention of lactase activity is variable and genetically controlled. Lactase activity usually decreases after 3 to 5 years to very low levels.[195,252] Significant lactase activity is retained primarily in individuals of northern European descent. Mucosal glucose transport is reduced until about 12 months.[187]

Fat absorption does not approach adult efficiency until about 6 months. Lipase reaches adult levels by 2 years, so infants are dependent on lingual-gastric and mammary lipase.[145] Lipolysis and micelle activity are minimal until 4 to 6 months; liver uptake of bile acids is decreased until 6 months.[277]

Introduction of Solid Foods

Maturation of the intestinal system in infancy may be stimulated by weaning and the introduction of solid foods in a manner somewhat similar to changes induced by enteral feedings after birth.[155] Timing for introduction of solids should be based on development of neuromuscular processes involved in the ability of the infant to handle solids. The infant's ability to handle foods can be divided into three physiologic stages: (1) nursing (birth to 6 months), when the infant has excellent suck-swallow coordination and does best if fed human milk or formula; (2) transitional (4 to 8 months), when neuromuscular processes needed to swallow pureed solids develop; and (3) modified adult (6 to 12 months), when chopped foods can be swallowed without choking.[20]

There are no particular advantages, and some disadvantages, to introducing solid foods before 3 to 4 months in formula-fed or before 5 to 6 months in breastfed infants. Before 3 to 4 months, an extrusion reflex is present (extrusion of material placed on the anterior tongue) and GER may still be present. Contrary to what many parents and professionals believe, feeding cereal before bedtime in young infants has not been demonstrated to reduce the incidence of night awakenings and may contribute to dental caries and obesity.[172]

Introduction of solid foods is generally recommended at 4 to 6 months for formula-fed infants and after 6 months for breastfed infants.[20] Infants fed foreign proteins before 6 months have a higher incidence of food allergies (see Chapter 12). Cereal is usually the initial solid food given to infants. Rice and barley cereals are of low antigenicity and contain iron in a relatively easy to digest form. Early introduction of high-caloric-density foods is associated with an increased risk of obesity.[20]

SUMMARY

Supporting nutritional needs and promoting nutritional status of infants are a challenge, but one that is critical for optimal outcome. Management of nutritional needs must be based on understanding of the anatomic and physiologic limitations of the GI system and the impact of these alterations on the infant's ability to consume, digest, and absorb various nutrients. Recommendations for clinical practice related to the GI system and perinatal nutrition are summarized in Table 11-24.

TABLE **11-24**   Recommendations for Clinical Practice Related to the Gastrointestinal System and Perinatal Nutrition in Neonates

Assess feeding reflexes, suck-swallow coordination, cardiorespiratory and gastrointestinal (GI) function before initiating oral feedings (pp. 443-445).

Observe for regurgitation and GI reflux (p. 461).

Observe respiratory status after feeding (pp. 458-459).

Monitor residuals and abdominal girth (pp. 461-462).

Evaluate for signs of dehydration and electrolyte imbalance (pp. 440, 445-446, 450).

Monitor stools for reducing substance, blood, and consistency (p. 461-462).

Record timing and appearance of first meconium stool (p. 444).

Know parameters used to measure growth and factors that alter accuracy of these parameters (pp. 451, 461).

Monitor growth parameters using appropriate curves (pp. 438-440, 451, 461).

Counsel women regarding nutritional advantages of breastfeeding (pp. 441-444, 457, and Chapter 5).

Support breastfeeding in mothers of term and preterm infants (pp. 443-444, 457 and Chapter 5).

Initiate early enteral feeding as appropriate (pp. 443-444).

Promote early breastfeeding and colostrum intake (pp. 443, 451-453 and Chapter 5).

Know limitations of gastrointestinal function in term and preterm infants (pp. 444-450 and Table 11-15).

Know the effects of health problems or surgery on digestion and absorption (pp. 458-459).

Monitor preterm, small for gestational age, and asphyxiated infants for hypoglycemia (p. 440 and Chapter 15).

Evaluate composition of feedings (formula or human milk) in relationship to an individual infant's GI system limitations (pp. 453-457 and Tables 11-19 and 11-20).

Avoid use of high solute load and caloric density formulas in immature infants (p. 456 and Chapter 10).

Evaluate renal function and fluid and electrolyte status in infants on high solute load or caloric density feedings (p. 456 and Chapter 10).

Recognize signs of liver dysfunction in infants (p. 450).

Know nutritional requirements for preterm and term infants (pp. 451-452 and Tables 11-17 and 11-18).

Monitor nutritional intake to ensure that nutritional requirements are met (pp. 451-452).

Know caloric requirements and factors that alter these requirements (pp. 451-452).

Monitor the caloric intake of infants (pp. 451-452, 456).

Monitor neonates for signs of excessive or inadequate protein, carbohydrate, and fat intake (pp. 451-452).

Monitor preterm infants for signs of late metabolic acidosis (p. 454 and Chapter 10).

Monitor intake and ratio of vitamin E and linoleic acid (pp. 455-456 and Chapter 7).

Ensure that term and preterm infants receive iron at the recommended times (p. 456 and Chapter 7).

Monitor intake of vitamins, minerals, and trace minerals (pp. 455-456).

Provide dietary supplementation (e.g., vitamins, minerals, trace elements, calories) as required (pp. 455-456).

Monitor infants for signs of vitamin, mineral, and trace element deficiencies (pp. 455-456).

Monitor preterm infants for signs of hypocalcemia (p. 456 and Chapter 16).

Monitor very-low–birth-weight infants for hyponatremia and hypokalemia (pp. 456-457 and Chapter 10).

Recognize the advantages and limitations of the use of human milk with preterm infants (p. 457).

Assist mothers of preterm and ill infants in providing breast milk for their infants (p. 457 and Chapter 5).

Recognize and monitor for signs of complications associated with parenteral nutrition (pp. 457, 460 and Table 11-23).

Recognize potential problems of infants with intrauterine growth restriction and the basis for these problems (pp. 438-440 and Table 11-11).

Know the effects of specific health problems on nutritional intake, feeding method, and gastrointestinal function (pp. 458-459 and Table 11-22).

Use feeding techniques that promote adequate intake and reduce stress in infants with cardiorespiratory problems (pp. 459-460).

Monitor infants following intestinal resection or with ostomies for adequacy of nutritional intake and excessive loss of nutrients (p. 459).

Know the advantages and disadvantages of different feeding methods and monitor infants for potential complications (pp. 459-460 and Table 11-23).

Select feeding methods appropriate for an individual infant's maturity, age, and health status (pp. 459-460 and Table 11-23).

Identify infants at risk for necrotizing enterocolitis and monitor for signs (pp. 461-463).

Counsel parents regarding introduction of solids (p. 463).

REFERENCES

1. Abrams, B. (1994). Weight gain and energy intake during pregnancy. *Clin Obstet Gynecol, 37,* 515.
2. Abrams, B. & Pickett, K.E. (1999). Maternal nutrition. In R.K. Creasy & R. Resnik (Eds.). *Maternal-fetal medicine* (4th ed.). Philadelphia: W.B. Saunders.
3. Abrams, B., et al. (2000). Pregnancy weight gain: still controversial. *Am J Nutr, 71*(suppl), 1233S.
4. Adams, M.D. & Keegan, K.A. (1998). Physiologic changes in normal pregnancy. In N. Gleicher (Ed.). *Principles and practice of medical therapy in pregnancy* (3rd ed.). Stamford, CT: Appleton & Lange.
5. Adamkin, D.H. (1986). Nutrition in very low birth weight infants. *Clin Perinatol, 13,* 419.
6. Aggett, P.J. (2000). Trace elements of the micropremie. *Clin Perinatol, 27,* 119.
7. Al-Tawul, Y.S. & Berseth, C.L. (1996). Gestational and postnatal maturation of duodenal motor responses to intragastric feeding. *J Pediatr, 129,* 374.
8. American Academy of Pediatrics Committee on Nutrition. (1993). *Pediatric nutrition handbook* (3rd ed.). Elk Grove, IL: American Academy of Pediatrics.
9. American Academy of Pediatrics, Work Group on Breastfeeding. (1997). Breastfeeding and the use of human milk. *Pediatrics, 100,* 1035.
10. Anderson, A.G. (1990). Nutrient requirements of the premature infants. In N.M. van Gelder, R.F. Butterworth, & B.D. Drujan (Eds.). *(Mal)nutrition and the infant brain.* New York: Wiley-Liss.
11. Anderson, D.M. & Kliegman, R.M. (1991). The relationship of neonatal alimentation practices to the occurrence of endemic necrotizing enterocolitis. *Am J Perinatol, 8,* 62.
12. Angelini, D.J. (1999). Obstetric triage: management of acute nonobstetric abdominal pain in pregnancy. *J Nurse Midwifery, 44,* 572.
13. Atkinson, S.A. (2000). Human milk feeding of the micropremie. *Clin Perinatol, 27,* 235.
14. Axelson, I., et al. (1989). Macromolecular absorption in preterm and term infants. *Acta Paediatr Scand, 78,* 532.
15. Aynsley-Green, A., et al. (1990). Gut hormones and regulatory peptides in relation to enteral feeding, gastroenteritis, and necrotizing enterocolitis in infancy. *J Pediatr, 117,* S24.
16. Badriul, H. & Vandenplas, Y. (1999). Gastro-oesophageal reflux in infancy. *J Gastroenterol Hepatol, 14,* 13.
17. Baker, J. & Berseth, C.L. (1995). Postnatal changes in inhibitory regulation of intestinal motor activity in human and canine neonates. *Pediatr Res, 38,* 133.
18. Baker, J.H. & Berseth, C.L. (1997). Duodenal motor responses in preterm infants fed formula with varying concentrations and rates of infusion. *Pediatr Res, 42,* 618.
19. Baker-Wills, E. & Berseth, C.L. (1996). Antenatal steroids enhance maturation of small intestine motor activity in preterm infants. *Pediatr Res, 39,* 193A.
20. Barness, L.E. (1989). Introduction of supplemental foods to infants. In E. Lebenthal (Ed.). *Textbook of gastroenterology and nutrition in infancy* (2nd ed.). New York: Raven.
21. Baron, T.H. & Richter, J.E. (1992). Gastroesophageal reflux disease in pregnancy. *Gastroenterol Clin North Am, 21,* 777.
22. Baron, T.H., Ramirez, B. & Richter, J.E. (1993). Gastrointestinal motility disorders during pregnancy. *Ann Intern Med, 118,* 366.
23. Bell, E.F. (1996). Nutritional support. In J.P. Goldsmith & E.H. Karotkin (Eds.). *Assisted ventilation of the neonate* (3rd ed.). Philadelphia: W.B. Saunders.
24. Berman, D.H. & Friedman, S. (2000). Disorders of the biliary tract and liver. In W.R. Cohen, S.H. Cherry, & I.R. Merkatz (Eds.). *Cherry & Merkatz's complications of pregnancy* (5th ed.). Baltimore: Williams & Wilkins.
25. Bernt, K.M. & Walker, W.A. (1999). Human milk as a carrier of biochemical messages. *Acta Paediatr Suppl, 430,* 27.
26. Berseth, C.L., et al. (1990). Postpartum changes in patterns of GI regulatory peptides in human milk. *Am J Clin Nutr, 51,* 985.
27. Berseth, C.L. (1992). Early feeding enhances maturation of the preterm small intestine. *J Pediatr, 120,* 947.
28. Berseth, C.L. & Nordyke, C. (1993). Enteral nutrients promote postnatal maturation of intestinal motor activity in preterm infants. *Am J Physiol, 264,* G1046.
29. Berseth, C.L. (1995). Minimal enteral feedings. *Clin Perinatol, 22,* 195.
30. Berseth, C.L. (1996). Gastrointestinal motility in the neonate. *Clin Perinatol, 23,* 179.
31. Berseth, C. (1998). Developmental anatomy and physiology of the gastrointestinal tract. In H.W. Taeusch & R.A. Ballard (Eds.). *Avery's Diseases of the newborn* (7th ed.). Philadelphia: W.B. Saunders
32. Berseth, C.L. & Abrams, S.A. (1998). Special gastrointestinal concerns. In H.W. Taeusch & R.A. Ballard (Eds.). *Avery's Diseases of the newborn* (7th Ed.; pp. 965-978). Philadelphia: W.B. Saunders.
33. Berseth, C.L. (1999). Assessment in intestinal motility as a guide in the feeding management of the newborn. *Clin Perinatol, 26,* 1007.
34. Blackburn, S. (1999). Understanding gastroesophageal reflux in infants. *NANN Central Lines, 15*(3), 1, 16-22.
35. Block, G. & Abrams, B. (1993). Vitamin and mineral status of women of childbearing potential. *Ann N Y Acad Sci, 678,* 244.
36. Bonapace, E.S. & Fisher, R.S. (1998). Constipation and diarrhea in pregnancy. *Gastroenterol Clin North Am, 27,* 197.
37. Brewer, M.M., Bates, M.R., & Vannoy, L.P. (1989). Postpartum changes in maternal weight and body fat depots in lactating and nonlactating women. *Am J Clin Nutr, 49,* 259.
38. Broach, J. & Newton, N. (1988). Food and beverages in labor. Part Cross-cultural and historical practices. *Birth, 15,* 81.
39. Broach, J. & Newton, N. (1988). Food and beverages in labor. Part The effects of cessation of oral intake during labor. *Birth, 15,* 88
40. Brock-Utne, J.G., et al. (1989). Influence of preoperative gastric piration on the volume and pH of gastric contents in obstetric tients undergoing caesarean section. *Br J Anaesth, 62,* 307.
41. Brooke, O.G. (1987). Nutritional requirements of low and ver birthweight infants. *Ann Rev Nutr, 7,* 91.
42. Broussard, C.N. & Richter, J.E. (1998). Nausea and vomiting o nancy. *Gastroenterol Clin North Am, 27,* 123.
43. Broussard, C.N. & Richter, J.E. (1998). Treating gastro-oeso reflux disease during pregnancy and lactation: what are th therapy options? *Drug Saf, 19,* 325.
44. Broussard, D.L. (1995). Gastrointestinal motility in the neor *Perinatol, 22,* 37.
45. Brown, J.E. & Carlson, M. (2000). Nutrition and multif nancy. *J Am Diet Assoc, 100,* 343.
46. Brown, P. (2000). Medical management of gastroesopha *Curr Opin Pediatr, 12,* 247.
47. Bucuvalas, J.C. & Balisteri, W.F. (1997). Neonatal gast system: Development in the fetus and neonate. In A.A R.J. Martin (Eds.). *Neonatal-perinatal medicine: Diseas and infant* (6th ed.). St. Louis: Mosby.
48. Bunin, G., et al. (1993). Relation between maternal d quent primitive neuroectodermal brain tumors in y *N Engl J Med, 329,* 536.

49. Calhoun, B.C. (1992). Gastrointestinal disorders in pregnancy. *Obstet Gynecol Clin North Am, 19,* 733.

50. Cappell, M.S. & Garcia, A. (1998). Gastric and duodenal ulcers during pregnancy. *Gastroenterol Clin North Am, 27,* 169.

51. Carlisle, W.R. (1987). The liver and pregnancy. *Ala Med, 57*(3), 32.

52. Carmichael, S., et al. (1997). The pattern of maternal weight gain in women with good pregnancy outcomes. *Am J Public Health, 87,* 1984.

53. Carver, J.D. & Barness, L.A. (1996). Trophic factors for the gastrointestinal tract. *Clin Perinatol, 23,* 265.

54. Catalano, P.M. (1999). Pregnancy and lactation in relation to range of acceptable carbohydrate and fat intake. *Eur J Clin Nutr, 53*(suppl), S124.

55. Chenger, P. & Kovacik, A. (1987). Dental hygiene during pregnancy: A review. *MCN, 12,* 342.

56. Christensen, M.L., et al. (1989). Plasma carnitine concentration and lipid metabolism in infants receiving parenteral nutrition. *J Pediatr, 115,* 794.

57. Christian, M., et al. (1999). Starch digestion in infancy. *J Pediatr Gastroenterol Nutr, 29,* 116.

58. Christie, D.L. (1981). Development of gastric function during the first month of life. In E. Lebenthal (Ed.). *Textbook of gastroenterology and nutrition in infancy.* New York: Raven.

59. Cohen, S.E. & Masse, R.I. (1985). Physiology of pregnancy. In J.M. Baden & J.B. Brodsky (Eds.). *The pregnant surgical patient.* New York: Futura.

60. Colley, J.R. & Creamer, B. (1968). Sucking and swallowing in infants. *Br Med J, 2,* 422.

61. Cripps, A.W. & Williams, V.J. (1975). The effect of pregnancy and lactation on food intake, gastrointestinal anatomy and the absorptive capacity of the small intestine in the albino rat. *Br J Nutr, 33,* 17.

62. Crowell, D.T. (1995). Weight change in the postpartum period. A review of the literature. *J Nurse Midwifery, 40,* 418.

63. Cunningham, F.G & Whitridge, W.J. (1997). *Williams obstetrics* (20th ed.). Stamford, CT: Appleton & Lange.

64. Cunningham, J.T. (1998). Upper gastrointestinal tract disease. Small and large bowel disease. In N. Gleicher (Ed.). *Principles and practice of medical therapy in pregnancy* (3rd ed.). Stamford, CT: Appleton & Lange.

65. Dawes, M., et al. (1992). Routine weighing in pregnancy. *Br Med J, 304,* 487.

66. de Groot, L.C. (1999). High maternal body weight and pregnancy outcome. *Nutr Rev, 57,* 62.

67. Deuchar, N. (1995). Nausea and vomiting in pregnancy: A review of the problem with particular regard to psychological and social aspects. *Br J Obstet Gynaecol, 102,* 6.

68. deVille, K.T., et al. (1993). Slow infusion feeding enhances gastric emptying in preterm infants compared to bolus feeding. *Clinical Res, 41,* 787A.

69. deVille, K., et al. (1998). Motor responses and gastric emptying in preterm infants fed formula with varying concentrations and rates of infusion. *Am J Clin Nutr, 68,* 103.

70. Devriendt, K. (2000). Genetic control of intra-uterine growth. *Eur J Obstet Gynecol Reprod Biol, 92,* 29.

71. Dilorio, C., et al. (1992). Patterns of nausea and vomiting during the first trimester of pregnancy. *Clin Nurs Res, 1,* 127.

72. Douglas, M.J. (1988). Commentary: The case against a more liberal food and fluid policy in labor. *Birth, 15,* 93.

73. Dumont, R.C. & Rudolph, C.D. (1994). Development of gastrointestinal motility in the infant and child. *Gastroenterol Clin North Am, 23,* 655.

74. Dunn, L., et al. (1988). Beneficial effects of early hypocaloric enteral feeding on neonatal gastrointestinal function: Preliminary report of a randomized trial. *J Pediatr, 112,* 622.

75. Edwards, R.K., et al. (2001). Surgery in the pregnant patient. *Curr Probl Surg, 38,* 213.

76. Everson, G.T., et al. (1982). Gallbladder function in the human female: Effect of the ovulatory cycle, pregnancy and contraceptive steroids. *Gastroenterology, 82,* 711.

77. Everson, G.T. (1992). Gastrointestinal motility in pregnancy. *Gastroenterol Clin North Am, 21,* 751.

78. Ewer, A.K., et al. (1994). Gastric emptying in preterm infants. *Arch Dis Child, 71,* F24.

79. Fagan, E.L. (1999). Diseases of the liver, biliary system, and pancreas. In R.K. Creasy & R. Resnik (Eds.). *Maternal-fetal medicine* (4th ed.). Philadelphia: W.B. Saunders.

80. Fanaroff, A.A. (1999). Nutrition and selected disorders of the gastrointestinal tract. 2: Selected disorders of the gastrointestinal tract. In M.H. Klaus & A.A. Fanaroff (Eds.). *Care of the high risk neonate* (5th ed.). Philadelphia: W.B. Saunders.

81. Fantz. C.R., et al. (1999). Thyroid function during pregnancy. *Clin Chem, 45,* 2250.

82. Faubion W.A. & Zein, N.N. 1998. Gastroesophageal reflux in infants and children. *Mayo Clinic Proceedings, 73*(2), 166-173.

83. Feig, D. & Naylor, C. (1998). Eating for two: are guidelines for weight gain during pregnancy too liberal? *Lancet, 315,* 1054.

84. Firstenberg, M.S. & Malangoni, M.A. (1998). Gastrointestinal surgery during pregnancy. *Gastroenterol Clin North Am, 27,* 73.

85. Fisher, R.S., Roberts, G.S. & Grabowski, C.J. (1978). Altered lower esophageal sphincter function during early pregnancy. *Gastroenterology, 74,* 1233.

86. Flaxman, S.M. & Sherman, P.W. (2000). Morning sickness: a mechanism for protecting mother and embryo. *Q Rev Biol, 75,* 113.

87. Food and Nutrition Board. (1989). *Recommended Dietary Allowances* (10th ed.). Washington, DC: National Academy of Sciences, National Research Council.

88. Forbes, G.B. (1989). Nutritional adequacy of human breast milk for premature infants. In E. Lebenthal (Ed.). *Textbook of gastroenterology and nutrition in infancy* (2nd ed.). New York: Raven.

89. Forsyth, J.S., Donnet, L., & Ross, P.E. (1990). A study of the relationship between bile salts, bile-salt stimulated lipase, and free fatty acids in breast milk: Normal infants and those with breast milk jaundice. *J Pediatr Gastroenterol Nutr, 11,* 205.

90. Fullman, H. & Ippoliti, A. (1986). Acid peptic disease in pregnancy. In V.K. Rustgi & J.N. Cooper (Eds.). *Gastrointestinal and hepatic complications in pregnancy.* New York: John Wiley & Sons.

91. Galbraith, R.M. (1998). Liver disease: General considerations. In N. Gleicher (Ed.). *Principles of medical therapy in pregnancy* (3rd ed.). Stamford, CT: Appleton & Lange.

92. Galeano, N.F. & Roy, C.C. (1985). Feeding of the premature infant. In F. Litshitz (Ed.). *Nutrition for special needs in infancy: Protein hydrolysates.* New York: Marcel Dekker.

93. Galtier-Dereure. F., et al. (2000). Obesity and pregnancy: complications and cost. *Am J Clin Nutr, 71*(suppl), 1242S.

94. Gao, S.S., et al. (1996). Weight-for-length reference data for preterm, low-birth-weight infants. *Arch Pediatr Adolesc Med, 150,* 964.

95. Gao, S.S., et al. (1997). Growth in weight, recumbent length and head circumference for preterm, low-birth-weight infants during the first three years of life using gestation-adjusted ages. *Early Hum Dev, 47,* 305.

96. Garnbica, A.D. & Chan, W.Y. 91996). The role of the placenta in fetal nutrition and growth. *J Am Coll Nutr, 15,* 206.

97. Georgieff, M.K. (1999). Nutrition. In G.B. Avery, M.A. Fletcher & M.G. MacDonald (Eds.). *Neonatology: Pathophysiology and management of the newborn* (5th ed.). Philadelphia: Lippincott, Williams & Wilkins.

98. Gingell, R.L., Pieroni, D.R. & Hornung, M.G. (1989). Growth problems associated with congenital heart disease in infancy. In E. Lebenthal (Ed.). *Textbook of gastroenterology and nutrition in infancy* (2nd ed.). New York: Raven.

99. Girling, J.C., et al. (1997). Liver function tests in pre-eclampsia: importance of comparison with a reference range derived for normal pregnancy. *Br J Obstet Gynaecol, 104,* 146.

100. Gluckman, P.D. & Harding, J.E. (1997). The physiology and pathophysiology of intrauterine growth retardation. *Horm Res, 48,* S11

101. Goldenberg, R.L., et al. (1995). The effect of zinc supplementation on pregnancy outcome. *JAMA, 274,* 463.

102. Goldman, A.S. (2000). Modulation of the gastrointestinal tract of infants by human milk: interfaces and interactions, an evolutionary perspective. *J Nutr, 130*(suppl), 426S.

103. Greer, F.R. (2000). Vitamin metabolism and requirements in the micropremie. *Clin Perinatol, 27,* 95.

104. Gross, T.L. & Sokol, R.J. (1989). *Intrauterine growth retardation: A practical approach.* Chicago: Year Book Medical.

105. Gross, T.L. & Kazzi, G.M. (1998). Maternal malnutrition and obesity. In N. Gleicher (Ed.). *Principles and practice of medical therapy in pregnancy* (3rd ed.). Stamford, CT: Appleton & Lange.

106. Gryboski, J.D. & Walker, W.A. (1983). *Gastrointestinal problems in the infant* (2nd ed.). Philadelphia: W.B. Saunders.

107. Hack, M., Estabrook, M. & Robertson, S. (1985). Development of sucking rhythm in preterm infants. *Early Hum Dev, 11,* 133.

108. Hack, M. (1987). The sensorimotor development of the preterm infant. In A.A. Fanaroff & R.J. Martin (Eds.). *Neonatal-perinatal medicine: Diseases of the fetus and infant.* St. Louis: Mosby.

109. Hamosh, M. (1987). Compensatory enzymatic digestive mechanisms in the very-low-birthweight infant. In M. Xanthou (Ed.). *New aspects of nutrition in pregnancy, infancy and prematurity.* New York: Elsevier.

110. Hamosh, M. (1994). Digestion in the premature infant: the effects of human milk. *Semin Perinatol, 18,* 485.

111. Hamosh, M. (1996). Digestion in the newborn. *Clin Perinatol, 23,* 191.

112. Hay, W.W., et al. (1999). Workshop summary: nutrition of the extremely low birthweight infants. *Pediatrics, 104,* 1360.

113. Heird, W.C. & Gomez, M.R. (1996). Parenteral nutrition in low-birth-weight infants. *Ann Rev Nutr, 16,* 471.

114. Herbst, J.J. & Mizell, L.L. (1990). Gastroesophageal reflux. In N.M. Nelson (Ed.). *Current therapy in neonatal-perinatal medicine* (2nd ed.). Philadelphia: B.C. Decker.

115. Howden, C.W. (1998). Small and large bowel disease. In N. Gleicher (Ed.). *Principles and practice of medical therapy in pregnancy* (3rd ed.). Stamford, CT: Appleton & Lange.

116. Huxley, R.R. (2000). Nausea and vomiting in early pregnancy: its role in placental development. *Obstet Gynecol, 95,* 779.

117. Hytten, F.E. & Chamberlain, G. (1980). *Clinical physiology in obstetrics.* Oxford: Blackwell Scientific.

118. Institute of Medicine. (1990). *Nutrition during pregnancy.* Washington, DC: National Academy Press.

119. Ittman, P.I., et al. (1992). Maturation of antroduodenal motor activity in preterm and term infants. *Digestive Dis Sci, 37,* 14.

120. James, D. (1990). Diagnosis and management of fetal growth retardation. *Arch Dis Child, 65,* 360.

121. Jansson, T. & Powell, T.L. (2000). Placental nutrient transfer and fetal growth. *Nutrition, 16,* 500.

122. Jarnfelt-Samsioe, A., et al. (1985). Some new aspects of emesis gravidarum. *Gynecol Obstet Invest, 19,* 174.

123. Jewell, D.J. & Young, G. (2000). Interventions for treating constipation in pregnancy. *Cochrane Database Sys Rev, 2,* CD001142.

124. Jewell, D.J. & Young, G. (2000). Interventions for nausea and vomiting in early pregnancy. *Cochrane Database Sys Rev, 2,* CD00145

125. Johnson, J.W., et al. (1992). Excessive maternal weight gain and pregnancy outcome. *Am J Obstet Gynecol, 167,* 253.

126. Johnson, J.W. & Yancey, M.K. (1996). A critique of the new recommendations for weight gain in pregnancy. *Am J Obstet Gynecol, 174,* 254.

127. Kalhan, S.C. & Price, P.T. (1999). Nutrition and selected disorders of the gastrointestinal tract. I: Nutrition for the high risk infant. In M.H. Klaus & A.A. Fanaroff (Eds.). *Care of the high risk neonate* (5th ed.). Philadelphia: W.B. Saunders.

128. Kalhan, S.C. & Iben, S. (2000). Protein metabolism in the extremely low-birth weight infant. *Clin Perinatol, 27,* 23.

129. Kazzi, G.M., et al. (1998). Vitamins and minerals. In N. Gleicher (Ed.). *Principles of medical therapy in pregnancy* (3rd ed.). Stamford, CT: Appleton & Lange.

130. Keen, C., et al. (1994). Should vitamin-mineral supplements be recommended for all women with childbearing potential? *Am J Clin Nutr, 59*(suppl), 532S.

131. Kelly, E.J., et al. (1993). Immunocytochemical localization of pareital cells and G-cells in the developing human stomach. *Gut, 34,* 1057.

132. Kelly, E.J. & Newell, S.J. (1994). Gastric ontogeny: clinical implications. *Arch Dis Child, 71,* F136.

133. Kelly, E.J., et al. (1994). Immunohistochemical localization of epidermal growth factor and its receptor in the developing human stomach. *Arch Dis Child, 71,* F69.

134. Kennedy, K.A. (1989). Dietary antioxidants in the prevention of oxygen-induced injury. *Semin Perinatol, 13,* 97.

135. Kennedy, K.A., et al. (2000). Rapid versus slow rate of advancement of feedings for promoting rapid growth and preventing necrotizing enterocolitis in parenterally fed low-birth-weight infants. *Cochrane Database Sys Rev, 2,* CD001241.

136. Kien, C.L., et al. (1989). Digestion, absorption and fermentation of carbohydrates. *Semin Perinatol, 13,* 78.

137. Kien, C.L. (1990). Colonic fermentation of carbohydrate in the premature infant: Possible relevance to necrotizing enterocolitis. *J Pediatr, 117,* S52.

138. Kien, C.L. (1996). Digestion, absorption, and fermentation of carbohydrates in the newborn. *Clin Perinatol, 23,* 211.

139. King, J.C., et al. (1994). Energy metabolism during pregnancy: influence of maternal energy status. *Am J Clin Nutr, 59*(suppl), 439S.

140. King, J.C. (2000). Determinants of maternal zinc status during pregnancy. *Am J Clin Nutr, 71,* 1334S.

141. Kleigman, R.M. (1990). Models of the pathogenesis of necrotizing enterocolitis. *J Pediatr, 117,* S2.

142. Kliegman, R.M. (103). Experimental validation of neonatal feeding practices. *Pediatrics, 103,* 492.

143. Klion, F.M. (1991). The liver in normal pregnancy. In S.H. Cherry & I.R. Merkatz (Eds.). *Complications of pregnancy: Medical, surgical, gynecological, psychosocial and perinatal* (4th ed.). Baltimore: Williams & Wilkins.

144. Knight, B., et al. (2001). Effect of acupuncture on nausea of pregnancy: a randomized, controlled trial. *Obstet Gynecol, 97,* 184.

145. Kolasa, K.M. & Weismiller, D.G. (1997). Nutrition during pregnancy. *Am Fam Physician, 56,* 205.

146. Kramer, F.M., et al. (1993). Breastfeeding reduces maternal lower-body fat. *J Am Diet Assoc, 93,* 429.

147. Kristal, A.R. & Rush, D. (1984). Maternal nutrition and duration of gestation: A review. *Clin Obstet Gynecol, 27,* 553.

148. Kuschel, C.A. & Harding, J.E. (2000). Multicomponent fortified human milk for promoting growth in preterm infants, *Cochrane, Database Sys Rev, 2,* CD000343.

149. Kuschel, C.A. & Harding, J.E. (2000). Protein supplementation of human milk for promoting growth in preterm infants., *Cochrane, Database Sys Rev, 2,* CD000433.

150. Kunz, C., et al. (1999). Nutritional and biochemical properties of human milk. I: General aspects, proteins, and carbohydrates. *Clin Perinatol, 26,* 307.

151. LaGamma, E.F., et al. (1985). Failure of delayed oral feeding to prevent necrotizing enterocolitis. *Am J Dis Child, 139,* 355.

152. Lapp, C.A., et al. (1995). Modulation by progesterone of interleukin-6 produced by gingival fibroblasts. *J Periodontol, 66,* 279.

153. Latham, P.S. (1998). Liver diseases. In N. Gleicher (Ed.). *Principles and practice of medical therapy in pregnancy* (3rd ed.). Stamford, CT: Appleton & Lange.

154. Lawson, M., Kern, F. & Everson, G.T. (1985). Gastrointestinal transit time in human pregnancy: Prolongation in the second and third trimesters followed by postpartum normalization. *Gastroenterology, 89,* 996.

155. Lebenthal, E. (1983). Impact of digestion and absorption in the weaning period on infant feeding practices. *Pediatrics, 75*(suppl.), 207.

156. Lebenthal, G., et al. (1983). Impact of development of the gastrointestinal tract on infant feeding. *J Pediatr, 102,* 1.

157. Lebenthal, E. & Leung, Y.K. (1988). Feeding the premature and compromised infant: Gastrointestinal considerations. *Pediatr Clin North Am, 35,* 215.

158. Lebenthal, E. & Tucker, N.T. (1986). Carbohydrate digestion: Development in early infancy. *Clin Perinatol, 13,* 37.

159. Lebenthal, E. (1995). Gastrointestinal maturation and motility patterns as indicators for feeding the premature infant. *Pediatrics, 95,* 207.

160. Lebenthal, A. & Lebenthal, E. (1999). The ontology of the small intestinal epithelium. *J Parenter Enteral Nutr, 23,* S3.

161. Lederman, S.A. (1993). Recent issues related to nutrition during pregnancy. *J Am Coll Nutr, 12,* 91.

162. Lederman, S.A. (2001). Pregnancy weight gain and postpartum loss: Avoiding obesity while optimizing growth and development of the fetus. *J Am Med Womens Assoc, 56,* 53.

163. Lefrak-Okikawa, L. (1988). Nutritional management of the very low birth weight infant. *J Perinat Neonat Nurs, 2,* 66.

164. Lucas, A., Bloom, S.R. & Aynsley-Green, A. (1986). Gut hormones and "minimal enteral feeding." *Acta Paediatr Scand, 75,* 719.

165. Lucas, A. & Cole, T.J. (1990). Breast milk and necrotizing enterocolitis. *Lancet, 336,* 1519.

166. Luder, A.S. & Greene, C.L. (1989). Maternal phenylketonuria and hyperphenylanemia: Implications for medical practice in the United States. *Am J Obstet Gynecol, 161,* 1102.

167. Ludka, L.M. & Riberst, C.C. (1993). Eating and drinking in labor. A literature review. *J Nurse Midwifery, 38,* 199.

168. Luke, B. (1994). Maternal-fetal nutrition. *Clin Obstet Gynecol, 37,* 93.

169. Lumey, L.H. (1998). Compensatory placental growth after restricted maternal nutrition in early pregnancy. *Placenta, 10,* 105.

170. Mabie, W.C. (1992). Obstetric management of gastroenterologic complications of pregnancy. *Gastroenterol Clin North Am, 21,* 923.

171. Macagno, F. & Dermarini, S. (1994). Techniques of enteral feeding in the newborn. *Acta Paediatr Suppl, 402,* 11.

172. Mackin, M.L. (1990). Infant sleep and bedtime cereal. *Am J Dis Child, 143,* 1066.

173. Mandel, L. & Tamari, K. (1995). Sialorrhea and gastroesophageal reflux. *J Am Dent Assoc, 126,* 1537.

174. Mannick, E. & Udall, J.N. (1996). Neonatal gestational mucosal immunity. *Clin Perinatol, 23,* 287.

175. Marcon, M.A. 1997. Advances in the diagnosis and treatment of gastroesophageal reflux disease. *Current Opinions in Pediatrics, 9*(5), 490-493.

176. Maxwell, K.B. & Niebyl, J.R. (1982). Treatment of nausea and vomiting in pregnancy. In J.R. Niebyl (Ed.). *Drug use in pregnancy.* Philadelphia: Lea & Febiger.

177. Mazzotta, P. & Magee, L.A. (2000). A risk-benefit analysis of pharmacological and nonpharmacological treatments for nausea and vomiting of pregnancy. *Drugs, 59,* 781.

178. McDonald, J.A. (1999). Cholestasis of pregnancy. *J Gastroenterol Hepatol, 14,* 515.

179. McKeown, R.E., et al. (1992). Role of delayed feeding and of feeding increments in necrotizing enterocolitis. *J Pediatr, 121,* 764.

180. McLaren, D.S. (1982). Nutritional assessment. In D.S. McLaren & D. Burman (Eds.). *Textbook of paediatric nutrition* (2nd ed.). Edinburgh: Churchill Livingstone.

181. Meetze, W.H., et al. (1992). Gastrointestinal priming prior to full enteral nutrition in very low birth weight infants. *J Pediatr Gastroenterol Nutr, 15,* 163.

182. Meier, P. (1990). Nursing management of breast feeding for preterm infants. In S.G. Funk et al. (Eds.). *Key aspects of recovery: Improving nutrition, rest, and mobility.* New York: Springer.

183. Menard, D., et al. (1995). Ontogeny of human gastric lipase and pepsin activities. *Gastroenterology, 108,* 1650.

184. Michaletz-Onody, P.A. (1992). Peptic ulcer disease in pregnancy. *Gastroenterol Clin North Am, 21,* 817.

185. Milla, P.J. (1996). The ontogeny of intestinal motor activity. In W.A. Walker, et al. (Eds.). *Pediatric gastrointestinal disease* (2nd ed.). St Louis: Mosby.

186. Mishkin, D.J., et al. (1998). Dental diseases. In N. Gleicher (Ed.). *Principles and practice of medical therapy in pregnancy* (3rd ed.). Stamford, CT: Appleton & Lange.

187. Mobassaleh, M., et al. (1985). Development of carbohydrate absorption in the fetus and neonate. *Pediatrics, 75*(suppl.), 160.

188. Mongelli, M. & Gardosi, J. (2000). Fetal growth. *Curr Opin Obstet Gynecol, 12,* 111.

189. Moore, K.L. & Persaud, T.V.N. (1998). *The developing human: Clinically oriented embryology* (6th Ed.). Philadelphia: W.B. Saunders.

190. Moore, T.R. (1997). Fetal growth in diabetic pregnancy. *Clin Obstet Gynecol, 40,* 771.

191. Morin, K.H. (1998). Perinatal outcomes of obese women: a review of the literature. *J Obstet Gynecol Neonatal Nurs, 27,* 431.

192. Murphy, M.S., et al. (1996). Regulatory peptides of the gastrointestinal tract in early life. In W.A. Walker et al. (Eds.). *Pediatric gastrointestinal disease* (2nd ed.). St Louis: Mosby.

193. Nathan, L. & Huddleston, J.F. (1995). Acute abdominal pain in pregnancy. *Obstet Gynecol Clin North Am, 22,* 55.

194. Nelson-Piercy, C. (1998). Treatments of nausea and vomiting in pregnancy. When should it be treated and what can be safely taken? *Drug Saf, 19,* 155.

195. Neu, J. (1996). Nutrient absorption in the preterm neonate. *Clin Perinatol, 23,* 229.

196. Neu, J. & Weiss, M.D. (1999). Necrotizing enterocolitis: pathophysiology and prevention. *J Parenter Enteral Nutr, 23,* S13.

197. Newell, S.J. (2000). Enteral feeding of the micropremie. *Clin Perinatol, 27,* 221.

198. Ohlin, R., et al. (1990). Maternal body weight development after pregnancy. *Int J Obes, 14,* 159.

199. Olson, M. (1970). The benign effects on rabbit's lungs of the aspiration of water compared with 5% glucose or milk. *Pediatrics, 46,* 538.

200. O'Reilly, S.A., et al. (1993). Low risk mothers: oral intake and emesis in labor. *J Nurse Midwifery, 38,* 228.

201. Orenstein, S.R. (1999). Gastroesophageal reflux. *Pediatr Rev, 20,* 24.

202. O'Sullivan, G.M., et al. (1987). Noninvasive measurement of gastric emptying in obstetric patients. *Anesth Analg, 66,* 505.

203. O'Sullivan, G. (1994). The stomach—fact and fantasy: eating and drinking during labor. *Int Anesthesiol Clin, 32,* 31.

204. Pauerstein, C. (1987). *Clinical obstetrics.* New York: John Wiley & Sons.

205. Pereira, G.R. & Barbosa, N.M. (1986). Controversies in neonatal nutrition. *Pediatr Clin North Am, 33,* 65.

206. Pereira, G.R. & Zucker, A. (1986). Nutritional deficiencies in the neonate. *Clin Perinatol, 13,* 175.

207. Pereira, G.R. (1995). Nutritional care of the extremely premature infant. *Clin Perinatol, 22,* 61.

208. Potter, S., et al. (1991).7 Does infant feeding method influence maternal postpartum weight loss? *J Am Diet Assoc, 91,* 441.

209. Premji, S.S. (1998). Ontology of the gastrointestinal system and its impact on feeding the preterm infant. *Neonatal Netw, 17,* 17.

210. Premji, S.S. & Paes, B. (2000). Gastrointestinal function and growth in premature infants: Is non-nutritive sucking vital? *J Perinatol, 20,* 46.

211. Prentice, A.M., et al. (1996). Energy requirements of pregnant and lactating women. *Eur J Clin Nutr, 50*(suppl), S82.

212. Putet, G. (2000). Lipid metabolism of the micropremie. *Clin Perinatol, 27,* 57.

213. Rassin, D.K. (1990). Quality of human milk versus formulas: Protein composition. In N.M. van Gelder, R.F. Butterworth, & B.D. Drujan (Eds.). *(Mal)nutrition and the infant brain.* New York: Wiley-Liss.

214. Resnik, R. (1999). The puerperium. In R.K. Creasy & R. Resnik (Eds.). *Maternal-fetal medicine* (4th ed.). Philadelphia: W.B. Saunders.

215. Riely, C.A. & Fallon, H.J. (1999). Liver diseases. In G.N. Burrow & T.P. Duffy (Eds.). *Medical complications during pregnancy* (5th ed.). Philadelphia: W.B. Saunders.

216. Rivera, A., et al. (1993). Effect of intravenous amino acids on protein metabolism of preterm infants during the first three days of life. *Pediatr Res, 33,* 106.

217. Robinson, J.S., et al. (2000). Origins of fetal growth restriction. *Eur J Obstet Gynecol Reprod Biol, 92,* 13.

218. Rodriguez-Palmero, M. (1999). Nutritional and biochemical properties of human milk. II: Lipids, micronutrients, and bioactive factors. *Clin Perinatol, 26,* 335.

219. Romero, R. & Kleinman, R.E. (1993). Feeding the very-low-birthweight infant. *Pediatr Rev, 14,* 123.

220. Rosso, P. (1987). Regulation of food intake during pregnancy and lactation. *Ann NY Acad Sci, 499,* 191.

221. Rosso, P.R. (1990). Prenatal nutrition and brain growth. In N.M. van Gelder, R.F. Butterworth, & B.D. Drujan (Eds.). *(Mal)nutrition and the infant brain.* New York: Wiley-Liss.

222. Rosso, P. (1990). *Nutrition and metabolism in pregnancy.* New York: Oxford University Press.

223. Rothman, K., et al. (1995). Teratogenicity of high vitamin A intake. *N Engl J Med, 333,* 1369.

224. Rouse, B., et al. (1997). Maternal Phenylketonuria Collaborative Study (MPCS) offspring: Facial anomalies, malformations, and early neurological sequelae. *Am J Med Genet, 69,* 89.

225. Rubin, P.H. & Janowitz, H.D. (1991). The digestive tract and pregnancy. In S.H. Cherry & I.R. Merkatz (Eds.). *Complications of pregnancy: medical, surgical, gynecological, psychosocial, and perinatal* (4th ed.). Baltimore: Williams & Wilkins.

226. Rushton, C.H. (1990). Necrotizing enterocolitis. I: Pathogenesis and diagnosis. *MCN, 15,* 296.

227. Sadler, T.W. (2000). *Langman's medical embryology* (8th ed.). Philadelphia: Lippincott, Williams & Wilkins.

228. Sanderson, I.R. (1999). The physiochemical environment of the neonatal intestine. *Am J Clin Nutr, 69,* 1028S.

229. Schandler, R.J., et al. (1998). Parenteral and enteral nutrition. In H.W. Taeusch & R.A. Ballard (Eds.). *Avery's Diseases of the newborn* (7th ed.). Philadelphia: W.B. Saunders.

230. Schanler, R.J., et al. (1999). The use of human milk and breastfeeding in premature infants. *Clin Perinatol, 26,* 379.

231. Schandler, R.J., et al. (1999). Feeding strategies for premature infants: randomized trial of gastrointestinal priming and tube feeding method. *Pediatrics, 103,* 434.

232. Schmitz, J. (1996). Digestive and absorptive function. In W.A. Walker et al. (Eds.). *Pediatric gastrointestinal disease* (2nd ed.). St. Louis: Mosby.

233. Schneider, R.E., et al. (2000). Dental complications. In W.R. Cohen, S.H. Cherry & I.R. Merkatz (Eds.). *Cherry & Merkatz's complications of pregnancy* (5th ed.). Baltimore: Williams & Wilkins.

234. Scholl, T.O., et al. (1996). Dietary and serum folate: Their influence on outcome of pregnancy. *Am J Clin Nutr, 63,* 520.

235. Scholl, T., et al. (1997). Use of multivitamin/mineral prenatal supplements: influence on outcome of pregnancy. *Am J Epidemiol, 146,* 134.

236. Schrade, R.R., et al. (1986). Gastric emptying time during pregnancy. *Gastroenterology, 86,* 1234.

237. Schreiber, R.A. (1996). Hepatobiliary system structure and function. In W.A. Walker et al. (Eds.). *Pediatric gastrointestinal disease* (2nd ed.). St. Louis: Mosby.

238. Schwitzgebel, V.M. & Gitelman, S.E. (1998). Neonatal hyperinsulism. *Clin Perinatol, 25,* 1015.

239. Scott, L.D. (1999). Gastrointestinal disease in pregnancy. In R.K. Creasy & R. Resnik (Eds.). *Maternal-fetal medicine* (4th ed.). Philadelphia: W.B. Saunders.

240. Seashore, M. (1999). Clinical genetics. In G.N. Burrow & T.P. Duffy (Eds.). *Medical complications during pregnancy* (5th ed.). Philadelphia: W.B. Saunders.

241. Sharp, H.T. (1994). Gastrointestinal surgical conditions during pregnancy. *Clin Obstet Gynecol, 37,* 306.

242. Shaw, B. (1995). Primary care for women. Comprehensive assessment of gastrointestinal disorders. *J Nurse Midwifery, 40,* 216.

243. Shaw, G., et al. (1995). Maternal preconceptional use of multivitamins and reduced risk for conotruncal heart defects and limb defects among offspring. *Am J Med Genet, 69,* 536.

244. Sherry, S.N. & Kramer, J.C. (1955). The time of passage of the first stool and first urine. *J Pediatr, 46,* 158.

245. Shulman, R.J., et al. (1998). Early feeding, antenatal corticosteroids, and human milk decrease intestinal permeability in preterm infants. *Pediatr Res, 44,* 519.

246. Skupski, D.W. (1998). Prenatal diagnosis of gastrointestinal anomalies with ultrasound. What have we learned? *Ann N Y Acad Sci, 847,* 53.

247. Smoleniec, J.S. & James, D.K. (1993). Gastro-intestinal crises during pregnancy. *Dig Dis, 11,* 313.

248. Snell, L.H., et al. (1998). Metabolic crisis: hyperemesis gravidarum. *J Perinat Neonatal Nurs, 12,* 26.

249. Sohaey, R., Woodward, P. & Zwiebel, W.J. (1996). Fetal gastrointestinal anomalies. *Semin Ultrasound CT MR, 17,* 51.

250. Steinlauf, A.F. & Traube, M. (1999). Gastrointestinal complications. In G.N. Burrow & T.P. Duffy (Eds.). *Medical complications during pregnancy* (5th ed.). Philadelphia: W.B. Saunders.

251. Suidan, J.S. & Young, B.K. (1986). The acute abdomen in pregnancy. In V.K. Rustgi & J.N. Cooper (Eds.). *Gastrointestinal and hepatic complications in pregnancy.* New York: John Wiley & Sons.

252. Sunshine, P. (1977). Absorption and malabsorption of carbohydrates. In *Selected aspects of perinatal gastroenterology* (Mead Johnson Symposium on Perinatal and Developmental Medicine, no. 11). Evansville, IN: Mead Johnson.

253. Sunshine, P. (1977). Digestion and absorption of proteins. In *Selected aspects of perinatal gastroenterology* (Mead Johnson Symposium on Perinatal and Developmental Medicine, no. 11). Evansville, IN: Mead Johnson.

254. Szabo, J.S., Hillemeier, A.C., & Oh, W. (1985). Effect of nonnutritive and nutritive suck on gastric emptying in premature infants. *J Pediatr Gastroenterol Nutr, 4,* 348.

255. Theron, G. & Thompson, M. (1993). The usefulness of weight gain in predicting pregnancy complications. *J Trop Pediatr, 39,* 269.

256. Thureen, P.J., et al. (1998). Protein balance in the first week of life in ventilated neonates receiving parenteral nutrition. *Am J Clin Nutr, 68,* 1228.

257. Thureen, P.J. (1999). Early aggressive nutrition in the neonate. *Pediatr Rev, 20,* 45.

258. Thureen, P.J. & Hay, W.W. (2000). Intravenous nutrition and postnatal growth of the micropremie. *Clin Perinatol, 27,* 197.

259. Tierson, F.D., Olsen, C.L. & Hook, E.B. (1986). Nausea and vomiting of pregnancy and association with pregnancy outcome. *Am J Obstet Gynecol, 155,* 1017.

260. Topper, W.H. (1981). Enteral feeding methods for compromised neonates and infants. In E. Lebenthal (Ed.). *Textbook of gastroenterology and nutrition in infancy.* New York: Raven.

261. Torfs, C., Curry, C., & Roeper, P. (1990). Gastroschisis. *J Pediatr, 116,* 1.

262. Trahair, J.F. (1993). Is fetal enteral nutrition important for normal gastrointestinal growth?: A discussion. *J Parenter Enteral Nutr, 17,* 82.

263. Tsang, R. (1993). *Nutritional needs of the preterm infant.* Baltimore: Williams & Wilkins.

264. Tsimoyiannis, E.C., et al. (1994). Cholelithiasis during pregnancy and lactation. *Eur J Surg, 150,* 627.

265. Tyson, J.E., et al. (1999). Vitamin A supplementation for extremely low birth weight infants. *N Engl J Med, 340,* 1962.

266. Uauy, R.D., et al. (1991). Necrotizing enterocolitis in very low birth weight infants. Biodemographic and clinical correlates. *J Pediatr, 119,* 630.

267. Uauy, R., et al. (2000). Essential fatty acid metabolism in the micro premie. *Clin Perinatol, 27,* 71.

268. Udall, J.N. (1990). Gastrointestinal tract host defense and necrotizing enterocolitis. *J Pediatr, 117,* S33.

269. Ulmsten, U. & Sundstrom, G. (1978). Esophageal manometry in pregnant and non-pregnant women. *Am J Obstet Gynecol, 132,* 260.

270. Vander, A.J., Sherman, J.H. & Luciano, D.S. (2001). *Human physiology: The mechanisms of body function* (8th ed.). Dubuque, IA: McGraw-Hill.

271. Vanderhoof, J.A., et al. (1999). Gastrointestinal disease. In G.B. Avery, M.A. Fletcher & M.G. MacDonald (Eds.). *Neonatology, pathophysiology and management of the newborn* (5th ed.). Philadelphia: J.B. Lippincott.

272. vanLingen, R.A., et al. (1992). Effects of early amino acid administration during total parenteral nutrition on protein metabolism in preterm infants. *Clin Sci, 82,* 199.

273. Van Thiel, D.H. & Schade, R.R. (1986). Pregnancy: Its physiologic course, nutrient cost, and effects on gastrointestinal function. In V.K. Rustgi & J.N. Cooper (Eds.). *Gastrointestinal and hepatic complications in pregnancy.* New York: John Wiley & Sons.

274. Vutyvanich, T., et al. (2001). Ginger for nausea and vomiting in pregnancy: randomized, double-masked placebo-controlled trial. *Obstet Gynecol, 97,* 577.

275. Walker, V., et al. (1989). Carbohydrate fermentation by gut microflora in preterm neonates. *Am J Dis Child, 64,* 1367.

276. Walker, W.A. (2000). Role of nutrients and bacterial colonization in the development of intestinal host defense. *J Pediatr Gastroenterol Nutr, 30,* S2.

277. Watkins, J.B. (1985). Lipid digestion and absorption. *Pediatrics, 75*(suppl.), 151.

278. Weaver, L.T. (1993). Development of bowel habit in preterm infants. *Arch Dis Child, 68,* 317.

279. Weaver, L.T. (1996). Anatomy and embryology. In W.A. Walker et al. (Eds.). *Pediatric gastrointestinal disease* (2nd ed.). St. Louis: Mosby.

280. Weigel, M.M. & Weigel, R.M. (1989). Nausea and vomiting of early pregnancy and pregnancy outcome: An epidemiological study. *Br J Obstet Gynaecol, 96,* 1304.

282. Weigel, M.M. & Weigel, R.M. (1989). Nausea and vomiting of early pregnancy and pregnancy outcome. A meta-analytical review. *Br J Obstet Gynaecol, 96,* 1312.

282. Wershil, B.K. (1996). Gastric function. In W.A. Walker et al. (Eds.). *Pediatric gastrointestinal disease* (2nd ed.). St. Louis: Mosby.

283. Wharton, B.A. (1987). *Nutrition and feeding of preterm infants.* Oxford: Blackwell Scientific Publications.

284. Widstrom, A.M., et al. (1988). Non-nutritive sucking in tube-fed preterm infants: Effects on feeding time and gastric contents of gastrin and somatostatin. *J Pediatr Gastroenterol Nutr, 7,* 517.

285. Wilson, D.C. (1995). Nutrition of the preterm baby. *Br J Obstet Gynaecol, 102,* 854.

286. Wolkind, S. & Zajicek, E. (1978). Psychosocial correlates of nausea and vomiting in pregnancy. *J Psychosom Res, 22,* 1.

287. Worthington-Roberts, B. (1989). Obesity and nutrition during pregnancy. In S.A. Brody & K. Ueland (Eds.). *Endocrine disorders in pregnancy.* Norwalk CT: Appleton & Lange.

288. Worthington-Roberts, B.S. & Williams, S.R. (1997). *Nutrition in pregnancy and lactation* (6th ed.). Madison, WI: Brown & Benchmark.

289. Worthington-Roberts, B.S. (2000). Nutrition. In W.R. Cohen, S.H. Cherry & I.R. Merkatz (Eds.). *Cherry & Merkatz's Complications of pregnancy* (5th ed.). Philadelphia: Lippincott, Williams & Wilkins.

290. Wright, L.I., et al. (1993). Rapid advances in feeding increase the risk of necrotizing enterocolitis in very low birth weight infants. *Pediatr Res, 33,* 313A.

291. Xu, R.J. (1996). Development of the newborn GI tract and its relation to colostrum/milk intake: a review. *Reprod Fertil Dev, 81,* 35.

292. Yip, D.M. & Baker, A.L. (1985). Liver diseases in pregnancy. *Clin Perinatol, 12,* 683.

293. Yu, V.Y. (1999). Enteral feeding in the preterm infant. *Early Hum Dev, 56,* 89.

294. Zachariasen, R.D. (1993). The effect of elevated ovarian hormones on periodontal health: oral contraceptives and pregnancy. *Women Health, 20,* 21.

295. Zeidenstein, L. (1998). Alternative therapies for nausea and vomiting of pregnancy. *J Nurse Midwifery, 43,* 392.

296. Zerzan, J. & O'Leary, M.J. (1997). Nutrition for the preterm and low-birth-weight infant. In C.M. Trahms & P.L. Pipes (Eds.). *Nutrition in infancy and childhood* (4th ed.). New York: McGraw-Hill.

297. Ziegler, E.E. (1994). Protein in premature feeding. *Nutrition, 10,* 69.

CHAPTER 19

Immune System and Host Defense Mechanisms

Host defense mechanisms consist of immunologic and nonimmunologic factors. Nonimmunologic factors include genetic susceptibility; skin and mucosal barriers; digestive enzymes; pH; temperature; proteins; and enzymes such as lysozyme, transferrin, and interferon. Immunologic factors consist of innate and adaptive immune responses. Innate immunity (Figure 12-1) includes the inflammatory response and phagocytosis by neutrophils and other cells (Figure 12-2). Adaptive immunity (Figure 12-3) involves specific immune responses as seen with cell- and antibody-mediated immunity. The immune system and host defense mechanisms are altered in both the pregnant woman and neonate. The interaction between the mother's host defense mechanisms and the fetus (who is antigenically unique from the mother) presents one of the more challenging questions in immunology: Why doesn't the mother reject the fetus? Current theories regarding this question—along with alterations in host defense mechanisms in the mother and neonate and implications for clinical practice—are examined in this chapter. Understanding of maternal, fetal, and neonatal immune physiology is still evolving, with conflicting or incomplete data for some parameters. Host defense mechanisms and terminology are summarized in Figures 12-1, 12-2, and 12-3 and in Table 12-1.

MATERNAL PHYSIOLOGIC ADAPTATIONS

Alterations in the immune system during pregnancy affect both innate (see Figure 12-1) and adaptive (see Figure 12-3) immunity. These alterations help the mother's host defense system tolerate the fetus but may also increase the risk of maternal infections and influence the course of chronic disorders such as autoimmune diseases.

Antepartum Period

"Pregnancy is an immunological balancing act in which the mother's immune system has to remain tolerant of potential major histocompatibility (MHC) antigens (Figure 12-4) and yet maintain normal immune competence for defense against microorganisms."[185,p. 643] Adaptations in the

maternal immune system during pregnancy include alterations in the inflammatory response, phagocytosis, and in B- and T-lymphocyte function. During pregnancy, Th2 helper responses increase and Th1 responses lessen. As a result, production of some cytokines (Table 12-2) is altered.[54] In addition, hormonal and serum factors that modulate various aspects of maternal host defense mechanisms are also modified. Alterations in host defense mechanisms during pregnancy and their implications are summarized in Table 12-3.

Alterations in Innate Immunity

Total white blood cell (WBC) volume increases slightly beginning in the second month and levels off during the second and third trimesters (see Table 7-2). The total WBC count in pregnancy varies with individual women, ranging from 5000 to 12,000 per mm^3, with values as high as 15,000 per mm^3 reported (see Chapter 7).[144,172] The increase is primarily due to increased polymorphonuclear neutrophils (PMNs).[144] A slight shift to the left may occur, with occasional myelocytes and metamyelocytes seen on the peripheral smear. Changes in other WBC forms are minimal (see Table 7-2). Functional alterations in the PMNs have also been reported.[56,63] Altered metabolic activity of maternal leukocytes along with both increased and decreased phagocytic and bacteriocidal activity has been reported, especially in response to gram-negative organisms.[56] PMN attachment, ingestion, and digestion of *Candida albicans* has been found to be increased, possibly secondary to the effects of human chorionic gonadotropin.[9] However, pregnant women have higher rates of fungal infection, probably due to the effects of estrogen on nutrient availability for fungal growth in the reproductive tract.[144] Chemotaxis (movement of neutrophils toward the site of infection) is decreased during pregnancy, which may delay initial maternal responses to infection.[57] Conversely, improved PMN antibody expression during pregnancy may enhance phagocyte recognition and destruction of antigen-antibody complexes.[169]

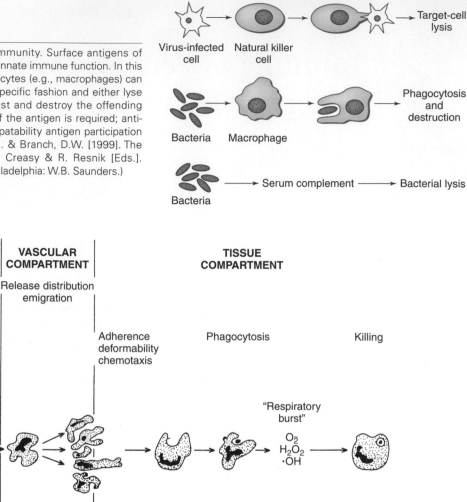

FIGURE **12-1** Summary of innate immunity. Surface antigens of viruses, bacterial, and tumors induce innate immune function. In this system, natural killer cells and phagocytes (e.g., macrophages) can recognize certain antigens in a nonspecific fashion and either lyse the offending infected cells or ingest and destroy the offending organism. Only the foreign nature of the antigen is required; antigen processing and major histocompatability antigen participation is not necessary. (From Silver, R.M. & Branch, D.W. [1999]. The immunology of pregnancy. In R.K. Creasy & R. Resnik [Eds.]. *Maternal-fetal medicine* [4th ed.]. Philadelphia: W.B. Saunders.)

MARROW COMPARTMENT	VASCULAR COMPARTMENT	TISSUE COMPARTMENT
Maturation	Release distribution emigration	

Adherence deformability chemotaxis

Phagocytosis

Killing

"Respiratory burst"

O_2^-
H_2O_2
$\cdot OH$

FIGURE **12-2** Overview of polymorphonuclear neutrophil (PMN) functions. PMNs are produced and mature in the bone marrow over a 2-week period. On release from the marrow, PMNs circulate for 6 to 8 hours before emigrating into tissues. At sites of infection, chemotactic factors enhance PMN adhesion to and emigration through vascular endothelium. PNMs migrate in a directed fashion (chemotaxis) toward the pathogens. Phagocytosis of the offending organisms stimulates an increase in production of oxygen metabolites (respiratory burst), which facilitates PMN killing of the ingested microbes. (From Kapur, R., et al. [2002]. Developmental immunology. In A.A. Fanaroff & R.J. Martin [Eds.]. *Neonatal-perinatal medicine: diseases of the fetus and infant* [7th ed.]. St. Louis: Mosby.)

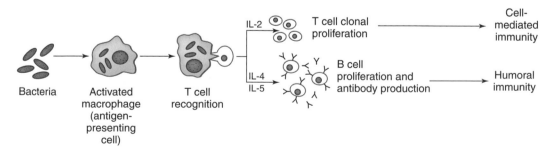

FIGURE **12-3** Summary of adaptive immunity. Adaptive immune responses initially require antigen processing and subsequent presentation in T cells. A T cell with a receptor specific for an inciting antigen will be activated and undergo clonal proliferation. In part, the type of cytokine produced by the activated T dictates the nature of the subsequent response. Interleukin-2 (IL-2) is the primary growth factor required for clonal proliferation of T cells; it stimulates the proliferation of cytotoxic and memory T-cells. IL-4 and IL-5 stimulate B-cell proliferation, differentiation, and antibody production. (From Silver, R.M. & Branch, D.W. [1999]. The immunology of pregnancy. In R.K. Creasy & R. Resnik [Eds.]. *Maternal-fetal medicine* [4th ed.]. Philadelphia: W.B. Saunders.)

TABLE 12-1   Definitions of Terms

Active immunity: Exposure to antigen (attenuated or inactivated/killed virus or bacterium) that leads to formation of antibodies and memory cells against that antigen.

Adaptive immunity: Involves specific antibody (humoral)-mediated and cell-mediated responses, which are mediated by B (antibody-mediated) and T (cell-mediated) lymphocytes.

Allograft: Graft taken from an organism that is the same species as the recipient but not genetically identical.

Antibody: Proteins (immunoglobulin) that react with specific antigens. The five classes are IgA, IgD, IgE, IgG, and IgM

Antibody (humoral)-mediated immunity: Specific host defense mechanisms mediated by B cells that provide protection through production of antibodies.

Antigen: Substances perceived by one's host defense mechanisms as "foreign" (e.g., bacteria, viruses, pollutants, dust, certain foods).

Cell-mediated immunity: Specific host defense mechanisms, mediated by T-helper, T-suppressor, and cytotoxic T cells, that provide protection against certain organisms, regulate B-cell function, defend against cancer, and mediate graft rejection.

Chemotaxis: Movement of neutrophils and other phagocytes in an organized fashion toward a site of antigenic invasion.

Complement: Sequential series of discrete plasma proteins and their fragments that when activated enhance other aspects of the immune system. Actions include attraction of various cell types to the initial site of invasion, promotion of chemotaxis and phagocytosis, enhancement of opsonization and the inflammatory response, and direct destruction of antigens by lysis of cell membranes.

Cytokines: Glycoproteins such as interleukins, interferon and tissue necrosis factor, produced by various components of the immune system, especially T lymphocytes and macrophages. Cytokines usually function in an autocrine or paracine manner to regulate immune processes and the inflammatory response.

Cytotoxic/killer T cell: Type of T lymphocyte acting directly on specific antigens or target cells with specific antigen resulting in cell lysis.

Fibronectin: Nonspecific opsonin, inhibitor of bacterial adherence to epithelial cells, and clot-stabilizing protein found in plasma and endothelial tissue.

Helper T (CD4+) cell: Type of T lymphocyte that acts to enhance the activity of B lymphocytes, other T cells, and macrophages via secretion of cytokines. Subsets include Th1 and Th2 cells.

Human leukocyte antigen (HLA): The major form of specific tissue antigens found on tissue surfaces that are unique to each person (includes HLA-A, HLA-B, HLA-C, HLA-D and HLA-G).

Immunoglobulin (Ig): Antibodies produced by B lymphocytes (includes IgG, IgM, IgA, IgD, and IgE).

Innate immunity: Initial nonspecific responses including the inflammatory response and phagocytosis, which result in either elimination of the foreign substance or antigen with cessation of the response or formation of a "processed antigen" while stimulating secondary mechanisms.

Major histocompatibility complex (MHC): Specific antigens found on tissue surfaces divided into three groups: MHC I (HLA-A, HLA-B, and HLA-C, which are found on most of a person's cells); MHC II (found on surface of immune cells); and MHC III (includes some components of complement).

Memory cell: Form of lymphocytes sensitized to specific antigens; with subsequent stimulation by the specific antigen, an exaggerated and accelerated response usually occurs.

Natural killer (NK) cells: A subpopulation of lymphoid cells that attack without previous immunization and independent of antibodies, phagocytosis, and complement; form a first line of defense against antigens until other defense mechanisms can be mobilized.

Opsonization: Processing and marking or altering the cell surface of an antigen by actions of immunoglobulin or complement; substances acting in this manner are called opsonins. This process is critical in allowing phagocytosis of organisms with a capsular polysaccharide coat such as group B streptococci.

Passive immunity: Transfer of antibodies from an actively immunized to a nonimmunized person.

Plasma cell: Form of B lymphocyte able to secrete immunoglobulins.

Suppressor T (T8) cell: Suppresses B-lymphocyte function including production of antibodies to autoantigens; may help to slow or terminate immune response once the antigens are destroyed.

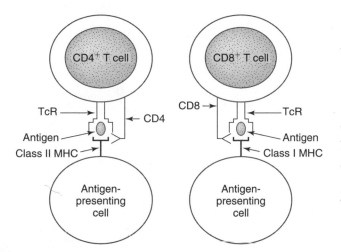

FIGURE 12-4 T-cell receptor *(TcR)* and antigen recognition, T cells recognize foreign antigen in the context of self major histocompatability antigen *(MHC)* when it is presented in this context by antigen-presenting cells (e.g., macrophages). Antigen presented with class II MHC molecules (left) is recognized by T cells bearing the CD4 adhesion molecule. Such cells usually act as T "helper" cells. Antigen processed with class I MHC molecules (right) is recognized by T cells bearing the CD8 adhesive molecule. Such T cells usually act as cytotoxic T cells or T "suppressor" cells. (From Silver, R.M. & Branch, D.W. [1999]. The immunology of pregnancy. In R.K. Creasy & R. Resnik [Eds.]. *Maternal-fetal medicine* [4th ed.]. Philadelphia: W.B. Saunders.)

TABLE **12-2** Cellular Sources, Target Cells, and Principal Activities of Cytokines Relevant to Reproductive Immunology

Cytokine	Cellular Sources	Target Cells	Principal Activities
INFLAMMATORY CYTOKINES			
Interleukin-1α	Macrophages	T and B cells	Lymphocyte activation, prostaglandin production
Interleukin-1β	Monocytes, B cells, fibroblasts, endothelial cells	Macrophages, endothelial cells, fibroblasts	Macrophage stimulation, pyrexia, enhanced leukocyte-endothelial interaction, tissue regeneration, enhanced MHC expression
Tumor necrosis factor	Macrophages, cytotoxic T cells, NK cells	Macrophages, neutrophils, fibroblasts	Cachexia, enhanced leukocyte-endothelial interaction, macrophage activation, enhanced cytotoxicity
Interleukin-6	Macrophages, fibroblasts, activated CD4$^+$ T cells	Macrophages, endothelial cells, hepatocytes, B cells	Acute phase response, T-cell activation, prostaglandin production, B-cell differentiation into plasma cells and antibody production
CHEMOKINES			
Interleukin-8	Macrophages, monocytes, endothelial cells, keratinocytes, fibroblasts	Neutrophils, T cells, basophils	Neutrophil activation and degranulation, chemotactic for neutrophils and T cells
T-CELL–DERIVED LYMPHOKINES			
Interleukin-2	Activated CD4$^+$ T cells, NK cells	CD4$^+$ and CD8$^+$ T cells	T-cell growth and proliferation
Interleukin-3	Activated CD4$^+$ T cells	Hematopoietic precursors, stem cells	Promotes growth and differentiation of myeloid progenitor cells
Interleukin-4	Activated CD4$^+$ T cells	B cells, eosinophils	B-cell growth and differentiation, IgE production, eosinophilia
Interleukin-5	Activated CD4$^+$ T cells	B cells	B-cell differentiation, antibody isotype switching
Interferon-γ	Activated CD4$^+$ T cells, NK cells	CD4$^+$ and CD8$^+$ T cells, macrophages	Enhances MHC class II expression, macrophage activation, enhances endothelial-leukocyte interaction
Interferon-α	Mononuclear phagocytes	Virus-infected cells, NK cells	Inhibits viral replication, inhibits cell proliferation, increases MHC expression, activates NK cells
COLONY-STIMULATING FACTORS (CSFS)			
Granulocyte-CSF	Mononuclear phagocytes, endothelial cells, fibroblasts	Granulocyte progenitors	Maturation of progenitors into granulocytes
Granulocyte-macrophage CSF	T cells, mononuclear phagocytes, endothelial cells, fibroblasts	Granulocyte and macrophage progenitors	Maturation of progenitors into granulocytes and macrophages
Macrophage CSF	Mononuclear phagocytes, endothelial cells, fibroblasts	Macrophage progenitors	Maturation of progenitors into macrophages
PEPTIDE GROWTH FACTORS			
Transforming growth factor-β	T cells, mononuclear phagocytes	T cells, mononuclear phagocytes, other cells	Inhibits the activation of mononuclear phagocytes, inhibits activation and proliferation of T cells

From Silver, R.M. & Branch, D.W. (1999). The immunology of pregnancy. In R.K. Creasy and R. Resnik (Eds.) *Maternal-fetal medicine* (4th ed.). Philadelphia: W.B. Saunders.
Ig, Immunoglobulin; *MHC*, major histocompatibility complex; *NK*, natural killer.

TABLE **12-3**   Alterations in Host Defense Mechanisms during Pregnancy

ALTERATION	RESULT	IMPLICATIONS
INNATE IMMUNITY		
Increased polymorphonuclear neutrophils (PMNs)	Increased available phagocytes	Protection of mother and fetus from infection
Altered metabolic activity and chemotaxis of PMN	Delay initial response to infection, especially gram negative organisms	Increase risk of colonization, urinary tract infection
Improved PMN antibody expression	Enhanced phagocyte recognition	Protect fetus and trophoblast from rejection Protect mother and fetus from infection
Decreased natural killer cell activity; lower cytolytic activity in third trimester	Delay initial response to infection	Increase risk of colonization, pathogens such listeria and toxoplasmosis Protect fetus and trophoblast from rejection
Increased fibronectin	Enhanced opsonization	Augmented maternal responses against bacterial infection
Increased estrogen and glycogen in reproductive tract	Altered local mucosal barrier function Nutrients for fungal growth	Increased risk of colonization Increased risk of yeast infection
CELL-MEDIATED IMMUNITY		
Reduction in Th1 responses and cytokines	Reduction in cell mediated responses and graft rejection	Increase risk of mycotic, fungal, and other opportunistic infections Protect fetus from rejection
Increased Th2 responses and cytokines	Enhanced antibody mediated responses	Protect mother and fetus from infection
Altered T-cell function and efficiency	Decrease graft rejection Depress reaction to tuberculin test	May alter diagnosis of infection in second half of pregnancy Increased risk of mycotic and viral infections
ANTIBODY-MEDIATED IMMUNITY		
Decreased responsiveness of B-cells in late pregnancy	Decreased responsiveness to antigen stimulation in late pregnancy	Increased risk of colonization with streptococci, staphylococci, other organisms
Reduction in circulating immunoglobulin G in late pregnancy	Due to transfer to fetus and hemodilution	Increased risk of colonization Protection of fetus/newborn
COMPLEMENT SYSTEM		
Increased total complement and C2, C3, C3 split products	Enhance chemotaxis and action of immunoglobulins through opsonization	Augment maternal defenses against bacterial infection Protect fetus from infection
Decreased C1, C1a, B, D	Delay initial activation of complement system	Protect fetus and trophoblast from rejection

Natural killer (NK) cell activity is downregulated during pregnancy.[41] NK cytolytic activity is normal in the first trimester but lower during the second and third trimesters and immediately after delivery.[31,75] This may assist in maternal tolerance of the fetus by protecting the trophoblast from destruction.[56,167] NK cells increase in the decidua early in pregnancy, but then they decrease, probably due to the effects of progesterone.[83] Pregnancy may induce formation of a blocking factor that decreases lymphocyte proliferation and NK activity.[143] Interleukin (IL)-4 and interferon-γ (IFN-γ) (Table 12-2) may also be decreased.[164,170] Fibro-

nectin, a glycoprotein with opsonic and clot-stabilizing properties, increases about 2.5 times. Further increases are seen in women with preeclampsia, probably due to vascular endothelial injury that is thought to be a primary event in the development of this disorder (see Chapter 8).

Alterations in the complement system. Alterations in the complement system (Figure 12-5) during pregnancy begin at 11 weeks with an increase (due to greater hepatic synthesis) in both total serum complement and specific proteins of the complement system, including C2, C3, and C3 split products.[56,93] These components enhance chemotaxis

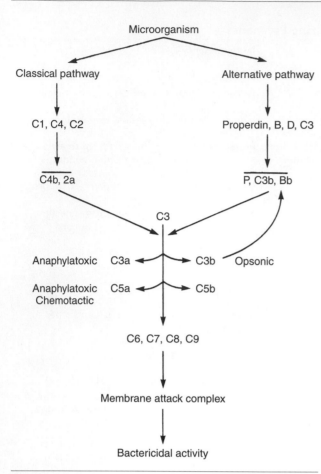

FIGURE **12-5** The complement system. The complement system involves a sequential series of discrete plasma proteins and their fragments that, when activated, enhance other parts of the immune system. Actions of complement include attraction of various cell types to the initial site of antigen invasion, promotion of chemotaxis and phagocytosis, enhancement of opsonization and other immunoglobulin functions, enhancement of histamine release and the inflammatory response, and direct destruction of antigens. Proteins of the complement system circulate in the plasma in an inactive state. Complement is activated through a sequential cascade. Activated molecules either act as enzymes to activate other proteins or fragments in the complement system or enhance actions of other parts of the immune system. There are two activation sequences. The classical pathway requires antibody or antigen-antibody complexes for activation, which occurs by C1 through C3. Complement activation and fixation are important for IgG and IgM function. Early in the immune response and during the initial inflammatory response, antibody may not be present, so an alternative activation sequence is needed. The alternative or properdin pathway is activated by factors B through C3 by substances such as bacterial products and circulating proteins. (From McLean, R.H. & Winkelstein, J.A. [1984]. Genetically determined variations in complement synthesis: Relationship to disease. *J Pediatr, 105,* 179.)

and actions of immunoglobulins through opsonization, thereby augmenting maternal defenses against bacterial infection. Other protein fragments of the complement system such as C1, C1a, B, and D are decreased.[60] Since these fragments are involved in activation of the complement system, through either the classical or the alternative pathway, activity of the complement system early in the immune response may be delayed. This may afford additional protection for the trophoblast and fetus, but it increases the risk of maternal infection.

Alterations in Adaptive Immunity

Pregnancy is characterized by a switch in the balance of Th1 and Th2 T-helper cell subsets with enhanced Th2 function. This change is probably mediated by progesterone and results in increased Th2 cytokines (e.g., IL-3, IL-4, IL-6, IL-10) and a reduction in Th1 cytokines (e.g., IL-2, IFN-γ, TNF-α).[54] Changes in Th1 cytokines may decrease the resistance of the pregnant woman to the spread of bacterial and viral organisms.[54] CD4[+] and CD8[+] expression is transiently down-regulated on cells specific for paternal MHC 1 antigens, reflecting a reduction in Th1 responses.[40] Because Th2 responses tend to enhance antibody-mediated and Th1 responses enhance cell-mediated immunity (Figure 12-6), this switch alters both cell-mediated and antibody-mediated response. Some investigators have reported an inversion of the usual B lymphocyte–to–T lymphocyte ratio of 1:3 at 10 to 13 weeks' gestation with a return to a normal ratio by 20 weeks.[56,83] However, most investigators have not noted this change.[63,154]

Alterations in cell-mediated immunity. The Th1 to Th2 switch alters cell-mediated immunity with changes in the function and efficiency of the T lymphocytes and in cytokine produciton.[41,54] Most investigators report that the total number of lymphocytes does not change significantly during pregnancy.[56,60] Others have found no change in the relative number but a reduction in the absolute number of T lymphocytes.[171] Some investigators have also reported a decrease in the T-helper to T-suppressor (CD4[+]/CD8[+]) ratio; however, others report no changes in this ratio.[63,83,186] The numbers of T-helper cells tend to decrease progressively to term, while T-suppressor cells tend to remain relatively unchanged.[56,104] A recent study reported an increase in T-suppressor cells (CD8[+], CD11b[+]) and NK cells in early pregnancy, followed by a later decrease in T-helper (CD4[+]) cells and NK cells in late pregnancy.[22]

Because T-helper cells normally augment the cytotoxic responses involved in graft rejection, a decreased number of these cells may help protect the fetus from rejection by the mother. T-suppressor cell function may increase in late

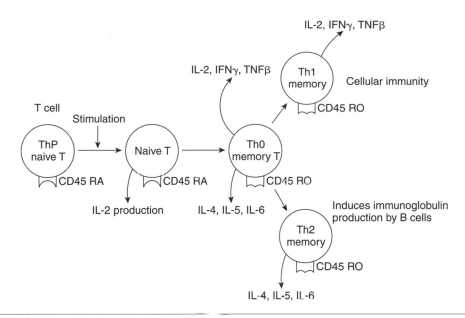

FIGURE **12-6** T-cell development from naive T cells to memory T cells. Cytokines released from different T cell types are indicated as follows: *IL,* interleukin; *IFN,* interferon; *TNF,* tumor necrosis factor. (From Saito, S. [2000]. Cytokine network at the feto-maternal interface. *J Reprod Immunol, 47,* 92.)

pregnancy and suppress or decrease B-cell function.[63] Decreased T-lymphocyte function and efficiency may increase the risk of viral and mycotic infections. In addition, the maternal reaction to the tuberculin test is depressed during the second half of pregnancy. As a result, diagnosis of tuberculosis in the pregnant woman may be more difficult.[56]

Alterations in antibody-mediated immunity. Antibody-mediated immunity is not significantly altered during pregnancy, although a decreased response of B-lymphocytes to antigen stimulation has been reported in late pregnancy and after delivery.[63] Most studies report no change in B cells during pregnancy, although a few have reported an increase.[63,83,164]

Changes in the antibody-mediated system are reflected primarily through changes in immunoglobulin G (IgG). Levels of maternal IgG fall as gestation progresses, with decreases ranging from 30% to 40% after 28 weeks reported.[56,113] However, others have found relatively little change.[113] A fall in IgG has been attributed to hemodilution, loss of IgG in the urine, and transfer of maternal IgG to the fetus in the last trimester. Higher maternal IgG levels have been noted in pregnancies complicated by intrauterine death and severe intrauterine growth restriction (IUGR). Maternal and cord blood IgG levels are lower in women with preeclampsia.[56] The decrease in IgG, along with alterations in WBCs, may increase the risk of streptococcal colonization.

Immunoglobulin A (IgA) decreases or remains stable during gestation, immunoglobulin M (IgM) remains stable or may decrease slightly, immunoglobulin E (IgE) change little, and immunoglobulin D (IgD) increases to term.[63,113] The slight decrease in serum IgA may reflect increased levels of IgA found in saliva and other mucosal fluids.[56] The specific role of IgD in pregnancy is unknown.

Influences of Nonimmune Serum and Hormonal Factors

Host defense mechanisms during pregnancy are also influenced by changes in nonimmunologic hormonal and serum factors that may modulate lymphocyte and macrophage synthesis, activation, or function.[57,164,195] Examples of these factors include estrogens, corticosteroids, progesterone, α-fetoprotein (AFP), human chorionic gonadotropin (hCG), human placental lactogen (hPL), prostaglandins, and serum proteins. The exact role of many of these factors in host defense during pregnancy is still unclear, although they probably act by suppressing cell-mediated immunity or by altering local mucosal barrier function.[164] Elevated levels of specific hormones in pregnancy depress various aspects of cell-mediated immunity. Estradiol inhibits graft rejection and enhances maternal tolerance of the fetus and placenta. Estrogens during pregnancy may stimulate growth of fungal organism, increasing the risk of infection.[164] Estrogens may also alter local mucosal barrier function in the genitourinary tract, allowing adherence of pathogenic organisms and increasing the risk of colonization.[164] Corticosteroids suppress activation of T-cell lymphokines, phagocytic activity, and lymphokine responsiveness of the macrophages.[195] Progesterone may enhance local immunosuppression of lymphocytes in the placenta.[56] The role of hCG in the maternal immune system is controversial. A localized function at the trophoblast site to prevent maternal rejection of the fetus has been proposed.[56,195] Prostaglandins (especially PGE_1 and PGE_2), hPL, and AFP also appear to have an immunosuppressive role during pregnancy. AFP may act by inducing production of suppressor T lymphocytes.[56,97]

Alterations in defense mechanisms may be mediated by a serum protein known as *pregnancy zone protein* (PZP), which has an inhibitory effect on the inflammatory process.[63] PZP decreases phagocytosis and suppresses inflammatory responses and IL-2, especially near the decidual-trophoblast interface.[63] PZP is a glycoprotein synthesized by the mother that increases during pregnancy and then gradually decreases after delivery. PZP also increases with use of estrogen-containing oral contraceptives.[63] An immunologic regulatory role has also been proposed for a unique group of pregnancy-associated plasma proteins (PAPPs) produced by the syncytiotrophoblast. Alterations in levels of specific PAPPs have been associated with pregnancies complicated by preeclampsia, diabetes, and multiple gestation.[56]

Intrapartum Period

The WBC count increases during labor and in the early postpartum period to values up to 25,000 to 30,000 per mm^3. This increase is primarily due to an increase in neutrophils and may represent a normal response to physiologic stress.[36] The rise in absolute numbers of WBCs and in neutrophils may complicate the diagnosis of infection during this time. Impairment in the functional activity of peripheral blood lymphocytes and a decrease in the absolute number of total, $CD4^+$, and $CD8^+$ lymphocytes immediately after delivery have been reported.[171]

Cytokines may have a role in the initiation of labor (see Chapter 4) and in reversing decreased maternal immune responsiveness at the decidual-trophoblast barrier at delivery.[54] IL-6 and IL-1 also increase with the onset of labor. Tumor necrosis factor–α (TNF-α) may assist in the initiation of contractions. IFN-γ may play a role in placental separation via activation of NK cells.[54]

Postpartum Period

The WBC count, which increases in labor and immediately after birth, gradually returns to normal values by 4 to 7 days. A recent study reported a postpartum increase in T-helper cells, cytotoxic T cells, and B cells.[22] It is unclear how quickly the immune system returns to prepregnant function after delivery, with various studies reporting time

lines from a few weeks to 3 to 9 months due to measurement differences.[59,174]

Immunologic Properties of Human Milk

Human milk contains many immunologic components, including leukocytes, immunoglobulins, and other proteins (Table 12-4). Reported immunologic benefits of human milk include decreases in asthma; cow's milk allergy; food allergy; gastrointestinal (GI) and respiratory infections; necrotizing enterocolitis; diabetes mellitus; and some immune disorders such as Crohn disease, celiac disease, and multiple sclerosis.[35,72,200]

Colostrum is especially rich in immunologic factors. Leukocytes in colostrum consist of 40% to 50% monocytic macrophages, 40% to 50% PMNs, and 5% to 10% lymphocytes.[199,201] Later in lactation, the leukocytes in human milk are primarily monocytic macrophages (85% to 90%) and lymphocytes (10% to 15%), with some neutrophils

TABLE **12-4** **Immunologic Properties of Human Milk**

Parameter	Immunologic Factors
Cellular components	PMN neutrophils
	Lymphocytes (T-cell and B-cell)
	Monocytic macrophages
Immunoglobulins	Secretory IgA (major immunoglobulin)
	IgM
	IgG
Complement	C3 and C4
Antibacterial factors	Lactoferrin
	Folic acid- and vitamin B_{12}-binding proteins
	Lysozyme
	Lactoperidase
	Bifidus factor
	Antistaphylococcal factor
Antiviral factors	Interferon
	Lipase
Antiinflammatory factors	Histaminase
	Antioxidants
	Vitamins C and E
	Prostaglandins (PGE$_2$ and PGF$_2$)
	Oligosaccharides and other factors that inhibit microbial attachment
Immunomodulators	Cytokines
	Nucleotides
Nonspecific factors	Low pH
	Lactose
	Low protein

and epithelial cells. Monocytic macrophages in human milk synthesize complement, lysozyme, and lactoferrin; transport immunoglobulin; and protect against necrotizing enterocolitis. These cells also have phagocytic activity against *Staphylococcus aureus*, *Escherichia coli*, and *Candida albicans* and may help to regulate T-cell function.[147,201]

Similar concentrations of B and T lymphocytes are found. B lymphocytes in human milk produce IgA, IgG, and IgM. T cells produce interferon, macrophage migration-inhibiting factor (MIF), and other cytokines. Human milk T cells respond to antigenic stimulation in a manner similar to those from an immunologically competent person, especially in response to *E. coli*. Since the neonate's own T cells are functionally immature, human milk may provide significant protection against gram-negative organisms. Human milk often contains antibodies against the O and K antigens of several *E. coli* serotypes, including K1, which has been associated with neonatal meningitis.[39]

All classes of immunoglobulins are found in colostrum and human milk.[91] However, the predominant immunoglobulin (90%) is secretory IgA (sIgA). The secretory component attached to the IgA monomer protects the IgA molecule from proteolytic digestion in the GI tract. The sIgA does not enter the circulation from the gut but provides localized gut barrier protection by attaching to the mucosal epithelium and preventing attachment and invasion by specific infectious agents.[58] Secretory IgA also neutralizes certain viruses and bacterial enterotoxins and inhibits intestinal absorption of proteins and other macromolecules found in foods.[28] The latter function may provide protection against the development of allergies. Levels of sIgA are highest in colostrum, fall gradually until 12 weeks, and then remain stable for the next 2 years of lactation.[58,109]

sIgA action is enhanced by complement. Human milk contains C3 and C4 and produces complement by the alternative pathway, which can be activated by factors such as bacterial products and circulating proteins. IgM and IgG are also present in human milk but in much lower concentrations than sIgA. Levels of IgG are consistent for at least the first 180 days; IgA and IgM are highest in colostrum, decreasing after 5 days and then remaining constant for at least 180 days.[91]

Most of the immunoglobulins in human milk are produced by sensitized plasma cells in the breast that have been transported to that site from gut-associated (i.e., maternal intestinal) lymphatic tissue (GALT) and bronchotracheal-associated lymphatic tissue (BALT). Specific sIgA against a wide variety of respiratory and enteric bacterial and viral organisms can be found in human milk.[58,91,195] The specificity in any woman is related to her previous antigenic exposure. Depending on the mother's immunologic experience, the immunoglobulins in human milk may provide the infant with protection against organisms such as diphtheria, pertussis, shigella, salmonella, polio virus, and echoviruses.

Human milk contains other nonspecific protective factors that act synergistically with each other and sIgA and include the following: [5,35,58,91,97,101,154,168,189,200,201]

1. Lactoferrin (an iron-binding protein synthesized by milk macrophages that restricts the availability of iron needed for growth by certain fungi and bacteria such as staphylococcus and *E. coli*). Lactoferrin also has antiviral properties. Lactoferrin, α-lactalbumin, and sIgA form the major whey proteins in human milk and constitute 60% to 80% of total human milk protein. Levels of lactoferrin decrease gradually to 12 weeks then remain stable over the next 2 years of lactation.
2. Folic acid and vitamin B_{12}-binding protein (restricts available folate and vitamin B_{12} for bacterial and fungal growth).
3. Lysozyme (bacteriocidal enzyme that lyses cell walls of many bacteria and enhances lactobacillus growth). Lysozyme acts with other substances to destroy *E. coli* and some strains of salmonella. Lysozyme falls in the first 2 to 4 postpartum months and then rises gradually to 6 months with stable levels to 2 years. Levels of lysozyme in human milk are several hundred times higher than in cow's milk.
4. Lactoperidase (inhibits bacterial growth).
5. Bifidus factor (nitrogen-containing polysaccharide that promotes growth of anaerobic lactobacilli that compete with invasive gram-negative organisms). This factor also limits growth of shigella and salmonella. Other factors in human milk that promote lactobacilli growth include lactose, low pH, and buffers.
6. Interferon (prevents viral replication).
7. Lipase (increases levels of free fatty acids and monoglycerides that may act against certain viruses).
8. Oligosaccharides (complex carbohydrates that prevent attachment of bacteria and other antigens to gut epithelial receptors).

Other components of human milk include macrophage-inhibiting factor and antiviral and antistaphylococcal factors.

Human milk produces acetic and lactic acid in the gut. These acids decrease stool pH and inhibit growth of shigella and *E. coli*. In addition to the intrinsic protective factors inherent in it, human milk may also induce the production of immune factors such as sIgA by the infant, although this remains controversial.[58]

Human milk may provide protection against infection and the development of allergies in the preterm infant. The preterm infant's GI tract lacks many intrinsic local defense factors including sIgA, lysozyme, and gastric acid, and there is immaturity of the intestinal mucosal barrier function.[28,147] As a result, the preterm infant is especially at risk for bacterial penetration through the intestines and development of sepsis and necrotizing enterocolitis. The lack of sIgA and immaturity of the intestinal mucosa increase the likelihood of foreign macromolecules entering the circulation, which may increase the risk of allergies in genetically susceptible infants.[28,147] Human milk may enhance maturation of the intestinal mucosal barrier, thereby reducing the risk of both infections and allergies. Increased levels of sIgA, lactoferrin, and lysozyme have been found in milk from mothers of preterm infants.[147] Thus mothers of preterm infants may have an important adaptation that provides additional protection from infection to their infants.

CLINICAL IMPLICATIONS FOR THE PREGNANT WOMAN AND HER FETUS

The maternal-fetal immunologic relationship is unique. Not only must the fetus be protected against a variety of potentially pathogenic organisms, but the mother must also protect the fetus from rejection as foreign tissue. Maternal adaptations also have the potential to interact with disorders of the immune system or other underlying alterations in host defense mechanisms that may complicate pregnancy and other infections; autoimmune disorders; and malignancy. Interactions between the normal pregnancy-induced changes in host defense mechanisms and pregnancy complications affecting these mechanisms are reviewed in this section along with issues and concerns related to maternal-fetal relationships, and immunization during pregnancy.

Maternal Tolerance of the Fetus

The fetus is an allograft; that is, foreign tissue from the same species but with a different antigenic makeup. Since the fetus has maternal, paternal, and embryonic antigens, major antigenic differences may exist between the fetus and mother, including blood group antigens and tissue antigens such as human leukocyte antigen (HLA). Yet the mother usually does not reject the fetus. Thus the major immunologic question regarding pregnancy is, "How does the pregnant mother continue to nourish within itself, for many weeks or months, a fetus that is an antigenically foreign body?"[16,p.256] The answer to this question is uncertain, although many theories have been proposed to explain maternal tolerance of the fetus and placenta.

Although the woman's immune system is altered during pregnancy, her system is still capable of responding to

and rejecting tissue transplants from the father and the fetus grafted onto areas other than the uterus.[185] Therefore protection of the fetus from rejection seems to be predominantly a localized uterine response, although there are also systemic responses mediated primarily by endocrine factors.[178] Maternal tolerance of the fetal-placental unit is generally thought to be secondary to elaboration of an immune "barrier" between the placenta and maternal tissue. Tolerance of the fetus by the maternal immune system is "an active mechanism whereby fetal tissues are prevented from being recognized as foreign and/or from being rejected by the cells of the maternal immune system."[178] Thellin et al. suggest that this tolerance is probably mediated by many factors acting in synergy. Factors that are currently thought to have a role in maternal tolerance of the fetus include HLA-G; leukemia inhibitory factor (LIF); indoleamine 2,3 dehydrogenase (INO); Th1/Th2 balance; suppressor macrophages; hormones, especially progesterone and placental growth hormone; CD95/CD95-ligand; annexin II; lowered complement activity; and possibly mechanisms that hide trophoblastic antigens from the mother.[178]

Major histocompatibility complex (MHC) antigens on the tissue surface classify specific antigenic characteristics of tissues. The MHC antigens in humans are HLA-A, HLA-B, HLA-C, and HLA-D/DR. HLA-A, HLA-B, and HLA-C (class I antigens) are found on most adult cells and are actively involved in graft rejection. HLA-D/DR (class II antigens) is associated with antibody-mediated immunity and found primarily on immune cells such as lymphocytes or macrophages. HLA-G, a unique antigen, is found only on trophoblast cells.

Sperm are MHC class I and II negative, which decreases their recognition as foreign, although sperm do carry other antigens, as does seminal fluid. Seminal fluid also contains immunosuppressors. Exposure to paternal antigens on sperm and seminal fluid may lead to decreased responsiveness and tolerance to paternal MHC antigens.[185]

The first direct contact between maternal and fetal tissues occurs 6 to 7 days after conception at the time of implantation. The trophoblast cells invade the maternal endometrial lining and erode endothelial tissue of the maternal spiral arteries (see Chapter 3). Recent evidence suggests that implantation is influenced primarily by NK cells. NK cells accumulate at the site of implantation and in the decidual during pregnancy.[45] NK cells may recognize HLA-G, HLA-C, and HLA-E on the invading trophoblast and subsequently influence production of cytokines and cytolytic factors to balance trophoblast growth and maternal resistance.[95] After the placenta is established, the two points of contact between maternal and fetal tissues are the syncytiotrophoblast lining the intervillous spaces, which is in direct contact with maternal blood, and the extravillous trophoblast (primarily cytotrophoblast), which is in direct contact with maternal decidual tissue. Beginning in early pregnancy, small quantities of trophoblast cells detach and enter maternal blood through the uterine veins. These cells form minute emboli that eventually lodge in pulmonary capillaries and are cleared by proteolysis. This appears to be a normal process that does not lead to a maternal inflammatory response or other respiratory distress.

The mother initially has a weak immune response to the fetus/placenta, as evidenced by production of antibody to paternal MHC antigens, production of specific T cells, and weak cellular sensitivity to paternal and fetal antigens.[186] The result is an activation (facilitation) reaction rather than rejection. This is mediated by Th2 helper cells with release of Th2 cytokines and growth factors. As a result, maternal immune responses are downregulated at the local level (i.e., maternal-placental interface) but not significantly at the systemic level.[134]

Trophoblast, the fetal tissue in direct contact with maternal tissues, does not have MHC class II antigens nor most MHC class I antigens, with the exception of HLA-G.[137,197] HLA-G is a nonclassical MHC I or Ib antigen expressed only on fetal tissues, especially the trophoblast at the maternal-fetal interface.[5,80,110,203] HLA-G has a role in maternal NK cell regulation and inhibition, although its exact function is still unclear. HLA-G may also have an antiviral function and may help prevent maternal rejection of the fetus by inducing apoptosis of activated maternal T cells.[5,80,110,137] Apoptosis may be mediated by CD95 and its ligand (CD95-L). For example, the CD95-L on the syncytiotrophoblast may bind to CD95 on the maternal immune cells, causing their destruction.[178] HLA-G synthesis may be stimulated by IL-10 from the placenta.[130] Figure 12-7 illustrates how HLA-G on the trophoblast may inhibit maternal NK cells and block NK cytotoxicity toward fetal cells.

Changes in the balance of the different T helper subsets (Th1/Th2) during pregnancy, mediated by progesterone, result in strengthening of Th2 (antibody mediated) responses and cytokines (IL-3, IL-4, IL-6, and IL-10) and a reduction in Th1 (cell-mediated and graft rejection) responses and cytokines (IL-2 , TNF-α, and IFN-γ).[142,178] Relaxin may balance the progesterone-induced Th2 enhancement to allow adequate Th1 responses to protect the mother against pathogens.[142]

Failure of Th2 responses to increase or Th1 responses to decrease leads increases the risk of recurrent abortion.[194] Voisin suggests that abortion before 3 months in primiparous women may be a defect in active maternal tolerance of the fetus, whereas rejection after the third month or with

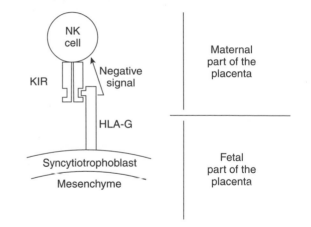

FIGURE 12-7 Potential role of human leukocyte antigen G (HLA-G) in maternal tolerance to the fetus. HLA-G, which is expressed specifically by the syncytiotrophoblast, may inhibit maternal natural killer (NK) cells by binding their killer-cell immunoglobulin-like receptors (KIRs). (From Thellin, O. [2000]. Tolerance to the foetoplacental "graft": Ten ways to support a child for nine months. *Curr Opin Immunol, 12,* 732.)

prior pregnancy may be due to excess rejection type responses with increased levels of Th1 inflammatory cytokines such as IFN-γ, TNF-α, and TNF-β.[186]

The cytokine (see Table 12-2) network at the maternal-fetal tissue interface (Figure 12-8) is important in implantation, pregnancy maintenance, and maternal tolerance of the fetus. Cytokines are produced by Th1 and Th2 cells as well as by the trophoblast.[41,178] The trophoblast produces Th2-specific cytokines, in particular IL-4, IL-5 and IL-10.[41,52] IL-10 is important in inducing adrenocorticotropins (see Chapter 18).[41]

Progesterone promotes production of IL-4 and IL-6 and the Th1-to-Th2 switch. IL-4 promotes production of LIF (which is needed for implantation) and embryonic development.[142] Following ovulation, LIF is secreted by the endometrium; the blastocyst has LIF surface receptors. Later LIF is synthesized by the decidua and Th2 lymphocytes, whereas LIF receptors are found on the syncytiotrophoblast.[178] Thellin et al suggest that binding of LIF to the LIF receptors might enhance trophoblast growth and differentiation. (Figure 12-9).[178] IL-4 and IL-10 inhibit development and function of Th1 responses and macrophages. This reduces cell-mediated responses and helps prevent fetal rejection.[142]

Another factor that may play a role in maternal tolerance of the fetus is INO. INO is an enzyme synthesized by the syncytiotrophoblast that catabolizes tryptophan. Destruction of tryptophan may inhibit maternal immune

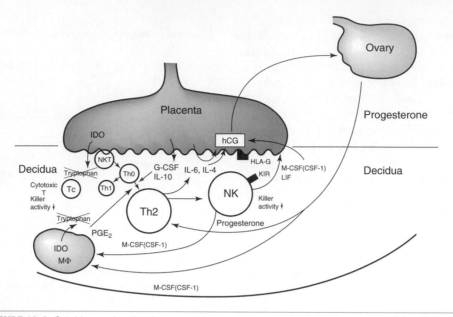

FIGURE **12-8** Cytokine and endocrine networks at the materno-fetal interface. (From Saito, S. [2000]. Cytokine network at the feto-maternal interface. *J Reprod Immunol, 47,* 97.)

cell function.[161] Placental macrophages produce IL-10 and other antiinflammatory molecules to further protect the fetus.[178] Placental growth hormone (see Chapter 18) may also alter the maternal immune system.[178] Annexin II, a glycoprotein that binds to phospholipids, is also produced by the placenta and may inhibit lymphocyte proliferation and IgG and IgM secretion at the placental site.[178]

Another mechanism proposed to reduce antigenicity of the trophoblast by "hiding" of its surface antigens is the binding of masking agents.[56] Potential masking substances are transferrin, antibodies, and antibody-antigen (immune) complexes.[178] Masking agents prevent recognition of fetoplacental antigens by maternal cells. An early phase of cytotoxic reactions with graft rejection involves allogenic recognition by the host. Blocking of this recognition by antibodies from B lymphocytes can inhibit subsequent activation of T lymphocytes and the succeeding steps in graft rejection.[121] The presence of blocking antibodies in maternal blood during pregnancy specific for paternal antigens has been demonstrated.[121] Blocking antibodies are thought to be IgG molecules and may be formed by binding of the Fc fragment of the IgG molecule to receptors on B lymphocytes. Blocking antibodies may protect the fetus by (1) binding to fetal or trophoblast cells that enter the maternal circulation so that fetal and trophoblast cell antigens and maternal T lymphocytes do not interact; (2) crossing the placenta

(if blocking antibodies are of the IgG class, which are the only immunoglobulins to cross the placenta in significant amounts) and binding to antigenic sites on fetal cells to protect fetal tissue from maternal lymphocytes that cross the placenta; or (3) binding with fetal antigens to produce antigen-antibody (or immune) complexes that bind to receptor sites on maternal T lymphocytes and interfere with maternal T-cell recognition of fetal cells as antigenic material.[17,185]

For the mother to protect the fetus, she must first recognize the antigens on the trophoblast as foreign. Thus HLA-incompatible fetuses are at an advantage, and recognition of HLA in the periphery may elicit protective responses in the pregnant woman.[137] Failure of or incomplete recognition can lead to failed or faulty implantation and pregnancy loss.[93,121] Contrary to experience with organ transplants, in which the best outcome is seen when patients receive HLA-matched organs, survival of the fetal allograft does not seem to depend on maternal-paternal antigenic similarity. This is demonstrated by the success of surrogate mothers in carrying infants conceived by in vitro fertilization from another woman and her partner. In fact, couples with similar HLA antigens have a higher rate of pregnancy loss, probably because of lack of stimulation of the maternal immune system. As a result, her system fails to recognize the fetus as foreign and to develop appropriate protective mechanisms.[57,121]

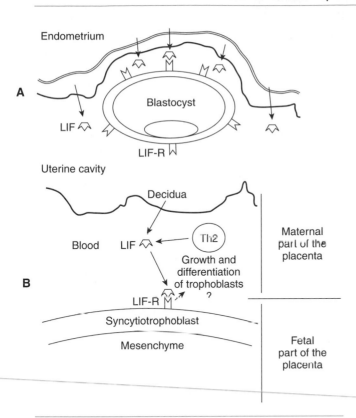

Endometrium

A

Blastocyst

LIF

LIF-R

Uterine cavity

B

Decidua

Blood   LIF   ← Th2

Growth and differentiation of trophoblasts ?

LIF-R

Syncytiotrophoblast

Mesenchyme

Maternal part of the placenta

Fetal part of the placenta

FIGURE **12-9** Potential role of leukemia inhibitory factor (LIF) and its receptor (LIF-R) in maternal tolerance to the fetus. **A,** During implantation, LIF is secreted by the endometrium and allows the LIF-R expressing blastocyst to implant. **B,** During pregnancy, LIF is synthesized by the decidua and Th2 cells. Its binding to syncytiotrophoblastic LIF-R could help the growth and differentiation of the trophoblast. (From Thellin, O. [2000]. Tolerance to the foetoplacental "graft": Ten ways to support a child for nine months. *Curr Opin Immunol, 12,* 732.)

Risk of Maternal Infection

In spite of alterations in host defense mechanisms, most women are not significantly immunocompromised during pregnancy. Most studies do not demonstrate significant increase in the severity of infection during pregnancy.[134] Other studies suggest an increased severity of some disorders such as genital papillomas and hepatitis A, which may be related to hormonal changes in pregnancy rather than immune limitations.[134] However, suppression of maternal Th1 cell-mediated immunity may increase the susceptibility (but not necessarily severity) of certain infections, especially viruses and certain opportunistic pathogens, including *C. albicans, Pneumocystis carinii, Toxoplasma gondii, Listeria monocytogenes, Streptococcus pneumoniae, Neisseria gonorrhoeae, Mycobacterium tuberculosis,* polio, rubella, influenza, varicella, cytomegalovirus, and herpes

simplex virus (HSV).[31,54,164] Alterations in neutrophil chemotaxis and function also contribute to the persistence of infections during pregnancy.[57] Changes in the frequency of infections during pregnancy are also due to other reasons. For example, the increased incidence of urinary tract infections and pyelonephritis during pregnancy is primarily due to anatomic alterations in the urinary tract that result in stasis (see Chapter 10).

Viral infections are seen more frequently during pregnancy, especially during the second and third trimesters; tend to be more severe; and take longer to resolve, with reactivation of subclinical infections.[56,83,164,175] Although methodologic limitations are prevalent, most studies of human immunodeficiency virus (HIV) infection find that pregnancy does not appear to significantly increase the risk of death, progression, or CD4 counts below 200, although there are suggestive trends in some studies.[3,113] Antiviral therapies during pregnancy has significantly reduced perinatal transmission and improved outcomes for HIV-infected women and their infants.[3] Infected women experience a greater reduction in CD4+ cells during pregnancy and a longer time to return to normal after pregnancy than noninfected women, but the effects are equivocal.[3,20]

The incidence of group B streptococci (GBS) colonization during pregnancy is 10% to 30%, with subsequent infection in 1% to 2% of infants.[96,132] The most common bacterial infection during pregnancy is urinary tract infection (see Chapter 10). Fungal infections are seen more frequently during pregnancy (30% of pregnant women versus 15% to 20% of nonpregnant women) with an increase in symptomatic vulvovaginitis during the third trimester.[164] The increase in fungal infections is related to increased *Candida* adherence in pregnancy, increased glycogen in the vagina, increased proliferation of *Candida* under the influence of estrogen, and alterations in cell-mediated immunity.[164] The incidence of infection with protozoa (e.g., malaria, amebiasis) and helminthic (intestinal parasites) organisms is increased, particularly in developing countries. During pregnancy, malaria is more frequent and more severe, with an increased risk of sequelae and a major cause of low birth weight in endemic areas.[54,164] The malaria parasite has an affinity for placental tissue, leading to stillbirth and preterm birth. Latent malaria can be reactivated by iron overload during pregnancy.

Infection and Preterm Labor

Inflammation (decidual, chorioamnionic, or systemic) is a major etiologic factor in preterm labor (see Chapter 4 and Figure 4-7). Both acute and chronic maternal infections are associated with preterm labor. Urinary tract infections have long been associated with preterm labor (see Chapter 10).

More recently there has been increasing evidence of the role of vaginal and cervical organisms and chorioamnionitis in the initiation of preterm labor and premature rupture of membranes.[114] Both these events are probably mediated via inflammatory cytokines that stimulate prostaglandin $E_{2\alpha}$ production.[68,110,114] Unrecognized infection may be an important etiologic factor when no apparent cause for preterm labor can be identified. In women with acute infections, high fever along with other stressors may lead to the release of catecholamines and corticotropin-releasing hormone and increase uterine irritability. Preterm labor is discussed further in Chapter 4.

Immunization and the Pregnant Woman

Ideally, immunization of women of childbearing age should occur at least 3 months before conception (or immediately after delivery) to reduce the risk of infection and adverse fetal effects.[51,155] At times, immunizations may need to be given during pregnancy after accidental or potential exposure to a preventable transmissible organism associated with significant maternal or fetal risks.[148] Alterations in the immune system during pregnancy do not seem to significantly alter the woman's responses to immunization.[51,52,54,148] Potential risks of immunization during pregnancy include fetal viremia, teratogenesis, interference with development of the infant's response to immunizations during childhood, and maternal side effects that might compromise uteroplacental function.[148,161]

Immunity can be achieved by either passive or active means. Passive immunity involves transfer of antibodies from an actively immunized to a nonimmunized person. Passive immunity provides short-term protection until the antibodies are catabolized by the nonimmunized person's system. Transfer of antibodies from mother to fetus during the third trimester and injection of γ-globulin are examples of passive immunity. Active immunity involves exposure to some form of the antigen (attenuated or live organisms rendered noninfectious, inactivated or killed organisms, inactivated exotoxins or toxoids) and the formation of antibodies and memory cells against that antigen by the nonimmunized person. Active immunization may take weeks or months for adequate protection to develop, but long-lasting or permanent immune responses are induced.[148,155,161]

Immunization of pregnant women with active viruses or bacteria is dangerous because of the risk of transfer of the antigen to the fetus.[51,176,181] Immunization with measles (rubeola), mumps, and rubella vaccines is specifically contraindicated because of potential adverse fetal consequences. This risk appears to be primarily theoretical at least with rubella. If a women is accidentally vaccinated early in pregnancy with live rubella vaccine, the risk of adverse fetal effects appears to be low, based on several series of women accidentally vaccinated before they realized they were pregnant.[25,51,69,148] Pregnant women who discover that they are pregnant after being immunized, especially with a live virus, must be counseled about possible risks.

Inactive viruses such as pneumococcal, influenza, diphtheria, tetanus, hepatitis B are considered safe in pregnancy.[51,176] Influenza vaccination is recommended for pregnant women who will be in their second or third trimesters during flu season or who are at high risk.[51] Other immunizations may occasionally be required during pregnancy. Data are available about the availability and safety of individual immunizations during pregnancy.[161] The risk of fetal and maternal infection must be compared with the risks of vaccination; passive immunization or an inactivated (killed) vaccine or toxoid should be used if available; and, if possible, vaccination should be delayed until the second trimester or later (i.e., after the period of organogenesis).[155,161] Both passive and active immunization (to provide immediate protection while the woman's endogenous protection is developing) can be used if safe and effective forms of immunization are available.[148]

Administration of immunizations during the first few days after delivery is often recommended. If live virus vaccines are used, the woman should be counseled to use methods to prevent conception for 3 months.[161] Blood and blood products given within 14 days of active immunization may interfere with the vaccine's effectiveness, because blood may contain antibodies against the antigens in the vaccine and therefore interfere with the woman's own immune response.[148] Rho(D) immune globulin (RhIG) does not seem to interfere with immunizations given at this time, probably because doses of RhIG are relatively small. Although there is a small theoretical risk of transfer of antigens through breast milk or nasopharyngeal secretions from a recently immunized woman to her infant, this is a rare event without significant reported morbidity.[148] Current recommendations regarding specific immunizations during pregnancy can be found in several reviews.[148,155,161,176]

Malignancy and Pregnancy

Theoretically, alterations in the maternal immune system could increase the risk of malignancy since cell-mediated immunity, which is suppressed in the pregnant woman, normally protects against virally-induced tumors. This finding is not supported by most reviewers, however.[15,22,85,122] Some investigators have specifically suggested an increase in rate and decreased survival for women with breast and cervical cancer during pregnancy, but this has generally not been supported.[85] Melanoma may intensify during pregnancy, then recede or disappear after delivery.[195] The basis for this change has been attributed to increased levels of melanocyte-stimulating hormone during pregnancy (see Chapter 13) and hormonal stimulation of estrogen receptors found on melanoma cells.[99,122]

Immunologic Aspects of Preeclampsia

Preeclampsia is a complex, multifaceted disorder involving alterations in many major body systems (see Chapter 8).There is increasing evidence that vascular endothelial cell injury is an early event in the pathogenesis of preeclampsia.[7,159] The exact cause of this damage is unclear but an immunologic role has been suggested. Factors that support an immunologic basis for preeclampsia include an increased incidence of the disorder in primigravidas, first pregnancies with a different father, and pregnancies with a large placental mass or hydatidiform mole; a decreased incidence in repeat pregnancies (even if the previous pregnancy ended in a miscarriage) with the same father and consanguineous marriages; a decrease with longer cohabitation with the father before pregnancy (and thus exposure to paternal antigens in semen); and pathologic changes in the uterine vessels near the placental site that are similar to those with allograft rejection.[7,159]

Specific alterations in the immune system have been observed in women with preeclampsia. Many of these changes are exaggerations of the changes normally found during pregnancy. Women with preeclampsia have a further reduction of NK cell activity, more T8 suppressor cells, decreased T4-to-T8 cell ratio, increased immune (antibody-antigen) complexes and fibronectin, and alterations in complement.[159] These women also have increased levels of inflammatory cytokines, including TNF-α and IL-2.[7,159] Alterations in placental HLA-G expression are also reported.[117] These changes may alter maternal tolerance of the fetus and increase the risk of vascular endothelial injury.

The Pregnant Woman with an Autoimmune Disease

The effect of pregnancy on autoimmune disorders is varied; individual women experience improvement, exacerbation, or no change depending on the disorder. These differences may be related to the immune mechanism involved in the specific disorder; that is, whether the disorder involves alteration in Th1 responses (which decrease during pregnancy) or Th2 responses (which increase).[54] Autoimmune disorders are thought to impair T-suppressor cell activity, resulting in hyperactive B-lymphocyte response and production of autoantibodies that form immune (antibody-antigen) complexes with their target antigens.[63] Autoantibodies damage tissue either by directly reacting with antigen on the surface of cells or by combining with antigen to form immune complexes.[63] The immune complexes activate the complement cascade, which in turn mediates phagocytosis, an inflammatory response, and tissue damage.

Because the usual changes in the immune system during pregnancy are the exact opposite of these events, women with autoimmune disorders may experience an improvement.[63] For example, 77% of women with rheumatoid arthritis (which is associated with increased Th1 mediators, which are decreased in pregnancy) experience improvement during pregnancy, generally beginning in the first trimester; 90% relapse between 6 weeks and 6 months after delivery.[24,54,63] Specific mechanisms underlying this improvement are unclear, but these changes are reported to parallel the rise in pregnancy zone protein, which has a suppressive effect on the inflammatory process.[63] Other changes during pregnancy that might lead to this amelioration include changes in maternal humoral factors, depression of cell-mediated immunity, and suppression of inflammatory reactions.

Conversely, systemic lupus erythematosus (SLE) has been associated with exacerbation in some studies, particularly in women with renal involvement or active SLE at the time of conception. SLE involves production of autoantibodies of the IgG class and increases in Th2 mediators, which are increased in pregnancy.[54] Women with mild involvement whose disease is under control for 6 to 12 months before and during pregnancy usually experience no exacerbation and a few may improve. Exacerbation has been reported to be more frequent in early pregnancy and during the first 6 to 8 weeks after delivery. Postpartum exacerbation may represent a rebound phenomenon as suppression of cell-mediated activity is terminated.[63] Several recent series have reported exacerbation rates of only 10 to 15% during pregnancy and no increase in flare ups after delivery.[24,63,180]

Women with SLE who have anticardiolipin antibodies or lupus anticoagulant antibodies have an increased risk of thrombosis, fetal loss, and thrombocytopenia.[180] SLE—especially if characterized by active renal disease, proteinuria, or the above two antibodies—is associated with an increased frequency of stillbirth, abortion, preterm birth, and IUGR.[63] These complications may result from a lupus anticoagulant factor, decidual vasculitis compromising the fetal blood supply, trophoblast-reactive lymphocytotic antibodies, or antibodies that destroy the fetal cardiac conducting system.[63] Lupus anticoagulant factor is an immunoglobulin that binds to prothrombin-activating complexes and predisposes the woman to recurrent thrombosis in the spiral arteries and placental infarction. SLE and other maternal autoimmune disorders are associated with passively acquired, transient fetal autoimmune manifestations due to transplacental passage of maternal antibody.

Transplacental Passage of Maternal Antibodies

Both protective and potentially damaging antibodies cross the placenta. Maternal IgG antibodies are the only ones to cross in significant amounts, primarily because of the size of the molecules and the presence of an IgG-specific carrier for active placental transport. All four IgG subclasses cross, although the IgG1 and IgG3 subclasses are the predominate ones. IgG1 crosses earliest in pregnancy and is the primary immunoglobulin transferred before about 28 weeks. IgG3 crosses later and does not reach maternal levels until after 32 to 33 weeks.[75,105] Fetal levels of IgG are low until 20 to 22 weeks' gestation, when passive and active transfer of IgG across the placenta increases. In some infants, IgG levels at term may be nearly twice maternal levels.[108,165]

A carrier attached to a trophoblast surface receptor that is specific for the Fc fragments of IgG (and does not bind other immunoglobulins) mediates active transfer of IgG across the placenta.[91,134] This receptor has the greatest affinity for IgG 1 and IgG3, followed by IgG4 with low affinity for IgG2; the receptor has no affinity for IgM or IgA.[105] Active transfer allows for transfer of IgG even when maternal levels are low.[28] Placental dysfunction seems to limit transfer of maternal IgG because lower levels are seen in small-for-gestational age (SGA) infants and in in-

fants born postterm. Maternal IgA, IgM, and IgE are not transferred.[105]

The fact that only IgG crosses the placenta is both an advantage and disadvantage to the fetus. Passage of IgG provides passive immunity against many disorders through passage of antibodies acquired by the mother from previous infection or immunization. Depending on maternal antibody complement, passive immunity against tetanus, diphtheria, polio, measles, mumps, GBS, *E. coli*, hepatitis B, salmonella, and other disorders may be acquired by the fetus (Table 12-5). Conversely, damaging antibodies in the IgG class, such as in Rh incompatibility, also cross the placenta.

Potentially damaging antibodies in other immunoglobulin classes, such as the ABO antigens, which are primarily IgM, and allergy-producing IgE antigen generally do not cross, so the fetus is protected. Conversely, transplacental passage of IgM would be an advantage in enhancing protection of the fetus and newborn from gram-negative bacteria and the TORCH organisms. (*TORCH* stands for *T*oxoplasmosis, *O*ther viruses, *R*ubella, *C*ytomegalovirus, and *H*erpes simplex.)

Potentially damaging maternal IgG antibodies may cross the placenta with several maternal chronic diseases as well as Rh incompatibility and lead to transient disorders in some neonates. Neonatal effects range from mild to severe. In general, if the disorder is not fatal during the perinatal period, manifestations are transient and regress as maternal antibody is catabolized.

TABLE **12-5**   Neonatal Passive Immunity: Placental Passage of Maternal Antibodies

Good Passive Transfer (IgG)	Poor Passive Transfer	No Passive Transfer
Tetanus antitoxin	*B. pertussis* Abs	*Salmonella somatic* (O) Abs
Diphtheria antitoxin	*Shigella flexneri* Abs	*Escherichia coli* H and O Abs
Bordetellia pertussi agglutinin	*Streptococcus* Mg Abs	Heterophile Abs
Antistreptolysin Abs		Wassermann Abs
Antistaphylolysin Abs		Natural (anti-A, anti-B) isoagglutinin
Poliomyelitis Abs		Rh saline (complete) agglutinins
Measles, mumps, rubella Abs		Reaginic Ab (IgE)
Herpes simplex Abs		
Haemophilus influenzae Abs		
Group B streptococcal Abs		
Salmonella flagellar (H) Abs		
Rh incomplete (Coombs') Abs		
Immune (anti-A, anti-B) isoagglutinin*		
Long-acting thyroid stimulator		
Antinuclear Abs		

Adapted from Miller, M.E. & Stiehm, E.R. (1983). Immunology and resistance to infection. In J.S. Remington & J.O. Klein (Eds.). *Infectious diseases of the fetus and newborn infant*. Philadelphia: W.B. Saunders.
*Mostly IgM
Abs, Antibodies.

Graves disease may involve transplacental passage of a thyroid-stimulating immunoglobulin that leads to transient neonatal hyperthyroidism in a few infants (about 1%), which lasts for 2 to 6 months. Myasthenia gravis is associated with passage of maternal IgG against acetylcholine receptors, resulting in transient myasthenia gravis in 10% to 20% of offspring. Symptoms last from a few hours to 2 to 4 weeks. Since symptoms usually develop at 1 to 2 days of age, infants who appear healthy at birth may later develop respiratory failure.[10,166]

Maternal antiplatelet antibodies induce fetal thrombocytopenia in up to 50% of the offspring of women with immune thrombocytopenia. The greatest neonatal risk is for severe hemorrhage in the perinatal period. In most infants, platelet levels reach lowest levels at 4 to 6 days after birth and return to normal by 1 to 2 months.[10,23,166]

In women with SLE, maternal autoantibodies to blood elements and cardiac tissue may result in transient fetal neutropenia, thrombocytopenia, skin lesions, and congenital heart block. These findings generally resolve by 8 to 9 months.[63,180] Many infants with congenital heart block have mothers with IgG antibodies to fetal heart tissue ribonucleoprotein. It is unclear if the antibodies are responsible for pathologic changes within the heart conduction system such as atrioventricular (AV) node absence, AV bundle lesions, or absent connections between the AV node and the atrial conduction system.[166] Not all mothers with these antibodies have infants with heart block. However, Gladman and Urowitz note that this association is "so striking that it is now probably wise to evaluate all children born to mothers with SLE for congenital heart block antibodies and, conversely, to investigate mothers of babies born with complete heart block for signs of SLE."[63] Congenital heart block is also associated with viral infections such as cytomegalovirus (CMV) and with latent or overt maternal connective tissue disorders. About 30% to 60% of mothers of infants with congenital heart block either have or eventually develop SLE.[166]

Rho(D) Isoimmunization and ABO Incompatibility

Rho(D) isoimmunization can be used as a model to examine the application of immunologic principles and to illustrate how the interaction of maternal and fetal host defense mechanisms can result in pathophysiologic processes during the perinatal period. Isoimmune hemolytic disease, hemolytic disease of the newborn, and erythroblastosis fetalis are all terms for a disorder caused by transplacental passage of maternal IgG antibody that reacts with antigens on the fetal red blood cell (RBC) and leads to cell lysis. The fetal-neonatal effects may be minimal or may include severe anemia, congestive heart failure, and death. Because

maternal antibody remains in the infant's circulation, the hemolytic process continues after birth.

The Rh system involves a group of at least 45 different antigens controlled by genes encoding Rh proteins (DCE). A related protein, Rh glycoprotein, is essential for expression of the Rh antigen.[8] Antigens of the D group are the ones usually involved in incompatibility between mother and fetus. Rho(D) isoimmunization occurs when a Rho(D)-negative mother carrying a Rho(D)-positive fetus produces antibody against the D antigen on the fetal RBC. Isoimmunization can occur with other RBC antigens such as Kell, Duffy, Kidd, MNS, and ABO.

Factors that influence whether a reaction between maternal antibody and fetal antigens will occur and the intensity of that reaction include the presence of antigens on fetal tissue that are not found on maternal tissue, distribution of the antigen in fetal tissue (if the antigen is widely distributed, competition for antibody is greater and the risk of tissue injury to specific body systems is reduced), strength and quantity of the antigen, efficacy of the maternal immune response, presence or absence of previous exposure and sensitization to the antigen, and the type of antibody produced by the mother.[18,107] In terms of Rho(D) isoimmunization, the D antigen is a potent antigen, is present in large amounts on the fetal RBC, appears as early as 6 weeks' gestational age, and stimulates formation of IgG-type antibody and memory cells in the mother.[73,82] The amount of antigen necessary to trigger an immune response in the mother varies for each person, as does the intensity of the response by the mother's immune system. The incidence of Rho(D) isoimmunization is actually relatively low, ranging from 10% to 14% (if Rho[D]) immune globulin [RhIG] is not given after delivery) to less than 2% if RhIG is given.[18] The R_2 phenotype (cDE) expresses the most D antigen and increases the risk of maternal sensitization.[181] Fetal Rh status can be determined by polymerase chain reaction (PCR) analysis of amniotic fluid or chorionic villous samples, (each of these PCR analyses requires an invasive procedure) and more recently by analysis of fetal cell-free deoxyribonucleic acid (DNA) in maternal plasma.[112]

Rho(D)-negative women are unlikely to have antibodies against the D antigen unless they have been immunized during a previous pregnancy or from a mismatched blood transfusion. As a result, isoimmunization is rare in first pregnancies. Normally during pregnancy the small amounts of fetal blood (<0.05 ml) that cross the placenta and enter the maternal circulation are too small to trigger production of antibodies by the mother's immune system. In a few women, however, as little as 0.01 ml of fetal blood has been reported to cause maternal immunization (sensitization).[18,107] Detectable fetal blood cells can be found in approximately 3% of pregnant women in the first trimester, 12% in the second trimester, and 45% in the third trimester.[73,182] Approximately 1% to 2% of Rho(D)-negative women develop anti-D antibodies during their first pregnancy.[18] This number can be reduced by prophylactic administration of RhIG during pregnancy.

With delivery and placental separation or with other traumatic events, larger quantities of fetal blood (0.5 ml or more) may enter the maternal circulation. This amount of fetal blood (if the fetus is Rho[D] positive) is sufficient to stimulate formation of both anti-D antibody and memory cells in many women (Figure 12-10, A). Formation of memory cells results in immunization. Once a woman is immunized, she is immunized for life. During subsequent pregnancies, even a very small amount of blood from a Rho(D)-positive fetus entering the mother's system may be enough to trigger memory cells to produce antibodies against the D antigen on the fetal RBC. The antibodies that are produced in this secondary response are predominantly of the IgG1 and IgG3 subclasses and are thus actively transported across the placenta to the fetal circulation and hemolyze fetal RBCs (Figure 12-10, B). With each subsequent exposure to this same antigen, the maternal immune system's response is as intense as previous responses, and it often responds more rapidly and intensely with each succeeding pregnancy.[18,73,107,182]

Intrauterine transfusions into the fetal abdominal cavity were used for many years as in utero therapy for the affected fetus. Currently intravascular transfusions are performed directly into the fetal vascular compartment through cordocentesis (see Chapter 1). Several other techniques involving alterations in the maternal and or fetal immune mechanisms have been tried to improve fetal outcome for Rho(D)-immunized women. These techniques include plasma exchange in the mother decreasing or removing maternal anti-D antibodies with albumin or crystalloid solution replacement and administration of intravenous immunoglobulins.[181]

With development of RhIG (a human γ-globulin concentrate of anti-D), initial immunization of most women can be prevented. RhIG is given in the postpartum period; prophylactically at 28 to 30 weeks (to prevent immunization during pregnancy); or after any potentially immunizing events such as an abortion, ectopic pregnancy, amniocentesis, or significant antepartal bleeding. A dose of RhIg given at 28 to 30 weeks provides protection for approximately 12 weeks (i.e., until term).[73] The incidence of immunization during pregnancy is 1.6%, decreasing to 0.18% with administration of both antenatal and postpartum RhIG.[73,182] RhIG does not cause hemolysis in the fetus even though the majority of the antibodies are transported across the placenta.[33,182]

RhIG acts by destroying fetal RBCs in the mother's system before the foreign D antigen on these cells can be recognized by her immune system and can trigger formation of antibodies and, more importantly, memory cells (Figure 12-10, C). RhIG is generally given within 72 hours of a potentially sensitizing event such as birth. The standard dose (300 μg) protects for up to 15 cc of fetal RBCs.[73] Since in the absence of previous sensitization, development of an adequate antibody response to a specific antigen can take days or weeks, RhIG can probably be given up to at least 2 weeks later (possibly longer) if omitted earlier for some reason.[73] After administration of RhIG during the antepartum period, some women may develop a low (1:4 or less) anti-D serum antibody titer. This positive titer reflects a passive immunity from the RhIG. The infant of a mother who received RhIG prophylaxis may have a weakly positive direct Coombs test due to placental transfer of RhIG antibodies. Neither of these responses indicates maternal immunization, and postpartum RhIG administration is indicated.[18,73,107]

Three potential mechanisms have been suggested for the action of RhIG: (1) clearance of antigen from the mother's system; (2) antigen-blocking by attaching to antigenic sites on the fetal cells, preventing interaction with maternal lymphocytes; or (3) central inhibition of antibody production.[18,73,107,182] The last theory suggests that RhIG forms immune complexes with the Rho(D) antigen. Immune complexes suppress the stimulating effect of helper T lymphocytes, which in turn suppresses antibody formation by B lymphocytes.[73,181]

The potential for isoimmunization also exists with ABO incompatibility, although severe hemolytic disease in the fetus and newborn is rare. ABO incompatibility is three times as common as Rho(D) incompatibility. Previous exposure and immunization are not necessary with ABO incompatibility because the mother already has naturally occurring antibodies against fetal RBC antigens. The most common situation in which ABO incompatibility occurs is with a type O mother and a type A (Figure 12-11, A) or, less frequently, type B infant (the A antigen seems to be more antigenic than B). The type O mother has naturally occurring anti-A and anti-B antibodies in her serum that can react against the A or B antigens on the fetal RBCs. ABO incompatibility could also occur with a type AB infant but never with a type O infant (type O RBCs have neither A nor B antigens for maternal anti-A or anti-B antibodies to react against).

Because the mother already has antibodies against fetal RBC antigens, why is ABO incompatibility a relatively mild

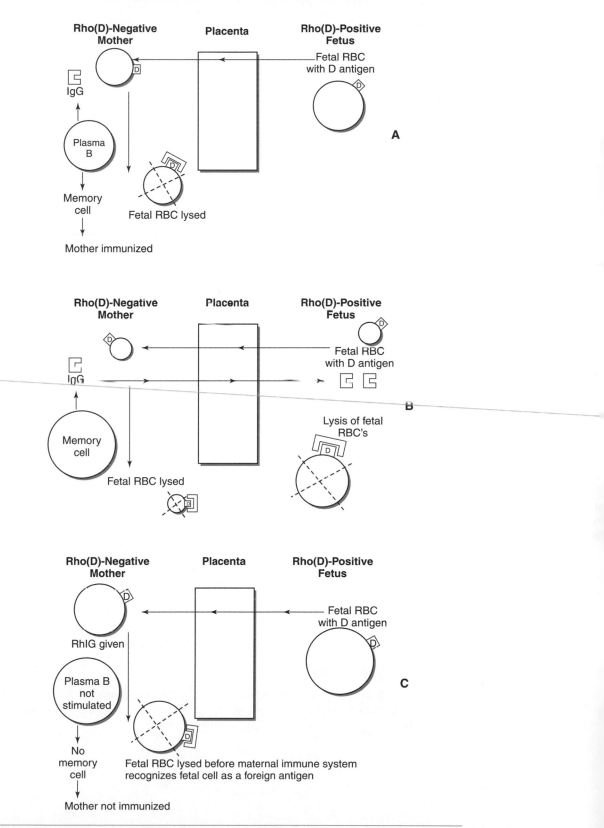

FIGURE **12-10** Rh isoimmunization. **A,** Process of immunization if Rho(D) immune globulin (RhIG) is not given to previously nonimmunized woman. **B,** Action of maternal immune system in subsequent pregnancies once the mother has been immunized. **C,** Role of RhIG in prevention of maternal immunization.

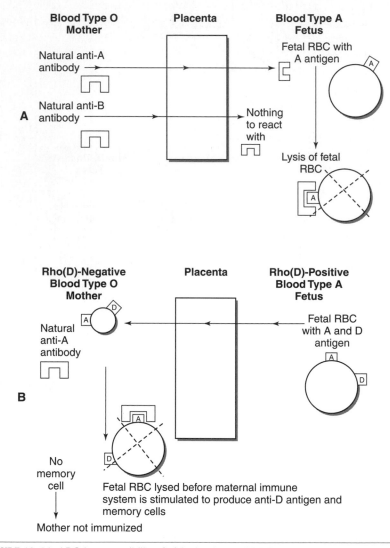

FIGURE **12-11** ABO incompatibility. **A,** Mechanisms of ABO incompatibility. **B,** Mechanism by which ABO and Rh incompatibility—occurring simultaneously—reduce the severity of Rh incompatibility.

disorder compared with Rho(D) isoimmunization? The major reason is that the primary antibodies of the ABO system are IgM, which does not cross the placenta. Some of these antibodies may be of the IgG type. IgG antibodies of the ABO system are more common in those with type O blood; hence ABO isoimmunization occurs most frequently with type O mothers. Because A and B antigens also appear on somatic cells and are secreted into body fluids in most people, there is a large quantity of antigen to compete with the fetal RBCs for any maternal antibody.[107] In addition, the fetus may have its own anti-A or anti-B antibodies that can neutralize maternal antibody; there are fewer A and B antigens on the fetal RBC (resulting in only a weakly positive Coombs test); and these antigens are relatively weak.[199] ABO isoimmunization and probably Rho(D) isoimmunization do not occur in the opposite direction (i.e., from baby to mother) because fetal antibodies tend to be in a macroglobulin form that cannot cross the placenta.

The simultaneous occurrence of Rho(D) and ABO isoimmunization has a protective effect that reduces the likelihood of maternal Rho(D) sensitization. This is illustrated in Figure 12-11, *B*, with a Rho(D)-negative, type O (naturally occurring anti-A and anti-B serum antibodies) woman with a Rho(D)-positive, type A (with A and D RBC antigens) fetus. The naturally occurring maternal anti-A antibody destroys fetal cells entering maternal circulation (during pregnancy or at delivery) before they can trigger the mother's immune system to produce anti-D antibodies and memory cells (see Figure 12-11, *B*). If anti-D antibodies and memory cells are not formed, the woman remains unimmunizaed.[18,181]

Protection of the Fetus from Infection

The fetus is at increased risk for infection throughout gestation because of developmental limitations in fetal host defense mechanisms. During gestation the potential for fetal exposure to pathogenic organisms from maternal bacterial colonization of the genital tract or primary or recurrent maternal viral infection and sexually transmitted diseases is an ongoing risk. Maternal, fetal, and placental factors play a role in protecting the fetus from infection.

Maternal factors include anatomic barriers such as maternal skin, respiratory mucosa, intestinal epithelium, and genitourinary tract surfaces. Maternal IgA enhances barrier function, whereas mucosal macrophages provide protection through phagocytic activity. Most viruses and many bacteria are capable of being transferred, although relatively few are.[58] It may be that immune factors that prevent maternal rejection of the fetus also protect the placenta from infectious agents.[134]

Organisms may occasionally reach the fetus by directly infecting placental tissue. The placenta allows transfer of maternal antibody to the fetus primarily through pinocytosis (see Chapter 3). Once the organism passes cytokines at the maternal-placental interface, it must interact with trophoblast receptors to pass through the placental stroma and enter fetal blood.[58] The main placental defense is the Hofbauer (macrophage) cells. The placenta also contains phagocytes and lymphocytes and produces cytokines such as interferon.[79] The organisms most commonly transferred across the placenta are *Listeria monocytogenes, Treponema pallidum,* HIV-1, parvovirus B19, rubella, *Toxoplasmas gondii,* and *Cytomegalovirus.*[134]

Amniotic fluid contains antibacterial and other protective substances similar to many of those found in human milk. These substances include transferrin, beta-lysin, peroxidase, fatty acids, immunoglobulins (IgG and IgA, but not IgM), and lysozyme.[172] The antibacterial capacity of amniotic fluid improves with advancing gestation.[79] The fetal membranes provide barrier protection against ascending infection, although some organisms can penetrate intact membranes.[108]

Premature rupture of membranes is associated with a significant increase in perinatal mortality from intrauterine infection as the length of time between rupture of the membranes and delivery increases. This is particularly apparent after 24 hours. The usual cause of infection is chorioamnionitis due to an ascending infection from the vagina and cervix.

Maternal responses to infection (particularly fever) may have a damaging effect on the fetus. Fever due to either maternal infection or hyperthermia secondary to sauna use or intense exercise may result in fetal anomalies (see Chapter 19). Maternal fever can increase uterine activity, which, along with elaboration of prostaglandins, may result in initiation of labor.

SUMMARY

Alterations in maternal host defense mechanisms are critical for maintenance of the pregnancy, ensuring that the mother does not reject the fetus and protecting the fetus against infection. Yet these same mechanisms may increase the risk of infection and other immune system disorders in the pregnant woman. Transplacental passage of maternal immunoglobulins provides protection against specific pathogens but can also lead to fetal disease. Concerns related to organisms that colonize the maternal genital tract and sexually transmitted diseases such as herpes, hepatitis B, and acquired immunodeficiency syndrome (AIDS) have increased interest in host defense mechanisms and maternal-fetal interrelationships in recent years and altered clinical

TABLE **12-6** Recommendations for Clinical Practice Related to Changes in Host Defense Mechanisms in Pregnant Women

Recognize normal parameters for immune system components and patterns of change during pregnancy and the postpartum period (pp. 471-476 and Table 12-3).

Obtain and evaluate the complete history for possible exposure to infectious organisms or potential for current illness (pp. 483-484).

Recognize risk factors for development of specific infections (pp. 483-484 and Table 12-3).

Monitor and counsel women regarding early signs and symptoms of infection and risk of prolonged hyperthermia (p. 491 and Chapter 19).

Recognize clinical and laboratory changes during labor and delivery and postpartum that may mask signs of infection (p. 478).

Monitor women with infections during the second and third trimesters for signs of initiation of labor (pp. 483-484 and Chapter 4).

Teach women regarding methods to prevent or reduce the risk of infection while pregnant (pp. 483-484).

Recognize that pregnancy may depress reactions to tuberculin tests (especially in the second half of pregnancy) (p. 477).

Counsel woman regarding the immunologic advantages of human milk and its potential role in preventing gastrointestinal infections and allergies (pp. 478-480 and Table 12-4).

Monitor iron intake and serum ferritin levels in women at risk for or with a history of malaria (p. 483).

Counsel women regarding risks of immunizations during pregnancy and to avoid pregnancy for 3 months after immunization (p. 484).

Avoid giving immunizations within 14 days of administration of blood or blood products (except RhIG) (p. 484).

Give RhIG to unsensitized Rho(D)-negative women prophylactically at 28 to 30 weeks' gestation and after potentially immunizing events (pp. 487-491).

Understand the implications of low antibody titers in some women who have received Rho(D) immune globulin (RhIG) during the prenatal period and the need for RhIG postpartum (p. 488).

Understand the implications of a weakly positive direct Coombs' test in some infants of women who have received RhIG during the prenatal period and the need for RhIG postpartum (p. 488).

Give RhIG postpartum to nonimmunized Rho(D)-negative women with a Rho(D)-positive fetus (pp. 487-491).

Counsel women with autoimmune disorders regarding potential effects of pregnancy (pp. 485-487).

Use standard precautions for blood and body fluids during the perinatal period (p. 483).

Recognize that women who are HBeAg or HBsAg positive are infectious and institute hepatitis precautions (pp. 506-507 and Table 12-14).

Counsel women with hepatitis B virus, herpes simplex, human immunodeficiency virus, and other viral infections regarding long-term effects on infant (including shedding of virus) and use of precautions to prevent spread of the infection (pp. 505-507).

Counsel women with chronic disorders associated with transplacental passage of antibodies regarding the potential impact on their fetus and neonate (pp. 486-487).

practice. Clinical recommendations for nurses working with pregnant women based on changes in host defense mechanisms are summarized in Table 12-6. By recognizing the changes in maternal host defense mechanisms, the nurse can identify women and infants at risk and initiate appropriate interventions and counseling.

DEVELOPMENT OF HOST DEFENSE MECHANISMS IN THE FETUS

Cellular components of the immune system arise from precursor cells within blood islands of the yolk sac. Multipotential stem cells arise in these islands and migrate into the liver and spleen and later to the bone marrow and thymus. Table 12-7 summarizes development of fetal host defense mechanisms.

Both B and T lymphocytes arise from common lymphoid stem cells. Pre–B cells are seen in the liver by 7 to 8 weeks; immature B lymphocytes with surface IgM receptors and complement are found by 10 to 12 weeks in the fetal liver.[91] By 12 weeks, B lymphocytes that have IgG and

IgA cell surface receptors are seen in peripheral blood and bone marrow, liver, and spleen, with numbers reaching adult values by 15 weeks.[134] Synthesis of immunoglobulins begins by 12 to 14 weeks; sIgA is not seen until after birth.[11,28] Levels of fetal immunoglobulins produced by the fetus normally remain low throughout gestation. Fetal serum IgG levels rise in the second and third trimesters with transplacental passage from the mother. Elevated IgM levels in cord blood (>20 mg/dl) suggest intrauterine infection and may be seen with pathogens such as cytomegalovirus, rubella, and toxoplasmosis. This IgM is of fetal origin since IgM does not cross from the mother.

Differentiation of the thymus begins at 6 to 7 weeks.[128] The thymus develops as an outgrowth of the third and fourth pharyngeal pouches. Stem cells from the liver and spleen migrate to the thymus to form thymocytes. T lymphocytes appear in the thymus by 8 to 9 weeks. Differentiation of CD4+ and CD8+ surface antigens begins around 10 weeks.[91] Mature CD4 and CD8+ T lymphocytes are detected in the liver and spleen by 14 weeks.[134] By

TABLE 12-7   Important Milestones in the Development of Fetal Immune Systems

NONSPECIFIC SYSTEMS

Event	Gestational Age (Weeks)
Leukocytes appear in the blood	6-8
Natural killer cells appear in liver and blood	6
Fetal complement synthesis begins	6-14
Macrophages and other antigen presenting cells are present and express class II MHC antigens	12*
Lymph nodes contain lymphocytes and other leukocytes	12-16
Mature neutrophils in circulation	14-16*
Eosinophils present	18
Tonsils contain primary nodules of lymphocytes (germinal centers appear 5 months after birth)	24

T CELLS

Event	Gestational Age (Weeks)
Stem cells enter the thymus	8
Thymus architecture defined-thymocyte differentiation occurs; Hassal's corpuscles appear	12
Post-thymic mature single positive CD4+ and CD8+ T cells found in liver and spleen	14*
TCR recombination increases and repertoire expands	18*
Gamma delta TCR genes rearranged	11-22
Proliferation of lymphocytes in unit volume of thymus reaches maximum	20
T cells able to secrete IL-2, TNF-α and TNF-β, and lower amounts of IFN-γ, IL-3, IL-4, IL-5, and IL-6	Midgestation*

B CELLS

Event	Gestational Age (Weeks)
Transplacental passage of maternal IgG begins	8
B cells expressing surface IgM detectable in fetal liver and spleen	10-12
B cells expressing surface IgA, IgG, IgD, and IgE	10-12*
Fetal B cells able to secrete immunoglobulin	12-14*
CD5+ B cells (B1a) are about 50% of fetal B cells in omentum and spleen	14
Stimulated B cells produce specific IgM	19-22*
IgG, IgA and IgM produced with intrauterine infections	22-26*
Lymphocytes show germinal centers	28
Efficient transport of maternal IgG begins	30
IgG1, IgG2, IgG3, IgG4, IgA, IgA2 produced	Within 1-2 months postnatally*
Secretory (polymeric) IgA produced	1 week to 2 months postnatally*

From Nahmias, A.J. & Kourtis, A.P. (1997). The great balancing acts: The pregnant woman, placenta, fetus, and infectious agents. *Clin Perinatol, 24,* 514.
*Many of these systems are activated earlier in utero by various transplacentally transmitted infectious agents and by many antigens after birth.
IFN, interferon; *IL,* interleukin; *TCR,* T cell receptor; *TNF,* tumor necrosis factor.

mid-gestation, T cells are capable of secreting IL-2; TNF-α; TNF-β; and, to a lesser extent, IFN-γ, IL-3, IL-4, IL-5, and IL-6.[134] Transplantation responses develop relatively early. Antigen recognition can be demonstrated by 12 weeks and graft-versus-host reactions by 13 weeks. Thus one potential form of fetal and neonatal therapy—transplantation of normal tissue into an infant with a specific congenital anomaly or inherited disorder—is difficult. Cell-mediated lympholysis can be detected by 18 to 20 weeks.[11,22,28,199]

WBCs arise initially from yolk-sac stem cells (see Chapter 7). Granulocytic cells from which neutrophils arise can be found in the blood by 6 to 8 weeks and mature neutrophils by 14 to 30 weeks.[134] After 5 months, neutrophils are produced primarily in the bone marrow. Neutrophils and macrophages arise from colony-forming unit–granulocyte-macrophage progenitor stem cells.[91] Myelopoiesis is 10 times more active in the fetus than in the adult. Few granulocytes are found in peripheral blood during the first half of gestation (for example, at 22 to 23 weeks the fetus has approximately 2% of the neutrophils found in cord blood), but by term numbers are similar to those in adults.[91,199] NK cells (which have a major role in surveillance against viral infection) are found in the liver and blood by 6 weeks, but basal activity of these cells is almost undetectable until after 20 weeks and does not increase significantly until after 32 weeks.[132] Complement synthesis by the fetal liver begins as early as 6 weeks, but individual components develop gradually; serum complement is seen after 20 to 22 weeks and increases rapidly after 26 to 28 weeks.[11,28,91] Complement is not transferred across the placenta.

In summary, a innate immune response can be identified in the fetus early in gestation, while adaptive immune functions remain inactive until term, although they may be activated in some infants in the face of fetal infection.[58] In terms of the functional development of the immune system, 32 to 33 weeks' gestation seems to be a critical time. Before this point the fetus or infant is compromised in comparison with the term neonate in terms of neutrophil, macrophage, and NK cell function and concentrations of complement and immunoglobulins.[132] After this time the preterm infant's immune system rapidly approaches that of the term infant.

NEONATAL PHYSIOLOGY

The increased rate and severity of infection in the fetus and neonate are well documented. The fetus and newborn are vulnerable to infection for two major reasons. The first reason is the immaturity-associated limitations of their host defense mechanisms, particularly in the preterm infant. The second reason is lack of experience and exposure to many common organisms, resulting in delayed or diminished responses to foreign antigens. Limitations in neonatal host defense mechanisms are found in the innate system and the inflammatory response, as well as in antibody- and cell-mediated immunity (adaptive immunity) and the complement system. The newborn is also at increased risk for entry of pathogenic organisms due to the breaks in mucosal or cutaneous barriers that may occur during delivery. Finally the neonate is at increased risk for GI infections and for later development of allergies due to immaturity of the gut host defense mechanism. The risk of infection in the preterm and ill neonate is also increased secondary to disruption of skin barriers because of the need for invasive procedures and tape and monitor lead abrasions, which create portals of entry for pathogenic organisms.

Transitional Events

With the transition to extrauterine life, newborns move from the usually sterile, protected environment of the uterus into an environment filled with potentially pathogenic organisms and other antigens that challenge their still immature host defense mechanisms. During the initial days after birth, the newborn's mucosal surfaces (skin, respiratory system, and GI tract) must develop normal microorganism flora and respond to bacterial colonization by potential pathogens, exposure to dietary proteins that are potential allergens, and exposure to other ingested or inhaled environmental agents.

Newborns are initially colonized with organisms from the maternal genital tract acquired during the birth process. This is followed by colonization with maternal skin flora and other organisms in the environment. The maternal genital tract flora at delivery normally includes *Lactobacillus*, *E. coli*, and protective anaerobes but may also contain potentially dangerous organisms such as GBS and *Chlamydia trachomatis*.[33] Colonization occurs initially on the skin, umbilical cord, and genitalia, followed by mucous membranes of the eyes, throat, and nares.[172]

The newborn's skin is usually sterile immediately after a cesarean birth; after a vaginal birth the skin flora reflects the organisms of the maternal genital tract. Skin flora is increased in infants with little or no vernix caseosa, which normally acts as a protective mechanical barrier.[172] With the use of common antiseptic preparations (triple dye, neomycin sulfate), colonization is reduced and the umbilicus remains sterile in most infants during the first week (see Chapter 13).[39]

Colonization of the GI system occurs in two stages. Before birth the gut is sterile. During the first stage (birth to 1 week) the infant is inoculated with organisms that he or she comes into contact with during and after birth. In the second stage (1 to 4 weeks) the infant's diet significantly influences the pattern of bacterial flora. The normal gut flora provides an important protective mechanism against GI infections by occupying potential pathogen-binding sites on intestinal mucosa. The upper small intestine is usually sterile or sparsely colonized, probably due to the gastric pH, or possibly due to the antibacterial properties of bile, secreted immunoglobulins, and normal intestinal motility. Coliform colonization of the upper small intestine is increased in very-low-birth-weight (VLBW) infants and infants who are intubated or fed by transpyloric tube.[39] Gut colonization occurs by attachment of organisms to glucoconjugate receptors in the intestinal mucosal surface.[184] Oligosaccharides in human milk help prevent colonization with pathogenic organisms by competing for mucosal bacterial receptors.[38]

Meconium is usually sterile at birth, except perhaps after prolonged ruptured membranes. Bacteria can be found in meconium within a few hours of birth and increase rapidly over the next few days. Use of antimicrobial drugs from birth partially suppresses but does not prevent colonization and may result in a shift in the dominant gut flora and an increase in resistant flora.[39]

In the first few days after birth, the neonate may be further protected from potentially pathogenic gut organisms by the acidity of gastric secretions (which inhibits growth of gram-positive and gram-negative bacteria) and by immaturity of the gut epithelium (which mediates attachment of pathogenic organisms). Infants for whom oral feedings are delayed are more likely to have no bacterial growth in fecal samples. The intestines of these infants are similar to the germ-free state. This state is associated with a slower mucosal cell turnover (which allows toxins to have a more profound effect), fewer lymphoid cells in the gut, and alterations in gut immune responses that may increase the risk of infection.[116,168]

Breastfed infants develop different colonization patterns than formula-fed infants. These different patterns may reflect physicochemical differences or the influence of antimicrobial factors in human milk.[114] The lower buffering capacity of human milk (due to lower concentrations of proteins and minerals) allows acids from bacterial metabolic end-products to increase. The resulting acidic environment is one in which *Lactobacillus* and *Bifidobacterium* thrive, preventing growth of acid-sensitive organisms such as bacteroides and enterobacteria. The low protein and phosphate and high lactose contents of human milk also promote growth of this flora. Protective substances in human milk (see Table 12-3) may stimulate sIgA, strengthen epithelial tight junctions, and possibly modify intestinal inflammatory and allergic responses.[85] Antimicrobial factors found in human milk may also al-

ter gut colonization patterns. For example, lactoferrin is an iron-binding protein that is only 9% saturated in human milk. As a result, lactoferrin can bind iron entering the gut that is not absorbed and reduce the availability of iron for bacteria metabolism.[109]

Formula feedings buffer the acid produced by gut bacteria. This leads to an alkaline environment in which the bifidobacteria cannot compete with gut enterobacteria. Gram-negative enterococci become the dominant gut organism. As formulas become more similar to human milk, differences in colonization, although present, are less apparent.[35,114]

Alterations in Innate Immunity

The inflammatory response and phagocytosis (see Figures 12-1 and 12-2) are altered in the newborn primarily because of functional limitations of the infant's PMNs that affect leukocyte metabolic activities, mobilization, chemotaxis, adhesion, opsonization, phagocytic activity, and intracellular killing. The neonate's PMNs are more rigid and less deformable (due to generation of less actin) and have a poorer response to chemotaxic stimulators and impaired receptor mobilization.[165] These limitations alter movement kinetics and orientation of the PMNs. The neonate's PMNs are less able to leave the blood vessel to reach the site of pathogen invasion because of the decreased deformability. The PMN limitations may also decrease adherence of the PMNs to the vascular epithelium, leading to poorer aggregation of PMNs along the vessel wall near the site of injury.[76] L-selectin—which is critical for initial neutrophil adhesion to vascular endothelium and migration—is low in neonates and remains low until adolescence, possibly due to large numbers of immature neutrophis.[165] Neonatal PMNs do not respond as readily as those of older individuals to chemotaxic factors.[27,91]

Chemotaxis is altered in the neonate and is about half that of adults, resulting in slower movement of neutrophils and monocytes to the site of antigenic invasion.[27] The decreased chemotaxis results from the structural and functional limitations of neonatal PMNs and from deficiency of chemotaxis-stimulating substances in the blood. In the fetus, chemotaxis is consistent from 24 weeks to term, decreases after birth, then increases to reach adult levels in term infants by about 2 weeks after birth.[27,49,156] In preterm infants, chemotaxis does not begin to increase until 2 to 3 weeks and increases slowly.[27] The reason for this is unclear. Achievement of adult chemotaxis is delayed in more immature preterm infants, with fewer than two thirds of them achieving adult values by 42 weeks.[156] Thus these infants remained at higher risk for infection even after reaching their due date.

Newborns and particularly preterm infants have decreased serum opsonic activity, resulting from low levels of immunoglobulins and complement components. (Opsonization is a process by which immunoglobulin or complement coats microorganisms. This enhances recognition of the antigen by PMNs and monocytes, leading to increased phagocytosis).[3,62] Neonates in particular have difficulty recognizing and destroying encapsulated bacteria unless the pathogen is first opsonized by coating with complement fragments and immunoglobulin.[165]

Most studies report that phagocytic activity in the healthy newborn is normal, although newborn phagocytic cells are less responsive to stimulation by chemotaxic factors.[25,28,39,91] Thus phagocytosis is altered to some extent by the decreased availability of neutrophils (the primary circulating phagocyte) at the invasion site due to altered chemotaxis. Macrophage (the primary tissue phagocyte) activity in response to cytokines (see Table 12-2) from T cells is also decreased. In general, however, the newborn's neutrophils seem to be as effective in killing bacteria as adult neutrophils when numbers of bacteria are relatively low or when numbers of bacteria and neutrophils are similar and the infant is not stressed.[28] Therefore phagocytic activity and intracellular bacteriocidal activity of PMNs are probably not significantly altered in most healthy infants and are similar to adult levels by 2 weeks.[10,27,91] However, others have reported that even healthy preterm infants of less than 33 weeks' gestational age have poorer phagocytosis for the first few months, possibly due to poor opsonization.[24,53]

Infants who are stressed either in utero or after birth (e.g., by perinatal asphyxia, respiratory distress, meconium aspiration, premature rupture of the membranes, sepsis, or hyperbilirubinemia) demonstrate significantly decreased bacteriocidal activity for both gram-positive and gram-negative organisms. Phagocytosis has been found to be normal in most stressed neonates, although decreased phagocytosis for some gram-negative bacteria has been reported. Bacteriocidal activity may be reduced even further in VLBW infants who weigh less than 600 grams.[10,28,39,89]

The cause of these alterations in stressed infants is unclear but may relate to intrinsic alterations or defects in leukocyte metabolic activity or result from perioxidative damage to the cell.[28,78] Changes in cellular metabolism associated with phagocytosis (i.e., the respiratory "burst" with a rapid increase in oxygen consumption, hexose monophosphate [HMP] shunt [involved with glycolysis] activity, and production of toxic oxygen metabolites necessary for bacteriocidal activity) are reduced in term infants with sepsis and in preterm infants of less than 34 weeks'

gestation.[27,89] In preterm infants these metabolic processes remain low for the first 1 to 2 months.[27]

The number of monocytes in infants is similar to that in adults but monocyte chemotaxis may be altered, although studies have yielded conflicting results, with decreased delivery of these macrophages to the infection site.[10,91,111] Production of IFN-γ and IL-6 by neonatal monocytic macrophages is reduced.[88] Monocytic bacteriocidal activity and processing of antigens are generally considered to be adequate. Phagocytic activity may be reduced and correlates with gestational age.

Fibronectin, a glycoprotein found in plasma and tissues, inhibits bacterial adherence to epithelial cells; enhances antibody binding of bacteria such as staphylococci and GBS; and is involved in opsonization and clearance of fibrin, immune complexes, and platelets. Levels of plasma fibronectin average 50% of adult values, with the lowest levels seen in preterm infants and those with perinatal asphyxia or respiratory distress.[10,91,111,199] Numbers of NK cells, which provide protection against tumors or virus-infected cells before the initiation of adaptive immune responses, are similar to those in adults, but activity is decreased 15% to 60% and averages 50% of adult activity.[91,98,111] Neonatal NK cells are especially deficient in binding to target cells and have decreased lytic ability.[98,111] The altered activity is probably due to decreased levels of interferon and other cytokines that augment NK cell function.[28]

The number of neutrophils varies during the first few days after birth, with an increase after birth to peak at 12 to 24 hours, followed by a fall to adult values by 72 hours.[91] Lower levels are seen in preterm infants. The increase after birth is probably due to movement of marginated neutrophils into the main circulation.[165] PMN levels below 3000 m³ in the first 3 days or below 1500 m³ after the first 3 days are unusual in term infants[91]; neutrophil levels may normally be as low as 1100 m³ in preterm infants.[91] Although low PMN levels are normally associated with neonatal infection, they are also seen with preterm birth, birth asphyxia, intraventricular hemorrhage, and Rh hemolytic disease.[91]

Bone marrow reserves (neutrophil storage pool [NSP]) are lower in the neonate, especially preterm infants. This is due to a reduction in granulocyte macrophage–colony stimulating factor (GM-CSF).[27] Approximately one third of preterm infants have a functional neutropenia.[64,140] Numbers of neutrophil precursors in the blood and marrow are increased. In neonates, especially preterm infants, the marrow is probably functioning at or near capacity for neutrophil proliferation. Therefore these infants are less able to increase production much further with infection and the NSP becomes exhausted more rapidly.[26,111,140]

adult cells to achieve full activity.[2,91,149,165] Development of necrotizing enterocolitis and bronchopulmonary dysplasia in preterm infants has been postulated to be related to unregulated cytokine production.[91,102]

Cell-mediated immunity is further depressed in SGA infants. These infants have a smaller proportion of T lymphocytes and altered lymphocyte function, perhaps sec-ondary to alterations in thymic activity. The thymus of SGA infants is smaller in weight and volume and demonstrates histologic alterations and decreased activity of thymic inductive factors.

Alterations in Antibody-Mediated Immunity

Alterations in antibody-mediated immunity are primarily due to the alterations in T-cell activity and cytokine production, which normally enhance B-cell function, and reductions in many of the immunoglobulins. B cells are activated by cytokines and antigens.[93] Many neonatal B cells have CD5 surface antigens (B1a cells). B1a cells are not dependent on T cell help for activation as are conventional B cells (B2) that require T-helper activation.[134] However, alterations in the neonatal T cells affect the ability of the B cells to switch production of immunoglobulins from IgM to IgG or IgA.[114] As a result, neonates produce primarily IgM and little IgG and IgA, even when exposed to bacterial with polysaccharide capsules.[83,165]

The total amount of immunoglobulin at birth is 55% to 80% of adult values and reflects IgG acquired from the mother.[125] Levels of serum immunoglobulins from birth to adulthood are presented in Table 12-11. Mean IgG levels at birth correlate with birth weight and gestational age, whereas levels of IgA and IgM do not. Immunoglobulin levels in the fetus and infant are illustrated in Figure 12-12.

IgG (especially IgG1 and IgG3) crosses the placenta from mother to fetus beginning in the third month (see Transplacental Passage of Maternal Antibodies) and increases progressively to term (see Figure 12-12). As a result, IgG1 and IgG3 are the predominate subclasses of IgG in the neonate versus IgG2 and IgG4 in adults.[165] Neonatal values depend on gestational age because placental transfer of IgG

TABLE **12-9**   Published Ranges of Complement Levels in Neonates

	MEAN % OF ADULT LEVELS (NUMBER OF STUDIES)	
COMPLEMENT COMPONENT	TERM NEONATE	PRETERM NEONATE
CH_{50}	56-90 (5)	45-71 (4)
AP_{50}	49-65 (4)	40-55 (3)
C1q	61-90 (4)	27-58 (3)
C4	60-100 (5)	42-91 (4)
C2	76-100 (3)	67-96 (2)
C3	60-100 (5)	39-78 (4)
C5	73-75 (2)	67 (1)
C6	47-56 (2)	36 (1)
C7	67-92 (2)	72 (1)
C8	20-36 (2)	29 (1)
C9	<20-52 (3)	<20-41 (2)
B	35-64 (4)	36-50 (4)
9	33-71 (6)	16-65 (3)
H	61 (1)	—
C3bi	55 (1)	—

From Lewis, D.B. & Wilson, C.B. (2001). Developmental immunology and role of host defenses in fetal and neonatal susceptibility to infection. In J.S. Remington & J.O. Klein (Eds.). *Infectious diseases of the fetus and newborn infant* (5th ed.). Philadelphia: W.B. Saunders.

TABLE **12-10**   Production of Selected Cytokines in the Newborn

CYTOKINE	SOURCE	ACTIVITY	NEWBORN PRODUCTION
IL-1	Macrophage	T and B proliferation; Ig synthesis	Normal
IL-2	T cell	T and B proliferation; induction of IL-2 receptors	Normal to low
IL-4	T cell	B cell proliferation; Ig switch	Low
IL-6	T and B cells, macrophages, endothelial cells	T and B activation; Ig production	Normal to low
IL-10	T cell	Inhibits T help; Ig production	
IL-12	T and B cells; macrophages	Promotes NK killing and antigen-dependent cytolysis	Low
IFN-γ	T cell	Inhibit Ig production; increase MHC expression, promotes antigen presentation	Low

From Schelonka, R.L. & Infante, A.J. (1998). Neonatal immunology. *Semin Perinatol, 22,* 7.
IFN, Interferon; *Ig,* immunoglobulin; *IL,* interleukin; *MHC,* major histocompatability complex; *NK,* natural killer cell.

TABLE **12-11** Levels of Serum Immunoglobulins from Birth to Adulthood

Age	Level of IgG*		Level of IgM*		Level of IgA*		Level of Total Immunoglobulin*	
	mg/100 ml (Range)	% of Adult Level	mg/100 ml (Range)	% of Adult Level	mg/100 ml (Range)	% of Adult Level	mg/100 ml (Range)	% of Adult Level
Newborn	1031 ± 200	89 ± 17	11 ± 5	11 ± 5	2 ± 3	1 ± 2	1044 ± 201	67 ± 13
1-3 mo	430 ± 119	37 ± 10	30 ± 11	30 ± 11	21 ± 13	11 ± 7	481 ± 127	31 ± 9
4-6 mo	427 ± 186	37 ± 16	43 ± 17	43 ± 17	28 ± 18	14 ± 9	498 ± 204	32 ± 13
7-12 mo	661 ± 219	58 ± 19	54 ± 23	55 ± 23	37 ± 18	19 ± 9	752 ± 242	48 ± 15
13-24 mo	762 ± 209	66 ± 18	58 ± 23	59 ± 23	50 ± 24	25 ± 12	870 ± 258	56 ± 16
25-36 mo	892 ± 183	77 ± 16	61 ± 19	62 ± 19	71 ± 37	36 ± 19	1024 ± 205	65 ± 14
3-5 yr	929 ± 228	80 ± 20	56 ± 18	57 ± 18	93 ± 27	47 ± 14	1078 ± 245	69 ± 17
6-8 yr	923 ± 256	80 ± 22	65 ± 25	66 ± 25	124 ± 45	62 ± 23	1112 ± 293	71 ± 20
9-11 yr	1124 ± 235	97 ± 20	79 ± 33	80 ± 33	131 ± 60	66 ± 30	1334 ± 254	85 ± 17
12-16 yr	946 ± 124	82 ± 11	59 ± 20	60 ± 20	148 ± 63	74 ± 32	1153 ± 169	74 ± 12
Adult	1158 ± 305	100 ± 26	99 ± 27	100 ± 27	200 ± 61	100 ± 31	1457 ± 353	100 ± 24

Adapted from Stiehm, E.R. & Fudenberg, H.H. (1966). Serum levels of immune globulins in health and disease: A survey. *Pediatrics, 37,* 715.
*Mean is ± 1 standard deviation (SD).

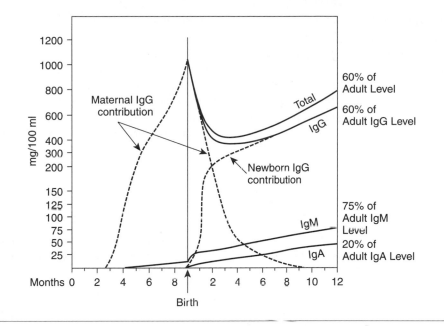

FIGURE **12-12** Immunoglobulin levels in the fetus, newborn, and infant. (From Stiehm, E.R. [1989]. *Immunologic disorders in infants and children* [3rd ed.]. Philadelphia: W.B. Saunders.)

increases during the third trimester. Thus preterm infants may have inadequate protection. For example, cord blood values are minimal in infants born at 24 to 25 weeks' gestation and average 400 mg/dl at 32 weeks and 1500 mg/dl at term.[134] Term IgG levels are 90% to 95% of adult values and 5% to 10% higher than maternal values.[28,91,156,199] As a result of IgG transfer, the neonate has antibodies against infectious agents for which the mother has circulating antibodies because of previous exposure or immunization (Table 12-5). IgG is primarily responsible for immunity to bacteria, especially gram-negative organisms, bacterial toxins, and virus.[91] Levels of IgG are lower in SGA infants, possibly due to impaired placental transport.[111] After birth, levels fall gradually as maternal IgG is catabolized. Because significant production of IgG by the infant does not occur until after 6 months, all infants experience a transient "physiologic hypogammaglobulinemia" in the first 6 months.

IgA is important for localized immunity in the GI and respiratory tracts. IgA does not cross the placenta in significant amounts. Neonatal (term and preterm) values are low (0.1 to 5 mg/dl, or less than 2% of adult values). Elevated IgA is found in cord blood after maternal-fetal transfusion and occasionally with intrauterine infection, although IgM is seen more commonly.[134,153] IgA occurs as a monomer or attached to a polypeptide chain (secretory component) in saliva; tears; colostrum; and human milk, which provides resistance to pH changes and protects the IgA molecule from proteolytic digestion in the GI tract. Secretory IgA is

not found at birth but can be detected in saliva, tears, and intestinal mucosa by 2 to 3 weeks.[168]

IgM is important for protection against bloodborne infections. IgM also does not cross the placenta. Neonatal values are low (5 to 15 mg/dl), with means of 6 mg/dl at 28 weeks and 11 mg/dl or about 10% of adult values at term.[91,111] The fetus is capable of producing significant IgM in response to exposure to certain antigens, such as the TORCH organisms, after 19 to 20 weeks' gestation. Neonatal CD5+ B lymphocytes secrete primarily IgM and some IgA. Increased IgM levels seen with intrauterine infection may be due to activation of the fetal B1a cells.[134] IgM is the major immunoglobulin synthesized in the first month of life.[2,140] Neonatal IgM has less specificity than adult IgM in responding to specific antigens, which may limit the initial recognition of pathogenic organisms. IgM levels increase rapidly after 2 to 4 days, probably secondary to stimulation from environmental antigens. IgE and IgD do not cross the placenta in significant amounts, and newborn values are less than 10% of adult values.[28,125,199]

Few immunoglobulin-secreting cells (IgSCs) are seen in the first 5 days after birth, and those that are found are mostly IgM-secreting cells. By a month of age, two thirds of neonates have IgSCs, most of which are IgA-secreting cells. Increased IgSCs are more common in both term and preterm infants with intrauterine infection.[177] In addition to alterations in immunoglobulin concentration, neonatal B lymphocytes are hyporesponsive, possibly due to the suppressor effects of T lymphocytes. The newborn's B cells also lack experience and exposure to many common organisms and thus have few memory cells. This delays the initial response of the immune system in producing antibodies to specific organisms. For example, with initial exposure to a specific foreign antigen, B cells are capable of producing specific antibody after 5 to 10 days. With repeated exposure, specific antibody is produced sooner (1 to 3 days), with a larger peak response due to immunologic memory.[91]

Alterations in Gut Host Defense Mechanisms

Host defense mechanisms in the gut involve both nonimmune and immune factors. Many of these factors are initially altered in the neonate, reducing the effectiveness of the gut mucosal barrier and increasing the risk of GI disorders, entry of pathogenic organisms into systemic circulation, and development of allergic reactions (Table 12-12). As defense mechanisms mature, GI barriers become more

TABLE 12-12 Alterations in Gut Host Defense Mechanisms in the Newborn

DEFENSE MECHANISM	MODE OF ACTION	ALTERATIONS IN NEWBORN
NONIMMUNE FACTORS		
Gastric acid	Decreased number of organisms entering intestines	Decreased in term and preterm infants until 4 weeks' postnatal age
Intestinal motility and peristalsis	Remove organisms and antigen	Decreased to 29 to 32 weeks postconceptual age
Intraluminal proteolysis	Determines amount of macromolecular transport across intestinal epithelium	Decreased pancreatic enzyme function in preterm infant; some decrease in response in both term and preterm infants to 2 years; result is an increased absorption of intact proteins across small intestine
Mucosal surface		
Mucous coat	Provides physical barrier to attachment, uptake, and penetration of organisms and other antigens. Carbohydrate moieties act as receptor inhibitors to protect against antigen penetration	Decreased and altered carbohydrate content and lack of mucus-specific receptor inhibition may interfere with surface defenses against organisms, toxins, and other antigens
Microvillous membrane	Carbohydrate composition influences specific adherence of organisms and other antigens to intestinal surface and prevents penetration	Altered membrane composition and incompletely developed surface leading to abnormal colonization, increased antigen penetration, and disease susceptibility
IMMUNOLOGIC FACTORS		
Secretory immunglobulin A (sIgA)	Complexes with antigens to impede absorption from intestinal lumen. Interferes with antigen attachment and uptake at mucosal surface	Low levels of IgA and especially sIgA resulting in increased transport of organisms, antigens, and other macromolecules across intestinal epithelium
Gut-associated lymphoid tissue (GALT)	Composed of Peyer's patches (aggregates of lymphoid tissue), plasma cells that are predominantly IgA producing, B and T lymphocytes, and specialized M epithelial cells. M cells bind and transport antigens to macrophages in lymphoid tissue	GALT develops more slowly than other lymphoid tissue and in newborns contains primarily T cells with few B cells. Paucity of IgA-producing plasma cells (requires weeks to months to establish protective levels). Low levels of IgA. Delayed response time to antigen penetration
Cell-mediated immunity	Includes activated T lymphocytes, mast cells, and macrophages along the intestinal lamina along with intraepithelial lymphocytes (cytotoxic T cells)	Immature and virginal T lymphocytes, altered T-suppressor function, and depression of responsiveness to specific antigens. Decreased intestinal and intraepithelial lymphocytes in small-for-gestational-age and nutritionally deprived infants. Respond to antigens with priming response versus tolerance

Compiled from references 39, 82, 116, 168, and 188.

impermeable, offering greater protection against uptake of antigenic substances. The development of gut defense mechanisms is called "gut closure."

A major task of the neonate is development of the mucosal barrier and other defense mechanisms to maintain the gut epithelial surfaces as an impermeable barrier against the uptake of antigens and antigenic fragments.[82,116,118,188] Neonatal GI mucosal immaturity is evidenced by its increased permeability to macromolecules (all potential antigens), altered tolerance, decreased sIgA, and decreased cytokine production.[118,202] Gut closure is influenced by ingestion of food, especially colostrum, which enhances maturation of the intestinal lining via factors such as thyroxine, transforming growth factor, insulin-like growth factors, neurotensin, cortisol, lactoferrin, bombesin, and epidermal growth factor.[136] Gut closure is delayed in preterm and SGA infants, who may absorb macromolecules across their intestinal epithelium for up to 8 to 12 months. Nonimmune factors include gastric acid, intestinal motility and peristalsis, intraluminal proteolytic activity, and the mechanical barrier properties of the gut mucosal surface. Hypoxia or hypotension further compromises integrity of the intestinal epithelial lining.

The major specific immune factors in gut closure are sIgA and cell-mediated immunity. Changes in cell-mediated immunity, especially a localized depression of T-lymphocyte suppressor activity, and the decreased IgA alter the response of the infant to antigens that can cross the intestinal barrier. This increases the incidence of antigen-induced disorders such as GI infection and allergies in infants.

The mature response to the presence of antigens in the gut is immune tolerance. With immune tolerance the absorbed antigen elicits a localized IgA response that destroys most of the antigen. As a result there is less antigen available to enter the systemic system. T-suppressor cell activity is also triggered, which interferes with and inhibits systemic responses to these antigens.[82,118] Immune tolerance appears to be enhanced by the presence of partially digested polypeptide fragments. These fragments may not be formed in the neonate with immature proteolysis. In the infant the absorbed antigens may actually prime the immune system and enhance rather than inhibit specific responses. With decreased IgA, greater amounts of antigen are absorbed. Decreased T-suppressor response can enhance systemic immune responses and lead to inflammatory or allergic responses.

Immaturity of gut defense mechanisms may have an etiologic role in the development of necrotizing enterocolitis (NEC). NEC is a multifactorial disorder that results in focal or diffuse ulceration and necrosis in the lower small intestine and colon (see Chapter 11). Factors involved in the development of NEC include intestinal ischemia, bacterial proliferation, and enteral feedings.[82] These factors may interact with the immature intestinal barrier to further increase mucosal permeability to enteric bacteria, toxins, and antigens.[82,114]

Human milk appears to reduce the incidence and severity of NEC.[67,114] Human milk, particularly colostrum, facilitates gut closure by reducing antigen penetration; providing sIgA; and enhancing maturation of the mucosal epithelial cells and development of brush border enzymes such as lactase, sucrase, and alkaline phosphatase.[67,188] Other factors contributing to the lower rate of GI infection in breastfed infants include antibacterial factors in human milk, stimulation of IgA, and the presence of ingested maternal antigen, which tends to promote immune tolerance responses.[35,82] With weaning and withdrawal of the immunosuppressive effect of human milk, the mucosal immune system is activated, with a physiologic inflammatory response followed by downregulation of responses.[35]

CLINICAL IMPLICATIONS FOR NEONATAL CARE

Alterations in host defense mechanisms in neonates and their inexperience as hosts place them at increased risk for sepsis and meningitis (due to the inability to localize infection) and for the development of specific types of bacterial and viral infections. Immunodeficiency diseases are rarely manifest in newborns since maternally acquired IgG and sIgA in breast milk usually mask the effects of these disorders. The inflammatory response and cytokines play a role in tissue damage seen with bronchopulmonary dysplasia and other disorders. There has been recent interest in the role of cytokines in response to intrauterine infection in the development of cerebral palsy.[61,136,138,190] Infection and cytokine-mediated injury to oligodendrites have also been proposed as having a role in the pathogenesis of periventricular leukomalacia and with brain injury following cerebral hypoxic-ischemic insults (see Chapter 14).[135,160]

Risk of Specific Infectious Processes

When examining limitations of the neonate's host defense system, the basis for an increased risk of infection with certain organisms becomes apparent (Table 12-8). Neonates are at increased risk of infection primarily because of their small NSP, reduced chemotaxis, decreased complement activity, decreased protective responses against capsular polysaccharide antigens, and large numbers of naive T cells, thus reducing cell-mediated responses.[165] The inability to localize infection increases the risk of sepsis from grampositive cocci such as GBS that often colonize the birth canal and can be transferred to the infant during delivery.

The risk of sepsis from gram-negative rods is increased because protection against these organisms is provided by IgM, IgA (against enteropathic *E. coli*), and T lymphocytes, which have decreased levels or altered activity in the neonate. Similarly, markedly low values of IgA and the lack of sIgA increase the risk of respiratory and GI infections, whereas low IgM levels increase the risk of rubella, toxoplasmosis, CMV, and syphilis. The risk of GI infections is increased because of immaturity of the intestinal mucosal barrier and lack of gut closure.

Decreased complement activity, particularly in relation to the alternative pathway, leads to decreased opsonic activity. This may be critical if the infant also lacks type-specific antibodies for organisms with a capsular polysaccharide coating, such as GBS or K1 *E. coli*. In this situation the infant's immune system is dependent on the (deficient) alternative pathway for opsonization of the organism in preparation for phagocytosis.

Altered activity of T lymphocytes along with their lack of antigen exposure increases the risk of infection due to herpes simplex virus, CMV, and *Candida*. Decreased production of IFN-γ (which inhibits viral replication) by the lymphocyte increases the risk of viral infection. In addition, IFN-γ is an important macrophage-activating factor that has an important role in destruction of intracellular pathogens such as *Toxoplasma* and *L. monocytogenes*.

Wilson examined the impact of altered neonatal host defense mechanisms on groups of infectious organisms, including GBS and HSV.[111] The response of the neonate to these organisms provides a model for examining the vulnerability of the newborn to bacterial and viral infections.

Immune Responses to Bacterial Infections

GBS and *E. coli* are currently the most common pathogens causing neonatal sepsis in North America. Neonatal infection generally occurs after exposure to organisms from the birth canal. Usually only a few infants exposed to these pathogens become infected. Both GBS and *E. coli* sepsis are more common with certain strains that contain specific capsular polysaccharide.

GBS can be divided into serotypes (Ia, Ib, Ic, II, III, IV, and V) based on their bacterial capsular polysaccharide and surface antigen. Type III accounts for two thirds of all GBS infection in infants, 90% of GBS meningitis, and 90% of late-onset GBS sepsis. One third of early-onset sepsis without meningitis is caused by types Ia, Ib, and Ic.[62] Similarly, infection with *E. coli* that results in neonatal meningitis occurs most often with organisms that have the K1 polysaccharide capsule. Capsular polysaccharide and the C protein protect the organism from destruction unless it is opsonized. The capsule contains sialic acid residues that increase the organism's virulence, perhaps by alternative pathway complement activation.[164] Opsonization and phagocytosis of type III and perhaps other GBS types require both type-specific immunoglobulins and complement.

The risk of neonatal sepsis from GBS is increased because of limitations in mucocutaneous barriers and humoral and cell-mediated defense mechanisms (Figure 12-13). The ability of organisms to penetrate human mu-

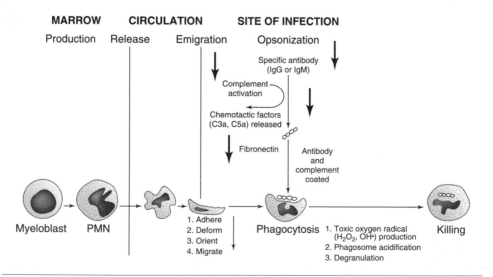

FIGURE **12-13** Limitations in neonatal defense mechanisms against group B streptococci. Limitations in the neonate are denoted by arrows. (Adapted from Wilson, C.B. [1986]. Immunologic basis for increased susceptibility of the neonate to infection. *J Pediatr, 108,* 1.)

cocutaneous barriers is facilitated by epithelial adherence, exposure to a high density of bacteria, and disruption of the skin or mucosal membranes.[111] Neonates whose mothers are colonized with GBS are likely to be exposed to dense concentrations of the organism. In addition, decreased levels of sIgA and fibronectin may alter bacterial adherence to the epithelium.[111] Type III organisms tend to adhere better to neonatal buccal epithelium, particularly in infected infants.[111]

GBS sepsis tends to occur only in infants deficient in type-specific IgG antibody. Neonates may lack these antibodies if their mother does not have the type-specific antibody to transfer to her infant, if the mother's antibody is in an immunoglobulin class that does not cross the placenta, or if the infant is born prematurely before maternal antibody is normally transferred to the fetus.[30] In the neonate, GBS antibody is acquired primarily from the mother (through transplacental transfer) if the mother has developed antibodies to specific GBS strains by previous exposure. Many women do have antibodies against type III GBS as well as types Ia, Ib, and II, and thus many term infants are protected.[4] This may partially explain why women who are colonized can have healthy infants even after prolonged ruptured membranes.[111] Maternal antibiotic prophylaxis in at-risk women during the intrapartum period reduces the risk of neonatal GBS sepsis.

Preterm infants are more vulnerable to GBS infection because these antibodies, like other IgG antibodies, do not cross the placenta in significant amounts until the latter part of the third trimester. Anti-K1 E. coli IgG antibodies are much rarer in the adult population, so the mother is less likely to provide protection to her fetus against this organism.[4]

Once infected, the neonate is often unable to mount an appropriate response to GBS. Optimal destruction of GBS depends on type-specific antibody, complement, and functional phagocytes. In infected neonates who do not have type-specific antibody, an increase in the time required for neutrophil migration to the invading organisms has been noted, along with a delay of 4 to 6 hours between the onset of infection and release of neutrophils from bone marrow storage pools (versus 2 hours in infants with type-specific antibodies).[30] This results in decreased complement activation (and thus opsonization and phagocytosis) and inability to localize the infection and increases the risk of a rapidly progressing overwhelming septicemia. When exposed to GBS, the B lymphocytes of most neonates do not produce adequate quantities of type-specific antibody critical for opsonization and phagocytosis.[111] Lower levels of complement in newborns, especially in preterm infants, further reduce opsonization of GBS and interfere with the

phagocytic ability of the PMNs. In infants with GBS sepsis, the number of lymphocytes is reduced. Factor B is also reduced by 30% to 35% and C3 by 40% to 60% from cord blood levels.[111,199]

Because of functional and structural alterations in PMNs that decrease chemotaxis, neonates are unable to rapidly deliver adequate numbers of phagocytes to the site of initial infection. Neutropenia, rarely seen in infected adults, is a frequent finding in neonatal septicemia. The reasons for this neutropenia include a small marrow storage pool of neutrophils and their precursors that is rapidly depleted with sepsis, inability of the marrow to increase production of neutrophils (stem-cell proliferation rate is already at maximal activity), failure of the marrow to release additional neutrophils, sequestration of neutrophils along vessel walls (margination), and the short circulating half-life (4 to 7 hours) of neutrophils in the neonate.[111]

PMNs of ill and stressed infants have decreased chemotaxis as well as decreased phagocytic and bacteriocidal activity. Neonates may also be deficient in local defense mechanisms in the lungs because of decreased numbers (and possibly altered function) of lung macrophages.[42] This deficit may predispose the infant to GBS pneumonia. In summary, the increased susceptibility of the neonate to bacterial pathogens results primarily from lack of type-specific antibody, alterations in the functional ability of PMNs (especially decreased chemotaxis), poor bone marrow response to maintain adequate numbers of neutrophils, and decreased complement, leading to ineffective opsonic activity necessary for phagocytosis and bacteriocidal activity (see Figure 12-13).[111]

Immune Responses to Viral Infections

Viral infections tend to be more serious and devastating disorders in neonates than in adults because of limitations in the infant's host defense mechanisms and lack of previous exposure to many organisms. The major defense mechanisms against viral infections (cell-mediated immunity, NK cells, IgM, and the ability to localize infection) are all altered in the neonate. In addition, most neonates have T lymphocytes that are not yet sensitized. This section examines immunologic aspects of neonatal herpes simplex and hepatitis B infection.

Herpes simplex virus infection. Neonatal HSV infection is a rapidly progressing disorder that usually involves multiple body systems and has high morbidity and mortality rates. Severe systemic HSV infection is an age-related phenomenon, with the morbidity, mortality, and severity of illness decreasing after the first 4 weeks of life. Neonates have an impaired immune response to HSV.[161]

Susceptibility of neonates to severe HSV infection is due to immaturity of the immune system, alterations in neutrophil function, T cell naiveté, reduction in NK cells, and cell-mediated cytolysis.[165,178] Alterations in the neonate's immune system that increase the risk of HSV infection include decreased NK-cell cytotoxicity, reduced ability of lymphocytes and monocytes to lyze HSV, decreased antibody-dependent cell-mediated toxicity, decreased or delayed production of and response to interferon, decreased diversity of specific receptors for HSV, delayed lymphocyte proliferation in response to antigens, and the inability of the neonate to generate a fever (HSV is a thermolabile organism).[111,165,178]

Eradication of HSV is dependent upon NK function and cell-mediated cytolysis, both of which are reduced in the newborn, probably as a result of decreased IL-12 and interferon activity.[165] Production of both IFN-γ and IFN-α is reduced and delayed in the neonate in response to HSV infection. IFN-α induces NK cells and other innate mechanisms.[178] Reduced complement and immature monocyte and macrophage responses to HSV also limit the infant's ability to respond to HSV. These changes allow dissemination of the virus in the neonate.[175]

Lack of maternal antibody also increases the risk of neonatal HSV infection. Maternal antibodies to HSV, which are capable of neutralizing the virus and mediating antibody-dependent cell-mediated cytotoxicity, are of the IgG class and can cross the placenta. These antibodies do not provide immunity to the neonate but are correlated with a lower infection rate in exposed newborns.[178] Women with primary HSV genital infection produce little IgG and their offspring are more likely to develop severe infection. A dose-dependent relationship has been observed between the amount of maternal anti-HSV antibody and the severity of neonatal infection, in which increasing levels of maternal antibody were associated with milder neonatal infection and a decreased incidence of disseminated infection or central nervous system involvement.[178]

Hepatitis B virus infection.   Another virus that has become increasingly prevalent in perinatal care is hepatitis B virus (HBV). HBV can be transmitted from the mother to the fetus and newborn by infected vaginal secretions, amniotic fluid, maternal blood, saliva, and possibly breast milk. Most infants who develop HBV infection acquire the organism late in the third trimester or at delivery. Up to 40% to 60% of infants of mothers with active, untreated infections late in the third trimester develop HBV infection.[97] Although many newborns exposed to HBV do not develop clinical infection, others develop fulminate neonatal disease. In addition, infants may be at risk for later disorders because HBV can cause acute and chronic hepatitis, cirrhosis, and hepatocellular carcinoma.[34,47]

HBV is a DNA virus associated with three distinct antigen forms (surface, core, and e) and their respective antibodies (anti-HBs, anti-HBc, and anti-HBe). The outer protein surface contains a surface antigen (HBsAg), whereas the inner core of the virus contains the DNA genome (circular DNA form) and the core antigen (HBcAg). The third antigen (HBeAg) is a soluble serum antigen usually seen in association with HBsAg. Table 12-13 summarizes characteristics of these antigens and antibodies.

HBeAg is a marker of infectivity and reflects ongoing viral replication. This antigen is usually seen in people with active disease and HBsAg-positive serum. HBsAg and HBeAg are detectable 1 to 3 weeks after HBV exposure but before onset of clinical symptoms.[48,97] HBeAg may also be present after the active disease subsides, indicating either chronic disease or a carrier state. Women with HBeAg are usually infectious, and appropriate blood and body-fluid precautions should be taken.

HBcAg is found only in hepatocytes and thus is not detectable in serum. Antibodies to this antigen (anti-HBc) are seen during both acute infection and convalescence, however, making anti-HBc a reliable indicator of HBV infection.[48] Anti-HBc during an acute infection is primarily IgM-type antibody, which may persist for 4 to 6 months and indicate recent infection. Anti-HBc antibodies, which are primarily IgG type, are also found in the carrier state.[97] Anti-HBc in HBsAg-positive serum indicates low infectivity.

HBsAg can be found in the serum of people who have acute or chronic HBV infections or are carriers for the virus. Infants who acquire the virus during birth are seronegative initially but develop elevated serum HBsAg within 2 to 4 months.[93] The woman who is HBsAg positive—regardless of whether she is a carrier or actively infected—can transmit the virus to her fetus and neonate and to others she comes in contact with. Therefore blood and body-fluid precautions are recommended for health care personnel caring for the woman and her infant. The appearance of antibody against HBsAg (anti-HBs), in response to either active infection or immunization, reflects immunity to HBV.[48,97]

The risk of maternal transmission to the neonate depends on the types of antigens and antibodies present. If the mother is positive for both HBsAg and HBeAg, there is a high likelihood of transmission to the fetus. Most of these infants will become HBV carriers.[4,97] Maternal anti-HBs antibodies do not provide significant protection of the infant from HBV infection because the amount of antibody transferred provides only transient protection.[97] Women who are chronic carriers of HBsAg can transmit HBV to

TABLE 12-13   Interpretation of the Presence of Combinations of Serologic Markers of Hepatitis B Virus

HbsAg	HBeAg	Anti-HBe	Anti-HBc	Anti-HBs	Interpretation	Infectivity*
+	+	−	−	−	Incubation period for early acute HB	High
+	+	−	+	−	Acute HB or chronic carrier	High
+	−	+	+	−	Late during HB or chronic carrier	Low
−	−	+	+	+	Convalescent from acute HB infection	Low
−	−	−	+	+	Recovered from past HB infection	None
−	−	−	−	+	Immunized without infection; repeated exposure to HBsAg without infection; recovered from past infection	None
−		−	+	−	Recovered from past HB infection with undetectable anti-HBs; early convalescence or chronic carrier	??

From Hanshaw, J.B., Dudgeon, J.A., & Marshall, W.C. (1985). *Viral diseases of the fetus and newborn*. Philadelphia: W.B. Saunders, using data from Deinhardt, F. & Gust, I.P. (1982). Viral hepatitis. *Bull World Health Organ, 60,* 661.
*Infectivity of blood.
HB, hepatitis B; *HBV*, hepatitis B virus.

their infants after birth especially if the woman's serum is both HBsAg and HBeAg positive (indicating high infectivity), versus HBsAg and anti-HBe positive (indicating lower infectivity) or anti-HBe positive (indicating minimal likelihood of transfer).[97] Patterns of antigens and antibodies in acute HBV are illustrated in Figure 12-14.

A combination of active and passive immunization is recommended for prevention of HBV infection in the neonate.[34,97] Thus HBV immune globulin (HBIG) and HBV vaccine are administered to infants of HBsAg-positive women. HBIG provides passive immunity by supplying antibodies to destroy HBV antigen that the infant may have acquired from the mother during the birth process. HBIG provides initial protection for the infant, although passive immunization may not completely suppress HBV infection.[34] Because infants of carrier mothers are at constant risk of reinfection, HBV vaccine is administered to provide immunization by stimulating the infant's system to produce its own antibodies against HBV.

Diagnosis of Neonatal Infection

Although microbiologic techniques are the basic tools used in the diagnosis of infection, other parameters that reflect

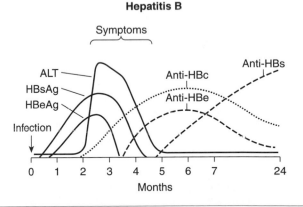

FIGURE 12-14 The course of acute hepatitis B infection. *HBsAg,* hepatitis B surface antigen; *anti-HBs,* antibody to HBsAg; *HBeAg,* hepatitis B e antigen; *anti-HBe,* antibody to HBeAg; *anti-HBc,* antibody to hepatitis B core antigen; *ALT,* alanine transferase. (From Klion, F.M. & Wolke, A. [1986]. Liver in normal pregnancy. In S.H. Cherry, R.L. Berkowitz, & N.G. Kase [Eds.]. *Rovinsky and Guttmacher's medical, surgical, and gynecological complications of pregnancy.* Baltimore: Williams & Wilkins.)

changes in components of the immune system can be useful. Newborns usually have low serum levels of IgM at birth. Thus, elevated IgM levels (over 20 mg/dl) in cord blood or in the first week are suggestive of an intrauterine or intrapartally acquired nonbacterial (fungal, viral, or parasitic) infection. Elevated IgM levels are not diagnostic of infection because an infant with an intrauterine infection may have normal IgM levels and a healthy infant may have elevated levels, especially if there was maternal bleeding into the fetal circulation. Generally IgM levels continue to rise in infected infants but remain stable or decrease in noninfected infants. Identification of specific IgM antibodies in cord blood to cytomegalovirus, rubella, or spirochetes is evidence of intrauterine infection.[91]

The total number of WBCs or percentages of individual WBC cell types are often not useful in diagnosing neonatal sepsis, but these values may provide evidence suggestive of infection. At birth the WBC count averages 15,000/mm³ (range of 9000 to 25,000, although some healthy infants may have lower or higher values), falling to about 12,000 by the end of the first week. Total WBC counts below 3000 to 4000/mm³ or above 25,000 to 30,000/mm³ suggest infection but are not diagnostic.

The neutrophil count varies significantly in normal newborns during the first few days, with lower counts seen in preterm infants. A transient neutrophilia usually occurs during this period, so moderately elevated neutrophil counts of 10,000 to 25,0000/μl are not suggestive of infection. Neutropenia can be a useful sign of sepsis in some neonates; however, a variety of clinical factors can also lead to neutropenia (Table 12-14). Mouzinho et al. have proposed reference ranges for absolute total neutrophil counts

TABLE **12-14**   Clinical Factors Affecting Neutrophil Counts

	NEONATES WITH ABNORMAL VALUES IN:[a]				
	TOTAL NEUTROPHILS		TOTAL IMMATURE	INCREASED	APPROXIMATE
COMPLICATIONS	DECREASE	INCREASE	INCREASE	I:T RATIO[b]	DURATION (HOURS)
Maternal hypertension	++++	0	+	+	72
Maternal fever, neonate healthy	0	++	+++	++++	24
≥6 hours of antepartum oxytocin	0	++	++	++++	120
Asphyxia (5 minute Apgar ≤5)	+	++	++	+++	24-60
Meconium aspiration syndrome	0	++++	+++	++	72
Pneumothorax with uncomplicated hyaline membrane disease	0	++++	++++	++++	24
Seizures: no hypoglycemia, asphyxia, or central nervous system hemorrhage	0	+++	+++	++++	24
Prolonged crying (≥4 minutes)	0	++++	++++	++++	1
Asymtomatic blood glucose (≤30)	0	++	+++	+++	24
Hemolytic disease	++	++	+++	++	7-28 days
Surgery	0	++++	++++	+++	24
High altitude	0	++++	++++	0	6[c]

From Weinberg, J.A. & Powell, K.R. (2001). Laboratory aids for diagnosis of neonatal sepsis. In J.S. Remington & J.O. Klein (Eds.). *Infectious diseases of the fetus and newborn infant* (5th ed.). Philadelphia: W.B. Saunders.
[a]+, 0%-25% of neonates affected; ++, 25%-50%; +++, 50%-75%; ++++, 75%-100%.
[b]Immature forms/total neutrophil count.
[c]Not tested after 6 hours.
I:T ratio, Immature neutrophils to total neutrophils ratio.

in VLBW infants (<1500 g and 30 weeks' gestational age) of 500 to 6000 at birth; 2200 to 14,000 at 18 hours; 1100 to 8800 at 60 hours; and 1100 to 5600 at 120 hours.[133]

The differential count can also be useful in the recognition of neonatal sepsis. Normally, in the first few days after birth, the majority of WBCs are PMN neutrophils (60%), with 20 to 40% of these neutrophils being band forms. Findings associated with infection include a relative absence of PMNs, an increased "shift to the left" (i.e., a predominance of immature forms of PMNs [bands, metamyelocytes, occasional myelocytes] due to an outpouring of immature cells from the bone marrow), an increase in toxic granulations in the PMNs, and an increase in the absolute number of bands or metamyelocytes (even with normal total neutrophil counts). Increased numbers of total immature neutrophils can be useful but are also influenced by infant variability and clinical factors (Table 12-14). The ratio of immature neutrophils to total neutrophils (I:T ratio) may also be useful. Maximum normal levels in term infants are 0.16 at 0 to 24 hours of age and 0.12 at 60 hours of age, with a maximum of 0.2 in preterm infants younger than 31 weeks' gestational age.[91] An increased I:T ratio suggests sepsis, but increases are also seen with clinical factors (see Table 12-14).

In some septic infants there is a marked decrease in the bone marrow NSP, which is normally reduced in the neonate. The decreased NSP probably arises from the release of stored neutrophils in response to sepsis, the increased need for phagocytes, and an inability of the bone marrow to significantly increase production of neutrophils because production is already near maximum capacity in the neonate.[30]

Acute phase reactions are proteins produced by the liver in response to inflammation due to sepsis, trauma, or other cell processes.[91] Examples of these substances are C-reactive protein (CRP), erythrocyte sedimentation rate, fibronectin, and fibrinogen. Most of these substances have not been useful due to low positive predictive values (if abnormal, the percentage with infection).[91] Other investigators have examined panels using combinations of these substances. Use of these panels has increased the negative predictive value (if normal, the percentage without infection) but has not significantly increased the positive predictive value.[91] The acute phase reactant used most often in the neonate is CRP. In many infants the CRP is normal at the onset of infection and then rises within the next day to peak at 2 to 3 days after infection onset. Levels remain high until the infection is controlled and the inflammatory response begins to resolve; levels then fall over the next 5 to 10 days.[172] A single CRP level generally has limited usefulness in initial diagnosis of infection, but serial levels may

be useful in determining antibiotic effectiveness and duration of therapy.[172]

MATURATIONAL CHANGES DURING INFANCY AND CHILDHOOD

Infants and children remain at greater risk for infection because of decreased levels of immunoglobulins. This risk is most marked during the first 6 months because of low levels of IgG associated with a physiologic hypogammaglobulinemia. Infancy is a time when hypersensitivity to food substances may develop because of immaturity of gut defense mechanisms. In this section, maturation of components of the host defense system is described and is followed by discussion of the physiologic hypogammaglobulinemia of infancy, immunizations, and the development of allergies.

Maturation of Host Defense Factors

By 1 year of life, total levels of immunoglobulins are 60% of adult values.[125] IgG production by the infant is minimal during the first few months but increases significantly after 6 months of age, with a gradual increase toward adult levels by 4 to 6 years.[91,140] The increase in IgG and other immunoglobulins is probably stimulated by exposure to environmental antigens. Maternally derived IgG reaches a nadir at 3 to 4 months and has generally disappeared by 9 months of age. IgG1 and IgG3 reach 50% of adult values by 1 year and 100% by 8 years; IgG2 and IgG4 are 50% by 2 to 3 years and 100% by 10 to 12 years. As a result, infants and toddlers are more susceptible to disorders such as infection with *Haemophilus influenzae* type B, which is dependent on IgG2 antibodies for opsonization of its capsular coating.[39,111]

IgA levels increase after birth and reach 20% of adult levels by 1 year.[125] Levels of sIgA reach adult values by 5 to 8; serum IgA levels attain adult values during adolescence.[91,140] Salivary and gut IgA may reach adult levels by 5 years.[116] Because IgA protects against many respiratory and GI infections, young children are more predisposed toward developing these disorders. IgM reaches 50% of adult values by 6 months and 75% to 80% by 1 year in both term and preterm infants. During the first year of life, the infant's B cells secrete primarily IgM. Adult levels of IgM are reached between 1 to 2 years.[91,140]

Serum complement levels gradually increase to adult values by 6 to 18 months.[11,91] T-cell function is relatively mature by 3 to 6 months or sooner.[165] Chemotaxis of neutrophils is decreased until 2 years, and monocyte chemotaxis is decreased until 6 to 12 years.[111] Responses to bacteria with capsular polysaccharide do not reach adult capabilities until 1.5 to 2 years.[132,151] As a result, infants are more susceptible to infections by organisms such as *H. influenzae* type B, pneumococci, and meningococci.[65] Fibronectin reaches low adult levels by 1 year.[111] The exact age at which other components of the immune system reach maturity is unknown, although the risk of infection with many of the pathogens associated with neonatal infection decreases after 2 to 3 months of age.

Physiologic Hypogammaglobulinemia

At term, IgG is 90% to 95% of adult values and greater than maternal values because of active placental transfer of maternal IgG. After birth, IgG levels fall gradually as maternal IgG is catabolized, with minimal production of new IgG by the infant. This results in a "physiologic hypogammaglobulinemia" during the first year of life. Lowest levels of IgG occur at 2 to 4 months and remain low until at least 6 months (see Figure 12-12).

The initial 6 to 12 months is therefore a period of heightened vulnerability to infection in all infants, with a higher risk in preterm infants. These infants have lower IgG levels at birth, reach lowest levels of IgG sooner, and remain at low levels longer because the ability to synthesize IgG is more closely related to conceptual age than to postbirth age.[72] Sasidharan found that 42.8% (18 of 42) of VLBW infants had IgG levels lower than 100 mg/dl by 2 to 3 months of age, with values of 22 mg/dl in one infant.[163] The lowest IgG levels during the first few months were directly proportional to gestational age and inversely proportional to postbirth age. The period of hypogammaglobulinemia is also exaggerated in SGA infants. These infants often have lower levels of maternal antibody, probably due to placental dysfunction.

Immunizations

Although immunizations have been part of well-baby care for many years, there is still controversy regarding timing, dosage, and side effects. Current recommendations for immunizations for infants and children are published each year by the Centers for Disease Control and Prevention and the American Academy of Pediatrics and can be found on their websites.

The American Academy of Pediatrics has recommended that immunizations be given to preterm infants at the same chronologic age as term infants.[11,28] Hospitalized infants may be receiving blood or blood products. Vaccinations should not be given within 14 days of these treatments because blood or blood products may contain specific antibodies against the vaccine's antigen and interfere with the development of an appropriate immune response.[148]

The ability to respond to antigens with production of specific antibodies improves with age and is influenced more by exposure to antigens than by maturation of the immune system per se.[11] Infant responses are not dependent on either birth weight or gestational age. Bernbaum et al. examined antibody responses of term and preterm infants to diphtheria-pertussis-tetanus vaccine injections at 2, 4, and 6 months after birth.[11] Before the first immunization, 84% of preterm and 100% of term infants had adequate antibody levels to diphtheria and tetanus (but only 16% of preterm infants and 86% of term infants to pertussis) from transplacental passage of maternal IgG. Thus the preterm infants would have had fewer antibodies to protect them if they were exposed to organisms that cause these disorders before immunization. Adequate immune responses to diphtheria and tetanus were noted in term infants after one dose and in preterm infants after two doses. Both groups required two doses to mount adequate responses to pertussis. Preterm infants have fewer febrile or local reactions to DPT injections, probably because of immature primary host defense mechanisms.[11,12]

Preterm infants should receive full-dose vaccines.[12,84] Bernbaum et al found that fewer than half of preterm infants who received half-dose immunizations were able to mount an appropriate serologic response after three doses and required a fourth full dose to achieve this response.[12] Thus use of half-dose immunizations with preterm infants leaves about half of these infants unprotected.

Pertussis vaccination is contraindicated in infants with progressive neurologic disorders or a history of severe reactions to earlier doses. Nonprogressive neurologic disorders such as cerebral palsy or a history of neonatal seizures that has occurred months earlier or that are well controlled is not a contraindication to this vaccination, nor is the use of pertussis with preterm infants who have had a severe intracranial hemorrhage or prolonged frequency of apnea of prematurity, although concerns have been raised.[11,28]

Passively acquired maternal antibody generally does not interfere with immunizations against diphtheria, pertussis, tetanus, or polio, perhaps because maternal antibody levels to these organisms are relatively low due to the length of time since vaccination. Term or preterm infants do not respond well to vaccination, except with tetanus, before 1 month.[28] After that time, infants respond adequately to tetanus and diphtheria at any age and to pertussis after 3 months, which is why several doses of pertussis may be required before an adequate antibody response is observed.

IgG acquired through placental transfer from the mother can interfere with live virus immunizations by neutralizing the viruses and preventing successful vaccination.

The predominance of T-suppressor versus T-helper cells in the neonate may also interfere with the ability of the infant to respond appropriately. Therefore vaccination with live viruses is usually delayed until after the first year. Vaccination with HBV vaccine is effective early in infancy because this is an inactivated protein antigen.

Development of Allergies

The etiology of allergic disorders is multifactorial. Hypersensitivity to cow's milk protein and foods is more frequent in infants than in older children. By 1 to 2 years, many children can tolerate substances to which they were "allergic" earlier.[82] However, exposure to potentially allergic substances in early infancy may sensitize susceptible infants to specific ingested proteins (a process similar to that described earlier for Rh isoimmunization). Later exposure to even small quantities of that protein may invoke an allergic response. Therefore food substances known to have strong antigenic potential, such as egg white and nuts, are usually not recommended for young infants.

Young infants are more likely to develop food allergies because of immaturity of gut defense mechanisms, lack of gut closure, and the ability of the immature gut to absorb intact protein macromolecules. Most infants fed cow's milk early develop IgG and IgA antibodies to cow's milk antigens. These antibodies are found from 3 to 9 months and then gradually decrease, but they may return (at lower levels) with later ingestion of cow's milk. Breastfeeding may reduce the risk of allergy by limiting ingestion of foreign antigens or, with early development of the IgA barrier in the gut, by binding foreign proteins with specific antibodies to prevent their absorption.[82,114,147] The American Academy of Pediatrics recommends delaying introduction of solids until 4 to 6 months in all children and until 6 months if there is a history of allergies in the family.[82]

SUMMARY

The fetus and neonate are immunocompromised hosts because of alterations in their host defense mechanisms that increase their risk of infection. This risk is particularly evident in relation to organisms that colonize the maternal genital tract, such as GBS and sexually transmitted diseases (e.g., herpes, hepatitis B, HIV infection). Clinical recommendations for nurses working with neonates based on changes in host defense mechanisms are summarized in Table 12-15. By understanding the limitations of the immune system in the neonate and infant, nurses can appreciate the vulnerabilities to infection from specific organisms

---

TABLE **12-15**   **Recommendations for Clinical Practice Related to Host Defense Mechanisms in Neonates**

Recognize normal parameters for immune system components and patterns of change during the neonatal period (pp. 494-503).

Obtain and evaluate maternal history of possible exposure to infectious organisms or potential for current illness (pp. 494-495).

Recognize the risk factors for development and clinical manifestations of specific infections (pp. 503-507 and Table 12-8).

Recognize the subtle signs of infection in the neonate and that fever is rarely a sign of infection (pp. 496-497).

Recognize laboratory findings associated with an increased likelihood of neonatal infection (pp. 507-509).

Monitor neonates for signs of infection, especially infants with disruption of their skin barrier; those who are preterm, ill, small for gestational age, or stressed; or those with delayed oral feedings (pp. 494-507).

Monitor for signs of necrotizing enterocolitis (p. 503 and Chapter 11).

Monitor for signs of group B stretoccoci (GBS) and *Escherichia coli* sepsis and meningitis in infants of mothers colonized with these organisms who do not have type-specific antibody (pp. 503-505 and Figure 12-13).

Teach parents regarding methods to prevent or reduce the risk of infection in their infant (pp. 503-507).

Monitor infants of women with chronic disorders associated with transplacental passage of antibodies for antibody-related clinical problems (pp. 486-487).

Monitor Rho(D)-positive infants of Rho(D)-negative women and A, B, or AB infants of type O mothers for hyperbilirubinemia (pp. 487-491).

Recognize antigens and antibodies associated with hepatitis B virus (HBV) infection and institute hepatitis precautions for infants born to mothers who are HBsAg or HBeAg positive (pp. 506-507, Table 12-13, and Figure 12-14).

Give hepatitis B immune globulin (HBIG) and HBV vaccine to infants of mothers who are HBsAg positive (pp. 506-507).

Use standard precautions for blood and body fluids during the perinatal period (pp. 503-507).

Know recommended schedule of immunizations (p. 510).

Monitor infants to ensure that they receive immunizations as scheduled, especially preterm infants and infants with chronic problems (pp. 510-511).

Avoid the use of live virus vaccines in infants who are hospitalized and in infants who are positive for human immunodeficiency virus (HIV) (pp. 510-511).

Avoid giving immunizations within 14 days of administration of blood or blood products (p. 510).

Counsel parents regarding practices to reduce risks of allergies (p. 511).

and the risk for developing sepsis, develop increased understanding of the rationales behind specific infection control policies, and provide appropriate parent teaching.

REFERENCES

1. American Academy of Pediatrics. (1991). *Report of committee on infectious diseases.* Elk Grove Village, IL: American Academy of Pediatrics.
2. Adkins, B. (1999). T-cell function in newborn mice and humans. *Immunol Today, 20,* 330.
3. Ahdieh, L. (2001). Pregnancy and infection with human immunodeficiency virus. *Clin Obstet Gynecol, 44,* 154.
4. Anthony, B.F. (1986). The role of specific antibody in neonatal bacterial infections. *Pediatr Infect Dis, 5,* S164.
5. Arck, P. (1999). From the decidual cell internet: trophoblast-recognizing T cells. *Biol Reprod, 60,* 227.
6. Arvin, A.N. & Whitley, R.J. (2001). Herpes simplex virus infections. In J.S. Remington & J.O. Klein (Eds.). *Infectious diseases of the fetus and newborn infant* (7th ed.). Philadelphia: W.B. Saunders.
7. August, P. (1999). Hypertensive disorders in pregnancy. In G.N. Burrow & T.P. Duffy (Eds.). *Medical Complications during pregnancy* (5th ed.). Philadelphia: W.B. Saunders.
8. Avent, N.D. & Reid, M.E. (2000). The Rh blood group system: a review. *Blood, 95,* 375.
9. Barriga, C., et al. (1994). Increased phagocytic activity of polymorphonuclear leukocytes during pregnancy. *Eur J Obstet Gynecol Reprod Biol, 57,* 43.
10. Bellanti, J.A., Zeligs, B.J. & Pung, H.Y. (1999). Immunology of the fetus and newborn. In G.B. Avery, M.A. Fletcher & M.G. MacDonald (Eds.). *Neonatology: Pathophysiology and management of the newborn* (5th ed.). Philadelphia: J.B. Lippincott.
11. Bernbaum, J., et al. (1984). Development of the premature infant's host defense mechanisms and its relationship to routine immunizations. *Clin Perinatol, 11,* 73.
12. Bernbaum, J., et al. (1989). Half-dose immunization for diphtheria, tetanus, pertussis: response of preterm infants. *Pediatrics, 83,* 471.
13. Bernbaum, J.C. (1999). Medical care after discharge. In G.B. Avery, M.A. Fletcher, & M.G.MacDonald (Eds.). *Neonatology: Pathophysiology and management of the newborn* (5th ed.). Philadelphia: J.B. Lippincott.
14. Bernt, K.M. & Walker, W.A. (1999). Human milk as a carrier of biochemical messages. *Acta Paediatr Suppl, 430,* 27.
15. Bernum, M.L., et al. (1999). Pelvic malignancies, gestational trophoblastic neoplasia and nonpelvic malignancies. In R.K. Creasy & R. Resnik (Eds.). *Maternal-fetal medicine* (4th ed.). Philadelphia: W.B. Saunders.
16. Billingham, R.E. & Head, J. (1981). Current trends in reproductive immunology: An overview. *J Reprod Immunol, 3,* 253.
17. Bjorksten, B. (1999). The intrauterine and postnatal environments. *J Allergy Clin Immunol, 104,* 1119.
18. Blackburn, S. (1985). Rho(D) isoimmunization: Implications for the mother, fetus, and newborn. In *NAACOG update series* (vol. 3). Princeton, NJ: Continuing Professional Education Center.
19. Blackwell, T.S., et al. (1996). Sepsis and cytokines: Current status. *Br J Anaesth, 77,* 110.
20. Boue, A. & Malbrunot, C. (1987). Fetal and neonatal viral infections. In L. Stern & P. Vert (Eds.). *Neonatal medicine.* New York: Masson.
21. Burns, D.N., et al. (1998). The influence of pregnancy on human immunodeficiency virus type 1 infection: Antepartum and postpartum changes in human immunodeficiency virus type 1 viral load. *Am J Obstet Gynecol, 178,* 355.
22. Burtness, B. (1999). Neoplastic diseases. In G.N. Burrow & T.P. Duffy (Eds.). *Medical complications during pregnancy* (5th ed.). Philadelphia: W.B. Saunders.
23. Bussel, J. & Kaplan, C. (1998). The fetal and neonatal consequences of maternal alloimmune thrombocytopenia. *Baillieres Clin Haematol, 11,* 391.
24. Buyon, J.P. (1998). The effects of pregnancy on autoimmune diseases. *J Leukoc Biol, 63,* 281.
25. Calame, A. & Vaudaux, B. (1987). Bacterial infections in the newborn. In L Stern & P. Vert (Eds.). *Neonatal medicine.* New York: Masson.
26. Carr, R. & Hulzinga, T.W.J. (2000). Low sFcRIII demonstrates reduced neutrophil reserve in preterm neonates. *Arch Dis Child Fetal Neonatal Ed, 83,* F160.
27. Carr, R. (2000). Neutrophil production and function in newborn infants. *Br J Haematol, 110,* 18.
28. Cates, K.L., Rowe, J.C. & Ballow, M. (1983). The premature infant as a compromised host. *Curr Prob Pediatr, 13,* 1.
29. Centers for Disease Control and Prevention. (1996). Prevention of perinatal group B streptococcal disease: A public health perspective. *MMWR, 45*(RR-7), 1.
30. Christensen, R.D. (1987). Intravenous immunoglobulin for prophylaxis or treatment of bacterial infections in neonates. *J Perinatol, 7,* 58.
31. Clark, D.A. (1999). Immunology of pregnancy. In G.N. Burrow & T.P. Duffy (Eds.). *Medical complications during pregnancy* (5th ed.). Philadelphia: W.B. Saunders.
32. Cline, M.K., Bailey-Dorton, C. & Cayelli, M. (2000). Maternal infections: Diagnosis and management. *Prime Care, 27,* 13.
33. Cohen, S.B., et al. (1999). Analysis of the cytokine production by cord and adult blood. *Hum Immunol, 60,* 331.
34. Crumpacker, C.S. (2001). Hepatitis. In J.S. Remington & J.O. Klein (Eds.). *Infectious diseases of the fetus and newborn infant* (7th ed.). Philadelphia: W.B. Saunders.
35. Cummins, A.G. & Thompson, F.M. (1997). Postnatal changes in mucosal immune response: physical perspective of breast feeding and weaning. *Immunol Cell Biol, 75,* 419.
36. Cunningham, F.G & Whitridge, W.J. (1997). *Williams obstetrics* (20th ed.). Stamford, CT: Appleton & Lange.
37. Curfs, J.H., et al. (1997). A primer on cytokines: sources, receptors, effects, and inducers. *Clin Microbiol Rev, 10,* 742.
38. Dai, D., et al. (2000). Role of oligosaccharides and glycoconjugates in intestinal host defense. *J Pediatr Gastroenterol Nutr, 30,* S23.
39. Davies, P.A. & Gothefors, L.A. (1984). *Bacterial infections in the fetus and newborn infant.* Philadelphia: W.B. Saunders.
40. de Vries, E., et al. (1999). Analyzing the developing lymphocyte system of neonates and infants. *Eur J Pediatr, 158,* 611.
41. Dekker, G.A. & Sibai, B.M. (1999). The immunology of preeclampsia. *Semin Perinatol, 23,* 24.
42. Delacourt, C., Harf, A. & Lafuma, C. (1997). Developmental aspects of alveolar macrophage function involved in pulmonary defenses. *Pediatr Pulmonol Suppl, 16,* 211.
43. Delespesse, G., et al. (1998). Maturation of human neonatal CD4[+] and CD8[+] T lymphocytes into Th1/Th2 effectors. *Vaccine, 16,* 1415.
44. Donaldson, J.O. (1999). Neurologic complications. In G.N. Burrow & T.P. Duffy (Eds.). *Medical complications during pregnancy* (5th ed.). Philadelphia: W.B. Saunders.
45. Duc-Goiran, P., et al. (1999). Embryo-maternal interactions at the implantation site: a delicate equilibrium. *Eur J Obstet Gynecol Reprod Biol, 83,* 85.

46. Dudley, D.J. (1999). Immunoendocrinology of preterm labor: the link between corticotrophin releasing hormone and inflammation. *Am J Obstet Gynecol, 180*(1 Pt. 3), 251S.

47. Duff, P. (1998). Hepatitis in pregnancy. *Semin Perinatol, 22,* 277.

48. Edwards, M.S. (1988). Hepatitis B serology-help in interpretation. *Pediatr Clin North Am, 35,* 503.

49. Eisenfield, I., et al. (1990). Longitudinal study of neutrophil adherence and motility. *J Pediatrics, 117,* 926.

50. Ellis, L.A., Mastro, A.M. & Picciano, M.F. (1997). Do milk-borne cytokines and hormones influence neonatal immune cell function? *J Nutr, 127,* 985S.

51. Englund, J., Glezen, W.P. & Piedra, P.A. (1998). Maternal immunization against viral disease. *Vaccine, 16,* 1456.

52. Fischer, G.W., Ottolini, M.G., & Mond, J.J. (1997). Prospect for vaccines during pregnancy and in the newborn. *Clin Perinatol, 24,* 231.

53. Falconer, A.E., et al. (1995). Impaired neutrophil phagocytosis in preterm neonates: Lack of correlation with expression of immunoglobulin or complement receptors. *Biol Neonate, 68,* 264.

54. Formby, B. (1995). Immunologic response in pregnancy. Its role in endocrine disorders of pregnancy and influence on the course of maternal autoimmune diseases. *Endocrinol Metab Clin North Am, 24,* 187.

55. French, R., et al. (1998). The effect of pregnancy on survival in women infected with HIV: A systematic review of the literature and meta-analysis. *Br J Obstet Gynecol, 105,* 827.

56. Gall, S.A. (1983). Maternal adjustments in the immune system in normal pregnancy. *Clin Obstet Gynecol, 26,* 521.

57. Gall, S.A. & Wenstrom, K.D. (1990). Maternal-fetal immunology. In R.D. Eden & F.H. Boehm (Eds.). *Assessment and care of the fetus.* Norwalk, CT: Appleton & Lange.

58. Garza, C., et al. (1987). Special properties of human milk. *Clin Perinatol, 14,* 11.

59. Gennaro, S. & Fehder, W.P. (1996). Stress immune function, and relationship to pregnancy outcome. *Nurs Clin North Am, 31,* 293.

60. Gibbs, R.S. & Sweet, R.L. (1999). Maternal and fetal infectious disorders. In R.K. Creasy & R. Resnik (Eds.). *Maternal-fetal medicine* (4th ed.). Philadelphia: W.B. Saunders.

61. Gilstrap, L.C. & Ramin, S.M. (2000). Infection and cerebral palsy. *Semin Perinatol, 24,* 200.

62. Givner, L.B. & Baker, C.J. (1988). The prevention and treatment of neonatal group B streptococcal infections. *Adv Pediatr Infect Dis, 3,* 65.

63. Gladman, D.D. & Urowitz, M.B. (1999). Rheumatic disease in pregnancy. In G.N. Burrow & T.P. Duffy (Eds.). *Medical complications during pregnancy* (5th ed.). Philadelphia: W.B. Saunders.

64. Glezen, W.P. & Alpers, M. (1999). Maternal immunization. *Clin Infect Dis, 28,* 219.

65. Goldenberg, R. L., et al. (2000). Intrauterine infection and preterm delivery. *N Engl J Med, 342,* 1500.

66. Goldman, A.S. (2000). Back to basics: host responses to infection. *Pediatr Rev, 21,* 342.

67. Goldman, A.S. (2000). Modulation of the gastrointestinal tract of infants by human milk. Interfaces and interactions. An evolutionary perspective. *J Nutr, 130,* 426S.

68. Gomez, R., et al. (1997), Pathogenesis of preterm labor and premature rupture of the membranes associated with intraamniotic infection. *Infect Dis Clin North Am, 11,* 135.

69. Hackley, B.K. (1999). Immunizations in pregnancy. A public health perspective. *J Nurse Midwifery, 44,* 106.

70. Hamai, Y., et al. (1997). Evidence for an elevation in serum interleukin-2 and tumor necrosis factor-alpha levels before the clinical manifestations of preeclampsia. *Am J Reprod Immunol, 38,* 89.

71. Hammer, A., Hutter, H. & Dohr, G. (1997). HLA class I expression on the materno-fetal interface. *Am J Reprod Immunol, 38,* 150.

72. Hanson, L.A. (1999). Human milk and host defense: immediate and long-term effects. *Acta Paediatr Suppl, 88,* 42.

73. Hartwell, E.A. (1998). Use of Rh immune globulin: ASCP practice parameter. *Am J Clin Pathol, 110,* 281.

74. Hiby, S.E., et al. (1997). Human uterine NK cells have a similar repertoire of killer inhibitory and activatory receptors to those found in blood, as demonstrated by RT-PCR and sequencing. *Mol Immunol, 34,* 419.

75. Hidaka, Y., et al. (1991). Changes in natural killer cell activity in normal pregnant and postpartum women: Increases in the first trimester and postpartum period and decreases in late pregnancy. *J Reprod Immunol, 20,* 73.

76. Hill, H.R. (1987). Biochemical, structural, and functional abnormalities of polymorphonuclear leukocytes in the neonate. *Pediatr Res, 22,* 375.

77. Hill, J.A., et al. (1995). T-helper 1-type immunity to trophoblast in women with recurrent spontaneous abortion. *JAMA, 273,* 1933.

78. Holt, P.G. & Jones, C.A. (2000). The development of the immune system during pregnancy and early life. *Allergy, 55,* 688.

79. Honkonen, E. & Erkkola, R. (1987). Antibacterial capacity in amniotic fluid in normal and complicated pregnancies. *Ann Chir Gynecol, 76*(suppl 202), 14.

80. Hutter, H. & Dohr, G. (1998). HLA expression on immature and mature human germ cells. *J Reprod Immunol, 38,* 101.

81. Hylander, M.A., et al. (1998). Human milk feeding and infection among very low birthweight infants. *Pediatrics, 102,* E38.

82. Israel, E.J. & Walker, W.A. (1988). Host defense development in gut and related disorders. *Pediatr Clin North Am, 35,* 1.

83. Iwatani, Y. & Watanabe, M. (1998). The maternal immune system in health and disease. *Curr Opin Obstet Gynecol, 10,* 453.

84. Izatt, S.D. (2002). Care of the newborn. In A.A. Fanaroff & R.J. Martin (Eds.). *Neonatal-perinatal medicine: diseases of the fetus and infant* (7th ed.). St. Louis: Mosby.

85. Jacob, J.H. & Stringer, C.A. (1990). Diagnosis and management of cancer during pregnancy. *Semin Perinatol, 14,* 79.

86. Jansson, M., et al. (1997). Role of immunity in maternal-infant HIV-1 transmission. *Acta Paediatr Suppl, 421,* 39.

87. Jenson, H.B. & Pollock, B.H. (1998). The role of intravenous immunoglobulin for the prevention and treatment of neonatal sepsis. *Semin Perinatol, 22,* 50.

88. Johnston, R.B. (1998). Function and cell biology of neutrophils and mononuclear phagocytes in the newborn infants. *Vaccine, 16,* 1363.

89. Kallman, J., et al. (1998). Impaired phagocytosis and opsonization towards group-B streptococci in preterm neonates. *Arch Dis Child Fetal Neonatal Ed, 28,* F46.

90. Kanellopoulos-Langevin, C. (1998). Tolerance of the fetus by the maternal immune system. *Rev Rhum Engl Ed, 65,* 603.

91. Kapur, R., et al. (2002). Developmental immunology. In A.A. Fanaroff & R.J. Martin (Eds.). *Neonatal-perinatal medicine: Diseases of the fetus and infant* (7th ed.). St. Louis: Mosby.

92. Kemp, A.S. & Campbell, D.E. (1996). The neonatal immune system. *Semin Neonatol, 1,* 67.

93. Kim, I.C. & Sabourin, C.L.K. (1987). Antigenic analysis of human trophoblast membrane: detection of a lymphocyte crossreactive antigen. *Am J Reprod Immunol Microbiol, 13,* 44.

94. Kim, K.S. (1991). Immune therapy in neonates and small infants. In T.F. Yeh (Ed.). *Neonatal therapeutics* (2nd ed.). St. Louis: Mosby.

95. King, A. & Loke, Y.W. (1999). The influence of the maternal uterine immune response on placentation in human subjects. *Proc NutrSoc, 58,* 69.

96. Klein, J.O. (2001). Bacterial sepsis and meningitis. In J.S. Remington & J.O. Klein (Eds.). *Infectious diseases of the fetus and newborn infant* (7th ed.). Philadelphia: W.B. Saunders.

97. Klion, F.M. (1991). The liver in normal pregnancy. In S.H. Cherry & I.R. Merkatz (Eds.). *Complications of pregnancy: Medical, surgical, gynecological, psychosocial and perinatal* (4th ed.). Baltimore: Williams & Wilkins.

98. Kohl, S. (1999). Human neonatal nature killer cell cytotoxicity function. *Pediatr Infect Dis J, 18,* 635.

99. Koren, G., et al. (1990). Cancer in pregnancy. *Obstet Gynecol Surv, 45,* 509.

100. Kovata, S. (1990). A class I antigen, HLA-G expressed in human trophoblasts. *Science, 248,* 220.

101. Kunz, C., et al. (1999). Nutritional and biochemical properties of human milk. I: General aspects, proteins, and carbohydrates. *Clin Perinatol, 26,* 307.

102. Lahrtz, F., et al. (1998). Chemokines and chemotaxis of leukocytes in infectious meningitis. *J Neuroimmunol, 85,* 33.

103. Landers, D.V., Martinez de Tejada, B. & Coyne, B.A. (1997). Immunology of HIV and pregnancy: the effects of each on the other. *Obstet Gynecol Clin North Am, 24,* 821.

104. Landesman, S. (1989). Human immunodeficiency virus infection in women: an overview. *Semin Perinatol, 13,* 2.

105. Landor, M. (1995). Maternal-fetal transfer of immunoglobulins. *Ann Allergy Asthma Immunol, 74,* 279.

106. Landry, M.L. (1999). In G.N. Burrow & T.P. Duffy (Eds.). *Medical complications during pregnancy* (5th ed.). Philadelphia: W.B. Saunders.

107. Laros, R.K. (1986). Erythroblastosis fetalis. In R.K. Laros (Ed.). *Blood disorders in pregnancy*. Philadelphia: Lea & Febiger.

108. Larsen, B. & Galask, R.P. (1977). Protection of the fetus against infection. *Semin Perinatol, 1,* 183.

109. Lawrence, R.A. & Lawrence, R.M. (1999). *Breastfeeding: A guide for the medical profession* (5th ed.). St. Louis: Mosby.

110. Le Bouteiller, P. (2000). HLA-G in the human placenta: Expression and potential functions. *Biochem Soc Trans, 28,* 208.

111. Lewis, D.B. & Wilson, C.B. (2001). Developmental immunology and role of host defenses in fetal and neonatal susceptibility to infection. In J.S. Remington & J.O. Klein (Eds.). *Infectious diseases of the fetus and newborn infant* (7th ed.). Philadelphia: W.B. Saunders.

112. Lo, Y.M. (1999). Fetal RhD genotyping from maternal plasma. *Ann Med, 31,* 308.

113. Lockitch, G. (1997). Clinical biochemistry of pregnancy. *Crit Rev Clin Lab Sci, 34,* 67.

114. Lockwood, C.J. & Kuczynski, E. (1999). Markers of risk for preterm delivery. *J Perinat Med, 27,* 5.

115. Maatan-Metzger, A., et al. (2000). Maternal anti-D prophylaxis during pregnancy does not cause neonatal hemolysis. *Arch Dis Child Fetal Neonatal Ed, 84,* F60.

116. MacDonald, T.T., et al. (1996). The ontogony of the mucosal immune system. In W.A. Walker, et al. (Eds.). *Pediatric gastrointestinal disease* (2nd ed.). St. Louis: Mosby.

117. Main, E., et al. (1994). Nulliparous preeclampsia (PE) is associated with placental expression of a variant allele of the new histocompatability gene HLA-G. *Am J Obstet Gynecol, 170,* 289.

118. Mannick, E. & Udall, J.N. (1996). Neonatal gastrointestinal mucosal immunity. *Clin Perinatol, 23,* 287.

119. Marshall-Clarke, S., et al. (2000). Neonatal immunity: How well has it grown up? *Immunology Today, 21,* 35.

120. Marzi, M., et al. (1996). Characteristics of type 1 and type 2 cytokine production profile in physiologic and pathologic human pregnancy. *Clin Exp Immunol, 106,* 127.

121. McIntyre, J.A. & Faulk, W.P. (1986). Trophoblast antigens in normal and abnormal human pregnancy. *Clin Obstet Gynecol, 29,* 976.

122. McManamny, D.S., et al. (1989). Melanoma and pregnancy: A long term follow-up. *Br J Obstet Gynaecol, 96,* 1419.

123. Mease, A.D. (1990). Tissue neutropenia: the newborn neutrophil in perspective. *J Perinatol, 10,* 55.

124. Michison, N.A., Schuhbauer, D. & Muller, B. (1999). Natural and induced regulation of Th1/Th2 balance. *Springer Semin Immunopathol, 21,* 199.

125. Miller, M.M. & Stiehm, E.R. (1983). Immunology and resistance to infection. In J.S. Remington & J.O. Klein (Eds.). *Infectious diseases of the fetus and newborn infant*. Philadelphia: W.B. Saunders.

126. Modi, N. & Carr, R. (2000). Promising stratagems for reducing the burden of neonatal sepsis. *Arch Dis Child Fetal Neonatal Ed, 83,* F150.

127. Mofenson, L.M. & McIntyre, J.A. (2000). Advances and research directions in the prevention of mother-to-child HIV-1 transmission. *Lancet, 24,* 2237.

128. Moore, K.L. & Persaud, T.V.N. (1998). *The developing human: Clinically oriented embryology* (6th ed.). Philadelphia: W.B. Saunders.

129. Moreau, P., et al. (1998). Molecular and immunologic aspects of the nonclassical HLA class I antigen HLA-G: Evidence for an important role in maternal tolerance of the fetal allograft. *Am J Reprod Immunol, 40,* 126.

130. Moreau, P., et al. (1999). IL-10 selectivity induces HLA-G expression in human trophoblasts and monocytes. *Int Immunol, 11,* 803.

131. Morgan, B.P. & Holmes, C.H. (2000). Immunology of reproduction: Protecting the placenta. *Curr Biol, 18,* R381.

132. Moriyama, I., et al. (1987). Infection and the functional immaturity of the fetal immune system. In K. Maeda (Ed.). *The fetus as patient '87* (proceedings of the Third International Symposium). Amsterdam: Excerpta Medica.

133. Mouzinho, A., et al. (1994). Revised reference ranges for circulating neutrophils in very-low-birth-weight neonates. *Pediatrics, 94,* 76.

134. Nahmias, A.J. & Kourtis, A.P. (1997). The great balancing acts: The pregnant woman, placenta, fetus, and infectious agents. *Clin Perinatol, 24,* 497.

135. Noetzel, M.J. & Burnstrom, J.E. (2001). The vulnerable oligodendrocyte, inflammatory observations on a cause of cerebral palsy. *Neurology, 66,* 1254.

136. Nelson, K.B. & Willoughby, R.E. (2000). Infection, inflammation, and the risk of cerebral palsy, *Curr Opin Neurol, 13,* 133.

137. Ober, C. (1998). HLA and pregnancy: the paradox of the fetal allograft. *Am J Hum Genet, 62,* 1.

138. O'Shea, T.M. & Dammann, O. (2000). Antecedents of cerebral palsy in very-low-birth weight infants. *Clin Perinatol, 27,* 285.

139. Pabst, H.F. (1997). Immunomodulation by breast-feeding. *Pediatr Infect Dis J, 16,* 991.

140. Pappas, B.E. (1999). Primary immunodeficiency disorders in infancy. *Neonatal Network, 18,* 13.

141. Piccinni, M.P., et al. (1998). Defective production of both leukaemia inhibitory factor and type 2 T-helper cytokines by decidual T-cells in unexplained recurrent abortions. *Nat Med, 4,* 1020.

142. Piccinni, M.P., Maggi, E. & Romagnani, S. (2000). Role of hormone-controlled T-cell cytokines in the maintenance of pregnancy. *Biochem Soc Trans, 28,* 212.

143. Pope, R.M. (1990). Immunoregulatory mechanisms present in the maternal circulation during pregnancy. *Baillieres Clin Rheumatol, 4*, 33.

144. Priddy, K.D. (1997). Immunologic adaptations during pregnancy. *J Obstet Gynecol Neonatal Nurs, 26*, 388.

145. Quan, R., et al. (1994). The effect of nutritional additives on anti-infective factors in human milk. *Clinical Pediatr, 33*, 325

146. Raghupathy, R. (1997). Th1-type type immunity is incompatible with successful pregnancy. *Immunol Today, 18*, 478.

147. Rassin, D.K et al (2001). Human milk. In J.S. Remington & J.O. Klein (Eds.). *Infectious diseases of the fetus and newborn infant* (5th ed.). Philadelphia: W.B. Saunders.

148. Rayburn, W. F. & Zuspan, F.P. (1991). *Drug therapy in obstetrics and gynecology.* St. Louis: Mosby.

149. Reen, D.J. (1998). Activation and functional capacity of human neonatal CD4 T cells *Vaccine, 16*, 1401.

150. Reinhard, G., et al. (1998). Shifts in the TH1/Th2 balance during human pregnancy correlate with apoptotic changes. *Biochem Biophys Res Commun, 245*, 933.

151. Rijkers, G.T., et al (1998). Infant B cell responses to polysaccharide determinants. *Vaccine, 16*, 1396.

152. Riviere, Y. & Buseyne, F. (1998). Cytotoxic T lymphocytes generation capacity in early life with particular reference to HIV. *Vaccine, 16*, 1420.

153. Robertson, S.A. (1997). Cytokine-leukocyte networks and the establishment of pregnancy. *Am J Reprod Immunol, 37*, 438.

154. Rodriguez-Palmero, M. (1999). Nutritional and biochemical properties of human milk. II: Lipids, micronutrients, and bioactive factors. *Clin Perinatol, 26*, 335.

155. Saballus, M.K., Lake, K.D. & Wager, G.P. (1987). Immunizing the pregnant woman: Risks versus benefits. *Postgrad Med, 81*, 103.

156. Sacchi, F., et al. (1982). Differential maturation of neutrophil chemotaxis in term and preterm newborn infants. *J Pediatr, 101*, 273.

157. Saji, F., et al. (2000). Cytokine production in chorioamnionitis. *J Reprod Immunol, 47*, 185.

158. Saito, S. (2000). Cytokine network at the feto-maternal interface. *J Reprod Immunol, 47*, 87.

159. Salas, S.P. (1999). What causes pre-eclampsia? *Balliere's Clin Obstet Gynecol, 13*, 41.

160. Saliba, E. & Henrot, A. (2001). Inflammatory mediators and neonatal brain damage. *Biol Neonate, 79*, 224

161. Samuel, B.U. & Barry, M. (1998). The pregnant traveler. *Infect Dis Clin North Am, 12*, 325.

162. Sanderson, I.R. (1999). The physicochemical environment of the neonatal intestine. *Am J Clin Nutr, 69*, 1028S.

163. Sasidharan, P. (1988). Postnatal IgG levels in very-low-birth-weight infants. *Clin Pediatr, 27*, 271.

164. Savoia, M.C. (1999). Bacterial, fungal and parasitic diseases. In G.N. Burrow & T.P. Duffy (Eds.). *Medical complications during pregnancy* (5th ed.). Philadelphia: W.B. Saunders.

165. Schelonka, R.L. & Infante, A.J. (1998). Neonatal immunology. *Semin Perinatol, 22*, 2.

166. Scott, J.R. (1985). Immunologic diseases in pregnancy. In J.R. Scott & N.S. Rote (Eds.). *Immunology in obstetrics and gynecology.* Norwalk, CT: Appleton-Century-Crofts.

167. Seaman, W.E. (2000). Natural killer cells and natural killer T cells. *Arthritis Rheum, 43*, 1204.

168. Sherman, P.M. & Lichtman, S.N. (1996). Mucosal barrier function and colonization of the gut. In W.A. Walker et al. (Eds.). *Pediatric gastrointestinal disease* (2nd ed.). St. Louis: Mosby.

169. Shibuya, T., et al. (1991). Study on non-specific immunity in pregnant women. II: Effect of hormones on chemiluminescense response of peripheral blood phagocytes. *Am J Reprod Immunol Microbiol, 26*, 76.

170. Shirahata, T. (1992). Correlation between increased susceptibility to primary *Toxoplasma gondii* infection and depressed production of gamma interferon in pregnant mice. *Microbiol Immunol, 36*, 81.

171. Shohat, B., et al. (1986). Cellular immune aspects of the human fetal-maternal relationship. *Am J Reprod Immunol Microbiol, 11*, 125.

172. Silver, R.M. & Branch, D.W. (1999). The immunology of pregnancy. In R.K. Creasy & R. Resnik (Eds.). *Maternal-fetal medicine* (4th ed.). Philadelphia: W.B. Saunders.

173. Silverstein, A.M. (1995). From the forehead of Zeus: the ontogeny of the immune response. *Eye, 9*, 147.

174. Stagnaro-Green, A., et al. (1992). A prospective study of lymphocyte initiated immunosuppression in normal pregnancy: Evidence of a T-cell etiology for postpartum thyroid dysfunction. *J Clin Endocrinol Metab, 74*, 645.

175. Stehm, E.R. (1996). Newborn factors in maternal-infant transmission of pediatric HIV infection. *J Nutr, 126*, 2632S.

176. Stevenson, A.M. (1999). Immunizations for women and infants. *J Obstet Gynecol Neonatal Nurs, 28*, 534.

177. Stoll, B.J., et al. (1993). Immunoglobulin secretion by the normal and the infected newborn infant. *J Pediatr, 122*, 780.

178. Thellin, O. (2000). Tolerance to the foeto-placental "graft": Ten ways to support a child for nine months. *Curr Opin Immunol, 12*, 731.

179. Trofatter, K.F., et al. (1990). Fetal immunology. In R.D. Eden & F.H. Boehm (Eds.). *Assessment and care of the fetus.* Norwalk, CT: Appleton & Lange.

180. Tseng, C.E. & Buyon, J.P. (1997). Neonatal lupus syndrome. *Rheum Dis Clin North Am, 23*, 31.

181. Urbaniak, S.J. & Greiss, M.A. (2000). RhD haemolytic disease of the fetus and the newborn. *Blood Rev, 14*, 44.

182. Urbaniak, S.J. (1998). The scientific basis of antenatal prophylaxis. *Br J Obstet Gynaecol, 105*, 11.

183. Vacchio, M.S. & Jiang, S.P. (1999). The fetus and the maternal immune system: Pregnancy as a model to study peripheral T-cell tolerance. *Crit Rev Immunol, 19*, 461.

184. van Rood, J.J. & Claas, F. (2000). Both self- and non-inherited maternal HLA antigens influence the immune response. *Immunol Today, 21*, 269.

185. Vince, G.S. & Johnson, P.M. (2000). Leukocyte populations and cytokine regulation in human uteroplacental tissues. *Biochem Soc Trans, 28*, 191.

186. Voisin, G.A. (1998). Immunology understood through pregnancy. *Am J Reprod Immunol, 40*, 124.

187. Wagner, C.L., Anderson, D.M. & Pittard, W.B. (1996). Special properties of human milk. *Clin Pediatr (Phila), 35*, 283.

188. Walker, W.A. (1987). Macromolecular transport in the neonatal gut: its role in milk allergy. In M. Xanthou (Ed.). *New aspects of nutrition in pregnancy, infancy and prematurity.* New York: Elsevier Science.

189. Walker, W.A. (2000). Role of nutrients and bacterial colonization in the development of intestinal host defense. *J Pediatr Gastroenterol Nutr, 30*, S2.

190. Wang, Y. & Walsh, S.W. (1996). TNF-alpha concentrations and mRNA expression are increased in preeclamptic placentas. *J Reprod Immunol, 32*, 157.

191. Warner, J. A., et al. (2000). Prenatal origins of allergic disease. *J Allergy Clin Immunol, 105*, S493.

192. Wantanabe, M., et al. (1997). Changes in t, B, and NK lymphocyte subsets during and after normal pregnancy. *Am J Reprod Immunol, 37,* 368.

193. Weetman, A.P. (1999). The immunology of pregnancy. *Thyroid, 9,* 643.

194. Wegmann, T.G., et al. (1993). Bi-directional cytokine interactions in the maternal-fetal relationship: is successful pregnancy a Th2 phenomena? *Immunol Today, 14,* 353.

195. Weinberg, E.D. (1984). Pregnancy associated depression of cell-mediated immunity. *Rev Infect Dis, 6,* 814.

196. Weinberg, J.A. & Powell, K.R. (2001). Laboratory aids for diagnosis of neonatal sepsis. In J.S. Remington & J.O. Klein (Eds.). *Infectious diseases of the fetus and newborn infant* (7th ed.). Philadelphia: W.B. Saunders.

197. Wolach, B. (1997). Neonatal sepsis: pathogenesis and supportive therapy. *Semin Perinatol, 21,* 28.

198. Wu, Y.W. & Colford, J.M. (2000). Chorioamnionitis as a risk factor for cerebral palsy. *JAMA, 284,* 1417.

199. Xanthou, M. (1987). Neonatal immunity. In L. Stern & P. Vert (Eds.). *Neonatal medicine.* New York: Masson.

200. Xanthou, M. (1998). Immune protection of human milk. *Biol Neonate, 74,* 121.

201. Xanthou, M., Bines, J. & Walker, W.A. (1995). Human milk and intestinal host defense in newborns: an update. *Adv Pediatr, 42,* 171.

202. Xu, R.J. (1996). Development of the newborn GI tract and its relation to colostrum/milk intake: a review. *Reprod Fertil Dev, 81,* 35.

203. Yokoyama, W.M. (1997). The mother-child union: the case of mission-self and protection of the fetus. *Proc Natl Acad Sci USA, 94,* 5998.

Integumentary System

The integumentary system consists of the skin and its appendages: eccrine, apocrine, apoeccrine, and sebaceous glands; hair; and nails. Functions of the skin include protection from physical and chemical injury, infection, and ultraviolet radiation; modulation of transepidermal water fluxes; prevention of fluid loss and fluid and electrolyte imbalances; and thermoregulation. The skin is also important in sensation (pain, pressure, touch, and temperature), contributes to maintenance of blood pressure by dilation or constriction of the peripheral capillaries, and contains precursor molecules for vitamin D.[19,142,55]

The skin and its associated structures are markedly altered during pregnancy. These changes are seen in most pregnant women, and although the changes themselves are seldom associated with serious physiologic consequences, they are of concern to most women because of the subsequent cosmetic alterations that may persist following delivery. In addition, there are several dermatologic disorders that are seen almost exclusively in pregnant women that can cause severe physical discomfort and may be associated with increased fetal morbidity. The skin is also an organ of considerable significance in the neonate. In addition, immaturity of the skin alters its permeability, immunologic capacity, bonding of the epidermis to the dermis, and role in thermoregulation and fluid balance. As a result, neonates, especially preterm and ill infants, are at risk for toxicity from topical substances, infection, skin excoriation, fluid loss, and thermal instability.

MATERNAL PHYSIOLOGIC ADAPTATIONS

Physiologic changes in the skin and its appendages during pregnancy and the postpartum period include alterations in pigmentation, connective and cutaneous tissue, integumentary vascular system, hair, nails, and secretory glands, and pruritus. Some integumentary alterations regress completely during the postpartum period; others recede but never completely disappear. Most of these alterations are secondary to the hormonal changes of pregnancy.

Antepartum Period

The basis for changes in the skin, hair, and secretory glands during pregnancy are thought to be hormonal—especially the effects of estrogen and adrenocortical steroids. Similar alterations are often seen in women using oral contraceptives. There also seems to be a familial tendency or genetic predisposition for many of the cutaneous and vascular changes.[125]

Alterations in Pigmentation

Alterations in pigmentation are common during pregnancy and include hyperpigmentation of specific areas of the body and melasma (chloasma). In early pregnancy, hyperpigmentation is probably due to estrogens and progesterone. This is also consistent with reports of alterations in pigmentation associated with use of oral contraceptives. Later progression is thought to be due to the effects of placental corticosteroid-releasing hormone and of pro-opiomelanocortin peptides such as adrenocorticotropic hormone (ACTH), melanocyte-stimulating hormone (MSH), and β-endorphin (see Chapter 18).[315,29,38,86,90,126]

Hyperpigmentation. Hyperpigmentation is the most frequent integumentary alteration during pregnancy. Changes in pigmentation are seen in 90% of pregnant women, tend to be more frequent in women with dark hair or complexions, and are progressive throughout pregnancy. Most women experience a mild, generalized increase in pigmentation that is especially prominent in areas of the body that tend to be naturally more intensely pigmented. These areas include the areolae, genital skin, axillae, inner aspects of the thighs, and linea alba.[1,18,27,29,62,80]

The linea alba is a tendinous median line that extends along the anterior of the abdomen from the umbilicus to the symphysis pubis and occasionally superiorly to the xiphoid process. Hyperpigmentation during pregnancy causes the linea alba to darken and become the linea nigra. Up to one third of women on oral contraceptives also develop a linea nigra. Pigmentary changes tend to fade during the postpartum period in fair-skinned women, but some pigmentary changes may remain in women with darker skin and hair. Hyperpigmentation may be exacerbated by sun exposure.[15,27,29,62,90,126]

Freckles, nevi, and recent scars may darken during pregnancy. Existing melanocytic nevi may also increase in size or new nevi may form with an increase in development of dendritic processes and in junctional activity of nevus cells. These changes may be similar to early melanoma but generally revert to their previous state following pregnancy. Prophylactic removal of these nevi following pregnancy may be considered. Any nevi showing signs suggestive of malignancy should be excised.[15,27,33,62,90,126]

Melasma (chloasma). Melasma (also known as *chloasma* or the "mask of pregnancy") occurs in 50% to 70% of pregnant women. Melasma is characterized by irregular, blotchy areas of pigmentation on the face. The areas of altered pigmentation are not elevated and can range in color from light to dark brown. Three distribution patterns have been described: centrofacial (63%), involving the cheeks, forehead, upper lip, nose, and chin; malar (21%), over the cheeks and nose; and mandibular (16%), over the ramus of the mandible.[101] Three histologic patterns have also been identified: epidermal (increased deposition of melanin in the melanocytes of the basal and suprabasal layers), which is seen in 70% of women; dermal (macrophages with large amounts of melanin can be found in both the papillary and reticular layers of the dermis), which is seen in 10% to 15%; and a mixed form, which is seen in 2%.[62,101] The pigmentary changes tend to fade completely within 1 year following pregnancy but may persist for years (especially in dark-haired individuals).[15,29,65,80,90,101,126]

There seems to be a genetic predisposition toward development of melasma. Melasma is seen most frequently in women with dark hair and complexions, is exacerbated by the sun, and tends to recur (often with increased intensity) in subsequent pregnancies or with use of oral contraceptives. Of women using oral contraceptives, 5% to 34% develop melasma. Melasma has also been reported occasionally in nonpregnant individuals who are not on oral contraceptives or other hormonal medications.[15,29,90,101,125]

Avoidance of suntanning during pregnancy and use of sunscreens with protective ratings greater than 15 may reduce the severity of melasma (Table 13-1). Since melasma often fades spontaneously following pregnancy, treatment is generally limited to individuals with persistent pigmentation. Various depigmenting formulas have been developed to treat persistent melasma, with varying success. These formulas tend to be relatively effective on epidermal type melasma but have little effect on the dermal type. Treatment may need to be continued for 5 to 7 weeks before satisfactory results are achieved. Topical 2% to 5% hydroquinone has also been used postpartum, again with varying success. This treatment can result in complications such as hypopigmentation, hyperpigmentation, and contact dermatitis.[15,29,90,101,125]

Changes in Connective Tissue

Striae gravidarum (often called linear striae, striae distensae, or linear "stretch marks") are linear tears in dermal collagen that are commonly seen during pregnancy. These markings initially appear as irregular, pink or purple, wrinkled linear streaks that gradually become white. Striae are most prominent by 6 to 7 months. They appear initially over the abdomen oriented in opposition to skin tension lines and then are found on the breasts, thighs, and inguinal area. Striae are seen more frequently in younger women with greater total weight gain and Caucasian women (90%) and less frequently in Asian and African-American women. In addition, there appears to be a familial tendency.[1,15,66,80,90,125]

Striae gravidarum usually fade following pregnancy but never completely disappear, remaining as depressed, irregular white bands. Some women report striae itching, although since both pruritus and striae formation are prominent over the abdominal area during pregnancy, these two phenomena may not be related. There is no effective treatment to prevent striae formation. Topical emollients and antipruritics may be used (see Table 13-1). However, the effectiveness of topical agents such as cocoa butter, vitamin E, tretinoin and olive oil, and massage to prevent striae formation have not been substantiated in controlled studies.[15,87,90,125,128]

The cause of striae is unclear. Striae gravidarum are believed to arise from hormonal alterations—especially of estrogens, relaxin, and adrenocorticoids—or perhaps a combination of hormonal changes and stretching. The increased levels of estrogens, corticosteroids, and relaxin relax the adhesiveness between collagen fibers and foster formation of mucopolysaccharide ground substance, which causes separation of the fibers and striae formation. The increased glucocorticosteroids may decrease dermal fibroblasts and collagen synthesis.[15,38] Mast cells, with hormonal receptors for estradiol, increase. Mast cells release enzymes to lyse collagen.[15,38,59,62,66,125]

Vascular and Hematologic Changes

Vascular changes during pregnancy related to the integumentary system include development of spider nevi or angiomas, palmar erythema, nonpitting edema, cutis marmorata, purpura, hemangiomas, and varicosities. Other alterations in the vascular and hematologic systems are de-

TABLE **13-1**   Nursing Management for Common Problems during Pregnancy Related to the Integumentary System

ALTERATION	INTERVENTION
All alterations	Provide anticipatory teaching regarding appearance of alteration.
	Counsel regarding basis for alteration and course.
	Evaluate effect on body image and relationship with partner and provide counseling.
Hyperpigmentation	Avoid suntanning during pregnancy and use broad spectrum (protective factor greater than 15) sunscreen.
	Use nonallergenic cover-ups.
Melasma	Avoid suntanning during pregnancy or when using oral contraceptives.
	Use broad-spectrum sunscreen (rating of 15 or greater).
	Use nonallergenic cover-ups.
	Counsel regarding the risk of similar changes with oral contraceptives.
	Counsel regarding alternative methods of birth control.
	Counsel regarding use of sunscreen and protection from sun with sunscreen use following pregnancy.
Striae gravidarum	Use topical emollients or antipruritics as required.
	Use supportive garments for breasts and abdomen.
Spider nevi	Reassure that most fade following pregnancy.
	Use cosmetic cover-up creams.
	Suggest considering electrocauterization if of great concern to patient.
Nonpitting edema	Elevate legs when sitting or lying down and sleep in the Trendelenburg position.
	Avoid prolonged standing or sitting.
	Rest in the left lateral decubitus position.
	Exercise.
	Avoid excessive added salt.
	Avoid tight clothing and girdles.
	Try elastic stockings (although their effectiveness is controversial).
Varicosities	Elevate legs when sitting or lying down and sleep in the Trendelenburg position.
	Avoid prolonged standing or sitting.
	Rest in the left lateral decubitus position.
	Exercise.
	Avoid tight clothing and girdles.
	Wear elastic stockings or support hose.
Increased eccrine gland activity	Wear light, loose clothing.
	Increase fluid intake.
	Bathe or shower regularly.
Pruritus	Wear loose nonsynthetic clothing.
	Use cool compresses and take baths or showers.
	Use oatmeal baths.
	Use adequate skin lubrication
	Consider topical antipruritics and emollients.

scribed in Chapters 7 and 8. Vascular changes are a result of distention, instability, and proliferation of blood vessels mediated by changes in pituitary, adrenal, and placental hormones with increased release of angiogenic growth factors.[15,38,62,65]

Cutis marmorata is a transient bluish mottling of the legs on exposure to cold that arises from vasomotor instability secondary to elevated estrogens. Persistence postpartally is abnormal and may suggest underlying pathology such as collagen vascular disorder, systemic lupus erythe-matosus, or vasculitis. Other changes due to vasomotor instability during pregnancy include pallor, facial flushing, and heat and cold sensations. Purpura secondary to increased capillary fragility and permeability occurs during the last months of pregnancy in many women.[15,125]

Spider nevi. Spider nevi (also called spider angiomas, spider telangiectases, or nevus araneus) are found in 10% to 15% of normal adults, in individuals with liver dysfunction, and in up to two thirds of pregnant women. These nevi are more common in Caucasian (14% at 2 months and 66% at 9 months) than African-American (8% at 2 months and 14% at 9 months) pregnant women.[27] Spider nevi consist of a central dilated arteriole that is flat or slightly raised with extensive radiating capillary branches. They are most prominent in areas of the skin drained by the superior vena cava (i.e., around the eyes, neck, throat, and arms). The basis for formation has been related to increased estrogen, since these structures are seen more frequently both during pregnancy and with use of oral contraceptives. However, many individuals with spider nevi associated with liver disorders do not have elevated estrogen levels.[1,62,125]

Spider nevi generally appear between months 2 and 5 of pregnancy and may increase in size and number as pregnancy progresses. These structures tend to regress spontaneously and fade within the first 7 weeks to 3 months following delivery, although they rarely completely disappear. They may recur or enlarge during subsequent pregnancies. Unresolved spider nevi can be treated by electrocauterization.[1,62,86,90,125]

Palmar erythema. Two patterns of palmar erythema are seen during pregnancy: erythema of hypothenar and thenar eminences, palms, and fleshy portions of the fingertips; and diffuse mottling of the entire palm. The latter form is more common and similar to changes seen with hyperthyroidism and cirrhosis. Palmar erythema generally appears during the first two trimesters and disappears by 1 week after delivery. This phenomenon has a familial tendency and is seen in approximately two thirds of Caucasian and one third of African-American pregnant women. Spider nevi and palmar erythema often occur together, suggesting a common etiology generally believed to be elevated estrogen levels with increased skin blood flow.[1,27,62,86,125]

Nonpitting edema. Increased vascular permeability and sodium retention due to the effects of estrogen result in transient nonpitting edema of the face, hands, and feet during late pregnancy. In the lower extremities this is aggravated by pressure from the growing uterus. This form of edema occurs in the face in approximately 50% of women and lower extremities in 70% and is not associated with preeclampsia.[80,125] Although generally present in the morning, it usually improves during the day (see Table 13-1). Vulvar edema may also be seen.

Capillary hemangiomas. Preexisting capillary hemangiomas may increase in size during pregnancy.[15] In about 5% of pregnant women, new hemangiomas appear by the end of the first trimester, with slight enlargement during the remaining trimesters.[125] New hemangiomas usually appear on the head and neck and are unusual elsewhere.[15] Enlarged existing hemangiomas and new hemangiomas

regress postpartum but may not completely disappear. Hemangioma development in pregnancy is related to elevated estrogen.[125]

Varicosities. Varicosities develop in approximately 40% of pregnant women. Varicosities occur most commonly in the legs but may also appear in the pelvic vessels, vulva, and anal area with hemorrhoid formation. Varicosities arise from estrogen-induced elastic tissue fragility, increased venous pressure in the lower extremities and pelvis from pressure of the gravid uterus, and familial tendency for valvular incompetence. Varicosities generally regress postpartum but do not completely disappear. Thrombi are rare with leg varicosities but are more frequent with hemorrhoids. Hemorrhoids are discussed in Chapter 11.[15,62,80,90,125]

Alterations in Cutaneous Tissue and Mucous Membranes

The most common mucous membrane alterations are changes in the vagina and cervix, which are seen in all pregnant women, and gingivitis, which is seen in many women. A less common oral finding is a cutaneous lesion of the gums known as angiogranuloma epulis. Epulis and gingivitis are discussed in Chapter 11. Jacquemier-Chadwick and Goodell signs are vascular changes that are early signs of pregnancy. Jacquemier-Chadwick sign is characterized by erythema of the vestibule and vagina; Goodell sign is characterized by increased vascularity of the cervix.[15,62,65]

Another cutaneous change during pregnancy is the development of skin tags called molluscum fibrosum gravidarum.[86] These are soft, flesh-colored or pigmented skin tags, which are small (usually 1 to 5 mm), pedunculated fibromas that appear during the second half of pregnancy, primarily on the lateral aspects of the face and neck, upper axillae, groin, and between and underneath the breasts. The cause of fibromata molle is unknown but is thought to be hormonal. These skin tags are more common in the second half of pregnancy, when they may increase in size and number. These growths may regress or clear spontaneously following delivery, although many remain. Remaining skin tags can be removed by electrocoagulation or clipping with sterile scissors.[15,38,62,65,86,90,125]

Alterations in Secretory Glands

Activity of the sebaceous, apocrine, and eccrine glands of the skin is altered during pregnancy. Sebaceous gland activity is generally reported to increase during pregnancy.[86,125] Many pregnant women report that their skin, especially on the face, feels "greasy." Some women may develop acne, often for the first time.[62] These changes are due to increased ovarian and placental androgens.[62,90]

Montgomery tubercles (small sebaceous glands on the areola) enlarge beginning as early as 6 weeks' gestation. Changes in Montgomery tubercles and in the breasts are described in Chapter 5.

Apocrine sweat gland activity decreases during pregnancy, possibly as a result of hormonal changes.[125] Eccrine sweat gland activity increases gradually during pregnancy, possibly because of increased thyroid activity along with increased body weight and metabolic activity.[86,125] Since eccrine glands are important (along with the cutaneous blood vessels) in thermoregulation at the skin surface (see Chapter 19), their increased activity reflects dissipation of excess heat produced by the increased metabolic activity of the pregnant woman and her fetus. Increased eccrine activity during pregnancy can lead to miliaria (prickly heat) or dyshidrotic eczema.[62,125] Palmar sweating is decreased in pregnancy, even though this is an area where eccrine glands are highly concentrated. The basis for this is unclear but may be related to increased adrenocortical activity. Interventions are listed in Table 13-1.[27,62]

Alterations in Hair Growth

Estrogen increases the length of the anagen (growth) phase of hair follicles during pregnancy (see the Hair Loss section under Postpartum Period). This results in increased hair loss postpartum. A mild hirsutism may develop early in pregnancy, with increased growth of hair on the upper lip, chin, and cheeks and in the suprapubic midline. Fine new hairs usually disappear by 6 weeks postpartum, but the coarser hairs usually remain.[15,62,90,125]

During late pregnancy and the early postpartum period, some women develop hair loss with frontoparietal recession of the hairline similar to changes seen in male-pattern baldness. This loss is rare and is usually associated with complete regrowth and not with later development of female-pattern alopecia.[15,62,122]

Alterations in the Nails

Changes in fingernails and toenails during pregnancy are uncommon and of unknown pathogenesis. Nail changes occur as early as 6 weeks and include transverse grooves (Beard lines), increased brittleness, distal separation of the nail bed (onycholysis), and subungual keratosis. Changes regress after delivery.[1,62,86,90,125]

Pruritus

Pruritus is the most common cutaneous symptom during pregnancy, occurring in approximately 14% to 20% of pregnant women. The itching may be localized, especially over the abdomen during the third trimester, or generalized. Abdominal pruritus at the end of the first trimester may be an isolated finding or an early sign of intrahepatic cholestasis of pregnancy with or without associated jaundice or one of the other specific dermatoses of pregnancy (Table 13-2). Pregnancy-associated pruritus always clears after delivery but may recur in subsequent pregnancies or with use of oral contraceptives. Pregnant women with pruritus should also be assessed for other skin disorders, including pregnancy dermatoses, contact dermatitis, and drug reactions.[37,90,93,125]

Postpartum Period

As noted earlier, some of the changes in the integumentary system and its associated structures clear spontaneously following delivery; other alterations may regress or fade but do not disappear completely. Hyperpigmentation and melasma fade in many; however, they may remain, especially in women with darker skin and hair. After delivery, striae gravidarum and spider nevi fade and capillary hemangiomas, varicosities, and skin tags regress. However these changes may not completely disappear.[15,62,90] Alterations in hair growth during pregnancy result in an increased hair loss during the postpartum period in many women.

Hair Loss

The scalp contains approximately 100,000 hair follicles. Hair fibers in each follicle independently cycle through three growth stages: anagen, catagen, and telogen. The anagen or growth stage lasts for 3 to 4 years and is characterized by intense metabolic activity. In this stage, hair grows an average of 0.34 mm/day. Catagen is a transitional stage that lasts several weeks. During this stage, metabolic activity and growth slow as the hair bulb is retracted upward into the follicle. Growth of the hair fiber stops during telogen (resting stage). Eventually a new hair bulb begins growing, which ejects the previous hair.[90,92] Normally about 80% of hair follicles are in the anagen stage and 15% to 20% of hair fibers are in the telogen stage, with about 50 to 100 hairs shed per day.[15,90]

Under the influence of estrogen during pregnancy, the rate of hair growth slows and the anagen stage is prolonged. This results in an increased number of anagen hairs and a decrease in telogen hairs to less than 10% during the second and third trimesters. During the postpartum period, these anagen hairs enter catagen and then telogen and are shed. Since there are more anagen hairs (and thus telogen hairs) than usual, most postpartum women experience an increased hair loss, beginning 4 to 20 weeks after delivery. During this time, 30% to 35% of the hairs may enter telogen. Generally, complete regrowth occurs by 6 to 15 months, although the hair may be less abundant than

TABLE **13-2**   Dermatoses of Pregnancy

Disorder*	Incidence	Onset and Etiology	Characteristics
Pemphigoid gestationis (herpes gestationis) (7, 15, 17, 28, 29, 38, 44, 56, 58, 59, 62, 90, 102, 106, 107, 108, 109, 110)	1/50,000-60,000 Seen most often in Caucasian women Has a familial tendency	Usually second and third trimesters Can appear as early as 2 weeks' gestation or up to 2 weeks postpartum May clear toward the end of pregnancy, then exacerbate postpartum Etiology: immunologic basis with production of anti-human leukocyte antigen (HLA) autoantibody against basal membranes that hold the epidermis and dermis together	Generalized, intense pruritus with erythematous urticarial plaques initially, followed by crops of fluid-filled vesicles and/or tense serum-filled bullae
Impetigo herpetiformis (54, 90, 117, 126)	Very rare	First to third trimesters, with peak incidence in third trimester Etiology unknown; associated with hypocalcemia and hypoparathyroidism May be a form of pustular psoriasis	Small (1-2 mm), sterile, white pustules on irregular erythematous plaques; central pustules become crusted as new pustules develop in periphery of plaque
Prurigo of pregnancy (44, 56, 62, 117, 126)	1/300	Any trimester May be due to hypersensitivity to placental antigens Includes several disorders, including prurigo gestationis of Besnier, Nurse's prurigo of late pregnancy, and papular dermatitis of pregnancy (Spangler's)	Severe pruritus with 3-5 mm papules that are not in crops or grouped; primary papules may be destroyed by scratching, leaving excoriated crusts as initial presentation
Pruritic urticarial papules and plaques of pregnancy (PUPPP), or polymorphic eruption of pregnancy (PEP) (9, 15, 29, 56, 62, 65, 90, 110, 117, 123, 126)	0.6% of pregnant women (more common in primiparas)	Third trimester (usually after 35 weeks) or postpartum Etiology unknown	Erythematous papules and urticarial plaques with excoriation usually absent
Intrahepatic cholestasis of pregnancy (27, 29, 32, 36, 44, 56, 62, 87, 90, 91, 117, 126)	0.02%-2.4% of pregnant women	Third trimester Cholestasis	Severe generalized pruritus without any skin lesions, although excoriation may result from scratching

*Numbers in parentheses refer to citations in reference list.

Location of Eruptions	Course	Other Maternal Findings	Effect on Fetus/Neonate
Initially around umbilicus, then spreads over abdomen to chest, back and extremities, and palms and soles	Spontaneous resolution, at delivery (75%) or usually within first month postpartum May regress in late pregnancy, then flare at delivery Often recurs in subsequent pregnancies (with earlier onset and increased severity) May reappear with menstrual cycle or with use of oral contraceptives	Pruritus, fatigue, fever, nausea, headache, and secondary infections May involve cyclic remissions and exacerbations	Severe forms have been associated with increased incidence of stillbirth, preterm birth, small for gestational age (SGA) infants, and transient neonatal skin lesions; in most SGA and preterm infants, probably due to effects of placental insufficiency
Often appears initially in femoral or perineal areas; spreads to lower abdomen, to medial aspects of the thighs, and around the umbilicus; occasionally involves hands, feet, under nails, and tongue	Spontaneous resolution postpartum Tends to recur in subsequent pregnancies, appearing earlier	Variable pruritus, associated with hypocalcemia, fever, lethargy, nausea and vomiting, and diarrhea	Increased incidence of abortion and stillbirth and possible placental insufficiency
Trunk (usually initial presentation) and/or extremities	Spontaneous resolution within 3-4 weeks after delivery May recur in subsequent pregnancies	Intense itching	None
Often appear initially in abdominal striae, then spread across abdomen to thighs, arms, and buttocks; rarely found above midthorax on chest	Spontaneous clearing within 2-3 weeks after delivery Little tendency to recur	May have mild pruritus	None
Pruritus usually begins on abdomen, then spreads to other areas	Clears rapidly after delivery May recur with subsequent pregnancy or use of estrogen medications (e.g., oral contraceptives)	May occur with or without jaundice If jaundice occurs, serum alkaline phosphatase, serum glutamate oxaloacetate transaminase, and serum bilirubin are elevated	If jaundice occurs, associated with decreased birth weight, increased incidence of meconium staining, increased stillbirth and fetal hypoxia secondary to placental insufficiency

before pregnancy. *Telogen effluvium* is the term used to describe the rapid transition of hair follicles into the telogen stage following delivery, surgery, or severe emotional or physical stress.[15,59,80,90,104,125]

CLINICAL IMPLICATIONS FOR THE PREGNANT WOMAN AND HER FETUS

The physiologic changes in the integumentary system during pregnancy and after delivery are common experiences for many women. These changes seldom significantly alter the function or structure of the integumentary system and are considered by some to be minor nuisances.[15] However, these changes may have significant psychologic and cosmetic implications for the pregnant woman and can contribute to alterations in body image. General interventions include anticipatory counseling, education, and reassurance (see Table 13-1). For example, postpartum hair loss can be devastating to the primipara who is unprepared for this event.

Dermatoses Associated with Pregnancy

In addition to the normal physiologic skin changes associated with pregnancy, there are several integumentary disorders that are unique to pregnancy. Specific dermatoses seen only during pregnancy include pemphigoid gestationis, impetigo herpetiformis, prurigo of pregnancy, pruritic urticarial papules and plaques of pregnancy (PUPPP) or polymorphic eruption of pregnancy (PEP), and intrahepatic cholestasis of pregnancy.[15,90] Several of these disorders have been associated with increased fetal morbidity and mortality (Table 13-2).

The etiology for many of these disorders is unclear, although they may have a hormonal or immunologic basis. For example, pemphigoid gestationis has an immunologic basis with production of anti–human leukocyte antigen (HLA) autoantibody against basal membranes that hold the epidermis and dermis together (see Table 13-2). There has often been confusion in classifying some of the rarer dermatoses, since much of the literature regarding these disorders involves reports of small numbers of women, which may represent different variations of the same disorder.[86] Treatment involves use of topical emollients, antipruritics, cold compresses, oatmeal baths (for relief of itching), and topical steroids. In women with moderate to severe eruptions, systemic steroids and antihistamines may be used.

Effects of Pregnancy on Preexisting Skin Disorders

The effects of pregnancy on preexisting skin disorders varies from no effect to marked improvement or worsening.[6,15,27,90,125] With disorders such as psoriasis, eczema, contact dermatitis, and acne vulgaris, this range of effects during pregnancy has been described within the same disease in different women.[15,27,90] Neurofibromas increase in size during pregnancy and new tumors may appear.[90] The effect of pregnancy on malignant melanoma is variable.[90] Pregnancy may have no adverse effects on stage I melanoma. However, decreased survival is reported with recurrent melanoma in some studies.[40] Other studies report an increased risk for appearance or exacerbation in pregnancy, especially in the second half, possibly due to the increased MSH and ACTH in later pregnancy. MSH may indirectly stimulate growth of the melanoma; ACTH enhances MSH activity.[40,90] Effects of pregnancy on other integumentary disorders are reviewed in the literature.[15,90]

SUMMARY

The effects of pregnancy on the integumentary system include physiologic changes in the skin and its appendages that are experienced by most pregnant women, skin disorders that are unique to pregnancy, and possible changes in preexisting skin disorders. Nursing management of the pregnant woman in relation to these effects includes preparation for the physiologic changes and their sequelae, and reassurance and support, as well as assessment for the specific dermatoses of pregnancy that are associated with maternal systemic symptoms and, if severe and untreated, with increased fetal mortality and morbidity. Clinical recommendations related to changes in the integumentary system during pregnancy are summarized in Table 13-3.

DEVELOPMENT OF THE INTEGUMENTARY SYSTEM IN THE FETUS

For the neonate the skin is a sophisticated and critical sensory organ for obtaining and receiving information about the environment. Since the neonate is an immunologically immature host, the integrity of the skin as a barrier to that same environment is essential to the survival and well-being of the infant. In order to understand the importance of this system to the infant, an overview of anatomic and functional development is needed.

Anatomic Development

The basic structure of the skin develops during the first 60 days of gestation. Around the time of transition from embryo to fetus, the skin undergoes a series of rapid morphologic changes, including keratinization of the epidermal appendages (around 15 weeks) and interfollicular epithelium (around 22 to 24 weeks).[52] By the third trimester, the structure of the skin is similar to that of the adult. However, its barrier properties are still immature, especially in the infant born before term.[52] Further maturation of the skin occurs within the first weeks after birth. Table 13-4 compares

TABLE **13-3**   Recommendations for Clinical Practice Related to Changes in the Integumentary System in Pregnant Women

Recognize the usual changes involving the skin, hair, nails, and sebaceous and sweat glands during pregnancy and the postpartum period (pp. 517-521).

Provide anticipatory teaching regarding the usual alterations in the skin and its appendages during pregnancy (pp. 517-521).

Counsel pregnant women regarding the basis for integumentary alteration and their usual course, including whether or not the change will regress postpartum (pp. 517-521).

Evaluate the effect of integumentary changes on the woman's body image and relationship with her partner and provide counseling (p. 524).

Counsel women regarding the potential for integumentary alterations during subsequent pregnancies or with use of oral contraceptives (pp. 517-521).

Recommend specific interventions to reduce or ameliorate the effects of integumentary changes (Table 13-1).

Recognize the specific dermatoses associated with pregnancy (p. 524 and Table 13-2).

Avoid use of isotretinoin in pregnant women or sexually active women of childbearing age who are not using a reliable, highly effective form of birth control (Chapter 6).

Counsel women with chronic integumentary disorders regarding the effect of pregnancy on their disorder (p. 524).

TABLE **13-4**   Comparison of the Structural Properties of the Skin of the Second-Trimester Fetus, Premature Infant (Third Trimester), Newborn Infant, and Older Child-Adult

CHARACTERISTIC	FETAL (SECOND TRIMESTER)	PREMATURE (THIRD TRIMESTER)	NEWBORN INFANT	CHILD-ADULT
Full thickness skin	0.5-0.9 mm	0.9 mm	1.2 mm	2.1 mm
Epidermal surface	Periderm	Cornified; some vernix caseosa	Cornified; may have some vernix caseosa	Dry, sebaceous lipids may be present
Epidermal thickness	50-60 μ	50-60 μ	~50-60 μ	>70 μ
Spinous cell content	Glycogen; fine bundles of keratin filaments	Glycogen; fine bundles of keratin filaments; lamellar granules	Little or no glycogen; larger bundles of keratin filaments; lamellar granules	No glycogen; prominent bundles of keratin filaments; lamellar filaments
Stratum corneum thickness	—	4-6 μ 5-6 cell layers	9-10 μ 15+ cell layers	9-10 μ 15+ cell layers
Stratum corneum barrier	Permeable	Permeable in the fetus and preterm infant; becomes similar to adult and full-term infants after 2-3 weeks postnatal maturation	Effective permeable barrier	Effective permeable barrier
Melanocytes	Dendritic melanocytes ~800 cells/mm^2	Dendritic melanocytes; melanosomes transferred to keratinocytes	Dendritic melanocytes; ~800-900 cells/mm^2; melanosomes transferred to keratinocytes	Dendritic melanocytes; ~600-700 cells/mm^2; melanosomes transferred to keratinocytes

From Holbrook, K.A. (1998). Structural and biochemical organogenesis of skin and cutaneous appendages in the fetus and newborn. In R.A. Polin & W.W. Fox (Eds.). *Fetal and neonatal physiology* (2nd ed.). Philadelphia: W.B. Saunders.   *Continued*

TABLE **13-4**   Comparison of the Structural Properties of the Skin of the Second-Trimester Fetus, Premature Infant (Third Trimester), Newborn Infant, and Older Child-Adult—cont'd

CHARACTERISTIC	FETAL (SECOND TRIMESTER)	PREMATURE (THIRD TRIMESTER)	NEWBORN INFANT	CHILD-ADULT
Langerhans cells	Adenosine triphosphatase (ATPase) positive, human leukocyte antigen-DR (HLA-DR)–positive, CD1-negative; small and truncated; ~50 cells/mm²*	ATPase positive, HLA-DR-positive, CD1-positive; small and truncated plus large and dendritic ; ~70 cells/mm²	ATPase positive, HLA-DR-positive, CD1-positive; large and highly dendritic; >160 cells/mm²	ATPase positive, HLA-DR-positive, CD1-positive; large and highly dendritic; >700 cells/mm²
Dermal-epidermal junction (DEJ)	Structurally complete; most of the antigens are expressed; no rete ridges	Structurally complete; number and size of adhesive junctions less than in adult; all known adult DEJ antigens are expressed; rete ridges lacking or poorly formed	Structurally complete and antigen expression similar to adult; rete ridges present	Well developed attachment and adhesive structure; well-developed rete ridges
Pilosebaceous structures	Bulbous hair peg; keratinization of the hair and follicle occurs	Lanugo follicles; sebaceous gland well developed; hairs present	Lanugo follicles, many have second hair pelage; large, active sebaceous gland	Follicles produce vellus or terminal hairs; sebaceous glands become quiescent until later childhood
Eccrine sweat glands	Formed only on palms and soles; primordia appear on other regions of the body surface late in this period	Sweat glands present; high in the dermis; sweating unlikely to occur	Sweat glands present; still high in dermis; not fully functional	Sweat glands become positioned deeper in dermis; most are inactive within the first few years
Dermis regions	Papillary and reticular regions defined	Papillary and reticular regions defined	Papillary and reticular regions defined	Papillary and reticular regions defined; greater distinction in fiber bundle size; an intermediate zone may also be evident
Cellularity	Cells abundant throughout dermis	Cells abundant throughout dermis	Cells abundant throughout dermis	Cells most abundant in papillary dermis
Collagen fibers	Small diameter; all biochemical types of adult skin are present; type III elevated compared with adult; high levels of enzymes for collagen processing	Diameter depends on region, but smaller than adult; elevated type III; active synthesis of all types present	Diameter depends on region, but smaller than adult; elevated type III	Distinct hierarchy of fibril and fiber diameter depending on region; types 1 and II present in ratio of 80%-85% to 15%-20%
Elastic fibers	Microfibrils present; elastin lacking but elastin messenger ribonucleic acid (mRNA) can be detected	Finer elastic fibers that are structurally immature	Finer elastic fiber networks; fibers are still structurally immature	Elastic fiber networks increase in size with postnatal age; fibers become structurally mature

From Holbrook, K.A. (1998). Structural and biochemical organogenesis of skin and cutaneous appendages in the fetus and newborn. In R.A. Polin & W.W. Fox (Eds.). *Fetal and neonatal physiology* (2nd ed.). Philadelphia: W.B. Saunders.
*Not statistically different than numbers of cells in embryonic epidermis

TABLE **13-4** Comparison of the Structural Properties of the Skin of the Second-Trimester Fetus, Premature Infant (Third Trimester), Newborn Infant, and Older Child-Adult—cont'd

Characteristic	Fetal (Second Trimester)	Premature (Third Trimester)	Newborn Infant	Child-Adult
Vascular structure	Two planar networks evident; differential wall structure of vessels implies segmentation; some capillary beds established; incomplete and variable	Incomplete and unstable	Incomplete and unstable; capillary loops formed in dermal papillae	Basic pattern is established; maturation of structure still occurs in accord with stabilization of function
Hypodermis	Fine connective tissue framework of lobules and adipocytes	Subcutaneous fat lobules	Subcutaneous fat layer; depends on nutritional status	Subcutaneous fat layer

characteristics of the skin in the fetus, preterm infant, term infant and adult.

The skin consists of three layers: epidermis, dermis, and subcutaneous layer (Figure 13-1). The epidermis consists of two parts: the outer stratum corneum and the living basal layer adjacent to the epidermal-dermal junction. The basal layer is subdivided into four strata containing melanocytes (pigment-producing cells) and keratinocytes. Keratinocytes, the major cell of the epidermis, develop from stem cells in the basal layer and migrate outward to cornify the outer layer.[24,75] The stratum corneum is the barrier layer and consists of keratinocytes linked by lipids. Underneath the epidermis lies the dermis, which is 2 to 4 mm thick at birth.[75] Fibrous protein, collagen, and elastin fibers are woven together to form this layer.[19] The dermis contains the nerves and blood vessels that nourish the skin cells and carry sensations from the skin to the brain (see Figure 13-1). Mechanical properties of the dermis include tensile strength, compressibility, resilience, and elasticity.[52] The subcutaneous layer is composed of fatty connective tissue that provides insulation and caloric storage.[69] The epidermis and dermis, along with their vascular and neural networks, develop concurrently. Major events in development of the skin and its appendages are summarized in Table 13-5.

Epidermis

Development of the epidermis "is characterized by coordinated establishment of increasing numbers of cell layers concomitant with expansion of skin surface area and cellular (keratinocyte) differentiation."[52] The epidermis initially consists of a single layer of cuboidal cells that develop from the outer germinal stratum (surface ectoderm) and can be identified during the third week of gestation (Figure 13-2, A). By 30 to 40 days, two layers are seen: the inner basal layer and the outer periderm (Figure 13-2, B).[19,24,75] The definitive epidermis develops from the basal layer.

The periderm is a transient layer that disappears during the second trimester.[24] The periderm serves as the protective barrier for the embryo. Until the underlying layers develop, active transport occurs across the periderm between the amniotic fluid and the embryo. The outer border of the cells has microvillous projections, which are coated with very fine filaments.[23,24] Development of the epidermis is under the influence of epidermal growth factor (EGF).[23,54] Cell surface receptors for EGF are found on both the basal layer and periderm.[52]

By 11 to 12 weeks, the epidermis has three layers (Figure 13-2, D): the basal layer, an intermediate layer, and the superficial periderm. The intermediate layer becomes more complex by the end of the fourth month, when the epidermis has stratified. The epidermal strata are the stratum germinativum (or stratum basale); the stratum spinosum, which is made up of large polyhedral cells connected by tonofibrils; the stratum granulosum, which contains small keratohyalin granules; and the stratum corneum, which is made up of dead cells packed full of keratin.[79,99] Peridermal cells are replaced continuously until regression begins around 18 weeks. Shedding of peridermal cells begins in the scalp, plantar surfaces, and face, areas where keratinization first begins.[13] The periderm gradually undergoes apoptosis as the stratum corneum develops. The epidermis is keratinized by the end of the second trimester.[12,24,52]

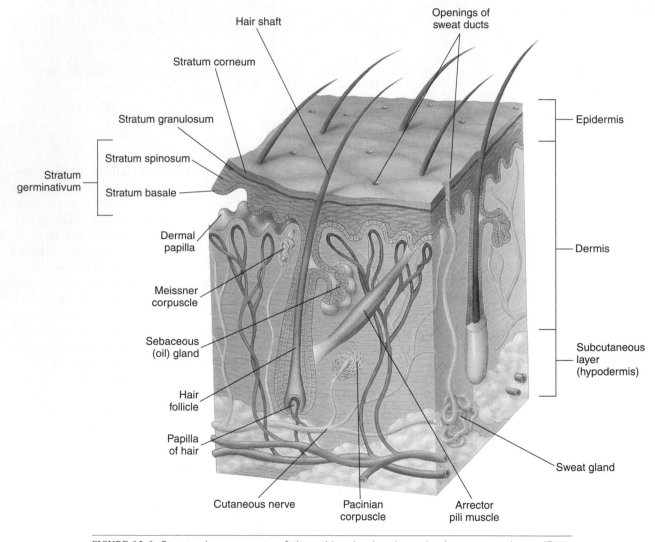

FIGURE **13-1** Structural components of the epidermis, dermis, and subcutaneous tissue. (From Thibodeau, G.A. & Patton, K.T. [1999]. *Anatomy and physiology* [4th ed.]. St. Louis: Mosby.)

TABLE **13-5**   **Embryonic and Fetal Development of Skin**

WEEKS OF GESTATION	DEVELOPMENT
3	Epidermis, which develops from surface ectoderm, consists of one layer of cells.
5	Cutaneous nerves are detectable in embryonic dermis.
6-7	Periderm, a thin protective layer of flattened cells, forms.
11	Collagen and elastic fibers develop in the dermis.
	Epidermal ridges (fingerprints) are forming.
	Nails begin to develop at the tips of the digits.
13-16	Scalp hair patterning is determined.
17-20	Melanocytes migrate to the epidermal-dermal junction and begin to produce melanin.
	Skin becomes covered with vernix caseosa and lanugo.
21-25	Skin is wrinkled, translucent, and pink to red because blood in the capillaries is visible.
26-29	Subcutaneous fat begins to be deposited and starts to smooth out the many wrinkles in the skin.
	Eccrine sweat glands are anatomically developed and located over the entire body. Their function is immature.
30-34	Skin is pink and smooth.
	Fingernails reach fingertips.
	Lanugo is shed.
35-38	Fetuses are usually round and plump with subcutaneous fat.
	Skin is white with pinkish hue.
	Toenails reach toe tips.

From Campbell, J.M. & Banta-Wright, S.A. (2000). Neonatal skin disorders: A review of selected dematologic abnormalities. *J Perinat Neonatal Nurs*, *14*(1), 66.

As stem cells in the stratum germinativum proliferate, they develop down growths (epidermal ridges) that extend into the dermis. Ridge pattern (future fingerprints) is genetically determined, although modified by the intrauterine fluid environment, and can be seen on the surface of the hands and soles of the feet.[78] These ridges are seen between 11 and 17 weeks in the hands and between 12 and 18 weeks in the feet.[12] Chromosomal abnormalities such as Down syndrome modify the ridge pattern.

Protoplasmic fibers and cellular bridges begin to form during this time. These make up the stratum spinosum, eventually protecting the neonate from dehydration and reducing permeability to noxious substances.[54] From 11 to 18 weeks, this layer has an abundance of glycogen to provide energy for growth.[12,19] Glycogen reserves decrease around 18 weeks.[23] Keratogenic structures are now evident, leading to regional differences in epidermal thickness. By 24 weeks, the skin has largely concluded its period of histogenesis and moves into a time of structural and functional maturation.[52]

Keratins are produced in the stratum germinativum by 2 months and increase rapidly as the epidermis stratifies. Keratinocytes are arranged in columnar fashion adjacent to the dermis.[52] Keratinocyte maturation is stimulated by several different growth factors, including EGF, transforming growth factor, insulin-like growth factors, and fi-broblast growth factor.[12] The first signs of keratinization are seen by 22 to 24 weeks.[13,52] The stratum corneum becomes thicker and more organized with increasing gestation, but it is not well defined until around 24 weeks' gestational age.[13]

As replacement keratinocytes mature, they rise and move through the stratum granulosum and acquire keratohyalin granules. As they continue to travel upward, the keratinocytes lose 85% of their water content and their organelles, which are replaced by keratin.[12,31,52] As the keratinocytes dehydrate and flatten, they adhere to each other to form a tough, resilient, and relatively impermeab[le] membrane—the stratum corneum.[86] Transit time for a ke[r]atinocyte from the basal layer to the uppermost strat[um] takes approximately 28 days.[78] By 5 months the perider[m] completely shed, mixing with secretions from the se[ba]ceous glands to form the vernix caseosa.[99]

During embryonic development, melanocytes [and] Langerhans cells migrate into the epidermis. Early i[n the] second trimester, the epidermis is invaded by cells fro[m] neural crest called melanoblast or dendritic melan[ocytes] because of their long processes much like dendrites. [These] cells come to lie adjacent to keratinocytes at the d[ermal-] epidermal junction. By mid-gestation the melan[ocytes] have been converted to melanocytes—with form[ation of] pigmentary granules—and gradually increase [in]

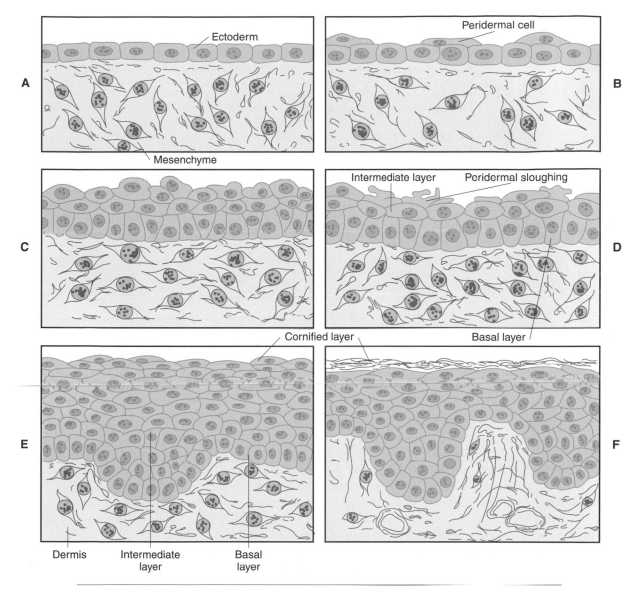

FIGURE **13-2** Stages in the histogenesis of human skin. **A,** At 1 month; **B,** at 2 months; **C,** at 2½ months; **D,** at 4 months; **E,** at 6 months; and **F,** after birth. (From Carlson, B.M. [1999]. *Human embryology & developmental biology* [2nd ed.]. St. Louis: Mosby, as modified from Carlson, B. [1996]. Patten's foundations of embryology [5th ed.]. New York: McGraw-Hill.)

numbers of cells.[52] Melanocytes transport melanin along their dendrites, from which it is taken up by the basal cells.[12,23]

Melanin synthesis begins by the end of the first trimester.[23] Production of melanin remains low in newborns, who have less pigmentation than older children.[23] Melanin is responsible for skin color; variations are due to the amount and color of the melanin. Prenatal pigmentation is seen in the nipples, axillae, and genitalia and around the anus.[19] Racial variations are seen not in the number of melanocytes, but rather in the number of pigmentary granules per cell.[12] Melanin protects deoxyribonucleic acid (DNA) from ultraviolet radiation damage.

Langerhans cells migrate into the epidermis later in the first trimester and increase markedly during the third trimester. Although their function is not entirely known, they do have phagocytic activity and are involved in skin host defense mechanisms.[7,12,23,52]

Dermis

Lying below the epidermis is the metabolically active dermis, which exerts a symbiotic and controlling influence on the epidermis. The dermis is composed of connective tissue, amorphous ground substance, free cells, nerves, blood vessels, and lymphatic vessels. The connective tissue consists of collagen (90%) and elastic and reticular fibers embedded in proteoglycans (ground substance). The fibroblasts are the most numerous cells, producing collagen and mucopolysaccharides. Mast cells, histiocytes, macrophages, lymphocytes, and neutrophils are all present in the dermis (Figure 13-1).

The dermis originates from the somatopleuric mesenchyme and the somites, which migrate ventrally.[6,24,78] Initially the dermis is a loose aggregate of interconnected mesodermal cells that secret a liquid intercellular matrix rich in glycogen and hyaluronic acid.[74] Hyaluronic acid is a protcoglycans that promotes cell migration.[52] The dermis in the eighth-week embryo has undifferentiated cells, appears myxedema-like (as seen in the umbilical cord), and contains no fibrils.[19,24] Eventually three layers form: superficial, papillary, and reticular.[23] The later two layers are present by 4 months' gestation. Between 8 and 12 weeks, the fibroblasts form, leading to differentiation of the connective tissues. During this time, fibrillae appear between dermal cells, which continue to grow, developing a network of collagenous and elastic fibers.[78,99] The fetal dermis contains all of the different types of collagen seen in the adult, although type III collagen is found in greater proportions in the fetus.[52]

With further maturation the dermal layer moves from an organ abundant in water, sugars, and hyaluronidase to one enriched with collagen and sulfated polysaccharides.[19] Neonatal skin is often edematous, a sign of the excess water and sodium contained within it and the continued immaturity of the system. Development of this fibrous matrix continues after birth, becoming thicker and more dense.[5]

Capillaries and lymph vessels form simultaneously. Initially the blood vessels are simple endothelium-lined structures from which new capillaries grow. The subcapillary vascular network is disorganized at birth. During the next 17 weeks the adult structures form and vasomotor tone control is refined. Vasomotor tone is achieved through a complex series of nervous and chemical control mechanisms. These involve the sympathetic nervous system, norepinephrine, acetylcholine, and histamine. Other possible chemical influences include serotonin, vasoactive polypeptides, corticosteroids, and prostaglandins.

The dermal-epidermal junction is critical for skin integrity. This junction begins to develop in the first trimester as the basal lamina, hemidesmosomes, anchoring fibrils, and anchoring filaments develop.[52] This junction is still immature in very-low–birth-weight (VLBW) infants (see Table 13-4). During the third and fourth months, the corium proliferates to form papillary projections that extend into the epidermis. These irregular structures are called the dermal papillae. Some contain capillary loops that nourish the epidermis, and others have sensory nerve endings.

Fat appears in the deeper portion of the dermis, becoming the subcorium (subcutaneous tissue). The major portion of the fat is laid down during the last trimester of pregnancy, to act as a heat insulator, shock absorber, and calorie storage area.[75]

Adipose Tissue

The hypodermis or subcutaneous tissue is a passive tissue that forms from mesenchymal cells. It has a lobar structure that is surrounded by connective tissue and has its own blood supply.[19] The first cells can be seen around 14 weeks; initially they are cytoplasmic and contain no fat droplets. With maturation, single or multiple fat granules develop.[19,78] Most adipose tissue is deposited in the third trimester.

Brown adipose tissue (BAT) is deposited in fetuses after 28 weeks' gestation, accumulating in the neck; underneath the scapulae; and in the axillae, mediastinum, and perirenal tissues. BAT differentiates from the hypodermal primitive cells between 26 and 30 weeks. Development of BAT continues after delivery, increasing by another 150% in the third to fifth week after delivery. BAT allows for nonshivering thermogenesis when the neonate is cold stressed (see Chapter 19).[19]

Cutaneous Innervation

In the third month of gestation, free nerve endings connect with the papillary ridges of the finger and toe pads. By term these nerve endings are exceptionally well developed around the lips, sucking pad, and perioral zone.[19] Specialized nerve endings are less well developed and continue their maturation throughout infancy.

The glands and muscles of the skin are innervated, and some are functional at birth; however, refinement of these responses continues after delivery. The arrector pili muscles, arterioles, and eccrine glands are innervated by the sympathetic nervous system in varying degrees. The sensory nerves may carry parasympathetic fibers to the vessel walls at birth; however, the vasodilatory abilities are reduced until further innervation takes place. The axon reflex (stimulus in one branch of a nerve cell that is transmitted to an effector organ down another branch of the cell) is poorly developed in the full-term infants, so sweating is an unusual occurrence.

Epidermal Appendages

The structures that result from either the downward growth of the epidermis into the dermis or the epidermis itself are the epidermal appendages. These include the eccrine sweat, sebaceous, and apocrine sweat glands; the lanugo and hair; and the nails.

Hair and nails. The hair is an epidermal derivative that develops under dermal induction. Hair is first seen at 12 weeks.[12] Initially the hairs develop from solid epidermal proliferations, cylindrical downward growths of the stratum germinativum into the dermis, where dermal cells condense into dermal papillae (inducer cells). The base of these growths becomes the club-shaped hair bulb. The epithelial cells of the hair bulb form the germinal matrix, which later gives rise to the hair itself. The lower part of the hair bulb becomes rapidly invaginated by the mesoderm, in which vessels and nerve endings develop. This is the pilary complex.[12,78,99]

The central cells of each downgrowth (germinal matrix) form the hair shaft. As the epithelial cells continue to proliferate, the hair shaft is pushed upward toward the epidermal surface. The peripheral cells (epithelial hair sheath) become cuboidal and form the wall of the hair follicle.[99] By the end of the third month, extensive fine hairs have developed. Hair on the eyebrows, upper lip, and chin regions develops first, appearing around 16 weeks.[12] Lanugo is shed before or after delivery and replaced by shorter, coarser hairs (vellus hairs) from new follicles.

Melanoblasts migrate into the hair bulb and differentiate into melanocytes. During the second half of gestation, melanogenesis is active in the fetal hair follicle. Hair patterning and growth is influenced by central nervous system (CNS) development. Infants with neurologic abnormalities may have abnormal hair whorls or alterations in the direction of hair growth or amount of hair. These differences may be related to tension on the epidermis during the period of hair follicle formation.[12]

Nails are the first tissue to keratinize, beginning around 11 weeks, and are completely formed by 5 months. During the remainder of gestation, nails continue to elongate.[23,52]

Sebaceous glands. The sebaceous glands form within the epithelial wall of the hair follicle, usually as a small outbudding of ectodermal cells that penetrate the surrounding mesoderm at the hair follicle neck. The outgrowths branch to form the primordia of the glandular alveoli and ducts. The center cells degenerate to form a fatlike substance (sebum), which is secreted into the hair follicle or directly onto the skin. The sebum mixes with the desquamated peridermal cells to help form the vernix caseosa.[23,99]

Most of the sebaceous glands differentiate at 13 to 15 weeks' gestation, immediately producing sebum in all hairy areas.[23] Each gland usually consists of several lobules filled with disintegrated cells that dump into an excretory duct. The rapid growth during gestation and immediately after birth is due to circulating maternal androgens and, possibly, endogenous steroid production by the fetus.

Arrector pili muscle. Some of the surrounding mesenchymal cells differentiate to form the arrector pili muscle, which is made up of smooth muscle fibers that attach to the connective tissue sheath of the hair follicle and dermal papillary layer. These muscles are located a short distance from the follicular wall in a region where the ground substance is metachromatic. The connection of the muscle root sheath is a secondary event, with innervation occurring later.[99]

Eccrine and apocrine glands. The sweat glands are also appendages of the epidermal layer. There are three types of sweat glands. Only two will be discussed here; little is known about the third type (apoeccrine), which develops in adolescence and is found only in adult axillae. The eccrine glands develop first and are distributed throughout the cutaneous barrier. The apocrine glands develop later and are more specialized. Both are downgrowths of solid cylindrical epidermal tissue that invade the dermal layer.

The eccrine glands appear in the sixth week of embryogenesis and are innervated by the sympathetic nervous system. The epidermal tissue for this gland is more compact than that of the hair primordia, and it does not develop mesenchymal papillae. Once the bud reaches the dermis, it elongates and coils, developing a lumen at around 16 weeks.[78] Eccrine glands retain two layers of cells once the lumen is formed. The inner layer is made up of the lining and gland cells; the outer layer is specialized ectodermal smooth muscle cells that aid in the expulsion of secretions. Eccrine glands are seen on the volar surface of the hand at 3.5 months and in the axillae by 5 months. All eccrine glands are present by 28 weeks, but their function is immature.[23,52]

The apocrine glands are large organs that develop after the eccrine glands. They are confined to the axillae, pubic area, and areolae of the mammary glands. Apocrine glands originate from and empty into the hair follicles, just above the sebaceous glands. At 7 to 8 months' gestation, they start to produce a milky white fluid containing water, lipids, protein, reducing sugars, ferric iron, and ammonia.[78] Decomposition of this fluid by skin bacteria produces a characteristic odor.

Functional Development

The skin is one of the organ systems in the fetus that begins to function before delivery. Intrauterine physiologic functioning of the skin is dependent upon the growth, development, and maturation of the fetus. The fluid environment of the uterus also has an impact on cutaneous functioning. The amniotic environment ensures an even distribution of temperature and protection from trauma and injury, allowing for symmetric development of the fetus, and providing a medium in which the fetus can move. Amniotic fluid composition and exchange is discussed in Chapter 3.

The longer the gestation, the more the skin contributes to the amniotic environment. As the fetus approaches 38 weeks, there is increased sloughing of anucleated cells and keratinized lipid-containing skin flakes. These changes can be used to assess fetal maturity. Increased numbers of lipid-laden cells are an indication of fetal maturation.[19] The periderm provides the embryo with a barrier to the amniotic environment but does not eliminate the exchange of water and electrolytes between the amniotic fluid and the embryo.

Fetal skin permeability is dependent upon morphologic changes and maturation in the epidermis related to sulfhydrylation and keratinization. Permeability therefore does not decrease until the third trimester. Vernix caseosa contributes to this change.[19] The decrease in permeability is also associated with a decrease in skin water content. A fetus at 22 weeks has a skin water content close to 100%, which reduces to 92% in the full-term infant and 77% in adults. This decrease in water is associated with an increase in connective tissue, especially collagen.[19]

Vernix Caseosa

Vernix caseosa forms as a superficial fatty film after 17 to 20 weeks. It is made up of sebaceous gland secretions and desquamated cells of the periderm or stratum corneum cells and is rich in triglycerides, cholesterol, and unsaponified fats. After 36 weeks, the vernix thins and begins to disappear. At term, the heaviest layers are found on the face, ears, shoulders, sacral region, and inguinal folds. The vernix has a tendency to accumulate at sites of dense lanugo growth.

The vernix covers the fetus until birth and provides insulation and protection from amniotic fluid maceration; it also prevents the loss of water and electrolytes from the skin to the amniotic fluid. In addition to providing insulation for the skin during gestation, the vernix also minimizes friction at delivery. It also optimizes stratum corneum hydration and may also play a role in fetal wound healing.[18,50]

NEONATAL PHYSIOLOGY

The physiology of the integumentary system in the neonate includes the barrier properties of the skin, permeability,

transepidermal water loss, heat exchange between the environment and the infant, collagen instability, and the protective mechanisms of the skin. Along with these functions, the skin is the major source of information about the environment for the infant, providing tactile perceptions of the immediate environment. The skin is the most sophisticated sensory organ system in the neonate. The neonate obtains the vast majority of its information about the environment through the skin. Tactile development is discussed in Chapter 14.

Transitional Events

During the birth process the skin is subjected to the mechanical stress of the delivery process, changes in blood circulation, and the bacterial flora of the maternal genital tract.[19] The skin also serves as a diagnostic barometer for systemic phenomena, especially those related to transition. Mechanical stresses include pressure from contractions, which alters blood flow to various regions and results in edema formation. Maternal structures (bony pelvis and musculature) can exert pressure on the presenting part, causing further edema and hematoma formation. Exertion of enough pressure may result in abrasions or cellular ischemia and tissue sloughing, threatening the integrity of the cutaneous barrier.

In addition to natural forces, epidermal breaks can also be caused by obstetric interventions such as internal fetal monitoring and fetal scalp sampling. Use of vacuum extraction and forceps can result in bruising, edema, tissue ischemia, tissue sloughing, subcutaneous fat necrosis, and nerve damage.

In the first hours following delivery, the infant develops an intense red color, which is characteristic of the newborn. This may remain for several hours; however, exposure to the cooler environment usually leads to a bluish mottling, which dissipates quickly upon warming. The preterm infant's skin is thinner, more transparent, and gelatinous, with more lanugo.

Newborns have less pigmentation than older children due to decreased melanin production. The increased pigment in the ear tips, scrotum, linea alba, and areolae are due to maternal and placental hormones.[23] Because of their lack of pigmentation, young infants are more susceptible to damage from ultraviolet light.[18]

Newborn skin is relatively transparent and smooth looking and is soft and velvety to touch. This appearance is due to the lack of large skin folds and skin texture. There is localized edema, especially over the pubis and the dorsa of the hands and the feet. Initially the skin is covered with the greasy yellow-white vernix caseosa. This insulating layer is lost with the bathing that occurs in the nursery. Removal

TABLE 13-6   Normal Neonatal Skin Variations

Condition	Characteristics
Milia	1-mm yellow-white cysts Appear on cheeks, forehead, nose, and nasolabial folds Frequently occur in clusters Affect 40% of all infants
Miliaria	Develops within the first 12 hours Caused by obstructed eccrine sweat ducts Appears on forehead and skin folds Superficial, thin-walled grouped vesicles *(M. crystallina)* or deep, grouped red papules *(M. rubra)*
Erythema toxicum	Most common transient lesion Irregular erythematous macules or patches with yellow or white central papule Can affect any area of body except palms and soles Appears between 24 and 72 hours after birth; continued eruption up to 3 weeks; dissipates in a few days More often affects full-term infants (30%-70%)
Mongolian spots	Macular, gray-blue without sharp borders Most frequently occur in lumbosacral region Cover an area 10 cm or greater Caused by delayed disappearance of dermal melanocytes Affect up to 70%-90% of African-American, Asian, and Native American infants and 5%-13% of Caucasian infants Gradually disappear over first few years of life
Harlequin color change	Transient color change usually appearing in first few days and sometimes up to 3 weeks of age, lasting a few minutes to ½ hour Midline demarcation; dependent side red; upper side pale Caused by temporary autonomic imbalance of cutaneous vasculature Nonsignficant More common in preterm infants
Ecchymoses	Subcutaneous hemorrhage Localized Usually seen over presenting part
Neonatal acne (cephalic pustulosis)	Small red papules and pustules on face Resolve spontaneously within 2 to 4 weeks Rarely associated with comedons or crysts
Café au lait spots	Brown macules or patches Less than 3 cm in diameter Occur occasionally in newborns; more common in African-American infants With six or more spots of greater than 0.5 cm diameter, the infant is at risk for underlying neurofibromatosis
Junctional (melanocytic) nevi	Flat, macular, purpura or plaque-like pigmented lesions Brown to black Less than 1 cm Most develop later in childhood Neonatal risk minimal, with aging, risk for later melanoma, especially with large lesions
Hemangiomas	Relatively common Developmental vascular anomaly Capillary hemangiomas: dilated vessels Cavernous hemangiomas: large, dilated, blood-filled cavities 65% are superficial; 15% are subcutaneous; 20% are mixed
Salmon patch hemangioma ("stork bites")	Occurs in up to 70%-75% of normal newborns Flat macular hemangioma Appears on nape of neck, eyelids, and glabella Indistinct borders Blanches with pressure Facial lesions disappear by 1 year of age; neck stains more permanent

TABLE **13-6**   Normal Neonatal Skin Variations—cont'd

CONDITION	CHARACTERISTICS
Nevus flammeus	Port-wine stain hemangioma
	Sharply delineated
	Blanches only slightly
	Purple to red, or jet black
	Does not involute
	If distributed over trigeminal territory of face, angiomatous malformation of the brain may occur (i.e., Sturge-Weber syndrome)
Strawberry hemangioma	Raised bright red capillary lesion with sharply demarcated borders
	Blanches with pressure
	Rarely seen immediately at birth; 90% manifest in neonatal period
	Increase in size for 4-9 months
	Most resolve spontaneously by early childhood
	Two times more frequent in females
Cavernous hemangioma	Deeper, less common
	Margins obscured by overlying epidermal tissue
	Reddish-blue
	Somewhat compressible
	Increases in size after birth
Cradle cap	Seborrheic eczema
	Reactive response to irritant
	Scaling lesions
	Greasy feeling

results in exposure of the stratum corneum to the much dryer postnatal environment. Desquamation of the upper layers of the stratum corneum results, leaving the skin with a grayish-white or yellowish cast. After the first week, visible desquamation gives way to normal proliferation and flaking, signaling adaptation. This drying out of the skin is part of the natural maturational process. Any interference in this keratinization (e.g., use of lotions or creams) only delays the development of an effective barrier and prolongs the difficulties associated with an immature cutaneous surface, such as increased water loss and thermal instability. Common neonatal skin variations are summarized in Table 13-6.

Once these initial stages are complete the skin takes on the adult protective functions by providing the needed environmental barrier. This development includes the discharge of water and electrolytes, an acid mantle, resorptive capacities, generalized pigmentation, and regulation of blood circulation and nerve supply.[19]

Barrier Properties

The skin acts as a barrier to limit transepidermal water loss (TEWL), prevent absorption of drugs and other chemicals, and protect from invasion by pathogens.[13] The barrier properties of the skin are located almost entirely in the stratum corneum. A component of barrier maturation is the thickness of the epidermal layer.

Epidermal thickness does not increase significantly until 24 weeks. From that point until term, there is progressive thickening, which is seen in dermoepidermal undulations.[31] In the full-term neonate the epidermis has marked regional variations in thickness, color, permeability, and surface chemical composition. As skin matures, the thickness of the stratum corneum increases. In the full-term infant this is a relatively well-developed barrier that may be 10 to 20 layers thick, as in the adult. However, in the preterm infant (especially those younger than 30 gestational weeks) the barrier is immature and may be only two to three layers thick. In infants younger than 24 gestational weeks, the stratum corneum may be nonexistent.[68,69]

For both the full-term and preterm infant, consequences of barrier immaturity include increased permeability and increased TEWL. Each of these properties is a function of gestational and postnatal age. The thinness of the barrier layer leaves the preterm neonate with an increased transepidermal loss, an increased skin permeability to chemical substances and microbes, and a decreased ability to withstand mechanical forces of friction.[96,97] Rapid barrier maturation occurs over the first 10 to 14 days after birth in the term infant and 2 to 4 weeks in the preterm infant. Barrier maturation may take up to 8 weeks in the infant born at 25 to 27 weeks' gestational age, or until the infant reaches a postconceptional age of 30 to 32 weeks.[57] Barrier maturation is mediated by exposure to the extrauterine environment. For example, an infant of 32 weeks' gestational age who is 2 weeks old has had striking epidermal development in the first 2 weeks of postnatal life. This infant may be better able to cope with the extrauterine environment at this age than the newly delivered full-term infant.[31,45,78]

Permeability

Skin permeability correlates with gestational age in the first few weeks of life. With decreasing gestational age, there is increasing permeability. Other factors increasing permeability are skin disease and injury.[13] Thus even though the newborn's skin may appear structurally similar to adult skin, it is more permeable to substances applied to the skin (e.g., drugs, chemicals) and more vulnerable to water fluxes. For example, antiseptics such as povidone-iodine, hexachlorophene and isopropyl alcohol applied to an infant's skin are absorbed to a much greater extent than in adults.[13]

Protective Mechanisms

Although there are many immaturities in the cutaneous system, the accelerated maturation (along with the pH of the infant's skin) results in a protective barrier to the environment as long as the skin stays intact. An acid skin surface with a pH lower than 5.0 has bacteriostatic properties.[19,68] The acid mantle is formed from the uppermost layer of the epidermis, sweat, superficial fat, metabolic by-products, and external substances (e.g., amniotic fluid, microorganisms). The acid mantel can be disrupted by bathing, soaps, and topical agents.[68]

Skin pH increases immediately after birth, from the fetal pH of 5.5 to 6 to a mean of 6.34 (range, 6.5 to 7.4), then decreases rapidly over the first week, but remains higher than values seen in adults.[23,127] Within 4 days skin pH drops to a mean of 4.95, then falls more slowly to adult values by 3 to 4 weeks.[18,34] The mechanism for this change remains unclear but may be due to changes in the composition of the surface lipids and the activity of the eccrine glands.[4,19,30] The acid mantle forms more slowly in preterm infants, especially those weighing less than 1000 grams.[34] Fox et al. reported that the skin pH in preterm infants (24 to 34 weeks' gestational age) increased to a mean of 6 on the first day after birth, then fell to 5.4 by 1 week and 5 by 1 month.[34]

Immediately following delivery, microbial colonization also begins. These bacteria grow in a state of equilibrium, providing protection against invading pathogenic organisms.[7] A rise in pH toward neutral (i.e., 7) causes an increase in the total number of bacteria and a change in the species present.[105] Skin colonization after birth is discussed in Chapter 12.

Transepidermal Water Loss

TEWL in term infants is 6 to 8 $g/ml^2/hr$, which is similar to that of a nonsweating adult.[13] TEWL decreases rapidly in term infants but more slowly in preterm infants. Due to the thinner stratum corneum, the higher water content, and the increased permeability, TEWL in the preterm infant is greatly increased, especially in the first 2 to 3 weeks after birth.[13] In infants less than 28 weeks' gestational age, there is a 10- to 15-fold increase in TEWL.[18,42,111] As a result, fluid losses of up to 30% of their total body weight can occur in a 24-hour period.[42] Even by 4 weeks of age, TEWL in immature infants is still twice that of term infants.[111] TEWL in infants older than 34 weeks' gestational age approaches that of term infants.[46] Other factors that increase TEWL in VLBW infants are their larger surface area in relation to body weight and increased blood supply that is closer to the skin surface.

These water losses can have a significant effect on fluid balance and the management and treatment of both preterm and full-term neonates (see Chapter 10). This may be compounded by environmental (e.g., radiant warmers) and therapeutic (e.g., phototherapy) modalities (see Chapters 17 and 19). Caloric needs increases due to the excessive TEWL may account for up to 20% of energy expenditure of infants younger than 30 weeks' gestational age.[18] Excess TEWL increases the risk of dehydration, intraventricular hemorrhage, hyperosmolar hypernatremia, and thermal instability due to evaporative heat loss (see Chapter 19).[18]

The degree of TEWL is dependent upon the hydration of the stratum corneum, the skin surface temperature, ambient humidity, and the neural capability for control of sweating. Factors that may contribute to these losses include basal metabolic rate, body temperature, activity, and phototherapy (see Table 10-15).[48] Term infants show little regional differences in TEWL, except for increased losses from the palms and soles secondary to sweating. TEWL in preterm infants is lowest on the forehead, cheeks, palms, and soles, areas where keratinization occurs early. These infants also do not sweat. TEWL is 50% higher in the abdomen of these infants and higher with warm (rather than cool) skin, increased ambient temperature, radiant heating, or skin damage.[13]

Reduction of TEWL losses can be achieved through the use of a thermal blanket, plastic blanket, plastic hood, or semiocclusive dressings (see Chapter 19). Semipermeable occlusive dressings and waterproof topical agents have been reported to reduce TEWL by 30% to 70%.[85]

Thermal Environment

Heat exchange between infant skin and the environment is dependent on the thermal gradient between the body surface and environment. Studies have found minimal oxygen consumption when the body surface and environmental temperature gradient does not exceed 1.5° C. Use of incubators, radiant warmers, and phototherapy modifies the environment, either reducing or accelerating oxygen consumption. The rate of thermal exchange between infant and environment is dependent upon relative humidity, wind velocity, radiant surfaces, and ambient air temperatures. In neonates, 50% to 75% of heat loss occurs through radiation and is therefore dependent upon both ambient (incubator) and environmental (room) temperature (see Chapter 19).[8]

Phototherapy (see Chapter 17) is an added radiant heat source. Infants receiving phototherapy have demonstrated increases in insensible water loss (IWL), respiratory rate, peripheral blood flow, and heel skin temperature. Absorption of the infrared bands increases kinetic energy, producing a degradation of the radiant energy to heat and leading to the clinical changes noted. The increased IWL is a compensatory mechanism to dissipate heat through hyperpnea and peripheral vasodilation. Careful temperature control can reduce some of these effects.

TEWL and heat loss via the skin are intimately linked (increased environmental temperature increases TEWL). Sweating is an important mechanism for heat regulation when thermal stress occurs and is a source of IWL.[24] However, the ability to sweat in response to thermal or emotional stressors is dependent upon gestational and postnatal age.[45]

Infants of 36 weeks' gestational age or older are able to generate sweat with a thermal stimulus. Term infants demonstrate emotional (palmar or plantar) sweating, although sweating is usually not seen until the third day.[23,45,73,98] The onset of sweating is delayed in preterm infants more than 30 weeks' gestation; sweating is minimal or nonexistent in infants less than 30 weeks' gestation, due to inadequate sweat gland development. In studies of infants less than 36 weeks' gestation, crying had to accompany thermal stimulus to yield sweating, and rectal temperatures had to be higher than in term infants before sweating was induced.[23,45,98]

Sweating appears first on the forehead, and that may be the only place where it does occur. There is a correlation between gestational age and the number of sites where sweating is found during the first week of life.[45,73] After that period, this correlation disappears. The amount of water loss varies with the state of arousal, the site of sweating, and the ambient and body temperatures, with the highest loss occurring from the forehead and then from the chest and the upper arms.[45,73]

Although density of sweat glands is greatest at birth, many glands are inactive; adult function is not achieved until 2 to 3 years of age.[52,73,75] The ability to respond to thermal stress matures between 21 and 33 days in more mature preterm infants and by 5 days in term infants. The actual water loss due to perspiration in the term infant is low, and although the preterm infant has greater losses, most are due not to perspiration but to direct TEWL.

Maturation of the sweat response may be a function of gland development (anatomic and functional) or maturation of the nervous system. In the 28-week fetus the full complement of sweat glands is in place, many having formed lumina. The cholinergic fibers of the sympathetic nervous system are also in place. Chemical maturation, however, has not occurred, contributing to the absence of the sweat response in these infants.[45]

Cohesion between Epidermis and Dermis

Increased fluid losses may occur due to stripping of the corneum stratum through the repeated removal of tape. This problem is due to decreased cohesion between the epidermis and dermis. The epidermis firmly adheres to the underlying dermis in the adult at the dermoepidermal junction. The basal layer is anchored to the basement membrane by hemidesmosomes, anchoring filaments, and fibers that protrude from the undersurface of the basal cells. The undulations encountered in its structure enhance resistance to shearing stress at the junction.[111]

In the preterm infant there is a combination of decreased anchoring structures, higher water content, and widely spaced collagen fiber bundles in the dermis. This structural liability makes the skin integrity fragile and more susceptible to skin trauma from shearing and frictional or adhesive forces.[25,52,68] For the preterm infant, cutaneous injury may occur with very little manipulation. The bond between the epidermis and the adhesive may be stronger than the bond between the infant's epidermis and dermis.[69] Denuded and damaged skin increases TEWL and may be a site of entry for bacterial infection until healing occurs. Extreme care when applying and removing tape or monitoring devices is therefore warranted, especially in the VLBW infant.[18,46,75]

Collagen and Elastin Instability

The connective tissue of the dermis is composed of collagen and elastin fibers embedded in a mucopolysaccharide gel. Collagen makes up more than 90% of the connective tissue, with fibroblasts being the most numerous cells. Like epidermal-dermal cohesion, collagen stability also increases with gestational and postnatal age.[75,79] Collagen maintains the tensile properties of skin, and the elastic fibers allow elastic recoil of the stretched skin. Because the elastin fibers are finer and less mature in the neonate, the skin stretches less and is more susceptible to damage from shearing forces. These liabilities are compounded in preterm infants.

Large amounts of glycosaminoglycans, proteoglycans, and glycoproteins in newborn skin bind large amounts of water. This provides a gel-like composition, which increases the compressibility of the newborn skin and decreases the potential for skin breakdown in the full-term infant.

Lack of connective tissue can result in increased trauma to the cutaneous layers in the VLBW infant. In addition, decreased collagen and elastic fibers may contribute to edema formation in the dermal layer, with concomitant increases in fluid loss due to increased fluid availability. This tendency toward water fixation decreases with gestational age as collagen stability increases. Heat loss may be enhanced, with thermal stability jeopardized, due to the decreased insulative capabilities of the fibrous elements of the dermal layer.[69]

CLINICAL IMPLICATIONS FOR NEONATAL CARE

There are numerous clinical implications for the neonate due to the limitations of the integumentary system. These implications include skin care, absorption of substances through the skin, the use of adhesives, and thermal stability. Thermal stability and evaporative water loss are discussed in Chapter 19.

Skin Care and Bathing

There is little consensus about the frequency of bathing. The first bath is delayed until the infant has stabilized. Standard precautions should be used before and during the first bath. Bathing is generally recommended only two to three times per week[18] Frequent baths are not needed for VLBW infants. Bathing can be a very stressful experience for these infants, with alterations in blood pH, hypoxemia, respiratory distress, increased oxygen consumption, crying, and behavioral stress cues.[18,83,84] Bathing may also alter the infant's skin barrier properties.[18]

Warm water baths are adequate; warm sterile water should be used on delicate or excoriated areas.[113] Soaps are not generally needed in infants because of the low output of their sebaceous glands.[18] Washing infants with alkaline soap destroys the acid mantle by neutralizing the

pH. For the full-term infant it takes 1 hour for the pH to return to baseline; for preterm infants this takes even longer.[19] Due to concerns about increased skin permeability to other solutions, warm water only is recommended for preterm infants younger than 32 weeks' gestation.[18,69]

Mild neutral pH soaps should only be used if needed for highly soiled areas. Because of concerns about human immunodeficiency virus and other pathogens, many institutions use a dilute antiseptic solution for the initial bath for term infants. The efficacy of this procedure is not clear.[69] The solution should be thoroughly rinsed off the infant's skin. Both antiseptic soaps and plain water decrease skin colonization of the infant, but only for about 4 hours, by which time the skin has recolonized.[69] No differences in skin bacterial colonization have been found after bathing with warm water versus mild soap and water.[77]

Creams, emollients, and lotions should not be used routinely. Not only do these substances affect the acid mantle; they may also be absorbed percutaneously.[19] Infants are exposed to many of these products. For example, one study of term newborns showed that an average of eight over-the-counter skin care products were used in the first month after birth.[14] As stated previously, the optimal skin condition for the neonate is dry and flaking, without cracks and fissures. If cracking does occur, a thin application of nonperfumed, preservative-free emollient can be used.

To facilitate rapid epidermal maturation following delivery, manipulation (handling) should be minimized, especially with preterm infants. Routine use of lubricants should be avoided and dry skin care practices instituted. Dry skin care includes the use of cotton sponges and water to remove blood from the face and head as well as meconium from the perineum. The remainder of the skin should be left untouched unless grossly soiled.[2]

Umbilical Cord Care

Cord care practices are often embedded in institutional tradition. Practices range from no care to cleansing with triple dye (brilliant green, gentian violet, and proflavine hemisulfate), providence-iodine, isopropyl alcohol, or antimicrobial ointments. There are little data on the most effective method.[18,63,69,111] Aseptic cord care decreases cord bacterial colonization but delays cord separation. For example, several recent studies comparing alcohol wipes with sterile water or no care found that with use of alcohol wipes the cord took longer to separate, with no umbilical infections in infants in any group.[22,76] The studies found that isopropyl alcohol is least effective. However, aseptic care was associated with decreased maternal concerns about the cord.[129]

Use of Adhesives

The epidermis is pulled off when adhesives are removed and can strip up to 70% to 90% of the stratum corneum in immature infants.[18] In adults it takes 10 adhesive removals to disrupt the skin barrier versus only one removal of plastic tape, pectin barrier, or adhesive tape to do so in the preterm infant.[67] Lund et al. recently compared plastic tape, pectin barrier, and hydrophilic gel use in the first week after birth in infants born at 24 to 40 weeks' gestation. They found that pectin barriers and plastic tape had the highest colorimeter and vaporimeter scores, suggesting greater epidermal injury with these products than with hydrophilic gels. Skin barrier function returned to baseline by 24 hours. Although gel adhesives seemed preferable, they did not adhere as well to the skin as other products and thus required more frequent replacment.[67] Other research suggests that increased TEWL seen with use of pectin barriers and plastic tape may be more due to occlusion and delay of barrier maturations rather than specific barrier injury per se.[124]

Denuded areas are a potential source of infection; they are also uncomfortable and are areas of increased fluid loss. Use of transparent semipermeable occlusive dressings, water-activated gel electrodes, and minimal tape to secure monitoring equipment and intravenous lines may reduce injury. Transparent dressings are impermeable to water and bacteria, while providing protection to abrasions and skin irritations, or can be used for dressings to cover line insertion sites or incision sites from invasive procedures. The advantages of this type of dressing include providing an optimal moist environment for healing, allowing serous exudate to form over the wound, facilitating migration of new cells across the wound area, and preventing cellular dehydration.[18,49]

The use of skin-bonding agents such as benzoin or Mastisol to promote adhesion should be avoided due to the already significant cohesion that occurs with tape.[69] These substances improve tape-epidermis adhesion and potentiate epidermal stripping upon tape removal. In addition, benzoin is absorbed through the skin, allowing acids to be released into the bloodstream. Adhesive removal products should also be avoided in immature infants because of concerns about increased skin permeability.

Protection from Infection

Protection from infection requires that the skin, as the first line of defense against infection, stay intact.[75] Current monitoring modalities require manipulation and attachment of equipment to the infant's epidermal layer. Careful handling can reduce shear damage and epidermal sloughing. Application of noninvasive monitoring equipment needs to be done such that pressure or constriction of blood flow does not occur. Use of heated electrodes can lead to local hyperthermia and erythema. Crater formation may occur in preterm infants with very thin skin. Increasing the frequency of site changes may also reduce skin damage; either use extreme care in removing the adherent ring or use equipment that allows for electrode site changes without moving the ring each time.

Transepidermal Absorption

Percutaneous absorption of substances can occur through two pathways: via the cells of the stratum corneum (the transepidermal route) and via the hair follicle–sebaceous gland complex (the transappendageal route). The major pathway is most likely the transepidermal route, with diffusion of a substance through the stratum corneum and epidermis into the dermis and microcirculation. In addition, the subepidermal circulation is readily accessible, enhancing rapid absorption.

Neonates are at increased risk for toxic reactions from absorption of topically applied substances for the reasons listed in Table 13-7. Along with these differences, skin metabolism is different in neonates, so drugs applied topically may result in the release of metabolites different from those that would occur if the drugs were given by other routes. This increases the risk of toxicity. Occlusion of the skin (e.g., placement against the mattress) permits more complete absorption, with longer contact enhancing absorption of the substance. In preterm infants, percutaneous

---

TABLE **13-7** **Factors Placing Neonates at Risk for Toxic Reactions Secondary to Absorption of Topically Applied Substances**

Increased permeability of the skin
Increased surface area-to-body weight ratio
Lower blood pressure
Variable skin blood flow patterns
Greater proportion of body weight being made up of brain and liver
Incomplete kidney development resulting in changes in drug excretion
Different body compartment ratios
Larger total body water content
Elevated ratio of intracellular to extracellular water
Decreased adipose tissue

From West, D., Worobec, S., & Solomon, L. (1981). Pharmacology and toxicology of infant skin. *J Invest Dermatol, 76,* 147.

absorption occurs even more rapidly and completely as a result of the increased permeability.[61]

The history of neonatal practice demonstrates the problems with the use of topical agents. For example, hexachlorophene was formerly used to prevent coagulase-positive staphylococci colonization; this practice was later found to increase the risk of CNS damage.[61] Eventually the Food and Drug Administration modified the allowable uses of hexachlorophene. Current practices also can lead to detrimental effects if not monitored carefully. Topical application of povidone-iodine yields significantly elevated levels of iodine in blood plasma if not removed completely from the skin after completion of invasive procedures (e.g., chest tube insertion, percutaneous line insertion).[88] Chlorhexidine at 0.5% has been reported to be superior to 10% povidone-iodine in decreasing colonization of peripheral catheters, possibly due to skin residues that prolong the half-life of the latter.[20,39] Gentle cleansing of the skin with water reduces this risk. In addition to risks of epidermal stripping with use of benzoin, this substance contains many different acids, all of which can be absorbed, causing either immediate or delayed reactions.

Isopropyl alcohol is also absorbed through the skin. Alcohol use can result in dry skin, skin irritation, and skin burns. The concentration of the solution, duration of exposure, and condition of the exposed skin determine the effects of alcohol use. Tissue destruction occurs with the de-esterifying of the skin and the disruption of the cell structure. Exposure, pressure, and decreased perfusion can contribute to the development of burns from alcohol, complicating fluid management and providing portals for infection.[47,103]

Limitations in Specific Infant Groups

For specific infant groups there are special conditions and circumstances that make integumentary integrity more difficult to maintain. For these infants, attention to preventive measures and careful monitoring and handling must be incorporated into nursing care activities.

Extremely Immature Infant

The extremely low–birth weight (ELBW) infant has edematous, friable, gelatinous skin that is covered with abundant lanugo. These infants have decreased subcutaneous tissue and increased water content. This is compounded by a greater ratio of surface area to body weight. All of these characteristics create difficulties in fluid balance and temperature control due to the high TEWL.[95] TEWL increases the risk of dehydration, hypothermia, and fluid and electrolyte imbalances. Double-walled incubators, heat shields, plastic or thermal blankets, preservative-free emollients,

and semiocclusive polyurethane dressings reduce TEWL and promote thermal stability (see Chapter 19).[60,81,85,119] Humidity also decreases TEWL. Increasing the ambient humidity to 85% eliminates almost all evaporative losses, although use of very high humidity is often accompanied by concerns of infection from water-borne organisms.

Preservative-free emollients are useful in increasing skin hydration and surface lipid content and reducing infection, as well as in reducing TEWL and promoting thermal stability.[3,18,64,81,115] Other products to prevent or manage barrier compromise in the preterm infant include gel-filled mattresses or pads, transparent semiocclusive dressings, and hydrocolloid dressings.[18,21,49,72,114,115,120]

The premature infant's skin is exceedingly sensitive because skin permeability and collagen instability decrease with gestational age. Cohesion at the dermoepidermal junction is also markedly reduced, which can cause stratum corneum and epidermal stripping with handling and attachment of monitoring devices. Careful handling and policies about skin adhesive practices should be employed. For example, use of adhesives (including hydrogel adhesives) and gauze wraps should be decreased, and when tape must be used, it should be left on for longer periods.[68] The maintenance of skin integrity should be the goal. Denuded areas may benefit from transparent dressings, thereby reducing further damage, providing protection from microbial invasion, and reducing fluid losses.

The stratum corneum is extremely thin; therefore cutaneous permeability is greater, providing little protection against topical substances. Percutaneous absorption occurs more rapidly and completely, placing these infants at greater risk for toxic reactions.[61,75] The use of harsh de-esterifying substances (soaps and alcohol) should be kept to an absolute minimum. The acid mantle is easily disrupted, and cellular destruction is possible. Avoid use of 70% isopropyl alcohol with these infants, since alcohol is more irritating and less effective than povidone-iodine and chlorhexidine.[68] Use of any of these products should be judicious and followed by complete removal with sterile water.

Collagen instability and incomplete dermal structures result in increased cutaneous edema and decreased resiliency. This may result in skin necrosis due to edema pressure within the dermis. The use of waterbeds, gentle handling with little compression force or friction, careful regular turning, and range-of-motion exercises may help to reduce this tendency.[75]

Postmature Infants

There are different categories of postmature infants, and the skin characteristics of these infants are unique, dictating distinctive care practices. For the postmature infant who is also dysmature, weight loss has occurred in utero secondary to placental insufficiency. This results in a loss of subcutaneous tissue, scaling, and parchment-like skin. There may also be a decrease in muscle mass, and bile staining of the skin may have occurred as the result of meconium passage.

Those infants who do not experience placental insufficiency continue to gain weight and may be quite large at the time of delivery. These infants have skin characteristics typical of the term neonate. However, because of their size, the possibility of cutaneous injury during passage through the birth canal or as the result of mechanical intervention (e.g., forceps or vacuum placement) to facilitate delivery is increased. The need to assess skin integrity and protect the infant from infection is high in the postmature infant.

The postmature-dysmature infant has special skin needs due to the loss of the protective covering of vernix caseosa in utero. This is accompanied by a change in skin turgor and consistency. Osmotic damage from the amniotic fluid occurs, leading to the development of abnormal skin folds, shedding of large patches of the stratum corneum, and formation of areas of maceration.[19]

Following delivery the skin shrinks and becomes wrinkled, almost parchment-like. There is general desquamation over the first few days. Cracks and fissures may develop in the joint areas, especially the joints of the fingers, toes, and ankles.

Special care to promote the maturation of the underlying epidermal tissue is warranted. Scrubbing and peeling of the sloughing skin are to be avoided, since damage to the underlying tissue is possible. Routine lubrication should not be used. Emollients may also interfere with the needed maturation of the "new" epidermis, while altering the desired pH of the acid mantle. A nonperfumed cream or a thin layer of antibiotic ointment may be used to moisten fissured skin and reduce discomfort in these areas. Allowing the normal desquamation, which is followed by epidermal and stratum corneum maturation, is recommended.

MATURATIONAL CHANGES DURING INFANCY AND CHILDHOOD

Although the full-term infant's skin is functionally comparable to the adult's, loss of water content, desquamation, and drying of the stratum corneum bring the skin to maturation within the first few days. In the premature infant this may take longer because body water content is higher and the barrier is more immature. The initial edema decreases within the first few days of life, after which the skin lies loosely over the entire body. Transfer from the intrauterine amniotic fluid environment to the external air environment results in accelerated maturation of skin function in the preterm infant. By 30 to 32 weeks' post-conceptional age, the integrity of the skin improves, approaching that of the term infant.[51,57] As the water content decreases, integrity and barrier function also improve.

Collagen stability results in a decreased ability to retain fluid within the dermis. This improves with increasing gestational age and in the early postnatal period. Most of the other components of the dermis are not formed until after birth and may not be mature until 3 years of age. Resiliency is therefore affected; it is low in full-term infants and even lower in premature infants.[105]

Melanin production and pigmentation are low during neonatal life, although high circulating maternal and placental hormones can lead to deep pigmentation of certain areas (i.e., linea alba, areolae, and scrotum). This decrease in production is even greater in the preterm infant. Given that melanin protects the skin from the ultraviolet rays of the sun by absorbing their radiant energy, neonates have an increased sensitivity to sunlight.[79] Sunburn can damage the barrier effectiveness of the skin by causing dehydration and desquamation and can promote the development of skin cancer.[33]

Although the sweat glands are functional within a short time of birth, activating influences are different in the infant than in the adult. For the first 2½ years of life, the sweat glands function irregularly and the total number of glands that are active is small. Emotionally induced eccrine sweating is much less marked in the prepubertal individual than in the adult. The sebaceous glands are also somewhat dormant until puberty.

The sebaceous glands are large and active in utero, contributing to the lipid content of the vernix caseosa. After birth, these glands rapidly decrease in size and remain so until puberty. At puberty, they once again become active structures. The free fatty acids in the gland secretions have a fungistatic effect and provide immunity against scalp infections from these pathogens.

The vasculature also changes over the first few months of life. Initially the cutaneous capillary network is imperfectly developed, and a progression to an orderly mature pattern occurs during infancy.

SUMMARY

The skin plays a major role in the protection of neonates from the atmospheric environment to which they are born. The development of the acid mantle and microbial colonization provide protection against pathogenic organisms. The thickness of the stratum corneum determines the effectiveness of this protection and reduces permeability to the loss of fluids and absorption of topical substances.

TABLE **13-8**   Recommendations for Clinical Practice Related to the Integumentary System in Neonates

GENERAL CONSIDERATIONS FOR SKIN CARE

Develop knowledge of normal development of the neonatal integumentary system (pp. 533-538).

Know the normal integumentary variations encountered in the neonate (pp. 533-535 and Table 13-6).

Monitor skin integrity on a routine basis (pp. 533-535).

Maintain a neutral thermal environment (p. 537).

Evaluate intake, output, and hydration status (pp. 535-537).

Avoid routine lubrication (p. 538).

Implement infrequent bathing using plain water (or neutral soaps if needed for highly soiled areas) (pp. 536, 538).

Counsel parents to use caution in exposing the infant to direct sunlight, especially if the infant is fair skinned (p. 541).

FLUID AND HEAT LOSS

Use thermal or plastic wrap blankets or plastic heat shields or barrier products (pp. 535-536).

Monitor phototherapy equipment use and position (pp. 536-537 and Chapter 17).

Monitor environmental and body temperature regularly (pp. 535-536 and Chapter 19).

Avoid removing vernix (pp. 533-535).

Assess skin for stratum corneum stripping and institute measures to reduce it (pp. 537-538).

Maintain appropriate humidity levels within the nursery (pp. 536-537).

BARRIER MAINTENANCE

Implement minimal tape-use policies (pp. 535-536; 539).

Avoid using adhesive bandages (pp. 535-539).

Remove tape carefully, using warm water to facilitate process (p. 538).

Use semipermeable occlusive dressings and water-activated gel electrodes (p. 539).

Avoid benzoin preparations (pp. 537-539).

Implement dry skin care practices for the first 2 weeks of postnatal life (pp. 538-539).

Avoid the use of gauze pads on premature skin (p. 540).

Implement plain-water bathing of premature infants (pp. 538-539).

Ensure appropriate positioning, avoiding pressure on bony prominences and friction stress points (pp. 540-541).

Use alcohol sparingly (p. 536).

Promote careful handling of preterm infants (pp. 540-541).

Recognize activities that produce friction, shearing, or stress, and implement interventions to reduce them (pp. 537-538).

PERMEABILITY

Avoid routine lubrication (p. 538).

Know the factors that place neonates at risk for toxic responses to topically applied substances (pp. 539-540 and Table 13-7).

Practice conservative treatment of integumentary disruptions (pp. 537-538).

Counsel parents regarding the use of topical emollients and powders (p. 538).

Avoid the use of benzoin (pp. 537-539).

Ensure immediate cleansing of skin prepped with povidone-iodine or chlorhexidine following invasive procedures (pp. 539-540).

Use alcohol sparingly (p. 536).

Gestational age is the major determinant of collagen and elastin stability, the thickness of the stratum corneum barrier, and thermal regulatory abilities. Delivery results in a rapid proliferation of the stratum corneum in the preterm infant in an attempt to compensate for some of the liabilities these infants must cope with. The fragility of the premature infant's skin results in denuded areas due to friction and shearing forces, as well as separation of the epidermis through adhesive stripping.

Understanding the normal developmental processes that the integumentary system undergoes as well as the goal of each of these processes provides the basis for nursing therapeutics. Careful assessment of skin integrity, knowledge of normal neonatal variations, and conservative therapeutics can result in appropriate and timely interventions. The care of the skin can enhance integumentary capabilities and contribute to the infant's ability to assimilate information from the environment.

Clinical implications for nursing practice are summarized in Table 13-8.

REFERENCES

1. Adams, M.D. & Keegan, K.A. (1998). Physiologic changes in normal pregnancy In N. Gleicher (Ed.). *Principles and practice of medical therapy in pregnancy* (3rd ed.). Stamford, CT: Appleton & Lange.

2. *American Academy of Pediatrics.* (1997). *Guidelines for perinatal care* (4th ed.). Elk Grove, IL: American Academy of Pediatrics.

3. Baker, S.F., et al. (1999). Skin care management practices for premature infants. *J Perinatol, 19,* 426.

4. Behrendt, H. & Green, M. (1971). *Patterns of skin pH from birth through adolescence.* Springfield, IL: Charles C. Thomas.

5. Bell, E.F. & Oh, W. 1999). Fluid and electrolyte management. In G.B. Avery, M.A. Fletcher, & M.G. MacDonald (Eds.). *Neonatology: pathophysiology and management of the newborn* (5th ed.). Philadelphia: J.B. Lippincott.

6. Bernum, M.L., et al. (1999). Pelvic malignancies, gestational trophoblastic neoplasia and nonpelvic malignancies. In R.K. Creasy & R. Resnik (Eds.). *Maternal-fetal medicine* (4th ed.). Philadelphia: W.B. Saunders.

7. Black, M.M. (1994). New observations on pemphigoid gestationis. *Dermatology, 189*(suppl 1), 50.

8. Blijham, A.O., Franz, W. & Bohn, E. (1982). Effects of forced convection of heated air on insensible water loss and heat loss in preterm infants in incubators. *J Pediatr, 101,* 108.

9. Borradori, L. & Saurat, J.H. (1994). Specific dermatoses of pregnancy: toward a comprehensive review. *Arch Dermatol, 130,* 778.

10. Brenner, S, & Politi, Y. (1995). Dermatologic diseases and problems of women throughout the life cycle. *Int J Dermatol, 34,* 369.

11. Campbell, J.M. & Banta-Wright, S.A. (2000). Neonatal skin disorders: A review of selected dematologic abnormalities. *J Perinat Neonatal Nurs, 14*(1), 63.

12. Carlson, B.M. (1999). *Human embryology & developmental biology* (2nd ed.). St. Louis: Mosby.

13. Cartlidge, P.H.T. & Rutter, N. (1998). Skin barrier function. In R.A. Polin & W.W. Fox (Eds.). *Fetal and neonatal physiology* (2nd ed.). Philadelphia: W.B. Saunders.

14. Cetta, F., et al. (1991). Newborn chemical exposure from over-the-counter skin care products. *Clin Pediatr, 30,* 286.

15. Chance Turner, M.E. (1999). The skin in pregnancy. In G.N. Burrow & T.P. Duffy (Eds.). *Medical complications during pregnancy* (5th ed.). Philadelphia: W.B. Saunders.

16. Cunningham, F.G, & Whitridge, W.J. (1997). *Williams obstetrics* (20th ed.). Stamford, CT: Appleton & Lange.

17. Daniel, Y., et al. (1995). Pregnancy associated with pemphigus. *Br J Obstet Gynecol, 102,* 667.

18. Darmstadt, G.L., et al. (2000). Neonatal skin care. *Pediatr Clin North Am, 47,* 757.

19. Dietel, K. (1978). Morphological and functional development of the skin. In U. Stave (Ed.). *Perinatal physiology.* New York: Plenum.

20. Dohil, M., et al. (2000). Vascular and pigmented birthmarks. *Pediatr Clin N Am, 4,* 783.

21. Donahue, M.L., et al. (1996). A seimipermeable skin dressing for low birth weight infants. *J Perinatol, 16,* 20.

22. Dore, S., et al. (1998). Alcohol versus natural drying for newborn cord care. *J Obstet Gynecol Neonatal Nurs, 27,* 621.

23. Drolet, B.A. & Esterly, N.B. (2002). The skin. In A.A. Fanaroff & R.J. Martin (Eds.). *Neonatal-perinatal medicine: Diseases of the fetus and infant* (7th ed.). St. Louis: Mosby.

24. Freinkel, R.K. & Woodley, D.T. (2001). *Biology of the skin.* New York: Parthenon.

25. Eichenfield, L.F. & Hardaway, C.A. (1999). Neonatal dermatology. *Curr Opin Pediatr, 11,* 471.

26. Elias, P.M. (1996). The stratum corneum revisited. *J Dermatol, 23,* 756.

27. Elling, S.V. & Powell, F.C. (1997). Physiological changes in the skin during pregnancy. *Clin Dermatol, 15,* 35.

28. Engineer, L., et al. (2000). Pemphigoid gestationis: a review. *Am J. Obstet Gynecol, 2,* 483.

29. Errickson, C.V. & Matus, N.R. (1994). Skin disorders of pregnancy. *Am Fam Physician, 49,* 605.

30. Esterly, N.B. (1998). pH patterns in newborns. In R.A. Polin & W.W. Fox (Eds.). *Fetal and neonatal physiology* (2nd ed.). Philadelphia: W.B. Saunders.

31. Evans, N.J. & Rutter, N. (1986). Development of the epidermis in the newborn. *Biol Neonate, 49,* 74.

32. Fagan, E.A. (1994). Intrahepatic cholestasis of pregnancy. *Br Med J, 309,* 1243.

33. Foucar, E., et al. (1985). A histopathologic evaluation of nevocellular nevi in pregnancy. *Arch Dermatol, 121,* 350.

34. Fox, C.E., et al. (1998). The timing of skin acidification in very low birth weight infants. *J Perinatol, 18,* 272.

35. Franck, L.S., et al. (2000). Effect of less frequent bathing of preterm infants on skin flora and pathogen colonization. *J Obstet Gynecol Neonatal Nurs, 29,* 584.

36. Furhman, L. (2000). Common dermatoses of pregnancy. *J Perinat Neonatal Nurs, 14,* 1.

37. Furhoff, A.K. (1974). Itching in pregnancy. *Acta Med Scand, 196,* 403.

38. Garcia-Gonzalez, E., et al (1999). Immunology of the cutaneous disorders of pregnancy. *Int J Dermatol, 38,* 721.

39. Garland, J.S., et al. (1995). Comparison of 10% povidone-iodine and 0.5% chlorhexidine gluconate for the prevention of peripheral intravenous catheter colonization in neonates: a prospective trial. *Pediatr Infect Dis, 14,* 510.

40. Grimes, P.E. (1995). Melanoma: Etiologic and therapeutic considerations. *Arch Dermatol, 131,* 1453.

41. Grubner, G., et al. (1989). Transepidermal water loss: The signal for recovery of barrier structure and function. *J Lipid Res, 30,* 323.

42. Hammarlund, K. & Sedin, G. (1979). Transepidermal water loss in newborn infants: Relation to gestational age. *Acta Dis Child, 54,* 477.

43. Hanley, K., et al. (1997). Acceleration of barrier ontogenesis in vitro through air exposure. *Pediatr Res, 41,* 293.

44. Hanno, R., et al. (1991). Disorders of pregnancy. In D.J. Demis (Ed.). *Clinical dermatology.* Philadelphia: J.B. Lippincott.

45. Harpin, V.A. & Rutter, N. (1982). Sweating in preterm babies. *J Pediatr, 100,* 614.

46. Harpin, V. & Rutter, N. (1983). Barrier properties of the newborn infant's skin. *J Pediatr, 102,* 419.

47. Harpin, V.A. & Rutter, N. (1982). Percutaneous alcohol absorption and skin necrosis in a premature infant. *Arch Dis Child, 57,* 477.

48. Hey, E. N. & Katz, G. (1969). Evaporative water in the newborn baby. *J Physiol, 200,* 605.

49. Hoath, S.B. & Narendran, V. (2000). Adhesives and emollients in the preterm infant. *Semin Neonatol, 5,* 289.

50. Hoath, S.B. (1997). The stickiness of newborn skin: bioadhesion and the epidermal barrier. *J Pediatr, 131,* 338.

51. Holbrook, K.A. (1982). A histological comparison of infant and adult skin. In H.I. Maibach & E.K. Boisits (Eds.). *Neonatal skin: Structure and function.* New York: Marcel Dekker.

52. Holbrook, K.A. (1998). Structural and biochemical organogenesis of skin and cutaneous appendages in the fetus and newborn. In R.A. Polin & W.W. Fox (Eds.). *Fetal and neonatal physiology* (2nd ed.). Philadelphia: W.B. Saunders.

53. Hsu, C.F., et al. (1999). The effectiveness of single and multiple applications of triple dye on umbilical cord separation time. *Eur J Pediatr, 158,* 144.

54. Hull, J.C. (2000). *Sauer's manual of skin diseases* (8th ed.). Philadelphia: Lippincott, Williams & Wilkins.

55. Johr, R.H. & Schachner, L.A. (1997). Neonatal dermatologic challenges. *Pediatr Rev, 18,* 86.

56. Jones, S.A.V. & Black, M.M. (1999). Pregnancy dermatoses. *J Am Acad Dermatol, 40,* 233.

57. Kalia, Y.N., et al. (1998). Development of skin barrier function in preterm infants. *J Invest Dermatol, 111,* 320.

58. Katz, S.I., et al. (1977). Immunopathologic study of herpes gestationis in mothers and infants. *Arch Derm, 113,* 1069

59. Kenkis, R.E., et al. (1993). Pemphigoid gestationis. *J Eur Acad Dermatol Venereol, 2,* 163.

60. Knauth, A., et al. (1989) A semipermeable polyurethane dressing as an artificial skin in premature neonates. *Pediatrics, 83,* 943.

61. Kopelman, A.E. (1973). Cutaneous absorption of hexachlorophene in low-birth-weight infants. *J Pediatr, 82,* 972.

62. Kroumpouzos, G. & Cohen, L.M. (2001). Dermatoses of pregnancy. *J Am Acad Dermatol, 45,* 1.

63. Lacour, J. (1998). Cord care: results of a survey from South-France and recommendations. *Eur J Pediatr Dermatol, 8,* 233.

64. Lane, A.T. & Drost, S.S. (1993). Effects of repeated application of emollient cream to premature neonates' skin. *Pediatrics, 92,* 415.

65. Lawley, T.J. & Yancy, K.B. (1999). Skin changes and diseases of pregnancy. In I.M. Freedberg, et al. (Eds.). *Fitzpatrick's dermatology in general medicine* (5th ed.), New York: McGraw-Hill.

66. Levin, W.M. (1995). Striae gravidarum: folklore and fact. *Arch Fam Med, 4,* 98.

67. Lund, C.H., et al. (1997) Disruption of barrier function in neonatal skin associated with adhesive removal. *J Pediatr, 131,* 367.

68. Lund, C. (1999). Prevention and management of infant skin breakdown. *Nurs Clin North Am, 34,* 907.

69. Lund, C., et al. (1999). Neonatal skin care: the scientific basis for practice. *J Obstet Gynecol Neonatal Nurs, 28,* 241.

70. Maki, D.G., et al. (1991). Prospective randomized trial of povidone-iodine, alcohol, and chlorhexidine for prevention of infection associated with central venous and arterial catheters. *Lancet, 338,* 339.

71. Malloy, M.B. (1995). Skin care for high-risk neonates. *J Wound Ostomy, Continence Nurs, 22,* 312.

72. Mancini, A.J., et al. (1994). Semipermeable dressings improve epidermal barrier function in premature infants. *Pediatr Res, 36,* 306.

73. Mancini, T.J. & Lane, A.T. (1998). Sweating in the neonate. In R.A. Polin & W.W. Fox (Eds.). *Fetal and neonatal physiology* (2nd ed.). Philadelphia: W.B. Saunders.

74. Margileth, A.M. (1999). Dermatologic conditions. In G.B. Avery, M.A. Fletcher, & M.G. MacDonald (Eds.). *Neonatology: Pathophysiology and management of the newborn* (5th ed.). Philadelphia: J.B. Lippincott.

75. McManus Kuller, J. (1984). Part I: Skin development and function. *Neonat Netw, 3,* 18.

76. Medves, J.M. & O'Brien, B.A. (1997). Cleaning solutions and bacterial colonization in promoting healing and early separation of the umbilical cord in healthy newborns. *Can J Pub Health, 88,* 380.

77. Medves, J.M. & O'Brien, B. (2001). Does bathing newborns remove potentially harmful pathogens from the skin? *Birth, 28,* 161.

78. Moore, K.L. & Persaud, T.V.N. (1998). *The developing human: clinically oriented embryology* (6th ed.). Philadelphia: W.B. Saunders.

79. Moschella, S.L. & Hurley, H.J. (1992). *Dermatology.* Philadelphia: W.B. Saunders

80. Murray, J.C. (1990). Pregnancy and the skin. *Dermatol Clin, 8,* 327

81. Nopper, A.J., et al. (1996). Topical ointment therapy benefits premature infants. *J Pediatr, 128,* 660.

82. Palmer, D.G. & Eads, J. (2000). Intrahepatic cholestasis of pregnancy: a critical review. *J Perinat Neonatal Nurs, 14*(1), 39.

83. Peters, K.L. (1996). Dinosaurs in the bath. *Neonatal Netw, 15*(1), 71.

84. Peters, K.L. (1998). Bathing premature infants: physiological and behavioral consequences. *Am J Crit Care, 7,* 90.

85. Porat, R. & Brodsky, N. (1993). Effect of Tegederm use on outcome of extremely low birth weight (ELBW) infants. *Pediatr Res, 33,* 231A.

86. Powell, F. & Powell, B. (1987). Cutaneous changes during pregnancy. *Ir Med J, 80,* 50.

87. Pribanich, S., et al. (1994). Low-dose tretinoin does not improve striae distensae: a double-blind placebo controlled study. *Cutis, 54,* 121.

88. Pyati, S.P., et al. (1977). Absorption of iodine in the neonate following topical use of povidone iodine. *J Pediatr, 91,* 825.

89. Randall, V.A. (1994). Androgens and hair human growth. *Clin Endocrinol, 40,* 439.

90. Rapini. R.P. (1999). The skin and pregnancy. In R.K. Creasy & R. Resnik (Eds.). *Maternal-fetal medicine* (4th ed.). Philadelphia: W.B. Saunders.

91. Reyes, N. (1997). Intrahepatic cholestasis: a puzzling disorder of pregnancy. *J Gastroenterol Hepatol, 12,* 211.

92. Robbins, C.R. (1988). *Chemical and physical behavior of human hair* (2nd ed.). New York: Springer-Verlag.

93. Rogers, D. (1994). Specific pruritic diseases of pregnancy: a prospective study of 3192 pregnant women. *Acta Dematol, 130,* 734.

94. Ross, M.H., Rumrell, R.J., & Kaye, G.I. (1995). *Histology: a textbook and atlas.* Baltimore: Williams & Wilkins.

95. Rutter, N. & Hull, D. (1979). Water loss from the skin of term and preterm babies. *Arch Dis Child, 54,* 858.

96. Rutter, N. (1996). The immature skin. *Eur J Pediatr, 155*(suppl 2), S18.

97. Rutter, N. (2000). Clinical consequences of an immature barrier. *Semin Neonatol, 5,* 281.

98. Rutter. N. (2000). The dermis. *Semin Neonatol, 5,* 297.

99. Sadler, T.W. (2000). *Langman's medical embryology* (8th ed.). Philadelphia: Lippincott, Williams & Wilkins.

100. Saijo, S. & Tagami, H. (1991). Dry skin of newborn infants: functional analysis of the stratum corneum. *Pediatr Dermatol, 8,* 155.

101. Sanchez, N.P., et al. (1981). Melasma: a clinical, light microscopic, ultrastructual and immunofluorescence study. *J Am Acad Dermatol, 4,* 698.

102. Satoh, S., et al. (1999). The time course of the change in antibody titers in herpes gestationis. *Br J Dermatol, 140,* 119.

103. Schick, J.B. & Milstein, J.M. (1981). Burn hazard of isopropyl alcohol in the neonate. *Pediatrics, 68,* 587.

104. Schiff, B.L. & Kern, A.B. (1963). A study of postpartum alopecia. *Arch Dermatol, 87,* 609.

105. Shalita, A. (1981). *Principles of infant skin care.* Skillman, NJ: Johnson & Johnson Baby Products.

106. Shornick, J.K. (1987). Herpes gestationis. *J Am Acad Dermatol, 17,* 539.

107. Shornick, J.K. (1992). Fetal risk in herpes gestationis. *J Am Acad Dermatol, 26,* 63.

108. Shornick, J.K., et al. (1993) Anti-HLA antibodies in pemphigoid gestationis. *Br J Dermatol, 129,* 257.

109. Shornick, J.K. (1996). Herpes gestationis. In K.A. Arndt et al. (Eds.). *Cutaneous medicine and surgery* (vol. 1). Philadelphia: W.B. Saunders.

110. Shornick, J.K. (1998). Dermatoses of pregnancy. *Semin Cutan Med Surg, 17,* 172.

111. Siegfried, E.C. (1998). Neonatal skin and skin care. *Dermatol Clin, 16,* 437.

112. Soll, R.F. & Edwards, W.H. (2000, January 1). Emollient ointment for preventing infection in preterm infants. *Cochrane Database Sys Rev, 2,* CD001150.

113. Storer, J. & Hawk, R. (1988). Neonatal skin disorders. In L.A. Schachner & R.C. Hansen (Eds.). *Pediatric dermatology* (vol. 1). New York: Churchill Livingstone.

114. Strickland, M.E. (1997). Evaluation of bacterial growth with occlusive dressing use on excoriated skin in the premature infants. *Neonatal Netw, 16,* 29.

115. Taquino, L. T. (2000). Promoting wound healing in the neonatal setting: process versus protocol. *J Perinat Neonatal Nurs, 14,* 104

116. Treadwell, P.A. (1997). Dermatoses in newborns. *Am Fam Physician, 56,* 443.

117. Vaughan-Jones, S.A. & Black, M.M. (1999). Pregnancy dermatoses. *J Am Acad Dermatol, 40,* 233.

118. Vaughan-Jones, S.A., et al. (1999). A prospective study of 200 women with dermatoses of pregnancy: correlating clinical findings for atopic dermatitis. *Br J Dermatol, 131,* 383.

119. Vernon, H.J., et al. (1990). Semipermeable dressing and transepidermal water loss in premature infants. *Pediatrics, 86,* 357.

120. Vohra, S., et al. (1999). Effect of polyethylene occlusive skin wrapping on heat loss in very low birth weight infants at delivery: a randomized trial. *J Pediatr, 3,* 547

121. Walker, N.P.J. (1999). Neonatal dermatology. In J.M. Rennie & N.R.C. Robertson (Eds.). *Textbook of neonatology* (3rd ed.). Edinburgh: Churchill Livingstone.

122. Wallace, M.L. & Smoller, B.R. (1998). Estrogen and progesterone receptors in androgenic alopecia versus alopecia areata. *Am J Dermatopathol, 20,* 160.

123. Weiss, R & Hull, P. (1992). Familial occurrence of pruritic urticarial papules and plaques of pregnancy. *J Am Acad Dermatol, 26,* 715.

124. Williams, M.L. & Feingold, K.R. (1998). Barrier function of neonatal skin. *J Pediatr, 3,* 467.

125. Wong, R.C. & Ellis, C.N. (1989). Physiologic skin changes in pregnancy. *Semin Dermatol, 8,* 7.

126. Yancey, B.K. & Lazarova, Z. (1996). Dermatoses of pregnancy. In K. Arndt, et al. (Eds.). *Cutaneous medicine and surgery.* Philadelphia: W.B. Saunders.

127. Yosipovitch, G., et al. (2000). Skin barrier properties in different body areas in neonates. *Pediatrics, 106,* 105.

128. Young, G.L. & Jewell, D. (2000). Creams for preventing stretch marks in pregnancy. *Cochrane Database Syst Rev, 2,* CD000066.

129. Zupan, J. & Garner, P. (2000). Topical umbilical cord care at birth. *Cochrane Database Sys Rev, 2,* CD001047.

Neuromuscular and Sensory Systems

The neuromuscular and sensory systems are two of the most complex systems in the human body. Normal function of the central nervous system (CNS) is critical for functioning of individual organs and integration of organ systems to achieve coordinated physiologic and neurobehavioral processes. Alterations in neuromuscular and sensory processes during pregnancy give rise to common experiences such as musculoskeletal discomforts, sleep disturbances, and alterations in sensation. Discomforts and pain during the antepartum, intrapartum, and postpartum periods influence maternal adaptations and the course of labor. Newborn and particularly preterm infants must respond to the extrauterine environment with neuromuscular and sensory systems that are still immature. Neurologic dysfunction during the neonatal period due to insults before, during, or after birth can affect the infant's ability to survive the perinatal and neonatal periods and has implications for later developmental and cognitive outcome. This chapter first examines physiologic adaptations in the mother and implications for healthy pregnant women and those with chronic health problems, and then discusses neurodevelopmental processes and clinical implications for the fetus and newborn.

MATERNAL PHYSIOLOGIC ADAPTATIONS

During pregnancy the neurologic and sensory systems are influenced by the altered hormonal milieu and by alterations in other systems. The effects of these changes on the sensory system are well documented. Many of the hormones of pregnancy have CNS activity, although their specific effects on neurologic function are not as well understood as their effects on other body systems. As a result, there is little known about specific changes in the function of the neurologic system, other than effects on endocrine glands (see Chapters 2, 5, and 18), during pregnancy. During the intrapartum period, maternal physiologic and psychologic responses are altered by the discomfort and pain of labor. These responses can have a significant impact on fetus homeostasis in addition to having important implications for management of the woman in labor.

Antepartum Period

This section examines specific alterations during pregnancy in ocular and otolaryngeal function, sleep, and the musculoskeletal system.

Ocular Changes

The eyes of the pregnant woman undergo several alterations during pregnancy that result from physiologic and hormonal adaptations. The pregnant woman develops a mild corneal edema, particularly during the third trimester. The cornea becomes slightly thicker, which (along with the fluid retention) changes its topography and may slightly alter the refractory power of the eye. Corneal hyposensitivity also develops during this period, probably because of the increased thickness and fluid retention.[142,205,226] A few women experience an increase in corneal epithelia pigmentation (known as *Krukenberg spindles*), possibly secondary to increases in estrogens, progesterone, adrenocorticotropic hormone (ACTH), and melanocyte-stimulating hormone.[226] The composition of tears changes slightly with an increase in secretion of lysozyme.[142]

Most studies report that intraocular pressure falls, especially during the second half of gestation after 28 weeks, although variations are seen between women in the degree of change.[74,173,174,175] This change is believed to be due to the effects of progesterone, relaxin, and human chorionic gonadotropin combined with an increase in aqueous outflow and decreased episcleral pressure.[205,226] Similar findings have been reported for women on oral contraceptives. The decrease in intraocular pressure is greater in multiparas than primiparas.[175] Changes in intraocular pressure are independent of changes in systemic blood pressure.[74] An increase in intraocular pressure has been reported in women with preeclampsia. This increase is not correlated with blood pressure, but may be due to increased extracellular fluid volume and decreased aqueous humor outflow in the preeclamptic woman.[74]

Ptosis occasionally develops for unknown reasons.[142,205] Ptosis may also occur as a complication of lumbar anesthesia, either as an isolated finding or as part of Horner syndrome. Horner syndrome is characterized by ptosis, miosis, and anhidrosis secondary to interruption of sympathetic innervation.[205,226] Some women experience an increased pigmentation of the face and eyelids known as *chloasma* (see Chapter 13).

During pregnancy there is a progressive decrease in blood flow to the conjunctiva, which is sensitive to estrogen.[216] This change is most marked in women with preeclampsia as a result of spasm and ischemia.[15] In these women, changes in the conjunctival vessels may occur earlier than in the retinal vessels.[226] Subconjunctival hemorrhages may occur spontaneously during pregnancy or in labor, with spontaneous resolution.

Otolaryngeal Changes

Changes in the ear, nose, and larynx are related to modifications in fluid dynamics and vascular permeability, increased protein synthesis, vasomotor alterations of the autonomic nervous system, and increased vascularity, along with hormonal (especially estrogen) influences.[55,121,185] As a result of these alterations, the nasal mucosa becomes congested and hyperemic. The pregnant woman experiences nasal stuffiness and obstruction associated with serous rhinorrhea or postnasal discharge.

Rhinitis is seen in up to 30% of all pregnant women and approximately two thirds of those who smoke.[55,56] These symptoms may appear anytime but usually begin in the second trimester and parallel increasing estrogen levels.[55,56,90,169,210] The symptoms may interfere with sleep and the sense of smell. Vascular congestion may result in epistaxis from rupture of superficial blood vessels. Chlorpheniramine is usually the antihistamine of choice in pregnancy.[185] Pseudoephedrine has been used frequently in the past, but recently has been reported to increase the risk of gastroschisis (from 1 to 2 to 2 to 6 per 10,000 births).[185,209] Thus women may want to defer use of this drug until after the first trimester. Prolonged use of topical sympathomimetic nasal sprays should be avoided because they can cause rebound congestion.[121,169,210]

The pregnant woman may also complain of ear stuffiness or blocked ears unrelieved by swallowing. This change is believed to result from estrogen-induced changes in mucous membranes of the eustachian tube, edema of the nasopharynx, and alterations in fluid dynamics and pressures of the middle ear.[121,169,210,229] There may be a transient, mild hearing loss, and an increased risk of serous effu-

sion. Management is usually supportive. Increased estrogen and progesterone leads to transient vertigo in some women.[210,229] Meniere's disease may be exacerbated during pregnancy because of fluid retention.[210]

Laryngeal changes during pregnancy are hormonally induced and include erythema and edema of the vocal cords accompanied by vascular dilation and small submucosal hemorrhages.[169,210] The woman may note hoarseness, deepening, or cracking of the voice; persistent cough; or other vocal changes. Laryngeal changes can complicate administration of endotracheal anesthesia. Similar changes are reported in women premenstrually and with use of progesterone-dominated oral contraceptives.[169]

The airway becomes hyperemic with mucosal edema (which may increase snoring) and sleep disorders.[57] Therefore snoring is more common during pregnancy.[72,132] An increase in hypertension, preeclampsia, and intrauterine growth restriction has been reported in snorers.[72]

Musculoskeletal Changes

Pregnancy is characterized by changes in posture and gait. Relaxin and progesterone affect the cartilage and connective tissue of the sacroiliac joints and the symphysis pubis. This, along with external rotation of the femurs, increases the mobility of these joints and leads to the characteristic "waddle" gait seen in many pregnant women.[69,107,233] Widening and increased mobility of the sacroiliac synchondroses and symphysis pubis begins by 10 to 12 weeks.[96] The symphysis pubis may widen up to 10 mm.[107]

Musculoskeletal changes during pregnancy may also be due to changes in gait to compensate for the increase in and redistribution of body mass.[69] The altered gait in pregnancy may increase the load on the lateral side of the foot and hindfoot, leading to lower limb pain.[152] Estrogen and progesterone receptors on fibroblasts in the blood vessels wall of the anterior cruciate ligaments increase during pregnancy, with decreased collagen synthesis and increased relaxin.[131,188] The risk of ligament injury is increased during pregnancy.[130,131,107,233] Muscle cramps are more frequent in pregnant women, especially during the second half of pregnancy and at night (see Chapter 16).[107]

Distention of the abdomen with growth of the infant tilts the pelvis forward, shifting the center of gravity. The woman compensates by developing an increased curvature (lordosis) of the spine that may strain muscles and ligaments of the back. Stretching and decreased tone of the abdominal muscles also contribute to the lordosis. Diastasis of the rectus abdominis muscles in the third trimester may persist after delivery. Breast tenderness, heaviness, tingling, and occasionally pain occur by 6 weeks. These changes are due to estrogens, progesterone, human placental lactogen (hPL), increased blood volume, and venous stasis.

Sleep

Sleep patterns are altered during pregnancy and the postpartum period. Sleep quality and insomnia worsen in the first and third trimester but tend to normalize in the second trimester (Table 14-1).[31,53,99,125,181] Both hormonal and mechanical factors alter the pregnant woman's sleep-wake patterns (Figure 14-1).[134,181,188] Sleep is divided into rapid eye movement (REM) and non–rapid eye movement (NREM) sleep, which is subdivided into four stages. Hormonal changes

TABLE 14-1   Changes in Sleep Parameters during Pregnancy

TRIMESTER	SUBJECTIVE (SURVEYS AND SLEEP LOGS)	OBJECTIVE (POLYSOMNOGRAPHY)
First	Increased total sleep time due to naps[187,203] Increased daytime sleepiness[187,203] Increased nocturnal insomnia[187,203] Increased total sleep time[125]	Increased total sleep time[125] Decreased stage 3 and 4 NREM sleep[125]
Second	Normalization of total sleep time[203] Increased awakening[187]	Normal total sleep time[125] Decreased stage 3 and 4 NREM sleep[125] Decreased REM sleep[125]
Third	Increased total sleep time[187,203] Increased insomnia[187,203] Increased nocturnal awakening[113] Increased daytime sleepiness[187,203]	Decreased total sleep time[53,125] Increased waking after sleep onset[31,99] Increased stage 1 NREM sleep[99] Decreased stage 3 and 4 NREM sleep[113,125] Decreased REM sleep[31,53,99,125]

Adapted from Santiago, J.R., et al. (2001). Sleep and sleep disorders in pregnancy. *Ann Intern Med, 134*, 399.
NREM, Non–rapid eye movement; *REM,* rapid eye movement.

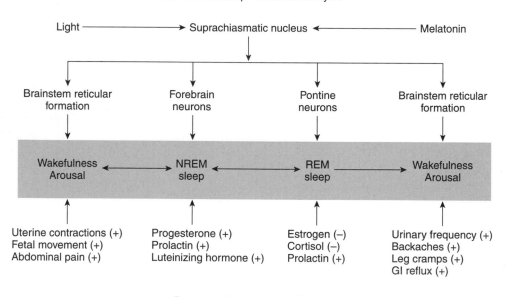

FIGURE 14-1 Central nervous system (CNS) structures involved in the sleep-wakefulness cycle and pregnancy influences on this cycle. The biological clock (suprachiasmatic nucleus), influenced by light and melatonin, interacts with neurons to generate a circadian timing for wakefulness and arousal and for rapid eye movement (REM) and non-REM (NREM) sleep. Bidirectional changes in physiologic states can occur, except in the REM and wakefulness stages. Physiologic and hormonal events in pregnancy promote (+) or reduce (−) time spent in each state through as yet unclear neural mechanisms. (From Santiago, J.R., et al. [2001]. Sleep and sleep disorders in pregnancy. *Ann Intern Med, 134*, 397.)

in pregnancy alter both REM and NREM sleep during pregnancy. Progesterone has a sedative effect and increases NREM sleep.[181] Estrogens and cortisol decrease REM, while prolactin increases both REM and NREM sleep.[181]

During the first trimester, total sleep time increases, as does napping. By the second half of gestation, pregnant women have less overall sleep time and more night awakenings than nonpregnant women do. The pregnant woman has decreased REM sleep in the third trimester along with increased awakenings, and napping and diminished alertness during the day.[31,53,99,125,181] Alterations in NREM sleep with an increase in stage 1 (sleep latency or transition between wakefulness and sleep) and a decrease in stages 2 and 4 (delta sleep or deep sleep stage) during late pregnancy have also been noted.[113,125,186] The decrease in stage 4 NREM sleep has implications for the pregnant woman's functioning, since this stage is important for basic biologic processes such as tissue repair and recovery from fatigue.[128] Sleep alterations during pregnancy are summarized in Table 14-1.

During pregnancy, night awakenings are often associated with nocturia, dyspnea, heartburn, uterine activity, nasal congestion, muscle aches, stress, and anxiety and can lead to sleep disturbances and insomnia. The major reasons given by women for sleep alterations include urinary frequency, backache, and fetal activity.[124,203] Interventions include establishing regular sleep-wake habit and periods, avoiding caffeine, relaxation techniques, massage, heat and support for lower back pain, modifying the sleep environment, and limiting fluids in the evening.[21,181] Sleep medications should be avoided because these drugs alter the physiologic mechanisms of sleep by suppressing REM and NREM stages 3 and 4 and may cross the placenta to the fetus. A pregnancy-associated sleep disorder has been described by the American Sleep Disorders Association.[13]

Intrapartum Period
Pain and Discomfort during Labor

The woman in labor experiences two types of pain: visceral and somatic. Visceral pain is related to contraction of the uterus and dilation and stretching of the cervix. Uterine pain during the first stage of labor results from ischemia caused by constriction and contraction of the arteries supplying the myometrium. Somatic pain is caused by pressure of the presenting part on the birth canal, vulva, and perineum. Visceral pain is experienced primarily during the first stage of labor; somatic pain is experienced during transition and the second stage.

Pain from uterine contractions and dilation of the cervix during the first stage of labor is transmitted by afferent fibers to the sympathetic chain of the posterior spinal cord at T10 to T12, and L1. In early labor, pain is transmitted primarily

to T11 to T12 (Figure 14-2 and Figure 14-3).[65,179,204] As activation of peripheral small A-delta and C afferent nerve fibers of these nerve terminals (by kinin-like substances released from the uterine and cervical tissues) intensifies, transmission spreads to T10 and L1. Pain during the first stage may be referred; that is, the nerve impulses from the uterus and cervix stimulate spinal cord neurons, innervating both the uterus and the abdominal wall. As a result, the woman experiences pain over the abdominal wall between the umbilicus and symphysis pubis, around the iliac crests to the gluteal area, radiating down the thighs, and in the lumbar and sacral regions.[194,204] During transition and the second stage, pain impulses from distention of the birth canal, vulva, and perineum by the presenting part are transmitted by the pudendal nerves through posterior roots of the parasympathetic chain at S2, S3, and S4.

As the A-delta and C nerve fibers enter the dorsal horn of the spinal cord, they synapse and ascend to the brain stem by the spinothalamic tract (see Figure 14-3). The pain impulses entering the brain stimulate a variety of neurons, including cortical neurons and those of the brain stem reticular formation (integrative function), thalamus, hypothalamus, and limbic system.[179] The result is a conscious sensation of pain as well as a variety of ventilatory, circulatory, and metabolic responses.[3,204] Spatial and temporal summation is processed in the cortex.[133,179] These responses include increases in ventilation,

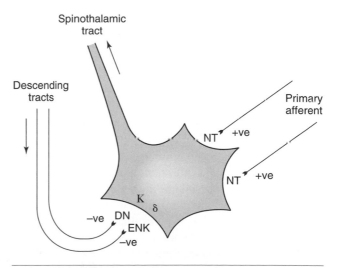

FIGURE 14-2 Pain pathways in the dorsal horn of the spinal cord. The dorsal horn receives excitatory impulses from primary nociceptive afferents mediated by the release of neurotransmitters (NTs) from the afferent terminal. Before the pain impulse ascends in the spinothalamic tract, it is modulated by inhibitory input from descending neural pathways, mediated by endogenous opioids, which bind to receptors on the dorsal horn cell. *DN*, Dynophin, *ENK*, enkephalin. (From Rowlands, S. & Permezel, M. [1998]. Physiology of pain in labour. *Baillieres Clin Obstet Gynaecol, 12*, 350.)

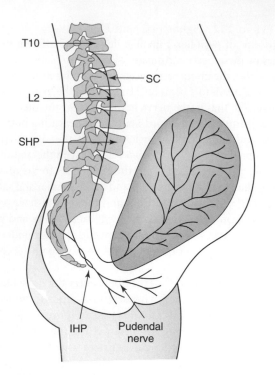

FIGURE **14-3** Neural pathways. The uterus, including the lower uterine segment and the cervix, is supplied by nociceptive afferents that pass to the spinal cord accompanying sympathetic nerves in the inferior hypogastric plexus (HP), the superior hypogastric plexus (SHP), and the hypogastric nerve. They then pass through the lumbar and lower thoracic sympathetic chain (SC) and enter the spinal cord through the posterior nerve roots of T10, T11, T12, and L1. The pudendal nerve supplies structures in the pelvis. (From Rowlands, S. & Permezel, M. [1998]. Physiology of pain in labour. *Baillieres Clin Obstet Gynaecol, 12,* 350.)

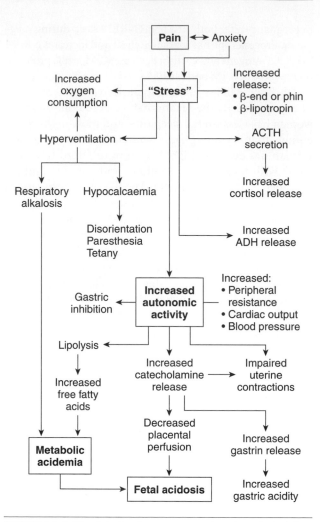

FIGURE **14-4** Physiologic changes secondary to pain in labor. (From Brownridge, P. & Cohen, S. [1988]. Neural blockade for obstetric and gynecologic surgery. In M.J. Cousins & P.O. Bridenbaugh [Eds.]. *Neural blockade* [2nd ed.]. Philadelphia: J.B. Lippincott.)

cardiac output, peripheral resistance, gastric acid secretion, metabolic rate, oxygen consumption, and catecholamine release.

The perception of pain is influenced by physiologic, psychologic, and cultural factors. Pain can lead to anxiety and influence maternal physiologic responses and the course of labor. For example, physical manifestations of anxiety may include muscular tension, hyperventilation, increased sympathetic activity, and norepinephrine release, which can lead to increased cardiac output, blood pressure, metabolic rate, and oxygen consumption, and impaired uterine contractility (Figure 14-4).[109,179] Anxiety can also increase fear and tension, reducing pain tolerance, which further decreases uterine contractility.[109,133] Relaxation techniques such as progressive muscle relaxation, touch, breathing, imagery, and autosuggestion help reduce anxiety and prevent or stop this cycle.[109]

Descending spinal tracts in the dorsal horn (see Figure 14-2) modulate nociception via input from the cortex and limbic system with release of endogenous opioids such as β-endorphins and enkephalin (see next section).[179] These modulating factors are produced by the placenta as well as the mother and may include an opioid enhancing factor.[179] Other modulating factors include analgesia induced by mechanical stimulation of the hypogastric (uterine mechanical stimulation) and pelvic (vaginal distension) nerves.[179] Exogenous modification of labor pain include both pharmacologic (opioids, sedative, analgesics, anesthetics) interventions and nonpharmacologic cognitive, behavioral, and sensory techniques. These techniques include relaxation, cognitive and behavioral childbirth preparation, hypnosis, movement, positioning, vocalizations, touch, massage, music, biofeedback, transcutaneous electrical nerve stimulation, and hydrotherapy.[109,139,179]

The gate control theory postulates that nervous stimuli can be inhibited at the level of the substantia gelatinosa and dorsal horn of the spinal cord from reaching the thalamus and cerebral cortex:

> [T]he theory proposes that a neural mechanism in the dorsal horns of the spinal cord acts like a gate which can increase or decrease the flow of nerve impulses from peripheral fibers to the central nervous system. Somatic input is therefore subjected to the modulating influence of the gate before it evokes pain perception and response. The degree to which the gate increases or decreases sensory transmission is determined by the relative activity in large-diameter (A-beta) and small diameter (A-delta and C) fibers and by descending influences from the brain. When the amount of information that passes through the gate exceeds a critical level, it activates the neural areas responsible for pain experience and response.[139]

Techniques to close the gate (inhibit) include stimulation of large nerve fibers to block impulses from the smaller pain fibers. This provides a basis for use of massage and effleurage during labor. With continued use of these techniques, the large nerve fibers become habituated and stimuli from smaller fibers are no longer blocked. Thus, as labor progresses, the woman needs to stimulate other fibers (using techniques such as heat, pressure with change of position, massage of other areas). Since descending fibers may also inhibit transmission to the brain, concentration techniques may also be useful.[109]

β-Endorphins

Pain during the intrapartum period may be modulated by endogenous opiate peptides such as β-endorphin (B-EP) and enkephalins. These substances are prohormones derived from precursor proteins such as preproopiomelanocortin (POMC) for B-EP and preproenkephalin for enkephalin.[75] POMC, found in the anterior pituitary gland, also contains the sequence for ACTH (see Chapter 18) and melanocyte-stimulating hormone (see Chapter 13). B-EP is also produced by the placenta. Endogenous opioids alter the release of neurotransmitters from afferent nerves and interfere with efferent pathways from the spinal cord to the brain (see Figure 14-2).[65] Thus, within the spinal cord, pain signals may be blocked at the level of the dorsal horns and never be transmitted to the brain. B-EP and other endogenous opioids, in addition to their analgesic role, may also alter mood during pregnancy and have a role in regulation of secretion of pituitary hormones.[75] For example, B-EP appears to modulate release of luteinizing hormones, prolactin, growth hormone, and follicle-stimulating hormone

by the anterior pituitary and arginine vasopressin from the posterior pituitary gland.[75]

Maternal plasma B-EP levels increase during pregnancy, especially from 28 weeks on, and are significantly elevated during late pregnancy and labor in both humans and animals.[34,65,75,228] Increased levels may be related to the increase in corticotropin-releasing hormone (see Chapters 4 and 18).[34] Maximum levels of B-EP are found during parturition and decrease postpartum.[239] Levels correlate with uterine muscle contraction and cervical effacement.[228] B-EP release may be stimulated by stress as an adaptive response. Endorphins may increase the pain threshold, are associated with feelings of euphoria and analgesia, and may enable the woman to tolerate the pain of labor and delivery.

The increased levels of B-EP during labor may contribute to the decreased doses of anesthetic drugs generally required in pregnant women.[65] The variable decrease in doses of local anesthetics for epidural and spinal blocks is also caused by vascular congestion within the spinal canal and progesterone as well as the altered neuronal sensitivity.[65] Increased progesterone levels also contribute to the decreased doses of inhalation anesthetics needed for pregnant women through their effect on the respiratory system.

Postpartum Period

During the postpartum period the ocular and otolaryngeal changes resolve as the physiologic and hormonal adaptations of pregnancy are reversed. Sensitivity of the cornea returns to usual parameters by 6 to 8 weeks postpartum.[142,226] Intraocular pressure returns to prepregnancy levels by 2 to 3 months postpartum, and possibly much earlier.[74] Both ptosis and subconjunctival hemorrhages disappear spontaneously.[142] Nasal congestion, ear stuffiness, and laryngeal changes and related discomforts usually disappear within a few days after delivery.[55,185]

B-EP levels decrease by 24 hours after birth.[61,228] Levels are higher after vaginal versus cesarean birth.[239] Levels of B-EP are twice as high in colostrum as in maternal plasma and may assist the newborn in the transition to extrauterine life and mediate the stressful events of labor and delivery.[239]

Headaches, generally bilateral and frontal, are a common discomfort in the first week after delivery. Postpartum headaches tend to begin around the time of postpartum weight loss and have been attributed to alterations in fluid and electrolyte balance.[198]

Sleep during the Postpartum Period

Sleep is also altered during the immediate postpartum period. Most of these changes normalize by 2 weeks postpartum. Stage 1 NREM sleep is longer immediately after birth than before birth. Stage 4 NREM sleep is also longer immediately after birth than before birth, with a gradual change to prepregnancy levels by about 2 weeks. REM sleep is decreased and awake time increased on the first postpartum night, with a reversal of these findings by 3 days.[113,114] These changes are probably related to the initial euphoria and discomfort after childbirth, followed by fatigue and restoration. Postpartum women have less overall sleep time and more night awakenings than nonpregnant women do. These night awakenings are often associated with urination, discomfort, activity by roommates or nursing staff, and infant feeding. Opportunities for restorative sleep after delivery and during the first postpartum night are often impeded by the environment and interruptions for nursing care activities.[128] The main reason for night wakening postpartum is for infant care.[124] Maternal night wakefulness decreases significantly from weeks 3 to 12.[148] This decrease is related to development of her infant's sleep-wake rhythm. Sleep medications alter sleep physiology and suppress REM sleep and NREM stages 3 and 4 and thus should be avoided.

Postpartum Discomfort

During the first few days to week of the postpartum period, the woman may experience considerable discomfort. The discomfort and pain can arise from a variety of sources, including an episiotomy, lacerations, perineal trauma, incisions, uterine contractions after delivery (afterpains), hemorrhoids, breast engorgement, and nipple tenderness. Breast engorgement initially occurs in both the lactating and nonlactating woman because of stasis and distention of the vascular and lymphatic circulations. In the breastfeeding woman, secondary engorgement occurs because of distention of the breast with milk as lactation is established. Alterations in comfort not only cause physical and emotional stress but can also interfere with the ability of the woman to interact with and care for her infant.

CLINICAL IMPLICATIONS FOR THE PREGNANT WOMAN AND HER FETUS

Changes in the neurologic, sensory, and musculoskeletal systems may result in common alterations and discomforts of pregnancy such as backache and contact lens intolerance. In addition, the physiologic and hormonal changes of pregnancy—along with mechanical forces during pregnancy, labor, and delivery—can lead to specific neurologic disorders in the pregnant woman. These disorders are primarily peripheral neuropathies and compression/entrapment disorders that arise late in gestation or during the intrapartum and postpartum periods. The usual physiologic and hormonal changes of pregnancy can also alter the course of preexisting neurologic disorders such as epilepsy, myasthenia gravis, and migraine headaches. Finally, pregnancy may occasionally be associated with the initial presentation of symp-

toms (brain tumors, arteriovenous malformations, multiple sclerosis) that can affect both the woman and her infant.

Ocular Adaptations

Although ocular alterations during pregnancy generally do not have major clinical significance, they can result in minor discomforts, particularly for women who wear contact lenses. Some women may be unable to tolerate their lenses and may occasionally develop corneal edema. The basis for this intolerance is believed to be retention of water by the cornea, changes in the composition of tears, and alterations in corneal topography.[158,226] Pregnancy may also alter healing following photorefractive keratectomy. Myopic regression and corneal haziness are reported in about 10% after delivery.[97,190] Changes in tear composition can make the contact lenses feel greasy shortly after insertion and cause blurring of vision.[142] Alterations in refractory power along with occasional transient insufficiency of accommodation can cause difficulty in reading and in near vision or blurred vision in someone who is farsighted.[142,205] These alterations resolve in the postpartum period. New prescriptions for glasses or contact lenses should be delayed until several weeks after delivery. Cycloplegic and mydriatic agents used for routine eye examinations should be avoided unless they are needed to evaluate retinal disease. These agents can cross the placenta or have systemic effects in the mother that affect the fetus.[205]

Women with specific disorders such as preeclampsia and diabetes mellitus may have ocular complications associated with their disease process. Preeclampsia is associated with vasospasm of the conjunctival vessels and narrowing of the retinal arterioles. The latter may progress to severe arteriolar spasm; multiple retinal hemorrhages; retinal hemorrhage; and, in severe disease, retinal detachment. Mild to moderate visual disturbances are most common; severe or complete loss of vision is rare.[205]

For many years it was believed that pregnancy significantly influenced the onset and progression of diabetic retinopathy, and pregnancy was discouraged for these women. It now appears that development and progression of retinopathy in both pregnant and nonpregnant women is more closely correlated with the duration of the disorder, severity of the diabetes, and degree of glycemic control. The pregnant diabetic (particularly those with proliferative retinopathy) demonstrates deterioration related to the metabolic and hormonal changes of pregnancy. Although remission usually occurs over the first 6 months postpartum, many women, especially those with preexisting retinopathy, do not experience complete return to their prepregnant status.[205]

Because intraocular pressure falls during pregnancy, the pregnant women with glaucoma may experience an improvement with a decreased need for medications.[205,226] This has an additional advantage of reducing fetal exposure to these agents.[117] Many ocular inflammatory disorders improve during pregnancy, possibly because of increased cortisol and other glucocorticosteroids, with exacerbation postpartum.[226]

Any symptoms of eye infections in the pregnant woman must be assessed, since some sexually transmitted organisms, including herpes simplex virus and chlamydia, may cause concurrent ocular infections. The presence of these organisms can have adverse consequences for the neonate if the mother also has a genital infection. For example, chlamydia can cause conjunctivitis and pneumonia in the newborn. Treatment of maternal ocular disorders during pregnancy should be done cautiously and with attention paid to the possible effects of the medication on the fetus. Even topical eye ointments must be used with caution because they can be absorbed systemically and cross the placenta to the fetus.[205] If these agents must be used, nasolacrimal occlusion after instillation may reduce systemic absorption.[117]

Musculoskeletal Discomforts

The pregnant woman may experience discomfort or pain associated with breast changes or stretching of the round ligament with growth of the uterus, pressure of the uterus nerve roots, or pressure of the presenting part on the perineum. The latter type of pain is most prominent close to the onset of labor and is aggravated by vascular engorgement of these tissues. Increased joint mobility can result in muscle and ligament strain and discomfort. Pregnant women have an increased risk of falls.[96]

Many pregnant women experience backache during pregnancy caused by exaggeration of the lumbar lordotic curve due to shifting of the center of gravity, weight gain, and relaxation of ligaments, or from muscle spasm due to pressure on nerve roots.[62] Backache occurs in up to 70% of women, most commonly after the fifth month of pregnancy, although high backache earlier may result from breast alterations.[50,62,96,107,155] Approximately 10% of these women experience severe back pain, peaking in intensity during the evening and night, and localized to the lower back or sacroiliac region.[62]

An increased frequency of backache is reported in multiparas, in individuals with a history of back pain prior to pregnancy or with a previous pregnancy, and with increasing maternal age.[96,107,156] Backache has not been associated with weight gain in pregnancy, maternal obesity, height, or infant birth weight.[96,107] Women tend to experience less pain if they are physically fit prior to pregnancy and have had education on postural adjustments (e.g., upright posture, tucking the pelvis, rotating shoulders) to reduce back pain.[2,157] Other recommendations include avoiding any-

thing that increases the lordosis (e.g., high-heeled shoes), application of local heat, exercises to increase lower abdominal and back muscle tone beginning early in pregnancy, abdominal pillows, back rubs, use of a firm mattress or bed board, pelvic tilt exercise, aerobic exercise such as swimming, and conditioning before subsequent pregnancies.[2,50,57,107,238] Backache, round ligament pain, or other discomfort should be assessed to distinguish "normal" discomfort from other processes such as preterm labor.

Exacerbation of intervertebral disc disorders is seen during pregnancy and the immediate postpartum period, probably because of postural changes and an increase in mechanical stress.[15,54] The most frequently affected areas are the fifth lumbar and first sacral nerve roots. Management usually involves bed rest.

During the third trimester, the woman may experience numbness and tingling of the arms, fingers, legs, and toes. Paresthesia of the upper extremities may be caused by marked lordosis along with anterior flexion of the neck and slumping of the shoulders, placing traction on the brachial, ulnar, and median nerves. In the legs and toes, paresthesia may be caused by pressure of the uterus on the blood vessels and nerves supplying the lower extremities. Painful legs are experienced by many pregnant women and arise either from the mechanical effects of the uterus or secondary to systemic alterations (Table 14-2).[126] These causes must be

---

TABLE 14-2   **Effects of Pregnancy on the Legs: Factors Increasing the Risk of Painful Legs**

Mechanical effects of the gravid uterus:
  Compression of the inferior vena cava and iliac veins, especially when supine
  Altered gait and posture
Systemic effects of pregnancy:
  Relaxation of cartilage and collagen; reduced pelvic girdle stability; altered gait and posture
  Reduced concentration of serum albumin causing increased colloid osmotic pressure and dependent edema
  Increased concentrations of clotting factors VII, VIII, IX, and X*
  Diminished activity of antithrombin III*
  Alterations in endocrine milieu (e.g., Does estrogen decrease production of tissue plaminogen factor?)*
  Physiologic hyperventilation and hypocapnia
  Alteration in calcium and phosphorus metabolism and diet
Iatrogenic effects of pregnancy:
  Lithotomy position with pressure problems secondary to stirrups
  Operative delivery

From Lee, R.V., McComb, L.E., & Mezzardi, F.C. (1990). Pregnant patients, painful legs: The obstetrician's dilemma. *Obstet Gynecol Surv, 45,* 290.
*Increases risk of thromboembolitic disorders.

differentiated from thromboembolitic disorders, which are also more prevalent during pregnancy (see Chapter 7). Leg cramps during the last few months of gestation are common. These cramps may be related to alterations in calcium and phosphorus metabolism (see Chapter 16) or to pressure of the enlarged uterus on pelvic blood vessels or nerves supplying the lower extremities.

Restless Legs Syndrome

Restless legs syndrome is an idiopathic disorder seen in 10% to 30% of pregnant women and may interfere with sleep.[33,80,143,208] This syndrome is often mistaken for leg cramps, and neuromuscular findings may be similar to those associated with excess caffeine consumption.[50] Restless legs syndrome usually occurs 10 to 20 minutes after the woman gets into bed. It is characterized by a "creeping, wormy, burning ache [that] develops within their legs. The more the urge to allow the legs to fidget is resisted, the greater the urge becomes until it can no longer be withstood."[50] This transient disorder generally appears after 20 weeks and disappears shortly after delivery.[208] The neurologic examination is negative.

The cause of restless legs syndrome is unknown. It may have a genetic basis or be related to the hormonal changes of pregnancy.[232] If the woman is iron deficient, improvement in the symptoms of restless legs syndrome may occur with treatment of the anemia. Women who are supplemented with folic acid have been reported to be less likely to develop this disorder.[50] Restless legs syndrome may also be associated with polyneuropathy and vascular insufficiency. Usually no treatment is indicated, although if the disorder is severe, dopaminergic agents may be used.[35,50,208] Walking may relieve some symptoms.

Chorea Gravidarum

Chorea gravidarum is a disorder involving rapid, brief, nonrhythmical, involuntary, jerky movements of the limbs and nonpatterned facial grimacing.[49,143,151] Mild cases may involve only persistent restlessness and clumsiness.[15] This disorder is seen both in pregnancy (incidence of 1 in 139,000) and in women on oral contraceptives.[15,49,50,80,151] Symptoms are most prominent in primiparas and during early pregnancy, late in the third trimester, and immediately postpartum. Approximately 30% of women with this disorder become asymptomatic by term; the remainder become symptomatic shortly after delivery.[49] About one third of women with this disorder are asymptomatic in the third trimester. The reason for this is unknown. A recurrence rate of 20% has been reported with subsequent pregnancies.[15]

The cause of chorea gravidarum is unknown, although it is related to streptococcal infection and is most common in woman with a history of rheumatic fever or heart disease.[15] This disorder has also been related to hormonal changes during pregnancy or contraceptive use, since estrogen can stimulate postsynaptic dopamine receptors (inhibitory transmitters with effects in the motor cortex and basal ganglia).[50] Chorea gravidarum may have a hematologic or immunologic basis. Changes in these systems during pregnancy may exacerbate a preexisting basal ganglia disturbance.[15] There are no fetal effects reported.

Headache

The most common form of headache in pregnant and breastfeeding women is caused by muscular contraction or tension.[32,92] This type of headache is characterized by a persistent bandlike or viselike pain extending from the base of the neck to the forehead. The woman often notices the headache on awakening, with worsening of symptoms during the evening.[15] The discomfort may be aggravated by postural changes or stress. Headaches during pregnancy may also be due to hormonal influences, especially estrogens, eye strain secondary to ocular changes, nasal congestion, emotional tension, muscle spasm, fatigue, altered cerebral fluid dynamics, or the mild respiratory alkalosis characteristic of pregnancy (see Chapter 9). Because headaches may also be a symptom of disorders such as preeclampsia, however, any pregnant woman complaining of headaches must be carefully evaluated. Management includes massaging neck and shoulder muscles, application of heat or ice to the neck, rest, warm baths, and minimal use of simple analgesics.[32,49,50] Sedatives and hypnotics are not recommended for routine use in pregnant or lactating women since they are ineffective and metabolites cross the placenta and the blood-milk barrier and are slowly excreted by the fetus.[15]

Migraine Headaches

Migraine headaches occur in 3% to 5% of the general population.[32] Migraines are more common in women and often occur with menses, with the initial development of migraine headaches associated with onset of menses.[92] Migraines may also occur for the first time during the first 2 to 3 months postpartum. Although the frequency of headaches decreases with age, migraines may flare up or start with menopause.[49] Headaches are also more frequent and severe in women on oral contraceptives, especially pills with higher estrogen content.[15]

Both classic and common migraines are vascular headaches caused by cerebral vasodilatation and cranial artery dilation. The severe throbbing during the initial phases is attributed to intense cerebral vasoconstriction with subsequent vasodilation.[49,116] Classic migraine is seen most frequently and is characterized by 20 to 30 minutes of sensorimotor prodromal symptoms followed by a severe unilateral headache accompanied by nausea. The prodromal symptoms usually involve visual phenomena but may also include aphasia, hemiplegia, and paresthesia. Common migraine is unilateral less often and not associated with prodromal symptoms.

During pregnancy, approximately 60% to 70% of women with a history of migraine headaches experience complete remission or decreased frequency, particularly during the second and third trimesters.[32,92,192,193] This change is particularly notable in women with a history of menstrual migraine (i.e., migraine associated with estrogen withdrawal). A small number of women will experience their first migraine during pregnancy, usually during the first trimester, and some women may experience a worsening of their migraines, also during the first trimester.[33,49,192,193] Migraines usually return within a few hours or days after delivery or with the first postpregnancy menses.[192]

The basis for remission of migraine headaches during pregnancy is unclear. Although the cause of migraines is unknown, migraines have been attributed to estrogen deficiency, excessive gonadotropins, fluid and salt retention, and increased red blood cell (RBC) mass.[92,116,192] Migraines are associated with periods of estrogen withdrawal such as menses or menopause and pregnancy, which involves changes in estrogen and progesterone levels and patterns of circulating estrogens.[15,92,116,192] Thus migraine remission during pregnancy may be related to changes in estrogen (particularly the sustained estrogen levels), progesterone, and aldosterone, or to hematologic and cardiovascular alterations.

Classic migraine headaches are often treated with ergot alkaloids. Since these compounds have oxytocic properties, they are generally not used during pregnancy because of the risk of preterm labor.[32,92,239] Analgesics and antiemetic suppositories are used for symptomatic relief. Other interventions include avoidance of triggers, biofeedback, analgesics, sedatives, and beta-blockers.[32] Propranolol has been used as a prophylactic treatment for frequent migraines, but its use is controversial since this drug has been associated with altered fetal growth and fetal and neonatal β-adrenergic blockade and subsequent decreased responsiveness to stress during asphyxia.[15,50,192]

The Pregnant Woman with a Chronic Neurologic Disorder

The physiologic and hormonal changes of pregnancy can influence the course of chronic neurologic and neuromuscular disorders such as epilepsy, myasthenia gravis, and multiple sclerosis. These disorders also have ramifications for the health and well-being of the mother and her infant.

Epilepsy is one of the most common neurologic disorders seen in pregnant women. The course of epilepsy is affected by the hormonal and physiologic changes of pregnancy, as well as psychologic stress. Estrogens and progesterone alter seizure thresholds—estrogens by activating seizure foci and progesterone by dampening activity. These responses may account for the exacerbation of seizure activity with menses in many women with severe epilepsy.[50] Increases in estrogens and progesterone during pregnancy may therefore alter the seizure threshold.[170] Seizure activity or susceptibility to seizures may also be affected by water and sodium retention, sleep alterations, and the mild respiratory alkalosis of pregnancy.[170] A major factor affecting the pregnant epileptic is the effect of the usual physiologic changes of pregnancy on the metabolism of anticonvulsant drugs. These changes are summarized in Table 6-7. The goal in managing the pregnant epileptic is to keep the mother free of seizures and to minimize the effects of epilepsy on both the pregnant woman and fetus, including fetal teratogenic effects.[50] Use and risks of antiepileptic drugs are discussed in Chapter 6. The implications of epilepsy and selected other neurologic and neuromuscular disorders during pregnancy are summarized in Table 14-3.

Peripheral Neuropathies

Pregnancy, labor and delivery, and lactation are associated with an increased incidence of a variety of peripheral neuropathies. Most of these disorders, although uncomfortable, do not alter the course of pregnancy, nor are they associated with maternal or fetal and neonatal complications. Other peripheral neuropathies develop secondary to trauma or pressure injury during the intrapartum or postpartum periods. Table 14-4 summarizes these disorders and their implications.

The Woman with a Spinal Cord Injury

Successful pregnancies are not uncommon for women who are paraplegic or quadriplegic. The usual physiologic changes of pregnancy place the woman with a spinal cord transection at increased risk for certain problems, however, including increased urinary incontinence, urinary tract and other infections, constipation, and pressure sores. Most of these problems can be prevented or minimized with good care. Management of the paralyzed pregnant women usually includes careful attention to bladder and skin care, high-bulk diet, adequate fluid intake, prevention of anemia, stool softeners, and acidification of the urine with vitamin C supplements.[15,50,104]

Labor and delivery present unique challenges and risks. Since contraction of the myometrium is relatively independent of neuronal influence (see Chapter 4), uterine

TABLE 14-3   Implications of Selected Neurologic and Neuromuscular Disorders for the Pregnant Woman and her Infant

DISORDER AND BASIS	IMPLICATIONS FOR THE PREGNANT WOMAN	IMPLICATIONS FOR THE FETUS/NEONATE
Epilepsy		
Heterogeneous disorder associated with sudden alterations in brain electrical activity, producing involuntary motor or sensory phenomena One of the most common neurologic disorders seen in pregnant women (incidence of 0.3% to 0.6%).	Effect of pregnancy on the course of epilepsy is variable and unpredictable. Seizure frequency may increase (~42%), decrease (~8%), or stay the same (~50%). Seizures may appear for the first time during pregnancy or reappear after many seizure-free years. Most women return to their prepregnant pattern after delivery. Usual physiologic changes of pregnancy alter the metabolism of anticonvulsant drugs (see Table 6-7) with subtherapeutic plasma concentrations and increased risk of seizures. May need increase in AED dosages (see Chapter 6), especially in during the second half of pregnancy (reverse by 6 weeks postpartum). Higher incidence of stillbirth and possibly preterm labor, but risks of other complications are not necessarily increased. Maternal bleeding may occur secondary to deficiency of vitamin K-dependent clotting factors, and is usually associated with phenytoin or phenobarbital use.	Major risks are from pathophysiologic consequences of maternal seizures and the use of antiepileptic drugs (AEDs). Each AED has potential fetal and neonatal risks (see Chapter 6), such as congenital anomalies, hemorrhagic disease of the newborn, folic acid deficiency, and neonatal addiction and withdrawal. Increased frequency of congenital anomalies in both epileptic women who are on AEDs and those who are not. The risk of anomalies is also increased if the father has epilepsy but the mother does not. Teratogenicity of specific AEDs is described in Chapter 6. Risk of hemorrhagic disease of the newborn is due to a deficiency of vitamin K-dependent clotting factors secondary to competitive inhibition of the formation of precursor molecules by AED (see Chapter 7).
Myasthenia Gravis		
Autoimmune disorder involving an immunoglobulin G (IgG) antibody against acetylcholine receptors on striated muscle. Reduction of available acetylcholine postsynaptic receptors at the neuromuscular junction.	May improve, worsen, stay the same (and effects are variable with each pregnancy). Most often exacerbates in first trimester, improves in second and third trimesters possibly due to effects of blocking of IgG antibodies by immunologic changes of pregnancy (see Chapter 12) or alpha-fetoprotein. Increased frequency of exacerbation in first few months postpartum. No effect on smooth muscle and myometrium, so labor is not prolonged, although the woman may have difficulty with expulsive efforts.	Fetal myasthenia gravis does not occur, possibly due to blocking of the IgG antibody by alpha-fetoprotein About 10% to 12% of neonates (up to 21%) develop transient myasthenia gravis due to passage of maternal IgG antibody against the acetylcholine receptors of striated muscle (see Chapter 12). Symptoms appear within 72 hours of birth and resolve spontaneously in 2 to 6 weeks.

Compiled from references 4, 15, 23, 24, 32, 33, 38, 41, 44, 50, 68, 116, 136, 165, 170, 207, and 236.

TABLE **14-3**   Implications of Selected Neurologic and Neuromuscular Disorders for the Pregnant Woman and her Infant—cont'd

DISORDER AND BASIS	IMPLICATIONS FOR THE PREGNANT WOMAN	IMPLICATIONS FOR THE FETUS/NEONATE
Myasthenia Gravis—cont'd		
Results in muscular weakness and fatigue.	Avoid use of muscle relaxants; magnesium sulfate for preeclampsia (can lead to apnea as hypermagnesemia inhibits release of acetylcholine); inhalation anesthetics and narcotics (because these pregnant women tend to hypoventilate if they have a bulbar muscle weakness); procaine if on pyridostigmine or neostigmine, which inhibit hydrolysis of procaine and can result in seizures (can use lidocaine); extensive regional blocks (may compromise respiration); and azathioprine owing to potential teratogenic effects.	Infants with transient myasthenia gravis often feed poorly, are hypotonic, and are at risk for respiratory difficulty and aspiration. Many infants require anticholinesterase therapy and some will need assisted ventilation. Neonatal effects do not correlate with maternal disease severity or antibody titer.
Myotonic Dystrophy		
Progressive autosomal dominant disorder that appears as a congenital form (possibly requiring an additional maternally transmitted factor) or, more commonly, with onset in young adulthood. Muscular weakness and myotonia affecting both striated and smooth muscle, including the myometrium.	Muscular weakness and myotonia may worsen, often in the second half of pregnancy (possibly due to effects of progesterone on cell membranes). Delayed gut motility with increased constipation in pregnancy. Increased risk of spontaneous and habitual abortion, and preterm labor. Abnormal uterine contractions, prolonged first stage, poor voluntary expulsive efforts in second stage, poor involution with postpartum hemorrhage. Avoid the use of inhalation anesthetics (often hypoventilate with chronic respiratory acidosis) and depolarizing muscle relaxants (succinylcholine) that can cause myotonic spasms and hyperthermia.	Presence of maternal disorder does not affect infant per se. If fetus has inherited myotonic muscular dystrophy, severe fetal and neonatal myotonia may occur. Fetal effects may include poor swallowing with hydramnios and arthrogryposis from inactivity; neonates may have respiratory distress and feeding problems.
Multiple Sclerosis (MS)		
Multifocal central nervous system demyelinating disorder with disseminated inflammatory lesions of cerebral myelin. Onset in early adulthood with unpredictable exacerbations and remissions over many years with increasing disability.	Rate of relapses decreases with each trimester, possibly owing to immunosuppressant effects of alpha-fetoprotein. Twofold to threefold increase in relapses in first 3 to 6 months postpartum. Usually minimal effect on course of pregnancy or incidence of complications. May experience worsening of bowel and bladder problems and urinary tract infection; for paraplegic or quadriplegic, care and risks similar to those for woman with spinal cord transection. Postpartum intravenous immunoglobulin therapy may reduce postpartum exacerbations.	None reported

TABLE **14-4**   Peripheral Neuropathies during Pregnancy and Lactation

DISORDER	DESCRIPTION	IMPLICATION
NEUROPATHIES ASSOCIATED WITH PREGNANCY		
Bell's palsy	Acute unilateral neuropathy of the seventh cranial nerve leading to facial paralysis with weakness of the forehead and lower face	Three times more frequent during pregnancy, possibly because of an inflammatory reaction Most often occurs in the third trimester or first 2 weeks postpartum Onset late in pregnancy usually associated with full recovery (but may take months) and generally requires no treatment if partial or mild.
Transient carpal tunnel syndrome	Entrapment and compression of the medial nerve at the wrist, more prominent in dominant hand	May develop in pregnancy because of excessive fluid retention. Onset usually in second or third trimester. Nocturnal hand pain reported by 20% to 40% of pregnant women, with electromyographic (EMG) evidence of this syndrome in about 5% Supportive treatment (splinting of wrist at night); a few may require surgery Most resolve by 3 months postpartum; may recur with later pregnancies
De Quervain tendosynovitis	Compression and irritation of tendons of extensor pollicis brevi and abductor pollicis longus of wrist	Seen in late pregnancy and lactation May be associated with fluid retention during pregnancy or child care activities postpartum Mild symptoms in late pregnancy increase after delivery and rapidly cease after weaning
Meralgia paresthesia (lateral femoral cutaneous neuropathy)	Unilateral or bilateral entrapment and compression of lateral femoral cutaneous nerve as it passes beneath the inguinal ligament	Associated with obesity and rapid weight gain in pregnancy; also related to trauma and stretch injury Lumbar lordosis in pregnancy may make nerve more vulnerable to compression Develops in third trimester, resolves spontaneously over first 3 months postpartum
NEUROPATHIES OCCURRING IN THE INTRAPARTUM AND POSTPARTUM PERIODS		
Postpartum foot drop	Compression of the lumbosacral trunk against the sacral ala by the fetal head or of the common peroneal nerve between leg braces and the fibular head	Most common intrapartum nerve injury Seen most often in women of short stature with large infants Clinical manifestations may not appear until 24 to 48 hours postpartum Prognosis is good if only the myelin sheath had been distorted, with improvement in 2 to 3 months
Other traumatic neuropathies	Compression of the lumbosacral plexus or obturator, femoral, or peroneal nerves against the pelvic wall, leading to muscular weakness and palsy	Associated with obstetric practices including use of lithotomy position, application of forceps, prolonged pressure from the fetal head, or trauma or hematomas from cesarean delivery Prognosis is good if only the myelin sheath had been distorted, with improvement in 2 to 3 months
Neuropathies associated with breastfeeding	Pressure on the nerves of the axilla Pain and tingling with flexion of the elbow Transient carpal tunnel syndrome	Occurs during engorgement with numbness and tingling of flexor surface of arms to ulnar distribution of hands that abates as the infant sucks Disappears as engorgement resolves Seen in women using a hand pump Develops about 1 month after delivery and resolves within a month of weaning

Compiled from references 15, 33, 37, 49, 50, 96, 116, 120, 178, 196, 200, 201, 210, 223, and 236.

contractions are usually normal. The level of the lesion influences the woman's perception of contractions, however. Sacral anesthesia is present in all of these women. Women with cauda equina lesions have relaxed perineal muscles. Women with lesions below T10 to T11—the level at which the uterine sensory nerves enter the spinal cord—experience labor pain.[50] Women with lesion at T10 and T11 may perceive contractions as abdominal discomfort or muscle spasm.[182]

If the lesion is above T9, labor will be painless, the onset of contractions will not be felt, and delivery may be precipitous.[107] These women need careful monitoring of the cervix and contractions from about 24 weeks' gestation on since preterm labor is common.[15] If the woman also has spasticity, local somatic reflex arcs may be activated by labor contractions. This may result in painful extensor and flexor muscle spasms and sustained ankle clonus.[15,50]

Autonomic hyperreflexia or dysreflexia (also called the autonomic stress syndrome) may occur during labor in women with complete cord lesions above T5 to T6 (above the outflow of the splanchnic autonomic nerves). This syndrome is characterized by hyperstimulation of the autonomic system with brief periods of severe hypertension, throbbing headaches, reflex bradycardia, sweating, nasal congestion, cutaneous vasodilatation with flushed skin, and piloerection above the level of the lesion.[15,33,50,107] Symptoms generally occur with uterine contractions and are most prominent immediately before delivery. Symptoms may be mistaken for preeclampsia.[15,50] Autonomic hyperreflexia occurs because of the sudden release of large amounts of catecholamines during uterine contractions. This syndrome can result in life-threatening complications including intracranial hemorrhage and cardiac arrhythmias. Treatment includes regional anesthesia and perhaps use of beta-blockers.[20,50,104,107]

Forceps may be required during delivery if the muscles used for expulsion during the second stage are paralyzed or if severe hyperreflexia occurs.[500] During the postpartum period, care involves prevention of complications of the elimination and integumentary systems. Poor wound healing is a concern and may be aggravated by anemia. Paraplegic and quadriplegic women have let-down reflexes and can successfully breastfeed.

The Woman with a Brain or Spinal Cord Tumor

Brain tumors, especially meningiomas, usually enlarge during pregnancy because of stimulation of tumor estrogen receptors that stimulate growth of neoplastic cells, increased vascularity and blood volume, and increased extracellular volume.[33,227,236] As a result of these changes, many tumors become symptomatic during the second half of pregnancy. Tumors may temporarily regress postpartum. About one third of women with brain tumors die during pregnancy, usually during the second half. Brain tumors account for approximately 10% of all maternal deaths.[15,49,50]

Spinal cord tumors tend to exacerbate with pregnancy and menstruation. The most common spinal cord lesions in pregnant woman are arteriovascular malformations (AVMs) and angiomas. An AVM is characterized by rapid shunting of blood between an artery and vein without any intervening capillaries, thus depriving adjacent areas of oxygen and nutrients. Exacerbations during pregnancy may be related to: (1) mechanical pressure of the gravid uterus on the vena cava, causing partial outflow obstruction with shifting of blood flow to vertebral and epidural veins and engorgement of the venous side of the malformation; (2) increased vascularity and blood volume; or (3) dilation of the shunt by estrogens.[33,49,50,227,236]

Cerebral Vascular Disorders

The physiologic and hormonal changes of pregnancy also increase the risk of certain cerebral vascular disorders with life-threatening consequences. Although most individual disorders are relatively rare, cerebral vascular disorders as a group are not uncommon during pregnancy.[15] The basis for and risks of subarachnoid hemorrhage, cerebral ischemia, and cerebral venous thrombosis during pregnancy are summarized in Table 14-5.

Preeclampsia and Eclampsia

CNS changes occur in both preeclamptic and eclamptic women. The more severe changes markedly increase the risk of fetal and maternal mortality. CNS manifestations of preeclampsia and eclampsia may include cerebral irritability (e.g., hyperreflexia, headache, clonus, altered consciousness), visual disturbances, cerebral edema, cerebral hemorrhage, and convulsions (with eclampsia). These events are the result of arteriolar vasospasm and vasoconstriction, fluid shifts from the vascular to intravascular space, and possibly a failure of cerebral autoregulation with localized capillary rupture.[50]

Eclampsia is the development of seizures in a pregnant woman with signs and symptoms of preeclampsia. Convulsions may be focal, multifocal, or generalized. Potential etiologic factors for seizures and coma in these women include cerebral vasospasm, hemorrhage, ischemia, edema, and hypertensive or metabolic encephalopathy. Donaldson[50] suggests that the cerebral manifestations of eclampsia are primarily due to severe vasoconstriction in association with failure of cerebral autoregulation. This leads to a pressure-induced rupture of thin-walled capillaries with vasogenic edema and hemorrhage. "In physiologic

TABLE **14-5** Cerebrovascular Disorders: Possible Basis for Increased Risk during Pregnancy

DISORDER	RISK	BASIS
Subarachnoid hemorrhage (SAH)	1 to 2 in 10,000 deliveries. Accounts for about 10% of all maternal deaths usually due to arteriovenous malformation (AVM) or berry aneurysm. Risk due to aneurysm increases with each trimester and postpartum. AVMs most often bleed in the second trimester or in the intrapartum period. One third of SAHs occur with bearing down and Valsalva maneuvers.	Bleeding during pregnancy may be associated with enlargement or increased shunting during pregnancy related to altered hemodynamics, increased cerebral blood flow (CBF), changes in coagulation, or hormonal influences altering integrity of blood vessels. Bleeding during labor in women with these anomalies may be initiated by rapid pressure and flow changes associated with Valsalva maneuver.
Cerebral ischemia	Fivefold to tenfold increase during pregnancy (a similar increase is noted with oral contraceptives). Most occur in second and third trimesters and during the first week postpartum.	Hormonal changes, anemia, and altered blood coagulation during pregnancy may be factors predisposing to emboli formation. Often occurs secondary to other disorders such as mitral valve prolapse, hypertension, subacute bacterial endocarditis, hypotension, or sickle cell anemia, or with use of anticoagulants.
Cerebral venous thrombosis	1 in 2500 to 1 in 10,000 deliveries. Most occur from 3 days to 1 month postpartum (most frequent at 2 to 3 weeks). May be arterial (most common in first week) or venous in origin.	Hematologic changes and alterations in blood coagulation in pregnancy may increase risk. Increased risk with preeclampsia and cesarean section.

Compiled from references 3, 15, 33, 49, 50, 116, 118, 137, 169, 202, 206, 224, and 236.

terms the upper limit of the autoregulation of cerebral perfusion by blood pressure has been exceeded. The upper limit of autoregulation is proportional to mean arterial blood pressure [and thus not standard diastolic or systolic values]. Cerebral eclampsia is hypertensive encephalopathy in previously normotensive women."[50] Hypertensive disorders in pregnancy are discussed in Chapter 8.

SUMMARY

The neurologic system and mediation of discomfort and pain are often of major concern for women during the intrapartum period. This system is probably the one about which least is known regarding specific effects of pregnancy. The pregnant woman experiences alterations in her neuromuscular and sensory systems related to the hormonal and physiologic adaptations of gestation. These changes may result in common experiences and discomforts of pregnancy—including back and headaches, ocular and voice changes, nasal stuffiness, epistaxis, sleep disturbances, postpartum blues, and peripheral neuropathies—and alter the course of neurologic disorders. Recommendations for clinical practice related to the neu-

romuscular and sensory systems during pregnancy are summarized in Table 14-6.

DEVELOPMENT OF THE NEUROMUSCULAR AND SENSORY SYSTEMS IN THE FETUS

The neuromuscular and sensory systems undergo a series of complex structural and functional changes to reach maturation. The CNS is one of the earliest systems to begin development and the latest to completely mature. Table 14-7 summarizes CNS development and timing of origin of specific anomalies. This section will examine anatomic and functional development of the fetal nervous, sensory, and motor systems and development of sensory abilities in preterm infants.

Anatomic Development
Embryonic Development

The development of the nervous system begins approximately 18 days after fertilization.[144] The process by which the beginnings of the nervous system are laid down is called primary neurulation and includes formation of the neural plate, neural folds, and neural tube (Figure 14-5). This process occurs on the dorsal surface of the em-

TABLE **14-6** Recommendations for Clinical Practice Related to the Neuromuscular and Sensory Systems in Pregnant Women

Recognize the usual ocular, otolaryngeal, and neuromuscular changes during pregnancy (pp. 546-548).

Provide anticipatory teaching regarding usual ocular, otolaryngeal, and neuromuscular changes during pregnancy (pp. 546-548).

Counsel women regarding intervention strategies for common problems related to ocular changes (pp. 552-553).

Counsel women, when possible, to delay getting new prescriptions for glasses or contact lenses until several weeks postpartum (p. 552).

Counsel women to avoid cycloplegic or mydriatic agents and topical ophthalmic ointments during pregnancy or, if necessary, to use nasolacrimal occlusion after use (pp. 552-553).

Counsel women regarding intervention strategies for common problems related to otolaryngeal changes (p. 547).

Counsel women regarding intervention strategies for common problems related to musculoskeletal changes (pp. 547-548, 553-554).

Assess posture and lifting techniques used by pregnant women (pp. 553-554).

Teach pregnant women relaxation techniques and exercises to reduce muscle strain and tension (pp. 553-554).

Recognize and assess for factors associated with painful legs during pregnancy (p. 554 and Table 14-2).

Assess sleep patterns of pregnant and postpartum woman and implement interventions to enhance rest and sleep (pp. 548-549, 551-552 and Table 14-1).

Avoid use of sleep medications during pregnancy (pp. 549, 552).

Assess women complaining of backache, headache, round ligament pain, or other discomfort for signs of other disorders (pp. 554-555).

Understand the basis for maternal feelings of pain and discomfort during labor and delivery and implement appropriate interventions (pp. 549-551 and Figure 14-4).

Counsel women during the postpartum period regarding alterations in comfort and implement appropriate interventions (pp. 551-552).

Assess and counsel women with diabetes mellitus and preeclampsia regarding potential ocular complications (pp. 552, 559-560).

Assess eye infections in pregnant women and evaluate for pathogenesis by organisms implicated with sexually transmitted disorders (p. 553).

Counsel women with migraine headaches regarding effects of pregnancy on their disorder and remission postpartum (pp. 554-555).

Know and counsel women regarding the side effects of drugs, including anticonvulsants, used to treat specific neurologic disorders and potential toxicity to the woman and fetus (p. 555 and Chapter 6).

Counsel women with chronic neurologic disorders, including epilepsy, regarding the impact of their disorder on pregnancy and of pregnancy on the disorder (p. 555 and Table 14-3).

Know the effects of physiologic alterations during pregnancy on metabolism of anticonvulsants (p. 555, Table 14-3, Table 6-7, and Chapter 6).

Monitor epileptic women during pregnancy and postpartum for levels of and responses to anticonvulsant (p. 555, Table 14-3, and Chapter 6).

Evaluate the infant of an epileptic woman for congenital anomalies, folate deficiency, drug withdrawal, bleeding, and feeding behavior (p. 555 and Table 14-3).

Ensure that vitamin K is administered to newborns of epileptic women who are on anticonvulsants (Table 14-3 and Chapter 7).

Recognize signs and symptoms of peripheral neuropathies and implement appropriate preventative and intervention strategies (p. 555 and Table 14-4).

Evaluate the woman with a spinal cord transection for bowel, bladder and integumentary complications and implement appropriate interventions (pp. 555, 559).

Monitor the woman with a spinal cord lesion for initiation of contractions, progression of labor, and autonomic hyperreflexia (p. 559).

Recognize the cerebral manifestations of preeclampsia and eclampsia and implement appropriate interventions (pp. 559-560).

TABLE **14-7**   Major Stages of Human Brain Development and Related Defects

Time of Occurrence (Weeks)	Stage of Human Development		Major Events	Major Anomalies During Stage
3 to 4	Neurulation	Notochord	Neural plate Neural tube	Anencephaly Exencephaly Meningocele Meningomyelocele Myeloschisis
			Neural tube Neural crest cells Brain differentiation of prosencephalon, mesencephalon, and rhombencephalon at 20 days Spinal cord	Arnold-Chiari malformation
			Neural crest cells	Dura Dorsal root ganglia Pia and arachnoid Schwann cells Autonomic ganglia
4 to 7	Caudal neural tube formation	Canalization followed by regressive differentiation		Spina bifida occulta
5 to 6	Ventral induction (prosencephalon development)	Precordal mesoderm Prosencephalon	Face and forebrain Cleavage of prosencephalon into cerebral vesicles to form two cerebral hemispheres at 33 days Differentiation of the hypothalamus Optic vesicles Olfactory bulbs and tracts First fibers in internal capsule at 41 days Thalamus and basal ganglia	Dermal sinus Faciotelencephalic malformations
8 to 16	Neuronal proliferation	Cellular proliferation in the ventricular and subventricular zones Proliferation of vascular tree, particularly venous Interkinetic nuclear migration Neuroblasts Glioblasts		Microencephaly (microencephaly vera and radial microbrain) Macrencephaly

12 to 20	Migration	Radial migration in cerebrum Radial tangential migration in the cerebellum	Cortical lamination Neuronal migration in the cerebral cortex is completed at about 5 months Neuronal migration in the cerebellum is completed at about 1 year postnatally	Schizencephaly Agenesis of the corpus callosum Hirschsprung's disease
24 to postnatal	Organization	Late neuronal migration in cerebrum and cerebellum Alignment, orientation, and layering of cortical neurons Synaptic contacts Proliferation of glia and differentiation		Mental retardation Down syndrome Perinatal insults
Peak at birth to years postnatal	Myelinization	Bulbospinal tracts Motor roots Medial lemniscus Pyramidal tract Frontopontine tract Corpus callosum	24 to postnatal 24 to postnatal 24 to postnatal 38 to 2 years postnatally 7 to 8 months to postnatal to 2 years 4 months postnatal to 16 years	Cerebral white matter hypoplasia

Adapted from Hill, A. & Volpe, J.J. (1989). *Fetal neurology.* New York: Raven.

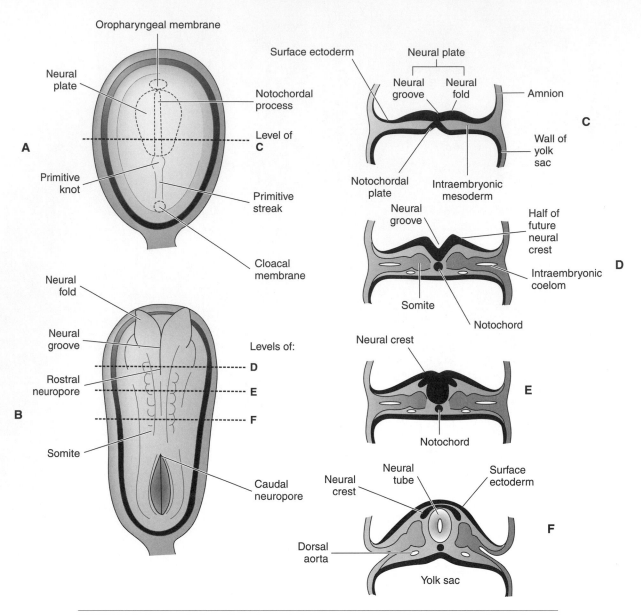

FIGURE **14-5** Embryonic formation of neural plate and neural tube. **A,** Dorsal view of an embryo of about 18 days, exposed by removing the amnion. **B,** Transverse section of this embryo, showing the neural plate and early development of the neural groove. The developing notochord is also shown. **C,** Dorsal view of an embryo of about 22 days. The neural folds have fused opposite the somites but are widely spread out at both ends of the embryo. The rostral and caudal neuropores are indicated. Closure of the neural tube occurs initially in the region corresponding to the future junction of the brain and spinal cord. **D** to **F,** Transverse sections of this embryo at the levels shown in **C,** illustrating formation of the neural tube and its detachment from the surface ectoderm. (From Moore, K.L. [1998]. *The developing human* [6th ed.]. Philadelphia: W.B. Saunders.)

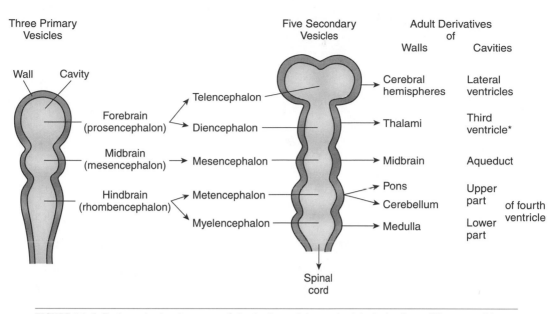

Three Primary Vesicles	Five Secondary Vesicles	Adult Derivatives of	
		Walls	Cavities

FIGURE **14-6** Embryonic development of the brain vesicles and adult derivatives. *The rostral (anterior) part of the third ventricle forms from the cavity of the telencephalon; most of the third ventricle is derived from the cavity of diencephalons. (From Moore, K.L. & Persaud, T.V.N. [1998]. *The developing human: Clinically oriented embryology* [6th ed.]. Philadelphia: W.B. Saunders.)

bryo and leads to formation of the brain and spinal cord (dorsal induction).[222]

The neural plate develops an invagination in its center, called the neural groove, beginning 22 to 23 days after fertilization. Bulges on both sides of the neural tube groove, called the neural folds, accompany the invagination process. The neural folds continue to enlarge, enveloping the neural groove, and fuse to form the neural tube, an entity separate from the overlying ectodermal layer.[144] The neural tube forms the CNS, with the rostral (anterior) portion developing into the brain (Figure 14-6) and the caudal (posterior) portion into the spinal cord. The ventricles and canal of the spinal cord are derived from the lumen of the neural tube.[144] Closure of the neural tube begins in the area of the future lower medulla at about 22 days and proceeds in cephalic and caudal directions. The rostral opening (neuropore) closes at 24 to 25 days; the caudal neuropore (at L1 to L2) closes 2 days later at 26 to 27 days.[144] Failure of these neuropores to close gives rise to neural tube defects.

Formation of the caudal portion of the neural tube in the lower sacral and coccygeal areas begins at 28 to 32 days. This process is known as secondary neurulation. Vacuoles develop in the caudal cell mass at the end of the neural tube. These vacuoles coalesce and fuse with the end of the neural tube. This process continues until 7 weeks, followed by regression of much of the caudal mass that continues until after birth.[222]

As the neural tube is forming, neuroectodermal cells migrate into the neural folds located on both sides of the developing neural groove, forming the neural crest. The neural crest develops into the peripheral nervous system, including the cranial and spinal nerve sensory ganglia, the autonomic nervous system, Schwann cells, the pia and arachnoid layers of the meninges, and the peripheral nerves (Figure 14-7).[144]

Ventral induction (prosencephalon development) refers to processes occurring on the ventral portion of the embryo, leading to formation of the face and forebrain, including eye formation, olfactory formation, and forebrain structures. Thus, errors of ventral induction often produce both facial and nervous system anomalies.[222] After closure of the rostral portion of the neural tube, three vesicles form that are the precursors of the brain. These vesicles, the forebrain (prosencephalon), midbrain (mesencephalon), and hindbrain (rhombencephalon), develop in the fourth week. With further differentiation the forebrain becomes the telencephalon and diencephalon, while the hindbrain becomes the metencephalon and myelencephalon, creating five vesicles. Adult derivatives of the vesicles are shown in Figure 14-6.

In the caudal portion of the neural tube, the alar (dorsal) and basal (ventral) plates develop (see Figure 14-7). These

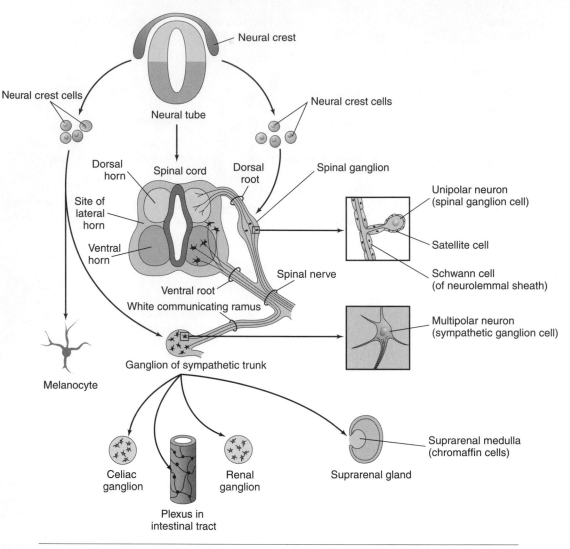

FIGURE **14-7** Selected derivatives of the neural crest. Neural crest cells also differentiate into the cells in the afferent ganglia and other structures. The formation of a spinal nerve is also illustrated. (From Moore, K.L. & Persaud, T.V.N. [1998]. *The developing human: Clinically oriented embryology* [6th ed.]. Philadelphia: W.B. Saunders.)

structures are the beginning formation of the motor and sensory tracts that form in the ventral and dorsal areas, respectively, of the cord.[144] In conjunction with formation of the spinal cord from the caudal neural tube, cells from the neural crest break into groups along the length of the cord, forming spinal and cranial ganglia, in addition to the ganglia of the autonomic nervous system. Further differentiation and migration of neural crest cells and their fibers form the peripheral nerves (somatic and visceral, sensory and motor) and their connections (Figure 14-8). The primitive brain structures also go through a series of flexures or foldings (see Figure 14-8, *A*).

Common Embryonic Anomalies of the Central Nervous System

The most common CNS anomalies arise in the embryonic period during the period of primary neurulation and result from failure of neural tube closure. These anomalies include anencephaly, myelomeningocele, encephalocele, and spina bifida occulta. Neural tube defects (NTDs) are usually accompanied by alterations in vertebral, meningeal, vascular, and dermal structures and arise from environmental or genetic factors. Folic acid supplementation significantly reduces the risk of NTDs in women with a history of a previous infants with an NTD and in the general public.[43,138,230]

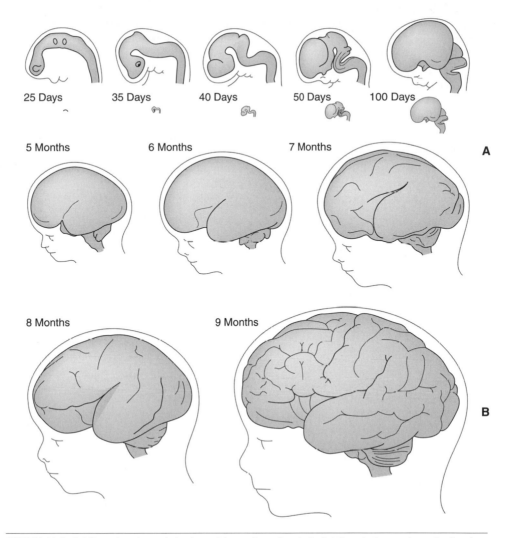

FIGURE **14-8** Folding of embryonic brain and formation of gyri. **A,** Folding during embryonic development. **B,** Development of sulci and gyri during fetal period. (From Cowan, W.M. [1979]. The development of the brain. *Sci Am, 241,* 116.)

Current recommendations are that women of childbearing age consume 0.4 mg of folic acid daily, with higher recommendations (4 mg beginning 3 months before pregnancy and lasting through the first trimester) for women who have previous had a child with an NTD.[12]

Anencephaly is due to failure of the neural tube to fuse in the cranial area. Since this area forms the forebrain, anencephalic infants have minimal development of brain tissue above the midbrain. Tissue that does develop is poorly differentiated and becomes necrotic with exposure to amniotic fluid. This results in a mass of vascular tissue with neuronal and glial elements and a choroid plexus with partial absence of the skull bones.[144] Since anencephaly arises from failure of the neural tube to close cranially, the insult must occur at or before 24 to 25 days.

Encephaloceles also arise from failure of closure of part of the caudal portion of the neural tube. About 70% to 80% of these defects occur in the occipital region, with the sac protruding from the back of the head or base of the neck.[27,222] Hydrocephalus occurs in up to 50% of occipital encephaloceles due to alterations in the posterior fossa. Hydrocephalus may be present at birth or develop after repair of the defect. Encephaloceles may occur in association with meningomyelocele. The protruding sac varies considerably in size, but the size does not correlate with the presence of neural elements. Ten percent to 20% of encephaloceles contain no neural elements.[222]

Spina bifida is a general term used to describe defects associated with malformations of the spinal cord and vertebrae that usually arise from defects in closure of the caudal neuropore. Approximately 80% occur in the lumbar area, which is the final area of neural tube fusion. Thus, spina bifida, arising from defects in primary neurulation, must occur at or before 26 to 27 days. Defects range from minor malformations to disorders that result in paraplegia or quadriplegia and loss of bladder and bowel control. The degree of sensory and motor neurologic deficit depends on the level and severity of the defect. The two major forms of spina bifida are spina bifida occulta and spina bifida cystica.

Spina bifida occulta (occult dysraphic states) is a vertebral defect at L5 or S1 that arises from failure of the vertebral arch to grow and fuse.[27] These are defects of secondary neurulation during formation of the caudal portion of the spinal cord (Figure 14-9, A). Most people with this defect have no problems and the defect may be unrecognized. A few have underlying abnormalities of the spinal cord or nerve roots, which are manifested externally by a hemangioma, dimple, tuft of hair, or lipoma in the lower lumbar or sacral area.

Spina bifida cystica describes neural tube defects characterized by a cystic sac, containing meninges or spinal cord elements, along with vertebral defects, covered by epithelium or a thin membrane, and usually occurring in the lumbar or lumbosacral area. Spina bifida cystica is usually due to alterations in primary neurulation. The three main forms of spina bifida cystica are meningocele, meningomyelocele, and myeloschisis (Figure 14-9, B, C, and D). Meningocele involves a sac containing meninges and cerebrospinal fluid (CSF) but with the spinal cord and nerve roots in their normal position. These infants usually have minimal residual neurologic deficit if the defect is covered with skin and is managed appropriately.

With a meningomyelocele, the most common form of spina bifida cystica, the sac contains spinal cord or nerve roots in addition to meninges and CSF. During development, nerve tissues become incorporated into the wall of the sac, impairing differentiation of nerve fibers.[27] These infants have a neurologic deficit below the level of the sac. Myeloschisis is a severe defect that occurs no later than 24 days.[222] With this disorder there is no cystic covering; the spinal cord is an open, exposed, flattened mass of neu-

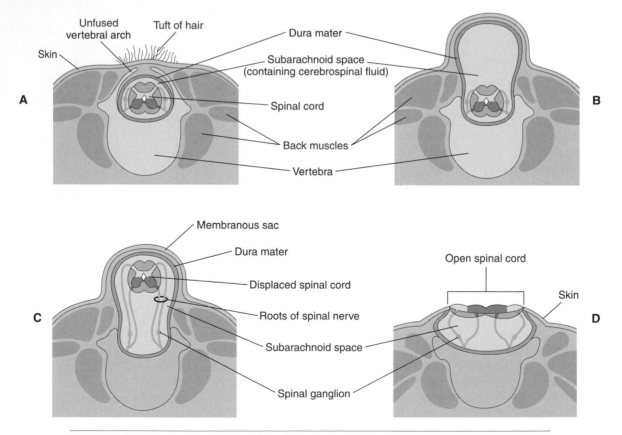

FIGURE **14-9** Different types of spina bifida. **A,** Spina bifida occulta; **B,** spina bifida with meningocele; **C,** spina bifida with meningomyelocele; and **D,** spina bifida with myeloschisis. (From Moore, K.L. & Persaud, T.V.N. [1998]. *The developing human: Clinically oriented embryology* [6th ed.]. Philadelphia: W.B. Saunders.)

ral tissue. These infants have significant neurologic deficits and are at great risk for infection. This defect can involve the entire length of the spinal cord and can occur in association with anencephaly.[27] Disorders of ventral induction are thought to arise no later than the fifth to sixth weeks of gestation. Disorders of forebrain development include holoprosencephaly and holotelencephaly (see Table 14-7).

Fetal Neurodevelopment

In the nervous system, structures continue to be elaborated beyond the embryonic period. The earliest growth of brain occurs in the lower-level structures, such as basal ganglia, thalamus, midbrain, and brain stem, whereas higher-level structures, such as the cerebrum and cerebellum, form somewhat later. Once the embryologic formations are established, CNS development is characterized by overlapping processes: neuronal proliferation, neuronal and glial cell migration, organization, and myelinization. These processes, especially organization and myelinization, continue past birth.

Neuronal proliferation. Neuronal proliferation (neuronogenesis) is a period of massive production of neurons and their precursors (Figure 14-10). The maximal rate of neuronal proliferation occurs between 12 and 18 weeks of gestational age, although neurons continue to proliferate until term and beyond.[222] Cerebellar neurons, in particular, proliferate after birth. During proliferation the walls of the neural tube thicken, forming layers. The ependyma is the lining of the neural tube interior that later becomes the lining of the ventricles and the central canal of the spinal cord. In the subependymal layer the neurons and glial cells of the CNS are formed in the ventricular and subventricular zones of the germinal layer (germinal matrix).[222] Neuronal proliferation thus occurs in the subependymal layer, producing neurons that become situated in the gray areas of the CNS.[144] In conjunction with the proliferation of neurons, glial cells also increase in number; however, the peak in glial cell numbers occurs roughly from 5 months' gestational age through the first year of life.[222] Thus a large proportion of the neuronal compliment is formed early in fetal life, but a few areas, notably the cerebellum, continue to acquire neurons during the early months after birth. This pattern of neuronal formation produces a particular vulnerability at time of birth, especially in the preterm infant, because the cerebellar neurons may be damaged by asphyxia and anoxia.

Alterations in neuronal proliferation can lead to increases or decreases in number and size of cells in the brain and associated structures. Micrencephaly arises from a decrease in size (micrencephaly vera) or number

(radial microbrain) of neuronal-glial stem cell units.[222] Micrencephaly vera may be due to unknown causes; have a familial basis; or be associated with teratogens such as alcohol, cocaine, radiation, and maternal phenylketonuria.[222] Excessive proliferation (macrencephaly) may also be due to unknown causes, have a familial basis, or occur with growth disturbances such as achondroplasia (or Beckwith syndrome) and chromosomal disorders (fragile X and Klinefelter syndromes). Macrencephaly is also seen with neurocutaneous syndromes (such as multiple hemangiomas and neurofibromatosis) that involve excessive proliferation of cells within the central nervous system and of mesodermal structures.[222]

Migration. Once formed, neurons travel from the germinal layer, near the ventricles in the subependymal layer, to the areas of the nervous system where they will further differentiate and take on unique and individual functions.[222] Neurons migrate from the ventricular area to the areas where gray matter is located. The bulk of migration occurs at 3 to 5 months' gestational age (see Figure 14-10).[222] Neuron migration is assisted by specialized glia, called *radial glia* (Figure 14-11).[105,222] The nuclei of the radial glia are in the germinal matrix. The basal process of each cell is attached to the ventricle and the apical process attached to the pia matter.[105] These processes extending from the radial glia guide the neuron to its respective site. This process is mediated by signaling proteins, surface molecules, and receptors on both the neurons and the radial glia.[222]

The early neurons migrate to areas deep within the cortex, whereas later neurons migrate further to the surface of the cortex. As a result, neurons formed early come to lie in deeper layers of cortex and subcortex; those formed later end at more superficial layers.[172,222] Most cortical neurons have reached their sites by 20 to 24 weeks' gestation.[222] The cortex generally has a complete component of neurons by 33 weeks' gestation.[172] The radial glia later develop into astrocytes.[22] Radial glial-assisted migration also occurs in the cerebellum.

Disorders of migration alter gyral development and lead to hypoplasia or agenesis of the corpus callosum. Gyral development is most prominent during the last 3 months of gestation (see Figure 14-8, *B*), with the most rapid increase between 26 and 28 weeks. The increased gyri result in a change in head shape (from oval to biparietal prominence). Gyral disorders arise secondary to inborn errors of metabolism, particularly proximal disorders and fatty acid oxidation defects; chromosomal anomalies; and exogenous insults, especially in preterm infants.[142,222]

Organization. Organization refers to the processes by which the nervous system takes on the capacity to operate

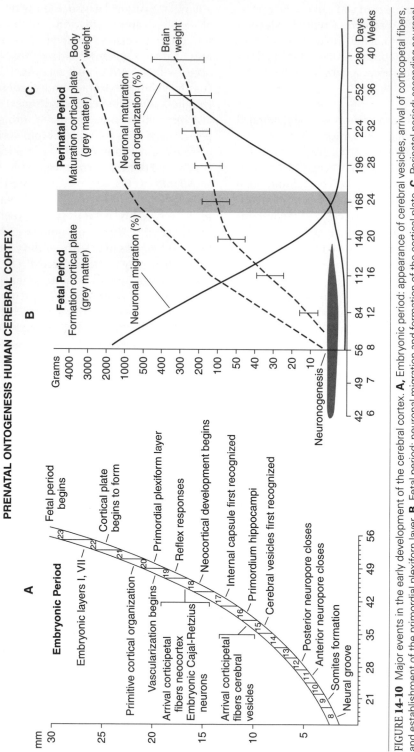

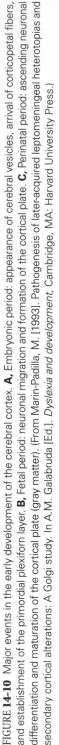

FIGURE **14-10** Major events in the early development of the cerebral cortex. **A,** Embryonic period: appearance of cerebral vesicles, arrival of corticopetal fibers, and establishment of the primordial plexiform layer. **B,** Fetal period: neuronal migration and formation of the cortical plate. **C,** Perinatal period: ascending neuronal differentiation and maturation of the cortical plate (gray matter). (From Marín-Padilla, M. [1993]. Pathogenesis of later-acquired leptomeningeal heterotopias and secondary cortical alterations: A Golgi study. In A.M. Galabruda [Ed.]. *Dyslexia and development,* Cambridge, MA: Harvard University Press.)

as an integrated whole. This phase of neurodevelopment begins at approximately 6 months' gestational age (see Figure 14-10) and extends many years after birth, and is believed to continue into adulthood. Neuron growth and connections lead to development of sulci and gyri (see Figure 14-8, *B*), with a brain growth spur seen from 26 to 30 weeks. With increasing organization, fetal and infant behaviors become more complex.[8,222] Alterations in organization are seen in infants with Down, fragile X, and Angelman syndromes; periventricular leukomalacia (PVL); and hypothryoxinemia.[222]

During the period of organization, six processes occur.[222] The first is differentiation and development of subplate neurons. These neurons migrate to cortex early and guide ascending and descending projections to target neurons. Subplate neurons provide a connection site for axons ascending from thalamus and other sites, until the neurons that these axons will eventually connect with have migrated from the germinal matrix. The subplate reaches its peak from 22 to 34 weeks.[222]

The second and third processes involve arrangement of cortical neurons in layers and arborization, wherein the dendrites and axons undergo extensive branching. This lat-

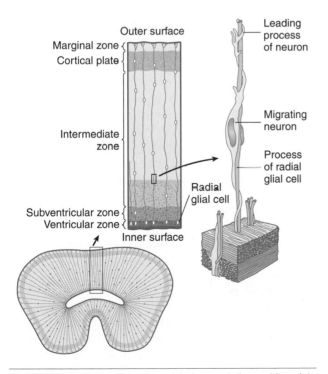

FIGURE 14-11 Radial glial cells and their associations with peripherally migrating neurons during the development of the brain. (Based on Rakic, P. [1975]. *Birth Defects Orig Article Series XI, 7,* 95-129.)

ter process is sometimes referred to as the "wiring of the brain" (Figure 14-12). The increase in cellular processes and in the size of the neuronal field is prerequisite for communication throughout the nervous system. This process is followed by the formation of connections or synapses between neurons, the fourth component of organization. The intracellular structures and enzymes that will produce neurotransmitters also develop at this time. Connections between cells are critical for integration across all areas of the nervous system. Throughout development, synapses continue to restructure; this process is believed to be the basis for memory and learning.

Synaptogenesis is mediated by excitatory neurotransmitters such as glutamate.[70] Glutamate acts on N-methyl-D-aspartate (NMDA) receptors to enhance neuronal proliferation, migration, and synaptic plasticity. During the brain growth spurt, NMDA receptors are hypersensitive. Blockage of these receptors by substances such as ethanol in animal models leads to apoptosis.[70,105,180] Other substances, such as erythropoietin, may also be important in enhancing brain organization.[112,180]

The fifth organizational process entails reduction in the number of neurons and their connections through the death of up to half of the original neurons as well as regression of many dendrites and synapses.[222] Neuronal survival has been likened to survival of the fittest, because neurons compete for resources such as nutrients, electrical impulses, and synapses.[29] Neuronal death assists in elimination of errors within the nervous system. The appropriate number of neurons and their connections are retained while neurons that are improperly located or fail to achieve adequate connections are eliminated.

The sixth organizational process is differentiation of glia from the general precursor cells into specific types (see Figure 14-7) and glia proliferation. There are three main types of glia: myelin-building (oligodendrites and Schwann cells), guiding (radial glia [for neuron migration] and Schwann cells), and "clean-up" (astroglia and microglia). The astroglia and microglia remove waste and dead tissue and occupy space left by neurons that have died.

Within the CNS, astrocytes also provide support for neurons. Oligodendrites produce myelin in the CNS. Schwann cells produce myelin for the peripheral nerves. Schwann cells also act as guiding glia following peripheral nerve injury to guide regenerating axons to their targets.[222] The increase in glia begins at approximately 30 weeks' gestational age and continues into the second year.

Myelinization. Myelinization refers to the laying down of myelin, the lipoprotein insulating covering of nerve fibers. This process occurs in both the central and peripheral nerve systems. Glia migrate to locations along the developing nerve

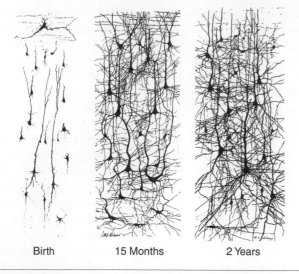

| Birth | 15 Months | 2 Years |

FIGURE 14-12 Dendritic growth. (From Dobbing, J. [1975]. Human brain development and its vulnerability. In *Biologic and clinical aspects of brain development*. [Mead Johnson Symposium on Perinatal and Developmental Medicine, no. 6.] Evansville, IN: Mead Johnson.)

fibers. Myelin is formed as the glia (either Schwann cells in the peripheral nervous system or oligodendroglia in the CNS) wrap around the nerve fiber. The glia's cellular membrane, once wrapped around the fiber, fuses to become myelin. Myelinization begins during the second trimester and continues into adulthood.[222]

The process of myelinization occurs at differing times in areas throughout the nervous system. For example, myelinization of the forebrain is most rapid after birth. Although incomplete myelinization does not prevent function, incomplete myelinization—because it affects nerve conduction—does alter the speed of impulse conduction. Generally, myelinization precedes mature function.[144] Myelinization first begins in the peripheral nervous system, with motor fibers becoming myelinated before sensory fibers. In the CNS, myelinization of sensory areas precedes that of motor areas, with the primary sensory areas becoming myelinated relatively early in development. The order of myelinization parallels overall nervous system functional development. Areas of the brain that support higher-level functions, such as cognition and learning, myelinate later in life.[222] Some brain areas continue to lay down myelin well into adulthood. Since myelin is a lipoprotein, dietary adequacy of fats and protein is important for normal myelinization. Disorders of myelinization are seen with amino and organic acidopathies, hypothyroidism, undernutrition, and possibly PVL.[222]

Electrical activity and impulse conduction. The earliest synapses appear at about 8 to 9 weeks' gestational age,

whereas cortical synapses are present at about 23 weeks' gestational age.[172] Impulse conduction provides for functional validation of connections. Evidence suggests that use of conduction pathways may increase or alter connections.[222] Characteristics of early neuronal activity include poor spontaneous neuronal activity, slow conduction velocity, slow synaptic potentials, and synaptic transmission uncertainty.[42] Immaturity of neurotransmitters and hypersensitivity of NMDA receptors increases the risk of receptor overstimulation with hypoxic-ischemic events.[110]

Development of Specific Systems

Autonomic nervous system. The autonomic nervous system has both central and peripheral components. Peripheral portions develop from neural crest cells (see Figure 14-7). Ganglia are formed from neural crest cells that migrate beyond the neural tube. Sympathetic ganglia are derived from neural crest cells that collect along either side of the developing spinal cord at about 5 weeks' gestational age.[144] The ganglia of the parasympathetic ganglia and plexi also form by migration.[144] Once they reach their respective sites, neurons in the autonomic ganglia continue to differentiate. Nerve fibers, originating in the cord, grow out and make connections with the ganglia. The autonomic nervous system regulates many endocrine functions through nerve impulses. The embryonic origins of some autonomic end organs demonstrate a structural basis for these regulatory actions. The pituitary, a primary source of autonomic regulation, is derived from two forms of tissue. The adenohypophysis is formed from ectoderm and the neurohypophysis is formed from neuroectoderm. Similarly, the adrenal gland is derived from two types of tissue. The adrenal cortex is derived from mesoderm, whereas the medulla, which secretes catecholamines, is derived from neuroectoderm (specifically neural crest cells) and is controlled by the sympathetic nervous system.

Peripheral nervous system. The peripheral nervous system is derived from the neural crest (see Figure 14-7). Through migration and specialization, cells of the neural crest develop into cranial, spinal, and visceral nerves and ganglia. Neural crest cells are precursors of the adrenal medulla chromaffin cells that secrete epinephrine.[144] Support cells of the peripheral nervous system also derive from the neural crest. Nerve fibers, which eventually innervate skeletal motor fibers, emerge from the spinal basal plate, combine into bundles to form the ventral root, and migrate to the developing motor fibers.[144] Similarly, sensory fibers form the dorsal root.

Functional Development

Studies of fetal neural activity in utero are limited to external monitoring of CNS electrical activity or noninvasive

TABLE **14-8**   Anatomic and Functional Development of the Different Parts of the Pain System

PART OF THE SYSTEM	DEVELOPMENTAL EVENT	TIMING (WEEKS)
Nociceptors	Nociceptors appear (starting around the mouth and later developing over the entire body).	7-20
Peripheral afferents	Synapses appear to the spinal cord.	10-30
Spinal cord	Stimulation results in motor movements.	7.5
	Spinothalamic connections are established.	20
	Pain pathways myelinize.	22
	Descending tracts develop.	Postnatally
Thalamocortical tracts	First axons appear to the cortical plate.	20-22
	Functional synapse formation of the thalamocortical occurs.	26-34
Cerebral cortex	Cortical neurons migrate (cortex develops).	8-20
	First electroencephgalogram (EEG) burst may be detected.	20
	Symmetric and synchronic EEG activity appears.	26
	Sleep and wakefulness patterns in EEG become distinguishable.	30
	Evoked potential becomes detectable.	29

From Vanhatalo, S. & van Nieuwenhuizen, O. (2000). Fetal pain? *Brain Dev, 22,* 146.

detection of fetal responses using measures of fetal movement or ultrasonography. The knowledge of fetal neural capabilities has been augmented by an accident of nature—preterm birth. Much of our understanding of fetal function comes from the study of preterm infants, who technically are not fetal. However, the behavior of these infants provides one means of appreciating fetal behaviors at various gestational ages. Studies of preterm infants have greatly increased information concerning operation of the fetal nervous system. The following section describes the neural function of the fetus, defined as gestational age less than 38 weeks. In many instances, information pertains to the "fetal infant" or preterm infant. Appreciation of fetal neural development provides a basis for anticipation of the many capabilities of the preterm and term infant.

Sensory Abilities

Generally the somatic sensory and special sensory systems develop in the following order chronologically: touch, proprioception, vestibular, chemoreception (smell and taste), hearing, and vision.[83,93] As noted in the previous section, in the periphery motor fibers myelinate before sensory fibers, whereas in the central nervous system sensory fibers myelinate before motor fibers. Thus, in terms of rate of impulse transmission, differences in myelinization are one basis for limited integration of sensory and motor actions in the fetus.

The early fetus has been shown to respond to touch around the mouth at around 2 months of gestational age; hands become touch sensitive by 10 to 11 weeks.[214] Touch in utero entails contact with amniotic fluid that is approximately at body temperature and contact with body parts or the wall of the uterus. Maternal movement and buoyant amniotic fluid provide rich vestibular stimulation for the fetus in utero.

Nociceptors appear at about 6 weeks' gestation, initially around the mouth, and by 20 weeks can be found throughout the fetus (Table 14-8).[214] The fetus can process pain at the subcortical level before cortical structures are in place.[214] Afferent synapses in the spinal cord develop from 10 to 30 weeks with spinothalamic connections by 20 to 25 weeks.[170,171] These connections are myelinated by 29 weeks.[214]

Proprioception, which is involved with perception of joint and body movement and the position of the body, develops next and is interrelated with tactile and vestibular receptors. Vestibular sensation is a form of proprioceptive sensation involved in balance and postural control. Vestibular sensation, mediated by receptors in ear, detects changes in direction and rate of head movement. Vestibular receptors mature by 14 to 15 weeks.[123]

Smell is mediated by three groups of receptors that bind fragrant molecules: (1) main ciliated neuroreceptors (seen by 11 weeks), (2) trigeminal nerve endings (respond by 7 to 10 weeks), and (3) vomeronasal (appear by 5 to 6 weeks and are maximal by 20 weeks).[123,231] Olfactory marker protein is present by 29 weeks.[231] Odor molecules in amniotic fluid stimulate the fetal smell receptors by the third trimester.[231] The fetus may detect aromatic substances from the maternal diet in amniotic fluid. This stimulation may have a role in later dietary preferences.[98] Responsiveness to odors is observed in preterm infants beginning at approximately 26 weeks and is readily documented by 32 weeks' gestation in most infants.

Taste occurs by activation of the taste buds and stimulation of the trigeminal nerve. Taste buds develop at 12 to 13 weeks. Taste receptors are present by 16 weeks, reaching adult numbers by term.[123] The fetus is known to ingest amniotic fluid (see Chapter 3). Although slight variations occur in the composition of the amniotic fluid, it is unknown to what extent the fetus experiences taste. Research with term infants, however, has documented the ability of infants to discriminate tastes.[123]

The structures of the auditory system, including the inner ear and cochlea, are mature enough to support hearing by approximately 20 weeks' gestation; fetal hearing begins at 24 to 25 weeks.[94,161] Auditory evoked potentials can be recorded as early as 25 to 26 weeks' gestation.[89,94] Responses to sound are observed in preterm infants at approximately 25 to 28 weeks.[89,97] The preterm infant can be observed to orient to sound, with evidence of arousal and attention.[83] The hearing threshold decreases with gestational age. For example, in infants of 28 to 34 weeks' gestation, the hearing threshold is approximately 40 decibels, whereas in term infants the hearing threshold is approximately 20 decibels.[119] Intrauterine recordings have revealed that sounds in the external environment are audible to the fetus; high-frequency sounds are attenuated, but low-frequency sounds are not.[98] The intrauterine auditory environment includes sounds within the mother such as breathing, movement of blood through the umbilical cord, and intestinal peristalsis. Hearing in preterm infants of different gestational ages is summarized in Table 14-9.

Formation of the eyes begins during embryonic development. Rod differentiation and retinal vascularization begin by 25 weeks' gestational age and myelinization of the optic nerve begins at 24 weeks.[78,89] The neurons forming the visual cortex are in place at 26 weeks. Between 28 and 34 weeks' gestation, visual neuronal connections and processes undergo rapid development.[89] Visual evoked potentials can be recorded between 25 and 30 weeks.[89,172] Visual attention begins at about 30 to 32 weeks' gestational age, although it is fleeting at this age. Development of vision in preterm infants at different gestational ages is summarized in Table 14-10.

The natural sensory environment of the uterus is developmentally appropriate for the fetus. This environment provides stimuli that are rich, varied, and rhythmical. Intrauterine sensory stimulation programs have not been studied extensively and cannot be assumed to be beneficial or without risk. Because the normal uterine sensory environment is already rich, the benefits of programs to supplement intrauterine stimulation are unclear at the present time.

Motor Abilities

The development of motor activity in the fetus is a function of both neural and muscle maturation. Muscle cells develop

TABLE **14-9**   Development of Hearing in Preterm and Term Infants

AGE	ANATOMIC AND FUNCTIONAL DEVELOPMENT
Preterm infants <28 weeks	Fetal hearing begins by 23 to 24 weeks Threshold about 65 db, with a range of 500-1000 Hz Auditory brain stem responses by 26 to 28 weeks
Preterm infants 28 to 30 weeks	Rapid maturation of cochlea and auditory nerve Responses rapidly fatigue Initial auditory processing by 30 weeks Threshold 40 db with an increased frequency range
Preterm infants 32 to 34 weeks	Outer hair cells mature by 32 weeks Rapid maturation of cochlea and auditory nerve
Preterm infants >34 weeks	Increased speed of conduction Ossicles and electrophysiology complete by 36 weeks Hearing threshold 30 db, with increasing range Increasing ability to localize and discriminate
Term infants	Localize and discriminate sounds Hearing threshold of 20 db, with a range of 500-4000 Hz

Compiled from references 28, 30, 78, 89, 93, 94,123, and 164.
db, Decibels; *Hz,* Hertz.

from mesoderm. Innervation during development is critical for muscle fiber development.[222] Muscle cells, as well as neurons, undergo migration and differentiation during development. Mature myocytes are present at approximately 38 weeks; muscle cells increase in size postnatally.[222] Gross motor movement appears as early as 7 weeks' gestation, whereas limb movement occurs at 9 weeks.[89] The earliest reflex is tilting of the head with perioral touch (7.5 weeks); legs demonstrate reflexive movement by 14 weeks.[214]

The pattern of fetal motor development includes differences in both emergence of muscle tone and the amount of movement over time.[89] Development of muscle tone follows a caudocephalad and distal-proximal pattern; that is, lower extremities precede upper extremities and extremities precede axial or truncal muscle tone.[2] Motor development is associated with increased flexor tone, with lower extremities demonstrating flexion before upper extremities. In the lower extremities, passive flexor tone is noticed at 29 weeks' gestation and active flexor tone becomes apparent at 31 weeks.[5] Tone in the upper extremities devel-

TABLE **14-10**   Development of Vision in Preterm and Term Infants

AGE	ANATOMIC AND FUNCTIONAL DEVELOPMENT
Preterm infants 24 to 28 weeks	Eyelid: unfuses at 24-26 weeks Lens: cloudy; second of four layers forming Cornea: hazy until 27 weeks Retina: rod differentiation by 25 weeks; vascularization begins Visual cortex: rapid dendritic growth No pupillary response Eyelid tightening to bright light but quickly fatigues VER to bright light but quickly fatigues Very myopic
Preterm infants 30 to 34 weeks	Lens: clearing, second layer complete, third forming Retina: rod complete except for fovea by 32 weeks; cone differentiation begins Visual cortex: rapid dendritic and synapse development VER more complex, latency decreases Bright light causes sustained pupil closure Abrupt reduction may cause eye opening Pupillary response sluggish but more mature Spontaneous eye opening, with brief fixation in low light
Preterm infants 34 to 36 weeks	Pupils: complete pupillary reflex by 36 weeks Retina: cone numbers in fovea increase Blood vessels reach nasal retina Visual cortex: morphologically similar to term Increased alertness; less sustained than for a term infant VER resembles that of term infant with longer latency Spontaneous orientation toward soft light Beginning to track and show visual preferences Less myopic
Term infants	Still immature, with much development from birth to 6 months Retinal vessels reach periphery of temporal retina Lens transmits more short-wave light than adult Acuity approximately 20/200 to 20/1600 Attend to form, object, and face; track horizontally and some vertically Can see objects to at least 2½ feet; attends best at 8-12 inches

Adapted from Glass, P. (1999). The vulnerable neonate and the neonatal intensive care environment. In G.B. Avery, M.A. Fletcher, & M.G. MacDonald (Eds.). *Neonatology: Pathophysiology and management of the newborn* (5th ed.). Philadelphia: Lippincott, Williams & Wilkins.
VER, Visual evoked response.

ops later, with flexor tone demonstrated in the upper extremities by 34 weeks.[14] Active tone develops before passive tone; that is, muscle tone is seen during movement or action before resting muscle tone. Both tone and flexion increase with gestational age. Motor movement also shows increasing coordination with gestational age, with less tremor, smoother movement, and more coordination.[89] More complex motor movements are observed after 24 weeks' gestation.[89] Muscle tone is used as one criteria in scoring gestational age.

Muscle tone is limited before 28 weeks' gestation. By 32 weeks, flexor tone can be observed in the lower extremities; it is observable in the upper extremities by 36 weeks. The term infant demonstrates flexion.[222] Movement changes with development. At 28 to 32 weeks' gestation, movement is slow, and may appear uncoordinated, with flailing or writhing-type movements.[222] By 32 weeks' gestation, flexion movements are somewhat more coordinated.[222] Neonates of this age can turn their head, but head control is lacking. With continued development there is increasing strength, alternating movements may be seen in lower extremities, and head control improves.[222]

During pregnancy the pattern of fetal movements is one of increasing frequency of movements, followed by a reduction in movement close to term. Spontaneous movements begin at 7 to 8 weeks' gestation with slow flexion-extension of the vertebral column and passive displacement of the extremities, followed by discrete limb movements at 9 weeks. The development of movement involves twitching type movement before 10 weeks, followed by independent limb movement (10 to 12 weeks); hand to face movement (12 to 13 weeks); limb, head, and torso

movement (12 to 16 weeks); sucking on fingers (15 weeks); and increasingly complex hand, face, and respiratory movements after 24 weeks.[222] All types of movements seen after birth are present by about 18 weeks' gestation. Maternal perception of fetal movement occurs at approximately 16 weeks' gestation in multiparas, and slightly later in primiparas. Before this time, fetal movements are too fine to be noticed. Fetal movements increase during gestation, reaching a maximum between 26 and 32 weeks; after this time the constraints of the uterine environment reduce fetal movement. Movements are largely spontaneous but can be stimulated.

The developing motor activity of the fetus reflects integration of nervous system activity as well as general fetal well-being. Changes in fetal movement may reflect placental insufficiency, hypoxemia, or other evidence of fetal distress. Daily fetal movement monitoring has been used as a screening tool for fetal well-being during the third trimester. In addition to changes in tone and frequency of movement during pregnancy, fetal movements provide evidence of fetal sleep-wake or state patterns.

Fetal State Patterns

Although the constancy of the uterine environment may suggest similar consistency in fetal behavior, this assumption is untrue. Fetal behaviors exhibit regular patterns of occurrence, particularly sleep-wake behaviors or behavioral states.[147] In the adult, sleep-wake behaviors demonstrate a diurnal pattern of activity and sleep. Sleep in the fetus and infant does not follow this pattern. Sleep changes with maturation of the central nervous system. Because sleep is qualitatively and quantitatively different in the young compared with adults, fetal and infant sleep-wake patterns are more commonly described as states. In the infant, state is determined by characteristics of heart and respiratory regularity, eyes open or closed, motor activity, and presence or absence of rapid eye movements (REM). Although not all of these parameters can be observed in the fetus, fetal state can be determined by regularity of heart rate, presence of eye movements, and fetal movement.[147]

In the fetus as well as the infant, motor activity and irregular heart rate occur during REM sleep. Motor movement also occurs during awake periods. During quiet sleep, regular heart rate and minimal motor movement are noted. Alteration of quiet and active periods in fetal movement have been reported as early as 21 weeks' gestation; however, there is little evidence of regular, rhythmic pattern and limited coordination among state parameters.[199] Fetal movement is largely continuous in early pregnancy, but with increasing maturation, quiet periods emerge. At 24 to 26 weeks' gestation there is almost continual motor activity of the fetal extremities.[52] By 32 weeks' gestation, alteration of activity and quiet periods becomes more regular and rhythmic. By 32 weeks' gestation, patterns of fetal heart rate, eye movement, and gross body movements also begin to show coordination.[217] This periodic function is credited with being a prenatal version of the alteration of REM and quiet sleep, representing a underlying rest-activity cycle.[174] The fetal state cycle is approximately 40 minutes long.[199] With continuing development the length of quiet periods and the integration among state behaviors increase.[159] These changes continue after birth.

NEONATAL PHYSIOLOGY
Transitional Events

At birth, the transition from intrauterine to extrauterine life entails a number of changes in the nervous system. The nervous system does not "turn on" at birth; rather, nervous system activity has increased steadily during pregnancy, producing a term gestation infant whose nervous system is prepared to receive and process information and respond in ways suited to neonatal development. In examining transition, it is useful to identify the behavioral abilities of the neonate, experiences of the fetus in the intrauterine environment, and differences between the intrauterine and extrauterine environments. The change in environment is the major challenge for the neonate's nervous system. The transitional characteristics of four areas of nervous system function will be examined: autonomic, motor, sensory, and state regulation.

Autonomic Regulation

During fetal life, placental circulation provides a steady flow of oxygen and nutrients supporting metabolic needs of the fetus. At birth, the first challenge faced by the neonate is initiating and sustaining respiration (see Chapter 9). In addition to an intact pulmonary and cardiovascular system, nervous system control of the respiration and heart activity is required. Although fetal respiratory movements are preparation for this action, the fetus has no experience breathing independently or in regulating cardiac and pulmonary functions to produce stable blood oxygen requirements in ambient air. The fetus has had experience monitoring autonomic functions and, to a degree, regulating vegetative behaviors. These capabilities are evidenced by fetal responses to hypoxemia or hypoglycemia, such as changes in activity, heart rate, and blood pressure.

In extrauterine life, nutrient intake must be derived independently from an outside source. Two primary changes in feeding occur: route of intake and pattern of intake. The neonate must switch to oral intake, which is achieved

through sucking. In the uterus the fetus has had sucking and feeding experiences in which amniotic fluid has been ingested, but the fetus has not needed to coordinate breathing with sucking and swallowing (see Chapter 11). Second, neonatal feeding is periodic, rather than the continuous supply of nutrients provided the fetus. Hunger, thirst, and satiety centers must regulate food intake and the neonate must exhibit appropriate hunger cues to elicit feeding from the caregiver and must also be able to end feeding with cues indicating satiety.

In the uterus the fetal temperature varied little. Thus, a major challenge at the time of birth is initiation of thermoregulation. Although thermoregulatory abilities begin at approximately 30 weeks' gestation, the fetus has not been required to independently monitor body temperature and adjust metabolic rate to meet thermal needs (see Chapter 19).

Motor Functions

Beginning early in fetal development, skeletal muscles are involved in movement. These experiences with motor activities provide a means of promoting motor development as well as an opportunity to test out motor innervation. Within the uterus, however, motor activities are enacted in an environment that reduces the effects of gravity and provides confinement. The buoyant amniotic fluid and uterine walls are replaced by the extrauterine environment, in which motion is not confined and gravity has a greater effect. Although movements of the fetus may have been smooth and limited in scale, movements of the neonate are often erratic, weak, or flailing. The neonate must exert energy to maintain body position against the pull of gravity.

Sensory Functions

The sensory input provided by the extrauterine environment is markedly different from that of the uterus. Before looking at these differences, however, it is important to recognize the sensory experience of birth itself. Although the fetus has experienced Braxton-Hicks contractions, the steady, rhythmic contractions of the uterus and resultant pressure changes are a new experience. The continuous flow of oxygen and nutrients through the placenta may be altered during contractions, providing intense autonomic input. The descent into the birth canal increases pressure, perhaps to the degree of being uncomfortable. During labor the mother's activity pattern may change and the sounds from the mother's body may be altered, such as rapid or heavy breathing or heart rate increase. Concurrent with the experiences of labor, changes in the extrauterine environment (e.g., noise) may be sensed by the infant. It would seem that the process of birth is one of being bombarded with stimuli. After birth a number of new sensory experiences await. In general sensations in the extrauterine environment are different in nature, more intense, and lack the pattern experienced in the intrauterine environment.

Whereas the uterus is dark, the extrauterine environment provides more, often intense light in the immediate postbirth period. In the uterus, the fetus was bathed in amniotic fluid that exhibited rare temperature variation, but the extrauterine environment is much cooler and can exhibit great variability. Until birth the fetus has never experienced cold stimulation. In the intrauterine environment, the sounds were relatively constant and rhythmical. Sounds from the mother's environment did reach the fetus, but were muted to a degree by body tissue and the amniotic fluid. The sounds in the external environment vary from silence to an overwhelming din and include many new sounds the neonate has not previously experienced.

For the fetus, touch consisted of warm amniotic fluid and the smooth wall of the uterus. After birth, for the first time the newborn infant has dry skin. Forms of touch increase dramatically after birth, including input from handling, stroking, rubbing, and possibly pain. The newborn has never worn clothing; even the touch of fabric against the skin is a new sensation. Taste sensations had been limited to amniotic fluid ingested in utero, and breast milk, formula, and possibly oral medications provide new taste experiences. Breast odors are preferred from birth.[168] Infants initially have a preference for amniotic fluid-treated breast versus a "natural" breast, but this changes to a "natural" breast preference within a few days.[215]

Sleep-Wake Pattern

After birth the neonate must manage sleep and activity patterns. Caregivers are important timekeepers for the neonate, but neonates and their mothers are frequently separated. In animals, the mother has an important influence on establishing biorhythms in her offspring. There is evidence that state organization is disturbed in the first few days after birth; there may be increased alertness in the first few days, followed by the infant's beginning to establish his or her own individual pattern.[89]

Neural Connections and Conduction of Impulses

Gestational age determines the level of brain maturation, including acquisition of neuronal component, dendritic and axonal branching, formation of connections between neurons, and myelinization. Although, at term gestation, most neurons have formed and migrated to their respective sites, a number of cerebellar neurons are completing this process and are at particular risk in terms of neonatal asphyxia or hypoxia. For the preterm infant, depending on the degree of prematurity, formation and migration of neurons bears even greater risk.

Although the elaboration of dendritic and axonal branches and connections between neurons begins in fetal life, these processes continue into adulthood. The ability of a neuron to change structure and function has been called plasticity. The more immature the infant is at birth, the greater the impact of CNS plasticity (see Neural [Brain] Plasticity). There is considerable evidence in animal studies that sensory input influences later neuronal structure and function; for instance, an enriched environment during infancy improves developmental outcome by maximizing brain potential. This plasticity is both an advantage and a liability. Although sensory input may increase cellular processes and interconnections, the sensory environment may also produce undesired changes in structure and function.[26,47] The preterm infant in the neonatal intensive care unit may be particularly vulnerable to these alterations.

Myelinization occurs predominantly in fetal and infant life but continues through the fourth decade and beyond. Brain areas governing high-level functions myelinate later in life. In the fetus and infant, myelinization involves both sensory and motor fibers and pathways. The primary effect of myelinization is on speed of transmission or conduction, since the presence of myelin insulates the nerve fiber, increasing conduction rate. Since myelin is being laid down at varying rates throughout the central and peripheral nervous system, rate of conduction potentially affects the integration of sensory information and effector response. In terms of sensory perception, the difference in conduction speed (msec) is not appreciable at the conscious level; however, even seemingly minor differences in transmission have an impact on integration of information. Speed of transmission is important in spatial (number of impulses coming into the CNS from various sites) and temporal (rapidity with which impulses are being sent) summation. Thus systems in which summation is required for neuronal firing may react less quickly. Conduction rate is inversely related to postconceptional age, becoming similar to that in adults by 3 to 4 years.[222]

Circulation in the Neonatal Brain

The brain of the neonate demonstrates differences in circulation compared with that of the adult. These differences produce vulnerability to damage by hypoxemia and pressure.

Brain Barriers

Early in embryonic life, circulation is conducted by a capillary network. Development is accompanied by proliferation of blood vessels, increasing the blood supply to meet the increasing metabolic demands of the growing CNS.

The complexity of the brain's vascular system increases in the last trimester. There is a rapid increase in the number and size of cerebral blood vessels after 26 weeks, peaking by 35 weeks.[95]

Sources of the brain barrier include the tight junctions between endothelial cells forming the capillaries, which limit diffusion of substances into the brain tissue; the basement membrane of the endothelial cells; and the astrocyte foot processes surrounding the capillary.[81] In the fetus and neonate, the tight junction between the capillary endothelial cells is not as well formed as that of the adult. However, the tight junctions develop early and are probably quite effective barriers to proteins, but are probably more permeable to small lipid-soluble molecules.[184] Endothelial tight junctions can be altered by hyposmolar conditions, hypercarbia, asphyxia, and intracranial infection leading to vasculitis with increased permeability and potential for rupture.[222] A second component of the blood-brain barrier is the basement membrane supporting capillary endothelial cells. In the neonate and infant this basement membrane is not fully developed.[81] Additionally, the astrocyte feet, which normally surround the capillary, are not completely developed in the neonate.[81] These three alterations in the blood-brain barrier predispose to capillary leakage and hemorrhage. Since cellular junctions are not well formed, the brain capillaries are sensitive to osmolar (and hence volume) changes of the blood.[81]

Cerebral Autoregulation

Cerebral autoregulation refers to the local control of brain blood flow, modifying resistance to compensate for changes in pressure, thus sustaining consistent flow. Cerebral autoregulation is mediated by vasoactive factors such as H^+ and K^+ ions, adenosine, prostaglandins, osmolality, and calcium.[222] These factors are all operative in the neonate.[222,225] The autoregulatory capabilities of the fetal and neonatal brain are limited, although pressure flow autoregulation is present even in very-low-birth-weight (VLBW) infants.[85] The range for cerebral autoregulation is narrower in the newborn, who is less able to limit cerebral blood flow (CBF) with hypertension.[95] In utero this is not a severe limitation, since metabolic demands of the brain are less and the cardiovascular system is not required to act independently. In the neonate, however, restriction of autoregulation predisposes the neonate to inadequate or excess pressure, resulting in too little or too much blood flow. Consequences are risk of bleeding from vascular rupture, increased intracranial pressure, and hypoxia/ischemia.

Cerebral perfusion pressure is a function of gestational age, and CBF increases with maturation.[212,222] Compared with the adult, however, cerebral perfusion pressure is low in the term infant and even lower in the preterm infant. Preterm infants have an extremely narrow range of autoregulation. Normal blood pressure in the preterm infant is slightly above the lower limit of autoregulation (~30 to 40 mgHg).[95,222] Thus, in the preterm infant, CBF is close to the level at which oxygen and nutrient delivery is potentially compromised.[85,222]

Low CBF and limited autoregulation combine to place the neonate in a position where there is a fine balance between cerebral ischemia and potential rupture of vessels or increased intracranial pressure.[95] The lower the gestational age, the greater the vulnerability is.[222] Autoregulation additionally exhibits a lag in responsiveness. A sudden intense rise or drop in cerebral blood pressure or flow may not be immediately controlled through autoregulatory efforts.[212]

By itself, autoregulation of CBF creates a high-risk situation that is magnified by the influence of hypoxemia. Hypoxemia (including asphyxia) abolishes autoregulation.[222] Thus during hypoxemia, CBF becomes pressure-passive. Auto-regulation is further influenced by hypercarbia and acidosis, conditions that frequently occur in conjunction with hypoxemia.[212] The nature of respiration in preterm infants predisposes to hypoxemia, hypercarbia, and acidosis. Because autoregulation exhibits a lag, even transient alterations in oxygen and carbon dioxide can have deleterious results as autoregulation is compromised.

Effects of autoregulation are a consequence of alterations in cerebral blood pressure and flow. Pressure, resistance, and flow are related physical processes. When blood flow is pressure-passive, a rise in blood pressure produces an increase in flow. The fragile capillaries of the immature brain possess neither tight junctions between endothelial cells nor a strong basement membrane; therefore increased blood pressure and flow increase intracranial pressure.[81] This increased pressure and flow may rupture the delicate capillaries, leading to bleeding.

Impairment of autoregulation may also produce damage through inability to respond to low blood pressure. Under normal circumstances, cerebral perfusion in the neonate is marginally adequate. Given any reduction in blood pressure, autoregulatory abilities do not support maintenance of blood flow. As a result, reduction in blood pressure may reduce cerebral perfusion, producing ischemia and hypoxia. Thus hypoxic damage of brain tissue may ensue. Hypoxia is therefore a critical concern since brain tissue may be injured by lack of oxygen as well as a reduction in CBF.

Certain areas of the brain are more sensitive than others to changes in blood flow. The nature of the distribution of the vascular system in the brain and the type of tissue (white or gray matter) are associated with risk for hypoxic damage. Vessels supplying blood to the brain have little overlap. The area defining margins between two vascular beds is called a boundary (or watershed) area. Boundary areas are particularly prone to disruptions of circulation and hypoxia because blood supply is limited.[212,222] The subependymal germinal matrix layer, located in ventricular and subventricular areas, is one such area.[81]

Blood flow is linked to metabolism. Gray matter has a higher metabolic rate than that of white matter; consequently, perfusion of gray matter exceeds that of white matter.[222] The lower blood flow in white matter predisposes this form of nervous tissue to the effects of limited autoregulation and hypoxemia.[212,222] One area particularly vulnerable to pressure- and hypoxia-related injury is the periventricular white matter.

Neonatal Sensory Function

In general the rate of nerve transmission continues to increase with postconceptional age. Evidence from animal experiments suggests that active use of sensory receptors and pathways is required for further development. Sensory deprivation results in degeneration of neural structures, leading to permanent damage and long-term implications for sensory function. In most circumstances, however, sensory deprivation does not occur. Rather, as discussed in later sections, sensory stimulation is more often excessive and the quality and pattern of stimulation may be inappropriate for the neonate.

A second consideration is the need for attention as a prerequisite for sensory input. The neonate's level of alertness and arousal determines attention to sensory stimulation. Thus any condition affecting neurologic control of alertness interferes with reception and processing of sensory input. The autonomic nervous system mediates responsiveness to external environment.[83] Alertness and arousal are functions of the infant's sleep-wake patterns or state, as well as the infant's physiologic status. Sensory input must always be considered in light of the infant's state.

Sensory Modalities

Neonates possess well developed sensitivity to vestibular and kinesthetic stimulation. Rocking motions produce soothing and quieting of the neonate and infant. Use of vestibular stimulation with preterm infants has been associated with increased rhythmicity and organization, decreased apnea, improved weight gain, sleep promotion, and increased alertness and attention.[127]

The term neonate can detect, localize, and discriminate various distinct odorants and respond to noxious odors. Neonates and infants can differentiate breast pads soaked with their mother's breast milk from those soaked with water or other substances. They habituate to repeated presentation of the same odor and show a preference for odors associated with positive reinforcements.[123,231] Term neonates exhibit a preference for sweet taste, showing aversion to sour or salty tastes, and can differentiate tastes.[217,231] Preterm infants respond to taste and smell by 26 to 27 weeks and possibly earlier, since this has not been extensively studied.

Term newborns can hear and discriminate sounds (see Table 14-9). Hearing acuity is best in the low and mid-range frequencies, with high-frequency hearing developing in later infancy.[164] Additionally, hearing sensitivity increases with development and hearing threshold decreases.[164] Term infants differentiate sounds, attending to sounds of interest and showing aversion to noxious sounds. They can distinguish their mothers' voices and readily turn toward the direction of the mother's voice. Neonates and infants demonstrate a preference for high intonation and the rhythmic, sing-song vocalization that is called "motherese." Auditory capabilities of VLBW infants are discussed in Development of the Neuromuscular and Sensory Systems in the Fetus (p. 474) and are summarized in Table 14-9.

Although vision in the term neonate is qualitatively different from that of the adult, the visual abilities of these infants are adept. Vision is functional at birth, but marked changes occur in the first 6 months of life.[78,93] The retina continues to mature after birth. The fovea, the most sensitive area of the retina associated with high-level discrimination, is not as sensitive in the neonate as in adults.[78,93] The neonate's limited accommodation ability decreases the ability to focus on objects that are extremely close to or far from the face. Accommodation improves during the first 3 months of life.[93] Infants see objects to a distance of at least 2½ feet but attend best to objects that are within 8 to 12 inches from their eyes and have high contrast or contours.[83,93] Neonates can follow movement of an object. Visual function in term infants is summarized in Table 14-10.

Preterm infants demonstrate pupillary light responses and blinking to light by 29 weeks' gestation with awake visual attention by 30 weeks. These infants fix on simple patterns by 30 weeks' gestation and demonstrate pattern preferences by 31 to 32 weeks. Visual scanning with cessation of sucking is seen from 30 weeks and is active after 36 weeks.[89,222] Preterm infants take longer to fixate on an object and are less responsive to visual stimuli than term infants and have poorer visual acuity and ability to accommodate. Most of the visual stimuli to which VLBW infants are exposed during their brief periods of awake are probably inappropriate to the infants' visual capabilities.[28,89] Visual capabilities of VLBW infants are discussed

further in Development of the Neuromuscular and Sensory Systems in the Fetus (p. 474) and are summarized in Table 14-10.

Sensory Processing

The neonate is readily capable of receiving sensory information. The neonate also demonstrates the ability to discriminate sensory information and to attend to sensory input. Knowledge of the neonate's sensory reception abilities must be balanced with appreciation of sensory processing abilities, since in this area the neonate demonstrates developmental differences of the nervous system that have implications for long-term outcomes. Although reception of sensory input is grossly intact, the ability to process information and respond in an organized fashion is limited. Adaptation, habituation, and inhibition limit responsiveness to stimuli; without these processes, people would be bombarded with input. In the brain of the neonate the structures and processes that underlie the ability to modulate sensory input are not well developed.

The neonate's brain continues to develop connections between neurons and lay down myelin. The degree of connectedness between neurons and speed of electrical conduction affect integration and organization of overall nervous system function. Behaviors of the neonate reflect these underlying maturational differences in the CNS. Neonates may exhibit differences in arousability, the extensiveness of responses, attention, tolerance to stimulation, soothability, regularity of state, motor tone, activity, synchrony, and rhythmicity.[8,52] Although stimulation is required for normal development, the neonate can also be overwhelmed by sensory input because of the level of brain development. Just as environmental temperature for the neonate must be neither too warm or too cool, so too the sensory input for a neonate must be balanced to the infant's individual needs and tolerance. Provision of a developmentally appropriate sensory environment is based on "stimuli that have sensory or affective properties that are consistent with developmental capabilities and thus most likely to be appropriately incorporated into neural processes"[47] For extremely immature infants, this means delaying auditory and visual input until the infants is stable and has more mature neurosensory capabilites.[28]

Neural (Brain) Plasticity

The brain changes in response to external experiences (plasticity). Development involves gene-environment interaction. The environment affects how genes work and genes affect how environment is interpreted. Neuronal differentiation and organization are controlled by the interaction of genes and the environment. Animal studies demonstrate that environmental input influences the fate and neural capabilities at the cellular level both before and after birth.[129] Each neuron has many synaptic connections that allow the brain to integrate and organize information. Initially there is an overproduction of neurons and nerve connections. Many of the extra neurons and connections are later eliminated based on early environment and experiences.[26,47] The brain is thought to strengthen and retain connections that are used repeatedly and is more likely to eliminate underused connections. Thus improper sensory input (too much or too little) or input that is inappropriate in terms of timing may alter brain development.[26]

Greenough and Black have postulated that there are two types of neural plasticity: experience-expectant and experience-dependent.[26,84] Experience-expectant plasticity is thought to be linked to the brain developmental timetable; that is, specific sensory experiences and input are needed at specific times for neural development and maturation. This stage requires appropriate timing and quality of input for normal development. Thus altered sequences or types of sensory input can alter or disrupt development. Experience-dependent plasticity involves interaction with the environment to develop specific skills for later use. This form of plasticity involves memory and learning and allows development of flexibility, adaptation, and individual differences in social and intellectual development.[26,84]

Neonatal Motor Function

Movement may be reflexive or volitional in nature. In adults, as in neonates, volitional motor activity entails movement under the control of the cortex and other higher-level control. In the neonate, however, control of motor function is emerging and demonstrates increasing integration and organization of the CNS. Reflexes in the neonates are somewhat different from those seen in the adult. Some of the reflexes exhibited by the neonate reflect both development of the muscles themselves as well as CNS control. Additionally, some reflexes normally observed only in the neonate and infant indicate the effects of development in motor control mechanisms. In general, motor activities include muscle tone, motor abilities, the quality of movement, and presence and strength of reflexes.[70] Motor control is critical to further development. Through movement and reflexes, infants are capable of expressing needs, eliciting care, taking in oral nutrients, and experiencing and manipulating the environment.

Muscle Development

The motor abilities of the neonate demonstrate a characteristic pattern of development that reflects underlying changes in both nervous system control and maturation of the muscle cells themselves. Muscle is derived from mesoderm. During embryonic development, formation of muscle cells is dependent on innervation by the nervous system. The full complement of muscle cells is generally achieved at approximately 38 weeks' gestational age, with formation of few muscle cells after this time. After birth, muscle cells increase in size by increasing the diameter of the muscle fibers and also grow in length.[144] Muscle strength in particular is an outcome of muscle enlargement and growth.

Developmental changes in the innervation of muscle include myelinization of afferent fibers and pathways; increasing activity in the motor cortex; and increasing coordination of system-modifying motor actions such as the cerebellum, basal ganglia, and reticular activating system. Myelinization improves the speed of motor nerve conduction. Maturation of the motor cortex allows conscious control of motor activities. The increasing integration of all levels of motor control results in smooth, coordinated movements; balance; and appropriate motor tone. Neonates exhibit a characteristic pattern of tone and flexion that undergoes predictable change throughout development.

The term neonate demonstrates strong muscle tone, which is largely passive.[222] After birth, active motor tone, which is the tone during use of muscles, increases and passive tone decreases. Alterations in muscle tone interfere with motor activities. Hypertonicity (excessive muscle tone) and hypotonicity (inadequate muscle tone) affect the underlying muscle tension that normally supports motor function. The predominant flexed position of the term neonate shows innervation of flexor muscles and reciprocal relaxation of extensor muscles. The flexed position is not only protective but also assists in conservation of energy by reducing motor movements and assists in thermoregulation by reducing the surface area for heat loss. Motor development entails inhibition of flexion and increasing extensor activity. These changes occur in part because of increasing control by the motor cortex. When cortical innervation is interrupted, as in many pathologic conditions, loss of extensor innervation results in flexion. Increasing sophistication of control by the CNS improves coordination of movement, control and accuracy of movement, and synchrony and rhythmicity of movement. These capabilities support ongoing motor development including head control, turning over, reaching, and grasping.

Neonatal Reflexes

Reflexes are automatic, built-in motor behaviors occurring at the spinal level. Reflexes therefore provide information about muscle tone and lower level motor function. In the neonate the presence of "built-in" behaviors is critical, since at birth the neonate has no experience in the extrauterine environment. Reflexes serve many neonatal needs and also provide valuable information regarding the neonate's motor and neural status. Although reflexes are automatic rather than volitional, the reflexive responses of the neonate provide evidence to parents and other caregivers of the neonate's motor capabilities, responsiveness, and individual needs. The development and strength of reflexes varies with gestational age.

Many reflexes characteristic to the neonate seemingly disappear with development. Some reflexes (such as the Babinski reflex) are masked by higher-order functions but are observed in the adult when pathologic conditions interfere with higher-level control. Other reflexes considered abnormal in the adult are seen in the neonate. For instance, clonus of the knee and ankle is commonly observed in the neonate, as is the Babinski reflex.[5]

The Moro reflex involves abduction of the arms at the shoulder with the elbows in extension and the hands open, followed by adduction of the arms at the shoulder into an embrace position with flexion of the elbows. Crying often accompanies the Moro reflex. Portions of the Moro reflex can be observed as early as 28 weeks' gestational age, with a mature reflex seen at approximately 36 to 37 weeks.[14]

Neonates exhibit a strong palmar grasp reflex with fingers tightly flexed and curled into the palm. The palmar grasp reflex is so strong that infants can grasp, although not consciously, items placed in the hand. The palmar grasp may also be assessed in the pull-to-sit maneuver. Although the palmar grasp is first observed at approximately 28 weeks' gestational age, full strength is not achieved until approximately 32 weeks.[14]

The tonic neck reflex (also termed the *fencing position*) is stimulated by rotation of the head to the side. The reflex movements include extension of the arm and leg on the side to which the head is turned, and flexion of the arm and leg on the side opposite to which the head is turned. The movements of the extremities are similar to the crossed extensor reflex. Portions of the tonic neck reflex appear during later fetal development, but the reflex is often not well established until 1 month after birth.[222] Like the Moro reflex, the tonic neck reflex stabilizes position, preventing rolling.

Neonates demonstrate a rhythmic stepping motion of their lower extremities. When the neonate is held upright with the feet touching a solid surface, an alternating stepping motion is observed. There is some evidence that coordination exhibited in the stepping reflex may be predictive of later developmental outcomes.

The sucking and rooting reflexes are essential for oral intake of nutrients by the neonate. Rooting assists the neonate in locating and latching on to the nipple and occurs at about 32 weeks' gestation.[5] Stimulation of the perioral region result in turning of the head in the direction of the stimulus and mouthing actions in search of the nipple. The sucking reflex is present at 28 weeks' gestation, but is weak and uncoordinated with swallowing. Some suck-swallow synchrony is seen by 32 to 34 weeks, and synchrony is complete by 36 to 38 weeks.[14]

Sleep-Wake Pattern

Fetal activity records document fluctuating periods of activity and quiescence, seen as early as 21 weeks' gestation.[199] After birth the infant exhibits alternating periods of sleep and wakefulness that initially reflect fetal activity/inactivity patterns.[122] Sleep in neonates and infants exhibits developmental differences from that of the adult. As a result, sleep is not as well defined and definitions are less precise than in the adult. Consequently, neonatal and infant sleep is described in terms of state—that is, a group of physiologic and behavioral characteristics that regularly recur together.[28]

Neonates and infants spend a large portion of the 24-hour day sleeping. Sleep therefore does not follow a light-dark pattern and is not diurnal, as in the adult. A major accomplishment in the development of the infant is the ability to sleep through the night and adapt to the diurnal pattern of activity and sleep-wake behaviors of the family. The sleep-wake pattern is an indicator of neurologic status and the neonate's ability to organize behavior.

Definition of Infant States

A number of systems have been developed to code or score neonatal and infant sleep-wake states. The major difference between conventional definitions of infant states is the number of subtypes of states and therefore the specificity and precision of the various states. Generally, the more immature the neonate is according to gestational and postconceptional age, the grosser or less precise the definitions of state, since the quality of state and consistency among indicators improve with age (Table 14-11). The six categories of infant state described by Wolff[234] will be discussed. Each state is complete unto itself, representing a particular form of neural control.[89] The six sleep-wake states are as follows: quiet (deep) sleep, active (light) sleep, drowsy, awake (quiet) alert, active alert, and crying (Table 14-12). The ability to clearly differentiate these states is dependent on the infant's postcon-

TABLE **14-11**   Infant State Parameters by Gestational Age

	GESTATIONAL AGE (WEEKS)					MONTHS PAST TERM	
	24	28	32	36	40	3	8
Body movements	±	+	++	+++	++++	++++	++++
Eye movements		+	++	+++	++++	++++	++++
Respiration pattern			±	++	+++	++++	++++
Electroencephalograph			±	++	+++	++++	++++
Chin electromyelograph				+	+++	++++	++++

From Parmelee, A.H. & Stern, E. (1972). Development of states in infants. In C.D. Clemente, D.P. Purpura, & F.E. Mayer (Eds.). *Sleep and the maturing nervous system.* New York: Academic Press.

ceptional age. The proportion of time spent in each of these states also varies with postconceptional age.

Quiet (deep or NREM) sleep is deep, restful sleep with the eyes closed, little body or facial movement, except for an occasional startle or twitch, regular respiration and heart rate, and no movement of the eyes.[159] Quiet sleep is restorative and anabolic. An increase in cell mitosis and replication occurs during this state. Oxygen consumption reaches the lowest levels during quiet sleep. In addition, the release of growth hormone is associated with quiet sleep, as are high levels of serotonin and low levels of glucocorticoid.

During active (light) sleep the eyes are closed but there are movements of the extremities and face, mouthing, grimacing, and sucking movements. Respiration and heart rate are irregular and penile erections occur. Active bouts of REM occur in association with dreaming; the fine, rapid movement of the eyes can be observed beneath the lid. Active sleep is also called paradoxical sleep or REM sleep and has been likened to "wide-awake asleep" because the level of brain activity is similar to that of the awake state. Information is processed during active sleep and entered into memory; thus active sleep has been linked to learning. Restructuring of synapses and changes in protein synthesis increase during active sleep.

During the drowsy state, the infant seems partially awake and partially asleep. Drowsiness usually indicates a state transition between awake and sleep states. In the quiet alert state, the infant is awake, the eyes are open, and there is little motor movement. The infant is alert and shows interest or attention by focusing on visual stimulation. The infant appears to be "drinking in" information from the surrounding environment and processing this information. This state is characterized by limited motion and activity associated with the infant attending to sensory information.

The neonate or infant's motor activity escalates in the active awake state. The eyes are less bright than in the quiet alert state. There may be spitting up or hiccoughing. Respiration often becomes increased and irregular and skin color changes may occur. The active alert state often precedes crying. In healthy infants, crying is easily recognizable. Crying behaviors include closed eyes with facial characteristics and the vocalization of cry sounds. In preterm infants the motor actions associated with cry sounds are evident, but because of the infant's immaturity and weakness, the sounds may not be produced.

Sleep-Wake States Related to Brain Maturation

Sleep is required for brain development. Sleep-wake patterns change with CNS maturation. Postnatal development of sleep-wake state pattern reflects the underlying maturation of the reticular activating system, brain stem, and related circadian rhythms. The developmental changes in state include both alterations in temporal pattern and the integration of variables within the state. Inhibitory ability increases with CNS maturation. Increased inhibitory ability results in smoother muscle movements, reduces global responses, improves habituation and adaptation, and generally acts to improve the infant's attentional abilities as well as bring about specific changes in sleep. These sleep changes include increasing duration of sleep periods, consolidation of sleep into nighttime hours, and maturation of the sleep states themselves.[40] Within each state, synchrony among the state variables increases.

Infant development entails increasing amounts of quiet sleep as well as increasing periods of quiet alertness. Both of these states reflect sophisticated neural control. Sustaining a state consistently or making a transition from one state to another requires tremendous neural organization. Thus sleep-wake patterns are an excellent window to the infant's neurologic status. Alterations in sleep-wake patterns are observed in infants with Down syndrome, biochemical disturbances, and brain malformations, and following asphyxia.[89]

TABLE **14-12** Infant State Chart (Sleep and Awake States)

State*	Body Activity	Eye Movements	Facial Movements
SLEEP STATES			
Quiet (deep) sleep	Nearly still, except for occasional startle or twitch	None	Without facial movements, except for occasional sucking movement at regular intervals
Active (light) sleep	Some body movements	Rapid eye movement (REM); fluttering of eyes beneath closed eyelids	May smile and make brief fussy or crying sounds
AWAKE STATES			
Drowsy	Activity level variable, with mild startles interspersed from time to time; movements usually smooth	Eyes open and close occasionally; are heavy-lidded with dull, glazed appearance	May have some facial movements, but often there are none and the face appears still
Quiet alert	Minimal	Brightening and widening of eyes	Faces have bright, shining, sparkling looks
Active alert	Much body activity; may have periods of fussiness	Eyes open with less brightening	Much facial movement; faces not as bright as in quiet alert state.
Crying	Increased motor activity with color changes	Eyes may be tightly closed or open	Grimaces

From Blackburn, S. & Kang, R. (1991). *Early Parent-Infant Relationships* (2nd ed.). White Plains, New York: March of Dimes Birth Defects Foundation.
*State is a group of characteristics that regularly occur together: body activity, eye movements, facial movements, breathing pattern, and level of response to external stimuli (e.g., handling) and internal stimuli (e.g., hunger).

Sleep is necessary for somatic and brain growth and development. As described earlier, restorative and growth processes are facilitated during quiet sleep. REM sleep is important for learning and memory. Attention behavior development parallels development of quiet sleep, indicating both inhibition and maturity.[159] The amount of quiet awake time parallels quiet sleep, and both increase with development.[89]

Development of Infant States

Before 28 to 30 weeks of gestational age, the preterm infant shows minimal pattern of state activity either by behavioral or electroencephalographic (EEG) characteristics. Active sleep or REM appears at 28 to 30 weeks' gestation with evidence of cycling of states at 32 weeks.[51,89] Quiet sleep appears much later in postconceptional devel-

BREATHING PATTERN	LEVEL OF RESPONSE	IMPLICATIONS FOR CAREGIVING
Smooth and regular	Threshold to stimuli very high so that only very intense and disturbing stimuli will arouse	Caregivers trying to feed infants in quiet sleep will probably find the experience frustrating. Infants will be unresponsive, even if caregivers use disturbing stimuli to arouse infants. Infants may arouse only briefly and then become unresponsive as they return to quiet sleep. If caregivers wait until infants move to a higher, more responsive state, feeding or caregiving will be much more pleasant.
Irregular	More responsive to internal and external stimuli; when these stimuli occur, infants may remain in active sleep, return to quiet sleep, or arouse to drowsy	Active sleep makes up the highest proportion of newborn sleep and usually precedes awakening. Because of brief fussy or crying sounds made during this state, caregivers who are not aware that these sounds occur normally may think it is time for feeding and may try to feed infants before they are ready to eat.
Irregular	Infants react to sensory stimuli, although responses are delayed; state change after stimulation frequently noted	From the drowsy state, infants may return to sleep or awaken further. To awaken, caregivers can provide something for infants to see, hear, or suck, as this may arouse them to a quiet alert state, a more responsive state. Infants who are left alone without stimuli may return to a sleep state.
Regular	Infants attend most to the environment, focusing attention on any stimuli that are present	Infants in this state provide much pleasure and positive feedback for caregivers. Providing something for infants to see, hear, or suck will often maintain a quiet alert state. In the first few hours after birth, most newborns commonly experience a period of intense alertness before going into a long sleep period.
Irregular	Increasingly sensitive to disturbing stimuli (hunger, fatigue, noise, excessive handling) Extremely responsive to unpleasant external or internal stimuli	Crying is the infant's communication signal. It is a response to unpleasant stimuli from the environment or within infants (e.g., fatigue, hunger, discomfort). Crying says that infants' limits have been reached. Sometimes infants can console themselves and return to lower states. At other times, they need help from caregivers. Caregivers may need to intervene at this state to console and bring the infant to a lower state.

opment, initially becoming apparent at approximately 36 weeks of gestational age.[159] With maturation, transitional sleep decreases.[222] General trends in sleep development include increasing quiet sleep, decreasing active sleep, and putting sleep cycles together consecutively, which yields longer sleep periods.[103]

The EEG of the infant is not always consistent with the behavioral expression of state. State is evidenced behaviorally before it is apparent on the EEG. Before 30 weeks' gestation, EEG activity is present but is discontinuous and of low amplitude. At 30 to 36 weeks of gestational age, active sleep can be determined by EEG.[222] Between 36 and 40 weeks of gestational age, both active and quiet sleep can be determined by EEG. Maturation of EEG activity includes differentiation of discontinuous activity into mature EEG wave forms and an increase in the amplitude of EEG waves.[58] The EEG of the newborn frequently shows paroxysmal activity, asymmetry of the left and right portions of the brain, and considerable individual variation.[91]

Continued development of sleep-wake patterns after birth also involves changes in the temporal pattern of sleep and the integration of variables within states. In the first month, neonates sleep an average of 12 to 16 hours per day.[22] Periods of sleep occur around the clock. Periods of sleep are short, typically not extending beyond 3 or 4 hours. The sleep cycle is roughly 50 minutes, compared with the 90-minute adult sleep cycle, and sleep is predominantly active in nature, with 50% to 90% of sleep time in active sleep, depending on postconceptional age. Circadian rhythmicity matures after birth with development of the sleep-wake rhythms and hormonal secretion prominent in the first 2 months.[176]

State Modulation

Some infants seem to "sleep like babies," whereas some are difficult to soothe, awaken easily, and sleep for short intervals and at unpredictable times. Other infants are overly drowsy, difficult to arouse, and sleep excessive periods of time. Differences in sleep-wake patterns reflect differences in neurologic development and the infant's ability to modulate state. State modulation refers to the infant's ability to make smooth transitions between states, arouse when appropriate, and sustain sleep states. By modulating or regulating state, the infant can control sensory input to some extent and the response to the environment.[30,83] In addition, the infant can use state behaviors to guide caregiving and to modify social interactions. Problems with state modulation, therefore, entail problems regulating sensory input and responses. Infants who cannot use state changes to turn stimulation on or off may be either missing important input or become sensorially overloaded. State modulation is therefore an asset in the infant's adaptation to the environment. Problems with state modulation may emanate from the infant or environment. Infant factors influencing state modulation include immaturity, pain, stress, maternal substance abuse, and illness. Environmental factors that affect state regulation and interfere with the infant's sleep-wake pattern include noise, light, temperature, and caregiver actions.

Neurobehavioral Organization

The concept of neurobehavioral organization is a means of holistically viewing the infant's response capabilities. The connectedness between elements of the nervous system is the basis for integration and organization of overall function. Neurobehavioral organization captures the essence of neonatal and infant function in the extrauterine environ-

ment and determines the infant's interaction with the surrounding physical and social environment.

What does neurobehavioral organization encompass? Als' synactive theory of development defines five subsystems governing the infant's interaction with the environment: autonomic/physiologic, motor, state organizational, attentional/interactive, and self-regulatory capacity.[6] These subsystems are interdependent and hierarchical; that is, the order of development begins with autonomic/physiologic stability, followed in succession by motor, state, and attentional/interactive, and finally development of self-regulatory capacity. The level of organization is determined by development and is largely dependent on postconceptional age; however, illness or injury may alter neurologic function and therefore neurobehavioral organization. In addition, organization at any level is determined by the previous levels. Thus, state organization is dependent on organization and stability of the motor and autonomic/physiologic subsystems; attentional/interactive behaviors require organization of the state, motor, and autonomic/physiologic subsystems. An infant's behavioral responses or cues are indicative of the level of organization.

Autonomic organization entails regulation of cardiorespiratory activity, gastrointestinal peristalsis, and peripheral skin blood flow. Motor organization includes skeletal muscle tone, posture, and quality of movement. State organization involves orderly progression of sleep-wake states, the ability to sustain a state, and smooth state transitions. The culmination of neurobehavioral organization is the infant's attentional/interactive and self-regulatory abilities. The attentional/interactive subsystem involves the infant's ability to orient and focus on stimuli and achieve well-defined periods of alertness. Self-regulatory capacity is the ability of the infant to maintain integrity and balance between the other subsystems, integrate all the subsystems, and modulate state.[6]

Neurobehavioral organization thus refers to the ability to modulate state, control internal reactions, control motor responses, self-regulate, respond to people and events in the external stressors, and maintain an appropriate degree of alertness.[30] Neurobehavioral organization is critical to energy consumption, oxygen and calorie requirements, and growth, as well as the foundation for development and interactions with parents and other caregivers. Examples of neurobehavioral organization include the ability to regulate sensory input, feed efficiently and effectively, coordinate sucking and swallowing, self-console, exhibit smooth coordinated movement, maintain muscle tone, and elicit caregiving through appropriate cues. Tools to asses neurobehavioral organization rely on observation of the infant in interaction with both the physical and social environments. The Brazelton Newborn Behavioral Assessment Scale (BNBAS) is an assessment of the infant's ability to organize and modulate states, habituate to external stimulation, regulate motor activity in the face of increasing sensory input, respond to reflexive testing, alert and orient to visual and auditory stimuli, interact with a caregiver, and self-console.[30] The Assessment of Preterm Infants' Behavior (APIB) is a neurobehavioral tool based on Als' synactive theory of development and geared to the assessment of the preterm infant and high-risk term infants. The purpose of the APIB assessment is to determine how the infant is coping with the intense environment of the neonatal intensive care unit (NICU) and the degree of CNS organization.[9]

CLINICAL IMPLICATIONS FOR NEONATAL CARE

During the neonatal period, glial proliferation, myelinization, cell differentiation, dendrite expansion, and synapse formation and remodeling are occurring. The developing CNS is vulnerable to a number of influences, including the effects of the environment, handling, and caregiving. In addition, the immature CNS produces variations in seizure activity and influences the diagnosis and treatment of pain. These concerns are particularly important when considering the infant born prematurely, since development of the nervous system is not consistent with demands posed by the extrauterine environment. The preterm infant is usually a third trimester fetus, and, with the increasing survival of extremely premature infants, viability is extending into the second trimester.

Risks Posed by the Caregiving Environment

Healthy term infants are well equipped to adapt to life outside the uterus. When neonates are compromised by illness or prematurity, adaptive abilities are challenged. The extrauterine environment is a critical factor in the development of the immature CNS and may alter developmental outcomes.[211] The hospital care environment has been viewed as providing a deficient or inappropriate sensory environment for the immature infants. Caregiving should always be individualized and be based on recognition of infant cues (Table 14-13).[6,8,28] Emphasis has been placed on controlling the physical environment, including noise and light, and caregiving interactions such as pacing and individualizing caregiving to fit the infant's level of neurobehavioral maturation.[6,8,28]

Stability or engagement cues demonstrate organization and reflect the infant's readiness for interaction (see Table 14-13). Distress or disengagement cues (see Table 14-13) indicate disorganization and signal the caregiver to provide

TABLE 14-13   Infant Neurobehavioral Cues

Distress/ Disengagement Cues	Stability/ Engagement Cues
Bradycardia, apnea	Facial gaze
Rapid heart or respiration rate	Smiling
	Vocalization
Grunting	Feeding posture
Stooling	Flexion of arms and legs
Mottled skin	Eyes alert
Dusky color	Stable heart rate
Cyanosis	Stable respiratory rate
Tremor	Smooth movements
Finger splay	Hand to mouth
Fingers interlaced	Finger folding
Arching	Smooth state transitions
Hyperalert face	Sucking and mouthing
Facial grimace	Consolable
Limb extension	"Ooh" face
Gaze aversion	Alert
Eyes closed	Eye-to-eye contact
Slack jaw	Grasping
Open mouth	
Tongue thrusting	
Sighing	
Regurgitation	
Jittery	
Flaccid	
Vomiting	
Hand to ear	
Worried face	
Rapid state change	
Eyes floating	
Staring	
Hyperextension	
Glassy eyed	
Tongue protrusion	
Flushed	
Hiccough	
Startle	
Yawn	
Flaccidity	
Sneezing	

Compiled from references 6, 8, 28, and 145.

supportive measures and time for recuperation. Supportive measures include interventions such as positioning, providing boundaries, swaddling, and reducing handling.[6,28,213] The Neonatal Individualized Developmental Care and Assessment Program (NIDCAP) is a specialized training program for high-risk infant care providers that focuses on sensitive recognition of infant behavioral cues and strategies and individualized intervention strategies to promote and support neurobehavioral organization.[8]

Vulnerability to Hypoxic and Pressure-Related Injury

Systemic hypoxemia and decreased cerebral perfusion leading to ischemia can lead to hypoxic-ischemic damage to the brain with hemorrhage and edema. The site of injury varies with maturational changes in the vascular anatomy and metabolic activity of the brain. In preterm infants of less than 32 to 34 weeks' gestation, injury is usually associated with periventricular-intraventricular hemorrhage or PVL. In older preterm and term infants, insults of this type result in hypoxic-ischemic encephalopathy in the cerebral cortex and other areas.

Periventricular and Intraventricular Hemorrhage

Periventricular hemorrhage (PVH) and intraventricular hemorrhage (IVH) are common forms of intracranial hemorrhage in the neonate. The consequences of intracranial hemorrhage include direct neuronal damage due to pressure and inflammation and potential hydrocephalus; severe hemorrhage often results in death.[220,221] Long-term outcomes are variable but include motor and sensory disabilities as well as cognitive delay.

The occurrence of PVH/IVH is related to structural and functional differences in the immature CNS, including the nature of the subependymal germinal matrix, differences in regulation of CBF, and venous pressure. The hemorrhage usually begins as microvascular event that spreads, presumably due to overperfusion of the area. The site of PVH/IVH is developmentally related. In term infants the hemorrhage is predominantly in the ventricular choroid plexus and trauma is more often a precipitating factor.[222] In preterm infants, bleeding occurs more often in the subependymal germinal matrix located adjacent the lateral ventricles in the subependymal layer (PVH), with subsequent extension of the hemorrhage into the ventricles (IVH).[221,222] PVH in preterm infants occurs most often in the area of the caudate nucleus and foramen of Monro. Blood may also be found in the white matter with severe IVH because of an associated hypoxic-ischemic insult. The highest risk of PVH/IVH is during the period of germinal matrix involution in infants less than 34 weeks of gestation.[81] Thus the more immature the neonate is, the greater the risk of PVH/IVH.[219]

The germinal matrix is a highly cellular, high metabolic area characterized as gelatinous in structure.[222] The germinal matrix receives a rich blood supply chiefly through a large bed of large, irregular vessels (immature vascular rete) that are fragile due to a thin basement membrane and prone to disruption.[95] In addition, the venous drainage in the area of the germinal matrix entails a distinctive U-shaped curve, and venous tributaries merge and flow into the vein of Galen, which is predisposed to stasis and increased venous pressure. After about 35 weeks, the germinal matrix involutes and the blood vessels become true capillaries.[95]

The physical characteristics of the germinal matrix, along with its highly vascular nature and potential limits in venous drainage, predispose to bleeding. These characteristics interact with cerebral autoregulation and the effects of hypoxia on autoregulation. During episodes of hypoxemia, autoregulation is abolished and blood flow becomes pressure-passive. Hypercarbia and acidosis also disrupt autoregulation. Thus any condition that reduces blood oxygen levels may alter autoregulation and contribute to the development of PVH/IVH. Although cardiorespiratory problems are easily recognized as sources of hypoxia, any factor that increases oxygen demand beyond the supply capabilities (i.e., increased metabolic rate) is also suspect in producing hypoxia, altered autoregulation, and PVH/IVH. Examples include thermoregulatory requirements, effects of handling, environmental disruptions, pain, or motor activity. During periods of pressure-passive flow, fragile capillaries of the germinal matrix may rupture if CBF or pressure increase. Once capillary disruption occurs, alterations in coagulation—which are thought to accompany perinatal complications—potentially perpetuate the hemorrhage.

Factors that produce fluctuating, decreased, or increased CBF also contribute to PVH/IVH.[219,221] If autoregulation of CBF is compromised, alterations in systemic blood pressure may also be causative factors. Examples of conditions thought to contribute to PVH/IVH include the pressure effects of ventilatory assistance, infusion of volume-expanding fluids, hypercarbia and other causes of cerebral vasodilatation, increase in central venous pressure, or respiratory distress.[222]

Many of the health care procedures experienced by preterm infants (e.g., handling or suctioning) alter oxygen level and blood pressure. Research on the effects of procedures has shown that blood pressure initially drops, followed by a rise; the more intensive the care is, the greater the initial drop and the greater the rebound.[153] Prevention of PVH/IVH requires sensitivity regarding the fragile nature of the capillaries within the CNS and recognition of the effects of hypoxemia on autoregulation, as well as the role of autoregulation and pressure in cerebral perfusion.[100]

Periventricular Leukomalacia

PVL is a condition in which necrotic changes subsequent to ischemia occur in the white matter in the area of the ventricles.[221] Blood flow is typically impaired by hypotension. Vascular structure and factors influencing CBF place the preterm infant at risk for PVL. Marginal (border or watershed) areas of blood flow occur near the lateral ventricles because of inadequate overlap in circulation.[222] Underperfusion of these areas leads to ischemia and necrosis. PVL is associated with two events. First, reduction of blood oxygen decreases delivery of oxygen to such vulnerable region, leading to hypoxic-ischemic injury. Second, the myelin-producing oligodendroglia are damaged by cytokines or free radicals, which alter cognitive, visual, and motor function.[108,163,222] Damage includes impairment of oligodendrocyte development and survival, thus altering myelinization and axonal damage and disruption. It is unclear if the oligodendrocyte damage leads to axonal disruption or vice versa.[45] Clinical implications for PVH/IVH and PVL entail recognition of the role of energy demands and oxygen level as well as regulation of both systemic blood pressure and cerebral flow. Infants with asphyxia, prolonged rupture of the membranes, and chorioamnionitis are at increased risk for PVL.[108,163]

Hypoxic-Ischemic Encephalopathy

After 33 to 34 weeks' gestation, blood flow and brain metabolic activity are less prominent in the periventricular area and shift to the cortical area. As a result, hypoxia and ischemia in older preterm and term infants is more likely to damage areas of the peripheral and dorsal cerebral cortex. The primary lesion in hypoxic injury is necrosis of neurons in the cortices of the cerebrum and cerebellum, and possibly the brain stem. The primary ischemic injury occurs in the posterior (boundary area) portion of the parasagittal region. This area is farthest from the original blood supply of the major cerebral vessels and with systemic hypotension or hypoperfusion receives the least blood. With asphyxia and systemic hypotension, cerebral perfusion is maintained at first by cerebral vasodilatation and redistribution of blood flow to the brain from other organs. If the asphyxia continues, brain water balance and CBF are altered and ischemia and edema develop.

The primary mechanisms for cell damage with HIE are excitoxicity, inflammation, and oxidation stress that deplete energy reserves in two phases. During the first phase, damage from the initial hypoxic insult leads to cell death secondary to: (1) depolarization and influx of sodium, chloride, and water leading to cell edema and lysis; (2) accumulation of calcium due to activation of NA/K channels and NMDA glutamate–mediated receptors; and (3) damage from oxygen free radicals.[11,106,135,162,183] The second phase involves cytotoxic damage and occurs 8 to 48 hours after the initial insult.[108] There is ongoing research on newer therapeutic strategies including head cooling, calcium channel blockers, antioxidants, xanthine oxidase inhibitors, free radical scavengers, and nitric oxide synthetase inhibitors.[135,150,183]

Neonatal Seizures

Seizure activity is the most frequent sign of neurologic problems in the neonate and infant.[222] Seizures result from an abnormal neuronal electrical discharge. Thus seizures are caused by a number of conditions in which the environment of neurons, which support normal electrical activity, is altered. These conditions include hypoxemia, ischemia, hypoglycemia, hypocalcemia, hyperkalemia, hypomagnesemia, hypo- or hypernatremia, acidosis, and meningitis.[140,222] In general, seizure activity may entail eye movements, oral movements, changes in posture, motor movements such as bicycling or rowing actions, and apnea. Types of seizures and their description are provided in Table 14-14. The timing of seizure onset and type of seizure are related to pathology and gestational age.[222]

Seizure activity is determined by brain maturation. Thus seizures are expressed differently based on gestational age and postmenstrual age and do not resemble the seizure activity of adults.[101,140,222] These differences in seizure activity result from the structural and functional differences in the immature CNS. Lower rate of nerve conduction, limited myelinization, and reduced connectivity between neurons reduce the threshold for and effect the propagation of the seizure.[101,222] Consequently, the signs of seizure in the neonate are often subtle and more localized than in the

---

TABLE 14-14 **Types of Neonatal Seizures**

Subtle Seizures

Premature and full-term infants

Ocular-tonic horizontal deviation of the eyes ± jerking; and sustained eye opening with ocular fixation

Eyelid blinking or fluttering

Sucking, smacking, drooling, or other oral-buccal-lingual movements

"Swimming," "rowing," and "pedaling" movements

Apneic spell

Generalized Tonic Seizures

Primarily premature infants

Tonic extension of upper and lower limbs (mimics decerebrate posturing)

Tonic flexion of upper limbs and extension of lower limbs (mimics decorticate posturing)

Multifocal Clonic Seizures

Primarily full-term infants

Multifocal clonic movements, either simultaneous or in sequence

Nonordered ("non-Jacksonian") migration

Focal Clonic Seizures

Full term more than premature infants

Well-localized clonic jerking

Infant usually not unconscious

From Volpe, J.J. (2001). *Neurology of the newborn* (4th ed.). Philadelphia: W.B. Saunders.

adult. In adults there is a balance between the excitatory (glutamate) and inhibitory (γ-amino butyric acid or GABA) neurotransmitter. In the neonate there is a mismatch, with increased glutamate and a delay in maturation of the inhibitory system.[101] GABA is altered in the early weeks after birth and may alter neonatal responses to AEDs (e.g., phenobarbital and phenytoin) that enhance GABA function.[180] In addition NMDA receptors, which respond to glutamate, are increased in the neonatal brain and spinal cord because glutamate is needed for synaptogenesis.[67,70]

Because seizures involve massive discharge of neurons, a seizure is associated with an intense increase in energy consumption by the neurons. Additionally, the seizure activity may interfere with adequate oxygenation of the blood. Hypoxia, as well as hypoglycemia and other metabolic changes, may occur within the CNS during seizures.[222] Although the neonatal brain is less susceptible than the adult brain to seizure-induced injury, seizures are related to developmental problems, particularly the effects of repeated seizures on the developing nervous system.[101,140,141]

Neonatal Pain

That pain occurs in the neonate and infant is unequivocal. In the history of infant care, the understanding of pain in infants was determined largely by conceptualization of brain function at this age. Since for many years the infant's central nervous function was believed to have minimal function above the level of the brain stem, the infant's ability to perceive and respond to pain was ignored. It was also believed that the infant's level of myelinization prevented reception of pain and therefore attenuated the effects of pain. Finally, discrediting of pain was further rationalized because it was assumed that the infant had no memory for painful experiences. Although a mass of data confirms the occurrence of pain in neonates and infants, many practices in the care of infants continue to be colored by previous thinking. In addition, the difficulty in objectively assessing pain in infants and the appropriate management are still challenges to neonatal care.

Pain Perception in Neonates and Infants

A number of reviews summarize studies that document the presence of pain in the fetus, neonate, and infant.[66,167,194,214] Because of the neurologic development of the neonate, pain may be qualitatively different from that experienced later in life, but it does exist. Table 14-8 summarizes anatomic and functional development of the different parts of the pain system. Pain receptors are in place and in fact the density of pain receptors or nociceptors is greater in the neonate.[16,79] The fibers that conduct pain stimuli to the

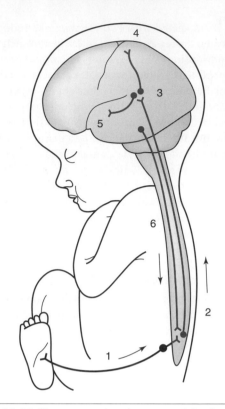

FIGURE **14-13** The neuronal pathways participating in pain. *(1)* Peripheral afferent nerve transmits signal to *(2)* the ascending tract neuron in the spinal cord dorsal horn, which synapses with *(3)* the next neuron in the hypothalamus. Here the pain impulse in distributed to two systems, which bring the signal to *(4)* somatosensory cortex (pain perception) and *(5)* limbic cortex (affective component). In addition there are *(6)* a number of descending neuronal pathways to the dorsal horn of the spinal cord, which modulate the ascending pain impulses. (From Vanhatalo, S. & van Nieuwenhuizen, O. [2000]. Fetal pain? *Brain Dev, 22,* 146.)

spinal cord are in place early in fetal life. Nociceptive receptors are among the first fibers to grow into the spinal cord in the fetus. The density of nociceptive nerve endings in the skin is similar to that in adults until 28 weeks' gestation and then increases to exceed adult density until approximately 2 years of age.[66,214]

In the neonate, transmission of pain occurs primarily along the C fibers, which are unmyelinated fibers, rather than along the A-delta myelinated fibers, as occurs in older individuals.[71] In the spinal cord the pathways (Figure 14-13) that carry pain stimuli to the brain (anterolateral pathways) are undergoing myelinization. Peripheral pain fibers are unmyelinated; therefore myelinization occurring with development does not alter transmission of pain messages to the spinal cord. The pain pathways are myelinated by 30 weeks' gestation, and thalamic fibers that relay information to the cortex are myelinated by 37 weeks' gestation.[222] Thus the rate of transmission may be altered (slower), but this is offset by the shorter distance that impulses must travel to reach the brain. These factors may be particularly important in temporal and spatial summation (see p. 578). Myelinization may have an effect on central processing and integration of pain information. Neonates, both term and preterm, have all the anatomic and functional requirements for pain perception.[66,163] Neonates possess the ability to produce endogenous opiates; increased levels of these substances are found after birth, and levels increase with difficult births and during times of stress (see Chapter 18).[66,167,214] However, levels of these endogenous opioids are still lower than needed to produce analgesia.[66,71]

Consequences of Pain in the Neonate

There is ample evidence to show that the physiologic response to pain is similar in the adult and the neonate (Table 14-15).[66] Neonates and infants feel pain, and pain may have severe consequences in terms of health status and outcomes. Although the infant's inability to verbally describe pain is limited, physiologic responses evidence distress. In general, responses to pain include release of catecholamines and cortisol. Heart rate changes and respiratory rate are linked to increased oxygen consumption. Blood glucose levels rise and the increase in metabolic rate increases energy requirements. A rise in blood pressure produces an elevation in intracranial pressure. Each of these responses may have adverse effects for the neonate, including increased oxygen and ventilatory requirements and changes in blood osmolarity.[167] Hypoxia and the risk of intracranial hemorrhage increase. Furthermore, the energy demands of the stress response to pain have implications for growth and wound healing.

There is further evidence that infants may be more vulnerable to the effects of pain because of their level of neurobehavioral organization and limited coping skills.[167] Neonates have virtually no control over the pain experience and cannot cognitively appreciate what is happening or why.

Of great concern are the long-term effects of early pain experiences on later development and psychologic outcomes. Although this area has not been thoroughly studied, evidence of memory capacities in the neonate augment this concern. Several reports suggest that early stress and pain in the fetus and neonate may alter pain thresholds and produce permanent changes in neural pathways, increasing the risk of later disorders such as adult psychopathology, altered pain sensitivity, altered responses to stress, and stress-related disorders.[10,16,17,36,46,88,166,195]

TABLE 14-15   Pain Responses of Neonates and Infants

MOTOR RESPONSES

Generalized motor activity	Reflexive withdrawal from pain
Swiping movements	Positioning
Increased/decreased motor tone	Fist clenching
Kicking	Wiggling
Guarding	Thrashing
Pulling away	

FACIAL EXPRESSIONS

Grimace	Furrowed brow
Chin quiver	Wincing
Frowning	Cry face
Tears in eyes	Gazing

VOCALIZATIONS

Cry	Whimper
Groan	

SLEEP-WAKE/ACTIVITY DISTURBANCE

Rapid state changes	Inability to sustain state
Increased or decreased activity	Fussiness
Decreased consolability	Irritability
Agitation	Restlessness
Lethargy	

AUTONOMIC RESPONSES

Pallor	Palmar sweating
Diaphoresis	Hyperglycemia
Dilated pupils	Shallow respirations
Increased/decreased heart rate	Apnea
Increased/decreased respiratory rate	Increased ventilatory needs
Decreased oxygen level	Increased/decreased carbon dioxide level
Increase in blood pressure	Increase in intracranial pressure
Cyanosis	Increase in serum cortisol
Flushing	

Compiled from references 66, 71, and 167.

MATURATIONAL CHANGES DURING INFANCY AND CHILDHOOD

Brain growth and maturation continue after birth into childhood and adolescence, with some processes continuing to mature into adulthood. The neonatal period and early infancy are periods of increased vulnerability to insults because of the rapid brain growth during this period. The brain reaches 90% of adult weight by 2 years because

TABLE **14-16** Recommendations for Clinical Practice Related to the Neuromuscular and Sensory Systems in Neonates

Know the major stages for development of the neuromuscular and sensory systems (pp. 560-576).

Provide parent counseling and teaching regarding development of central nervous system (CNS) defects (pp. 560-572 and Table 14-7).

Recognize the stages of CNS development and vulnerabilities in preterm infants (pp. 560-572, 577-578 and Table 14-10).

Recognize the processes of fetal neurosensory development (pp. 573-576).

Recognize the sensorimotor capabilities of the term infant and provide appropriate interventions (pp. 579-582 and Tables 14-9 and 14-10).

Recognize the sensorimotor capabilities of the preterm infant and provide appropriate interventions (pp. 573-576, 580, and Tables 14-9 and 14-10).

Promote neurosensory adaptations during transition to extrauterine life (pp. 576-577).

Protect term and preterm infants from overstimulation (pp. 580-581, 586-587).

Recognize implications of differences in cerebral blood flow and autoregulation within the neonate (pp. 578-579).

Implement interventions to prevent or minimize changes in oxygenation and intracranial pressure (pp. 587-589).

Position term and preterm infants to enhance motor development (pp. 574-575, 581).

Assess reflexes, motor tone, and sensory capabilities (pp. 573-576, 579-582, Figures 14-13 and 14-14, and Tables 14-9 and 14-10).

Recognize normal and abnormal neonatal reflex responses (pp. 581-582).

Recognize different states and their implications (pp. 582-586 and Table 14-12).

Interact with infants appropriate to their state (pp. 582-586 and Table 14-12).

Promote state modulation in term and preterm infants (p. 586).

Promote neurobehavioral organization in term and preterm infants (pp. 586-587).

Recognize stress, stability, engagement, and disengagement cues and respond appropriately (pp. 586-587 and Table 14-13).

Modify the neonatal intensive care unit environment to reduce sensory overload (pp. 580-581, 586-587).

Teach parents to recognize infant states, stress, stability, engagement, disengagement cues, and sensorimotor capabilities (pp. 582-587 and Tables 14-12 and 14-13).

Recognize factors that may increase the risk of periventricular hemorrhage (PVH) and intraventricular hemorrhage (IVH) (pp. 579, 588).

Implement interventions to reduce the risk of PVH and IVH (p. 588).

Recognize signs of seizure activity (pp. 589-590 and Table 14-14).

Recognize consequences of pain in the neonate (pp. 590-591).

Assess infants for signs of pain (p. 591 and Table 14-15).

Use pharmacologic and nonpharmacologic interventions to treat neonatal pain (pp. 590-591).

of increases in nerve fibers and development of nerve tracts. Synaptic density is greatest at 3 years of age. The rate of synapse development differs between brain regions. For example, synaptogenesis in the prefrontal lobe increases form 8 months to a maximum at 2 years; the cortex from 2 years to 12 to 13 years.[47]

Myelinization continues through late adolescence and early adulthood. Nociceptive receptor density gradually decreases to adult levels by 2 years.[66] The cerebellar growth spurt begins later (about 30 weeks' gestation) and ends earlier (about 1 year) than in other areas and thus is particularly vulnerable to nutritional and other insults during infancy. CBF and metabolism increase to 6 years, then decline.[95]

The cranial bones are not fully fused until 16 to 18 months of age. With increasing gestational age, conduction rates increase. The speed of transmission becomes similar to adults by 3 to 4 years of age.[222] At 8 months, electrical responses after stimulation become like those observed in the adult.[197] By 8 months of age, the six EEG patterns observed in the mature brain are found in the EEG of the infant.[159] The

Moro reflex disappears by 6, palmar grasp by 2, and tonic neck reflex by 7 months of age.

Sensory abilities are similar to those of the adult at approximately 2 years of age. Visual acuity is adultlike at 6 months of age. Depth perception matures sometime after 3 months of age. Color vision is present to some degree by 2 months of age and increases at 3 months.[93] By 4 to 5 months, visual-motor neuroconnections begin to develop, although the prehensile stage is not reached until 6 to 7 months. By 5 to 6 months, visual impulses begin to be retained (memory), with recognition of familiar and strange objects and faces.

Infants sleep a mean of 14 hours per day by 1 month of age.[22] As the infant develops, total sleep time (the total number of hours spent asleep) per day decreases to a mean of 13 hours per day by 12 months.[22] Sleep cycles increase in length, reaching the adult length in roughly the late school-age years. The infant is increasingly capable of linking together two or more sleep cycles, leading to increased duration of sleep periods.[102] Sleep first exhibits longer periods and then gradually becomes consolidated into the night-time hours. The percentage of sleep time spent in active sleep decreases and the percentage of time in quiet sleep increases.[102] The reduction in active sleep is paralleled by an increase in wakefulness.[39] By the first year, 30% to 40% of sleep time is active sleep. This proportion becomes adult-like in the early teen years.

SUMMARY

Transition from intrauterine to extrauterine life involves numerous changes in the nervous system as the infant adapts to his or her new environment and caregivers. The term newborn has the ability to receive and process information and respond in ways suited to neonatal development. These abilities are less well developed in the preterm infant. In the past two decades our knowledge of response patterns, interactive abilities, and cues used by term and preterm infants to communicate with caregivers has expanded dramatically. An understanding of the level of maturation and organization of these systems in the neonate is critical for providing appropriate environments, promoting neurobehavioral organization, and influencing parent teaching. Recommendations for clinical practice related to the neuromuscular and sensory systems in the neonate are summarized in Table 14-16.

REFERENCES

1. Ababd, K.J.S. (1998). Clinical importance of pain and stress in preterm neonates. *Biol Neonate, 73,* 1.
2. Adams, M.D. & Keegan, K.A. (1998). Physiologic changes in normal pregnancy. In N. Gleicher (Ed.). *Principles of medical therapy in pregnancy* (3rd ed.). Stamford, CT: Appleton & Lange.
3. Alahuta, S., et al. (1990). Visceral pain during caesarian section under spinal and epidural anesthesia with bupivacaine. *Acta Anaesthesiol Scand, 34,* 95.
4. Allbert, J.R. & Morrison, J.C. (1992). Neurologic diseases in pregnancy. *Obstet Gynecol Clin North Am, 19,* 765.
5. Allen, M.C. & Capute, A.J. (1990). Tone and reflex development before term. *Pediatrics, 85,* 393.
6. Als, H. (1986). A synactive model of neonatal organization: Framework for the assessment of neurobehavioral development in the premature infant and for support of infants and parents in the neonatal intensive care unit. *Phys Occup Ther Pediatr, 6,* 3.
7. Als, H. (1998). Developmental care in the neonatal intensive care unit. *Curr Opin, Pediatr, 10,* 138.
8. Als, H. (1999). Reading the premature infant. In E. Goldson (Ed.). *Nurturing the premature infant: developmental interventions in the neonatal intensive care nursery.* New York: Oxford University Press.
9. Als, H., et al. (1982). Toward a research instrument for the assessment of preterm infants' behavior (APIB). In H.B. Fitzgerald, B.M. Lester, & M.W. Yogman (Eds.). *Theory and research in behavioral pediatrics* (vol. 1.). New York: Plenum Press.
10. Alves, S.E., et al. (1997). Neonatal ACTH administration elicits long-term changes in forebrain monoamine innervation. *Ann N Y Acad Sci, 814,* 226.
11. Amato, M. & Donati, F. (2000). Update on perinatal hypoxic insult: mechanism, diagnosis and interventions. *Europ J Paediatr Neurol, 4,* 203.
12. American Academy of Pediatrics Committee on Genetics. (1999). Folic acid for the prevention of neural tube defects. *Pediatrics, 104,* 325.
13. American Sleep Disorders Association. (1997). *The international classification of sleep disorders, revised: diagnostic and coding manual.* Rochester, MN: American Sleep Disorders Association.
14. Amiel-Tison, C. (1977). Evaluation of the neuromuscular system of the infant. In A. Rudolph (Ed.). *Pediatrics.* New York: Appleton-Century-Crofts.
15. Aminoff, M.J. (1999). Neurologic disorders. In R.K. Creasy & R. Resnik (Eds.). *Maternal–fetal medicine* (4th ed.). Philadelphia: W.B. Saunders.
16. Anand, K.J.S. (2000). Effects of perinatal pain and stress. *Prog Brain Res, 122,* 117.
17. Anand, K.J. & Scalzo, F.M. (2000). Can adverse neonatal experiences alter brain development and subsequent behavior? *Biol Neonate, 77,* 69.
18. Andrews, K. & Fitzgerald, M. (1994). The cutaneous withdrawal reflex in human neonates: sensitization, receptive fields, and the effects of contralateral stimulation. *Pain, 56,* 95.
19. August, P. (1999). Hypertensive disorders in pregnancy. In G.N. Burrow & T.F. Ferris (Eds.). *Medical complications during pregnancy* (5th ed.). Philadelphia: W.B. Saunders.
20. Baker, E.R., et al. (1992). Risks associated with pregnancy in spinal cord-injured women. *Obstet Gynecol, 80,* 425.
21. Baratte-Beebe, K.R. & Lee, K. (1999). Sources of midsleep awakenings in childbearing women. *Clin Nurs Res, 8,* 386.
22. Barnard, K.E. (1999). *Beginning rhythms: The emerging process of sleep-wake behaviors and self-regulation.* Seattle: Nursing Child Assessment Satellite Training, University of Washington.
23. Batocchi, A.P., et al. (1999). Course and treatment of myasthenia gravis during pregnancy. *Neurology, 52,* 447.
24. Benito-Leon, J. & Aguilar-Galan, E.V. (2001). Recurrent myotonic crisis in a pregnant woman with myotonic dystrophy. *Eur J Obstet Gynecol Reprod Biol, 95,* 181.
25. Berger-Sweeney, J. & Hohmann, C.F. (1997). Behavioral consequences of abnormal cortical development: insights into developmental disabilities. *Behav Brain Res, 86,* 121.
26. Black, J.E. (1998). How a child builds its brain: some lessons from animal studies of neural plasticity. *Prev Med, 27,* 168.
27. Blackburn, S. (In press). Assessment and management of the neurological system. In C. Kenner & J.W. Lott (Eds.). *Comprehensive neonatal nursing care. A physiologic perspective* (3rd ed.). Philadelphia: W.B. Saunders.
28. Blackburn, S. & VandenBerg, K. (1997). Assessment and management of neonatal neurobehavioral development. In C. Kenner, J.W. Lott, & A.A. Flandermeyer (Eds.). *Comprehensive neonatal nursing care: A physiologic perspective.* Philadelphia: W.B. Saunders.
29. Borsellino, A. (1980). Neuronal death in embryonic development: A model for selective cell competition and dominance. *Dev Neurosci, 9,* 495.
30. Brazelton, T.B. & Nugent, J.K. (1995). *Neonatal behavioral assessment scale* (3rd ed.). London: MacKeith.
31. Brunner, D.P., et al. (1994). Changes in sleep and sleep electroencephalogram during pregnancy. *Sleep, 17,* 576.
32. Burke, M.E. (1993). Myasthenia gravis and pregnancy. *J Perinat Neonatal Nurs, 7*(1), 11.
33. Cartilidge, N.E.F. (2000). Neurologic diseases. In W.M. Barron, M.D. Lindheimer, & J.M. Davison (Eds.). *Medical disorders during pregnancy.* St. Louis: Mosby.

34. Chan, E.C., et al. (1993). Plasma corticotropin-releasing hormone, beta-endorphin and cortisol inter-relationships during human pregnancy. *Acta Endocrinol (Copenh), 128*, 339.

35. Chesson, A.L., et al. (1999). Practice parameters for the treatment of restless legs syndrome and periodic limb movement disorder: An American Academy of Sleep Medicine report. Standards of Practice Committee of the American Academy of Sleep Medicine. *Sleep, 22*, 961.

36. Clark, P.A. (1998). Programming of the hypothalamic-pituitary-adrenal axis and the fetal origins of adult disease hypothesis. *Eur J Pediatr, 157*, S7.

37. Cohen, Y., et al. (2000). Bell palsy complicating pregnancy: A review. *Obstet Gynecol Surv, 55*, 184.

38. Confavreux, C., et al. (1998). Rate of pregnancy-related relapse in multiple sclerosis: Pregnancy in Multiple Sclerosis Group. *N Engl J Med, 339*, 285.

39. Coons, S. (1987). Development of sleep and wakefulness during the first 6 months of life. In C. Guilleminault (Ed.). *Sleep and its disorders in children.* New York: Raven.

40. Coons, S. & Guilleminault, C. (1984). Development of consolidated sleep and wakeful periods in relation to the day/night cycle in infancy. *Dev Med Child Neurol, 26*, 169.

41. Crawford, P., et al., (1999). Best practice guidelines for the management of women with epilepsy. The Women with Epilepsy Guidelines Development Group. *Seizure, 8*, 201.

42. Crepel, F. (1980). Electrophysiological correlates of brain development. *Dev Neurosci, 9*, 155.

43. Czeizel, A.E. & Dudas, I. (1992). Prevention of the first occurrence of neural tube defects by periconceptual vitamin supplementation. *N Engl J Med, 327*, 1832.

44. Dalessio, D.J. (1990). Epilepsy in pregnancy. In N.M. Nelson (Ed.). *Current therapy in neonatal-perinatal medicine 2.* Toronto: B.C. Decker.

45. Dammann, O., et al. (2001). Is periventricular leukomalacia an axonopathy as well as an oligopathy? *Pediatr Res, 49*, 453.

46. De Lima, J., et al. (1999). Sensory hyperinnervation after neonatal skin wounding: Effect of bupivacaine sciatic nerve block. *Br J Anaesth, 83*, 662.

47. DiPietro, J.A. (2000). Baby and the brain: Advances in child development. *Annu Rev Public Health, 21*, 455.

48. Dommisse, J. (1990). Phenytoin Na and magnesium sulfate in the management of eclampsia. *Br J Obstet Gynaecol, 97*, 104.

49. Donaldson, J.O. (1989). *Neurology of pregnancy* (2nd ed.). Philadelphia: W.B. Saunders.

50. Donaldson, J.O. (1998). Neurologic complications. In G.N. Burrow & T.P. Duffy (Eds.). *Medical complications during pregnancy* (5th ed.). Philadelphia: W.B. Saunders.

51. Dreyfus-Brisac, C. (1968). Sleep ontogenesis in early human prematurity from 24 to 27 weeks of conceptional age. *Dev Psychobiol, 1*, 162.

52. Dreyfus-Brisac, C. (1975). Neurophysiological studies in human premature and full-term newborns. *Biol Psychol, 10*, 485.

53. Driver H.S. & Shapiro, C.M. (1992). A longitudinal study of sleep stages in young women during pregnancy and postpartum. *Sleep, 15*, 449.

54. Edwards, R.K., et al. (2001). Surgery in the pregnant patient. *Curr Probl Surg, 4*, 223.

55. Ellegard, E. & Karlsson, G. (1999). Nasal congestion during pregnancy. *Clin Otolaryngol, 24*, 307.

56. Ellegard, E et al. (2000). The incidence of pregnancy rhinitis. *Gynecol Obstet Invest, 49*, 98.

57. Elkus, R. & Popovich, J. (1992). Respiratory physiology in pregnancy. *Clin Chest Med, 13*, 555.

58. Ellingson, R.J. (1972). Development of wakefulness-sleep cycles and associated EEG patterns in mammals. In C.D. Clemente, D.P. Purpura, & F.E. Mayer (Eds.). *Sleep and the maturing nervous system.* New York: Academic Press.

59. Fajardo, B., et al. (1990). Effect of nursery environment on state regulation in very-low-birth-weight premature infants. *Infant Behav Dev, 13*, 287.

60. Fajardo, B., et al. (1992). Early state organization and follow-up over one year. *J Dev Behav Pediatr, 13*, 83.

61. Fajardo, M.C., et al. (1994). Plasma levels of beta-endorphin and ACTH during labor and immediate puerperium. *Eur J Obstet Gynecol Reprod Biol, 55*, 105.

62. Fast, A., et al. (1990). Low-back pain in pregnancy: abdominal muscles, sit-up performance, and back pain. *Spine, 15*, 28.

63. Faucher, M.A. & Brucker, M.C. (2000). Intrapartum pain: pharmacologic management. *J Obstet Gynecol Neonatal Nurs, 29*, 169.

64. Fielder, A.R. & Moseley, M.J. (2000). Environmental light and the preterm infant. *Semin Perinatol, 24*, 291-298.

65. Fisher, S. (1989). Obstetrical analgesia and anesthesia. In W.R. Cohen, D.B. Acker, & E. Friedman (Eds.). *Management of labor* (2nd ed.). Rockville, MD: Aspen.

66. Fitzgerald, M. & Anand, K.J.S. (1993). Developmental neuroanatomy and neurophysiology of pain. In N.L. Schechter, C.B. Berde, & M. Yaster (Eds.). *Pain infants, children and adolescents.* Baltimore: William & Wilkins.

67. Fitzgerald, M. & Jennings, E. (1999). The postnatal development of spinal sensory processing. *Proc Natl Acad Sci USA, 96*, 7719.

68. Foldvary, N. (2001). Treatment issues for women with epilepsy. *Neurol Clin N Am, 19*, 409.

69. Foti, T., et al. (2000). A biomechanical analysis of gait during pregnancy. *J Bone Joint Surg Am, 82*, 625.

70. Fox, K., et al. (1996). Glutamate receptor blockage at cortical synapses disrupts development of thalamocortocal and columnar organization in somatosensory cortex. *Proc Nat Acad Sci USA, 93*, 5584.

71. Franck, L.S., et al. (2000). Pain assessment in infants and children. *Pediatr Clin N Am, 47*, 487.

72. Franklin, K.A., et al. (2000). Snoring, pregnancy-induced hypertension, and growth retardation of the fetus. *Chest, 117*, 137.

73. Franklin, M. E. & Conner-Kerr, T. (1998). An analysis of posture and back pain in the first and third trimesters of pregnancy. *J Orthop Sports Phys Ther, 28*, 133.

74. Giannina, G., et al. (1997). Comparison of intraocular pressure between normotensive and preeclamptic women in the peripartum period. *Am J Obstet Gynecol, 176*, 1052.

75. Gianoulakis, C. & Chretien, M. (1998). Endorphins in fetomaternal physiology. In N. Gleicher (Ed.). *Principles of medical therapy in pregnancy* (3rd ed.). Stamford, CT: Appleton & Lange.

76. Gilleard, W. L. & Brown, J. M. (1998). Structure and function of the abdominal muscles in primigravid subjects during pregnancy and the immediate postbirth period. *Phys Ther, 76*, 750.

77. Gladman, D.D. & Urowitz, M.B. (1999). Rheumatic disease in pregnancy. In G.N. Burrow & T.P. Duffy (Eds.). *Medical complications during pregnancy* (5th ed.). Philadelphia: W.B. Saunders.

78. Glass, P. (1999). The vulnerable neonate and the neonatal intensive care environment. In G.B. Avery, M.A. Fletcher, & M.G. MacDonald (Eds.). *Neonatology: Pathophysiology and management of the newborn* (5th ed.). Philadelphia: Lippincott, Williams & Wilkins.

79. Gleiss, J. & Stuttgen, G. (1970). Morphologic and functional development of the skin. In U. Stave (Ed.). *Physiology of the perinatal period* (vol. 2). New York: Appleton & Lange.

80. Golbe, L.I. (1994). Pregnancy and movement disorders. *Neurol Clin, 12,* 497.

81. Goldstein, G.W. & Donn, S.M. (1984). Periventricular and intraventricular hemorrhages. In H.B. Sarnat (Ed.). *Topics in neonatal neurology.* New York: Grune & Stratton.

82. Gordon, N. (1998). Some influences on cognition in early life: A short review. *Eur J Paediatr Neurol, 1,* 1.

83. Gorski, P.A., Lewkowicz, D.J. & Huntington, L. (1987). Advances in neonatal and infant behavioral assessment: Toward a comprehensive evaluation of early patterns of development. *Dev Behav Pediatr, 8,* 39.

84. Greenough, W.T., et al. (1987). Experience and brain development. *Child Dev, 58,* 539.

85. Greisen, G. (1997). Cerebral blood flow and energy metabolism in the newborn. *Clin Perinatol, 24,* 531.

86. Gressens, P. (2000). Mechanisms and disturbances of neuronal migration. *Pediatr Res, 48,* 725.

87. Grunau, R.V.E., et al. (1994). Early pain experience, child and family factors as precursors of somatization: A prospective study of extremely premature and full-term children, *Pain, 56,* 353.

88. Grunau, R.V.E., et al. (1994). Pain sensitivity and temperament in extremely low-birth-weight premature toddlers and preterm and full-term controls. *Pain, 58,* 341.

89. Hack, M. (1987). The sensorimotor development of the preterm infant. In A.A. Fanaroff & R.J. Martin (Eds.). *Behrman's neonatal-perinatal medicine* (4th ed.). St. Louis: Mosby.

90. Haeggstrom, A., et al. (2000). Nasal mucosal swelling and reactivity during a menstrual cycle. *ORL J Otorhinolaryngol Relat Spec, 62,* 39.

91. Hagne, I. (1972). Development of the EEG in normal infants during the first year of life. *Acta Paediatr Scand, 232*(suppl), 1.

92. Hainline, B. (1994). Headache. *Neurol Clin, 12,* 443.

93. Haith, M.M. (1986). Sensory and perceptual processes in early infancy. *J Pediatr, 109,* 158.

94. Hall, J.W. (2000). Development of the ear and hearing. *J Perinatol, 20,* S12.

95. Hardy, P., et al. (1997). Control of cerebral and ocular blood flow autoregulation in neonates. *Pediatr Clin North Am, 44,* 137.

96. Heckman, J. D. & Sassard, R. (1994). Current concepts review: musculoskeletal considerations in pregnancy. *J Bone Joint Surg, 76.*

97. Hefetz, L., et al. (1996). Influence of pregnancy and labor on outcome of photorefractive keratectomy. *J Refract Surg, 12,* 511.

98. Hepper, P.G. (1995). Human fetal "olfactory" learning. *Int J Prenatal Perinatal Psychol Med, 7,* 147.

99. Hertz, G., et al. (1992). Sleep in normal late pregnancy. *Sleep, 15,* 246.

100. Hill, A. (1998). Intraventricular hemorrhage: emphasis on prevention. *Semin Pediatr Neurol, 5,* 152.

101. Holmes, G.L. & Ben-Ari, Y. (2001). The neurobiology and consequences of epilepsy in the developing brain. *Pediatr Res, 49,* 320.

102. Hoppenbrouwers, T. (1987). Sleep in infants. In C. Guilleminault (Ed.). *Sleep and its disorders in children.* New York: Raven.

103. Hoppenbrouwers, T., et al. (1988). Sleep and waking states in infancy: Normative studies. *Sleep, 11,* 387.

104. Hughes, S.J., et al. (1991). Management of the pregnant woman with spinal cord injuries. *Br J Obstet Gynaecol, 98,* 513.

105. Ikonomidou, C., et al. (2001). Neurotransmitters and apoptosis in the developing brain. *Biochem Pharmacol, 62,* 401.

106. Inder, T.E. & Volpe, J.J. (2000). Mechanisms of perinatal brain injury. *Semin Neonatol, 5,* 3.

107. Ireland, M.L. & Ott, S.M. (2000). The effects of pregnancy on the musculoskeletal system. *Clin Orthop, 372,* 169.

108. Jacobson, L.K. & Dutton, G.N. (2000). Periventricular leukomalacia: an important cause of visual and ocular motility dysfunction in children. *Surv Ophthalmol, 45,* 1.

109. Jimenez, S.L.M. (1983). Application of the body's natural pain relief mechanisms to reduce comfort in labor and delivery. *NAACOG Update Series, 1*(1), 1.

110. Johnston, M.V. (1995). Neurotransmitters and vulnerability of the developing brain. *Brain Dev, 17,* 301.

111. Jones, B.E. (2000). Basic mechanisms of sleep-wake states. In M.H. Kryger, T. Roth & W.C. Dement (Eds.). *Principles and practice of sleep medicine* (3rd ed.). Philadelphia: W.B. Saunders.

112. Juul, S.E. (2000). Nonerythropoietic roles of erythropoietin in the fetus and neonate. *Clin Perinatol, 27,* 527.

113. Karacan, I., et al. (1968). Characteristics of sleep patterns during late pregnancy and the postpartum periods. *Am J Obstet Gynecol, 10,* 579.

114. Karacan, I., et al. (1969). Some implications for the sleep pattern for postpartum emotional disorder. *Br J Psych, 115,* 929.

115. Killien, M. & Lentz, M. (1985). Sleep patterns and adequacy during the postpartum period. *Commun Nurs Res, 18,* 56.

116. Kohn, N.V. (1998). Neurologic diseases. In N. Gleicher (Ed.). *Principles of medical therapy in pregnancy* (3rd ed.). Stamford, CT: Appleton & Lange.

117. Kooner, K.S. & Zimmerman, T.J. (1988). Antiglaucoma therapy during pregnancy. *Ann Ophthalmol, 166,* 208.

118. Lanska, D.J. & Kryscio, R.J. (2000). Risk factors for peripartum and postpartum stroke and intracranial venous thrombosis. *Stroke, 31,* 1274.

119. Lary, S., et al. (1985). Hearing threshold in preterm and term infants by auditory brainstem response. *J Pediatr, 107,* 593.

120. Lawrence, R. A. & Lawrence, R.M. (1999). *Breastfeeding: A guide for the medical profession* (5th ed.). St Louis: Mosby.

121. Lawson, W., Reino, A.J., & Biller, H.F. (2000). Ear, nose & throat disorders in pregnancy. In Cohen, W.R., Cherry, S.H., & Merkatz, I.R. (Eds.). *Cherry and Merkatz's complications of pregnancy* (5th ed.). Philadelphia: Lippincott, Williams & Wilkins.

122. Leake, P. (1990). Comparing fetal activity patterns with newborn wake and sleep cycles. *NCAST National News, 6,* 2.

123. Lecanuet, J.P., & Schaal, B. (1996). Fetal sensory competencies. *Eur J Obstet Gynecol, 68,* 1.

124. Lee, K.A. & DeJoseph, J.F. (1992). Sleep disturbances, vitality, and fatigue among a select group of employed childbearing women. *Birth, 19,* 208.

125. Lee, K.A., et al. (2000). Parity and sleep patterns during and after pregnancy. *Obstet Gynecol, 95,* 14.

126. Lee, R.V., McComb, L.E., & Mezzardi, F.C. (1990). Pregnant patients, painful legs: The obstetrician's dilemma. *Obstet Gynecol Surv, 45,* 290.

127. Leners, D. (1989). Vestibular stimulation. In M. Craft & J. Denehy (Eds.). *Nursing interventions for infants and children.* Philadelphia: W.B. Saunders.

128. Lentz, M.J. & Killien, M.G. (1991). Are you sleeping? Sleep patterns during postpartum hospitalization. *J Perinatal Neonatal Nurs, 4*(4), 30.

129. Levitt, P., et al. (1998). The critical impact of early cellular environment on neuronal development. *Prev Med, 27,* 180.

130. Liu, S.H., et al (1996). Primary immunolocalization of estrogen and progesterone target cells in the human anterior cruciate ligament. *J Orthop Res, 14,* 526.

131. Liu, S.H., et al. (1997). Estrogen affects the cellular metabolism of the anterior cruciate ligament: A potential explanation for female athletic injury. *Am J Sports Med, 25,* 704.

132. Loube, D.I., et al. (1996). Self-reported snoring in pregnancy: Association with fetal outcome. *Chest, 109,* 885.

133. Lowe, N.K. (1996). The pain and discomfort of labor and birth. *J Obstet Gynecol Neonatal Nurs, 25,* 82.

134. Manber, R. & Armitage, R. (1999). Sex, steroids and sleep: a review. *Sleep, 22,* 540.

135. Marret, S., et al. (2001). Fetal and neonatal cerebral infarcts. *Biol Neonate, 79,* 236.

136. Martins, M.E. (1998). Diseases of the striated muscles. In N. Gleicher (Ed.). *Principles of medical therapy in pregnancy* (3rd ed.). Stamford, CT: Appleton & Lange.

137. Maymon, R. & Fejin, M. (1990). Intracranial hemorrhage during pregnancy and puerperium. *Obstet Gynecol Surv, 45,* 157.

138. Medical Research Council Vitamin Study Research Group. (1991). Prevention of neural tube defects: Results of the Medical Research Council Vitamin Study. *Lancet, 338,* 131.

139. Melzack, R. & Wall, P.D. (1983). *The challenge of pain.* New York: Basic Books.

140. Mizrahi, E.M. (2001). Neonatal seizures and neonatal epileptic syndromes. *Neurol Clin, 19,* 427.

141. Mizrahi, E.M. & Clancy, R.R. (2000). Neonatal seizures: Early-onset seizure syndromes and their consequences for development. *Ment Retard Dev Disabil Res Rev, 6,* 229.

142. Mogil, L.G. & Friedman, A.H. (2000). Ocular complications of pregnancy. In W.R. Cohen, S.H. Cherry, & I.R. Merkatz (Eds.). *Cherry and Merkatz's complications of pregnancy* (5th ed.). Philadelphia: Lippincott, Williams & Wilkins.

143. Montplaisir, J., et al. (1992). The treatment of the restless legs syndrome with or without periodic leg movements in sleep. *Sleep, 15,* 391.

144. Moore, K.L. & Persaud, T.V.N. (1998). *The developing human: Clinically oriented embryology* (6th ed.). Philadelphia: W.B. Saunders.

145. *NCAST learning resource manual.* (1987). Seattle: Nursing Child Assessment Satellite Training, University of Washington Child Development and Mental Retardation Center.

146. Nelson, C.A. & Carver, L.J. (1998). The effects of stress and trauma on brain and memory: A view from developmental cognitive neuroscience. *Dev Psychopathol, 10,* 793.

147. Nijhuis, J.G. (1986). Behavioral states: Concomitants, clinical implications and the assessment of the condition of the nervous system. *Eur J Obstet Gynecol Reprod Biol, 21,* 301.

148. Nishihara, K., et al. (2000). Mothers' wakefulness at night in the post-partum period is related to their infants' circadian sleep-wake rhythm. *Psychiatry Clin Neurosci, 54,* 305.

149. Nissenkorn, A., et al. (2001). Inborn errors of metabolism: a cause of abnormal brain development. *Neurology, 56,* 1265.

150. Noetzel, M.J. & Brunstrom, J.E. (2001). The vulnerable oligodendrocyte: Inflammatory observations on a cause of cerebral palsy. *Neurology, 56,* 1254.

151. Nyman, M., et al. (1997). Chorea gravidarum. *Acta Obstet Gynecol Scand, 76,* 885.

152. Nyska, M., et al. (1997). Plantar foot pressures in pregnant women. *Isr J Med Sci, 33,* 139.

153. Omar, S.Y., et al. (1985). Blood pressure responses to care procedures in ventilated preterm infants. *Acta Paediatr Scand, 74,* 920.

154. Orvieto, R., et al. (1999). Pregnancy and multiple sclerosis: A 2-year experience. *Eur J Obstet Gynecol Reprod Biol, 82,* 191.

155. Ostgaard, H. C., et al. (1991). Prevalence of back pain in pregnancy. *Spine, 16,* 549.

156. Ostgaard, H.C. & Andersson, G. (1991). Previous back pain and risk of developing back pain in a future pregnancy. *Spine, 16,* 432.

157. Ostgaard, H.C., et al. (1994). Reduction of back and posterior pelvic pain in pregnancy. *Spine, 19,* 894.

158. Park, S.B., et al. (1992). The effect of pregnancy on corneal curvature. *CLAO J, 18,* 256.

159. Parmelee, A.H. & Stern, E. (1972). Development of states in infants. In C.D. Clemente, D.P. Purpura, & F.E. Mayer (Eds.). *Sleep and the maturing nervous system.* New York: Academic Press.

160. Paulson, G.W. (1995). Headaches in women, including women who are pregnant. *Am J Obstet Gynecol, 173,* 1734.

161. Peck, J.E. (1994). Development of hearing. Part II embryology. *J Am Acad Audiol, 5,* 359.

162. Peeters, C. & van Bel, F. (2001). Pharmacotherapeutical reduction of post-hypoxic-ischemic brain injury in the newborn. *Biol Neonate, 79,* 274.

163. Perlman, J.M. (1990). White matter injury in the preterm infant: An important determination of abnormal neurodevelopment outcome. *Early Hum Dev, 53,* 99.

164. Philbin, M.K. & Klaas, P. (2000). Hearing and behavioral responses to sound in full-term newborns. *J Perinatol, 20,* S68.

165. Pimentel, J. (2000). Current issues on epileptic women. *Curr Pharm Des, 6,* 865.

166. Porte, F.L., et al. (1999). Long-term effects of pain in infants. *J Dev Behav Pediatr, 20,* 253.

167. Porter, F. (1989). Pain in the newborn. *Clin Perinatol, 16,* 549.

168. Porter, R.H. & Winberg, J. (1999). Unique salience of maternal breast odors for newborn infants. *Neurosci Biobehav Rev, 23,* 439.

169. Portugal, L.G. & Applebaum, E.L. (1998). Otolaryngology: Head and neck problems in pregnancy. In N. Gleicher (Ed.). *Principles of medical therapy in pregnancy* (3rd ed.). Stamford, CT: Appleton & Lange.

170. Patterson, R.M. (1989). Seizure disorders in pregnancy. *Med Clin North Am, 73,* 661.

171. Popovic, R.M. & White, D.P. (1998). Upper airway muscle activity in normal women: Influence of hormonal status. *J Appl Physiol, 84,* 1055.

172. Purpura, D.P. (1975). Neuronal migration and dendritic differentiation: Normal and aberrant development of human cerebral cortex. *Biologic and clinical aspects of brain development* (Mead Johnson Symposium on Perinatal and Developmental Medicine, no. 6). Evansville, IN: Mead Johnson.

173. Qureshi, I.A. (1997). Measurements of intraocular pressure throughout the pregnancy in Pakistani women. *Chin Med Sci J, 12,* 53.

174. Qureshi, I.A., et al. (1997). Effect of third trimester of pregnancy on diurnal variation of ocular pressure. *Chin Med Sci J, 12,* 240.

175. Qureshi, I.A., et al. (2000). The ocular hypotensive effect of late pregnancy is higher in multigravidae than in primigravidae. *Graefes Arch Clin Exp Ophthalmol, 238,* 64.

176. Rivkees, S.A. & Hao, H. (2000). Developing circadian rhythmicity. *Semin Perinatol, 24,* 232.

177. Robinson, J. & Fielder, A.R. (1992). Light and the immature visual system. *Eye, 6,* 166.

178. Rosenbaum, R.B. & Donaldson, J.O. (1994). Peripheral nerve and neuromuscular disorders. *Neurol Clin, 12,* 461.

179. Rowlands, S. & Permezel, M. (1998). Physiology of pain in labour. *Baillieres Clin Obstet Gynaecol, 12,* 347.

180. Sanchez, R.M. & Jensen, F.E. (2001). Maturational aspects of epilepsy mechanisms and consequences for the immature brain. *Epilepsia, 42,* 577.

181. Santiago, J.R., et al. (2001). Sleep and sleep disorders in pregnancy. *Ann Intern Med, 134*, 396.

182. Sauer, P.M. & Harvey, C.J. (1993). Spinal cord injury and pregnancy. *J Perinat Neonatal Nurs, 7*(1), 22-34.

183. Saugstad, O.D. (2001). Resuscitation of the asphyxic newborn infant: new insight leads to new therapeutic possibilities. *Biol Neonate, 79*, 258.

184. Saunders, N.R. (1999). Barrier mechanisms in the brain. II: Immature brain. *Clin Exp Pharmacol Physiol, 26*, 85.

185. Schatz, M. (1998). Special considerations for the pregnant woman and senior citizen with airway disease. *J Allergy Clin Immunol, 101* (2 pt 2), S373.

186. Schorr, S.J., et al. (1998). Sleep patterns in pregnancy: a longitudinal study of polysomnographic recordings during pregnancy. *J Perinatol, 18*, 427.

187. Schweiger, M.S. (1972). Sleep disturbance in pregnancy: A subjective survey. *Am J Obstet Gynecol, 114*, 879.

188. Seron-Ferre, M., et al. (1993). Circadian rhythms during pregnancy. *Endocr Rev, 14*, 594.

189. Seror, P. (1998). Pregnancy-related carpal tunnel syndrome. *J Hand Surg, 23*, 98.

190. Sharif, K. (1997). Regression of myopia induced by pregnancy after photorefractive keratectomy. *J Refract Surg, 13*(suppl), S445.

191. Sibai, B.M. (1990). Magnesium sulfate is the ideal anti-convulsant in pre-eclampsia. *Am J Obstet Gynecol, 162*, 1141.

192. Silberstein, S.D. (1997). Migraine and pregnancy. *Neurol Clin, 15*, 209.

193. Silberstein, S.D. (2000). Sex hormones and headache. *Rev Neurol (Paris), 156*(suppl 4), S30.

194. Smith, R.P., et al. (2000). Pain and stress in the human fetus. *Eur J Obstet Gynecol Reprod Biol, 92*, 161.

195. Smyth, J.W., et al. (1996). Median eminence corticotropin-releasing hormone content following prenatal stress and neonatal handling. *Brain Res Bull, 40*, 195.

196. Solomon, D.H., et al. (1999). Nonoccupational risk factors for carpal tunnel syndrome. *J Gen Intern Med, 14*, 310.

197. Starr, A., et al. (1977). Development of auditory function in newborn infants revealed by auditory brainstem potentials. *Pediatrics, 60*, 831.

198. Stein, G.S. (1981). Headaches in the first postpartum week and their relationship to migraines. *Headache, 21*, 201.

199. Sterman, M.B. (1972). The basic rest-activity cycle and sleep: Developmental considerations in man and cats. In C.D. Clemente, D.P. Purpura, & F.E. Mayer (Eds.). *Sleep and the maturing nervous system.* New York: Academic Press.

200. Stevens, J.C., et al. (1992). Conditions associated with carpal tunnel syndrome. *Mayo Clin Proc, 67*, 541.

201. Stolp-Smith, K.A., et al. (1998). Carpal tunnel syndrome in pregnancy: Frequency, severity, and prognosis. *Arch Phys Med Rehabil, 79*, 1285.

202. Stoodley, M.A., et al. (1998). Pregnancy and intracranial aneurysms. *Neurosurg Clin N Am, 9*, 549.

203. Suzuki, S., et al. (1994). Sleeping patterns during pregnancy in Japanese women. *J Psychosom Obstet Gynecol, 15*, 19.

204. Taylor, H.J. (1985). Choice of analgesia and anaesthesia during labour and delivery. *Clin Invest Med, 8*, 345.

205. Teich, S.A. (1998). Common disturbances of vision and ocular movement and surgery of the eye. In N. Gleicher (Ed.). *Principles of medical therapy in pregnancy* (3rd ed.). Stamford, CT: Appleton & Lange.

206. Terhaar, M.F. & Kaut, K. (1993). Perinatal superior sagittal sinus venous thrombosis. *J Perinat Neonatal Nurs, 7*(1), 35-48.

207. Thompson, D.S., et al. (1986). The effects of pregnancy in multiple sclerosis: A retrospective study. *Neurology, 36*, 1097.

208. Thorpy, M., et al. (2000). Restless legs syndrome: Detection and management in primary care: National Heart, Lung, and Blood Institute Working Group on Restless Legs Syndrome. *Am Fam Physician, 62*, 108.

209. Torfs, C.P., et al. (1996). Maternal medications and environmental exposures as risk factors for gastroschisis. *Teratology, 54*, 84.

210. Torsiglieri, A.J., et al. (1990). Otolaryngologic manifestations of pregnancy. *Otolaryngol Head Neck Surg, 102*, 293.

211. Touwen, B.C.L. (1980). The preterm infant in the extrauterine environment: Implications for neurology. *Early Hum Dev, 4*(3), 287.

212. Vannucci, R.C. & Hernandez, M.J. (1981). Perinatal cerebral blood flow. In *Perinatal brain insult* (Mead Johnson Symposium on Perinatal and Developmental Medicine, no. 17.) Evansville, IN: Mead Johnson.

213. VandenBerg, K.A. (1995). Behaviorally supportive care for the extremely premature infant. In L.P. Gunderson & C. Kenner (Eds.). *Care of the 24-25 week gestational age infant (small baby protocol)* (2nd ed.). Petaluma, CA: NICU Ink.

214. Vanhatalo, S. & van Nieuwenhuizen, O. (2000). Fetal pain? *Brain Dev, 22*, 145.

215. Varendi, H., et al. (1997). Natural odour preferences of newborn infants change over time. *Acta Paediatr, 86*, 985.

216. Vavilis, D., et al. (1995). Conjunctiva is an estrogen-sensitive epithelium. *Acta Obstet Gynecol Scand, 74*, 799.

217. Visser, G.H.A., et al. (1987). Fetal behavior at 30 to 32 weeks' gestation. *Pediatr Res, 22*, 655.

218. Volpe, J.J. (1997). Brain injury in the premature infant. Neuropathology, clinical aspects, pathogenesis, and prevention. *Clin Perinatol, 24*, 567.

219. Volpe, J.J. (1997). Brain injury in the premature infant—from pathogenesis to prevention. *Brain Dev, 19*, 519.

220. Volpe, J.J. (1998). Neurologic outcome of prematurity. *Arch Neurol, 55*, 297.

221. Volpe, J.J. (1998). Brain injury in the premature infant: Overview of clinical aspects, neuropathology, and pathogenesis. *Semin Pediatr Neurol, 5*, 135.

222. Volpe, J.J. (2001). *Neurology of the newborn* (4th ed). Philadelphia: W.B. Saunders.

223. Wand, J.S. (1990). Carpal tunnel syndrome in pregnancy and lactation. *J Hand Surg, 15B*, 93.

224. Wiebers, D.O. (1985). Ischemic cerebrovascular complications of pregnancy. *Arch Neurol, 42*, 1106.

225. Weindling, A.M. & Kissack, C.M. (2001). Blood pressure and tissue oxygenation in the newborn baby at risk of brain damage. *Biol Neonate, 79*, 241.

226. Weinreb, R.M., et al. (1987). Maternal ocular adaptations during pregnancy. *Obstet Gynecol Surv, 42*, 471.

227. Weintraub, H.J. (1994). Demyelinating and neuropastic disorders in pregnancy. *Neurol Clin, 12*, 509.

228. Weissberg, N., et al. (1990). The relationship between beta-endorphin levels and uterine muscle contractions during labor. *Int J Gynaecol Obstet, 33*, 313.

229. Weissman, A. (1993). Eustachian tube function during pregnancy. *Clin Otolaryngol, 18*, 212.

230. Werler, M.M., et al. (1993). Periconceptual folic acid exposure and risk of occurent neural tube defects. *JAMA, 269*, 1257.

231. Winberg, J., et al. (1998). Olfaction and human neonatal behaviour: clinical implications. *Acta Paediatr, 87*, 6.

232. Winkelmann, J., et al. (2000). Clinical characteristics and frequency of the hereditary restless legs syndrome in a population of 300 patients. *Sleep, 23,* 597.

233. Wojtys, E.M., et al. (1998). Association between the menstrual cycle and anterior cruciate ligament injuries in female athletes. *Am J Sports Med, 26,* 614.

234. Wolff, P.H. (1966). The causes, controls, and organization of behavior in the neonate. *Psychol Issues, 5*(monogr 17), 1.

235. Xiang, M., et al. (2000). Long-chain polyunsaturated fatty acids in human milk and brain growth in early infancy. *Acta Paediatr, 89,* 142.

236. Yahr, M.D., et al. (1991). Neurological complications of pregnancy. In S.H. Cherry & I.R. Merkatz (Eds.). *Complications of pregnancy: medical, surgical, gynecologic, psychosocial, and perinatal* (4th ed.). Baltimore: Williams & Wilkins.

237. Young, B.K. & Kirshenbaum, N.W. (1987). Neurologic disorders in pregnancy. In C.J. Pauerstein (Ed.). *Clinical obstetrics.* New York: John Wiley & Sons.

238. Young, G. & Jewell, D. (2000). Interventions for preventing and treating backache in pregnancy. *Cochrane Database Syst Rev, 2,* CD001139.

239. Zanardo, V., et al. (2001). Labor pain effects on colostral milk beta-endorphin concentrations of lactating mothers. *Biol Neonate, 79,* 87.

CHAPTER 15

Carbohydrate, Fat, and Protein Metabolism

Metabolism comes from the Greek word meaning "to change." It is essentially the totality of chemical reactions within a living organism.[121] Cahill, as cited by Hare, identified four principles that underlie and guide metabolic functions in humans:[61]

1. Plasma glucose must be maintained within normal limits.
2. An optimal source of glycogen must be maintained as an emergency fuel.
3. An optimal supply of protein must be maintained for use in enzymatic mechanisms of metabolism as well as muscular mobility. Excess protein is converted to fat and the nitrogen released is excreted in urine.
4. Protein must be conserved when it is scarce and stored fat used in time of caloric need.[61,p.2]

Metabolic processes in the pregnant woman, fetus, and neonate are closely linked with and mediated by the function of various endocrine glands. Major alterations in metabolic processes arise during pregnancy. These changes are essential for the mother to provide adequate nutrients to support fetal growth and development. Maternal metabolic changes also alter the course of pregnancy in women with chronic disorders such as diabetes mellitus. After birth, major changes occur in both the sources of nutrients and the use of substrates by the neonate. Limitations in metabolic processes and related endocrine function during this period can compromise extrauterine adaptations and health. This chapter examines alterations in carbohydrate, fat, and protein metabolism and related endocrinology during pregnancy and in the fetus and neonate.

MATERNAL PHYSIOLOGIC ADAPTATIONS

Metabolic adaptations during pregnancy are directed toward the following:

1. Ensuring satisfactory growth and development of the fetus
2. Providing the fetus with adequate stores of energy and substrates needed for transition to extrauterine life
3. Meeting maternal needs to cope with the increased physiologic demands of pregnancy

4. Providing energy and substrate stores for the demands of pregnancy, labor, and lactation[7]

The first two demands compete with the third and fourth demands. As a result, alterations in maternal metabolic processes can significantly affect maternal and fetal health status.

Pregnancy involves a "coordinated series of physiologic adjustments which act in concert to preserve maternal homeostasis while at the same time providing for fetal growth and development."[61] Pregnancy is primarily an anabolic state in which food intake and appetite are increased, activity is decreased, approximately 3.5 kg of fat is deposited, energy reserves of approximately 30,000 kcal are established, and 900 g of new protein is synthesized (by the mother, fetus, and placenta). The overall energy cost of reproduction is estimated at 75,000 to 85,000 kcal.[7,99,107] Anabolic aspects are most prominent during the first half to two thirds of pregnancy, when accumulation of maternal fat and increased blood volume lead to maternal weight gain. Insulin increases in response to glucose with a normal or slight increase in peripheral insulin sensitivity and serum glucose levels.[15] This results in uptake of nutrients and maternal fat accumulation. During the second half to last third of pregnancy, the woman's metabolic status becomes more catabolic as stored fat is used; counterinsulin hormones increase, leading to insulin resistance (Figure 15-1). During this phase, weight gain is primarily due to the growing fetus and placenta; the fetus gains 90% of its growth in the last half of pregnancy.[15,78,99,107]

Antepartum Period

Pregnancy is associated with major changes in metabolic processes and endocrine function. Hare characterizes pregnancy as a metabolic "tug of war" between the competing needs of the mother and the fetus.[61] The fetus and placenta influence maternal metabolic alterations since these tissues become an additional site for metabolism of maternal hormones as well as a new site for hormonal biosynthesis. Many of these changes are aimed at providing substances (especially glucose and amino acids) for the growth and development of the fetus. As the fetus and placenta grow, maternal fuel economy is altered.[50,156]

Human placental lactogen (hPL), estrogen, progesterone, and possibly leptin influence metabolic processes during pregnancy primarily by altering glucose utilization and insulin action. These changes contribute to the diabetogenic effects of pregnancy, stimulate alterations in lipid and protein metabolism, and increase the availability of glucose and amino acid for transfer to the fetus, while providing an alternative energy substrate (free fatty acids) to meet maternal needs and maintain homeostasis. The changes in carbohydrate and lipid metabolism parallel the energy needs of the mother and fetus, whereas the changes in maternal nitrogen and protein metabolism occur early in pregnancy, before fetal demand.[144]

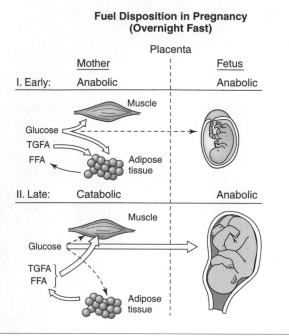

FIGURE **15-1** Fuel disposition in pregnancy during early (I) and late (II) gestation. (From Knopp, R.H., Childs, M.T., & Warth, M.R. [1979]. *Dietary management of the pregnant diabetic*. In M. Winick [Ed.]. *Nutritional management of genetic disorders*. New York: Wiley-Interscience.)

Basal Metabolic Rate

The basal metabolic rate (BMR) increases during pregnancy (Figure 15-2). The rate of change varies with maternal prepregnant nutritional status and fetal growth with significant variations, with up to an eightfold difference reported. Similar variations are reported for fat accretion.[98,105] If a woman has low energy reserves at conception, there is less of an increase in the BMR and energy is conserved. The total energy required for pregnancy can be divided into three parts: (1) obligatory energy needed for the fetus, placenta, uterus, and breasts (which is the smallest part); (2) energy for maternal fat storage; and (3) energy maintenance of these new tissues.[88,98] If a woman has lower energy stores, less of the maternal energy intake is needed to maintain new tissues and energy is conserved for maternal basic needs and the fetal-placental unit.[41,62,98,99,114,154,156] For example, in undernourished women, fetal weight accounts for 60% of the pregnancy weight gain, versus 25% in a well-

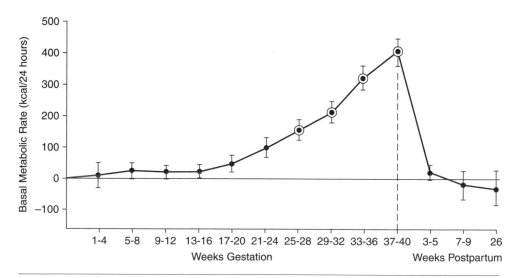

FIGURE **15-2** Changes in basal metabolic rate (BMR) throughout pregnancy and during the first 6 months postpartum for 96 women (means and confidence intervals). (From Durnin, J.V.G.A. [1991]. Energy requirements of pregnancy, *Diabetes*, 40[suppl 2], 152.)

nourished women.[156] This energy-sparing response may allow the woman to sustain the pregnancy but is often at the expense of fetal growth, with decreased birth weight and risk of intrauterine growth restriction (IUGR).[156] Prentice and Goldberg suggest that leptin might monitor a woman's prepregnancy energy stores and adjust or coordinate maternal metabolic resources.[156] Women with large-for-gestational-age (LGA) infants tend to have markedly increased BMR with less maternal energy storage.[98,156]

The pregnant woman meets the energy demands of pregnancy by increasing her intake, decreasing her activity, or limiting fat storage.[99,153] King et al propose three examples of how women in different situations might alter their energy to sustain pregnancy.[98] First, an underweight impoverished woman with limited food, poor fat stores, and need for physical work cannot increase food intake or limit physical activity during pregnancy. Her body responds by decreasing basal energy expenditures so that pregnant energy needs are similar to nonpregnant needs. Second, a normal weight woman in a developed country with fat stores prior to pregnancy and an adequate nutrition during pregnancy increases fat stores in pregnancy and increases her BMR slightly. Finally, an overweight woman in a developed country increases her BMR by 20% or more, perhaps to reduce additional fat deposition.[98] Figure 15-3 compares the total energy costs of pregnancy in women from affluent and poor countries.

Carbohydrate Metabolism

Basal endogenous hepatic glucose production remains sensitive to insulin and increases 15% to 30% during pregnancy to meet fetal and placental needs.[15,18,90,93] Endogenous glucose production increases with gestational age, paralleling fetal and maternal needs.[90,93] Hepatic glucose production remains sensitive to insulin.[18] Blood glucose levels in pregnancy are generally 10% to 20% lower than in nonpregnant women. In addition, during the overnight fasting period, maternal plasma glucose values fall to levels 15 to 20 mg/dl lower than in nonpregnant women.[115] This decrease in glucose leads to lower insulin levels during the postabsorptive state (between meals and overnight) and a tendency toward hypoglycemia and ketosis. The tendency toward hypoglycemia in the postabsorptive state is due to continued placental transport of glucose to the fetus and increases with increasing gestation as fetal glucose needs increase.[139]

During early pregnancy, insulin secretion increases with increased peripheral glucose use ("accelerated starvation"), without increases in insulin resistance.[13,81] As pregnancy progresses, peripheral glucose use by the mother decreases because of increasing insulin resistance. This reduces maternal glucose utilization and makes glucose more readily available to the fetus. The mother compensates by using her fat stores to meet her energy needs with breakdown of glycerol to glucose.[78] The mechanisms underlying the insulin resistance of pregnancy are not completely understood. Insulin resistance is believed to be a result of a

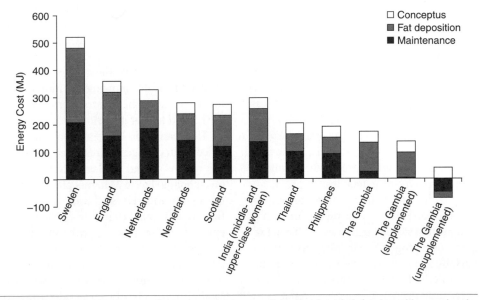

FIGURE **15-3** Total energy costs of pregnancy (conceptus [including fetal fat], fat deposition, and maintenance) in women from affluent and poor countries. The energy cost of the conceptus was estimated pro rata according to birth weight. The supplemented women from Gambia received balanced protein-energy supplements. (From Prentice, A.M. & Goldberg, G.R. [2000]. Energy adaptations in human pregnancy: limits and long-term consequences. *J Clin Nutr*, 71[suppl], 1228S.)

decrease in sensitivity of cell receptors that results from the insulin antagonism effects of hPL, progesterone, and cortisol.[18,61] The insulin antagonism is partially modulated by pancreatic beta-cell hyperplasia and hypertrophy with increased insulin availability after a meal.[8,18] Pregnancy is also characterized by greater oscillations in insulin and glucagon levels.[61] A reduction in the extraction of insulin by the liver may contribute to peripheral hyperinsulinemia. Variations in hepatic insulin binding may contribute to alterations in the ratio of insulin to glucagon.[7]

Progesterone augments insulin secretion, decreases peripheral insulin effectiveness, and increases insulin levels after a meal. Estrogen increases the level of plasma cortisol (an insulin antagonist), stimulates beta-cell hyperplasia (and thus insulin production), and enhances peripheral glucose utilization. Increased levels of both bound and free cortisol decrease hepatic glycogen stores and increase hepatic glucose production. These changes further increase glucose availability for the fetus.[115,139]

hPL levels correlate with fetal and placental weight and are higher in multiple pregnancies.[18] hPL increases synthesis and availability of lipids. Lipids can be used by the mother as an alternative fuel, enhancing availability and transfer of glucose and amino acids to the fetus. A mild form of the metabolic changes seen during pregnancy can be induced by giving hPL to nonpregnant women. However, there is no consistent relationship between hPL levels and insulin requirements in the pregnant diabetic.

Protein Metabolism

Decreased serum amino acid and serum protein levels are found in pregnancy.[92,93] This decrease is related to increased placental uptake, increased insulin levels, hepatic diversion of amino acids for gluconeogenesis, and transfer of amino acids to the fetus for use in glucose formation. Maternal plasma levels of glucogenic amino acids (e.g., those that can be converted into glucose) such as alanine, threonine, glutamate, and serine are reduced due to placental transfer of amino acids.[93] Maternal plasma alanine levels, in particular, are lower because alanine is a key precursor for glucose formation (gluconeogenesis) by the fetal liver.[93]

Alterations in protein metabolism during pregnancy seem to have a biphasic pattern.[93,147] During the first half of gestation, maternal protein storage increases, with a net retention of 1.3 g/day of nitrogen.[99] Most of this is transported to the fetus, but some is retained in maternal tissues. During the second half, maternal protein use is more economic, with decreased urinary nitrogen excretion, thus conserving protein.[99] The early changes may be mediated by decreased activity of hepatic enzymes involved in amino acid deamination and urea synthesis.[147]

Lipid Metabolism

Pregnancy results in marked alterations in lipid metabolism. Lipid metabolism in pregnancy is characterized by two phases and is analogous to the patterns of change in carbohydrate and protein metabolism.[78] During the first two trimesters, triglyceride synthesis and fat storage increase. By 12 weeks, high-density lipoproteins (HDLs) have increased 20% and remain high. Low-density lipoproteins (LDLs) increase by 18 weeks. Triglycerides increase 40% by 18 weeks and 250% by term.[115,119] Phospholipids and cholesterol levels also increase; the triglyceride-to-cholesterol level remains stable.[135] These changes enhance the availability of substrates for the fetus.[78]

Maternal fat storage is most prominent from 10 to 30 weeks, before the peak of fetal energy demands.[99] Promotion of lipogenesis and suppression of lipolysis in this anabolic storage phase are mediated by the progressive increase in insulin and enhanced by estrogen, progesterone, and cortisol.[7,18,76] During this period the pregnant woman experiences a physiologic ketosis with a twofold to threefold increase in baseline ketone body production, with an acute increase after fasting, suggesting enhanced fat utilization.[109,147]

The third trimester is characterized by both lipogenesis and lipolysis, with increased breakdown of fat deposits.[78] Fat is broken down into free fatty acids and glycerol (Figure 15-4). The increased lipolysis is due to the rise of hPL levels with its antiinsulinogenic and lipolytic effects, as well as the effects of cortisol, glucagon, and prolactin.[18,78] Accelerated ketogenesis in the liver is a consequence of increased oxidation of free fatty acids for energy, which increases the risk of maternal ketosis. The fat mobilization is associated with increased glucose and amino acid uptake by the fetus. Thus fats are used by the mother as an alternative maternal energy substrate, allowing the mother to conserve glucose for the fetus and her central nervous system (CNS) during the second half of gestation.[7,18,76,147]

The changes in lipid metabolism during pregnancy are reflected in changes in maternal serum free fatty acid concentrations as well as plasma triglyceride, cholesterol, and phospholipid levels. Maternal plasma free fatty acid levels are not significantly elevated until after about 30 weeks' gestation. The minimal change in free fatty acids during the first part of pregnancy is probably due to increased fat storage and augmented fat utilization. As maternal fat stores are mobilized, serum levels of free fatty acids increase and peak at term. Since elevations in free fatty acids are due to catabolism of stored triglycerides (into free fatty acid and glycerol), changes in free fatty acids are mirrored by changes in glycerol.[7,147] Hypertriglyceridemia during the third trimester is due primarily to increases in very–low-density

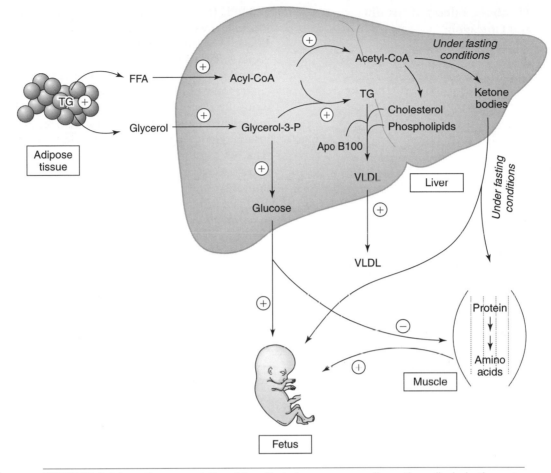

FIGURE **15-4** Schematic representation of the effect of pregnancy on adipose tissue lipolysis, the metabolic fate of the lipolytic products and liver production of glucose, very–low-density lipoproteins (VLDLs) and ketone bodies, and the availability of substrates to the fetus. *FFA,* Free fatty acid; *TG,* triglyceride. (From Herrera, E. [2000]. Metabolic adaptations in pregnancy and their implications for the availability of substrates to the fetus. *Eur J Clin Nutr,* 54, S49.)

lipoproteins (VLDLs) (see Figure 15-4).[18,51] The increase is due to reduced VLDL clearance secondary to decreased activity of lipoprotein lipase in the liver and adipose tissue, increased gastrointestinal absorption of lipids, and increased hepatic triglyceride production.[18,76] Near term, lipoprotein lipase activity increases in the mammary glands. This enhances availability of triglycerides for milk production.[78]

Changes in lipid metabolism are accompanied by functional and morphologic changes in the adipocytes. Hypertrophy of these cells accommodates the increased fat storage during the first two thirds of pregnancy. In the last trimester, maximal glucose transport, glucose oxidation, and lipogenesis within the adipocytes decrease.[79] The number of insulin receptors on the adipocytes increases in the first part of pregnancy and returns to nonpregnant levels

by term.[7] Since responsiveness of adipose tissue to insulin is not diminished as much as that of other tissues, these changes in the adipocytes facilitate fat storage. After a meal, maternal fat stores are replenished by increased glucose uptake, incorporation of glucose into glycerol, and esterification of fatty acids by adipocytes.[7]

Insulin

Insulin levels and responsiveness of tissues to insulin change dramatically during pregnancy. Actions of insulin are summarized in Table 15-1. Insulin production and sensitivity during pregnancy differ in early compared to later pregnancy.[18,20,21] During early pregnancy (up to 12 to 14 weeks), insulin responses are enhanced, sending glucose to the embryo and young fetus. The pregnant woman has a

TABLE 15-1   Metabolic Effects of Insulin and Glucagon

HORMONE	METABOLIC ACTIONS
Insulin	Acts in the liver to: 　Increase glycogen synthesis from carbohydrate (glycogenesis) or fat and protein (glyconeogenesis) 　Decrease formation of glucose from fats and protein (gluconeogenesis) 　Increase protein synthesis Acts in muscle to: 　Increase glucose uptake 　Increase glycogen and protein synthesis 　Retard proteolysis Acts in adipose cells to: 　Increase glucose uptake 　Increase conversion of carbohydrate to fat 　Decrease lipolysis 　Increase uptake of free fatty acids
Glucagon	Acts in the liver to: 　Decrease glycogen synthesis and increase conversion of glycogen to glucose (glycogenolysis) 　Increase uptake of amino acids 　Increase conversion of alanine to glucose 　Increase ketogenesis Acts in adipose tissue to: 　Increase lipolysis

Compiled from Guyton, A.C. & Hall, J.E. (1996). *Textbook of medical physiology* (9th ed.). Philadelphia: W.B. Saunders; and Vander, A., Sherman, J., & Luciano, D. (2000). *Human physiology: The mechanism of body function* (8th ed.). New York: McGraw-Hill.

normal glucose tolerance, basal glucose production, and peripheral muscle sensitivity to insulin.[18,20,21] Adipose tissue is more sensitive to insulin during this period, resulting in lipogenesis and fat storage.[80]

In late pregnancy (from 20 weeks to term), insulin secretion and resistance increase with decreased glucose uptake by muscle and adipose tissue.[8,18,20,21,192] Maternal insulin levels increase 30% or more by the third trimester.[61,139] Increased insulin secretion ensures adequate maternal protein synthesis in the face of increasing resistance of peripheral tissues to the effects of insulin.[147] Mean insulin sensitivity decreases 40% to 80% with increasing gestation.[20,21,90,115,169] Tissue resistance is most prominent in liver, adipose, and muscle cells, and is further altered in women with preeclampsia.[13,21,177]

Insulin antagonism is mediated by the increasing levels of placental hormones, especially estrogens, progesterone, and hPL, to a lesser extent by prolactin and cortisol, and is minimally affected by changes in blood glucose levels. In late pregnancy, although basal insulin levels are elevated, maternal blood glucose values are similar to nonpregnant levels.[7] Increased insulin secretion after a meal (in response to the higher blood glucose) offsets the contrainsulin effects of the placental hormones and facilitates movement of nutrients to the fetus. As a result, changes in insulin response are most noticeable in the postabsorptive state.[18,61] If the pregnant woman is not able to elevate her insulin secretion to overcome the increasing pregnancy-induced insulin resistance, maternal and fetal hyperglycemia will result and metabolic abnormalities such as gestational diabetes may develop or existing metabolic problems such as diabetes will be aggravated.

Alterations in insulin production and responsiveness are critical in integrating changes in carbohydrate and fat metabolism throughout the course of pregnancy. Baird summarizes these interactions as follows: During early pregnancy, increased insulin in response to glucose, minimal changes in insulin sensitivity, and increased number of insulin receptors on the adipocytes result in normal or slightly enhanced carbohydrate tolerance. The increased hepatic synthesis and secretion of triglycerides during this period, along with a normal or slightly elevated removal of triglycerides from the circulation, lead to a net storage of fat. During late pregnancy the elevated plasma insulin, decrease in numbers of adipocyte insulin receptors to nonpregnant levels, and increasing insulin resistance result in reduced assimilation of glucose and triglycerides by maternal tissues, greater transfer of these substances to the fetus, and increased lipolysis. The net result is a decrease in maternal blood glucose, increased glucose turnover, and greater maternal reliance on lipid catabolism for energy.[7] Changes in lipid, carbohydrate, and protein metabolism are summarized in Table 15-2.

Absorptive Versus Postabsorptive States

In addition to phasic changes in metabolic processes in early versus late pregnancy, metabolism of amino acids, carbohydrates, and fats also varies on a daily basis depending on whether the mother is in the absorptive (fed) or postabsorptive state (Figures 15-5 and 15-6). As a result of these changes, pregnancy has been characterized as a time of both "accelerated starvation" and "facilitated anabolism" (described in Clinical Implications for the Pregnant Woman and Her Fetus).

The absorptive state. During the absorptive (fed) state, ingested nutrients (amino acid, glucose, triglyceride) are entering the blood from the gastrointestinal tract (see Chapter 11) and must be oxidized for energy, used for pro-

TABLE **15-2**   **Maternal Metabolic Processes during Pregnancy: Relationship Between Hormonal and Metabolic Changes**

HORMONAL CHANGE	EFFECT	METABOLIC CHANGE
Increased hPL	Diabetogenic	Facilitated anabolism during feeding
	Decreased glucose tolerance	Accelerated starvation during fasting
Increased prolactin	Insulin resistance	Facilitated anabolism during feeding
		Accelerated starvation during fasting
Increased bound and free cortisol	Decreased hepatic glycogen stores	Ensures glucose and amino acids to fetus
	Increased hepatic glucose production	
Increased estrogen, progesterone, and insulin during early pregnancy	Increased fat synthesis	Anabolic fat storage during early pregnancy
	Fat cell hypertrophy	
	Inhibition of lipolysis	
Increased hPL in late pregnancy	Lipolysis	Catabolic fat mobilization in late pregnancy

Adapted from Hollingsworth, D.R. & Moore, T.R. (1989). Diabetes and pregnancy. In R.K. Creasy & R. Resnik (Eds.). *Maternal-fetal medicine: Principles and practice* (2nd ed.). Philadelphia: W.B. Saunders.

hPL, Human placental lactogen.

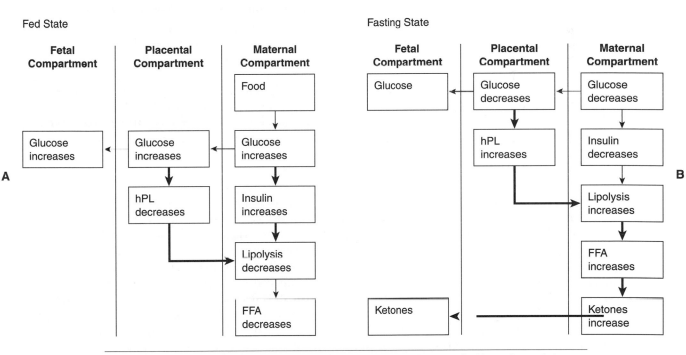

FIGURE **15-5** The absorptive and postabsorptive states during pregnancy. **A,** Absorptive or fed state. **B,** Postabsorptive or fasting state. (From Speroff, L., Glass, R.H., & Kase, N.G. [1999]. *Clinical gynecologic endocrinology and fertility* [6th ed.]. Baltimore: Williams & Wilkins.)

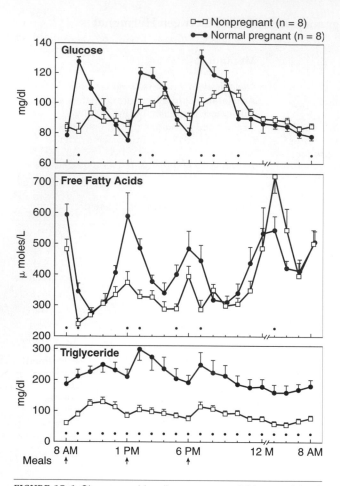

FIGURE **15-6** Glucose and insulin response to 24 hours of feeding and fasting in the third trimester of pregnancy *(closed circles)* and the nonpregnant state *(open squares)*. In the fed state, pregnancy is associated with elevated levels of both circulating glucose and insulin. In the fasting state, pregnancy is associated with decreases in glucose below those seen in the nonpregnant state. (From Phelps, R.L., et al. [1981]. Carbohydrate metabolism in pregnancy. *Am J Obstet Gynecol*, 140, 730.)

tein synthesis, or stored. The average meal takes about 4 hours for complete absorption. In this state anabolism exceeds catabolism and glucose is the major energy source. Small amounts of amino acid and fat are converted into energy or used to resynthesize body proteins or for structural fat. Most of the amino acid and fat and any extra carbohydrate are transformed into adipose tissue; carbohydrate is also stored as glycogen.

The absorptive state during pregnancy (see Figure 15-5, *A*) is characterized by relative hyperinsulinemia (related to decreased insulin sensitivity), hyperglycemia (due to failure of liver glucose uptake), and hypertriglyceridemia and lipogenesis (more glucose is converted to triglyceride

for storage).[18,86,177,183,187] Maternal blood glucose levels may rise transiently to 130 to 140 mg/dl (see Figure 15-6).[39] Gluconeogenesis and circulating free fatty acids are decreased. The hyperinsulinemic response is most marked during the third trimester because of hypertrophy and hyperplasia of islet beta cells. These cells become more responsive to alterations in blood glucose and amino acid levels. Under the influence of placental hormones, resistance of the liver and peripheral tissues to insulin is reduced by as much as 60 to 80%.[141,177,183] The increased insulin levels after eating overcome the insulin resistance to allow glucose uptake by muscles for storage as glycogen.[177] Even with increased production of insulin, however, overall glucose levels are maintained, although at a relatively lower level than in the nonpregnant woman because of the counterbalancing effects of estrogen, progesterone, and hPL.

The postabsorptive state. In the postabsorptive (i.e., when nutrients are not entering the blood from the intestines) or fasting state, energy must be supplied by body stores. Most energy is produced by catabolism of fat. In this state, fat and protein synthesis are decreased and catabolism exceeds anabolism. Plasma glucose levels are maintained during the postabsorptive state by use of alternate sources of glucose and glucose-sparing or fat-utilization reactions.[18] In the postabsorptive state the CNS continues to use glucose, while other organs and tissues become glucose sparing, depending on fat as the primary energy source. Fatty acids are liberated by breakdown of triglycerides by the Krebs cycle, with production of ketone bodies that can produce ketoacidosis if allowed to accumulate.

Maternal responses during the fasting or postabsorptive state are exaggerations of normal postabsorptive responses. These responses are influenced by: (1) continuous placental uptake of glucose and amino acids from the maternal circulation; (2) decreased peripheral utilization of glucose as plasma concentrations of ketones and free fatty acids increase; (3) decreased renal absorption of glucose; and (4) decreased hepatic glucose production. Thus, the postabsorptive state in pregnancy is characterized by a relative hypoglycemia (due to the fetal siphon, increased renal losses, and decreased liver production), hyperketonuria (ketones used as an alternative energy source), hypoaminoacidemia (due to placental transfer for use in fetal glucose production), and hypoinsulinemia (see Figures 15-5, *B*, and 15-6).[15,18,78,86,93] Levels of lipoprotein lipase are increased, enhancing triglyceride breakdown with release of free fatty acids and glycerol (which is broken down into glucose) and production of ketone bodies to provide energy when plasma glucose supply is low.[18] Glycerol is a source for hepatic gluconeogenesis. The elevated free fatty acids prevent glucose uptake and oxidation by maternal cells, thus preserving glucose for the maternal CNS and the fetus.[15] In the nonpregnant woman this switch to fat oxidation occurs after 14 to 18 hours of fasting; during pregnancy the switch occurs after 2 to 3 hours and is termed "accelerated starvation" (see Clinical Implications for the Pregnant Woman and her Fetus).[15]

During the first half of pregnancy, glucose metabolism in the fasting postabsorptive state is an exaggeration of normal responses and leads to lower plasma glucose, blood glucose, and insulin levels. During the second half of pregnancy, effectiveness of insulin in translocating glucose into cells is reduced.[86] Since insulin is the ultimate arbitrator of both the absorptive and postabsorptive states, alterations in insulin secretion alter substrate availability to the mother and fetus.[61] The insulin antagonism in pregnancy is progressive, paralleling the growth of the fetoplacental unit, and disappears immediately after delivery. Placental hormones are probably major factors in producing this insulin antagonism.

Effects of Placental Hormones

The phasic changes in carbohydrate, lipid, and protein metabolism during pregnancy are due to the interplay of placental hormones, especially estrogen, progesterone, and hPL and probably leptin. During the first half of pregnancy, metabolism is affected primarily by estrogens and progesterone. In late pregnancy the influences of increasing concentrations of hPL and leptin become more prominent. Maternal metabolic changes are also influenced by prolactin and cortisol.[15]

Estrogen stimulates islet beta-cell hyperplasia and insulin secretion; enhances glucose utilization in peripheral tissues; and increases plasma cortisol, an insulin antagonist. As a result, particularly in the first half of gestation, estrogen decreases fasting glucose levels, improves glucose tolerance, and increases glycogen storage.[9,86,130] Progesterone augments insulin secretion, increases fasting plasma insulin concentrations, and diminishes peripheral insulin effectiveness. Cortisol mediates these changes by inhibiting glucose uptake and oxidation, increasing liver glucose production, and possibly augmenting glucagon secretion.[15] Cortisol increases to 2.5 times normal levels by late pregnancy.[15,192] Prolactin increases five- to tenfold and stimulates insulin production and, at least in animal models, increases in the number of beta-cell receptors.[144,192]

hPL, a polypeptide hormone produced by the syncytiotrophoblast (see Chapter 3), is the most potent insulin antagonist of the placental hormones. This hormone is secreted primarily into the maternal circulation although some is also secreted into fetal circulation after around 6 weeks.[58] Levels of hPL increase markedly after 20 weeks. Since effects of hPL are similar to those of growth hormone, it has been called the "growth hormone" of the second half of pregnancy.[15] hPL action increases availability of maternal glucose and amino acids to the fetus. Other effects of hPL include diminished tissue response to insulin; increasing beta-cell mass; lipolysis, which increases plasma free fatty acids; enhanced nitrogen retention; decreased urinary potassium excretion; and increased calcium excretion. The major effect is sparing of maternal carbohydrate (glucose) by providing alternative energy sources such as free fatty acids (see Figure 15-4) for the mother.[14,18,147]

Leptin, a protein product of the obese (ob) gene, was identified in 1994. It is produced and secreted by adipose tissue (and, during pregnancy, by the placenta). Leptin is involved in regulating appetite and food intake and enhancing energy expenditure and may also be important in signaling readiness for sexual maturation at puberty.[192] Leptin receptors are found in the hypothalamus, placenta, muscle, liver, lymphoid tissue, uterus, pancreas, ovary, and adipose tissue.[192] Leptin is thought to play a role in maturation and regulation of reproduction and "may serve as a detector of long-term metabolic fuel availability signaling the presence of significant maternal fat stores to initiate reproduction."[18] Other roles of leptin in pregnancy may be to mediate changes in appetite, thermogenesis, and lipid metabolism.[18,62] Leptin may also modulate fetal growth. Figure 15-7 illustrates the roles of leptin in reproduction. Concentrations of leptin increase from 6 to 8 weeks' gestation, rising further in the second and (especially) third trimesters.[80,106,127] The increase is probably due primarily to increased placental leptin production.[80] Levels in early pregnancy correlate with maternal weight and body mass index; this correlation is not found in later pregnancy.[106] Since appetite also increases in pregnancy and food intake does not generally decrease as might be expected, this may reflect a form of leptin resistance (similar to that seen with obesity).[18,80,106,127] Low leptin levels are associated with spontaneous abortion.[110] Elevated leptin levels with a decrease in sensitivity have been reported in preeclamptic women.[111]

Intrapartum Period

The processes of parturition are dependent on an available supply of glucose and triglycerides as energy sources. In addition, essential fatty acids are important as precursors of prostaglandins (arachidonic acid is a derivative of essential fatty acid), which are critical to the onset of labor. These relationships are described in Chapter 4.

During labor and delivery, maternal glucose consumption increases markedly to produce the energy required by the uterus and skeletal muscles.[51,61,88] As a result, maternal insulin requirements fall. Oxytocin may augment or supplant insulin during this period. In animals, oxytocin has

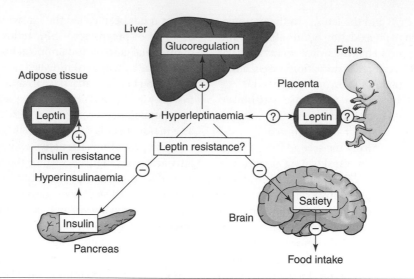

FIGURE **15-7** Possible roles of leptin in pregnancy. Maternal leptin levels are elevated in late pregnancy and the placenta and fetal tissues express leptin. Leptin may have a role in placental-fetal physiology, maintenance of maternal glucose homeostasis, and modulation of maternal insulin secretion. Maternal hyperleptinemia is not associated with a decreased food intake, suggesting maternal leptin resistance. (From Holness, M.J., et al. [1999]. Current concepts concerning the role of leptin in reproductive function. *Mol Cell Endocrinol*, 157, 13.)

been demonstrated to act similarly to insulin; that is, oxytocin stimulates glucose oxidation, lipogenesis, glycogen synthesis, and protein formation.[59,61]

Postpartum Period

With removal of the placenta, concentrations of placental hormones such as hPL, estrogens, and progesterone fall rapidly within hours after delivery (see Chapter 5).[46] The postpartum woman is in a state of relative hypopituitarism with blunted production of gonadotropins and growth hormone.[27,61] This hypopituitarism may result from the feedback effects of elevated hPL and prolactin levels during pregnancy on the pituitary gland. hPL is similar to growth hormone, and its disappearance with removal of the placenta leaves the woman without its contrainsulin effects during a period of relative deficiency of growth hormone.[61] Plasma leptin levels decrease by 24 hours after delivery.[110,127]

Plasma free fatty acids fall during the first postpartal week then increase to late pregnancy levels by 6 weeks, followed by a decrease to nonpregnant levels by 3 to 6 months.[7] The initial decrease during the first week coincides with the fall in hPL. The increasing levels of fatty acids from 1 to 6 weeks postpartum may reflect maternal use of other nutrients for milk production.[7] Maternal plasma amino acid levels return to nonpregnant values of approximately 4.3 mg/dl (versus pregnant values of 3.5 mg/dl) by several days after birth.[1,47]

CLINICAL IMPLICATIONS FOR THE PREGNANT WOMAN AND HER FETUS

The metabolic adaptations of pregnancy safeguard against variations in maternal caloric intake through decreased activity (assumed but not well documented), increased metabolic efficiency, and changes in the metabolism of carbohydrates, fats, and proteins.[7,147] These metabolic changes occur in a phasic pattern—probably programmed by placental hormones—that spreads the energy costs and protein requirements of pregnancy over the entire 9 months of gestation. In early pregnancy, energy is conserved (facilitated anabolism), followed by later redirection of energy (glucose) to the fetus ("accelerated starvation"), whereas throughout pregnancy the mother uses protein more economically to provide adequate amino acids for development of the fetal brain and other organs.[7,61]

Pregnancy has also been characterized as a diabetogenic state. This state is reflected in the elevated blood glucose levels in association with increasing insulin resistance. These states are described in this section along with the basis for alterations in the glucose tolerance test (GTT) and the effects of the normal metabolic changes of pregnancy on the diabetic woman and her fetus.

Pregnancy as a State of Facilitated Anabolism

Pregnancy has been called a state of facilitated anabolism to describe metabolic alterations that conserve energy during early pregnancy and help offset the accelerated starvation (described below). After a meal (absorptive state) the pregnant woman has higher glucose, insulin, and triglyceride levels and suppression of glycogen. These changes increase glucose availability for transport to the fetus; increase availability of an alternate energy source (triglycerides) for maternal needs; and provide fewer stimuli for maternal gluconeogenesis, glycogenolysis, and ketogenesis.[61]

Pregnancy as a State of "Accelerated Starvation"

During the postabsorptive state, when glucose is not being continuously supplied from the gastrointestinal tract, plasma glucose levels fall. The magnitude of the decline is greater in pregnant women than in nonpregnant women, due to the continuous transfer of glucose to the fetus, and is associated with a more rapid conversion to fat metabolism. This response is an exaggeration of the changes normally seen in the postabsorptive (fasting) state in nonpregnant women and similar to changes that occur during starvation ketosis. This state, seen primarily in late pregnancy, is characterized by lower fasting glucose and amino acid levels; increased blood glucose levels after eating; and increased plasma free fatty acids, triglycerides, ketones, and insulin secretion in response to glucose.[9,15,86,151]

Maternal metabolic changes associated with this state of "accelerated starvation" include increased lipolysis due to hPL with increased free fatty acids, which increases ketogenesis in the liver and liver gluconeogenic potential. These changes would normally raise blood glucose levels, but in the pregnant woman the fasting glucose level tends to be lower because of the limited availability of substrate for gluconeogenesis. For example, as early as 15 weeks' gestation, maternal glucose levels after a 12- to 14-hour overnight fast are 15 to 20 mg lower than levels in nonpregnant women. The decrease in glucose during the overnight "fasting" period is especially prominent during the second and third trimesters.[7,86] Hypoalaninemia also develops because maternal protein stores can provide only limited substrate, which is insufficient to meet both maternal and fetal amino acid needs.[61]

Thus the accelerated starvation of pregnancy is characterized by hypoglycemia, hypoalaninemia, hyperketonemia, and increased levels of free fatty acids (see Figure 15-5, *B*) after a normal overnight (12- to 16-hour) fast. These changes are similar to those seen in insulin-dependent diabetics with ketoacidosis except that a diabetic woman would be hyperglycemic rather than hypoglycemic. This disparity is due to differences in tissue sensitivity to insulin.[61]

Metabolic changes characteristic of this state are primarily due to hPL, which promotes lipolysis to increase free fatty acid levels and opposes insulin action, thus increasing glucose availability to the fetus. Other factors influencing this response include increased glucose utilization by the fetus ("the fetal siphon") and mother, along with an increase in the volume of distribution for glucose (i.e., hemodilution).[86]

Drainage of glucose and amino acids by the fetus may lead to increased maternal appetite and a feeling of faintness sometimes experienced in pregnancy. Pregnant women may experience more rapid development of ketosis and fasting hypoglycemia after food deprivation or in the postabsorptive state. With greater maternal reliance on fat utilization during pregnancy, production of ketone bodies and risks of abnormalities such as acidosis are increased. Ketones readily cross the placenta and have been associated with neurologic deficits in infants, although all studies have not confirmed this finding.[161] Dieting and caloric restrictions during pregnancy should be considered potentially dangerous to both the mother and fetus.[55]

Pregnancy as a Diabetogenic State

The diabetogenic effects of pregnancy are reflected by alterations in the GTT, with higher glucose values after a meal reflecting an acquired resistance to insulin. The alterations in carbohydrate metabolism are most evident during late pregnancy in the absorptive state (see Figure 15-5, *A*). When the woman is in this state and glucose is being added to the plasma, her blood glucose levels do not drop as rapidly as usual, even in the face of higher circulating insulin levels. This response results from decreased maternal sensitivity to insulin due to the action of hormones such as hPL, progesterone, and cortisol. Secretion of these hormones increases during the second half of pregnancy; therefore diabetogenic effects are most prominent during this period. Insulin resistance is somewhat compensated for by increased plasma insulin concentrations.[86]

The changes in insulin sensitivity tend to protect the fetus if the mother is fasting by keeping glucose in the blood and thus available for placental transfer. hPL decreases insulin effectiveness (and thus movement of glucose out of the blood into cells) by decreasing tissue sensitivity and mobilizes free fatty acids and amino acids. The result is an increase in available glucose and amino acid for transfer to the fetus and increased free fatty acids for maternal energy.

Effects of Metabolic Changes on Glucose Tolerance Tests

The alterations in carbohydrate metabolism in the absorptive state during pregnancy result in an elevated blood glucose response to a carbohydrate load. This progressive decrease in glucose tolerance is reflected in the criteria for an abnormal GTT in pregnancy. These changes are most marked in the second and third trimesters.[19,141]

Two methods are used to evaluate glucose tolerance in pregnancy: (1) a 75-g, 2-hour test (recommended by the

TABLE **15-3**   Criteria for Glucose Tolerance Test for Diagnosis of Gestational Diabetes Mellitus

| | CRITERIA* | | |
TIME	NATIONAL DIABETES DATA GROUP (100 g) (≥2 ABNORMAL RESULTS)	CARPENTER AND COUSTAN (100 g) (≥2 ABNORMAL RESULTS)	WORLD HEALTH ORGANIZATION (75 g) (≥1 ABNORMAL RESULT)
0 hour (fasting)	≥105 mg/dl (5.8 mmol/L)	≥95 mg/dl (5.3 mmol/L)	≥140 mg/dl (7.8 mmol/L)†
1 hour	≥190 mg/dl (10.6 mmol/L)	≥180 mg/dl (10.0 mmol/L)	
2 hours	≥165 mg/dl (9.2 mmol/L)	≥155 mg/dl (8.6 mmol/L)	≥200 mg/dl (7.8 mmol/L)†
3 hours	≥145 mg/dl (8.1 mmol/L)	≥140 mg/dl (7.8 mmol/L)	

Data from National Diabetes Data Group. (1979). Classification and diagnosis of diabetes mellitus and other categories of glucose intolerance. *Diabetes, 28,* 1039; Carpenter, M.W. & Coustan, D.R. (1982). Criteria for screening tests for gestational diabetes. *Am J Obstet Gynecol, 144,* 768; and World Health Organization. (1985). *Diabetes mellitus: Report of a WHO study group* (tech rep ser no 727). Geneva: World Health Organization. Table from Inzucchi, S.E. (1999). Diabetes mellitus. In G.N. Burrow & T.P. Duffy (Eds.). *Medical complications during pregnancy* (5th ed.). Philadelphia: W.B. Saunders.
*All criteria based on venous plasma determination.
†If the fasting result is <140 mg/dl and the 2-hour is 140-199 mg/dl, the diagnosis is "impaired glucose tolerance", and, during pregnancy, the patient should be treated in the same aggressive fashion as if she had "frank" diabetes.

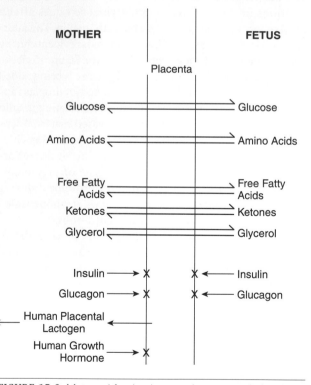

FIGURE **15-8** Maternal-fetal substrate, hormone relationships. (From Kalhan, S., et al. [1997]. Disorders of carbohydrate metabolism. In A.A. Fanaroff & R.J. Martin [Eds.]. *Neonatal-perinatal medicine, diseases of the fetus and infant* [6th ed.]. St. Louis: Mosby.)

World Health Organization); and (2) a two-step test with a 50-g glucose challenge followed by a 100-g, 3-hour oral glucose tolerance test (OGTT) if challenge levels are greater or equal to 135 mg/ml.[139] The latter test is used most commonly in the United States, the former in countries outside the United States. Moore indicates that in the United States the 75-g test is an acceptable alternative for the challenge.[139]

As can be seen from values on the OGTT in Table 15-3, the initial fasting blood glucose value is lower because of decreased glucose utilization and increased fat utilization by the mother (making increased glucose available to the fetus) and the subsequent effects of the fetal siphon. Blood glucose levels tend to remain high after ingestion of carbohydrates for a longer period of time secondary to insulin antagonism and decreased insulin sensitivity. Normally the magnitude of the increase in blood glucose after a carbohydrate feeding is a refection of failure in glucose uptake by the liver. During pregnancy the increased glucose response in the face of increased endogenous insulin confirms the relative insensitivity and resistance of the liver (as well as peripheral tissues such as muscle and adipose tissue) to insulin.[86,139]

Maternal-Fetal Relationships

Growth and development of the fetus is dependent on the availability of a constant supply of glucose, amino acids, and lipids from the mother for energy, protein synthesis, and production of new tissues. The fetus must also develop adequate stores of these substances to meet the demands of the intrapartum period and transition to extrauterine life. Placental transfer of selected nutrients and hormones is summarized in Figure 15-8. Fetal requirements for sub-

TABLE **15-4**   Potential Advantages and Disadvantages to the Fetus of Alterations in Maternal Metabolism during Pregnancy

Maternal Parameter	Potential Fetal Advantages	Potential Fetal Disadvantages
Diabetogenic effects	Increased availability of glucose for the fetus since the mother stores glucose less readily	Increased tendency to maternal and subsequent fetal hyperglycemia with increased risk of fetal hyperinsulinemia and macrosomia
Accelerated starvation		May lead to maternal ketosis; ketones cross the placenta and have been associated with impaired neurologic development by some investigators
Increased availability of free fatty acids	Free fatty acids are not transferred to the fetus in significant amounts and serve as an alternate maternal energy source, especially during the postabsorptive state, conserving maternal glucose for transfer to the fetus	Ketones from metabolism of free fatty acids are probably transferred to the fetus when maternal glucose levels are reduced (as an alternate fetal energy source) and have been associated with neurologic deficits by some investigators

strates involved in carbohydrate, fat, and protein metabolism are discussed in the next section.

Alterations in maternal metabolic processes or in placental transfer of essential nutrients reduce or increase the availability of specific substrates and can be both an advantage and a potential disadvantage to the fetus (Table 15-4). For example, since fetal energy requirements are met almost exclusively by glucose, the diabetogenic state increases availability of glucose in maternal plasma for placental transfer by reducing efficiency of maternal glucose storage. If the usual metabolic changes of pregnancy or placental function are altered, however, variations in fetal growth—such as occur in the infant of a diabetic mother or infant with intrauterine growth restriction—may develop. Maternal glucose infusions during the intrapartum period can lead to a fetal hyperglycemia that stimulates insulin and inhibits glucagon secretion. This may delay gluconeogenesis after birth and increase the risk of neonatal hypoglycemia.[95]

The placenta is a highly metabolic organ with its own substrate needs. Placental metabolic activities include glycolysis, gluconeogenesis, glycogenesis, oxidation, protein synthesis, amino acid interconversion, triglyceride synthesis, and lengthening or shortening fatty acid chains.[66] Glucose uptake by the placenta is similar to that of the brain. Cholesterol from the mother is essential for placental synthesis of estrogens and progesterone. Fatty acids are needed by the placenta for oxidation and membrane formetion.[18] Leptin may have a role in coordinating placental metabolism.[80,106]

Glucose is the nutrient that crosses the placenta in highest concentrations. The fetal-placental unit uses approximately 50% of the total maternal glucose needed for pregnancy.[78] Amino acids are transferred via active transport since levels are higher in the fetus than mother. Amino acids are removed from maternal circulation and concentrated in the placental intercellular matrix. As fetal amino acids levels fall, these stores are transferred to the fetus. Mechanism for amino acid transfer include direct transfer from mother to fetus without modification in the placenta, metabolism by the placenta to produce other amino acids that are then transferred to the fetus, and production of amino acids by the placenta for fetal transfer.[78,84] Lipids are transferred to the fetus according to maternal-fetal concentration gradients mediated by specific fatty acid carriers. The pattern of essential and other fatty acids in the fetus reflect maternal concentrations.[78,84] Maternal triglycerides do not cross the placenta.[26] Placental lipoprotein lipase and other lipases hydrolyze triglycerides, releasing fatty acids when they cross.[78]

The Pregnant Diabetic Woman

The metabolic changes during pregnancy contribute to alterations in insulin requirements in insulin-dependent pregnant diabetic women. Since the metabolic changes in pregnancy normally lead to increased insulin availability by the end of pregnancy, it is not surprising that pregnant diabetic women experience an increase in insulin requirements by this time.[16,61,86,139]

The classification system for diabetes proposed by the National Diabetes Data Group—consisting of type I (insulin-dependent), type II (non–insulin-dependent), type III (gestational diabetes), and type IV (secondary diabetes)—has been modified.[16,141] The revised system includes four types and two risk categories. The types are as follows: *type 1*, absolute insulin deficiency secondary to beta-cell destruction (insulin-dependent diabetes mellitus); *type 2*, relative insulin deficiency with insulin resistance (non–insulin-dependent diabetes mellitus); *type 3*, other types (genetic defects, pancreas alterations, or endocrine, drug-induced or infectious etiologies); and *type 4*, gestational diabetes mellitus. The risk categories are as follows: I, impaired fasting glucose; and II, impaired glucose tolerance.[16]

Gestational diabetes mellitus (GDM) is defined as the onset or first recognition of carbohydrate intolerance in pregnancy.[2] GDM occurs in 2% to 3% of pregnancies in the Unites States.[16] Women with GDM have a pronounced peripheral insulin resistance, decreased numbers of insulin receptors and decreased binding of insulin to target cells, which results in a progressive alteration in glucose tolerance.[18,39] Fasting, postprandial and 24-hour glucose, and lipid and amino acid concentrations are altered.[18] Possible etiologies include a autoimmune defect in the beta cells, impaired beta-cell function, increased insulin degradation, and decreased tissue sensitivity to insulin either due to impaired insulin-receptor binding or intracellular insulin signalling.[108] In late pregnancy the pregnant woman normally increases insulin secretion, but the woman with GDM cannot do so even in the face of increasing insulin resistance.[13,101] Women with GDM have an increased risk for later development of diabetes, primarily type 2 with a risk of approximately 50% by 5 years postpartum.[18,101] The risk is greater with weight gain after pregnancy or GDM in a subsequent pregnancy.[18,20,150]

Pregnant women with type 1 diabetes may experience no change or decreased insulin requirements during the first trimester because of increased glucose siphoning by the fetus, which decreases maternal blood glucose levels. Maternal food intake may also decrease during this period because of the nausea and vomiting of pregnancy. Since circulating glucose levels are reduced, maternal insulin requirements are also lowered. As pregnancy progresses, the diabetogenic actions of increasing amounts of placental hormones and the increasing insulin insensitivity outweigh the effects of the fetal siphon. Thus maternal insulin requirements usually increase during the second half of gestation to levels two to three times higher than prepregnancy values.[61,86,139]

The diabetic woman may have altered insulin requirements during labor, probably because of an increase in energy needs (and thus glucose utilization) and the presence of oxytocin, with its insulin-like effects.[51,88] After delivery and removal of the placenta, levels of estrogens, progesterone, and hPL fall rapidly. This quickly reverses the insulin insensitivity of pregnancy. Maternal insulin requirements usually fall rapidly to prepregnancy levels or even below (due to a rebound phenomenon). Oxytocin may also contribute to these changes. As a result, the insulin-dependent diabetic woman may need little or no exogenous insulin the first few days after delivery. Insulin requirements generally return to prepregnancy levels by 4 to 6 weeks postpartum.[55]

Levels of glycosylated hemoglobin and other glycosylated proteins are useful in monitoring glucose concentrations over time and in genetic counseling and have been used to evaluate fetal and maternal risks for complications in a pregnancy complicated by maternal diabetes.[9,17,43,146,152,186] Glycosylated hemoglobin is formed slowly over the life span of the red blood cell and represents an overall measure of glycemia. The parameters used most frequently are hemoglobin A_{1c} (the most abundant component of hemoglobin A) and total amounts of hemoglobin A. Levels of glycosylated hemoglobin A reflect ambient glucose concentrations over the previous 4 to 6 weeks and have been used to monitor maternal glycemic control on a monthly basis. Hemoglobin A_{1c} is higher in pregnant diabetics than in other pregnant women, but lower than in nonpregnant diabetics.[17] Levels of hemoglobin A_{1c} correlate with development of fetal anomalies with women, with lowest levels having the least risk.[43]

Hemoglobin A_{1c} is not as useful as an independent measure of glycemic control in pregnancy, since these levels may not be a good predictor of capillary blood glucose levels in the woman.[112,113] The use of verified glucose data (i.e., a glucose reflectance meter with memory capability) collected by the pregnant woman (using protocols for self-monitoring of blood glucose) has been shown to provide more reliable data.[112]

Fetus of a Diabetic Mother

Maternal metabolic abnormalities, particularly hyperglycemia during the period of embryonic organogenesis (3 to 8 weeks), have been associated with an increased risk of congenital anomalies.[1,9,24,43,52,106,125] Rigid glycemic control before conception and during early pregnancy has been associated with a reduction in the frequency of congenital anomalies, but the risk is still higher than in the nondiabetic woman.[85,112,113,134,135] Preconceptional counseling and glycemic control are critical for improving pregnancy outcome in a diabetic mother.

The basis for the increase in anomalies is not completely understood. Possible etiologies include excessive formation of free oxygen radicals in the mitochondria; inhibition of prostacyclin formation resulting in an excess of thromboxane A_2, as compared to prostacyclin (thromboxane A_2 is a potent vasoconstrictor that alters vascularization of tissues); altered levels of arachidonic acid and myoinositol; accumulation of sorbitol and trace metals; and hyperglycemia-induced apoptosis with exaggerated programmed cell death (glucose alters the expression of regulating genes).[62,136,139,148,165]

Although the exact basis for development of macrosomia and other problems in the fetus of a diabetic woman has not been completely determined, this phenomenon is generally thought to arise from increased fetal production of insulin and other growth factors (especially insulin-like growth factors [IGFs] and leptin) in response to fetal hyperglycemia.[9,132] Since maternal insulin does not cross the placenta (see Figure 15-8), fetal hyperinsulinemia arises as a response to increased placental transfer of substrates, particularly glucose. Maternal hyperglycemia increases fetal insulin, IGFs, and leptin, which increase glucose transporters (GLUT) that move glucose across the placenta and into fetal cells.[85] Hyperglycemia in pregnant diabetic women results in fetal hyperglycemia and subsequent hyperplasia of the fetal islet cells, with increased production of insulin, enhanced glycogen synthesis, lipogenesis, and increased protein synthesis.[31,39,167] Increased levels of other substances ("mixed nutrients"), particularly amino acids and fatty acids, are also thought to be important in the development of fetal macrosomia.[31,167]

Levels of endogenous insulin in the fetus are correlated with the development of macrosomia.[9] Insulin is the major fetal growth hormone; therefore fetal hyperinsulinemia leads to increased body fat and organ size. The major organs affected are the heart, lungs, liver, spleen, thymus, and adrenal gland. The brain and kidney are not significantly affected. The organomegaly probably arises from increased protein synthesis.[9] Even short-term fetal hyperinsulinemia promotes storage of excess nutrients.[138] Stringent maternal glucose control, especially during the third trimester, when fetal growth peaks, reduces the risk of macrosomia.[12,39,159] The accelerated growth velocity seen in these infants may continue into childhood and adulthood.[138]

Maternal diabetes also alters lipid metabolism and transfer of fatty acids to the fetus. In diabetic women, transfer of fatty acids to the fetus is increased, as is the amount of triglyceride stored in the placenta. These changes are secondary to alterations in several factors that influence fatty acid transfer, including maternal and fetal blood flow and concentrations of serum proteins and placental fatty acid-binding protein.[25]

The placenta is also affected, especially in women whose diabetes is poorly controlled, with increased peripheral and capillary surface area and intervillous space volume.[39,132] These changes may result from the increased glucose load and abnormal metabolic environment with fetal hyperinsulinemia (a fetal "growth" hormone), or as a compensatory mechanism to increase oxygen delivery. The fetus of a diabetic mother shows increases in metabolic rate and oxygen consumption due to metabolism of excessive glucose and other substrates.[7,132]

SUMMARY

Maternal adaptations during pregnancy alter the woman's metabolic processes. These changes are critical for protection of the mother and promote her ability to adapt to pregnancy. Maternal adaptations are essential to ensure that the fetus obtains an adequate supply of nutrients to support growth and development. Alterations in metabolic processes in the mother also interact with the course of disorders such as diabetes mellitus. An understanding of the normal metabolic changes during pregnancy increases understanding of the alterations seen in the pregnant diabetic, the fetus, and the newborn. Implications for clinical practice are summarized in Table 15-5.

TABLE **15-5**   **Recommendations for Clinical Practice Related to Changes in Carbohydrate, Protein, and Fat Metabolism in Pregnant Women**

Recognize the usual changes in carbohydrate, protein, and fat metabolism during pregnancy (pp. 600-603 and Table 15-2).

Assess and monitor maternal nutrition in terms of carbohydrate, protein, and fat intake (p. 610 and Chapter 11).

Counsel women regarding nutrient and energy requirements to meet maternal and fetal needs during pregnancy (p. 610 and Figure 15-11).

Monitor maternal glucose and ketone status (pp. 601-602, 610-611).

Monitor fetal growth (pp. 600-601, 610 and Figure 15-11).

Understand the implications of changes in the absorptive and postabsorptive states for the pregnant woman and her fetus (pp. 604-609 and Figure 15-5).

Monitor maternal energy status during the intrapartum period (pp. 607-608).

Counsel women regarding changes in appetite and weight during pregnancy (pp. 599-601 and Chapter 11).

Counsel women regarding the risks of dieting and caloric restriction during pregnancy (p. 599-601, 609, and Chapter 11).

Know the usual parameters for the glucose tolerance test during pregnancy (pp. 609-610 and Table 15-3).

Recognize the effects of metabolic changes on insulin requirements of diabetic women during the prenatal, intrapartum, and postpartum periods (pp. 611-612).

Evaluate and monitor metabolic and insulin status in the pregnant diabetic woman (pp. 611-612).

Counsel diabetic women regarding the effects of diabetes on pregnancy and the fetus and of pregnancy on diabetes (pp. 611-613 and Figure 15-14).

Counsel diabetic women regarding prepregnancy strategies to optimize maternal and fetal outcomes (pp. 612-613, 624, and Figure 15-14).

Recognize the potential effects of diabetes on the fetus and newborn (pp. 612-613, 624 and Figure 15-14).

FETAL DEVELOPMENT OF CARBOHYDRATE, FAT, AND PROTEIN METABOLISM

The placenta and fetal liver function as a "coordinated multiorgan system for the exchange of nutrients and for ensuring the production of nutrients sufficient to meet fetal requirements."[10] Fetal metabolic processes are dominated by anabolism and governed primarily by glucose with little oxidation of fat. The fetus must produce energy and maintain oxidative phosphorylation in the face of a low-oxygen environment. Although energy is produced in the fetus under aerobic conditions, the fetus has a greater capacity for anaerobic metabolism and is efficient in using lactate. Oxygen consumption in the fetus is 8 ml/kg/min. Glucose contributes more than half of the substrate for oxygen consumption.[10,96]

The fetal caloric requirement has been estimated to average 90 to 100 kcal/kg/day. Almost all of the fetal fuel requirements are met by metabolism of glucose; lactate; and amino acids such as alanine, glutamate, and serine.[10,11,68] The fetus also uses these substrates as major precursors for storage of fuels (e.g., fatty acids, glycogen). The stored fuels are critical energy sources during the intrapartum period and transition to extrauterine life. By term, the fetus has increased its weight 175-fold, protein content 400-fold, and fat content 5000-fold.[188] Fetal nutrient uptake and growth is influenced by maternal nutrition and health, uterine blood flow, placental nutrient uptake, metabolism and transfer, umbilical blood flow, and fetal endocrine status.[50]

Fetal leptin may be important in controlling fetal growth. Leptin may act by modulating growth hormone secretion and may also have a role in hematopoiesis and angiogensis.[43] Leptin has been found in immature subcutaneous fat cells by 6 to 10 weeks' gestation.[4] Circulating levels of leptin, an adipostatic hormone, increase after 32 to 34 weeks' gestation, around the time of increasing body fat mass.[128,143] Levels of leptin decrease rapidly after birth and may help limit energy expenditure and conserve the infant's nutrient reserves for later growth and development.[75] Concentrations of leptin are 3 times higher in LGA infants than in infants of appropriate size for gestational age; concentrations are 12 times higher in LGA infants than in small-for-gestational-age (SGA) infants.[62]

Carbohydrate Metabolism

The fetus, who has been described as a "glucose-dependent parasite," uses glucose from the mother as the major substrate for energy production.[96,107] Fetal glucose utilization rates (4 to 6 mg/kg^{-1}/min^{-1}) are higher than in adults (2 to 3 mg/kg^{-1}/min^{-1}).[31,68] Even with fetal growth restriction, maternal glucose is the major energy substrate for the fetus, although the placenta can produce alternate substrates such as lactate and ketone bodies for use as energy and for glycogen synthesis.

The placenta has a high facility for glucose uptake and transport via membrane transport proteins (GLUTs, or the gene symbol for facilitated glucose transporter) on the microvillous facing maternal blood and fetal facing basal membrane of the placenta.[70,85] GLUT-1 is the major placental glucose transporter. There is a fivefold greater increase in GLUT-1 on the microvillous facing maternal blood than on the fetal facing basal membrane (Figure 15-9).[85] This increases the movement of maternal glucose into the placenta, where approximately 40% to 50% is used by the placenta for oxidation or converted to glycogen and lactate to meet its energy needs.[85,91] Basal membrane GLUT-1 is the rate-limiting step in fetal glucose transfer. In the second half of pregnancy, basal membrane GLUT-1s increase and their activity increases 50% to meet increasing demands with fetal growth in late pregnancy.[85] If the uteroplacental nutrient supply is diminished, the fetus consumes nutrients and oxidizes them at the usual rate, but the placenta reduces consumption of both nutrients and oxygen.[103]

During the first few days after fertilization, the zygote has a limited ability to metabolize glucose. After the embryonic genome is activated, glucose metabolism increases. Both glucose and pyruvate uptake increase initially; glucose uptake remains high throughout pregnancy, while pyruvate uptake falls.[38] The major regulators of fetal growth are IGF-I and IGF-II (Figure 15-10), which stimulate cell proliferation, differentiation, and metabolsim.[50,163] IGFs act via cell membrane receptors and are modulated

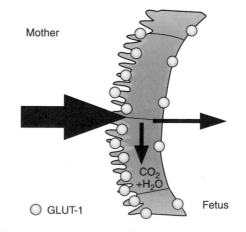

FIGURE **15-9** Relative magnitude of transmembrane glucose fluxes across the maternal-facing microvillous membrane into the synsytium, across the fetal-facing basal membrane into the fetus and the loss of glucose to placental metabolism. *GLUT-1,* Glucose transporter. (From Illsley, N.P. [2000]. Placental glucose transport in diabetic pregnancy. *Clin Obstet Gynecol, 43,* 120.)

by a group of binding proteins.[163] The liver is the main source of IGFs, which have autocrine, paracrine, and endocrine functions.[163,191] Both IGF-I and IGF-II increase with gestational age. In early gestation, IGF-II activity, which is not significantly affected by nutritional factors, is predominant. In late pregnancy IGF-I, which is regulated by nutrient availability, is predominant.[191] Fetal growth in later gestation is regulated by the interaction of glucose,

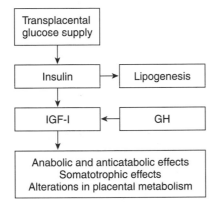

```
┌─────────────────────┐
│   Transplacental    │
│   glucose supply    │
└─────────────────────┘
          │
          ▼
┌──────────┐      ┌──────────────┐
│ Insulin  │─────▶│ Lipogenesis  │
└──────────┘      └──────────────┘
          │
          ▼
┌──────────┐      ┌──────────────┐
│  IGF-I   │◀─────│      GH      │
└──────────┘      └──────────────┘
          │
          ▼
┌─────────────────────────────────────┐
│  Anabolic and anticatabolic effects  │
│       Somatotrophic effects          │
│  Alterations in placental metabolism │
└─────────────────────────────────────┘
```

FIGURE **15-10** Schema of the major fetal endocrine factors influencing fetal growth and metabolism in late gestation. (From Gluckman, P.D. [1997]. Endocrine and nutritional regulation of prenatal growth. *Acta Paediatr Suppl, 423,* 155.)

insulin, and IGF-I (see Figure 15-10).[50] Glucose transfer across the placenta stimulates fetal insulin release. Insulin in turn stimulates lipogenesis and IGF, which increases fetal anabolism and placental uptake of glucose and other nutrients for fetal (versus placental) use.[191] Low levels of IGF-I are seen in growth restricted infants.[191] Poor fetal nutrition may alter the ability to produce and respond to insulin in adulthood, increasing the risk of type 2 diabetes, or may alter fetal LDL metabolism, increasing the risk of coronary artery disease.[37,40,118,157]

Under basal, nonstressed conditions, the fetal glucose pool is in equilibrium with the maternal pool and almost all fetal glucose is of maternal origin.[183] Fetal glucose levels are generally 10 to 20 mg/dl less than maternal levels (or 70% to 80% of maternal values) and increase slightly toward the end of gestation.[9,91,96,103,189] This gradient is regulated by the placenta and favors transfer of glucose across the placenta from the mother through carrier-mediated facilitated diffusion (GLUTs) (Figure 15-11). If fetal glucose supply decreases, then placental glucose uptake increases.[48,69,70] The levels at which these carriers become saturated is significantly above the usual maternal blood glucose level, which promotes a constant supply of glucose to the fetus.[107] There is no net transfer of insulin or glucagon to the fetus (see Figure 15-8).[31,69,70] With adequate maternal nutrition, gluconeogenesis and ketogenesis are not seen in

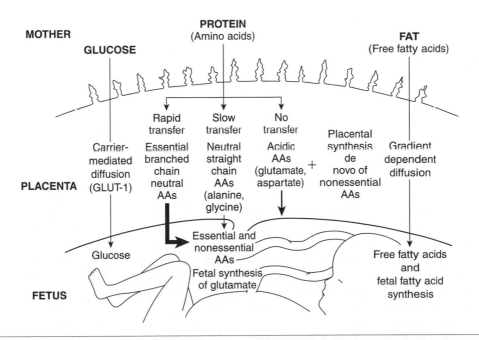

FIGURE **15-11** Placental transport of maternal fuels. (From Hollingsworth, D.B. [1983]. Alterations of maternal metabolism in normal and diabetic pregnancies in insulin-dependent, noninsulin-dependent, and gestational diabetes. *Am J Obstet Gynecol, 146,* 420.)

the fetus.[123] However, with prolonged glucose deprivation, the fetus can produce some glucose and ketones, probably mediated by cortisol.[68]

Fetal glucose utilization is independent of maternal glucose availability. The mother meets this demand by an increasing reliance on fat metabolism for her own fuel needs. If the maternal system is not able to meet the fetal demand for gluconeogenic precursors, hypoglycemia can result. Since fetal blood glucose levels are 70% to 80% of maternal values, maternal hypoglycemia leads to even lower fetal blood glucose levels.[86] Placental glucose transfer increases with increasing gestational age not only by increases in GLUT, but also secondary to increases in insulin receptors on fetal tissues such as adipose tissue and skeletal muscle.[69,70]

Glucose is also needed by the fetus for protein synthesis, as a precursor for fat synthesis, for conversion to glycogen for storage, and as the primary substrate for oxidative metabolism. Most of the transferred glucose is oxidized to carbon dioxide and water by the Krebs cycle and oxidative phosphorylation.

The fetus has an active capacity for anaerobic metabolism, which has a greater role in fetal metabolic processes than it does in adults.[185] The fetus has increased amounts of glycolytic isoenzymes such as hexokinase, glucose-6-phosphate dehydrogenase (G6PD), and pyruvate dehydrogenase, which favor anaerobic glycolysis.[96,185] Fetal and, especially, placental tissues actively metabolize glucose to lactate. The greater amount of lactate generated by the placenta serves as an important fuel for the fetus.[68,69] Lactate rather than glucose may be the major precursor of fetal hepatic glycogen and fatty acid synthesis.[96] Under aerobic conditions the fetus is a net consumer of lactate. The placenta produces large amounts of lactate and ammonia, which may help in regulating metabolic activities in the fetal hepatocytes.[67]

Glycogen synthesis is greater than glycogenolysis in the fetus. Glycogen synthetase and other gluconeogenic enzymes can be found in the liver from the eighth week and increase to term.[96,123] Deposition of hepatic glycogen during the perinatal period is regulated by glucocorticoids and insulin. Glucocorticoids may induce glycogen synthetase, which is then activated by insulin. Fetal cells have increased insulin receptors, greater receptor affinity for glucose, and delayed maturation of hepatic glucagon receptors. These changes promote storage of glucose as glycogen and fat. Glycogen can also be synthesized from lactate, pyruvate, alanine, and glycerol as well as glucose.[189]

Glycogen is stored in fetal tissues from 9 weeks' gestation on and increases significantly during the third trimester. Until 20 to 24 weeks, the fetal liver is the main glycogen storehouse; after that time, glycogen is stored in heart and skeletal muscle. Compared with adults, the term fetus has 2 to 3 times more liver glycogen, 3 to 5 times more skeletal muscle glycogen, and 10 times more cardiac muscle glycogen stores.[147] The placenta has enzymes for gluconeogenesis and glycolysis and also accumulates glycogen, with greatest storage at 8 to 10 weeks' gestation.

Insulin is present in fetal islet tissue from about 9 to 11 weeks' gestation and can be found in plasma by 13 weeks' gestation. GLUT-1 and GLUT-2 are expressed early in development and are found on both the trophoblast and blastocyst.[145] GLUT-1 is the major fetal glucose transporter and is found on most fetal cells; fetal GLUT-2 levels remain low.[168] Insulin levels are dependent on fetal glucose levels. Insulin production is stimulated by increasing glucose and amino acid concentrations, especially after 20 weeks.[189] Fetal glucose metabolism is relatively independent of the insulin-glucagon regulatory mechanisms seen after birth, however. Acute changes in glucose concentrations leading to hypo- or hyperglycemia do not significantly alter fetal insulin or glucagon secretion.[168] However, secretion of these hormones is markedly altered by chronic changes such as long-term hyperglycemia in a diabetic woman, which augments insulin secretion by beta-cell hyperplasia and suppresses glucagon, or by chronic maternal malnutrition, which depresses insulin and stimulates release of fetal glucagon.[183] Since insulin is a fetal growth hormone, fetal hyperinsulinemic states are associated with fetal and neonatal macrosomia.[52,78]

Glucagon is found in fetal plasma by 15 weeks' gestation and reaches peak concentrations at 24 to 26 weeks. In comparison with adults, the number of fetal hepatic glucagon receptors is decreased and insulin receptors are increased. The fetal liver, erythrocyte, monocyte, and lung have an increased affinity for insulin. These attributes promote insulin-mediated anabolic processes such as glycogen formation and decrease glucagon-mediated catabolism.[183]

The fetal liver receives the highest net flux of maternal glucose because it is the first organ system encountered by blood returning from the placenta (see Chapter 8). Fetal hepatic enzymes for glycogenesis (carbohydrate to glycogen) are increased, whereas enzymes for glycolysis (carbohydrate to pyruvate and lactate) and gluconeogenesis (fat and protein to glucose) are present but decreased. For example, glucose-6-phosphatase, an enzyme involved in gluconeogenesis and inhibited by glucose and amino acids, is at 20% to 50% of adult levels at mid-gestation.[96] These relationships are maintained until birth, when decreased glucose availability and onset of high-fat feedings stimulate decreases in glycogenolytic enzymes.[185]

Lipid Metabolism

Fetal fat content increases during gestation from 0.5% of body weight in early gestation to approximately 3.5% by 28 weeks and 16% by term or by approximately 3.5 g/kg/day in the third trimester.[71] This increase is due to transfer of fatty acids from the mother and active lipogenesis in the fetal liver and other tissues. Lipogenesis is primarily through the fatty acid synthetase pathway, which is highly active in the fetus.[25,97,185] Maternal lipoproteins do not cross the placenta but are taken up by the placenta, where they are broken down and their products used for energy or steroid hormone production or released to the fetus; free fatty acids, ketone bodies, and glycerol cross the placenta.[76] Free fatty acids cross by diffusion in limited amounts, with a net flux of unesterified fatty acids to the fetus.[9,96,104,182] These fatty acids are derived primarily from maternal circulating free fatty acids or cleavage of maternal triglycerides by lipoprotein lipase.[77,147] The maternal diet is reflected in the fatty acid content of fetal tissues.[25,96]

Because transport of fatty acids is partly controlled by maternal concentrations, increased maternal levels are associated with increased transfer and fetal storage.[18,182] Other factors influencing free fatty acid transfer include serum albumin level, fatty acid chain length, uteroplacental and umbilical blood flow, α-fetoprotein, fetulin (placental protein that binds fatty acids), and binding affinity.[25,182] The essential fatty acids, linoleic and α-linolenic acids, cannot be synthesized by the fetus and must be transported across the placenta. These substances can be desaturated by the fetus to form other fatty acids. Transfer of essential fatty acids increases in late pregnancy, when demand for brown and white adipose tissue development and for vascular and neural growth increase; however, some early transfer is needed for uteroplacental vascular development.[181,182]

Increased fat deposition during the third trimester is associated with increasing fetal weight and decreased serum triglycerides because these are used in fat deposition.[30] Most (80%) of the fetal fat accretion during this period is due to de novo synthesis from acetyl coenzyme A (CoA) (Figure 15-12, *A*) with formation of palmitic acid, especially in the brain and liver.[77,97,181] Fetal and maternal cholesterol levels are not correlated.[76]

Fetal lipid metabolism is characterized by early development of mechanisms for lipogenesis (see Figure 15-12, *A*) with decreased lipolytic activity (Figure 15-12, *B*) throughout gestation, except in the liver.[147] Fetal fatty acid synthesis occurs through lipogenesis and desaturation of essential fatty acids. Lipogenesis is dependent on substrate availability. Lipogenic precursors include glucose, lactate, and ketone bodies; the latter two are the most important.[77,97,96]

The rate of synthesis is primarily controlled by the ratio of plasma insulin-to-glucagon levels. Insulin stimulates and glucagon inhibits fatty acid synthesis. The action of glucagon is mediated by cyclic adenosine monophosphate (cAMP), which inhibits acetyl CoA enzymes.[77,97] The high insulin-to-glucagon ratio in the fetus promotes

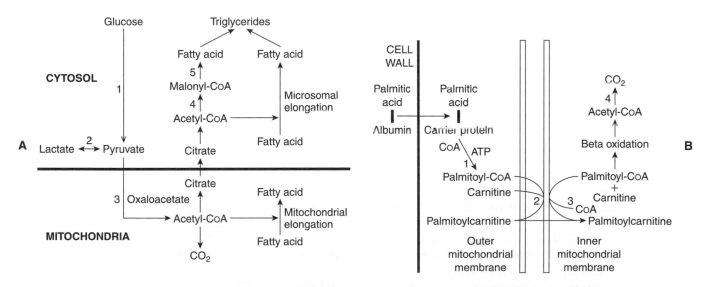

FIGURE **15-12** Fatty acid synthesis and oxidation. **A,** Metabolic pathways involved in fatty acid synthesis: *1,* glycolysis; *2,* lactate dehydrogenase; *3,* pyruvate dehydrogenase; *4,* acetyl-coenzyme A (CoA) carboxylase; *5,* fatty acid synthase complex. **B,** Metabolic pathways involved in fatty acid oxidation: *1,* palmitoyl-CoA synthetase; *2,* carnitine palmitoyl transferase I; *3,* carnitine palmitoyl transferase II; *4,* citric acid cycle. (From Kimura, R.E. (1989). Fatty acid metabolism in the fetus. *Semin Perinatol, 13,* 202.)

fatty acid synthesis. Lipogenesis is increased by glucose, fatty acids, and T_4 (see Chapter 18) and reduced by catecholamines.[96,181] The fetal liver and brain contain enzymes for ketone oxidation as an alternative energy substrate.[9] Lipolytic activity becomes active after delivery, when the infant can no longer rely on a constant glucose supply from the mother and must cope with relatively high fat intake.

By 15 weeks the fetus has developed enzymes to convert acetate or citrate to fatty acid and thus the potential to use fat as an alternative source of energy.[147] Blood lipid and free fatty acid levels are relatively stable after about 26 weeks but remain low until after delivery. The free fatty acids that cross the placenta are used by the fetus in organ development; synthesis of pulmonary surfactant, other phospholipids, bile, and serum lipoprotein; formation of cell membranes; precursors for prostaglandins; and as second messenger precursors. Fatty acids needed by developing neuronal and glial cells and in formation of the myelin sheath are synthesized within the brain.[77,185]

Activity of the pentose phosphate intermediary metabolic pathway is also high in the fetus. Activity of this pathway is associated with cell proliferation and an increased requirement for ribose phosphate precursors of nucleic acids and provision of nicotinamide-adenine dinucleotide (NADH) for synthesis of long-chain fatty acids.[185]

Protein Metabolism

At least 10 amino acids are essential for the fetus, including those essential for adults plus cysteine and histidine, with a dependency on arginine and tyrosine. Arginine and leucine are insulin secretogogues; arginine may also enhance vascular development. Taurine helps regulate metabolism and is needed in development of the heart, eye, and brain.[69] Because of the relative inactivity of hepatic enzymes such as cystathionase and phenylalanine hydroxylase, the fetus cannot synthesize tyrosine and cysteine from phenylalanine and methionine.[60] The fetus uses amino acids for protein synthesis or oxidation since organ development involves continuous remodeling (breakdown and resynthesis) of tissue. The availability of glucose and other substances influences fetal amino acid catabolism and protein accretion.[72,116]

There is a net flux of most amino acids from the mother to the fetus (see Figure 15-11).[73,107] Since concentrations of most amino acids are higher in fetal than maternal blood, amino acids are actively transported across the placenta. Fetal-to-maternal amino acid nitrogen ratios average 1.03 to 3.0, with a net active transfer of nitrogen to the fetus of 54 nmol/day and a total accumulation of about 400 g of protein by term.[7,107,147]

Placental transport proteins regulate amino acid transfer. Amino acids are supplied to the fetus in greater amounts than are needed for nitrogen accretion. The fetus uses the carbon from excess amino acids for oxidation and to make nonessential amino acids.[69,72,73] Some critical amino acids are not transferred across the placenta but are, rather, produced in the placenta. For example, glutamate, which is needed for neurotransmitters, is not transferred from mother to fetus. Instead glutamine is transferred from the mother to the placenta, where it is used to produce glutamate. Similarly asparagine is used by the placenta to produce aspartate, another neurotransmitter. Both glutamate and aspartate are toxic, so by transferring precursors, the placenta can produce only the amounts that are needed by the fetus.[67,69] The placenta also produces ammonia that is used by the fetal liver for additional protein synthesis.[67,69]

Levels of most amino acids remain higher in fetal than in maternal blood until near term, when fetal blood amino acid levels—particularly those of nonessential amino acids—fall. Levels of gluconeogenetic amino acids such as alanine are the only ones that remain elevated in late gestation. In the third trimester, alanine is the most common amino acid transferred across the placenta; transfer of glutamine, glycine, and serine also remains high.[96,147] The urea cycle is decreased or absent until mid-gestation.[107]

Until about 26 weeks' gestation most of the increase in fetal weight is due to accumulation of protein; after that time, weight gain is due to fat accumulation. During the last weeks before term, fetal uptake of nitrogenous compounds falls and fetal nitrogen levels decrease with the increased deposition of fat.[147]

NEONATAL PHYSIOLOGY

Neonates must develop a homeostatic balance between energy requirements and the supply of substrates as they move from the constant glucose supply of fetal life to the normal intermittent variations in the availability of glucose and other fuels that characterize the absorptive and postabsorptive states. The development of this homeostasis is dependent on substrate availability and maturation of hormonal, neuronal, and enzymatic systems and is influenced by gestational age, health status, and intake.[31] Alterations in metabolic substrates and hormones in the fetus and neonate are summarized in Table 15-6.

Transitional Events

Metabolic transition is characterized by a shift from the anabolic-dominant fetal state to the catabolic state of the neonate. This transition is influenced by genetic, environmental, and endocrine factors as well as by major alter-

TABLE **15-6**   **Alterations in Metabolic Substrates and Hormones in the Fetus and Neonate**

	FETUS	NEWBORN
Hormone concentration:		
Insulin	Low	Low
Glucagon	Low	High
Epinephrine	Low	High
Hormone receptors:		
Insulin:		
Density	High	Decrease
Affinity	High normal	Decrease
Structure	Normal	Normal
Functional kinase	Present	Present
Glucagon:		
Density	Low	Rapid increase
Structure	??	Normal
Functional linkage to cAMP	Absent to low	Rapid increase
Epinephrine:		
β-receptor	Present	Present
Functional linkage	Present	Present
Liver enzymes:		
Phosphorylase	Low	High
PEPCK	Low	High
Source of nutrients	Mother	Endogenous
Endogenous glucose production	Minimal	Highly active
Lipolysis/ketogenesis	Minimal	Highly active
	Anabolic	Catabolic

From Sperling, M.A. (1988). Glucose homeostasis after birth. In C.T. Jones (Ed.). *Research in perinatal medicine. VII: Fetal and neonatal development*. Ithaca, NY: Perinatology Press.
cAMP, Cyclic adenosine monophosphate; *PEPCK*, phosphoenolpyruvate carboxykinase.

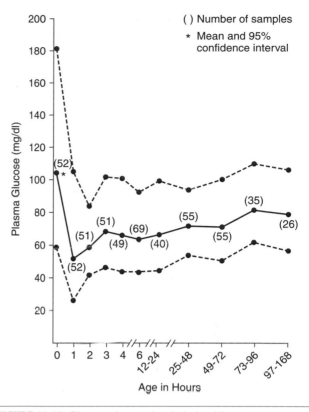

FIGURE **15-13**   Plasma glucose levels in healthy term neonates delivered vaginally with birth weights between 2.5 and 4 kg. (From Srinivansan, G., et al. [1986]. Plasma glucose values in normal neonates: a new look. *J Pediatr*, 109, 114.)

ations in energy metabolism within the mitochondria.[185] The ability of the fetus to use glucose anaerobically and to readily metabolize lactate may be important in maintaining homeostasis during the stresses of labor and delivery. The fetus prepares for this transition during the last weeks of gestation by increasing fuel storage in the form of glycogen and lipids. Glycogen is critical in order to maintain glucose homeostasis immediately after birth, whereas the fat stores, through lipolysis of fatty acids and ketone bodies, serve as an alternate energy source.[189] Postnatal changes in metabolism involve the transition from the almost exclusive reliance on glucose for energy production in the fetus to markedly increased use of fatty acid oxidation and ketone body use for energy production in the neonate.[147] The

changes in metabolism with birth are due to expression of genes that regulate various enzymes.[30]

Carbohydrate Metabolism

Birth results in the loss of the maternal glucose source. As a result, neonatal blood glucose normally falls after birth, reaching a nadir at 60 to 90 minutes after birth (Figure 15-13).[30,120] These values generally stabilize at levels of 50 to 60 mg/dl during the first few hours after birth. Steady-state hepatic release of glucose at 4 to 6 mg/kg^{-1}/min^{-1} is seen by 3 to 4 hours in term infants.[89] Earlier data that demonstrated a longer period for the glucose nadir to be reached were based on infants in whom feeding was delayed after birth.[189] The basis for the fall in blood glucose is summarized in Table 15-7.

The newborn responds to the decrease in blood glucose in several ways. The rapid glycogenolysis (liberation of glucose from glycogen) after birth is stimulated by a fall in the insulin-to-glucagon ratio and sluggish insulin secretion (because of the decreased blood glucose with removal of

TABLE 15-7   **Basis for Changes in Glucose Levels in the First Few Hours after Birth**

Characteristic	Basis
Immature liver enzyme systems	Promotes glucose storage rather than release
Larger brain in proportion to body size	Obligatory glucose user
Increased red blood cell volume	Obligatory glucose user
Decreased liver response to glucagon	Limits release of glucose from glycogen stores
Increased energy needs	Increased metabolic and motor activity with birth

the placenta), increased serum glucagon, stimulation of the sympathetic nervous system with catecholamine release, and increases in hepatic cAMP.[30,168,189] Since insulin promotes transfer of glucose out of the blood into cells, the lowered levels decrease transfer and elevate blood glucose levels. Glucagon stimulates conversion of glycogen into glucose, also raising blood glucose levels.[175]

Hepatic glycogen stores decrease markedly during this period. An estimated 90% of liver and 50% to 80% of muscle glycogen are used within the first 24 hours after birth. As glycogen falls, the newborn responds by mobilizing fat stores with release of free fatty acids. This response is stimulated by the catecholamine release associated with cooling at birth (see Chapter 19). Catecholamines tend to stimulate glucagon, suppress insulin, and augment growth hormone secretion.[183] Healthy infants are able to readily mobilize free fatty acids and ketones to maintain their blood glucose. Breastfed infants have lower blood glucose levels and thus higher ketone bodies than bottle-fed infants.[17,63] The elevated ketone bodies may provide an alternate fuel during the period of lower nutrient intake as breastfeeding is being established.[30] Ketone bodies and lactate increase in late fetal and early neonatal life, providing other alternative fuel sources if glucose levels are low (e.g., hypoglycemia).[184] Production of glucose from amino acids, especially alanine, increases and accounts for 4% to 10% of the glucose used for energy in term infants. Glycogen stores remain low for several days before rising.

Gluconeogenic enzyme activity develops after birth. By 12 to 24 hours after birth, both gluconeogenesis and ketogenesis are active.[123] From late fetal life to 3 days after birth, blood glucose regulation is glucose dominant. As a result, gluconeogenesis is diminished during this period. After this period, blood glucose regulation becomes insulin dominant (the adult pattern).[96] The increased gluconeogenesis

after birth is regulated by changes in the serum insulin-to-glucagon ratio, catecholamine secretion, fatty acid oxidation, and activation of hepatic enzyme systems.[96]

After birth, GLUT-1 transporters on fetal cells decrease, whereas GLUT-2 (uptake of glucose by liver), GLUT-3 (uptake by neurons) and GLUT-4 (uptake by muscle) increase.[47,170] GLUT-1, although lower than in the fetus, remains active and needed for transfer of glucose into red blood cells and across the blood brain barrier.[184]

Increased secretion of catecholamines at birth, stimulated by postbirth cooling, increases glucagon secretion and reverses the fetal insulin-to-glucagon ratio. Increased glucagon concentrations and norepinephrine are important in subsequent activation of the hepatic gluconeogenic enzymes.[129] The predominant enzymes activated during this period are hepatic glycogen phosphorylase, G6PD, and phosphoenolpyruvate carboxykinase (PEPCK). Hepatic glycogen phosphorylase is activated by norepinephrine and glucagon and stimulates glycogenolysis. G6PD activity increases markedly after birth, increasing hepatic release of glucose. This is probably due to surges of glucagon and cAMP, which help to shift the activity of the liver from glycogen to glucose production. PEPCK is the rate-limiting enzyme for gluconeogenesis. PEPCK is inhibited by insulin. With changes in the insulin-to-glucagon ratio after birth, this enzyme increases about 20-fold, thus increasing gluconeogenesis.[96] Concentrations of these enzymes continue to increase over the first 2 weeks after birth in both term and preterm infants.[126]

The resumption of a carbohydrate source (i.e., feeding) generally stabilizes the infant's glucose concentration, and most neonates achieve a steady state in their glucose concentrations by about 5 days.[96] The first enteral feeding immediately increases blood glucose levels. This increase is accompanied by an increase in plasma insulin levels in term infants and development of cyclic changes in insulin and blood glucose levels.[5] In preterm infants the initial feeding is not accompanied by similar hormonal changes and the cyclic responses in insulin and blood glucose take 2 to 3 days to develop (and longer in VLBW infants or infants who are not fed). Enteral feeding stimulates production of digestive hormones and secretion of peptides critical for induction of gastrointestinal tract maturation and development of the enteroinsular axis. These changes lead to additional modifications of hepatic metabolism.[175]

Basal glucose production in newborns is 4 to 6 mg/kg^{-1}/min^{-1} versus 2 to 3 mg/kg^{-1}/min^{-1} in adults and approximately 6 to 10 mg/kg^{-1}/min^{-1} in preterm infants (<1000 g).[47] The high glucose needs in neonates reflect the increased brain-to-body mass, since the brain has a high obligatory glucose use.[85] For infants weighing less than

1000 g, glucose is the major energy source for most of the neonatal period.[47] Newborns are able to produce and use ketone bodies and lactate for brain energy metabolism when glucose levels are low.[34,149] This mechanism is present in term, large preterm, and term SGA infants but is absent VLBW infants and other intrauterine growth–restricted infants who are at risk for hypoglycemia.[34,65,149] In addition glycogen stores in astrocytes may provide another alternative source of glucose for the neurons during periods of low glucose.[45,65]

Lipid Metabolism

The inability of the fetus to oxidize fatty acids is rapidly reversed at birth because of changes in the functional ability of enzymes such as carnitine palmitoyltransferase (see Figure 15-12, *B*).[185] During this period the levels of glucose and free fatty acids are mirror images of each other.[96] Lipolysis increases quickly after birth, reaching a maximum within a few hours.[77,185,190] This increase is reflected in changes in plasma free fatty acid levels, which rise rapidly beginning 4 to 6 hours after birth and reach adult levels by 24 hours. At this time, two thirds of the infant's energy is produced from oxidation of fat.[96,147]

Fat is the major form of stored calories in the newborn and the preferred energy source for tissues such as the heart and adrenal cortex, which have high energy demands.[96] After birth, mobilization of fatty acids from these stores is reflected in the rise in serum levels over the first few hours. This process is initiated by the increase in catecholamines and glucagon, resulting in increased cAMP followed by an increase in protein kinases, phosphorylation, and activation of adipose tissue lipase with release of fatty acids.[77,96,190]

The transition from glucose to fatty acid oxidation after birth is reflected in the fall of the respiratory quotient from 1.0 to 0.5 by 2 hours.[89] This indicates that the infant has moved from obtaining nearly two thirds of its energy from oxidation of glycogen immediately after birth, to deriving most of its energy from fat metabolism.[89] This transition reflects increasing dependence on oxidative metabolism and is associated with an increase in the number of mitochondria and enzymes of the Krebs cycle and changes in blood free fatty acid levels. This shift to fat metabolism is delayed in infants of diabetic mothers with hyperinsulinemia.[89] The neonate's brain may use free fatty acids, along with branched-chain amino acids and ketones, as additional energy sources.[96,185]

The increase in fatty acid oxidation and ketogenesis after birth is related to increased enzyme activity, especially of carnitine palmitoyltransferase (see Figure 15-12, *B*), which reaches adult values by 30 days.[96,185] Carnitine activity enhances fatty acid oxidation. Concentrations of carnitine are

high in human milk for 2 to 3 days after delivery. Another factor influencing this change is alteration in the insulin-to-glucagon ratio with increased glucagon. This increases the availability of substrates such as acetyl-CoA and carnitine for fatty acid oxidation in the mitochondria.[97]

Protein Metabolism

Serum amino acid levels are higher during the first few weeks of life.[122] Urinary amino acids are elevated immediately after birth, with excretion of 8.8 mg/day in preterm and 7.6 mg/day in term infants versus 2.5 mg/day in older children. The average body nitrogen content at birth is 2%.[122]

The newborn has a limited capacity to synthesize protein, primarily because of the relative inactivity of several hepatic enzymes.[60] This limitation is especially marked in preterm infants, whose capacity to use excess amino acid is reduced. Preterm infants who receive excess protein or an unbalanced amino acid intake are at risk for hyperammonemia, azotemia, metabolic acidosis, and altered plasma amino acid profiles. The latter changes are associated with altered protein synthesis and growth, CNS function, and bile acid uptake. The ability to metabolize excess amino acids may also be altered in the newborn depending on maturity of enzyme systems in the liver and skeletal muscle and activity of the urea cycle to eliminate nitrogen.[96]

CLINICAL IMPLICATIONS FOR NEONATAL CARE

The newborn's transitional state in relation to glucose homeostasis can result in problems even for healthy newborns as they attempt to provide adequate energy for maintenance and growth. Alterations in metabolic processes in the newborn can result in clinical problems, most notably hypoglycemia. The status of metabolic function in the newborn also influences nutritional needs (see Chapter 11).

Neonatal Hypoglycemia

The neonate may develop hypoglycemia if glycogen stores are insufficient to provide fuel during transition and until production of energy by fat oxidation is adequate or if the infant fails to adequately mobilize available glycogen stores.[185] There is no clear consensus on the definition of hypoglycemia. Blood glucose levels below 40 (and some investigators suggest <47) mg/dl are uncommon in the first few hours after birth with early feeding.[29,54,103,123,193] Aynsley-Green and Hawdon conclude that there is no evidence that the preterm is able to tolerate low glucose better than term infants.[6] Infants who are very immature or ill (hypoxia, ischemia, sepsis) may have greater glucose needs and be more vulnerable to the effects of hypoglycemia.[29]

Four approaches have been used to define hypoglycemia.[30] These include approaches based on appearance of clinical manifestations, measured glucose value ranges, acute metabolic changes and endocrine responses, and long-term neurologic outcomes.[30] None have been satisfactory. Recently, Aynsley-Green and Hawdon noted that "hypoglycemia is a continuum, no single blood glucose concentration reflecting functional changes in every infant at that level."[6] Similarly, in 1990 an expert panel concluded that the "rational definition of hypoglycemia is clearly not a specific value but a continuum of falling blood glucose values, creating thresholds for neurologic dysfunction, which may vary from one cause of hypoglycemia or clinical circumstance to another."[27] Cornblath and others recommended that the concept of "cutoff" blood glucose values be discarded and the focus be on promoting normoglycemia for all infants with prompt intervention for values less than 40 mg/dl.[27,145] The optimal glucose value and risk for neurologic sequelae probably varies from infant to infant depending on their brain maturity, glycogen stores, presence of hypoxia or ischemia, activity of gluconeogenic pathways, glucose transport status, and brain glucose demand.[29]

Clinical signs of hypoglycemia include tremors, jitteriness, irregular respiration, hypotonia, apnea, cyanosis, poor feeding, high-pitched cry, lethargy, irritability, hypothermia, and seizures. Since hypoglycemic infants may be symptomatic or asymptomatic and signs of hypoglycemia are often nonspecific, careful monitoring of infants at risk for development of hypoglycemia is critical. Multiple factors influence the outcome of infants with hypoglycemia, including severity and duration of the episode, cerebral blood flow and CNS glucose levels, rates of glucose uptake, maturity, availability of alternative substrates, response to intervention, and type of clinical manifestation.[27,29,123] Infants with symptomatic hypoglycemia and seizures have been reported to have a high incidence of later neurologic impairment.[171,173] Most infants with short-term asymptomatic hypoglycemia were reported to have generally good outcomes in earlier studies, although recently this finding has been challenged by several investigators.[27,28,30,65,173] Prolonged or recurrent hypoglycemia may lead to neurologic sequelae.[30] Many studies on the outcome of infants with hypoglycemia have significant methodologic limitations and there have been no controlled prospective studies.

Monitoring of blood glucose values is also an issue. Glucose oxidase reagent sticks are difficult to use in newborns because these sticks are dependent on the hematocrit; have great variance; and lack reproducibility, especially at levels less than 40 to 50 mg/dl.[26,27,29,117,189] Reagent strips are unreliable (levels may vary by ± 5 to 15 mg/dl) and tend to overestimate hypoglycemia.[103,160,173,189] Glucose reflectance meters are also reported to be unreliable in evaluation of capillary blood glucose concentrations in high-risk neonates (i.e., hematocrits over 55% tend to reduce readings, hematocrits below 35% tend to result in falsely high readings).[26,57] Glucose analysis with non–ion-selective electrodes are more reliable (±1.5 mg/dl) but are still limited in that they cannot show trends.[27,57]

Neonatal hypoglycemia can arise from an inadequate supply of glucose, alterations in endocrine regulation, or increased glucose regulation.[29,33,129] Preterm and SGA infants tend to develop hypoglycemia because of insufficient glycogen and fat stores and a decreased rate of gluconeogenesis. Normally with hypoglycemia, brain glucose utilization decreases by up to 50%, with increased reliance on ketones and lactate for energy. Preterm infants may be limited in their ability to mobilize these responses and thus more vulnerable to the effects of hypoglycemia.[47] Infants of diabetic mothers usually have sufficient stores, however, but glycogenolysis is prevented by their high insulin levels and inability to secrete glucagon despite falling blood glucose levels.[185] Infants at risk for neonatal hypoglycemia and associated mechanisms are summarized in Table 15-8.

The Low-Birth-Weight Infant

Hypoglycemia is a common problem of low-birth-weight (LBW) infants, including both appropriate-for-gestational-age (AGA) preterm infants and infants with IUGR. AGA preterm infants usually develop hypoglycemia secondary to inadequate intake or decreased hepatic glucose production. These infants have decreased glycogen and fat stores, (since accumulation of these stores occurs during the third trimester) and immature hepatic function, with low levels of gluconeogenic and glycogenolytic enzymes, especially glucose-6-phosphatase, which is important in glycogenolysis and gluconeogenesis.[82] Preterm infants are less able to produce alternate substrates such as ketone bodies.[189] These infants may also have altered metabolic demands from tachypnea, respiratory distress syndrome, hypoxia, hypothermia, or other events that increase glucose use. Infants of mothers treated with β-adrenergic agonists for preterm labor may develop hypoglycemia secondary to hyperinsulinemia. These agents rapidly cross the placenta and stimulate beta receptors on the fetal pancreas, with subsequent insulin release and altered glucose, homeostasis in the fetus and newborn. β-Adrenergic agents may also blunt normal responses to falling glucose levels.[57]

SGA infants are at risk for hypoglycemia primarily because of alterations in hepatic glucose production and increased glucose utilization.[129,189] These infants may have reduced glycogen stores due to altered placental

TABLE **15-8**   Causes and Time Course of Neonatal Hypoglycemia

MECHANISM	CLINICAL SETTING	EXPECTED DURATION
Decreased substrate availability	Intrauterine growth restriction	Transient
	Prematurity	Transient
	Glycogen storage disease	Prolonged
	Inborn errors of metabolism	Prolonged
Endocrine disturbances: hyperinsulinemia	Infant of a diabetic mother	Transient
	Beckwith-Wiedemann syndrome	Prolonged
	Erythroblastosis fetalis	Transient
	Exchange transfusion	Transient
	Islet cell dysplasia	Prolonged
	Maternal β-sympathomimetics	Transient
	Improperly placed umbilical artery catheter	Transient
Other endocrine disorders	Hypopituitarism	Prolonged
	Hypothyroidism	Prolonged
	Adrenal insufficiency	Prolonged
Increased utilization	Perinatal asphyxia	Transient
	Hypothermia	Transient
Miscellaneous or multiple factors	Sepsis	Transient
	Congenital heart disease	Transient
	Central nervous system abnormalities	Prolonged

From McGowan, J.E., et al. (1998). Glucose homeostasis. In G.B. Merenstein & S.L. Gardner (Eds.). *Handbook of neonatal care* (4th ed.). St. Louis: Mosby.

transport of substrates during fetal life, delayed maturation of gluconeogenesis, and a tendency toward hyperinsulinemia.[123,189] SGA infants have increased energy demands due to their greater brain-to-body mass size, increased metabolic rate, and a tendency toward polycythemia. Since the brain and red blood cells are obligatory glucose users, these factors can markedly increase glucose needs even in nonstressed infants. Glucose utilization may be further increased by chronic or acute perinatal hypoxia. Secretion of hepatic gluconeogenic enzymes (especially PEPCK) is impaired in SGA infants, further limiting their ability to increase glucose production to meet metabolic demands.

The Infant of a Diabetic Mother

Although improved preconceptional care and careful metabolic control of pregnant diabetic women have reduced the incidence of significant macrosomia and improved perinatal mortality, these infants continue to be at risk for a variety of health problems. The cause of these problems relates to fetal and neonatal responses to maternal metabolic alterations and consequences to the neonate of cessation of placental transfer of substrates after birth. Many infants of diabetic mothers are LGA, lethargic, poor feeders, and at risk for the problems summarized in Figure 15-14. Infants born to mothers with significant vascular involvement are often SGA; however,

with more mature liver enzyme systems and lungs due to the effects of intrauterine stress. This group of infants is at particular risk for problems associated with chronic hypoxia such as perinatal asphyxia and polycythemia.

A prominent problem seen in these infants is hypoglycemia. Hyperinsulinemia and a blunted glucagon response, aggravated by decreased hepatic responsiveness to glucose, are responsible for the hypoglycemia.[9,168,185] Levels of epinephrine and norepinephrine are also elevated, suggesting that hypoglycemia in these infants may also be related to adrenal medullary exhaustion.[33,123]

The Infant with Perinatal Asphyxia

Hypoxia and asphyxia alter glucose production and utilization with an increase in glycogenolysis to meet the increased metabolic and energy demands. Since oxygen availability is compromised, the infant switches from aerobic to anaerobic glycolysis. Anaerobic metabolism is less efficient than aerobic metabolism, producing a net increase of only two molecules of adenosine triphosphate (ATP) per molecule of glucose oxidized (versus 36 molecules of ATP per glucose molecule under aerobic conditions). These changes rapidly deplete glucose (glycogen) reserves, with decreased energy production that may be inadequate to maintain normal cell biologic processes and accumulation of lactic acid.[33,185] Hypoxic-ischemic damage to the liver may further impair glucose production and delay the postnatal

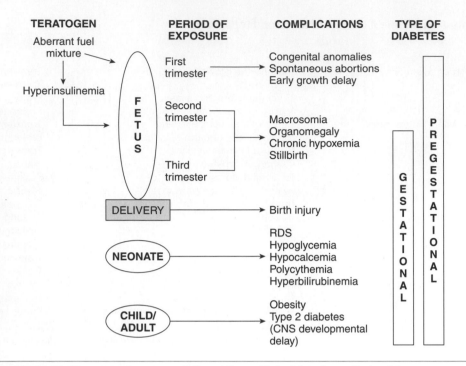

FIGURE **15-14** Diagrammatic representation of the multiple deleterious effects of the pregnancy of a diabetic patient on the offspring during the various periods of fetal and postnatal life. *CNS*, central nervous system; *RDS*, respiratory distress syndrome. (Adapted from Hod, M., et al. [1995]. Gestational diabetes mellitus: Is it a clinical entity? *Diabetes Rev, 3*, 605.)

increase in gluconeogenesis.[74] These infants may have a transient hyperinsulinemia.[33,123]

Because the fetus normally produces large amounts of lactate, intermediary pathways to metabolize lactate are relatively mature and efficient in the fetus and the newborn. As a result, metabolic acidosis with birth and perinatal asphyxia—if it is not severe enough to overwhelm these pathways or associated with postnatal alterations in oxygenation—is often reversed without administration of sodium bicarbonate. Even with moderate to severe perinatal asphyxia, this ability is probably an advantage.

The ability of the infant to mobilize fat stores may be impaired in hypoxia. During hypoxia, release of catecholamines and fatty acids is impaired and oxidation of fats is inhibited.[64,185] These changes impair the ability of the infant to generate the energy necessary for normal cell functions and to meet the increased demands of the hypoxic state. The infant of a diabetic woman may be further compromised, since although this infant has adequate (or excessive) fat stores, the concomitant hyperinsulinemia and reduced glucagon secretion result in inadequate lipolysis.[120]

Neonatal Hyperglycemia

Neonatal hyperglycemia is a blood glucose level greater than 125 mg/dl (whole blood) or 145 to 150 mg/dl (plasma). Hyperglycemia occurs less frequently than hypoglycemia but has the potential for significant alterations in neurodevelopmental outcome.[27,47,129] Hyperglycemia is seen predominantly in preterm infants, especially those weighing less than 1000 g and receiving parenteral glucose infusions.[33,47] Hyperglycemia is negatively correlated with birth weight and positively correlated with the rate of glucose infusion.[69] Markedly increased blood glucose levels can lead to osmotic changes and fluid shifts within the CNS (with a risk of intraventricular hemorrhage) and to glycosuria (with increased fluid and electrolyte loses and subsequent dehydration).

Neonatal hyperglycemia is believed to arise primarily from an inability of the immature infant to suppress endogenous glucose production while receiving a glucose infusion.[33,47,102] This inability may be due to a decrease in expression of GLUT-2 on hepatocytes, decreased sensitivity and response to glucose and insulin with hyperglycemia, and decreased ability of the pancreatic beta cells to adequately increase insulin in response to increased glucose.[47] Stressed

16. Borg, W.P. & Sherwin, R.S. (2000). Classification of diabetes mellitus. *Adv Intern Med, 45,* 279.

17. Brownlee, M., Vlassara, H. & Cerami, A. (1984). Nonenzymatic glycosylation and the pathogenesis of diabetic complications. *Ann Intern Med, 101,* 527.

18. Butte, N.F. (2000). Carbohydrate and lipid metabolism in pregnancy: normal compared with gestational diabetes mellitus. *Am J Clin Nutr, 71*(suppl), 1256S.

19. Carpenter, M.W. & Coustan, D.R. (1982). Criteria for screening tests for gestational diabetes. *Am J Obstet Gynecol, 144,* 768.

20. Catalano, P.M., et al. (1991). Longitudinal changes in insulin release and insulin resistance in nonobese pregnant women. *Am J Obstet Gynecol, 165,* 1667.

21. Catalano, P.M. (1993). Carbohydrate metabolism during pregnancy in control subjects and women with gestational diabetes. *Am J Physiol, 264,* E60.

22. Catalano, P.M., et al. (1996). Relationship between reproductive hormones/TNF-alpha and longitudinal changes in insulin sensitivity during gestation. *Diabetes, 45*(suppl 2), 175a.

23. Chugani, H.T. (1992). Functional brain imaging in paediatrics. *Pediatr Clin N Am, 39,* 777.

24. Coetzee, E.J. & Levitt, N.S. (2000). Maternal diabetes and neonatal outcome. *Semin Neonatol, 5,* 221.

25. Coleman, R.A. (1989). The role of the placenta in lipid metabolism and transport. *Semin Perinatol, 13,* 180.

26. Conrad, P.D., et al. (1989). Clinical application of a new glucose analyzer in the neonatal intensive care unit: Comparison with other methods. *J Pediatr, 114,* 281.

27. Cornblath, M., et al. (1990). Hypoglycemia in infancy: The need for a rational definition. *Pediatrics, 85,* 834.

28. Cornblath, M. (1997). Neonatal hypoglycemia 30 years later: does it injure the brain? Historical summary and present challenges. *Acta Paediatr Jpn, 39,* S7.

29. Cornblath, M. & Ichord, R. (2000). Hypoglycemia in the neonate. *Semin Perinatol, 24,* 136.

30. Cornblath, M., et al. (2000). Controversies regarding definition of neonatal hypoglycemia: Suggested operational thresholds. *Pediatrics, 105,* 1141.

31. Cowett, R.M. (1986). Metabolism in the fetus and infant of the diabetic mother. *In infant of the diabetic mother: Report of the 93rd Ross conference on pediatric research.* Columbus, OH: Ross Laboratories.

32. Cowett, R.M., et al. (1988). Ontogeny of glucose homeostasis in low birth weight infants. *J Pediatr, 112,* 462.

33. Cowett, R.M. (1998). Hypoglycemia and hyperglycemia in the newborn. In R.A. Polin & W.W. Fox (Eds.). *Fetal and neonatal physiology* (2nd ed.). Philadelphia: W.B. Saunders.

34. deBoissieu, D., et al. (1995). Ketone body turnover at term and in premature newborns in the first two weeks after birth. *Biol Neonate, 67,* 84.

35. DeLucchi, C., et al. (1987). Effects of dietary nucleotides on the fatty acid composition of erythrocyte membrane lipids in term infants. *J Pediatr Gastroenterol, 6,* 568.

36. Desci, T., Molnar, D. & Klujber L. (1990). Lipid levels in VLBW preterm infants. *Acta Paediatr Scand, 29,* 577.

37. Desai, M., et al. (1995). Adult glucose and lipid metabolism may be programmed during fetal life. *Biochem Soc Trans, 23,* 331.

38. Devreker, F. & Englert, Y. (2000). In vitro development and metabolism in the human embryo up to the blastocyst stage. *Eur J Obstet Gynecol Reprod Biol, 92,* 51.

39. Dickson, J.E. & Palmer, S.P. (1990). Gestational diabetes: Pathophysiology and diagnosis. *Semin Perinatol, 14,* 2.

40. Dorner, G. & Plagemann, A. (1992). Perinatal hyperinsulinism as possible disposing factor for diabetes mellitus, obesity, and enhanced cardiovascular risk in later life. *Horm Metab Res, 26,* 213.

41. Durnin, J.V.G. (1991). Energy requirements of pregnancy, *Diabetes, 40*(suppl 2), 152.

42. Economides D.L., et al. (1990). Hypertriglyceridemia and hypoxemia in SGA fetuses. *Am J Obstet Gynecol, 162,* 382.

43. Eriksson, U.J., et al. (1991). Diabetic embryopathy: studies with animal and in vitro models. *Diabetes, 40*(suppl), 94.

44. Evain-Brion, D. (1999). Maternal endocrine adaptation to placental hormones in humans. *Acta Paediatr Suppl, 428,* 12.

45. Eyre, J.A., et al. (1994). Glucose export from the brain in man: Evidence for a role of astrocyte glycogen as a reservoir of glucose for neural metabolism. *Brain Res, 635,* 349.

46. Falcone, T. & Little, A.B. (1994.) Placental polypeptides. In D. Tulchinsky & A.B. Little (Eds.). *Maternal-fetal endocrinology.* Philadelphia: W.B. Saunders.

47. Farrag, H.M. & Cowett, R.M. (2000). Glucose homeostasis in the micropremie. *Clin Perinatol, 27,* 1.

48. Freinkel, N. (1980). Of pregnancy and progeny. *Diabetes, 29,* 1023.

49. Garner, P.R. (1995). Glucose metabolism assessment in pregnancy. *Clin Biochem, 28,* 499.

50. Gluckman, P.D. (1997). Endocrine and nutritional regulation of prenatal growth. *Acta Paediatr Suppl, 423,* 153.

51. Golde, S.H., et al. (1982). Insulin requirements during labor: A reappraisal. *Am J Obstet Gynecol, 144,* 556.

52. Goldman, J.A., et al. (1986). Pregnancy outcome in patients with insulin-dependent diabetes mellitus with preconceptual diabetic control: A comparative study. *Am J Obstet Gynecol, 155,* 293.

53. Grasso S., et al. (1990) Glucose and insulin secretion in low birth weight preterm infants. *Acta Paediatr Scand, 79,* 280.

54. Gregory, J.W. & Aynsley-Green, A. (1993). The definition of hypoglycemia. *Baillieres Clin Endocrinol Metab, 7,* 587.

55. Gross, T.L. & Kazzi, G.M. (1985). Effects of maternal malnutrition and obesity on pregnancy outcome. In N. Gleicher (Ed.). *Principles of medical therapy in pregnancy.* New York: Plenum.

56. Guyton, A.C. & Hall, J.E. (1996). *Textbook of medical physiology* (9th ed.). Philadelphia: W.B. Saunders.

57. Halamek, L.P., Benaron, D.A. & Stevenson, D.K. (1997). Neonatal hypoglycemia, Part I: background and definition. *Clin Pediatr (Phila), 36,* 675.

58. Handwerger, S. & Freemark, M. (2000). The roles of placental growth hormone and placental lactogen in the regulation of human fetal growth and development. *J Pediatr Endocrinol Metab, 13,* 343.

59. Hanif, K., et al. (1982). Oxytocin action: Mechanisms for insulin-like activity in isolated rat adipocytes. *Mol Pharmacol, 22,* 381.

60. Hanning, R.M. & Zlotkin, S.H. (1989). Amino acid and protein needs of the neonate: Effects of excess and deficiency. *Semin Perinatol, 13,* 131.

61. Hare, J.W. (1989). *Diabetes complicating pregnancy: The Joslin Clinic method.* New York: Alan R. Liss.

62. Harigaya, A., et al. (1997). Relationship between concentrations of serum leptin and fetal growth. *J Clin Endocrinol Metab, 82,* 3281.

63. Hawdon, J.M., et al. (1992). Patterns of metabolic adaptation for preterm and term infants in the first neonatal week. *Arch Dis Child, 67,* 357.

64. Hawdon, J.M. & Ward Platt, M.P. (1992). Metabolic and hormonal interrelationships in perinatal asphyxia. *Biol Neonate, 62,* 300.

TABLE **15-9** Recommendations for Clinical Practice Related to Carbohydrate, Protein, and Fat Metabolism in Neonates

Know the usual changes in carbohydrate, protein, and fat metabolism during the fetal and neonatal periods (pp. 614-621 and Table 15-6).

Monitor neonates for alterations in metabolic processes (pp. 618-625).

Monitor newborn glucose status during transition and in the early neonatal period (pp. 619-621 and Table 15-7).

Initiate early enteral feeding as appropriate (p. 620 and Table 15-7).

Monitor neonates for signs of excessive and inadequate intake of carbohydrates, protein, and fat (pp. 617-621).

Recognize infants at risk for hypoglycemia (pp. 621-624 and Table 15-8).

Know the clinical signs of hypoglycemia (p. 622).

Assess and monitor infants at risk for neonatal hypoglycemia (pp. 621-624 and Table 15-8).

Recognize infants at risk for hyperglycemia (pp. 624-625).

Assess and monitor infants at risk for hyperglycemia (pp. 624-625).

Monitor infants at risk for hyperglycemia for alterations in fluid and electrolyte balance (pp. 624-625).

Recognize and monitor for problems for which the infant of a diabetic mother is at increased risk (p. 623 and Figure 15-14).

infants seem to be at particular risk for hyperglycemia because of the simultaneous increase in catecholamine release (as a stress response), which further increases glucose levels by inhibiting insulin release and glucose utilization.[32,120] Other infants at risk for hyperglycemia include infants treated with methylxanthines for apnea or with lipid infusions given at rates greater than 0.25 g/kg/hour, infants with sepsis or after surgery, and term newborns with severe growth restriction who develop a transient neonatal diabetes. The latter disorder may a result of partial insulin insensitivity and the effects of stress on glucose homeostasis.[32]

MATURATIONAL CHANGES DURING INFANCY AND CHILDHOOD

Energy and calorie requirements per unit of body weight remain higher in children than in adults because of their higher metabolic rate and growth needs. The relative requirement for carbohydrates is similar for children and adults. For infants, generally not more than 40% of the total calories should be carbohydrates; for children and adults this value is 40% to 60%.[122] Cerebral glucose utilization is increased until chldhood.[23]

Serum amino acid levels decrease and urinary exc increases until early childhood. Total body prote creases and reaches adult proportions (3%) by 4 Retention of nitrogen decreases during this time to values (11 mg/kg/day).[122] Diet alters the fatty acid co sition of adipose tissue during periods of rapid weigh in the first year of life and possibly the compositic structural lipids. This may affect functional ability o sues and structures.[186]

SUMMARY

Growth "is an accretion of materials brought together synergism involving anabolism and catabolism."[107] Gro involves increases in cell size and in the complexity of c tissues, and organs. Alterations in growth during the p natal period arise from maternal, fetal, or placental fact that alter the availability, accretion, or use of substrates nutrients. When this occurs the fetus or neonate may unable to adapt to environmental stress and is at increas risk for morbidity and mortality.[107] Implications for clir cal practice are summarized in Table 15-9.

REFERENCES

1. Aberg, A., et al. (2001). Congenital malformations among infan whose mothers had gestational or preexisting diabetes. *Early Hum Dev, 61,* 85.
2. ACOG Technical Bulletin. (1995). Diabetes in pregnancy. *In J Gynaecol Obstet, 48,* 331.
3. Alsat, E., et al. (1998). Physiological role of human placental growth hormone. *Mol Cell Endocrinol, 140,* 121.
4. Atanassova, P. & Popova, L. (2000). Leptin expression during the differentiation of subcutaneous adipose cells of human embryos in situ. *Cells Tissues Organs, 166,* 15.
5. Aynsley-Green, A. (1985). Metabolic and endocrine interrelations in the human fetus and neonate. *Am J Clin Nutr, 41,* 399.
6. Aynsley-Green, A. & Hawdon, J.M. (1997). Hypoglycemia in the neonate: current controversies. *Acta Paediatr Jpn, 39,* S12.
7. Baird, J.D. (1986). Some aspects of the metabolic and hormonal adaptation to pregnancy. *Acta Endocrinol, 112*(suppl 277), 11.
8. Barbieri, R.L. (1999). Endocrine disorders in pregnancy. In S.S.C. Yen, R.B. Jaffe, & R.L. Barbieri (Eds.). *Reproductive endocrinology* (4th ed.). Philadelphia: W.B. Saunders.
9. Barss, V. (1989). Diabetes and pregnancy. *Med Clin North Am, 73,* 685.
10. Battaglia, F.C. & Thureen, P.J. (1997). Nutrition of the fetus and premature infant. *Nutrition, 13,* 903.
11. Battaglia, F.C. (1992). Metabolic aspects of fetal and neonatal growth. *Early Hum Dev, 29,* 99.
12. Berk, M.A., et al. (1989). Macrosomia in infants of insulin-dependent diabetic mothers. *Pediatrics, 83,* 1029.
13. Berkowitz, K.M. (1998). Insulin resistance and preeclampsia. *Clin Perinatol, 25,* 873.
14. Bernard-Karger, C. & Ktorza, A. (2001). Endocrine pancreas plasticity under physiological and pathological conditions. *Diabetes, 50*(suppl 1), S30.
15. Boden, G. (1996). Fuel metabolism in pregnancy and in gestational diabetes mellitus. *Obstet Gynecol Clin North Am, 23,* 1.

65. Hawdon, J.M. (1999). Hypoglycemia and the neonatal brain. *Eur J Pediatr, 158*, S9.

66. Hay, W.W. (1991). The placenta. Not just a conduit for maternal fuels. *Diabetes, 40*(suppl 2), 44.

67. Hay, W.W. (1994). Placental transport of nutrients to the fetus. *Horm Res, 42*, 215.

68. Hay, W.W. (1994). Placental supply of energy and protein substrates to the fetus. *Acta Paediatr Suppl, 405*, 13.

69. Hay, W.W. (1995). Metabolic interrelationships of placenta and fetus. *Placenta, 16*, 19.

70. Hay, W.W. (1995). Regulation of placental metabolism by glucose supply. *Reprod Fertil Dev, 7*, 365.

71. Hay, W.W. (1998). Nutritional and metabolism needs of the fetus and very small infants: A comparative approach. *Biochem Soc Trans, 26*, 75.

72. Hay, W.W. (1998). Fetal requirements and placental transfer of nitrogen compounds. In R.A. Polin & W.W. Fox (Eds.). *Fetal and neonatal physiology* (2nd ed.). Philadelphia: W.B. Saunders.

73. Hay, W.W. (1998). Prologue: placental-fetal metabolic inter-relationships. *Biochem Soc Trans, 26*, 67.

74. Hendrickse, W., Stammers, J.P. & Hull, D. (1989). The transfer of free fatty acids across the human placenta. *Br J Obstet Gynaecol, 92*, 945.

75. Henson, M.C. & Castracane, V.D. (2000). Leptin in pregnancy. *Biol Reprod, 63*, 1219.

76. Herrera, E., et al. (1998). Maternal-fetal transfer of lipid metabolites. In R.A. Polin & W.W. Fox (Eds.). *Fetal and neonatal physiology* (2nd ed.). Philadelphia: W.B. Saunders.

77. Herrera, E. (2000). Lipid metabolism in the fetus and the newborn. *Diabetes Metab Res Rev, 16*, 202.

78. Herrera, E. (2000). Metabolic adaptations in pregnancy and their implications for the availability of substrates to the fetus. *Eur J Clin Nutr, 54*, S47.

79. Hjollund, E., et al. (1986). Impaired insulin receptor binding and postbinding defects of adipocytes from normal and diabetic pregnant women. *Diabetes, 35*, 598.

80. Holness, M.J., et al. (1999). Current concepts concerning the role of leptin in reproductive function. *Mol Cell Endocrinol, 157*, 11.

81. Homko, C.J., et al. (1999). Fuel metabolism during pregnancy. *Semin Reprod Endocrinol, 17*, 119.

82. Hume, R. & Burchell, A. (1993). Abnormal expression of glucose-6-phosphatase in preterm infants. *Arch Dis Child, 68*, 202.

83. Hytten, F. & Chamberlain G. *Clinical physiology in obstetrics.* Oxford: Blackwell Scientific.

84. Illsley, N.P. (2000). Glucose transporters in the human placenta. *Placenta, 21*, 14.

85. Illsley, N.P. (2000). Placental glucose transport in diabetic pregnancy. *Clin Obstet Gynecol, 43*, 116.

86. Inzucchi, S.E. (1999). Diabetes mellitus. In G.N. Burrow & T.P. Duffy (Eds.). *Medical complications during pregnancy* (5th ed.). Philadelphia: W.B. Saunders.

87. Jansson, T. & Powell, T.L. (2000). Placental nutrient transfer and fetal growth. *Nutrition, 16*, 500.

88. Jovanovic, L. & Peterson, C.M. (1983). Insulin and glucose requirements during the first stage of labor in insulin-dependent diabetic women. *Am J Med, 75*, 607.

89. Kalhan, S., et al. (1997). Disorders of carbohydrate metabolism. In A.A. Fanaroff & R.J. Martin (Eds.). *Neonatal-perinatal medicine, diseases of the fetus and infant* (6th ed.). St. Louis: Mosby.

90. Kalhan, S., et al. (1997). Glucose turnover and gluconeogenesis in human pregnancy. *J Clin Invest, 100*, 1775.

91. Kalhan, S.C. & Robinson, C.V. (1998). Metabolism of glucose in the fetus and newborn. In R.A. Polin & W.W. Fox (Eds.). *Fetal and neonatal physiology* (2nd ed.). Philadelphia: W.B. Saunders.

92. Kalhan, S. & Devapatla, S. (1999). Pregnancy, insulin resistance, and nitrogen accretion. *Curr Opin Clin Nutr Metab Care, 2*, 359.

93. Kalhan, S.C. (2000). Protein metabolism in pregnancy. *Am J Clin Nutr, 71*(suppl), 1249S.

94. Kalhan, S. (2000). Gluconeogenesis in the fetus and neonate. *Semin Perinatol, 24*, 94.

95. Kenepp N.S., et al. (1980). Fetal and neonatal hazards of maternal hydration with 5% dextrose before caesarian section. *Lancet, 1*, 1150.

96. Kimura, R.E. & Warshaw, J.B. (1983). Metabolism during development. In J.B. Warshaw (Ed.). *The biological basis of reproductive and developmental medicine.* New York: Elsevier Biomedical.

97. Kimura, R.E. (1989). Fatty acid metabolism in the fetus. *Semin Perinatol, 13*, 202.

98. King, J.C., et al. (19994). Energy metabolism during pregnancy: influence of maternal energy status. *Am J Clin Nutr, 59*(suppl), 439S.

99. King, J.,C. (2000). Physiology of pregnancy and nutrient metabolism. *Am J Clin Nutr, 71*(suppl), 1218S.

100. Kitzmiller, J.L., et al. (1991). Preconception care of the diabetic: Glycemic control prevents congenital anomalies. *JAMA, 265*, 731.

101. Kjos, S.L. & Buchanan, T.A. (1999). Gestational diabetes mellitus. *N Engl J Med, 341*, 1749.

102. Kliegman, R.M. (1993). Problems in metabolic adaptation: Glucose, calcium and magnesium. In M.H. Klaus & A.A. Fanaroff (Eds.). *Care of the high risk neonate* (4th ed.). Philadelphia: W.B. Saunders.

103. Koh, T.H. (1996). Glucose and the newborn baby: sweet justice? *J Paediatr Child Health, 32*, 281.

104. Koletzko, B., Demmelmair, H. & Socha, P. (1998). Nutritional support of infants and children: supply and metabolism of lipids. *Baillieres Clin Gastroenterol, 12*, 671.

105. Kopp-Hoolihan, L.E., et al. (1999). Longitudinal assessment of energy balance in well-nourished pregnant women. *Am J Clin Nutr, 69*, 697.

106. Kratzscm J. Y., et al. (2000). Leptin and pregnancy outcome. *Curr Opin Obstet Gynecol, 12*, 501.

107. Kretchmer, N., Schumacher, L.B. & Silliman, K. (1989). Biological factors affecting intrauterine growth. *Semin Perinatol, 13*, 169.

108. Kuhl, C. (1998). Etiology and pathogenesis of gestational diabetes. *Diabetes Care, 21*, B19.

109. Laffel, L. (1999). Ketone bodies: A review of physiology, pathophysiology and application of monitoring to diabetes. *Diabetes Metab Res Rev, 15*, 412.

110. Lage, M., et al. (1999). Serum leptin levels in women throughout pregnancy and the postpartum period and in women suffering spontaneous abortion. *Clin Endocrinol, 50*, 211.

111. Laivuori, H., et al. (2000). Leptin during and after pre-eclamptic or normal pregnancy: its relation to serum insulin and insulin sensitivity. *Metabolism, 49*, 259.

112. Langer, O. (1990). Critical issues in diabetes and pregnancy: Early identification, metabolic control, and prevention of adverse outcome. In I.R. Merkatz & J.E. Thompson (Eds.). *New perspectives on prenatal care.* New York: Elsevier.

113. Langer, O. & Mazze, R.S. (1986). The relationship between glycosylated hemoglobin and verified self-monitored blood glucose among pregnant and non-pregnant women with diabetes. *Practical Diabetes, 4*, 32.

114. Lawrence, M., et al. (1987). Energy requirements of pregnancy in Gambia. *Lancet, 2*, 1072.

115. Lesser, K.B. & Carpenter, M.W. (1994). Metabolic changes associated with normal pregnancy and pregnancy complicated by diabetes mellitus. *Semin Perinatol, 18,* 399.

116. Liechty, E.A. & Denne, S.C. (1998). Regulation of fetal amino acid metabolism: substrate or hormonal regulation. *J Nutr, 128,* 342S.

117. Lin, H.C., et al. (1989). Accuracy and reliability of glucose reflectance meters in the high-risk neonate. *J Pediatr, 115,* 998.

118. Lithell, H., et al. (1996). Relation of size at birth to non-insulin dependent diabetes and insulin concentrations in men aged 50-60 years. *BMJ, 312,* 406.

119. Lockitch, G. (1997). Clinical biochemistry of pregnancy. *Crit Rev Clin Lab Sci, 34,* 67.

120. Lorenz, J.M. (1997). Assessing fluid and electrolyte status in the newborn. National Academy of Clinical Biochemistry. *Clin Chem, 43,* 205.

121. Louik, C., et al. (1985). Risk factors for neonatal hyperglycemia associated with 10% dextrose infusion. *Am J Dis Child, 139,* 783.

122. Lowrey, G. (1986). *Growth and development of children.* Chicago: Yearbook.

123. Lteif, A.N. & Schwenk, W.F. (1999). Hypoglycemia in infants and children. *Endocrinol Metab Clin North Am, 28,* 619.

124. Marconi, A.M., et al. (1993). An evaluation of fetal glucogenesis in intrauterine growth retarded pregnancies. *Metabolism, 42,* 860.

125. Maresh, M. (2001). Diabetes in pregnancy. *Curr Opin Obstet Gynecol, 13,* 103.

126. Marsac, C., et al. (1976). Development of gluconeogenic enzymes in the liver of human newborns. *Biol Neonate, 28,* 317.

127. Masuzaki, H., et al. (1997). Nonadipose tissue production of leptin: leptin as a novel placenta-derived hormone. *Nat Med, 3,* 1029.

128. Matsuda, J., et al. (1999). Dynamic changes in serum leptin concentrations during fetal and neonatal periods. *Pediatr Res, 45,* 71.

129. McGowan, J.E., et al. (1998). Glucose homeostasis. In G.B. Merenstein & S.L. Gardner (Eds.). *Handbook of neonatal care* (4th ed.). St. Louis: Mosby.

130. Metzger, B.E., et al. (1995). Prepregnancy weight and antepartum insulin secretion predict glucose tolerance five years after gestational diabetes mellitus. *Diabetes Care, 16,* 1598.

131. Metzger, B.E. & Coustan, D.M. (1998). Summary and recommendations of the Fourth International Workshop-Conference on Gestational Diabetes Mellitus. *Diabetes Care, 21*(suppl 2), B161.

132. Meyer, B.A. & Palmer S.A. (1990). Pregestational diabetes. *Semin Perinatol, 14,* 12.

133. Milley, J.R. (1989). Fetal protein metabolism. *Semin Perinatol, 13,* 192.

134. Mills, J.L., et al. (1988). Lack of relation of increased malformation rates in infants of diabetic mothers to glycemic control during organogenesis. *N Engl J Med, 318,* 672.

135. Miodovinik, M., et al. (1988). Major malformations in infants of IDDM women: Vasculopathy and early first-trimester poor glycemic control. *Diabetes Care, 11,* 713.

136. Moley, K.H. (2001). Hyperglycemia and apoptosis: Mechanisms for congenital malformations and pregnancy loss in diabetic women. *Trends Endocrinol Metab, 12,* 78.

137. Molina, R.D., et al. (1991). Gestational maturation of placental glucose transfer capacity in sheep. *Am J Physiol, 261,* R697.

138. Moore, T.R. (1997). Fetal growth in diabetic pregnancy. *Clin Obstet Gynecol, 40,* 771.

139. Moore, T.R. (1999). Diabetes and pregnancy. In R.K. Creasey & R. Resnik (Eds.). *Maternal-fetal medicine: Principles and practice* (4th ed.). Philadelphia: W.B. Saunders.

140. Morris, M.A., Grandis, A.S., & Litton, J.C. (1986). Longitudinal assessment of glycosylated blood protein concentrations in normal pregnancy and gestational diabetes. *Diabetes Care, 9,* 107.

141. National Diabetes Data Group. (1979). Classification and diagnosis of diabetes mellitus and other categories of glucose intolerance. *Diabetes, 28,* 1039.

142. Neville, M.C. (1999). Adaptation of maternal lipid flux to pregnancy: research needs. *Eur J Clin Nutr, 53,* S120.

143. Ng, P.C., et al. (2000). Leptin and metabolic hormones in preterm newborns. *Arch Dis Child Fetal Neonatal Ed, 83,* F198.

144. Nielsen, J.H., et al. (1999). Beta cell proliferation and growth factors, *J Mol Med, 77,* 62.

145. Ogata, E.J. (1999). Carbohydrate homeostasis. In G.B. Avery, M.A. Fletcher, & M.G. Macdonald (Eds.). *Neonatology-pathophysiology and management of the newborn* (5th ed.). Philadelphia: Lippincott, Williams & Wilkins.

146. Oski, F.A. & Komazaw, M. (1975). Metabolism of the erythrocytes of the newborn infant. In F.A. Oski, R.F. Jaffee, & P.A. Miescher (Eds.). *Current problems in pediatric hematology.* New York: Grune & Stratton.

147. Page, E.W., Villee, C.A. & Villee, D.B. (1981). *Human reproduction: Essentials of reproductive and perinatal medicine* (3rd ed.). Philadelphia: W.B. Saunders.

148. Pampfer, S. (2000). Peri-implantation embryopathy induced by maternal diabetes, *J Reprod Fertil Suppl, 55,* 129.

149. Patel, D. & Kalhan, S. (1992). Glycerol metabolism and triglyceride-fatty acid cycling in the human newborn: Effect of maternal diabetes and intrauterine growth retardation. *Pediatr Res, 31,* 52.

150. Peters, R.K., et al. (1996). Long-term diabetogenic effect of a single pregnancy in women with prior gestational diabetes mellitus. *Lancet, 347,* 227.

151. Phelps, R.L., Metzger, B.E. & Freinkel, N. (1981). Carbohydrate metabolism in pregnancy. XVII: Diurnal profiles of plasma glucose, insulin, free fatty acids, triglycerides, cholesterol and individual amino acids in late normal pregnancy. *Am J Obstet Gynecol, 140,* 730.

152. Phelps, R.L., et al. (1983). Biphasic changes in hemoglobin A_{1c} concentration during normal human pregnancy. *Am J Obstet Gynecol, 147,* 651.

153. Pitkin, R.M. (1999). Energy in pregnancy. *J Clin Nutr, 69,* 583.

154. Poppitt, S.D., et al. (1993). Evidence of energy-sparing in Gambian women during pregnancy: a longitudinal study using whole-body calorimetry. *Am J Clin Nutr, 57,* 353.

155. Prentice, A.M. (1996). Energy requirements of pregnant and lactating women. *Eur J Clin Nutr, 50,* S82.

156. Prentice, A.M. & Goldberg, G.R. (2000). Energy adaptations in human pregnancy: limits and long-term consequences. *J Clin Nutr, 71*(suppl), 1226S.

157. Pribylova, H. & Dvorakova, L. (1996). Long-term prognosis of infants of diabetic mothers. *Acta Diabetol, 33,* 30.

158. Ramirez, I., et al. (1998). Lipoprotein lipase. In R.A. Polin & W.W. Fox (Eds.). *Fetal and neonatal physiology* (2nd ed.). Philadelphia: W.B. Saunders.

159. Reece, E.A., et al. (1990). A longitudinal study comparing growth in diabetic pregnancies with growth in normal gestations: I. Fetal weight. *Obstet Gynecol Rev, 45,* 160.

160. Reynolds, G.J. & Davis, S.M. (1993). A clinical audit of cotside blood glucose measurement in the detection of neonatal hypoglycemia. *J Paediatr Child Health, 4,* 289.

161. Rizzo, T., et al. (1991). Correlations between antepartum maternal metabolism and intelligence of offspring. *N Engl J Med, 325,* 911.

162. Rosenn, B.G.M. & Miodovnik, M. (2000). Glycemic control in the diabetic pregnancy: is tighter always better? *J Matern Fetal Med, 9,* 29.

163. Rutanen, E.M. (2000). Insulin-like growth factors in obstetrics. *Curr Opin Obstet Gynecol, 12,* 163.

164. Ryan, E.A., et al. (1985). Insulin action during pregnancy: studies with euglycemic clamp technique. *Diabetes, 34,* 380.

165. Sadler, T.W., Denno, K.M. & Hunter, E.S. (1993). Effects of altered maternal metabolism during gastrulation and neurulation stages of embryogenesis. *Ann N Y Acad Sci, 15*(678), 48.

166. Sauer, P.J. (1994). Substrate utilization during the first weeks of life. *Acta Paediatr Suppl, 405,* 49.

167. Schwartz, R. & Teramo, K.A. (2000). Effects of diabetic pregnancy on the fetus and newborn. *Semin Perinatol, 24,* 120.

168. Schwitzgebel, V.M. & Gitelman, S.E. (1998). Neonatal hyperinsulinism. *Clin Perinatol, 25,* 1015.

169. Simmons, M.A., Battaglia, F.C. & Meschia, G. (1979). Placental transfer of glucose. *J Dev Physiol, 1,* 227.

170. Simmons, R.A. (1998). Cell glucose transport and glucose handling during fetal and neonatal development. In R.A. Polin & W.W. Fox (Eds.). *Fetal and neonatal physiology* (2nd ed.). Philadelphia: W.B. Saunders.

171. Sinclair, J.C. (1997). Approaches to the definition of neonatal hypoglycemia. *Acta Paediatr Jpn, 39,* 17S.

172. Singhi, S. (1988). Effect of maternal intrapartum glucose therapy on neonatal blood glucose levels and neurobehavioral status of hypoglycemic term newborns. *J Perinat Med, 16,* 217.

173. Singh, M., et al. (1991). Neurodevelopmental outcome of asymptomatic and symptomatic babies with neonatal hypoglycemia. *Ind J Med Res, 94,* 6.

174. Skouby, S.O., et al. (1990). Mechanisms of action of oral contraceptives on CHO metabolism at the cellular level. *Am J Obstet Gynecol, 163,* 343.

175. Sperling, M.A. (1988). Glucose homeostasis after birth. In C.T. Jones (Ed.). *Research in perinatal medicine. VII: Fetal and neonatal development.* Ithaca, NY: Perinatology Press.

176. Sperling, M.A. (1994). Carbohydrate metabolism: insulin and glucagon. In D. Tulchinsky & A.B. Little (Eds.). *Maternal-fetal endocrinology* (2nd ed.). Philadelphia: W.B. Saunders.

177. Sugden, M.C. & Holness, M.J. (1998). Fuel selection: the maternal adaptation to fetal nutrient demand. *Biochem Soc Trans, 26,* 79.

178. Swenne, I., et al. (1994). Inter-relationship between serum concentrations of glucose, glucagon and insulin during the first two days of life. *Acta Paediatr, 83,* 915.

179. Swislocki, A. & Kraemer, F.B. (1989). Maternal metabolism in diabetes mellitus: Pathophysiology of diabetes in pregnancy. In S.A. Brody & K. Ueland (Eds.). *Endocrine disorders in pregnancy.* Norwalk, CT: Appleton & Lange.

180. Takeda, Y. (1988). Metabolic adjustment in perinatal period. In G.H. Wiknjosastro, W.H. Prakoso, & K. Maeda (Eds.). *Perinatology.* Amsterdam: Elsevier.

181. Uauy, R., Treen, M. & Hoffman, D.R. (1989). Essential fatty acid metabolism and requirements during development. *Semin Perinatol, 13,* 118.

182. Uauy, R., Mena, P. & Rojas, C. (2000). Essential fatty acid metabolism in the micropremie. *Clin Perinatol, 27,* 71.

183. Vander, A., Sherman, J. & Luciano, D. (2000). *Human physiology: The mechanism of body function* (8th ed.). New York: McGraw-Hill.

184. Vannucci, R.C. & Vannucci, S.J. (2000). Glucose metabolism in the developing brain. *Semin Perinatol, 24,* 107.

185. Warshaw, J.B. & Maniscalco, W.M. (1978). Perinatal adaptations in carbohydrate and lipid metabolism. In L. Stern, W. Oh, & B. Friis-Hansen (Eds.). *Intensive care of the newborn II.* New York: Masson.

186. Warshaw, J.B. & Terry, M.L. (1976). Cellular energy metabolism during fetal development. VI: Fatty acid oxidation by developing brain. *Dev Biol, 52,* 161.

187. Weiss, P.A.M. (1988). *Gestational diabetes.* New York: Springer-Verlag.

188. Widdowson, E.M. (1981). The demands of the fetal and maternal tissues for nutrients, and the bearing of these on the needs of the mother to "eat for two." In J. Dobbing (Ed.). *Maternal nutrition in pregnancy—eating for two?.* London: Academic Press.

189. Williams, A.F. (1997). Hypoglycemia of the newborn: a review. *Bull World Health Organ, 75,* 261.

190. Williamson, D.H. (1998). Ketone body production and metabolism in the fetus and newborn. In R.A. Polin & W.W. Fox (Eds.). *Fetal and neonatal physiology* (2nd ed.). Philadelphia: W.B. Saunders.

191. Wollmann, H.A. (2000). Growth hormone and growth factors during perinatal life. *Horm Res, 53*(suppl 1), 50.

192. Yamashita, H., Shao, J. & Friedman, J.E. (2000). Physiologic and molecular alteration in carbohydrate metabolism during pregnancy and gestational diabetes mellitus. *Clin Obstet Gynecol, 43,* 87.

193. Yamauchi, Y. (1997). Hypoglycemia in healthy, full term, breast-fed neonates during the early days of life: preliminary observation. *Acta Paediatr Jpn, 39,* S44

Calcium and phosphorus are critical in cardiovascular, nervous, homeostatic, and muscular processes and in the function of many hormones and enzyme systems. Maternal calcium metabolism during pregnancy and lactation undergoes a series of hormone-mediated adjustments to enhance transport of this mineral to the fetus without long-term alterations in the maternal skeleton.[48] Calcium, phosphorus, and other minerals are transported across the placenta for fetal bone mineralization and skeletal growth. After birth the neonate loses the placental supply of calcium and must quickly establish homeostasis of this system to avoid metabolic derangements. This chapter discusses alterations in these substances and related hormones during pregnancy and the neonatal period. Calcium and phosphorous homeostasis in nonpregnant individuals is summarized in Figure 16-1 and the box on p. 631. The roles of the major calcitropic hormones (parathyroid hormone, calcitonin, and vitamin D) are summarized in Table 16-1.

MATERNAL PHYSIOLOGIC ADAPTATIONS

Calcium and phosphorus metabolism is altered during pregnancy, with an increase in the amount and efficiency of intestinal calcium absorption. During pregnancy, absorption increases to 50%, versus 20% to 25% in nonpregnant individuals.[33] The increased absorption is mediated primarily by increased 1,25-dihydroxyvitamin D (1,25-[OH]$_2$D).[64] Calcium accumulation in the fetus by term totals 28 to 30 g.[64] Most of this accretion occurs in the third trimester and is used for fetal bone formation and mineralization. Calcium metabolism undergoes further changes during lactation to meet the calcium needs of the growing infant. Understanding of changes in maternal calcium metabolism in pregnancy and lactation has grown in recent years with improved assay techniques and recognition of the roles of parathyroid hormone–related protein (see the box on p. 632).[4,8,69]

Antepartum Period

Calcium homeostasis during pregnancy is interrelated with changes in extracellular fluid volume, renal func-

tion, and fetal needs. The mother meets the fetal requirement for calcium primarily by increasing intestinal calcium absorption. These change are mediated by increased production of 1,25-(OH)$_2$D and under the influence of hormones such as estrogens, prolactin (PRL), and human placental lactogen (hPL) as well as parathyroid hormone–related protein (PTHrP). PRL and hPL may increase intestinal absorption of calcium in pregnancy, decrease urinary excretion, and stimulate synthesis of both PTHrP and 1,25-(OH)$_2$D.[48,69] Changes in substances involved in calcium and phosphorus homeostasis during pregnancy are summarized in Table 16-2 and Figures 16-2 and 16-3.

Calcium

Maternal total serum calcium levels fall progressively beginning soon after fertilization and decrease by an average of 1 to 1.5 mg/dl. Calcium reaches its lowest levels at 28 to 32 weeks, followed by a plateau or slight rise to term (see Figure 16-2).[64,65,72,96] Serum calcium levels during pregnancy average 9 to 10 mg/dl—a decrease of 5 to 6%.[64] The decrease in serum calcium is a relative decrease, since it is primarily related to and parallels the fall in serum proteins, especially albumin, with a decrease in both total and bound calcium. Other factors that contribute to alterations in serum calcium include increased plasma volume and hemodilution, increased urinary calcium excretion, and fetal transfer (primarily in the third trimester).[39,64,66,86] Ionized calcium does not change significantly and is stable or in the low normal range.[15,25,48,82,83]

Calcium absorption occurs by active transport in the duodenum and proximal jejunum and by passive mechanisms in the distal jejunum and ileum.[7] Intestinal absorption of calcium doubles during pregnancy, with a positive calcium balance noted by as early as 12 weeks' gestation, and continues to the third trimester.[11,48] The early increase allows the mother to store calcium throughout pregnancy to meet the high fetal demands in the latter part of the third trimester.[11,26] The rise in calcium absorption follows and

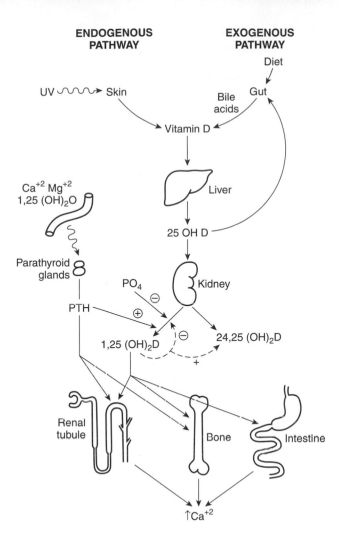

ENDOGENOUS PATHWAY   EXOGENOUS PATHWAY

Diet

UV ⤳ Skin

Bile acids   Gut

Vitamin D

Ca^{+2} Mg^{+2}
$1,25\ (OH)_2O$

Liver

Parathyroid glands

25 OH D

PO_4 ⊖   Kidney

PTH   ⊕

$1,25\ (OH)_2D$ ⊖ $24,25\ (OH)_2D$

＋

Renal tubule   Bone   Intestine

$\uparrow Ca^{+2}$

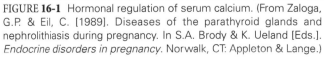

FIGURE **16-1** Hormonal regulation of serum calcium. (From Zaloga, G.P. & Eil, C. [1989]. Diseases of the parathyroid glands and nephrolithiasis during pregnancy. In S.A. Brody & K. Ueland [Eds.]. *Endocrine disorders in pregnancy.* Norwalk, CT: Appleton & Lange.)

Calcium and Phosphorus Homeostasis

Serum calcium is present in three forms: (1) bound to albumin and other proteins (40%), (2) completed to bicarbonate and other buffers (10%), and (3) ionized (50%). Calcium is also found in extracellular fluid (ECF) and cytoplasm. Parathyroid hormone (PTH) and vitamin D are the major hormones involved in calcium homeostasis. Calcitonin also influences calcium but appears to be less important. Actions of PTH and intestinal absorption of vitamin D are enhanced by magnesium. Hormonal regulation of calcium metabolism is summarized in Figure 16-1. Calcium and phosphorus are absorbed in the small intestine under the influence of 1,25-dihydroxyvitamin D (1,25-[OH]_2D), which stimulates a calcium-binding protein. PTH mobilizes calcium and phosphorus in bone by stimulating osteolysis. This process is vitamin D–dependent and releases calcium and phosphorus into ECF. In the kidneys, PTH inhibits proximal tubular reabsorption of phosphate, leading to increased urinary loss and decreased ECF levels. PTH increases distal tubular reabsorption of Ca^{2+} to conserve calcium by decreasing renal excretion. Thus PTH increases the release of both calcium and phosphorus from the bones, increasing ECF levels. Since concentrations of Ca^{2+} and PO_4 in ECF are closely tied to each other (i.e., $[Ca^{2+}] \times [PO_4]$ is a constant of sol-

ubility), if ECF PO_4 levels increase, further release of calcium from the bones would normally be decreased to keep the total concentration of calcium and phosphorus constant. If the kidneys increase PO_4 excretion, however, extracellular phosphorus decreases and more calcium is released from bone. The net result is increased serum and ECF calcium and decreased phosphorus. Decreased serum PO_4 occurs because the phosphaturic actions of PTH exceed serum phosphate–elevating activities. Release of PTH is regulated by concentrations of serum calcium. Even small changes in serum ionized calcium stimulate PTH release.

Vitamin D also enhances PTH action to increase calcium release from bone and tubular reabsorption of these minerals (see Figure 16-1). Vitamin D can be produced endogenously in the epidermal layer of skin by ultraviolet light irradiation of 7-dehydrocholesterol to D_3 (cholecalciferol) or ingested as D_2 (ergocalciferol) or D_3. Ingested vitamin D requires bile salts for intestinal absorption. Vitamin D is converted to serum 25-hydroxyvitamin D (25-[OH]D) (major circulating metabolite) in the liver. In the kidneys, 25-(OH)D is hydroxylated to 1,25-(OH)_2D (see Figure 16-1). Regulation of vitamin D is through negative feedback from 25-(OH)D levels.

TABLE **16-1**   Hormonal Actions Controlling Calcium and Phosphorus Levels

HORMONE	BONE	INTESTINE	KIDNEY
Parathyroid hormone	Increased calcium release Increased phosphorus release		Increased calcium reabsorption Decreased phosphorus reabsorption
Calcitonin	Decreased calcium release Decreased phosphorus release	May inhibit calcium and phosphorus reabsorption	Increased calcium excretion Increased phosphorus excretion
Vitamin D	Increased calcium release	Increased calcium absorption Increased phosphorus absorption	Increased calcium reabsorption Increased phosphorus reabsorption

Roles of Parathyroid Hormone–Related Protein

Parathyroid hormone–related protein (PTHrP), which is thought to be a prohormone, was first isolated in 1987. It is produced from a single gene similar in origin and sequencing to the parathyroid (PTH) gene.[103] PTHrP is produced in most tissues of the body and has a broad range of functions. Since few of these functions directly relate to calcium, the name is somewhat a misnomer. PTHrP is divided into three peptides that can each produce a family of peptides, each with differing functions.[38,103] The major functions of PTHrP are as follows: (1) stimulation of transepithelial calcium transport, especially in the kidneys, placenta, and breast; (2) smooth muscle (uterus, bladder, stomach, intestines, arterial wall) relaxation; and (3) regulation of cellular proliferation, differentiation, and apoptosis (see Chapter 3).[103] Critical perinatal functions of PTHrP include milk production (see Chapter 5), labor onset (see Chapter 4), fetal-maternal calcium gradient and placental calcium transport.[99,103] Disruption of the PTHrP gene in the fetus or neonate is lethal.[99]

TABLE **16-2**   Changes in Calcium and Phosphorus Metabolism in Pregnancy and Lactation

PARAMETER	PREGNANCY	LACTATION
Total serum calcium	Relative decrease because of decreased albumin and hemodilution	Slightly increased
Ionized calcium	Stable to low normal	Slightly increased
Phosphorus	Stable to low normal	Increased
1,25-dihyroxyvitamin D	Increased from early pregnancy, peaking at twice normal	Decreased
Serum 25-hydroxyvitamin D	No change or slightly lower	No change
Parathyroid hormone	Decreased or low normal	Decreased
Calcitonin	Increased or high normal	Decreased
Parathyroid hormone–related protein	Increased, especially in the second half	Increased
Intestinal calcium reabsorption	Doubles	No change
Urinary calcium excretion	Relative increase	Decreased to conserve calcium
Bone reabsorption	Increased toward the end of pregnancy	Increased

Compiled from references 42, 48, 68, 69, and 76.

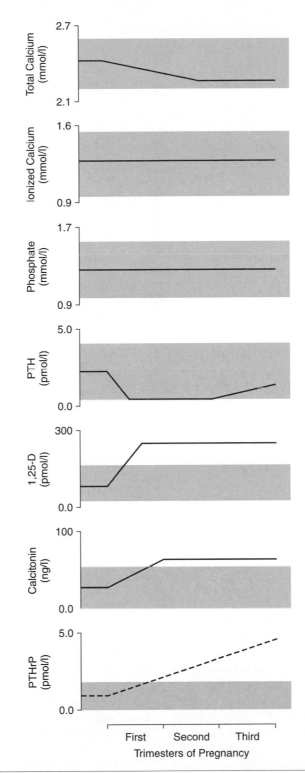

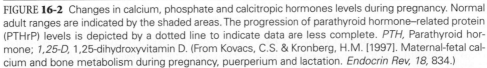

FIGURE **16-2** Changes in calcium, phosphate and calcitropic hormones levels during pregnancy. Normal adult ranges are indicated by the shaded areas. The progression of parathyroid hormone–related protein (PTHrP) levels is depicted by a dotted line to indicate data are less complete. *PTH,* Parathyroid hormone; *1,25-D,* 1,25-dihydroxyvitamin D. (From Kovacs, C.S. & Kronberg, H.M. [1997]. Maternal-fetal calcium and bone metabolism during pregnancy, puerperium and lactation. *Endocrin Rev, 18,* 834.)

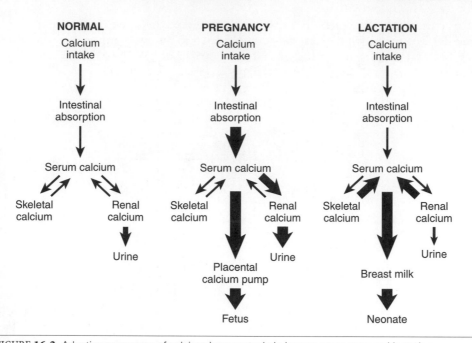

FIGURE **16-3** Adaptive processes of calcium homeostasis in human pregnancy and lactation as compared with the normal nonpregnant state. The thickness of the arrows indicates the relative increase or decrease with respect to the normal, nonpregnancy state. (From Kovacs, C.S. & Kronberg, H.M. [1997]. Maternal-fetal calcium and bone metabolism during pregnancy, puerperium and lactation. *Endocrin Rev, 18,* 859.)

parallels the rise in 1,25-(OH)$_2$D, which is the primary mediator of this change.

Bone mass is not normally lost in pregnancy.[46] The rate of bone turnover is low in the first half of pregnancy when maternal bone stores are increasing. The change in intestinal absorption begins early in pregnancy, thus preceding fetal bone calcium demand. Maternal bone formation also increases early with increased storage of calcium in maternal bones. Maternal bone growth is associated with increases in bone alkaline phosphatase and procollagen peptides in the blood.[74] Osteocalcin, which normally increases with bone formation, is lower in pregnancy, although some increase is noted in late pregnancy. This may be due to increased placental calcium uptake.[74,76,103] Bone turnover increases in the third trimester at the time of peak calcium transfer to the fetus. During this time, maternal bone stores are mobilized to meet fetal demands.[48,66,82] There does not appear to be a large change in maternal skeletal mass or bone density during pregnancy, probably because the fetal calcium accumulation of 28 to 30 g represents only a small proportion of maternal skeletal stores.[66,106]

Urinary calcium excretion rises by 12 weeks, but falls near term.[11,15,65,106] This change is due to the increased glomerular filtration rate and occurs even when the maternal diet is calcium deficient.[33] The increased urinary excretion probably also reflects the increased intestinal calcium absorption.[26,48] After 36 weeks, urinary calcium excretion decreases by about 35%, increasing calcium availability by approximately 50 mg/day. Since fetal needs at this point are approximately 350 mg/day, however, other maternal calcium sources (i.e., dietary sources or the maternal skeleton) are essential.[64,94,106] Increased urinary excretion of calcium has been reported in women with good dietary calcium intake who are given calcium supplements.[26]

Phosphorus and Magnesium

Serum inorganic phosphate levels are generally stable during pregnancy, as is renal tubular reabsorption of this mineral (see Figure 16-2).[15,48] Magnesium is at or below the lower reference range limit.[14] These changes are related to hemodilution and decreased serum albumin.

Parathyroid Hormone

Early studies reported that PTH production increases during pregnancy.[20,48,64] However, newer immunoreactive and bioreactive assays demonstrate low normal parathyroid hormone (PTH) levels in pregnancy.[15,48,82] Several recent prospective studies have reported that PTH is decreased in the first trimester but in the midnormal range by term.[11,15,48] The initial decrease may be a response to increased PTHrP derived from the fetus and placenta.[38] Others have reported little change in values over the course of pregnancy.[11,74] The increased levels of PTHrP may contribute to suppression of parathyroid function during pregnancy.[46,48,103]

Vitamin D

Both free and bound levels of 1,25-$(OH)_2D$ rise early in pregnancy, double by 10 weeks' gestation, and remain high to term.[48,69,82,98] Vitamin D–binding protein also increases possibly due to the increased estrogen.[46] Changes in 1,25-$(OH)_2D$ are probably not mediated by PTH, since levels are low or normal during the first trimester, but are under the influence of estrogens, PTHrP, and possible PRL and hPL.[48] The increased 1,25-$(OH)_2D$ comes from increased production by the maternal kidney and decidua as well as the fetoplacental unit.[69,76,103] The doubling of 1,25-$(OH)_2D$ is paralleled by a twofold increase in intestinal calcium absorption. Serum 25-hydroxyvitamin D (25-[OH]D) levels do not change significantly during pregnancy.[84] The increase in 1,25-$(OH)_2D$ after 34 to 36 weeks has been associated with an increase in a vitamin D–binding protein and bound vitamin D. Thus intestinal absorption of vitamin D is enhanced throughout gestation (see Figure 16-3).[26]

Calcitonin

Calcitonin levels are generally reported to increase during pregnancy (see Figure 16-2), with about 20% of women having values outside the normal range, although some report little change.[11,15,48,74] During pregnancy calcitonin is synthesized by the breast and placenta in addition to the usual synthesis by the C cells of the thyroid gland. The increase in calcitonin with advancing pregnancy may stimulate the proximal renal tubule to increase 1,25-$(OH)_2D$ production.[38] Increased calcitonin inhibits calcium and phosphorus release from the bones, counteracting the action of PTH (Table 16-1). This may help prevent excessive reabsorption of bone calcium and conserve the maternal skeleton while simultaneously permitting the intestinal and renal actions of PTH and 1,25-$(OH)_2D$ to provide the additional calcium needed by the fetus.[17,91] The adaptive processes in calcium homeostasis in pregnancy and lactation are summarized in Figure 16-3.

Intrapartum Period

Calcium is essential for activation of myosin light chain kinase in smooth muscle and thus myometrial contraction. Without calcium, much of which comes from extracellular sources, myometrial contraction does not occur. PTHrP levels in the myometrium and amnion decrease at the onset of labor.[23,102] The role of calcium in uterine contraction is discussed in Chapter 4.

Postpartum Period

Serum calcium, PTH, and calcitonin gradually return to prepregnant values by 6 weeks postpartum in nonlactating women.[64] In lactating women, changes in calcium metabolism continue in order for the mother to provide adequate calcium for infant growth and development.[49,69] Lactation is a greater challenge to calcium homeostasis than pregnancy. During lactation the woman must provide 220 to 349 mg/day of calcium.[61,68] PTHrP and maternal bone reabsorption are increased. Levels of 1,25-$(OH)_2D$ fall from the high pregnancy values but may be increased during lactation in women with multiple pregnancy.[48,69] PTH decreases to low normal values.[48] Serum total and ionized calcium levels are slightly increased but within normal limits; phosphorus levels are high normal or increased (Figure 16-4).[42,48,61,68] Intestinal calcium absorption is not increased in lactation as it was during pregnancy. However, renal calcium excretion is reduced, thus conserving calcium for milk production.[42,61] Changes in calcium metabolism during lactation are summarized in Figure 16-4 and Table 16-2.

Thus the calcium demands of lactation are met primarily through reabsorption of maternal skeletal calcium and reduction in renal excretion of calcium. Maternal bone density decreases during lactation, with up to 7% of the maternal bone mass lost by 9 months' lactation.[46,52] These changes are most prominent in the axial skeleton (e.g., there is a 3% to 5% loss of bone mass in the spine and hip), with wide individual variation.[1,43,46,49] These are reversible changes with no long-term adverse effects in most women. Very rarely bone reabsorption may be excessive, with fractures and a clinical diagnosis of osteoporosis.[48,69]

Changes in the maternal skeleton are reversed in the later stages of lactation and with weaning. Markers of bone reabsorption increase in the first 5 to 12 months of lactation then decrease.[69] During weaning, there is decreased suckling and milk volume and increase in estradiol levels. Resumption of menses is associated with increases in calcium absorption, PTH, and, in most studies, 1,25-$(OH)_2D$.[11,69] By 3 to 5 months after lactation, bone status is similar in lactating women and nonlactating women, regardless of the length of lactation.[69]

The mechanisms leading to the changes in calcium metabolism during lactation are unclear since the changes are not associated with significant changes in the calcitropic hormones.[69] These changes may be mediated by PTHrP, since

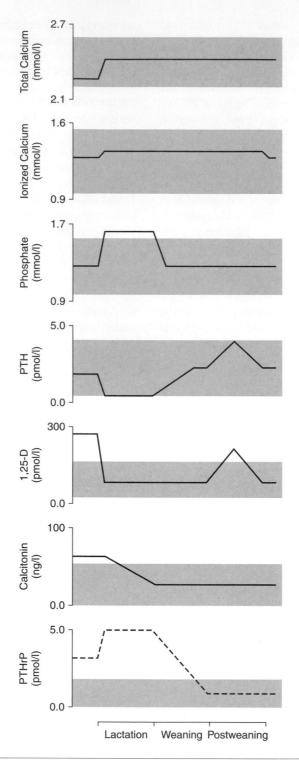

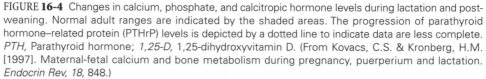

FIGURE **16-4** Changes in calcium, phosphate, and calcitropic hormone levels during lactation and post-weaning. Normal adult ranges are indicated by the shaded areas. The progression of parathyroid hormone–related protein (PTHrP) levels is depicted by a dotted line to indicate data are less complete. *PTH,* Parathyroid hormone; *1,25-D,* 1,25-dihydroxyvitamin D. (From Kovacs, C.S. & Kronberg, H.M. [1997]. Maternal-fetal calcium and bone metabolism during pregnancy, puerperium and lactation. *Endocrin Rev, 18,* 848.)

levels are very high in breast milk and in the lactating woman's circulation.[48,69,102] The increases in PTH and 1,25-(OH)$_2$D after weaning help restore the maternal skeleton.[69,74] Lactation physiology is discussed further in Chapter 5.

CLINICAL IMPLICATIONS FOR THE PREGNANT WOMAN AND HER FETUS

Changes in calcium and phosphorus metabolism are essential to provide adequate substrate for fetal growth and development and to simultaneously ensure maternal homeostasis. To support these changes, maternal calcium and phosphorus intake must increase during pregnancy and lactation. This section considers these needs as well as implications of alterations in calcium, phosphorus, and magnesium in relation to leg cramps and selected disorders complicating pregnancy.

Maternal Calcium and Phosphorus Needs

During pregnancy an additional 400 mg/day of both calcium and phosphorus is recommended, especially during the second and third trimesters. This results in a total calcium intake of 1200 mg/day in the pregnant woman (or 1600 mg/day in the pregnant adolescent).[42,102] The effect of supplemental calcium intake on bone density during pregnancy is unclear. The changes in bone metabolism occur even with increased calcium intakes.[11,69,99] There is no consistent correlation between dietary calcium intake or 1,25-(OH)$_2$D bioavailability and intestinal calcium absorption.[46] Additional supplementation above this level is not needed in most woman, although it may be needed by pregnant adolescents, especially those with low dietary intakes (less than 600 mg/day).[46,53] Current evidence does not suggest that pregnant women over age 35 have special needs for calcium supplementation nor that depletion of maternal stores over multiple pregnancies increases the risk of osteoporosis in later life.[48,69] Hoskings notes that since the fetal skeleton contains only 28 to 30 g of calcium (far less than the average 1000 g of calcium in the adult skeleton), it is unlikely that fetal calcium needs cause clinical bone disease in the mother, but these needs may exacerbate the effects of existing low peak bone mass.[38] However, there is some evidence that women with low calcium intakes may benefit from increased calcium intake during pregnancy.[70] The role of calcium and calcium supplementation and hypertension is discussed in Maternal Calcium Metabolism and Pregnancy Complications.

Prentice summarizes the effects of calcium supplementation during lactation and pregnancy: "There is no evidence that the changes observed during lactation reflect inadequacies in calcium intake. Supplementation studies have shown that neither the bone response nor breast milk calcium excretion is modified by increases in calcium supply during lactation, even in women with a low calcium intake. The situation in pregnancy is less clear. Calcium nutrition may influence the health of the pregnant woman, her breast milk calcium concentration, and the bone mineralization and blood pressure of her infant, but these possibilities require formal testing."[69] Calcium and phosphorus needs during lactation are discussed further in Chapter 5.

Vitamin D intake is critical in maintaining calcium homeostasis. Vitamin D intakes of 400 IU (10 µg) per day are recommended in pregnancy. Vitamin D helps ameliorate fluctuations in the calcium-to-phosphorus ratio and enhances calcium absorption. Alterations in calcium and bone metabolism, including increased risk of maternal osteomalacia and neonatal hypocalcemia, tend to occur primarily in women who have diets that are low in both calcium and vitamin D.[42] Supplementation is recommended for women with low dietary intakes and for those who live in northern latitudes during the winter, where sunlight exposure is minimal.

Milk is an excellent source of calcium, vitamin D, and phosphorus. Alternatives for women who are lactose intolerant include cheese, yogurt, lactose-free milks, sardines, whole or enriched grains, and green leafy vegetables. Some substances alter calcium absorption. For example, lactose increases calcium absorption, possibly by decreasing luminal pH or through chelate formation. Excessive fats, phosphate, phytates (found in many vegetables), or oxalates interfere with calcium absorption by forming insoluble calcium salts within the intestinal lumen. High sodium concentrations may also decrease calcium absorption by interfering with active transport mechanisms.[10,106]

Adequate intake of phosphorus is as important as that of calcium since these two minerals exist in a constant of solubility in the blood (see the box on p. 631). Excess dietary phosphorus binds calcium in the intestine, limiting absorption; excess blood phosphorus leads to increased urinary excretion of calcium. Therefore it is essential for the pregnant and lactating woman's diet to be balanced in regard to these substances. Foods such as processed meats, snack foods, and cola drinks have high phosphorus but low calcium levels.[102]

Leg Cramps

Sudden tonic or clonic contraction of the gastrocnemius muscles and occasionally the thigh and gluteal muscles is experienced by up to half of all pregnant women.[95] These cramps are felt most frequently at night or on awakening and are most common after 24 weeks' gestation.[19,105] Leg cramps are also more common in sedentary versus active pregnant women.[37]

Cramps may be associated with increased neuromuscular irritability due to decreased serum ionized calcium levels combined with increased serum inorganic phosphate levels.[64] The incidence of leg cramps is not correlated with ionized calcium levels, however. Some women who drink more than 1 quart of milk per day report relief from leg cramps after a decrease in milk intake.[19] Muscular irritability in pregnancy also arises from the lowered calcium levels and mild alkalosis caused by changes in the respiratory system (see Chapter 9).[102] Interventions have included reducing milk intake (although milk is rich in calcium, it also contains large amounts of phosphate); supplementation with nonphosphate calcium salts; or use of aluminum hydroxide antacids to promote formation of insoluble aluminum phosphate salts in the gut, thus reducing absorption of phosphorus.[64] Oral magnesium is reported to decrease leg cramps but not increase serum magnesium levels; excess magnesium increases urinary magnesium excretion.[14] Treatment with oral calcium versus a placebo has not been reported to significantly reduce the incidence of leg cramps.[32] Thus the specific basis for leg cramps in pregnant women and the most effective interventions remain unclear.

Maternal Calcium Metabolism and Pregnancy Complications

Women with acute and chronic hypertension during pregnancy tend to have lower serum calcium and higher magnesium levels.[48,61] Decreased calcium increases vascular resistance.[68] The incidence of preeclampsia has been reported to vary inversely with calcium intake.[47] Preeclampsia is associated with hypocalciuria and low 1,25-$(OH)_2$D levels.[48] Some studies report that calcium supplementation decreased the risk of this disorder; however, a recent large clinical trial did not find any effect, at least in a population of healthy women with good calcium intakes before and during pregnancy.[54,68,87] Since calcium supplements did not prevent preeclampsia in these women, the changes in calcium were thought to be due to renal alternations rather than changes in calcium metabolism.[54] However, other studies suggest that calcium supplements may decrease the risk of preeclampsia in women with chronically low calcium intakes.[55]

Women on long-term heparin therapy for thromboembolism during pregnancy may occasionally develop heparin-induced osteopenia.[64] Heparin inhibits 1α-hydroxylation of 25-(OH)D, decreasing levels of 1,25-$(OH)_2$D; altering calcium homeostasis; and increasing bone calcium absorption.[42,61] Calcium status should be monitored carefully in women receiving this therapy.

Disorders of the parathyroid glands are rare. The diagnosis of primary hyperparathyroidism may be obscured by pregnancy changes in calcium metabolism. Pregnancy may provide some protection to women with this disorder, with 39% to 80% becoming asymptomatic during pregnancy. This is often followed by an acute increase in calcium postpartum. Moderate to severe forms of this disorder may lead to maternal hypercalcemia with fetal parathyroid suppression and hypocalcemia and risk for neonatal tetany.[42,48,61,68,104] In women with hypoparathyroidism the normal replacement dose of vitamin D may need to be increased due to the increased vitamin D–binding hormone in pregnancy.[42,48,61,68,104]

Osteoporosis is a rare complication of pregnancy and seems to be associated with various factors—such as chronic heparin, anticonvulsant, or steroid use, or excessive reabsorption secondary to chronic inadequate calcium intake, low 1,25-$(OH)_2$D stores, or excessive PTHrP—rather than pregnancy-induced alteration in calcium metabolism.[11,17,46,48] Similarly the also rare pregnancy-associated osteoporosis of the hip is also thought to be unrelated to alterations in mineral balance in pregnancy.[11,17,48]

Maternal-Fetal Interactions

Maternal-placental-fetal calcium metabolism is interrelated. As noted earlier, fetal calcium accumulation is mediated by increased maternal absorption of calcium. Calcium is actively transported across the placenta, mediated primarily by PTHrP.[9,48,64,103] Calcium transport increases from 50 mg/day (20 weeks) up to 350 mg/day (mean 200 mg/day) at term.[24,48] About 80% of fetal mineral accretion occurs after 25 weeks, with peak accretion occurring from 34 to 38 weeks' gestation coinciding with bone development.[47] Total fetal calcium accretion increases during pregnancy from 100 mg (4 months) to 28 to 30 g at term.[41,68] Fetal serum calcium (10 to 11 mg/dl) is about 1 mg/dl above maternal values. The higher fetal values are primarily due to increased ionized calcium.[71]

Fetal calcium accretion and active transport across the placenta are independent of maternal calcium levels and stores. Calcium movement across the placenta involves three phases: (1) passive bidirectional movement across the maternal-facing microvillous trophoblast membrane into the syncytiotrophoblast cytosol; (2) binding of calcium to calcium-binding protein such as calmodulin for transport through the syncytiotrophoblast cytosol (binding buffers the calcium so that it does not disrupt cellular processes in the trophoblast); and (3) active transport across the fetal-facing basolateral trophoblast membrane into fetal circulation.[28,38,40] Calcium levels in the cytosol are 1000 times higher than in the maternal circulation.[40]

PTHrP (see the box on p. 632) regulates control of calcium transport across the placenta. PTHrP may also be the major factor in maintaining the fetal calcium level higher than maternal levels. PTHrP is produced by the fetal parathyroid glands, skeletal growth plate, umbilical cord, amnion, chorion, and placenta.[38,103] PTHrP levels are higher in the fetus than in adults.[103] Fetal calcium levels are set at a specific level and appear to be maintained at that level regardless of maternal calcium level, even with maternal hypocalcemia.[48] Although fetal calcium levels are maintained primarily by placental calcium transport, movement of calcium in and out of fetal bone, fetal renal tubular reabsorption and excretion of calcium, and swallowing of amniotic fluid also have a role in maintaining fetal homeostasis.[48]

Fetal phosphorus and magnesium levels are also higher than maternal levels; these minerals are actively transported across the placenta.[22,28,52,64] Magnesium is transported to the fetus in increasing amounts after the fifth month.[13] Fetal magnesium levels depend on adequate placental function and maternal stores. Placental insufficiency and inadequate nutritional intake increase the risk of neonatal hypomagnesemia.[84] Transplacental passage of magnesium is influenced by maternal level; for example, administration of large amounts of magnesium sulfate to the mother leads to elevated magnesium on both mother and fetus.[28]

Placental transport of 1,25-$(OH)_2$D is low.[64,89] The placenta is the primary source of this metabolite and contains 1,25-$(OH)_2$D receptors and enzymes such as 1-hydroxylase.[27,106] The fetus is dependent on maternal 25-(OH)D, which is readily transported across the placenta, since fetal hepatic enzyme processes are limited. The 25-(OH)D can be 1α-hydroxylated to 1,25-$(OH)_2$D in the fetal kidneys.[48] Maternal vitamin D deficiency is associated with an increased incidence and severity of neonatal hypocalcemia. PTH and calcitonin do not appear to cross the placenta.[64]

SUMMARY

Calcium and phosphorus are essential minerals for many body processes and growth. Alterations in metabolic processes related to these elements during pregnancy can alter maternal, fetal, and infant health status. Health can be promoted by careful assessment and monitoring of maternal and fetal status and initiation of appropriate interventions. Recommendations for clinical practice related to calcium and phosphorus metabolism during pregnancy are summarized in Table 16-3.

DEVELOPMENT OF CALCIUM AND PHOSPHORUS METABOLISM IN THE FETUS
Anatomic Development

Calcium and phosphorus metabolism is regulated by a variety of hormones, including PTH, vitamin D, and calcitonin. This section reviews development of the parathyroid glands; development of the thyroid glands (site of calcitonin synthesis) is discussed in Chapter 18. Because calcium and phosphorus are critical for bone mineralization processes, skeletal growth is also considered.

Parathyroid Glands

Many structures of the head and neck—including the maxillary process, mandibular arch, several muscles of the jaw, hyoid and ear bones, thyroid, and cricoid cartilage—develop from the branchial or pharyngeal arches. These are bars of mesenchymal tissue separated by pharyngeal clefts. The pharyngeal pouches are outpouchings along the lateral walls of the pharyngeal gut (Figure 16-5). Structures that develop from these pouches include the palatine tonsil, thymus, primitive tympanic cavity, and (from the third and fourth pouches) the parathyroid glands.[60]

The third and fourth pharyngeal pouches develop bulbar and ventral portions. The inferior parathyroid glands differentiate from the dorsal bulbar portion of the third pharyngeal pouch during the sixth week. The ventral portion of this pouch forms the thymus. The parathyroid glands initially migrate caudally and medially with the thymus, later separating and attaching to the inferior portion of the dorsal surface of the descending thyroid gland (see Chapter 18). The superior parathyroid glands develop from

TABLE **16-3** **Recommendations for Clinical Practice Related to Changes in Calcium and Phosphorus Metabolism in Pregnant Women**

Recognize the usual changes in calcium and phosphorus metabolism during pregnancy (pp. 630-635, Figures 16-2 and 16-3, and Table 16-2).

Assess and monitor maternal nutrition in terms of calcium, phosphorus, and vitamin D intake (p. 637).

Counsel women regarding calcium, phosphorus, and vitamin D requirements to meet maternal and fetal needs during pregnancy (p. 637).

Monitor fetal growth (pp. 640-641).

Know usual parameters for serum calcium during pregnancy (p. 630).

Evaluate diet of women complaining of leg cramps (pp. 637-638).

Counsel women regarding leg cramps and appropriate interventions (p. 637-638).

Recognize usual changes in calcium and phosphorus metabolism during lactation (pp. 635-637, Figures 16-3 and 16-4, and Table 16-2).

Assess and monitor nutrition during lactation in terms of calcium, phosphorus, and vitamin D intake (pp. 635-637).

Counsel women regarding calcium, phosphorus, and vitamin D requirements to meet maternal needs during lactation (pp. 635-637 and Chapter 5).

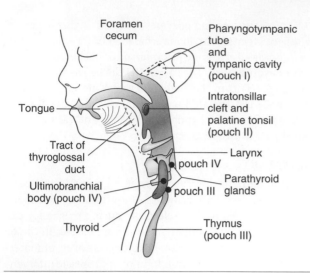

FIGURE **16-5** Schematic sagittal section of the head and neck of a 20-week-old fetus showing the adult derivatives of the pharyngeal pouches and descent of the thyroid gland. (From Moore, K. [1998]. *The developing human* [6th ed.]. Philadelphia: W.B. Saunders.)

the dorsal bulbar portion of the fourth pharyngeal pouch by the sixth week and attach to the superior portion of dorsal side of the caudally migrating thyroid gland.[60]

Skeletal Development and Growth

Skeletal growth occurs in two phases. During fetal life a cartilage anlage (primordium) is formed that is later replaced by bone. Bone formation also occurs by differentiation of mesenchyme directly into bone cells. Later, linear growth depends on cartilaginous growth in the endochondral ossification centers at the epiphyses; appositional growth of the skeleton depends on laying down of new bone by bone-forming cells with subsequent remodeling (reabsorption of existing bone followed by formation of new bone).[18] Bone formation and remodeling is a cyclic process that occurs continuously throughout life. During growth, bone formation is greater than remodeling. Once maximal growth is achieved, the skeletal mass is stable for 10 to 15 years and remodeling and bone formation occur at the same rate. With aging, remodeling is greater than bone formation, with a gradual loss of bone mass. Excessive differences between bone formation and remodeling can lead to osteoporosis and compromised skeletal integrity.[18] Stress, such as subjecting bone to heavy loads or that occurs with strenuous exercise, stimulates osteoblastic deposition of new bone, leading to thickening of bones.[31,73]

Skeletal development begins in early embryonic life and continues into postnatal life. Bone consists primarily of organic matrix and bone salts. Compact bone is 30% organic matrix and 70% bone salts; newer bone has more organic matrix. The organic matrix is composed primarily of collagen fibers that give the bone its tensile strength. The rest of the matrix is ground substance, consisting of extracellular fluid and proteoglycans, which may assist in controlling deposition of calcium salts. Crystalline bone salts (hydroxyapatites) give bone compressional strength and consist primarily of calcium and phosphorus with small deposits of sodium, potassium, magnesium, and carbonate salts.[31,73]

Bone is formed by either intramembranous or endochondral ossification. Intramembranous ossification is the process involved in formation of bones such as the skull, mandible, and maxilla.[73] With intramembranous ossification, the fibrous mesenchyme condenses to form a collagenous membrane in which some cells differentiate into osteoblasts. Osteoblasts produce a collagenous material and ground substance to fill the extracellular spaces. The collagen polymerizes to form collagen fibers and the tissue becomes osteoid and similar to cartilage.[73] Osteoblasts later secrete alkaline phosphatase, which leads to deposition of calcium salts in the form of calcium hydroxyapatite crystals, with gradual conversion of the osteoid to bone. Some osteoblasts are trapped within lacunae in the bone matrix to form osteocytes. The bone matrix grows in all directions as spicules and ossification centers are established.

The osteoblasts deposit spongy bone first, followed by plates of compact bone (periosteal ossification). Spongy bones are filled with fibrous and cellular mesenchymal derivatives that later differentiate into elements characteristic of red bone marrow (reticular tissue, fat cells, sinusoids, and developing blood cells). Bone growth is accompanied by remodeling in which much of the original matrix is reabsorbed by osteoclasts simultaneously with formation of new bone by osteoblasts. During this process the osteoclasts project villi that secrete proteolytic enzymes to dissolve the organic matrix and citric, lactic, and other acids that cause solution of bone salts.[31]

The long bones of the appendicular and axial skeleton form by endochondral ossification in which the condensed mesenchymal cells give rise to hyaline cartilage models that are shaped like the eventual bone. This cartilage is eroded locally and destroyed as bone is formed. Endochondral ossification involves the progressive destruction of cartilage, deposition of calcium salts, and formation of a central area of spongy bone (that will develop a red marrow matrix) surrounded by compact bone. This process begins in the middle of the bone shaft and progresses toward the epiphysis. At birth the long bones consist of central ossification centers and bony shafts with cartilaginous ends. Secondary areas of ossification later appear in the epiphyses.[18,60,73,90]

Bone growth is mediated by a variety of regulating hormones and growth factors including calcitropic hormones (e.g., PTH, vitamin D, calcitonin); PTHrP ; systemic growth-

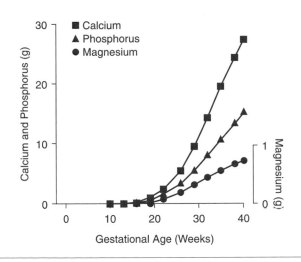

FIGURE **16-6** Total fetal content of calcium, phosphorus, and magnesium with increasing gestational age. (From Husain, S.M. & Mughai, M.Z. [1992]. Mineral transport across the placenta. *Arch Dis Child, 67*(spec no 7], 874.)

regulating hormones (e.g., growth hormone, insulin, glucocorticoids, thyroid hormones, sex steroids); circulating growth factors (e.g., somatomedin, insulin-like growth factor [IGF], epidermal growth factor, platelet-derived growth factor, fibroblast growth factor); and local factors (e.g., osteoclast activity factor, cartilage-derived growth factor).[18,73] Factors such as growth hormone, thyroid hormones, cortisol, and estrogen do not seem to be as important in regulating bone development in the fetus as in older individuals.

Functional Development

Fetal mineral requirements are met by transport of calcium, phosphorus, magnesium and other minerals across the placenta (see Maternal-Fetal Interactions). From 25 weeks' gestation to term, bone mineralization increases fourfold and fetal calcium acquisition ranges from 92 to 119 mg/kg/day or higher and phosphorous from 2.51 to 3.44 mg/kg/day. (Figure 16-6).[47,97] In contrast, calcium accretion immediately after birth increases from 15 mg/kg on day 1 to 45 mg/kg on day 3.[13] Phosphate levels peak at mid-gestation (15 mg/dl), then decrease to 5.5 to 7 mg/dl by term.

1,25-$(OH)_2$D and PTH levels are low in the fetus and probably have a limited role in fetal calcium physiology.[48] The parathyroid gland contains PTH by 10 to 12 weeks and actively secretes PTH by 25 to 26 weeks in response to decreased extracellular fluid calcium.[60,84] The fetal parathyroid is less responsive to decreased serum calcium, perhaps because of suppression of the parathyroid by the relative fetal hypercalcemia or placental PTH production.[67] The predominant hormone regulating fetal calcium homeostasis is PTHrP rather than PTH as occurs after birth and in adults.[38]

Cord concentrations of vitamin D metabolites are lower than maternal levels.[76] 25-(OH)D is transferred from the mother since fetal liver processes for vitamin D metabolism are limited.[48] Renal 1α-hydroxylation to form 1,25-$(OH)_2$D occurs in the fetal kidneys and probably in the placenta and decidua.[101] The fetus needs to store vitamin D to cope with the relatively high calcium requirements of the early postbirth period. Fetal vitamin D synthesis is described further in Maternal-Fetal Interactions.

Calcitonin-containing cells appear in the thyroid at about 14 weeks' gestation and secrete immunoreactive calcitonin from 28 weeks.[84] Calcitonin levels are high in the fetus, with increasing concentrations during the third trimester. The role of calcitonin in the fetus is unclear.[48]

NEONATAL PHYSIOLOGY

The newborn is hypercalcemic and hyperphosphatemic when compared with the mother. The infant must quickly move from the intrauterine dependence on maternal calcium sources and placental hormones to independent extrauterine control of calcium and phosphorus metabolism and homeostasis with reliance on oral intake and bone stores. Failure to do so may lead to hypocalcemia or other metabolic abnormalities.

Transitional Events

At birth, maternal supplies of calcium and other minerals are no longer available to the infant. Within 48 hours of birth, the infant moves from the hypercalcemic, PTHrP-dominated calcium metabolism to a PTH and 1,25-$(OH)_2$D environment. In this environment, the infant must mobilize bone calcium and increase intestinal absorption to maintain serum calcium levels.[48] Total and ionized calcium levels are higher in cord blood than in maternal serum; PTH is decreased, but PTHrP is increased.[48,64,71] Cord blood magnesium levels are slightly increased and related to maternal levels, whereas phosphorus levels are markedly increased.[44,80] Cord blood levels of calcitonin are reported to be 68% to 108% of maternal levels and correlate with maternal levels.[30]

Maternal serum 25-(OH)D levels at term correlate with cord blood levels, although cord blood values are 20% to 30% lower; 1,25-$(OH)_2$D levels are about half maternal values.[76] At birth serum osteocalcin levels are two to three times higher than in adults. This reflects the rapid rate of fetal bone formation in the last weeks of pregnancy. Osteocalcin is a noncollagenous bone-specific protein that is released into the blood in proportion to the amount of bone formation.[76] Levels increase from birth to 1 to 5 days then decrease. Osteocalcin levels are correlated with 23-(OH)D levels in cord blood and at 5 days after birth.[76] Changes in blood levels of calcium, PTH, magnesium, and phosphorus with birth are summarized in Figure 16-7.

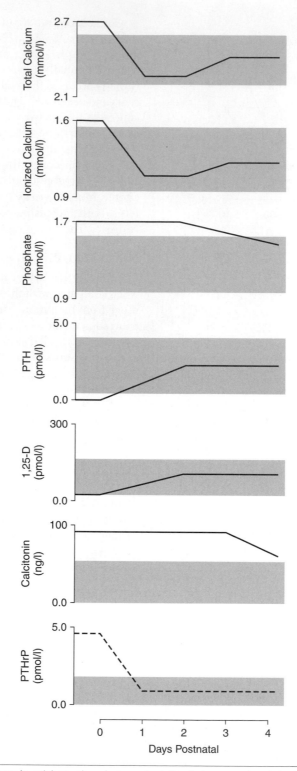

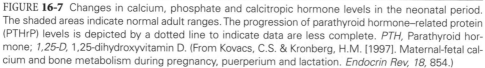

FIGURE **16-7** Changes in calcium, phosphate and calcitropic hormone levels in the neonatal period. The shaded areas indicate normal adult ranges. The progression of parathyroid hormone–related protein (PTHrP) levels is depicted by a dotted line to indicate data are less complete. *PTH,* Parathyroid hormone; *1,25-D,* 1,25-dihydroxyvitamin D. (From Kovacs, C.S. & Kronberg, H.M. [1997]. Maternal-fetal calcium and bone metabolism during pregnancy, puerperium and lactation. *Endocrin Rev, 18,* 854.)

Calcium

The relative hypercalcemia at birth is followed by a physiologic hypocalcemia over the next 24 to 48 hours as both total and ionized calcium fall (see Figure 16-7) to levels lower than those found in older infants and about 1 mg/dl lower than birth values.[10,64] There is a rapid decrease in ionized calcium in the first 4 to 6 hours after birth.[48,62] Calcium levels generally stabilize in the next 48 hours then increase along with increases in PTH and $1,25\text{-}(OH)_2D$.[48] The fall in calcium is probably due to parathyroid suppression in late gestation from elevated calcium levels and loss of placental calcium.[48] In term infants, values average 8 to 9 mg/dl (total), with a range of 8 to 11, and 3.5 to 4 mg/dl (ionized) calcium using older methods and 1.1 to 4.5 to 5.6 mg/dl using newer ion-selective electrodes.[47] Calcium levels at birth correlate inversely with gestational age.[47,64] The length and degree of the postbirth physiologic hypocalcemia is also correlated inversely with gestational age.[29] In very-low–birth-weight (VLBW) infants this hypocalcemia may persist in spite of increasing levels of PTH and $1,25\text{-}(OH)_2D$.[29,30]

Intestinal absorption of calcium is correlated with both gestational and postbirth age, but the major factor in determining absorption is postnatal age.[35] Immature intestinal function and decreased intake may limit calcium absorption. Renal calcium excretion is relatively efficient in both term and preterm infants, although increased renal sodium losses in VLBW infants may also increase calcium loss.[10] Renal calcium excretion increases with gestational and postbirth age, ranging from 60 to 88 mg/day during the first 2 weeks to 180 mg/day by 3 to 12 weeks in the term infant and from less than 8 to 80 mg/day to 120 mg/day by 2 weeks of age in the preterm infant.[13]

Phosphorus

Phosphorus levels may decrease slightly during the first 1 to 2 days after birth but remain higher than those of adults (4 to 7.1 versus 2.7 to 4 mg/dl) (see Figure 16-7).[64] Endogenous stores of calcium are released after birth, leading to elevated serum phosphorus in the first 3 days. Renal excretion of phosphorus is delayed because of decreased glomerular filtration rate and increased tubular reabsorption of phosphorus. Increased energy demands during birth with conversion of adenosine triphosphate (ATP) to adenosine diphosphate (ADP) lead to additional phosphorus release. Delayed feeding further elevates phosphorus levels because of tissue catabolism. Levels are lower in small-for-gestational-age (SGA) infants and correlate with the degree of growth restriction.[62]

Parathyroid Hormone

Most studies of PTH in the neonate are based on older assay methods.[48] As serum calcium levels decrease over the first few days after birth, PTH levels gradually increase (Figure 16-7) by about 48 hours.[76] Although the neonatal parathyroid gland can respond to a hypocalcemic stimulus by increasing PTH output, in many infants these glands remain functionally immature for the first 48 hours after birth.[10,48] However, other studies suggest that levels may reach the adult range by 24 hours after birth.[4] Neonate parathyroid glands respond less readily to decreased serum calcium, leading to a "functional hypoparathyroidism." This state is observed more frequently in VLBW infants and infants of diabetic mothers. Renal responsiveness to PTH is also decreased during the first 48 hours. Neonatal parathyroid gland responsiveness is dependent on gestational and postnatal age.[10] By 3 to 4 days of age, the preterm infant's parathyroid gland generally responds effectively to calcium.[44] PTH levels do not appear to change with oral administration of calcium supplements, but intravenous bolus administration of calcium can suppress parathyroid function.[10,29] PTHrP decreases rapidly after birth to the low levels normally seen in adults. Its role in neonatal calcium homeostasis is unclear, but PTH is the major calcitropic hormone by 48 hours of age.[48]

Vitamin D

Plasma concentrations of 25-(OH)D in term infants correlate with maternal serum values.[2] With elimination of 25-(OH)D from maternal sources after birth, the neonate must metabolize and hydroxylate vitamin D. Term infants are able to effectively metabolize vitamin D in the liver and kidneys. The kidneys can convert 25-(OH)D to $1,25\text{-}(OH)_2D$ by 28 to 32 weeks. However, vitamin D metabolism remains limited in the preterm infant because 25-hydroxylation by the liver does not occur at significant rates until 36 to 38 weeks' gestation.[89] Absorption of exogenous vitamin D may also be limited because of immature fat absorption. Serum $1,25\text{-}(OH)_2D$ levels increase during the first 48 hours, probably because of decreased serum calcium or increased PTH. This helps to maintain calcium levels within physiologic limits by stimulating bone and intestinal reabsorption.[29,48]

Calcitonin

Calcitonin levels may be normal or slightly elevated at birth, followed by a surge that is reported to peak anywhere from two- to tenfold over cord blood levels in the first 24 to 48 hours of age, then plateau.[10,58] The elevated calcitonin may be accompanied by an increase in plasma glucagon, a hypocalcemic agent.[10] After 36 to 48 hours, calcitonin levels gradually fall, but they remain elevated for 1 to 2 weeks in term infants.[36] Calcitonin levels are inversely correlated with gestational age. Calcitonin is also higher in infants with asphyxia.[44]

Increased calcitonin may protect the infant from excessive bone reabsorption and promote mineralization during a period of active bone growth and in the face of increased PTH and 1,25-$(OH)_2$D.[10,35,89] High calcitonin levels may contribute to the lower serum calcium levels and increased risk of hypocalcemia seen in preterm infants. Calcitonin levels remain high in preterm infants for a longer period of time, slowly decreasing over the first 2 to 3 months to reach normal levels by about 40 weeks' postconceptional age.[35] Oral calcium supplementation does not stimulate (and may decrease) calcitonin secretion, although early oral supplementation decreases the postdelivery calcitonin surge. Intravenous calcium does not appear to affect calcitonin levels.[10,35]

Magnesium

Serum magnesium levels increase initially after birth, then fall to levels similar to those in adults (range, 1.5 to 2.8 mg/dl) by 2 weeks.[10] Urinary excretion of magnesium may be low for the first few days after birth.

CLINICAL IMPLICATIONS FOR NEONATAL CARE

Bone mineralization and synthesis of new tissues continue after birth and are dependent on adequate substrate. Alterations in calcium and phosphorus metabolism in the neonatal period have implications for nutritional needs of term and preterm infants and are critical in ensuring adequate postnatal growth and development. In addition, these alterations may increase the risk for disorders such as hypocalcemia. This section examines postnatal nutritional needs related to calcium and phosphorus metabolism and the demands of bone mineralization and the basis for common disorders.

Nutritional Needs

Recommended dietary allowance for calcium, phosphorus, and magnesium in term infants are summarized in Table 11-17. Suggested parenteral and enteral intakes for these minerals in preterm infants are summarized in Table 11-19. A calcium-to-phosphorus ratio of 2:1 is thought to be ideal for human infants.[13]

The ratio of calcium to phosphorus can have a significant impact on mineral homeostasis. Hyperphosphatemia may lead to hypocalcemia by blunting the responsiveness of the bone to PTH and vitamin D. Conversely, low serum phosphorus levels can lead to reduction of calcium entry into bone, bone demineralization, and hypercalcemia.[13] Infant formulas have higher phosphorus and lower ionized calcium concentrations than does human milk. The calcium-to-phosphorus ratio of 1.3:1 found in some formulas may result in an excessive phosphorus load for some infants. Many commercial formulas currently have ratios that more closely approximate those of human milk.[89] Nutritional needs are discussed further in Chapter 11.

Infants Fed Human Milk

Levels of calcium are lower in human milk than in cow's milk formulas. Human milk averages 24 to 35 mg/dl of calcium and 11 to 16 mg/dl of phosphorus.[13,72,78] The 2:1 ratio of calcium to phosphorus promotes calcium-phosphorus homeostasis. The efficiency of intestinal calcium absorption increases up to twofold with human milk feedings. Vitamin D supplementation of infants fed human milk increases 25-(OH)D levels with no difference in 1,25-$(OH)_2$D values.[34,89] Calcium and phosphorus levels of human milk are not adequate initially for VLBW infants, and supplementation is recommended (see Chapter 11).

Calcium Intake in Preterm Infants

Preterm infants may have difficulty maintaining an adequate calcium intake because of increased growth needs and a low intake. Calcium levels in mature breast milk and standard formulas are significantly below daily intrauterine calcium accretion rates in the third trimester.[10,100] As a result, bone mineralization is reduced in infants fed these feedings.[35] Preterm infants fed breast milk do have increased calcium absorption (60% to 70% versus 35% to 60% with formulas).[73] Initially, extremely-low–birth-weight (ELBW) infants will need parenteral nutrition to supply enough calcium and phosphorus to meet intrauterine excretion rates.[73] Increased levels of calcium and phosphorus can be delivered with newer formulations containing calcium glycerophosphate and monobasic phosphate (up to 86 mg/dl calcium and 46 mg/dl of phosphorus). Fortification of human milk can increase calcium retention up to 60 mg/kg/day, and if the fortifier contains calcium glycerophosphate, up to 90 mg/kg/day.[73] If supplementation is used for preterm infants fed human milk, calcium-to-phosphorus ratios of 1.7:1 are recommended to maximize intake and retention.[73] Ratios should not be greater than 2:1 to prevent hyperphosphatemia.[77]

Preterm formulas, which average 140 mg/kg/day of calcium and 75 mg/kg/day of phosphorus, come closer to duplicating intrauterine calcium accretion rates during the last weeks of the third trimester (120 to 150 mg/kg/day).[6,47] Vitamin D levels are increased in these formulas to enhance intestinal calcium absorption. Medium-chain triglycerides (MCTs) are also added to increase fat absorption and thus absorption of vitamin D and calcium.[85]

Bone Mineralization

After birth the neonatal skeleton continues to accrete calcium at a rate of approximately 150 mg/kg/day.[48] In order to accomplish this, the infant must have adequate vitamin D and intestinal absorption of calcium. This may be difficult to achieve in VLBW and ELBW infants.[3,73,79] Rigo et al. note that the goal for VLBW infants is postnatal growth similar to the intrauterine rate, with a slightly higher rate in ELBW infants.[75] In order to reach this goal, these infants need not only adequate supplies of calcium, phosphorus and other minerals, but also protein and energy for formation of the collagen matrix synthesis.[73] VLBW infants have been reported to have decreased postnatal bone mineralization and a significant delay in completing bone development in comparison with intrauterine rates.[59]

LBW infants given a calcium and phosphorus intake similar to intrauterine accretion rates mineralize their bones at rates similar to those of the fetus.[85] These infants tend to have more stable calcium, phosphorus, magnesium, PTH, and 25-(OH)D concentrations, with a lower than expected calcitonin level. This suggests that the major problem in bone mineralization for the preterm infant is a lack of calcium and phosphorus.[10,89] Mineralization can also be altered in preterm infants by decreased absorption of fat-soluble vitamin K, an important factor in osteoclast formation.[35]

Preterm infants are at risk for both rickets and osteopenia (demineralization of the bone with or without signs of rickets). By term-corrected age, VLBW infants are still of lower weight and length than term infants with linear growth retardation seen in up to 22% of AGA preterm infants.[5] Significant bone mineralization problems, ranging from osteopenia to rickets, are seen in over 30% of ELBW infants.[3,47,73,79] Mineralization may also be delayed in SGA infants. Longitudinal follow-up is important after discharge to promote catch-up growth and optimal bone mineralization.[73] Factors leading to inadequate bone mineralization are illustrated in Figure 16-8.

Alterations in Neonatal Calcium Homeostasis
Neonatal Hypocalcemia

The serum calcium level below which an infant is considered to be hypocalcemic varies in the literature from 7 to 8 mg/dl.[41,44,47,64] Most sources use a lower limit of 7 in preterm and 7.8 to 8 in term infants.[3,6,47] Ideally determination of hypocalcemia should be based on the ionized calcium fraction (less than 3 to 4.4 mg/dl) (the limit varies with the method of measurement), since this is the biologically active form.[13,47] These determinations are becoming increasingly accurate even with small amounts of blood.

Hypoproteinemia or acid-base changes can alter calcium levels. Serum calcium is either ionized (physiologi-

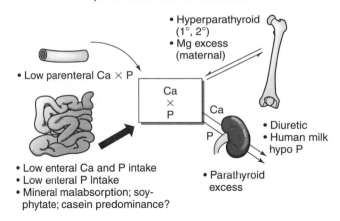

Osteopenia-Rickets in Preterm Infants

FIGURE **16-8** Possible mechanisms for inadequate bone mineralization leading to osteopenia and rickets in infants. (From Venkataraman, P.S. & Tsang, R.T. [1995]. Calcium, magnesium and phosphorus in the nutrition of the newborn. *J Am Col Nutr, 14,* 443.)

cally active form) or undissociated and bound to protein or complexed to anions. Since these two forms of serum calcium are in equilibrium, hypoproteinemia lowers serum calcium levels. This equilibrium is influenced by acid-base status. Acidosis increases the movement of calcium from bone and decreases the amount of protein-bound calcium. As a result, levels of ionized calcium increase. Opposite effects are seen during alkalosis.[13]

Infants at greatest risk for hypocalcemia are preterm infants, those born to diabetic mothers, or those born after perinatal asphyxia.[63] Possible pathogenic mechanisms are discussed below and summarized in Table 16-4. Hypocalcemia due to decreased ionized calcium may occur after exchange transfusion, with renal dysfunction, after furosemide therapy, or with magnesium deficiency.[44] Hypocalcemia with a decrease in ionized calcium but without a decrease in total calcium can occur with alkalosis, after exchange transfusion with citrated blood, or with elevated serum free fatty acids after lipid infusion.[13] Generally there is no increase in the incidence of hypocalcemia in infants with intrauterine growth restriction (IUGR) unless these infants are also preterm and/or experience birth asphyxia.[47]

The usual physiologic course of neonatal hypocalcemia involves a decrease in serum calcium to a nadir at 24 to 48 hours of age in term infants and slightly earlier in preterm infants. This is associated with a concomitant increase in phosphorus levels. Magnesium levels may be normal or low. Infants can be asymptomatic or symptomatic. Symptoms may include tremors, twitching, hyperexcitability, irritability, high-pitched cry, laryngospasm, tachycardia,

TABLE 16-4   Possible Pathogenic Mechanisms in Early Neonatal Hypocalcemia

CLINICAL PARAMETER	POSSIBLE PATHOGENIC MECHANISMS
Prematurity	Decreased calcium and phosphorus intake
	Decreased parathyroid hormone responsiveness altering ability to move calcium out of bone
	Increased calcitonin
	Immature absorption
	Immature renal function with decreased phosphorus excretion
	Decreased vitamin D intake and absorption
	Interference with calcium metabolism by acidosis
	Increased needs
Infant of a diabetic mother	Prematurity (see above)
	Transient hypoparathyroidism due to fetal parathyroid suppression by maternal hyperparathyroidism
Perinatal asphyxia	Increased tissue breakdown with phosphorus release
	Effects of pH and bicarbonate on protein binding of calcium and levels of ionized calcium
	Impaired parathyroid function
	Increased calcitonin

apnea, and (rarely) seizures. Early and late forms of hypocalcemia are seen.

Hypocalcemia in the preterm infant. Hypocalcemia is seen frequently in preterm infants, with serum calcium levels lower than 7 mg/dl (total) or 3 to 3.5 mg/dl (ionized) reported in 30% to 40% of preterm infants and up to half of VLBW infants.[44,47] The hypocalcemic preterm infant is often asymptomatic. The hypocalcemia usually occurs early (beginning by 12 to 24 hours after birth). Preterm infants are at greater risk since the rapid skeletal accretion of calcium seen in the fetus in the last weeks of gestation continues after birth, but in an environment without the benefit of the placental calcium pump and with immature intestinal absorption.[48] Possible causes of hypocalcemia in preterm infants include lack of available calcium due to decreased early intake, decreased PTH response to move calcium out of the bones (although some recent studies do not support immaturity in parathyroid function in these infants), immature absorption, interference with calcium metabolism by acidosis, increased calcitonin levels, decreased vitamin D intake and absorption, and 1,25-$(OH)_2D$ in VLBW infants.[13,47,57,75,84]

Hypocalcemia in preterm infants may not be due to parathyroid immaturity as was once thought, since PTH increases appropriately as serum calcium decreases after birth in these infants.[75,76] By 24 hours of age, most preterm infants have elevated PTH levels that are sustained for 2 to 3 days, falling with correction of the hypocalcemia. There may be an imbalance between calcium needs and PTH production, however, with increased calcium needs due to growth and a decreased supply.[84] The preterm infant also has a limited renal response to PTH during the first 48 hours.

A refractory response to PTH or alterations in calcitonin may be important in the etiology of this disorder.[84] The preterm infant has a marked elevation of calcitonin at 2 to 5 hours that reaches a plateau at 12 to 24 hours. Serum calcium values are negatively correlated with calcitonin at 12 to 24 hours of age, possibly impeding resolution of the hypocalcemia.[2] Alterations in vitamin D metabolism or availability may also impede resolution. Hyperphosphatemia has also been observed, along with an occasional transient decrease in magnesium at 24 to 48 hours.[47] The decrease in magnesium can be prevented by calcium, suggesting that hypomagnesemia is a consequence and not a cause of this hypocalcemia.[47]

Hypocalcemia in the infant of a diabetic mother. Hypocalcemia occurs in about 50% of infants of insulin-dependent diabetic women.[47,57] A decreased incidence is seen in infants of women with tight maternal glycemic control during pregnancy.[16] This form of hypocalcemia tends to appear within the first 24 hours of age and to be more severe and last longer than hypocalcemia seen in preterm infants.[23] The decrease in calcium level is directly correlated with the severity of the maternal diabetes.[76,57,88,92]

Cord blood of these infants contains decreased total and ionic calcium and PTH. The cause of this form of hypocalcemia may be related to suppression of the fetal parathyroid by maternal hypomagnesemia or by the relative maternal hyperparathyroidism seen in many diabetic women. These metabolic disorders in diabetic women are believed to be caused by increased urinary losses and lead to chronic fetal hypomagnesemia and decreased PTH secretion.[13] This results in a transient neonatal hypoparathyroidism.[63] The pregnant diabetic woman has lower magnesium levels and a failure of the usual increase in PTH, although serum total and ionic calcium values are often within normal limits for pregnancy.[17] Hypocalcemia in the infant of a diabetic mother (IDM) may also be related to immaturity since it is seen more frequently in infants who are also immature. Since these infants are often hypomagnesemic also, magnesium therapy may be needed to correct both the hypocalcemia and hypomagnesemia.[64] No consistent alterations in vitamin D metabolism are seen in IDMs.[76] The increased bone mass is secondary to the effects of insulin and IGF-I on bone formation in the IDM.[76] Because the increased bone mass increases calcium needs, this may also be a factor in the neonatal hypocalcemia in these infants.

Hypocalcemia and perinatal asphyxia. With birth asphyxia, there is increased tissue breakdown with release of phosphorus as well as accelerated conversion of ATP to ADP (to meet the increased energy demands), with subsequent phosphorus release. Administration of bicarbonate increases pH, which alters protein binding and decreases ionized calcium.[84] Alkalosis from bicarbonate therapy reduces the flux of calcium from bone and reduces serum ionized calcium.[13] Birth asphyxia is also associated with an impairment of parathyroid function, increased calcitonin levels, and decreased serum levels of magnesium and phosphorus.[44,57]

Late neonatal hypocalcemia. Late hypocalcemia is seen infrequently and primarily in formula-fed term infants with increased phosphate intake at 3 to 30 days of age.[44,84] Other less frequent causes are malabsorption of calcium, hypomagnesemia, and hypoparathyroidism. Late hypocalcemia may be asymptomatic but is associated with tetany. Symptoms range from mild tremors to seizures.

These infants demonstrate hypoparathyroidism in the face of decreased serum calcium and a reduction in efficient parathyroid activity that extends the usual postnatal decrease in calcium beyond 72 hours. The cause of persistent hypoparathyroidism is unknown. These changes may be aggravated by other factors such as vitamin D deficiency or high phosphorus loads from cow's milk formulas.[47,84] Late hypocalcemia was seen more often in the past, when higher phosphate formulas were more common. The disorder is uncommon with current formulas and essentially nonexistent in breastfed infants. Late hypocalcemia is occasionally seen in preterm infants secondary to immature renal function; transient parathyroid dysfunction; or altered responsiveness to 1,25-(OH)$_2$D.[44]

Neonatal Hypercalcemia

Hypercalcemia is rare in the neonate and is generally defined as a serum calcium level over 11.0 mg/dl, or ionized calcium over 5.6 mg/dl.[47] Infants may be asymptomatic or symptomatic (hypotonia, poor feeding, lethargy, vomiting, seizures, polyuria, and hypertension). Neurologic manifestations arise from the effects of calcium on nerve cells and cerebral ischemia. Polyuria is due to interference with the action of arginine vasopressin on the collecting ducts and can lead to dehydration. Hypertension is related to the vasoconstrictive effects of calcium and subsequent increased activity of the renin-angiotensin system.[2]

Hypercalcemia may be idiopathic, iatrogenic, or due to hypervitaminosis (vitamin A or D) or underlying metabolic or genetic disorders.

Alterations in Neonatal Magnesium Homeostasis

Hypomagnesemia in the neonate (less than 1.5 mg/dl) occurs most often in infants who are SGA, preterm, or born to insulin-dependent diabetic women. Less frequent causes of neonatal hypomagnesemia include decreased intake due to malabsorption or short-bowel syndrome, increased losses with frequent exchange transfusions or loop diuretic use or aminoglycosides, maternal hyperparathyroidism, neonatal hypoparathyroidism, and hyperphosphatemia from cow's milk formula.[10,17] Occasionally tissue hypomagnesemia may be present with normal serum magnesium levels.[47] Hypocalcemia and hypomagnesemia usually occur simultaneously and symptoms are similar. Magnesium plays an important role in bone-serum calcium homeostasis and intestinal absorption of calcium (see Figure 16-1 and the box on p. 631). Decreased magnesium leads to decreased PTH secretion, with subsequent reduction in calcium levels.

Hypermagnesemia (greater than 2.5 mg/dl) is most often associated with administration of magnesium sulfate to the mother for treatment of preeclampsia or preterm labor prevention. This can lead to elevated neonatal magnesium levels during the first 48 hours and respiratory depression, hypotonia, flaccidity, ileus, and poor feeding (magnesium has a curare-like effect). These infants have lower calcium levels, although they are not necessarily hypocalcemic. Hypermagnesemia may be treated with calcium, which increases magnesium excretion.[44,84]

Neonatal Rickets

Rickets occurs because of a deficiency of calcium or phosphorus in extracellular fluid, usually associated with inadequate vitamin D to ensure adequate intestinal absorption of these minerals (see Figure 16-8). This results in increased secretion of PTH, which stimulates osteoclastic breakdown and absorption of bone. Additional calcium is then available to maintain serum levels and prevent hypocalcemia. After a time the bone weakens and becomes stressed. Osteoblast activity is stimulated to replace the absorbed bone, leading to production of large amounts of osteoid (organic bone matrix) that never becomes completely calcified because of lack of calcium and phosphorus.

In preterm infants, rickets develops from inadequate intake of calcium or phosphorus over an extended period of time during which the infant is growing rapidly.[8,50,51] In these infants, rickets is associated with increased levels of 1,25-(OH)$_2$D, a finding consistent with inadequate calcium and phosphorus.[10] The second month of life seems to be an especially vulnerable period for development of rickets in VLBW infants. Rickets may be treated by providing a supplemental elemental calcium intake of 100 mg/kg/day, phosphorus intake of 50 mg/kg/day, and 400 IU vitamin D per day (provided a calcium- and phosphorus-fortified formula is not already being used).[41] Infants on total parenteral nutrition, with chronic health problems such as bronchopulmonary dysplasia, or on long-term diuretic therapy have higher mineral requirements and are at greater risk to develop rickets. Acidosis increases urinary calcium losses and interferes with synthesis of 1,25-(OH)$_2$D.[35] Factors predisposing to osteopenia rickets in infants are summarized in Figure 16-8.

Rickets has been reported in breastfed infants, but in most cases appears to be related more to lack of ultraviolet (sunlight) exposure of the mother than nutritional deficiencies per se. The greatest risks to the infant seem to occur if the mother's diet is deficient in vitamin D and she also does not get enough sun exposure.[89]

MATURATIONAL CHANGES DURING INFANCY AND CHILDHOOD

Age-related changes in calcium and phosphorus and their regulating hormones reflect needs of the infant and child to maintain calcium stability while providing for skeletal growth. Phosphorus levels decrease during the first year. With increasing exposure to ultraviolet light, 25-(OH)D levels increase during this same period. Levels of 1,25-(OH)$_2$D are higher than adult values for the first year.[81] Levels of this biologically active metabolite may remain even higher in preterm infants for up to 3 months, perhaps to compensate for immature calcium absorption.[77] Levels of 1,25-(OH)$_2$D tend to be elevated during periods of growth. Serum magnesium levels tend to remain slightly higher that adult values in infants and young children.[47]

From 3 weeks to 6 months, serum calcium values in exclusively breastfed infants gradually increase, leading to a transient physiologic hypercalcemia.[47] This increase may be related to decreased phosphorus intake due to the lower levels of phosphorus in human milk.[84,89] Serum calcium levels do not change significantly in formula-fed infants from birth to 18 months. Serum calcium levels gradually decrease from 6 to 20 years. Intestinal absorption of calcium tends to be passive until after weaning. Absorption is mediated by high lactose levels that increase absorptive efficiency.[38]

Infants on standard formulas experience a progressive fall in serum PTH during the neonatal period that reaches a nadir at about 3 months, at which time bone mineralization increases. This is analogous to the lowered PTH levels

TABLE **16-5** Recommendations for Clinical Practice Related Calcium and Phosphorus Metabolism in Neonates

Know the usual changes in calcium, phosphorus, and magnesium metabolism during the neonatal period (pp. 641-644 and Figure 16-7).

Monitor newborn calcium, phosphorus, and magnesium status during transition and in the early neonatal period (pp. 641-644).

Recognize factors that influence bone mineralization and growth (pp. 643, 647-648).

Initiate early enteral feeding as appropriate (pp. 644-645).

Monitor the nutritional intake of calcium, phosphorus, and vitamin D in infants (pp. 644-645).

Monitor neonates for signs of excessive and inadequate intake of calcium, phosphorus, and magnesium (pp. 644-648).

Recognize infants at risk for hypocalcemia (pp. 645-647 and Table 16-4).

Know clinical signs of hypocalcemia (pp. 645-646).

Assess and monitor infants at risk for hypocalcemia (pp. 645-647).

Recognize infants at risk for hypomagnesemia and hypermagnesemia (p. 647).

Know the clinical signs of hypomagnesemia and hypermagnesemia (p. 647).

Assess and monitor infants at risk for hypomagnesemia and hypermagnesemia (p. 647).

Recognize and monitor infants at risk for late neonatal hypocalcemia (p. 647).

Recognize and monitor infants at risk for neonatal rickets (pp. 647-648 and Figure 16-8).

seen in utero and may promote extrauterine bone development.[10] By 2 to 4 months, the renal response to exogenous PTH is similar to that seen in adults.[45]

SUMMARY

Calcium and phosphorus are essential minerals for many body processes and normal growth and development. Alterations in metabolic processes related to these elements can significantly alter the infant's health status. Many of these problems can be prevented and normal growth and development promoted by careful assessment and monitoring of neonatal nutritional status and initiation of appropriate interventions. Recommendations for clinical practice related to calcium and phosphorus metabolism are summarized in Table 16-5.

REFERENCES

1. Affinito, P., Tommaselli, G.A., DiCarlo, C., et al. (1996). Changes in bone mineral density and calcium metabolism in breast-feeding women: A one-year follow-up study. *J Clin Endocrinol Metab, 81,* 2314.

2. Anast, C.S. & David. L. (1983). The physiology of calcium in the human neonate. In M.F. Holick, C.S. Anast, & T.K. Gray (Eds.). *Perinatal calcium and phosphorus metabolism*. Amsterdam: Elsevier.

3. Backstrom, M.C., Kuusela, A.L. & Maki, R. (1996). Metabolic bone disease of prematurity. *Ann Med, 28,* 275.

4. Bagnoli, F., Bruchi, S., & Garosi, G. (1990). Relationship between mode of delivery and neonatal calcium homeostasis. *Eur J Pediatr, 149,* 800.

5. Berry, M.A., Abrahamowicz, M., & Usher, R.H. (1997). Factors associated with the growth of extremely premature infants during initial hospitalization. *Pediatrics, 100,* 640.

6. Bishop, NJ (1999). Metabolic bone disease. In J.M. Rennie & N.R.C. Robertson (Eds.). *Textbook of neonatology* (3rd ed.). Edinburgh: Churchill Livingstone.

7. Bringhurst, F.R. (1995). Calcium and phosphate distribution, turnover, and metabolic actions. In L.J. De Groot (Ed.). *Endocrinology.* Philadelphia: W.B. Saunders.

8. Campbell, D.E. & Fleischman, A.R. (1988). Rickets of prematurity: Controversies in causation and prevention. *Clin Perinatol, 15,* 879.

9. Care, A.D. (1991). The placental transfer of calcium. *J Dev Physiol, 15,* 253.

10. Chan, G.M., Venkataraman, P. & Tsang, R.C. The physiology of calcium in the human neonate. In M.F. Holick, C.S. Anast, & T.K. Gray (Eds.). *Perinatal calcium and phosphorus metabolism*. Amsterdam: Elsevier.

11. Cross, N.A., Hillman, L.S., Allen, S.H., et al. (1995). Calcium homeostasis and bone metabolism during pregnancy, lactation and post-weaning: a longitudinal study, *Am J Clin Nutr, 61,* 514.

12. Cruikshank, D.P., et al. (1979). Effects of magnesium sulfate on perinatal calcium metabolism; I. Maternal and fetal responses. *Am J Obstet Gynecol, 134,* 243.

13. Cruz, M.L. & Tsang, R.C. (1991). Disorders of calcium and magnesium homeostasis. In T.F. Yeh (Ed.). *Neonatal therapeutics* (2nd ed.). St. Louis: Mosby.

14. Dahle, L.O., Berg, G., Hammar, M., et al. (1995). The effect of oral magnesium substitution on pregnancy-induced leg cramps. *Am J Obstet Gynecol, 173,* 175.

15. Dahlman, T., Sjoberg, H.E., & Bucht, E. (1994), calcium homeostasis in normal pregnancy and puerperium: A longitudinal study, *Acta Obstet Gynecol Scand, 73,* 393.

16. Demarini, S., Mimouni, F., Tsang, R.C., et al. (1994). Impact of metabolic control of diabetes during pregnancy on neonatal hypocalcemia: A randomized study. *Obstet Gynecol, 83,* 918.

17. Dettos, L.J. (1993). Calcitonin. In M.J. Favus (Ed.). *Primer on the metabolic bone diseases and disorders of mineral metabolism.* NY: Raven.

18. Disousa, S.M. & Mundy, G.R. (1983). Hormonal regulation of fetal skeletal growth and development. In M.F. Holick, C.S. Anast, & T.K. Gray (Eds.). *Perinatal calcium and phosphorus metabolism.* Amsterdam: Elsevier.

19. Donaldson, J.O. (1999). Neurologic complications. In G.N. Burrows & T.P. Duffy (Eds.). *Medical complications during pregnancy* (5th ed.). Philadelphia: W.B. Saunders.

20. Drake, T.S., Kaplan, R.A., & Lewis, T.A. (1979). The physiologic hyperparathyroidism of pregnancy: Is it primary or secondary? *Obstet Gynecol, 53,* 46.

21. Dunne, F., Walters, B., Marshall, T., et al. (1993). Pregnancy associated osteoporosis, *Clin Endorinol, 39,* 487.

22. Fawcett, W.J., Haxby, E.J., & Male, D.A. (1999). Magnesium: physiology and pharmacology. *Br J Anaesth, 83,* 302.

23. Ferguson, J.E., Gorman, J.V., Bruns, D.E., et al. (1992)., Abundant expression of parathyroid hormone-related protein in human amnion and its association with labor. *Proc Nat Acad Sci, 89,* 8384.

24. Forbes, G.B. (1976). Calcium accumulation by the human fetus. *Pediatrics, 57,* 976.

25. Frolich, A., Rudnicki, M., Fischer-Rasmussen, W., et al. (1991). Serum concentrations of intact parathyroid hormone during late human pregnancy: A longitudinal study. *Eur J Obstet Gynecol Reprod Biol, 42,* 85.

26. Gertner, J.M., et al. (1986). Pregnancy as a state of physiologic absorptive hypercalciuria. *Am J Med, 81,* 451.

27. Gray, T.K., Lesaer, G.F., & Lorene, R.S. (1979). Evidence for extrarenal 1α-hydroxylation of 25OHD3 in pregnancy. *Science, 204,* 1311.

28. Greer, F.R. (1994). Calcium, phosphorus, magnesium and the placenta. *Acta Paediatr Suppl, 405,* 20.

29. Greer, F. (2000) Vitamin metabolism and requirements in the micropremie, *Clin Perinatol, 27,* 95.

30. Greer, F.E. & Zachman, R.D. (1998). Neonatal vitamin metabolism: Fat-soluble. In R.M. Cowert (Ed.). *Principles of perinatal-neonatal metabolism.* New York: Springer.

31. Guyton, A.C. & Hall, J.E. (1996). *Textbook of medical physiology* (9th ed.). Philadelphia: W.B. Saunders.

32. Hammar, M., et al. (1987). Calcium and magnesium status in pregnant women: A comparison between treatment with calcium and vitamin C in pregnant women with leg cramps. *Int J Vitamin Nutr Res, 57,* 179.

33. Harum, K., Thordarson, H., & Hervig, T. (1993). Calcium homeostasis in pregnancy and lactation. *Acta Obstet Gynecol Scand, 72,* 509.

34. Hayashi, T., Takeuchi, T., Itabashi, K., et al. (1994). Nutrient balance, metabolic response, and bone growth in VLBW infants fed fortified human milk. *Early Hum Dev, 39,* 27.

35. Hillman, L.S., et al. (1977). Serial measurements of serum calcium, magnesium, parathyroid hormone, calcitonin and 25-dihydroxyvitamin D in premature and term infants during the first week of life. *Pediatr Res, 11,* 739.

36. Hillman, L.S. (1983). Mineralization and late mineral homeostasis in infants: Role of mineral and vitamin D sufficiency and other factors. In M.F. Holick, C.S. Anast, & T.K. Gray (Eds.). *Perinatal calcium and phosphorus metabolism.* Amsterdam: Elsevier.

37. Horns, P.N., Ratcliffe, L.P., Legett, J.C., & Swanson, M.S. (1996). Pregnancy outcomes among active and sedentary primiparous women, *J Obstet Gynecol Neonatal Nurs, 25,* 49.

38. Hoskings, D.J. (1996). Calcium homeostasis in pregnancy. *Clin Endocrinol (Oxf), 45,* 1.

39. Howarth, A.T., Morgan, D.B. & Payne, R.B. (1977). Urinary excretion of calcium in late pregnancy and its relation to creatinine clearance. *Am J Obstet Gynecol, 129,* 499.

40. Husain, S.M. & Mughai, M.Z. (1992). Mineral transport across the placenta. *Arch Dis Child, 67*(spec no 7), 874.

41. Itani, O. & Tsang, M.B.B.S. (1991). Calcium, phosphorus, and magnesium in the newborn: Pathophysiology and management. In W.W. Hay (Ed.). *Neonatal nutrition and metabolism.* St. Louis: Mosby.

42. Jubanyik, K.J. (1999). Calcium and parathyroid glands. In G.N. Burrows & T.P. Duffy (Eds.). *Medical complications during pregnancy* (5th ed.). Philadelphia: W.B. Saunders.

43. Kent, G.N., Price, R.I., Gutteridge, D.H., et al. (1990). Human lactation: forearm trabecular bone loss, increased bone turnover, and renal conservation of calcium and inorganic phosphate with recovery of bone mass following weaning. *J Bone Miner Res, 5,* 361.

44. Kleigman, R.M. & Wald, M.K. (1986). Problems in metabolic adaptation: Glucose, calcium and magnesium. In M.H. Klaus & A.A. Fanaroff (Eds.). *Care of the high risk neonate* (3rd ed.). Philadelphia: W.B. Saunders.

45. Kodama, S., et al. (1975). Etiologic analysis of neonatal hypocalcemia. Relationship with reactivity to parathyroid hormone. *Kobe J Med Science, 21,* 69.

46. Kohlmeier, L. & Marcus, R. (1995). Calcium disorders of pregnancy. *Endocrinol Metab Clin North Am, 24,* 15.

47. Koo, W.W.K. & Tsang, R.C. (1999). Calcium and magnesium homeostasis. In G.B. Avery, M.A. Fletcher & M.G. Macdonald (Eds.). *Neonatology-pathophysiology and management of the newborn* (5th ed.). Philadelphia: J.B. Lippincott.

48. Kovacs, C.S. & Kronberg, H.M. (1997). Maternal-fetal calcium and bone metabolism during pregnancy, puerperium and lactation. *Endocrin Rev, 18,* 832.

49. Krebs, N.F., Reidinger, C.J., Robertson, A.D., et al. (1997). Bone mineral density changes during lactation: maternal, dietary, and biochemical correlates. *Am J Clin Nutr, 65,* 1738.

50. Laing, I.A., et al. (1985). Rickets of prematurity: Calcium and phosphorus supplementation. *J Pediatr, 106,* 265.

51. Lapillonne, A., Glorieux, F.H., Salle, B.l., et al. (1994). Mineral balance and whole body bone mineral content in very low birth weight infants. *Acta Paediatr Suppl, 405,* 177.

52. Laskey, M.A. & Prentice, A. (1999). Bone mineral changes during and after lactation. *Obstet Gynecol, 94,* 608.

53. Lenders, C.M., McElrath, C.M., & Scholl, T.O. (2000). Nutrition in adolescent pregnancy. *Curr Opin Pediatr, 12,* 291.

54. Levine, R.J., Hauth, J.C. & Curet, L.B. (1997). Trial of calcium to prevent preeclampsia. *N Eng J Med, 337,* 69.

55. Lopez-Jaramillo, P. (2000). Calcium, nitric oxide and preeclampsia. *Semin Perinatol, 24,* 33.

56. Loughead, J.L., Mimouni, F., & Tsang, R.C. (1988). Serum ionized calcium concentrations in normal neonates. *Am J Dis Child, 142,* 516.

57. Mimouni, F. & Tsang, R.C. (1987). Disorders of calcium and magnesium metabolism. In A.A. Fanaroff & R.J. Martin (Eds.). *Neonatal-perinatal medicine: Diseases of the fetus and infant.* St. Louis: Mosby.

58. Mimouni, F., Loughead, J.L., Tsang, R.C., & Khoury, J.C. (1991). Postnatal surge in serum calcitonin concentrations: no contribution to neonatal hypocalcemia in infants of diabetic mothers. *Pediatr Res, 28,* 493.

59. Minton, S.D., Steichen, J.J., & Tsang, R.C. (1979). Bone mineral content in term and preterm appropriate-for-gestational-age infants. *J Pediatr, 95,* 1037.

60. Moore, K., Persaud, T.V.N., & Schmitt, W. (1998). *The developing human: Clinically oriented embryology* (6th ed.). Philadelphia: W.B. Saunders.

61. Nader, S. (1999). Other endocrine disorders of Pregnancy. In Creasy, R.K. & Resnik, R. (Eds.). *Maternal-fetal medicine* (4th ed.). Philadelphia: W.B. Saunders.

62. Nelson, N., et al. (1989). Plasma ionized calcium, phosphate and magnesium in preterm and SGA infants. *Acta Paediatr Scand, 78,* 351.

63. Noguchi, A., Eren, M., & Tsang, R.C. (1980). Parathyroid hormone in hypocalcemic and normocalcemic infants of diabetic mothers. *J Pediatr, 97,* 112.

64. Pitkin, R.M. (1985). Calcium metabolism in pregnancy and the perinatal period: A review. *Am J Obstet Gynecol, 151,* 99.

65. Pitkin, R.M. & Gebhardt, M.P. (1977). Serum calcium concentrations in human pregnancy. *Am J Obstet Gynecol, 127,* 775.

66. Pitkin, R.M., et al. (1979). Calcium metabolism in pregnancy: A longitudinal study. *Am J Obstet Gynecol, 133,* 781.

67. Pitkin, R.A., et al. (1980). Fetal calcitropic hormones and neonatal calcium homeostasis. *Pediatrics, 66,* 77.

68. Power, M.L., Heaney, R.P., & Kalkwarf, H.J. (1999). The role of calcium in health and disease. *Am J Obstet Gynecol, 181,* 1560.

69. Prentice, A. (2000). Maternal calcium metabolism and bone mineral status. *Am J Clin Nutr, 71*(suppl), 1312S.

70. Prentice, A., Dibba, B., Jarjou, L.M., et al. (1994). Is breast milk calcium concentration influenced by calcium intake during pregnancy? *Lancet, 344,* 144.

71. Reitz, R.E., et al. (1977). Calcium, magnesium, phosphorus and parathyroid hormone interrelationships in pregnancy and newborn infants. *Obstet Gynecol, 50,* 701.

72. Repke, J.T. (1994). Calcium homeostasis in pregnancy. *Clin Obstet Gynecol, 37,* 59.

73. Rigo, J., DeCurtis, M., Pieltain, C., et al. (2000). Bone mineralization in the micropremie. *Clin Perinatol, 27,* 147.

74. Ritchie, L.D., Fung, E.B., Halloran, B.P., et al. (1998). A longitudinal study of calcium homeostasis during human pregnancy and lactation and after resumption of menses. *Am J Clin Nutr, 67,* 693.

75. Saggese, G., Baroncelli, G.I., & Bertelloni, S. (1991). Intact parathyroid hormone levels during normal pregnancy, in healthy term neonates and in hypocalcemic preterm infants. *Acta Paediatr Scand, 50,* 36.

76. Salle, B.L., Devlin, E.E., Lapillonne, A., et al. (2000). Perinatal metabolism of vitamin D. *Am J Clin Nutr, 71*(suppl), 1317S.

77. Salle, B.L., et al. (1987). Vitamin D metabolism in preterm infants. *Biol Neonate, 52*(suppl), 119.

78. Salle, B., et al. (1986). Effects of calcium and phosphorus supplementation on calcium retention and fat absorption in preterm infants fed pooled human milk. *J Pediatr Gastroenterol Nutr, 5,* 638.

79. Schanler, R.J. & Rifka, M. (1994). Calcium, phosphorus and magnesium needs for the low-birth-weight infant. *Acta Paediatr Suppl, 405,* 111.

80. Schauberger, C.W. & Pitkin, R.M. (1980). Maternal-perinatal calcium relationships. *Obstet Gynecol, 53,* 74.

81. Schilling, R., et al. (1990). High total and free 1,25-dihydroxyvitamin D concentrations in the serum of preterm infants. *Acta Paediatr Scand, 79,* 36.

82. Seely, E.W., Brown, E.M., DeMaggio, D.M., et al. (1997). A prospective study of calcitropic hormones in pregnancy and postpartum: Reciprocal changes in serum intact parathyroid hormone and 1,25-dihydroxyvitamin D. *Am J Obstet Gynecol, 176,* 214.

83. Seki, K, Makimura, N, Nitsuim C., et al. Calcium-regulating hormones and osteocalcin levels during pregnancy: a longitudinal study. *Am J Obstet Gynecol, 164,* 1248.

84. Senterre, J. & Salle, B. (1987). Calcium, phosphorus, magnesium and vitamin D. In L. Stern & P. Vert (Eds.). *Neonatal medicine.* New York: Masson.

85. Shaw, J.C.L. (1976). Evidence for defective skeletal mineralization in low-birth-weight infants: The absorption of calcium and fat. *Pediatrics, 57,* 16.

86. Shenolikar, I.S. (1970). Absorption of dietary calcium in pregnancy. *Am J Clin Nutr, 23,* 63.

87. Sibai, B.M. (1998). Prevention of preeclampsia: A big disappointment. *Am J Obstet Gynecol, 179,* 1275.

88. Specker, B.L. (1994). Do North American women need supplemental vitamin D during pregnancy or lactation? *Am J Clin Nutri, 59*(suppl), 484S.

89. Specker, B.L. & Tsang, R.C. (1986). Vitamin D in infancy and childhood: Factors determining vitamin D status. *Adv Pediatr, 33*, 1.

90. Tassinari, M.S. & Holtrop, M.E. (1983). Development of the fetal skeleton: Factors determining normal and abnormal growth. In M.F. Holick, C.S. Anast, & T.K. Gray (Eds.). *Perinatal calcium and phosphorus metabolism.* Amsterdam: Elsevier.

91. Taylor, T.G., Lewis, P.E., & Balderstone, O. (1975). Role of calcitonin in protecting the skeleton during pregnancy and lactation. *J Endocrinol, 66*, 297.

92. Tsang, R.C., Chen, I.W., Friedman, F.A., et al. (1975). Parathyroid function in infants of diabetic mothers. *J Pediatr, 86*, 399.

93. Tsang, R.C., et al. (1976). Hypomagnesemia in infants of diabetic mothers. *J Pediatr, 89*, 115.

94. Tulchinsky, D. & Little, A.B. (1994). *Maternal-fetal endocrinology* (2nd ed.). Philadelphia: W.B. Saunders.

95. Valbo, A. & Bohmer, T. (1999). Leg cramps in pregnancy—how common are they? [English abstract], *Tidsskr Nor Laegeforen, 119*, 1589

96. Vander, A., Sherman, J., & Luciano, D. (2000). *Human physiology: The mechanism of body function* (8th ed.). New York: McGraw-Hill.

97. Venkataraman, P.S. & Tsang, R.T. (1995). Calcium, magnesium and phosphorus in the nutrition of the newborn. *J Am Col Nutr, 14*, 439.

98. Verhaeghe, J. & Bouillon, R. (1992). Calcitropic hormones during reproduction, *J Steroid Biochem Mol Biol, 41*, 469.

99. Villar, J. & Belizan, J. (2000). Same nutrient, different hypotheses: Disparities in trial of calcium supplementation during pregnancy. *Am J Clin Nutr, 71*(suppl), 1375S.

100. Wauben, I.P., Atkinson, S.A., Grad, T.L., et al. (1998). Moderate nutrient supplementation of mother's milk for preterm infants supports adequate bone mass and short-term growth: a randomized, controlled trial. *Am J Clin Nutr, 67*, 465.

101. Weisman, Y., et al. (1979). 1,25-dihydroxyvitamin D3 and 24,25-dihydroxyvitamin D in vitro synthesis by human decidua and placenta. *Nature, 281*, 317.

102. Worthington-Roberts, B.S. & Williams, S.R. (1996). *Nutrition during pregnancy and lactation* (6th ed.). St. Louis: Mosby.

103. Wysolmerski, J.J. & Stewart, A.F. (1998). The physiology of parathyroid hormone-related protein: an emerging role as a developmental factor. *Ann Rev Physiol, 60*, 431.

104. Yamaga, A., Taga, M, Minaguchi, H., & Sato, K. (1996). Changes in bone mass as determined by ultrasound and biochemical markers of bone turnover during pregnancy and puerperium: A longitudinal study, *J Clin Endocrinol Metab, 81*, 752.

105. Young, G.L. & Jewell, D. (2000). Interventions for leg cramps in pregnancy. *Cochrane Database Sys Rev 2*, CD000121.

106. Zaloga, G.P. & Eil, C. (1989). Diseases of the parathyroid glands and nephrolithiasis during pregnancy. In S.A. Brody & K. Ueland (Eds.). *Endocrine disorders in pregnancy.* Norwalk, CT: Appleton & Lange.

Bilirubin Metabolism

Physiologic jaundice is a common problem in term and preterm infants during the first week after birth. For most of these infants, this phenomenon is mild and resolves without treatment. A small group of infants develop neonatal hyperbilirubinemia, which may be an exaggeration of normal physiologic processes or may herald underlying disorders such as hemolytic disease of the newborn or sepsis. When any infant develops significant hyperbilirubinemia, concerns arise about possible sequelae in the form of bilirubin encephalopathy. This chapter focuses on bilirubin metabolism and its pattern in the fetus and neonate along with issues related to neonatal hyperbilirubinemia and its management. Maternal adaptations are discussed only briefly, since bilirubin metabolism is not normally significantly altered in pregnancy. Bilirubin synthesis, transport, and metabolism are summarized in Figures 17-1 and 17-2 and the boxes on pp. 653 and 655.

MATERNAL PHYSIOLOGIC ADAPTATIONS

Alterations in the liver and hepatic function during pregnancy are described in Chapter 11. Bilirubin metabolism is not significantly altered in the pregnant woman, with bilirubin levels generally reported to be similar to those in nonpregnant women with upper limits of 0.4 to 0.5 mg/dl for total and 0.2 mg/dl for direct values.[11,16,45,101] However, recently, others report that both total and free bilirubin levels are lower in all three trimesters, with a slight decrease in direct bilirubin in the third trimester.[7] This discrepancy may be because of differences in the reference ranges used. Recently, new reference ranges for liver function tests during pregnancy have been proposed, with the upper limit of normal values lower than previous values for both pregnant and nonpregnant women of childbearing age.[7,52] Using these new references, Girling et al reported that approximately half of women with preeclampsia had abnormal liver function tests versus 20% using previous values.[52] Fallon reports that slight increases in serum bilirubin levels may be seen in approximately 5% of healthy pregnant women, possibly secondary to hormonal influences. Elevated serum bilirubin levels in pregnancy warrant further evaluation for liver or hematologic disfunction.[46]

CLINICAL IMPLICATIONS FOR THE PREGNANT WOMAN AND HER FETUS

A major difference between fetal and adult handling of bilirubin is that the fetus uses the placenta rather than its own intestines as the major elimination pathway. Most of the bilirubin produced by the fetus remains in the indirect state, a form that can be readily cleared by the placenta. The indirect fetal bilirubin eliminated across the placenta is conjugated and excreted by the maternal liver. Even with severe hemolysis, infants are rarely born jaundiced since the placenta efficiently clears excess fetal indirect bilirubin. However, these infants may have an accumulation of direct bilirubin and are often severely anemic. The maternal system efficiently handles the fetal bilirubin load and has sufficient reserve so maternal hyperbilirubinemia secondary to fetal hemolysis is rare.[11] Immunologic aspects of hemolytic disorders secondary to blood group incompatibility are discussed in Chapter 12.

Maternal Hyperbilirubinemia

Elevated total and direct serum bilirubin levels during pregnancy may occur with viral hepatitis, hyperemesis gravidarum (usually less than 5 mg/dl), intrahepatic cholestasis of pregnancy (usually less than 5 mg/dl), preeclampsia/eclampsia (often normal but if increased levels are generally less than 5 mg/dl), acute fatty liver of pregnancy (usually less than 10 mg/dl), cholelithiasis, and hepatic rupture.[64,136] The most common cause of jaundice in the first two trimesters of pregnancy is viral hepatitis.[45] Other causes of jaundice in early pregnancy include drug-induced hepatotoxicity, septicemia, or cholelithiasis, with biliary tract disease becoming more prominent in the second trimester. Causes of jaundice in the third trimester include intrahepatic cholestasis of pregnancy, viral hepatitis, gallstone disease, HELLP syndrome, acute fatty liver of pregnancy, and disseminated herpes. Postpartum jaundice

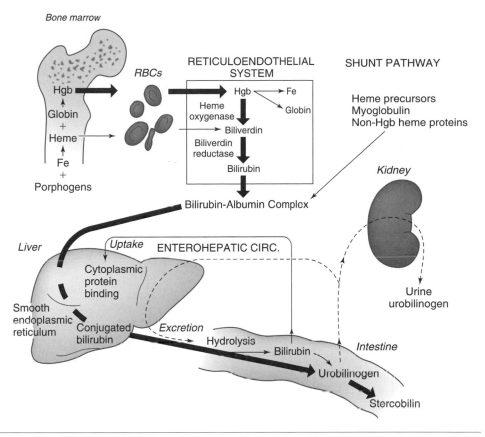

FIGURE **17-1** Bilirubin synthesis, transport, and metabolism. (From Gartner, L.M. & Hollander, M. [1972]. Disorders of bilirubin metabolism. In N.S. Assali [Ed.]. *Pathophysiology of gestation* [vol. 2]. New York: Academic Press.)

Bilirubin Synthesis, Transport, and Metabolism

Bilirubin is an end product of hemoglobin catabolism. Hemoglobin is broken down into heme iron–porphyrin complex and globin in the reticuloendothelial system (see Figure 17-1). The iron is released and stored. Heme is further degraded by macrophages to carbon monoxide and biliverdin under the influence of heme oxygenase. Heme oxygenase is a microsomal enzyme found primarily in the spleen, liver, and bone marrow. Biliverdin is a water soluble, nontoxic, blue-green pigment. It is catabolized to indirect (unconjugated) bilirubin (4Z-15Z-bilirubin-IXa) by action of nicotinamide adenine dinucleotide phosphate (NADPH)–dependent biliverdin reductase. Most of the heme comes from catabolism of senescent red blood cells (RBCs) and ineffective erythropoiesis (each gram of hemoglobin produces 34 to 35 mg of unconjugated bilirubin). Some bilirubin also comes from catabolism of nonhemoglobin heme proteins and free heme in the liver. Indirect bilirubin is orange-yellow, fat soluble, and not readily excreted in bile or urine. Indirect bilirubin is transported in plasma—bound to albumin (1 g albumin binds 8.5 to 10 mg of bilirubin) with a small amount of free bilirubin—to the liver for metabolism and excretion. Direct (conjugated) bilirubin is a water-soluble complex that has been metabolized by the liver to form bilirubin monoglucuronides or diglucuronides (see Figure 17-2). Direct bilirubin is excreted through the biliary tree into the intestines and forms a major component of bile and feces; small amounts may also be excreted through the kidneys (increases with elevated direct bilirubin).[16,25,44,58,59,106]

In the intestines, conjugated bilirubin is further catabolized by intestinal bacterial flora into urobiloids. Urobilinogen is oxidized by intestinal bacteria to stercobilin, which is excreted in stool. Stercobilin has a characteristic brown-orange color that contributes to the color of feces. Direct bilirubin is unstable and can by hydrolyzed by the relatively alkaline environment of the duodenum and jejunum or by specific enzymes such as β-glucuronidase or bacteria back into indirect bilirubin. Some urobilinogen is unconjugated in the small intestine by β-glucuronidase, absorbed across the intestinal mucosa, and returned to the circulation and portal venous system through enterohepatic circulation (see Figure 17-1). Recirculated bilirubin eventually is reconjugated by the liver.[17,18,19,20,39,59,68]

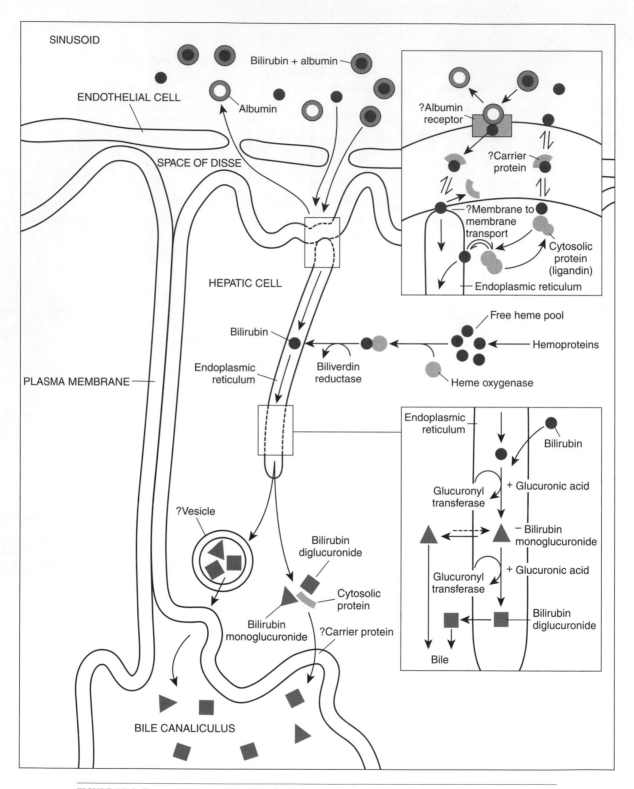

FIGURE **17-2** Transport and conjugation of bilirubin by the hepatocyte. The upper box illustrates bilirubin uptake by the hepatocyte by two proposed mechanisms: membrane-to-membrane transport or a carrier protein. The lower box illustrates proposed mechanisms for conjugation of bilirubin. (From Gollan, J.L. & Knapp, A.B. [1985]. Bilirubin metabolism and congenital jaundice. *Hosp Pract, 20*[2], 87.)

Bilirubin Transport and Conjugation by Hepatocytes

Cell membranes of hepatocytes have receptor sites for bilirubin. Bilirubin is also removed from albumin and transported into the hepatocyte bound to intracellular carrier proteins (Y and Z) that bind organic anions (see Figure 17-2). Protein Y (ligandin) is the major intracellular carrier protein for bilirubin. Protein Z is used when levels of bilirubin are high. Indirect bilirubin is conjugated in the smooth endoplasmic reticulum of the liver to form bilirubin monoglucuronide or diglucuronide. The major conjugation pathway involves action of the enzyme uridine diphosphoglucuronyl (UDP-glucuronyl) transferase. There are at least four forms of this liver enzyme, including a bilirubin-specific form. Other forms are involved in conjugation of various drugs and hormones and may provide alternative methods for bilirubin conjugation in the immature liver.

Conjugation of each bilirubin molecule involves a two-step process and two molecules of UDP-glucuronic acid (see Figure 17-2). In the first step the bilirubin is converted to a monoglucuronide. In children and adults, about two thirds of the monoglucuronides are conjugated to form diglucuronides. In neonates, most of the conjugated bilirubin is monoglucuronide. The glucuronyl-conjugating system is dependent on adequate supplies of glucose and oxygen for proper functioning. Most conjugated bilirubin passes into the intestines in bile and is excreted in feces. A small amount is reabsorbed in the colon and subsequently excreted in urine. The excretion of bilirubin into the biliary tree is by carrier-mediated active transport. These carriers may become saturated at high bilirubin levels. This is a rate-limiting step in clearance of bilirubin from the blood. If these carriers become saturated (as occurs with hepatocellular disorders such as hepatitis), direct hyperbilirubinemia develops.[17,18,19,20,59,68]

---

is most often a result of septicemia, drug use, transfusion (viral hepatitis) or cholelithiasis.[45] Liver function in pregnancy is discussed further in Chapter 11.

The effects of excessive maternal bilirubin production on the fetus depend on whether the woman has direct or indirect hyperbilirubinemia. Direct (conjugated) bilirubin is not transferred across the placenta in either direction.[46] Therefore the fetus of a woman with direct hyperbilirubinemia and jaundice secondary to hepatitis or other functional liver disorders does not have an elevated direct bilirubin level. Indirect (unconjugated) bilirubin can be transferred across the placenta in both directions and may increase the risk of neurologic complications in the infant.[16,46,133] HELLP syndrome is associated with an increase in indirect bilirubin, although levels in the mother are usually less than 5 mg/dl.[136] Neonatal hyperbilirubinemia is seen in about half of the infants in pregnancies complicated by this syndrome.[41] Isolated indirect hyperbilirubinemia is rare in adults; however, several cases of elevated indirect bilirubin levels in cord blood have been reported in infants of women with end-stage cirrhosis.[16,32,78] It is unclear whether this increase results from maternal-to-fetal transfer or whether the elevated maternal bilirubin levels prevented the normal fetal-to-maternal transfer of indirect bilirubin.

DEVELOPMENT OF BILIRUBIN METABOLISM IN THE FETUS

Because the placenta transfers only unconjugated (indirect) bilirubin, fetal bilirubin must remain in this state.[11,26] This is facilitated by immaturity of the liver and intestine, decreased hepatic blood flow as a result of shunting of blood away from the fetal liver by the ductus venosus, and increased recirculation of bilirubin by the enterohepatic shunt (see the box on p. 653 and Figure 17-1). Hepatic uptake is reduced by very low levels of the Y intracellular carrier protein ligandin.[119] Conjugation of indirect bilirubin by the fetal liver is reduced because of immaturity of uridine diphosphoglucuronyl (UDP-glucuronyl) transferase and other liver enzyme systems and decreased hepatocyte uptake and excretion of bilirubin (see the box above and Figure 17-2). UDP-glucuronyl transferase can be detected by 16 weeks' gestation.[47,71] Activity of this enzyme remains low in the fetus (Figure 17-3) and is 0.1% of adult activity at 17 to 30 weeks, increasing to 1% by term.[71]

Elevated concentrations of β-glucuronide in the fetal small intestine lead to increased deconjugation of direct bilirubin with recirculation to the blood for removal by the placenta. Limited intestinal motility also promotes intestinal reabsorption of bilirubin by lengthening the time available for β-glucuronide to act. Fetal bilirubin levels are slightly higher than maternal values (averaging 1.5 ± 0.3 mg/L), which may facilitate diffusion across the placenta.[99,109] Bilirubin and its conjugates can be detected in fetal bile by 22 to 24 weeks' gestation.[54] Fetal total and direct bilirubin increase with increasing gestational age, probably due to increasing numbers of red blood cells (RBCs) that then undergo physiologic hemolysis.[61,99] Bilirubin production increases about 150% per unit of body weight in late gestation as RBCs formed earlier in gestation undergo normal degradation.

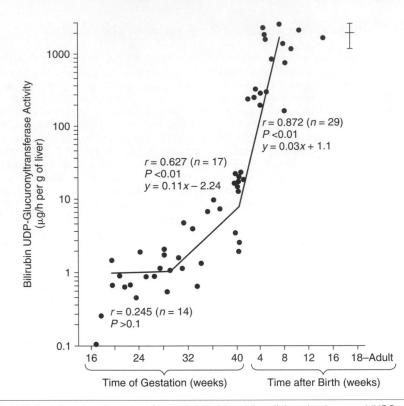

FIGURE **17-3** Developmental pattern of hepatic bilirubin uridine diphosphoglucuronyl (UDP-glucuronyl) transferase activity from fetal life to adulthood. (From Kawade, N. & Onishi, S. [1981]. The prenatal and postnatal development of UDP-glucuronyl transferase activity towards bilirubin and the effect of premature birth on this activity in the human liver. *Biochem J, 196,* 257.)

Indirect bilirubin can be found in the amniotic fluid beginning at about 12 weeks' gestation.[59] Amniotic fluid bilirubin levels initially rise, plateau between 16 and 25 weeks, then decrease, essentially disappearing by about 36 weeks.[59,109] This pattern has been plotted on graphs used to monitor and manage the fetus in pregnancies complicated by Rh sensitization and other blood group incompatibilities.

The mechanism by which bilirubin reaches amniotic fluid is uncertain. Bilirubin may be transferred directly across placental tissue from the mother or across the amnion or umbilical cord from fetal blood vessels.[71] The lipid-soluble indirect bilirubin may enter the amniotic fluid dissolved in phospholipids from tracheobronchial secretions. In animal studies, serum bilirubin concentrations correlate with concentrations of bilirubin in tracheal fluid.[92] Failure of amniotic fluid bilirubin levels to decrease during gestation is associated with hemolytic disease or disorders that interfere with the normal production and turnover of amniotic fluid (see Chapter 3), such as high intestinal obstruction or anencephaly with decreased fetal swallowing.

Heme oxygenase, an enzyme involved in bilirubin production, has recently been identified in the placenta.[94]

Heme oxygenase catabolizes heme into carbon monoxide and biliverdin, which is subsequently catabolized to bilirubin (see the box on p. 653). Carbon monoxide is a potent vasodilator and bilirubin a potent antioxidant. These substances may have a local role in control of placental vascular tone and protection of fetal-placental endothelium and syncytiotrophoblast from oxidative injury.[94]

NEONATAL PHYSIOLOGY

Before birth, bilirubin clearance is handled efficiently by the placenta and mother. After birth the liver of the newborn must assume full responsibility for bilirubin metabolism. Immaturity of liver and intestinal processes for metabolism, conjugation, and excretion can result in physiologic jaundice and interact with other factors to increase the risk of neonatal hyperbilirubinemia.

Transitional Events

Cord blood bilirubin levels are normally less than 2 mg/dl and range from 1.4 to 1.9 mg/dl.[83] With clamping of the umbilical cord, blood flow and pressure in the venous circulation decrease, the ductus venosus constricts, and flow of rel-

TABLE **17-1** Types of Jaundice in the Neonate

	PHYSIOLOGIC JAUNDICE	BREASTFEEDING-ASSOCIATED JAUNDICE	BREAST MILK JAUNDICE
Time of onset (serum total bilirubin >7 mg/dl)	After 36 hours	2-4 days	4-7 days
Usual time of peak bilirubin	3-4 days	3-6 days	5-15 days
Peak serum total bilirubin	5-12 mg/dl	>12 mg/dl	>10 mg/dl
Age when total bilirubin <3 mg/dl	1-2 weeks	>3 weeks	9 weeks
Incidence in full-term neonates	50%-60%	12%-13%	2%-4%

Adapted from American Academy of Pediatrics, Provisional Committee for Quality Improvement and Subcommittee on Hyperbilirubinemia. (1995). Practice parameter: Management of hyperbilirubinemia in the healthy term newborn. *Pediatrics, 94,* 588; Clarkson, J.E., et al. (1984). Jaundice in full-term healthy neonates: a population study. *Aust Pediatr J, 20,* 303; Gartner, L.M. & Auerbach, K.G. (1987). Breast milk and breastfeeding jaundice. *Adv Pediatr, 34,* 249; Maisels, M.J. & Gifford, K. (1986). Normal serum bilirubin levels in the newborn and the effect of breastfeeding. *Pediatrics, 78,* 837; Odell, G.B. (1980). Normal metabolism of bilirubin during neonatal life. In Odell, G. (Ed.). *Neonatal hyperbilirubinemia.* New York: Grune & Stratton; Schneider, A.P. (1986). Breast milk jaundice in the newborn: a real entity. *JAMA, 255,* 3270; and Winfield, C.R. & MacFaul, R. (1978). Clinical study of prolonged jaundice in breast- and bottle-fed babies. *Arch Dis Child, 53,* 506.

atively unoxygenated blood to the liver increases. Persistent or fluctuating patency of the ductus venosus, which occurs in some immature or ill infants, results in shunting of portal blood past the liver sinusoidal circulation (reducing the amount of blood perfusing the liver) and may interfere with normal clearance of bilirubin from the plasma.[93,119]

At birth the meconium in the intestines may contain 100 to 200 mg of bilirubin.[54] About half of this is unconjugated bilirubin and equals 5 to 10 times the daily bilirubin production rate from heme catabolism in the term neonate. Meconium passage usually occurs within 6 to 12 hours (69% of infants); it occurs in 94% of term infants by 24 hours of age (see Chapter 11). Any delay in passage of meconium through the intestinal tract increases the likelihood that conjugated bilirubin will be unconjugated (see the box on p. 655) and returned to the circulation.

Bilirubin is a potent antioxidant that binds to membranes to prevent their peroxidation.[8,59,60] Highly reactive metabolites of oxygen or free radicals are a by-product of oxidative phosphorylation. Cellular enzymes normally scavenge for and destroy these radicals before they can interfere with cell metabolic functions and destroy cell lipid membranes. Bilirubin accumulation after birth may augment other antioxidant systems and help protect the fetus in moving from the lower oxygenation of the intrauterine environment to oxygen-rich extrauterine environment.[28,122] Bilirubin has also been suggested to have a protective role in prevention of retinopathy of prematurity (ROP), again because of its activity in scavenging and detoxifying oxygen radicals; however, studies have not supported this role.[19,26,38]

Bilirubin Production in the Neonate

Usual destruction of circulating RBCs accounts for about 75% of the bilirubin produced in the healthy term newborn. Catabolism of nonhemoglobin heme, ineffective erythropoiesis, and enterohepatic recirculation (enterohepatic shunt) account for 20% of the bilirubin produced in the term and 30% in the preterm infant.[83] In newborns the amount of nonhemoglobin heme is increased by heme from the large pool of hematopoietic tissue that ceases to function after birth.[59] Bilirubin produced by catabolism of nonhemoglobin heme and immature RBCs is sometimes referred to as "early" bilirubin.

The newborn produces up to 8 to 10 mg/kg/day of bilirubin (which is more than twice as much as adults).[39,83] Bilirubin production is inversely correlated with gestational age and remains higher (per kilogram) for 3 to 6 weeks.[59] Increased bilirubin production in the newborn is due to a greater circulating RBC volume per kilogram (and subsequent breakdown of senescent cells), decreased RBC life span (80 to 100 days in term, 60 to 80 days in preterm, and 35 to 50 days in extremely low–birth weight [ELBW] infants, versus 120 days in adults), increased numbers of immature or fragile cells, and an increase in early bilirubin.[67,83]

Levels of unbound bilirubin are also higher in the newborn, and more so in the preterm infant, because of lower albumin concentrations, decreased albumin binding capacity, and decreased affinity of albumin for bilirubin.[27,28,59] The reasons for these alterations are unclear. There may be a maturational defect in albumin structure, or endogenous metabolic products produced during periods of stress or abnormal metabolism may block or interfere with albumin-binding sites.[26]

Physiologic Jaundice

Physiologic jaundice in the newborn is seen in 50% to 60% of term and up to 80% of preterm infants during the first days after birth (Table 17-1).[4,39,59,83] Visible jaundice usually appears as the bilirubin levels reach 5 to 7 mg/dl.[83,119] Up to 90% of term infants develop bilirubin levels over 2 mg/dl in the first week.[83] Neonatal jaundice accounts for 75% of hospital readmissions in the first week after birth.[21,95]

Patterns of Physiologic Jaundice

The usual pattern of bilirubin change is a two-phase process.[49,51,59] These general phases are seen in term and preterm infants and in breastfed and formula-fed infants, although characteristics of the phases vary depending on gestation and method of feeding. During phase I in term Caucasian and African-American formula-fed infants, bilirubin levels increase to around 5 to 6 mg/dl by 60 to 72 hours of age, then gradually fall to 2 to 3 mg/dl by day 5 (Table 17-1).[59] Asian and Asian-American infants usually reach levels of 10 to 14 mg/dl between 72 and 120 hours of age, falling to 2 to 3 mg/dl by 7 to 10 days.[59] The reason for the increased bilirubin levels in Asian infants is not known, although there is some evidence to suggest that their rate of bilirubin synthesis may be slightly elevated.[59] In addition, alterations in the gene for UDP-glucuronyl transferase that alter activity of this enzyme are seen with greater frequency in Asian populations.[59] During phase II, bilirubin remains relatively stable for several days, then gradually decreases to less than 1 mg/dl by 11 to 14 days. Patterns of physiologic jaundice in term breastfed infants are similar to phases in term formula-fed infants, except that the peak is higher (8 to 9 mg/dl) and later (4 to 6 days) and phases I and II are longer. In these infants, bilirubin levels generally decrease over 2 to 4 weeks, although it may take up to 6 weeks.[39,67,83] Approximately one third of these infants have bilirubin levels over 12 mg/dl.

Preterm formula-fed infants also have similar phases to term formula-fed infants; however, these patterns are only seen if early, prophylactic phototherapy is not used. In preterm infants the peak is higher (10 to 12 mg/dl) and reached later (5 to 6 days) and decreases over 2 to 4 weeks.[15] Phase II is also altered and bilirubin levels may not fall to less than 1 mg/dl until the end of the first month.[83] In preterm infants, mean peak concentrations reach 10 to 12 mg/dl by 5 days, then gradually fall over several weeks.[28,59] The greater the immaturity of the infant, the greater the alterations in phases and risk of hyperbilirubinemia. Patterns of physiologic jaundice in preterm breastfed infants have not been well described. Normal patterns of jaundice in preterm infants treated with early prophylactic phototherapy are also not well defined. Maisels suggests that the term *physiologic jaundice* has little usefulness with preterm and especially very-low–birth-weight (VLBW) infants, since these infants are treated with phototherapy even at "physiologic" levels.[83]

Causes of Physiologic Jaundice

Physiologic jaundice is not caused by a single factor, but rather reflects a combination of factors related to the newborn's physiologic maturity (Table 17-2 and Figure 17-4). The increased levels of circulating indirect bilirubin in the newborn are due to the combination of increased bilirubin availability and decreased clearance from the plasma. Phase I bilirubin elevations are primarily due to a sixfold increase in bilirubin load, decreased bilirubin-specific hepatic UDP-glucuronyl transferase activity (see Figure 17-3), and increased enterohepatic circulation.[51] Phase II elevations are primarily due to the continuing high bilirubin load from increased reabsorption of bilirubin by the enterohepatic shunt (see Figure 17-1) and increased bilirubin production, and decreased hepatic uptake of bilirubin.[51] Table 17-3 lists other factors associated with development of increased bilirubin levels in newborns.

Increased bilirubin availability results from greater bilirubin production (with more RBCs per kilogram), decreased RBC life span, and greater early bilirubin. Active recirculation of bilirubin by the enterohepatic shunt also raises serum indirect bilirubin levels (see the box on p. 653 and Figure 17-1). Increased recirculation of bilirubin is promoted by absent bacterial flora (which normally fur-

TABLE **17-2**   Factors Associated with the Development of Physiologic Jaundice

Increased bilirubin availability	Increased bilirubin production	Increased RBCs Decreased RBC lifespan Increased early bilirubin
	Increased recirculation through the enterohepatic shunt	Increased β-glucuronidase activity Absent bacterial flora Delayed passage of meconium
Decreased clearance of bilirubin	Decreased clearance from plasma Decreased hepatic metabolism	Deficiency of carrier proteins Decreased uridine diphosphoglucuronyl (UDP-glucuronyl) transferase activity

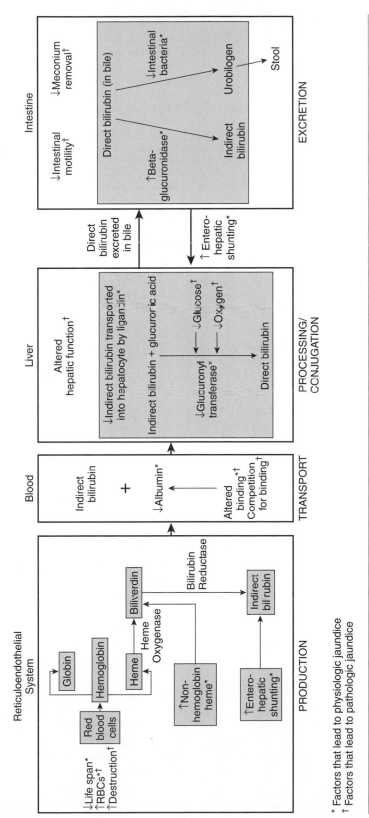

FIGURE **17-4** Basis for increased bilirubin levels in the newborn.

* Factors that lead to physiologic jaundice
† Factors that lead to pathologic jaundice

TABLE 17-3 Epidemiologic Factors Associated with the Development of Neonatal Jaundice

EFFECT ON SERUM BILIRUBIN LEVELS	FACTOR	SPECIFIC PARAMETERS
Increase	Race	East Asian,* Native American, Greek
	Genetic or familial	Previous sibling with jaundice*
	Maternal	Older mothers, diabetes,* hypertension, oral contraceptive use at time of conception, first trimester bleeding
	Drugs administered to mother	Diazepam, oxytocin,* epidural anesthesia, promethazine
	Labor and delivery	Premature rupture of membranes, forceps delivery, breech delivery, vacuum extraction
	Infant	Low birth weight, decreasing gestation,* male gender,* delayed cord clamping, elevated cord blood bilirubin level, delayed meconium passage, breastfeeding,* caloric deprivation,* larger weight loss after birth*
	Drugs administered to infant	Chloral hydrate, pancuronium
	Other	Altitude, short hospital stay after birth*
Decrease	Race	African American
	Maternal	Smoking
	Drugs administered to mother	Phenobarbital, meperidine, reserpine, aspirin, chloral hydrate, heroin, phenytoin, antipyrine, alcohol
No association	Drugs administered to mother	β-Adrenergic agents
	Labor and delivery	Fetal distress, low Apgar scores

From Maisels, M.J. (1999). Jaundice. In G.B. Avery, M.A. Fletcher, & M.G. MacDonald (Eds.). *Neonatology, pathophysiology and management of the newborn* (5th ed.). Philadelphia: J.B. Lippincott.
*Most common clinically important factors.

ther metabolizes direct bilirubin for excretion in feces), high levels of β-glucuronidase activity (which unconjugates direct bilirubin), and decreased intestinal motility. β-Glucuronidase concentrations in the newborn are 10 times higher than in adults, in whom little bilirubin is normally reabsorbed from the intestines.[39,67]

The longer direct bilirubin remains in the small intestine, the greater the likelihood it will be unconjugated. Thus infants who are fed earlier (before 4 hours of age versus after 24 hours) or fed more frequently and infants with meconium staining or early passage of meconium tend to have a lower incidence of physiologic jaundice.[17,49,138] Formula-fed infants tend to excrete more bilirubin in their meconium during the first 3 days after birth than breastfed infants. Among breastfed infants, bilirubin levels tend to be lower in those who defecate more frequently.[36] Infants with delayed passage of meconium, meconium ileus, or intestinal obstructions are more likely to develop physiologic jaundice. Recirculated bilirubin puts an additional load on an already stressed and functionally immature liver.

Decreased clearance of bilirubin from the plasma and metabolism by the liver are impaired in the newborn because of deficient Y intracellular carrier protein (ligandin), reduced UDP-glucuronyl transferase activity, and diminished excretion by a liver overloaded with bilirubin. Levels of ligandin reach adult values by 5 days of age.

UDP-glucuronyl transferase activity is minimal during the first 24 hours after birth. Activity is lower in preterm than term infants; however, increases in activity after birth are related more to postbirth age than to gestational age. Activity of this enzyme increases rapidly after the first 24 hours but does not reach adult levels for 6 to 14 weeks (see Figure 17-3).[71,83] This increase is independent of gestational age. The increase in bilirubin levels in the newborn infant may help induce UDP-glucuronyl transferase activity and conjugation in the liver after birth.[28] The major bilirubin conjugate formed in the newborn infant is monoglucuronide rather than diglucuronide as in older individuals (see the box on p. 655). Monoglucuronide is more easily hydrolyzed to indirect bilirubin than diglucuronide, and only indirect bilirubin can be reabsorbed across the intestinal mucosa via enterohepatic shunting.[51]

Hypoglycemia or hypoxemia may interfere with bilirubin conjugation. Decreased liver perfusion due to persistent patency of the ductus venosus may also impede clearance of bilirubin from plasma, particularly in preterm infants.[83,119] Hypoxemia further alters blood flow to the liver and hepatocyte function. The ability of the newborn's liver to excrete conjugated bilirubin may also be decreased. This may be critical in disorders with large bilirubin loads (e.g., severe erythroblastosis fetalis) and accounts for the direct hyperbilirubinemia in these infants.[83]

The preterm infant is more likely to develop physiologic jaundice and hyperbilirubinemia than the term infant. All of the factors described previously that contribute to physiologic jaundice in the term infant are more prominent in the preterm infant and are magnified with decreasing gestational age. RBC life span is related to gestational age and may be only 35 to 50 days in the ELBW infant. Some ELBW infants may have an ongoing low-grade hemolysis.[28] The lower serum albumin levels in the ELBW infant may limit extracellular binding and transport of bilirubin when concentrations are high.[28] These infants often have delayed feeding, with a low caloric intake initially and slower intestinal transit time. Feeding provides substrate for intestinal flow and bacterial colonization. A major factor contributing to the increased risk in the preterm infant is decreased UDP-glucuronyl transferase activity (see Figure 17-3).[96] Stable preterm infants achieve adequate bilirubin clearance by 1 to 2 weeks after birth.[28] Postnatal maturation of UDP-glucuronyl transferase and ligandin and canalicular transportation for bile may be slower in ELBW infants.[28]

CLINICAL IMPLICATIONS FOR NEONATAL CARE

Alteration in bilirubin metabolism is a relatively common event during the first week after birth. Neonatal jaundice results from either physiologic or pathologic causes. Physiologic jaundice is a normal process in the first days after birth and is due to normal physiologic adaptations. Physiologic jaundice is usually associated with a bilirubin level below 5 to 7 mg/dl and is seen in 50% to 60% of term infants and up to 80% of preterm infants. Pathologic jaundice is due to pathologic factors, such as Rh or ABO incompatibility, polycythemia, intestinal obstruction, sepsis, and other factors that alter normal bilirubin metabolism. Neonatal jaundice reflects an increase in bilirubin. At times these increases may reach levels that characterize hyperbilirubinemia. The risk of this disorder is increased in breastfed infants and preterm infants. Hyperbilirubinemia can be due to physiologic or pathologic causes or may be due to a combination of physiologic and pathologic causes. Neonatal hyperbilirubinemia is of concern because it may be a sign of an underlying pathologic problem, such as hemolysis or sepsis, and because of its association with bilirubin encephalopathy or kernicterus.[15] This section addresses these issues and discusses the basis for phototherapy and other methods of managing hyperbilirubinemia.

Neonatal Hyperbilirubinemia

Neonatal hyperbilirubinemia is usually defined as jaundice within the first 24 hours after birth or persistence of visible jaundice after 1 week of age in term infants (or after 2 weeks in breastfed term infants or 2 to 3 weeks in preterm infants), or bilirubin values that exceed any of the following parameters: (1) rise in total bilirubin over 5 mg/dl per day; (2) total bilirubin over 12.9 mg/dl in a term infant or over 15 mg/dl in a preterm infant; or (3) direct bilirubin over 1.5 to 2 mg/dl.[83,95] Maisels and Gifford suggest that for breastfed infants the upper limit might more appropriately be 15 mg/dl.[85] Bilirubin levels over 12.9 mg/dl are reported in approximately 3.6% and over 15 mg/dl in 0.3% of term formula-fed infants. Levels over 12.9 mg/dl are reported in 13% and over 15 mg/dl in 2% of breastfed term infants.[26,89] Jaundice associated with other abnormal findings such as feeding problems, irritability, hepatosplenomegaly, acidosis, or metabolic abnormalities is also of concern. A specific pathologic cause for hyperbilirubinemia is identified in only about 30% of term infants with bilirubin levels over 12.9 mg/dl.[83]

Investigators have attempted to predict the risk of later significant hyperbilirubinemia in healthy term infants prior to early hospital discharge.[2,12,117] Alpay reported that a serum bilirubin level of 6 mg/dl or greater in the first 24 hours after birth predicted nearly all healthy term infants who later developed significant hyperbilirubinemia and all who required phototherapy for bilirubin levels greater than 20 mg/dl.[2] Bhutani et al developed a nomogram by plotting total serum bilirubin levels with age in hours to identify infants at high, intermediate, and low risk of later requiring phototherapy.[12] They reported that no baby who fell into the low-risk graph later required phototherapy.

Neonatal hyperbilirubinemia is due to increased production or decreased hepatic clearance of bilirubin (Table 17-4; also see Figure 17-4) and occurs more frequently in immature infants. Significant hyperbilirubinemia within the first 36 hours after birth is usually due to increased production (primarily from hemolysis), since hepatic clearance is rarely altered enough during this period to produce bilirubin values over 10 mg/dl.[59,83] An increase in the hemoglobin destruction rate by 1% leads to a fourfold increase in the bilirubin production rate.

Direct or conjugated hyperbilirubinemia (obstructive jaundice), which is common in adults with jaundice, is rare in the neonate. Elevations of direct bilirubin involve cholestasis and are associated with alterations in hepatic function and interference with excretion of bilirubin into bile or obstruction of bile flow in the biliary tree. In neonates this can occur with hepatitis, severe erythroblastosis, sepsis, biliary atresia, and inborn errors of metabolism, including galactosemia, α_1-antitrypsin deficiency, tyrosinemia, prolonged parenteral alimentation, and cystic fibrosis.

TABLE **17-4**   Causes of Neonatal Indirect Hyperbilirubinemia

BASIS	CAUSES
INCREASED PRODUCTION OF BILIRUBIN	
Increased hemoglobin destruction	Fetomaternal blood group incompatibility (Rh, ABO)
	Congenital red blood cell abnormalities
	Congenital enzyme deficiencies (G6PD, galactosemia)
	Enclosed hemorrhage (e.g., cephalhematoma, bruising)
	Sepsis
Increased amount of hemoglobin	Polycythemia (maternal-fetal or twin-twin transfusion, SGA)
	Delayed cord clamping
Increased enterohepatic circulation	Delayed passage of meconium, meconium ileus, or plug
	Fasting or delayed initiation of feeding
	Intestinal atresia or stenoses
ALTERED HEPATIC CLEARANCE OF BILIRUBIN	
Alteration in glucuronyl transferase production or activity	Immaturity
	Metabolic/endocrine disorders (e.g., Criglar-Najjar disease, hypothyroidism, disorders of amino acid metabolism)
Alteration in hepatic function and perfusion (and thus conjugating ability)	Asphyxia, hypoxia, hypothermia, hypoglycemia
	Sepsis (also causes inflammation)
	Drugs and hormones (e.g., novobiocin, pregnanediol)
Hepatic obstruction (associated with direct hyperbilirubinemia)	Congenital anomalies (biliary atresia, cystic fibrosis)
	Biliary stasis (hepatitis, sepsis)
	Excessive bilirubin load (often seen with severe hemolysis)

G6PD, Glucose-6-phosphate dehydrogenase; *SGA,* small for gestational age.

Breastfeeding and Neonatal Jaundice

Most studies have shown clear differences in patterns of bilirubin production between breastfed and formula-fed term infants (see Table 17-1).[11,57,68,83,85,115] Breastfed infants are three times more likely to develop total serum bilirubin levels greater than 12 mg/dl and six times more likely to develop levels greater than 15 mg/dl than term formula-fed infants.[115] The increased incidence of hyperbilirubinemia in the United States over the past 25 years has been attributed to the increase in breastfeeding. Approximately 50% to 80% of infants with hyperbilirubinemia for which no specific cause can be found are breastfed.[85,95] Two forms or phases of neonatal jaundice are seen in breastfed infants: the more common early (breastfeeding-associated) jaundice, and late (breast milk) jaundice (see Table 17-1). However, these forms do overlap and in some infants may not be readily distinguishable from each other.[52,67]

Breastfeeding-Associated Jaundice

The early-onset form, referred to as *breastfeeding-associated jaundice,* is believed to be related to the process of feeding.[42,49,76] Factors leading to breastfeeding-associated jaundice include increased enterohepatic shunting due to lower fluid intake and/or less frequent feedings. The decreased caloric intake results in increased fat breakdown for energy

and fatty acid production that may indirectly interfere with glucuronyl transferase and ligandin. Breastfed infants excrete less bilirubin in stools than formula-fed infants because more conjugated direct bilirubin is changed back to indirect bilirubin by β-glucuronidase.[36] Breastfed infants produce lower weight individual stools, have a lower initial stool output, and have stools that contain less bilirubin than formula-fed infants.[83] Greater weight loss after birth and less stooling are associated with higher bilirubin production.[127] These infants also have slower urobilinogen formation, possibly due to different intestinal colonization patterns after birth (see Chapter 12). Human milk has been reported to contain β-glucuronidase that converts direct bilirubin back to indirect bilirubin, although no increase in this enzyme was found in a recent study.[65] There is no evidence in infants with this form of jaundice of increased bilirubin production or abnormal hepatic uptake or conjugation of bilirubin, suggesting that the most likely mechanism is increased enterohepatic shunting.[51]

Breast Milk Jaundice

Breastfed infants also develop a late-onset, prolonged hyperbilirubinemia. The late-onset form is believed to be related to attributes of breast milk that interfere with normal conjugation and excretion.[42,49,76] This syndrome is seen in approximately 1 in 100 to 200 breastfed infants.[42,59] Many of these infants also have a history of the early-onset form of jaundice. Late-onset jaundice is characterized by increasing bilirubin levels from day 4 on, peaking at 10 to 30 mg/dl by 10 to 15 days, followed by a slow decrease in bilirubin values to normal limits over the next 3 to 12 weeks.[49,61] If breastfeeding is interrupted for 48 hours (generally not currently recommended unless bilirubin levels are above 20 to 25 mg/dl), bilirubin levels fall rapidly, followed by a slight increase (1 to 3 mg/dl) with resumption of breastfeeding.[59,83] These infants do not have any signs of hemolysis or abnormal liver function.

The cause of late-onset (breast milk) jaundice in breastfed infants is unknown but has been attributed to the presence of specific factors in breast milk that appear to be minimal or absent in colostrum but appear in transitional and mature milk.[51] Although the specific factor or factors have not been identified, these may include the following: 3α-20β-pregnanediol (which may interfere with UDP-glucuronyl transferase activity or release of conjugated bilirubin from the hepatocyte); increased lipoprotein lipase activity with subsequent release of free fatty acids in the intestines; inhibition of conjugation by the increased amounts of unsaturated fatty acids such as palmitic, stearic, oleic, and linoleic acid found in breast milk; or β-glucuronidase or other factors in breast milk that may increase enterohepatic shunting.[51,54,55,59,65,83,108] Most studies have demonstrated an increase in β-glucuronidase, although others have not.[54,65] Inhibition of conjugation by the increased amounts of free fatty acids that are released in the duodenum of breastfed infants may occur as these fatty acids are absorbed into the circulation. When fatty acids reach the liver, they may inhibit glucuronyl transferase activity or saturate the hepatic protein carrier system.[35,100] The increased absorption of fat from breast milk may also increase intestinal bilirubin absorption. In vitro levels of free fatty acids are increased in milk stored over 3 to 5 days or frozen.[102,105]

Prevention of Breastfeeding-Associated Jaundice in Breastfed Infants

Breastfeeding-associated jaundice in breastfed infants may be reduced by preventative interventions. Gartner and Lee have suggested that breastfeeding-associated jaundice is an iatrogenic phenomenon and preventable.[49,51] Encouraging feeding soon after delivery will increase intestinal activity and begin establishing gut flora. Frequent feeding stimulates intestinal activity and meconium removal (less bilirubin for enzymes to convert back to indirect form) and reduce enterohepatic shunting and stimulate maternal milk production.[15] Infants fed in the first 1 to 3 hours after birth

pass meconium sooner than infants fed after 4 hours.[17] Feeding stimulates the gastrocolonic reflex, increases intestinal motility, and stimulates meconium (colostrum acts as a laxative) passage. This removes conjugated bilirubin from the small intestine, thus reducing the likelihood that this bilirubin will be recirculated by the enterohepatic shunt.

A critical factor in reducing the risk of jaundice in breastfed infants seems to be enhancing breast milk intake.[49,50] Bilirubin levels in these infants tend to correlate negatively with breast milk intake; that is, as intake decreases, bilirubin levels tend to rise. Supplements should be avoided as they can interfere with establishment of breastfeeding.[4] If supplementation is required for medical reasons, supplementation with formula provides more calories. Supplementation of breastfeeding with water or dextrose water does not lower bilirubin levels in healthy breastfeeding infants. Supplemental feedings with dextrose water have been found to decrease breast milk intake and increase bilirubin levels and may increase the risk of hyponatremia.[77,105] Dextrose water supplementation may satiate the infant but lead to inadequate caloric intake; caloric deprivation increases bilirubin levels.[49] Use of any form of supplementation can alter intake of breast milk and establishment of the mother's milk supply (see Chapter 5). Use of supplementation was also associated with a significant decrease in the number of infants still breastfeeding at 3 months.[62]

A linear relationship between the number of feedings per day and bilirubin levels has been reported.[35,36] Bilirubin levels were lowest in infants who were breastfed more than eight or nine times in 24 hours during the first 3 days after birth.[141] Increasing the frequency of feedings may stimulate gut motility and decrease intestinal absorption of bilirubin.[35] Current recommendations are to encourage breastfeeding of 8 or 10 to 12 times per 24 hours initially to ensure adequate milk intake.[5,51] Signs of inadequate milk intake include delayed meconium passage, fewer bowel movements (less than 3 per day), decreased urine output (less than 6 wet diapers per day after the third day), and weight loss greater than 7%.[39,51]

Initial and continuing support of the mother and other family members is essential to enhance breastfeeding success.[86,98] The American Academy of Pediatrics (AAP) recommends evaluation of breastfeeding in term infants in the first 24 to 48 hours after birth and again 48 to 72 hours after discharge.[5] Follow-up and monitoring of bilirubin levels before and after hospital discharge using recommended protocols is also essential.[4,6,104]

Management of Jaundice in Breastfed Infants

Management of jaundice in breastfed infants is often problematic. Multiple issues and concerns, including maternal desire to breastfeed, advantages of breastfeeding to both mother and infant, effects on maternal-infant interaction, parental stress with the potential for bilirubin toxicity, and legal implications related to "safe" bilirubin values must be balanced.[49,59,73] This has been further complicated by recent reports of an increase in the incidence of hyperbilirubinemia and kernicterus (although both remain rare) in term infants.[24,56,69,86,87,88,95,104,135] In the early 1990s, less aggressive treatment of hyperbilirubinemia in term infants was advocated and reflected in guidelines released by the AAP in 1994.[4,103] One of the bases for these guidelines was the estimate that the risk of kernicterus in well term infants with bilirubin levels of 20 to 25 mg/dl was lower than the risks associated with exchange transfusion.[104] Newman and Maisels suggest that the increase in hyperbilirubinemia and kernicterus could be a result of early discharge, the AAP guidelines, or the possibility that the guidelines were not being followed, especially since cases have been primarily breastfed infants admitted with bilirubin levels over 30 mg/dl, higher than recommended standards.[104]

Amato et al report no difference in the time needed to reduce bilirubin levels with jaundice managed by discontinuing breastfeeding versus the use of phototherapy and continued breastfeeding.[3] Martinez and associates compared four interventions (continue breastfeeding and observe; discontinue breastfeeding and begin formula feeding; discontinue breastfeeding, begin formula feeding, and start phototherapy; and continue breastfeeding and start phototherapy) once bilirubin levels reached 17 mg/dl.[90] They found that if an adequate dosage of phototherapy was provided, there was no significant advantage to stopping breastfeeding.[90] Maisels recommends that any interruption of breastfeeding be avoided, unless the infant develops bilirubin levels above 25 mg/dl, and rather to continue frequent breastfeeding (10 or more times/day) while using intensive phototherapy.[83]

Lawrence emphasizes a more proactive approach, focusing on prevention and modifying factors (particularly inadequate frequency of feeding) that are associated with early-onset jaundice in breastfed infants (Table 17-5).[77] Interruption of breastfeeding must be accompanied by parental emotional support and facilitation of breast pumping or manual expression of milk. Elander and Lindberg measured maternal stress with urinary cortisol levels.[42] They found that separating the mother and infant for phototherapy increased both maternal stress and the likelihood that she would stop breastfeeding.

Measurement of Serum Bilirubin

Serum bilirubin levels are measured by laboratory and transcutaneous methods. Clinical estimations of serum

TABLE 17-5 Management Outline for Early Jaundice while Breastfeeding

1. Monitor all infants for initial stooling. Consider stimulating stooling if no stool in 24 hours.
2. Initiate breastfeeding early and frequently. Frequent short feeding more effective than infrequent prolonged feeding, although total time may be the same.
3. Discourage water, dextrose water, or formula substitutes.
4. Monitor weight, voidings, stooling in association with breastfeeding pattern.
5. When bilirubin level approaches 15 mg/dl, augment feeds, stimulate breast milk production with pumping, and use phototherapy if this aggressive tack fails.
6. There is no evidence that early jaundice is associated with an "abnormality" of the breast milk; therefore withdrawing breast milk as a trial is only indicated if jaundice persists longer than 6 days or rises above 15 mg/dl or the mother has a history of a previously affected infant.

Modified from Lawrence, R.A. & Lawrence, R.M. (1999). *Breastfeeding: A guide for the medical profession* (5th ed.). St. Louis: Mosby.

bilirubin levels by the cephalopedal progression of jaundice are correlated with serum bilirubin concentrations in most but not all studies.[74,75,81,97,142] Cephalopedal progression is most useful at low bilirubin levels and is less reliable at levels over 12 mg/dl.[83] Knudsen suggests that the basis for this progression may be due to conformational changes in the bilirubin-albumin complex and in the binding affinity of bilirubin for albumin.[74,75] Indirect bilirubin leaving the reticuloendothelial system, where it is produced, binds to albumin. Initially binding affinity is lower with less effective binding, so bilirubin is more likely to be deposited in this area (i.e., in more proximal tissues). By the time bilirubin reaches more distal areas, it is more tightly bound and less likely to be deposited in the peripheral tissues unless bilirubin levels are high (overwhelming the available albumin binding capacity).[74,75]

These observations only approximate actual serum bilirubin values, so laboratory assessments are also necessary. Laboratory methods involve measurement of total and direct bilirubin and calculation of indirect values. Alternatives to laboratory measurement are reference devices to assess color (icterometer) and transcutaneous measurements.[14,116] Transcutaneous bilirubinometry is most appropriate for screening and monitoring healthy term infants with physiologic jaundice because it avoids repeated heel sticks.[116,140,142] Both icterometer and transcutaneous measurements are correlated with total serum bilirubin levels.[14,81,116,126]

Transcutaneous measurements provide a quantification of skin color by an arbitrary "bilirubin index." This index is obtained by measuring color as a function of light wavelength over the visible portion of the light spectrum.[83,116] These instruments are placed over the infant's skin, and pressure is applied to blanch the skin. Light is reflected through the skin to the subcutaneous tissues and back into the instruments through fiberoptic filaments. The intensity of the yellow skin coloration is calculated within the spectrophotometric module.

Transcutaneous bilirubin is linearly related to laboratory measurements of total serum bilirubin.[83] These measurements are affected by gestation, skin color differences, and birth weight, so different standards must be used.[116,142] This may limit its use in heterogenous populations. Transcutaneous measurements are also altered by phototherapy. Variations may be reduced by covering the area of the skin used for measurement by an opaque patch.[83] Other factors altering the reliability of transcutaneous bilirubin measurements include interoperator differences, using an angle other than 90 degrees between the instrument and the skin surface, the presence of unevaporated isopropyl alcohol on the probe, and exchange transfusion.[83,116]

Recent techniques include a colorimeter that uses a xenon flash tube and light sensors connected to a computer to examine skin luminosity and changes in the yellow component of the light spectrum and a handheld device using multiwavelength spectral analysis to examine the reflectance of light within 400 to 700 nm.[13,126] Initial studies with these devices report good correlations with total serum bilirubin—with diverse populations and in infants under phototherapy.

Management of Neonatal Hyperbilirubinemia

Various techniques have been used to manage neonates with indirect hyperbilirubinemia. Strategies have included prevention, use of pharmacologic agents, exchange transfusion, and phototherapy. Prevention has focused on early initiation of feedings and frequent breastfeeding to decrease enterohepatic shunting, promote establishment of normal bacterial flora, and stimulate intestinal activity. Specific pharmacologic agents have been used to prevent hyperbilirubinemia or reduce bilirubin levels.

Pharmacologic Agents

Pharmacologic agents have been used in the management of hyperbilirubinemia to stimulate the induction of hepatic enzymes and carrier proteins, to interfere with heme degradation, or to bind bilirubin in the intestines to decrease enterohepatic reabsorption. Inert nonabsorbable substances such as charcoal and agar have been tried for the latter purpose with equivocal results and are not recommended.[72,129] Intravenous immunoglobulin has been used with infants with severe Rh and ABO incompatibility to suppress isoimmune hemolysis and decrease the number of exchange transfusions.[67]

Phenobarbital has been demonstrated to be effective in stimulating activity and concentrations of hepatic glucuronyl transferase and Y carrier proteins and may increase the number of bilirubin-binding sites.[79,83] Postbirth use of phenobarbital is controversial and generally not recommended. Several days of therapy may be required before a significant change is seen, which makes postbirth use undesirable since phototherapy is effective much earlier.[129] Phenobarbital has been used primarily with Rh incompatibility to reduce the number of exchange transfusions.[129] Long-term effects of this therapy are unclear.[84,129]

Recently, prevention of hyperbilirubinemia with the use of synthetic metalloprotoporphyrins has been investigated.[31,67,70,91,121,128,132] These substances are synthetic heme analogues. Protoporphyrin has been shown to be an effective competitive inhibitor of heme oxygenase, the enzyme necessary for catabolism of heme to biliverdin (see Figure 17-1) and the rate-limiting step in formation of bilirubin. With use of these substances, the heme that is prevented from being catabolized does not accumulate but is excreted intact in bile.[67] In studies with both term and preterm infants, and in infants with and without hemolytic diseases, tin-protoporphyrin (Sn-PP) and tin-mesoporphyrin (Sn-MP) have significantly decreased serum bilirubin levels.[31,67,70,91,128,132] Use of phototherapy after administration of Sn-PP in particular has been associated with phototoxic erythema. Sn-MP is a less toxic variant, especially when used in conjunction with phototherapy. In recent studies, Sn-MP use has been associated with no need for phototherapy in term infants and a marked decreased in phototherapy in preterm infants.[31,91,128] These agents are still experimental; long-term outcomes have not been established.

Exchange Transfusion

Exchange transfusions are used in the management of indirect hyperbilirubinemia and hemolytic disease of the newborn. An exchange transfusion removes antibody-coated blood cells and bilirubin and helps to correct the anemia associated with hemolytic disease. A two-volume exchange replaces 85% of the circulating RBC volume and reduces the bilirubin by approximately 50%. This rebounds up to 60% of preexchange values over the next hours as bilirubin diffuses into the vascular space from extravascular tissues. The frequency of exchange transfusions has been significantly reduced with the availability of Rho(D) immune globulin (see Chapter 12) and phototherapy.

Phototherapy

Phototherapy was first introduced in 1958 and has been used extensively and effectively in treating neonatal indirect hyperbilirubinemia since the late 1960s.[33,98] Over 60 studies have documented the effectiveness of phototherapy in preventing and treating neonatal hyperbilirubinemia.[84] Protocols are available to guide initiation of phototherapy in healthy term infants and in preterm infants (Tables 17-6 and 17-7).

Physics of phototherapy. Light reduces bilirubin by photoisomerization and photooxidization (Figure 17-5). Indirect bilirubin (IXa) is composed of four pyrrole rings. Photoisomerization involves conversion of poorly soluble indirect bilirubin into water-soluble reversible configurational (rearrangement of chemical groups in the molecule) or irreversible structural (rearrangement of the atoms) photoisomers (i.e., photobilirubin, lumirubin). The photoisomers can be excreted into bile without conjugation. Formation of configurational isomers (4Z,15E or 4E,15Z or 4E,15E) is rapid, but these isomers are excreted slowly in bile, with a serum half-life of 12 to 21 hours.[44,67,96] Configurational isomers are unstable and may be changed back into unconjugated bilirubin and recirculated via en-

TABLE 17-6 American Academy of Pediatrics' Guidelines for the Management of Hyperbilirubinemia in the Healthy Term Newborn

	TOTAL SERUM BILIRUBIN LEVEL IN mg/dl (μmol/l)			
AGE (HOURS)	CONSIDER PHOTOTHERAPY	PHOTOTHERAPY	EXCHANGE TRANSFUSION IF INTENSIVE* PHOTOTHERAPY FAILS†	EXCHANGE TRANSFUSION AND INTENSIVE PHOTOTHERAPY*
25-48	≥12 (170)	≥15 (260)	≥20 (340)	≥25 (430)
49-72	≥15 (260)	≥18 (310)	≥26 (430)	≥30 (510)
>72	≥17 (290)	≥20 (340)	≥25 (430)	≥30 (510)

Modified by Halamek, L.P. & Stevenson, D.K. (1997). Neonatal jaundice and liver disease. In A.A. Fanaroff & R.J. Martin (Eds.). *Neonatal-perinatal medicine: Diseases of the fetus and infant* (6th ed.). St. Louis: Mosby, from American Academy of Pediatrics, Provisional Committee for Quality Improvement and Subcommittee on Hyperbilirubinemia. (1994). Practice parameter: Management of hyperbilirubinemia in the healthy term newborn. *Pediatrics, 94,* 558.

*Intensive phototherapy includes utilizing more than one bank of lamps, employing units containing "special blue" lamps, maximizing the surface areas illuminated by the use of phototherapy blanket or other means, and delivery on a continuous, uninterrupted schedule.
†Intensive phototherapy failure is defined as: (1) an inability to produce a decline of total serum bilirubin of 1 to 2 mg/dl within 4 to 6 hours after the initiation, or (2) subsequent failure to produce a steady decrease in total bilirubin to levels remaining below exchange transfusion threshold.

TABLE 17-7 Guidelines for Management of Hyperbilirubinemia Based on the Gestational Age and Relative Health of the Newborn

	HEALTHY*		SICK*	
	PHOTOTHERAPY	EXCHANGE TRANSFUSION	PHOTOTHERAPY	EXCHANGE TRANSFUSION
PREMATURE				
<1000 g	5-7	Variable	4-6	Variable
1001-1500 g	7-10	Variable	6-8	Variable
1501-2000 g	10-12	Variable	8-10	Variable
2001-2500 g	12-15	Variable	10-12	Variable
TERM				
>2500 g	15-18	20-25	12-15	18-20

From Halamek, L.P. & Stevenson, D.K. (2002). Neonatal jaundice and liver disease. In A.A. Fanaroff & R.J. Martin (Eds.). *Neonatal-perinatal medicine: Diseases of the fetus and infant* (7th ed.). St. Louis: Mosby.
*Quantities represent the total serum bilirubin level in mg/dl.

terohepatic shunting. Lumirubin, a structural nonreversible isomer, is formed at a slower rate but is excreted in bile more rapidly with a serum half-life of 2 hours. Lumirubin is the major pathway through which bilirubin is eliminated during phototherapy. There is a dose-response relationship between lumirubin formation and phototherapy irradiance.[67] Formation of lumirubin is irreversible; it is excreted in bile or, to a lesser extent, in urine. Excretion of these isomers increases bile flow, which may stimulate intestinal activity and more rapid removal of bilirubin. As a result, phototherapy is often more effective in infants being fed and less effective in infants who are not being fed or infants with bowel obstruction.

Photooxidization probably has a minor role in elimination of bilirubin with phototherapy.[44] In this process the bilirubin molecule absorbs light energy from the phototherapy lights. Some of this energy is transferred to oxygen, leading to the formation of a highly reactive oxygen molecule (singlet oxygen). This molecule aids in oxidation and breakdown of bilirubin into water-soluble breakdown products (e.g., monopyrroles, dipyrroles) that are excreted primarily in urine.[96] Decomposition of bilirubin under phototherapy occurs in the skin in the superficial capillaries and interstitial spaces.[29,92]

Side effects of phototherapy. Although many concerns have been raised about the safety of phototherapy and possible short-term and long-term effects, significant side effects are rare. Short-term concerns focus on complications of photoisomerization and photooxidation; long-term concerns focus on irradiation damage, retinal damage, and neurodevelopmental issues.[59] Studies done in vitro and in animals have demonstrated adverse effects of phototherapy, including altered cell growth, damage to cell membranes, breaks in deoxyribonucleic acid (DNA), and alterations in hormonal and enzyme release.[10,53,83,138] However, investigations have generally failed to demonstrate any significant problems with phototherapy usage in human infants and side effects are usually transient.[114] These transient effects include thermal and metabolic changes, hemodynamic changes, increased insensible water loss, altered physiologic function and weight gain, skin and ocular effects, behavioral alterations, and hormonal changes (Table 17-8).[9,138,143]

There are also a variety of psychobehavioral concerns associated with the use of phototherapy, including the potential effect of isolation and the lack of usual sensory experiences, behavioral and activity changes (including lethargy, irritability, and altered feeding behavior), and alterations in state organization and biologic rhythms as well as effects of parental stress (see Table 17-8).[100,107] These concerns may alter parental perceptions of their infant and parent-infant interactions.

Methods of providing phototherapy. Currently phototherapy is usually provided using a bank of fluorescent lights, tungsten halogen or quartz halide spotlights, and fiberoptic blankets. These blankets are woven fiberoptic pads. Halogen light beams are transmitted through a cord of fiberoptic filaments to a flexible pad that is placed

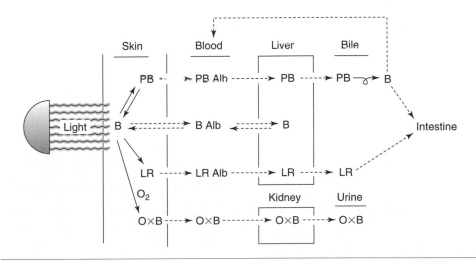

FIGURE **17-5** Mechanisms of action for phototherapy. (*Solid arrows* illustrate chemical reactions; *dotted arrows* illustrate transport processes.) *Alb,* Albumin; *B,* bilirubin (Z,Z isomer); *LR,* lumirubin (E and Z isomers); *O × B,* bilirubin oxidation products; *PB,* photobilirubin (E,E and E,Z isomers). (From McDonagh, A.F. & Lightner, D.A. [1985]. "Like a shriveled blood orange"—Bilirubin, jaundice and phototherapy. *Pediatrics, 75,* 452. Reproduced by permission of *Pediatrics.*)

TABLE 17-8   Side Effects of Phototherapy

SIDE EFFECT	SPECIFIC CHANGES	IMPLICATIONS
Thermal and other metabolic changes	Increased environmental and body temperature Increased oxygen consumption Increased respiratory rate	Influenced by maturity, caloric intake (energy to respond to thermal changes), adequacy of heat dissipation from phototherapy unit, distance of unit from infant and incubator hood (related to space for air flow and radiant heat loss), use of servocontrol
Cardiovascular changes	Increased skin blood flow Transient changes in cardiac output and decrease in left ventricular output Hemodynamic changes are seen primarily in the first 12 hours of phototherapy use; after that, return to previous levels or higher	Reopening of ductus arteriosus Possible due to photorelaxation; usually not hemodynamically significance
Fluid status	Increased peripheral blood flow Increased insensible water loss	Increase fluid loss May alter uptake of intramuscular medications Due to increases in evaporative water loss, metabolic rate, and possibly respiratory rate Influenced by environment (e.g., air flow, humidity, temperature); characteristics of phototherapy unit (e.g., heat dissipation, distance from infant); ambient temperature alteration; infant alterations in skin and core temperature, heart rate, respiratory rate, metabolic rate, caloric intake; type of bed (increased with radiant warmer and incubator)
Gastrointestinal function	Increased number, frequency of stools Watery, greenish-brown stools Decreased time for intestinal transit Decreased absorption; retention of nitrogen, water, electrolytes Altered lactose activity, riboflavin	May be related to increased bile flow, which stimulates gastrointestinal activity Increases stool water loss Increases stool water loss and risk of dehydration Temporary lactose intolerance with decreased lactase at epithelial brush border and increased frequency and water content of stools
Altered activity	Lethargy or irritability Decreased eagerness to feed	May impact on parent-infant interaction May alter fluid and caloric intake
Altered weight gain	Decreased initially but generally catches up in 2 to 4 weeks	Due to poor feeding and increased gastrointestinal losses
Ocular effects	Not documented in humans, but continued concerns about effects of light versus effects of eye patches	Lack of appropriate sensory input and stimulation Eye patches increase risk of infection, corneal abrasion, increased intracranial pressure (if too tight)
Skin changes	Tanning Rashes Burns Bronze baby syndrome	Due to induction of melanin synthesis or dispersion by ultraviolet light Due to injury to skin mast cells with release of histamine; erythema from ultraviolet light From excessive exposure to short-wave emissions from fluorescent light Due to interaction of phototherapy and cholestasis jaundice, producing a brown pigment (bilifuscin) that stains the skin; reversible change which may take months to resolve.
Hormonal changes	Alterations in serum gonadotropins (increased luteinizing hormone and follicle-stimulating hormone)	Significance unclear May also affect circadian rhythms (unclear)

TABLE **17-8**   Side Effects of Phototherapy—cont'd

SIDE EFFECT	SPECIFIC CHANGES	IMPLICATIONS
Hematologic changes	Increased rate of platelet turnover	May be a problem in infants with low platelets and sepsis
	Injury to circulating red blood cells with decreased potassium and increased adenosine triphosphate activity	May lead to hemolysis, increased energy needs
Psychobehavioral concerns	Isolation or lack of usual sensory experiences, including visual deprivation	Impact can be mediated by provision of appropriate nursing care
	Alteration in state organization and neurobehavioral organization	May interfere with parent-infant interaction and increase parental stress

beneath or wrapped around the infant. These pads remain at room temperature and deliver light within the 425- to 475-nm wavelength.[13,144] The fiberoptic pads have been shown in most studies to be as effective as single conventional phototherapy (in both term and preterm infants) in reducing bilirubin levels in infants with mild to moderate hyperbilirubinemia and are associated with fewer side effects.[40,48,113,130] A disadvantage of these pads is lower spectral power due to small surface area—making them less useful in treating infants with severe hyperbilirubinemia, unless used in conjunction with overhead lights to provide double phototherapy. Tungsten-halogen spotlights cover a smaller infant surface area; therefore they also provide less spectral power than fluorescent bank lights.[83] A new method for providing phototherapy is use of high-intensity blue gallium nitride light-emitting diodes (LEDs).[118] With these devices the amount of blue-green light can be customized. Since these units generate little heat, the unit can be placed a short distance from the infant to deliver irradiances over 200 μW/cm^2/nm, thus enhancing lumirubin formation.[118] To date, there have been limited trials of these devices.

An issue in caring for infants under phototherapy is whether to turn off the "lights" or remove the infant from under them during feeding and other caregiving. The benefits to both the infant and the parents of removing the eye shields and holding the infant during feeding seem to outweigh concerns regarding the effectiveness of bilirubin reduction in most situations.[119] Intermittent phototherapy has been shown to be effective in some studies, although other studies demonstrate increased effectiveness for continuous treatment.[83,137] However, most studies of intermittent phototherapy have been with infants with mild to moderate hyperbilirubinemia, not infants with severe hy-

perbilirubinemia who require continuous phototherapy.[67,83] The most rapid catabolism of bilirubin appears to take place within the first few hours after the start of each phototherapy period. It takes bilirubin about 3 hours to return to the skin after removal of photoisomers.[67] Thus, for infants with mild to moderate hyperbilirubinemia, the irradiance, area of skin exposed, and initial effects of phototherapy on bilirubin in the skin seem to have more influence than whether the infant is removed for short periods of feeding or holding.[26]

Intensive phototherapy is used for infants with severe hyperbilirubinemia. By using multiple (fluorescent or halogen) phototherapy units or combining overhead phototherapy with fiberoptic blankets or using special blue lights on an uninterrupted schedule, the intensity and thus effectiveness of phototherapy can be increased.[59] Simultaneous use of overhead phototherapy and fiberoptic blankets increases the surface area exposed to light and spectral irradiance, which can also increase effectiveness.[63] As compared to single phototherapy, double phototherapy has been reported to be twice as effective in preterm infants and 50% more effective in term infants.[113,124] Use of special blue fluorescent bulbs placed 15 cm above the infant's surface have been reported to reduce bilirubin levels of term infants by 43% to 45% in the first 24 hours of use (compared with a 15% decrease using traditional methods).[82] Exposure can also be increased by using a reflective surface (such as white sheets or aluminum foil) around the incubator or bassinet or two to three fiberoptic blankets to cover more surface area.[37,83] The spectral irradiance can also be increased by placing the lights at the minimum safe distance from the infant's surface.[37,67,82] Care must be taken to keep halogen lights in particular at the manufacturer's recommended distance from the infant's skin, since these lights can cause burns if too close.[37,67,82,83]

Equipment issues. Effective phototherapy requires sufficient illumination over an adequate area of exposed skin at a sufficiently short distance to produce the desired effect of light on bilirubin molecules.[119] Therefore the effectiveness of phototherapy depends on the spectrum of light delivered by the phototherapy unit, intensity of the energy output (power output) or irradiance, and the surface area of the infant exposed to the light.[82] The surface area of exposure can be increased with the use of intensive phototherapy.

Irradiance is the radiant power of light on a surface per unit of surface area (W/m^2). Irradiance is directly related to the distance of the light source from the infant.[82] Spectral irradiance—which is the irradiance of the light source (radiant power per unit area) within the therapeutic wavelength of maximum light absorbance by the bilirubin molecule (425 to 550 nm), not the intensity (i.e., illumination or brightness)—determines effectiveness.[82,83] The intensity of the light is inversely related to the distance between the light source and the skin surface.[95] There is a significant linear relationship between the spectral irradiance received by the infant and the decrease in serum bilirubin levels over a 24-hour period.[82,123]

Initially it was thought that the effective range was at a spectral irradiance of 4 to 5 $\mu W/cm^2$ in the 425- to 475-nm waveband.[67,96] However, this irradiance is only for production of configurational isomers. For production of the structural isomer lumirubin, a higher spectral irradiance is required.[67] Because phototherapy units vary in effectiveness, light emission may decrease over time. Irradiance levels can be monitored with a radiometer using the instructions in equipment manuals or unit protocol. The radiometer has a wide bandwidth so that the effective irradiance of the phototherapy unit (as amount of blue light) can be measured. Measurement is in $\mu W/cm^2/nm$ and called the spectral irradiance. In comparing different devices, spectral power (mW/nm) may be a more useful measure since it measures the average spectral irradiance across the skin surface area of the infant.[82]

For phototherapy to be effective, light photons must penetrate the skin and be absorbed by bilirubin molecules. Only certain wavelengths are absorbed by bilirubin; longer waves penetrate deeper into the skin.[43] Light wavelengths in the blue-green spectrum (425 to 550 nm) are most effective in reducing bilirubin levels. Green, daylight white, blue, and special blue (super blue) fluorescent bulbs have been used. Special blue (narrow spectrum) bulbs are the most effective since they provide more irradiance at 450 nm (maximal blue wavelength absorbance).[83,112] Difficulty in deter-

mining infant skin color and side effects in staff such as nausea and headaches have been reported with the use of blue bulbs. Green lights have been reported to be less effective than special blue bulbs by many but not all investigators.[43,44,83,85,111] Green light favors formation of lumirubin, and its longer waves penetrate farther into the skin.[67,95] Thus use of a blue-green light (as found in new LED devices) may be advantageous.[118] Considerations regarding phototherapy equipment are summarized in Table 17-9.

Competition for Albumin Binding

Most indirect bilirubin is transported in plasma bound to albumin (1 g albumin binds 8.5 to 10 mg of bilirubin). Two terms used to describe albumin binding are capacity and affinity. Each molecule of albumin has a certain number of binding sites available (the binding capacity). The tightness by which bilirubin is bound to sites available for binding is the affinity.

In adults each molecule of albumin can bind at least two molecules of bilirubin.[59] The binding sites may be primary (tight or high affinity) or secondary (weak affinity). Each albumin molecule has one primary binding site and one or more secondary sites. If the primary site is saturated, there is a rapid increase in loosely bound or free bilirubin.[83] Albumin binding capacity is lower in the neonate due to lower albumin levels and decreased albumin binding capacities.[59] Unbound bilirubin can leave the vascular system and enter the skin, brain, and other organs. Various techniques have been developed to measure albumin binding of bilirubin but none of them are acceptable for widespread clinical management in terms of either application or interpretation.[26,59,83]

Competing substances easily displace bilirubin bound to secondary sites. Drugs such as sulfonamides, salicylate, chlorothiazide, ceftriaxone, rifampicin, certain x-ray contrast substances, and sodium benzoate (a preservative used in multiple injection vials for drugs such as diazepam and plasma expanders) may displace bilirubin.[22,23,26,67] Bilirubin also displaces some drugs (including ampicillin, phenobarbitol, and phenytoin) from albumin (see Chapter 6). Albumin binding and actions of selected drugs used in neonates in competing with bilirubin for binding sites have been reported.[110]

Albumin binding of bilirubin can be altered by pathologic events. Plasma free fatty acids compete with bilirubin for albumin-binding sites.[106] Hypothermia increases metabolism and catabolism of fatty acids, which may displace bilirubin from albumin. However, risk is minimal if the concentrations of free fatty acids are less than 4:1.[67] Concerns have been raised about risks with the use of emulsified lipid solutions (e.g., Intralipid) in neonates.[120]

TABLE **17-9**   Equipment Considerations with Phototherapy

PARAMETER	CONSIDERATIONS
Energy output	Intensity of energy output of light source, not light intensity (i.e., illumination or brightness), determines effectiveness; adequate spectral irradiance.
Distance of light from infant	Amount of radiant energy delivered to infant is related to distance (increasing distance decreases irradiance [i.e., twofold increase in distance produces a fourfold decrease in irradiance]).
Wavelength	Wavelengths in the blue-green spectrum (450 to 550 nm) most effective. Special blue (narrow spectrum) bulbs provide more irradiance at 450 nm (maximal blue wavelength absorbance. Green light favors formation of lumirubin and its longer waves penetrate farther into the skin. Use of blue-green light such as occurs with the new LED devices may be advantageous.
Ultraviolet irradiation	This may be reduced by placing a Plexiglas shield (¼" thick) between the light source and the infant.
Electrical hazards	Phototherapy units should be checked regularly for grounding and electrical leakage.
Effectiveness	Light emission may decrease over time; therefore energy levels (irradiance) should be monitored and kept in the effective wavelength range. Bulbs should be replaced as recommended by the manufacturer.
Thermal hazards	The risk for overheating or hyperthermia may be reduced by monitoring the infant's thermal status and maintaining a space of about 2" between the incubator hood and lamp cover to allow a free flow of air. Halogen lights in particular should not be placed closer to the infant than the manufacturer specifications state because of the risk of burns. The risk of overheating is increased for infants in radiant warmers with three-sided lights because these prevent radiant heat loss
Alteration in blood samples	Phototherapy should be discontinued while blood for bilirubin values is drawn.

Dosages below 1 to 2 g/kg every 15 hours had no significant effect on bilirubin levels, but at higher levels, increased dosages were correlated with increased levels of free fatty acids and decreased binding of bilirubin, especially in preterm infants.[27,120] The amount of unbound indirect bilirubin may also be increased if there is more bilirubin than available albumin because of excess production of bilirubin or decreased albumin (e.g., with malnourishment). Serum pH per se may not alter binding but may influence deposition of unbound bilirubin in the central nervous system.[83]

Bilirubin Encephalopathy

Development of bilirubin encephalopathy, commonly called kernicterus, is a concern for any infant with elevated bilirubin levels. Bilirubin encephalopathy involves permanent brain damage secondary to deposition of bilirubin in brain cells, with yellow staining and neuronal necrosis. Although the specific toxic effects are still unclear, acidic forms of bilirubin act as mitochondrial poisons that uncouple oxidative phosphorylation in the mitochondria, interfering with cellular respiration, blocking adenosine triphosphate (ATP) production, inhibiting cellular enzymes, and altering water and electrolyte transport.[25,26,30,67,83] Areas of the brain most often affected include the basal ganglia, brain stem auditory pathways, and oculomotor nuclei. The reason for the increased risk in these area may be related to increased blood flow and metabolic activity in these areas.[67] Some infants (30% to 50%) with this disorder also have extraneural lesions, primarily in the renal tubular cells and gastrointestinal system.[59]

Early signs of acute bilirubin encephalopathy include progressive lethargy, poor feeding, vomiting, temperature instability, hypotonia, and a high-pitched cry. Many infants, especially VLBW infants, are asymptomatic in the neonatal period. Later signs include ataxia, opisthotonos, extrapyramidal disturbances, dental enamel hypoplasia, deafness, seizures, and developmental and motor abnormalities. The neurotoxic effects of bilirubin are exacerbated by other pathologic conditions such as hypoxia, asphyxia, and hypercapnia.[61,66,83]

Current theories regarding the mechanisms by which bilirubin passes into neural tissue include the free bilirubin theory and a hypothesis that suggests an opening of the blood-brain barrier.[20,96] The blood brain barrier has tight junctions between endothelial cells of the cerebral blood vessels. These junctions are permeable to lipid-soluble substances but usually impermeable to water-soluble substances, proteins, and other large molecules.[67] For many years, bilirubin encephalopathy was believed to be caused

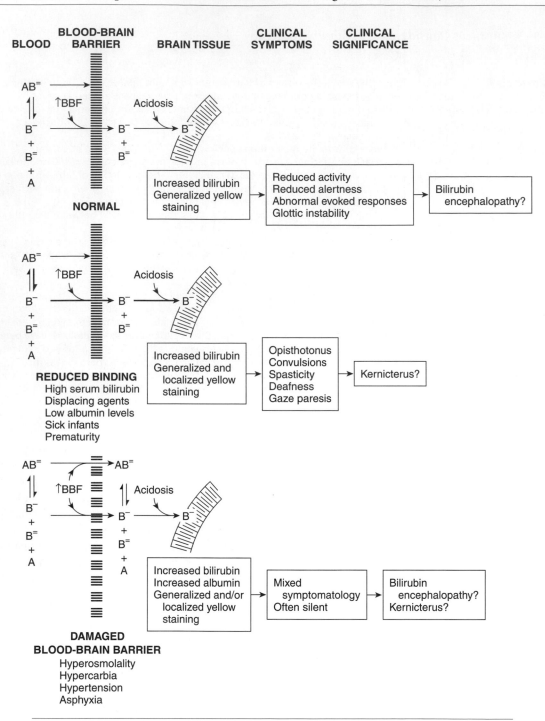

FIGURE **17-6** Schematic of possible mechanisms for bilirubin entry into the brain and binding to neuronal cell membranes. The different factors affecting this process are also indicated. *A*, Albumin; *AB=*, albumin-bilirubin complex; *B−*, bilirubin monoanion; *B=*, bilirubin dianion; *BBF*, brain blood flow. (From Bratlid, D. [1990]. How bilirubin gets into the brain. *Clin Perinatol, 17,* 460.)

by passage of unbound indirect bilirubin across the blood-brain barrier (free bilirubin theory), with deposition of this fat-soluble form of bilirubin in the basal ganglia and other areas of the brain with a high lipid content. Some bilirubin does cross into the brain, but it is not considered harmful.[20] More recently a hypothesis was proposed suggesting that reversible alterations ("opening") in the blood-brain barrier (caused by infection, dehydration, hyperosmolality, or hypoxemia) allow entry of albumin-bound bilirubin as well (Figure 17-6).[26]

The critical level of bilirubin beyond which brain damage occurs is not certain.[102] Most healthy term infants with kernicterus in the recent resurgence (see the section on Management of Jaundice in Breastfed Infants) have had bilirubin levels greater than 30 mg/dl.[83] Reanalysis of data from the Collaborative Perinatal Project showed little correlation between bilirubin levels, hearing loss, and neurologic abnormalities.[101] Low bilirubin values are not "safe" for all infants, since pathologic changes associated with bilirubin encephalopathy have clearly been demonstrated on autopsy at much lower values.[83] Factors associated with the greatest risk for developing kernicterus at lower bilirubin levels are prematurity, respiratory distress syndrome, hypoxia, and acidosis.[26,28] However, there has not been a consistent pattern of hazardous bilirubin levels related to birth weight or gestational age with low-bilirubin-level kernicterus nor have serum bilirubin concentrations or treatment been significant independent variables affecting long-term neurodevelopmental outcome.[28,134]

MATURATIONAL CHANGES DURING INFANCY AND CHILDHOOD

The bilirubin load tends to remain higher in infants for 3 to 6 weeks after birth. Bilirubin-specific UDP-glucuronyl transferase activity increases to adult values by 6 to 12 weeks of age (see Fig. 17-3).[71]

SUMMARY

Alterations in bilirubin metabolism that occur with birth result in one of the more frequent problems seen in the neonate: physiologic jaundice. These changes also interact with pathologic factors in the development of hyperbilirubinemia. Hyperbilirubinemia is of concern because it may be a sign of underlying pathologic processes, such as hemolysis or sepsis, and may lead to adverse consequences—namely, kernicterus. Therefore it is essential for caregivers to appreciate the processes involved in bilirubin metabolism and its maturation to understand the basis for physiologic jaundice and hyperbilirubinemia and to recognize infants at risk for these disorders. Clinical recommendations are summarized in Table 17-10.

TABLE **17-10**   **Recommendations for Clinical Practice Related to Bilirubin Metabolism in Neonates**

Know the usual cord blood values for serum bilirubin (p. 656).	Teach parents to monitor for hyperbilirubinemia and importance of health care following early hospital discharge (pp. 663-664, 673).
Know the usual patterns for serum bilirubin in term and preterm neonates, as well as breastfed infants (pp. 657-658 and Table 17-1).	Plan with parents of term infants for follow-up care with the primary care provider after discharge (pp. 663-664, 673).
Recognize infants at risk for physiologic jaundice (pp. 658-661 and Tables 17-2 and 17-3).	Assess and monitor infants at risk for hyperbilirubinemia (pp. 661-663 and Table 17-4).
Monitor fluid intake and stooling patterns (pp. 658-659).	Know the methods of monitoring serum bilirubin levels and factors that can alter accuracy of measurement (pp. 664-665).
Assess and monitor infants at risk for physiologic jaundice (pp. 658-661).	
Recognize infants at risk for hyperbilirubinemia (pp. 661-663 and Table 17-4).	Monitor infants during and after exchange transfusion for alterations in fluid, electrolyte, and acid—base status (pp. 665-666).
Know the substances and pathophysiologic events that may compete with bilirubin for albumin-binding sites and monitor status of exposed infants (pp. 670-671).	Recognize and monitor for physiologic and psychobehavioral side effects associated with phototherapy (pp. 666-670 and Table 17-8).
Counsel and support the family of a jaundiced infant (pp. 667-669 and Table 17-8).	Provide a safe environment for the infant under phototherapy (pp. 667-670 and Tables 17-8 and 17-9).
Monitor breastfed infants for early and late hyperbilirubinemia (pp. 662-663).	Recognize infants at risk for bilirubin encephalopathy (pp. 671-673).
Institute interventions to prevent early-onset jaundice in breastfed infants (pp. 663-664 and Table 17-5).	Monitor for signs of bilirubin encephalopathy (p. 671).
Counsel and support parents of a jaundiced breastfed infant (pp. 663-664, 667-669).	

REFERENCES

1. Abrol, P. & Sankarasubramanian, R. (1998). Effect of phototherapy on behavior of jaundiced neonates. *Indian J Pediatr, 65,* 603.

2. Alpay, F. (2000). The value of first-day bilirubin measurement in predicting the development of significant hyperbilirubinemia in healthy term newborns. *Pediatrics, 106,* E6.

3. Amato, M., Howald, H., & van Murah, G. (1985). Interruption of breastfeeding versus phototherapy as treatment of hyperbilirubinemia in full term infants. *Helv Paediatr Acta, 40,* 127.

4. American Academy of Pediatrics, Provisional Committee for Quality Improvement and Subcommittee on Hyperbilirubinemia. (1994). Practice parameter: Management of hyperbilirubinemia in the healthy term newborn. *Pediatrics, 94,* 558.

5. American Academy of Pediatrics. (1997), Policy Statement: Breastfeeding and the use of human milk. *Pediatrics, 10,* 1035.

6. Augustine, M.C. (1999). Hyperbilirubinemia in the healthy term newborn, *Nurse Pract, 24,* 24.

7. Bacq, Y., et al. (1996). Liver function tests in normal pregnancy: A prospective study of 103 pregnancy women and 103 matched controls. *Hepatology, 23,* 1030.

8. Belanger, S., Lavoie, J.C. & Chessex, P. (1997). Influence of bilirubin on the antioxidant capacity of plasma of newborn infants. *Biol Neonate, 71,* 233.

9. Benders M., Bel F.V., & Bor M.V., (1999). Cardiac output and ductal reopening during phototherapy in preterm infants. *Acta Paediatrica, 88,* 1014.

10. Benders, M. J. N. L., van Bel, F. & van de Bor, M. (1999). Haemodynamic consequences of phototherapy in term infants. *Eur J Pediatr, 158,* 323.

11. Bergstein, N.A.M. (1973). *Liver and pregnancy.* Amsterdam: Excerpta Medica.

12. Bhutani, V.K., Johnson, L. & Silvieri, E.M. (1999). Predictive ability of a predischarge hour-specific serum bilirubin for subsequent significant hyperbilirubinemia in healthy term and near-term newborns. *Pediatrics, 103,* 6.

13. Bhutani, V.K., et al. (2000). Noninvasive measurement of total serum bilirubin in a multiracial predischarge newborn population to assess risk of severe hyperbilirubinemia. *Pediatrics, 106,* E17

14. Bilgen, H., et al. (1998). Transcutaneous measurement of hyperbilirubinemia: comparison of the Minolta jaundice meter and the Ingram icterometer. *Ann Trop Pediatr, 18,* 325.

15. Blackburn, S. (1995). Back to basics: Neonatal jaundice and hyperbilirubinemia. *Neonatal Net, 14(7).*

16. Blanco, J.D. (1987). Gastrointestinal problems and jaundice. In C.J. Pauerstein (Ed.). *Clinical obstetrics.* New York: John Wiley & Sons.

17. Boyer, D.B. & Vidyasagar, D. (1987). Serum indirect bilirubin levels and meconium passage in early fed normal newborns. *Nurs Res, 36,* 174.

18. Boylan, P. (1976). Oxytocin and neonatal jaundice. *Br Med J, 3,* 564.

19. Bracci, R., et al. (1988). Neonatal hyperbilirubinemia: Evidence for a role of the erythrocyte enzyme activities involved in the detoxification of oxygen radicals. *Acta Paediatr Scand, 77,* 349.

20. Bratlid, D. (1990). How bilirubin gets into the brain. *Clin Perinatol, 17,* 449.

21. Britton, J.R., Britton, H.L., & Beebe, S. A. (1994). Early discharge of the term newborn: a continued dilemma. *Pediatrics, 94,* 291.

22. Broderson, R. (1978). Free bilirubin in blood plasma of the newborn: Effects of albumin, fatty acids, pH, displacing drugs, and phototherapy. In L. Stern, W. Oh & B. Friis-Hansen (Eds.). *Intensive care of the newborn II.* New York: Masson.

23. Brown, A.K., Kim, M.H., & Bryla, D. (1983). Report on the NIH Cooperative Study of Phototherapy: Efficacy of phototherapy in controlling hyperbilirubinemia and preventing kernicterus. *In Hyperbilirubinemia in the newborn: Report of the 85th Ross Conference on Pediatric Research.* Columbus, OH: Ross Laboratories.

24. Brown, A.K. & Johnson, L. (1996). Loss of concern about jaundice and the reemergence of kernicterus in full-term infants in the era of managed care. In A.A. Fanaroff & M.H. Klaus (Eds.). *Yearbook of neonatal and perinatal medicine.* St. Louis: Mosby.

25. Cashore, W.J. (1990). The neurotoxicity of bilirubin. *Clin Perinatol, 17,* 437.

26. Cashore, W.J. & Stern, L. (1987). Neonatal hyperbilirubinemia. In L. Stern & P. Vert (Eds.). *Neonatal medicine.* New York: Masson.

27. Cashore, W.J., et al. (1977). Influence of gestational age and clinical status on bilirubin-binding capacity in newborn infants. *Am J Dis Child, 131,* 898.

28. Cashore, W.J. (2000). Bilirubin and jaundice in the micropremie. *Clin Perinatol, 27,* 171.

29. Christensen, T. & Kinn, G. (1993). Bilirubin bound to cells does not form photoisomers. *Acta Paediatr, 82,* 22.

30. Connolly, A.M. & Volpe, J.J. (1990). Clinical features of bilirubin encephalopathy. *Clin Perinatol, 17,* 371.

31. Cooke, R.W. (1999). New approach to prevention of kernicterus. *Lancet, 353,* 1814.

32. Cotton, D.B., Brock, B.J. & Schifrin, B.S. (1981). Cirrhosis and fetal hyperbilirubinemia. *Obstet Gynecol, 57,* 25s.

33. Cremer, R.J., Perryman, P.W. & Richards, D.H. (1958). Influence of light on the hyperbilirubinemia of infants. *Lancet, 1,* 1094.

34. De Carvalho, M., Holl, M. & Harvey, D. (1981). Effects of water supplementation on physiological jaundice in breastfed babies. *Am J Dis Child, 56,* 568.

35. De Carvalho, M., Klaus, M. & Merkatz, R.B. (1982). Frequency of breast-feeding and serum bilirubin concentration. *Am J Dis Child, 136,* 737.

36. De Carvalho, M., Robertson, S., & Klaus, M. (1985). Fecal bilirubin excretion and serum bilirubin concentrations in breast-fed and bottle-fed infants. *J Pediatr, 107,* 786.

37. DeCarvalho M.D., et al. (1999). Intensified phototherapy using daylight fluorescent lamps. *Acta Paediatr, 88,* 768.

38. DeJonge M.H., et al. (1999). Bilirubin levels and severe retinopathy of prematurely in infants with estimated gestational ages of 23 to 26 weeks. *J Pediatr, 135,* 102.

39. Dixit, R. & Gartner, L.M. (1999). The jaundiced newborn: Minimizing the risks. *Contemporary Pediatr, 16,* 166.

40. Donzelli, G.P., et al. (1996). Fiberoptic phototherapy in the management of jaundice in low birthweight neonates. *Acta Paediatr, 85,* 366.

41. Eeltink, C., et al. (1993). Maternal haemolysis, elevated liver enzymes and low platelets syndrome: specific problems in the newborn. *Eur J Pediatr, 152,* 160.

42. Elander, G. & Lindberg, T. (1986). Hospital routines in infants with hyperbilirubinemia influence the duration of breastfeeding. *Acta Paediatr Scand, 75,* 708.

43. Ennever, J.F. (1990). Blue light, green light, white light, more light: Treatment of neonatal jaundice. *Clin Perinatol, 17,* 467.

44. Ennever, J.F. (1998). Phototherapy for neonatal jaundice. In R.A. Polin & W.W. Fox (Eds.). *Fetal and neonatal physiology* (2nd ed.). Philadelphia: W.B. Saunders

45. Everson, G.T. (1998). Liver problems in pregnancy: Distinguishing normal from abnormal hepatic changes. *Medscape Women's Health, 3(2).* Available online at www.medscape.com/Medscape/WomensHealth1998/v03.n02/wh3096.ever/wh3096.ever.html.

46. Fallon, H.J. & Riely, C.A. (1995). Liver diseases. In G.N. Burrow & T.F. Ferris (Eds.). *Medical complications during pregnancy* (4th ed.). Philadelphia: W.B. Saunders.

47. Felsher, B.F., et al. (1978). Reduced hepatic bilirubin uridine diphosphate glucuronyl transferase and uridine diphosphate glucose dehydrogenase activity in the human fetus. *Pediatr Res, 12,* 838.

48. Gale, R., et al. (1990). A randomized, controlled application of the Wallaby phototherapy system compared with standard phototherapy. *J Perinatol, 10,* 239.

49. Gartner, L. M (1994). On the question of the relationship between breastfeeding and jaundice in the first five days of life. *Sem Perinatol, 18,* 502.

50. Gartner, L. (1998). Practice patterns in neonatal hyperbilirubinemia. *Pediatrics, 101,* 25.

51. Gartner, L.M. & Lee, K.S. (1999). Jaundice in the breastfed infant. *Clin Perinatol, 26,* 431.

52. Girling, J.C., Dow, E. & Smith, J.H. (1997). Liver function tests in pre-eclampsia: Importance of comparison with a reference range derived for normal pregnancy. *Br J Obstet Gynaecol, 104,* 246.

53. Gounaris, A., et al. (1998). Gut hormone levels in neonates undergoing phototherapy. *Early Hum Dev, 51,* 57.

54. Gourley, G.R. (1998). Pathophysiology of breast-milk jaundice. In R.A. Polin & W.W. Fox (Eds.). *Fetal and neonatal physiology* (2nd ed.). Philadelphia: W.B. Saunders.

55. Gourley, G.R. & Arend, R.A. (1986). Beta-glucuronidase and hyperbilirubinemia in breast-fed and formula-fed babies. *Lancet, 22,* 644.

56. Grupp-Phelan, J., et al. (1999). Early newborn hospital discharge and readmission for mild and severe jaundice. *Arch Pediatr Adolesc Med, 153,* 1283.

57. Gutcher, G. (1981). Breast milk jaundice: An evolving tale. *Wis Med J, 80,* 26.

58. Guyton, A.C. & Hall, J.E. (1996). *Textbook of medical physiology* (9th ed.). Philadelphia: W.B. Saunders

59. Halamek, L.P. & Stevenson, D.K. (2002). Neonatal jaundice and liver disease. In A.A. Fanaroff & R.J. Martin (Eds.). *Neonatal-perinatal medicine: Diseases of the fetus and infant* (7th ed.). St. Louis: Mosby.

60. Hammerman, C., et al. (1997). Antioxidant potential of bilirubin in the premature infant. *Pediatr Res, 41,* 157A.

61. Harmon, C.R. (1999). Percutaneous fetal blood sampling. In R.K. Creasy & R. Resnik (Eds.). *Maternal-fetal medicine* (4th ed.). Philadelphia: W.B. Saunders.

62. Herrera, H.A. (1984). Supplemented versus unsupplemented breastfeeding. *Perinatol Neonatal, 8*(3), 70.

63. Holtrop, P.C., et al. (1992). Double versus single phototherapy in low birth weight infants. *Pediatrics, 90,* 674.

64. Hunt, C.M. & Sharara, A.I. (1999). Liver disease in pregnancy. *Am Fam Physician, 59,* 829.

65. Ince, A., et al. (1995). Breast milk beta-glucuronidase and prolonged jaundice in the neonate. *Acta Paediatr, 84,* 237.

66. Ives, N.K., et al. (1988). The effects of bilirubin on brain energy metabolism during normoxia and hypoxia: An in vitro study using 31P nuclear magnetic resonance spectroscopy. *Pediatr Res, 23,* 569.

67. Ives, N.K. (1999). Neonatal jaundice. In JM Rennie & N.R.C. Robertson (Eds.). *Textbook of neonatology* (3rd ed.). Edinburgh: Churchill Livingstone.

68. Johnson, C.A., Lieberman, B., & Hassanein, R.E. (1985). The relationship of breastfeeding to third-day bilirubin levels. *J Fam Pract, 20,* 147.

69. Johnson, L. & Bhutani, V.K. (1998). Guidelines for management of the jaundiced term and near-term infant. *Clin Perinatol, 25,* 555.

70. Kappas, A., et al. (1988). Sn-Protoporphyrin use in the management of hyperbilirubinemia in term newborns with direct Coombs-positive ABO incompatibility. *Pediatrics, 81,* 485.

71. Kawade, N. & Onishi, S. (1981). The prenatal and postnatal development of UDP-glucuronyl transferase activity towards bilirubin and the effect of premature birth on this activity in the human liver. *Biochem J, 196,* 257.

72. Kemper, K., Horowitz, R.I., & McCarthy, P. (1988). Decreased neonatal serum bilirubin with plain agar: A meta-analysis. *Pediatrics, 82,* 631.

73. Kemper, K., Forsyth, B. & McCarthy, P. (1989). Jaundice, terminating breastfeeding, and the vulnerable child. *Pediatrics, 84,* 773.

74. Knudsen, A. (1990). The cephalocaudal progression of jaundice in newborns in relation of transfer of bilirubin from plasma to skin. *Early Hum Dev, 22,* 23.

75. Knudsen, A. (1991). The influence of the reserve albumin concentration and pH on the cephalocaudal progression of jaundice in newborns. *Early Hum Dev, 25,* 37.

76. Lascari, A.D. (1986). "Early" breast-feeding jaundice: Clinical significance. *J Pediatr, 108,* 156.

77. Lawrence, R.A. & Lawrence, R.M. (1999). *Breastfeeding: A guide for the medical profession* (5th ed.). St. Louis: Mosby.

78. Lee, W.M. (1992). Pregnancy in patients with chronic liver disease. *Gastroenterol Clin North Am, 21,* 889,

79. Lee, K., Moscioni, A.D., & Choi, J. (1991). Jaundice. In T.H. Yeh (Ed.). *Neonatal therapeutics* (2nd ed.). St. Louis: Mosby.

80. Lucey, J.F. (1989). Bilirubin and brain damage—a real mess. *Pediatrics, 69,* 381.

81. Madlon-Kay, D.J. (1997). Recognition of the presence and severity of newborn jaundice by parents, nurses, physicians, and icterometer. *Pediatrics, 100,* E3.

82. Maisels, M.J. (1996). Why use homeopathic doses of phototherapy? *Pediatrics, 98,* 283.

83. Maisels, M.J. (1999). Jaundice. In G.B. Avery, M.A. Fletcher & M.G. MacDonald (Eds.). *Neonatology, pathophysiology and management of the newborn* (5th ed.). Philadelphia: J.B. Lippincott.

84. Maisels, M.J. (1992). Neonatal jaundice. In J.C. Sinclair & M.B. Brocker (Eds.). *Effective care of the newborn infant.* Oxford: Oxford University Press.

85. Maisels, M.J. & Gifford, K.L. (1986). Normal serum bilirubin levels in the newborn and the influence of breastfeeding. *Pediatrics, 78,* 837.

86. Maisels, M.J. & Kring, E. (1998). Length of stay, jaundice, and hospital readmission, *Pediatrics, 101,* 995.

87. Maisels, M.J. & Newman, T.B. (1995). Kernicterus in otherwise healthy, breast-fed term newborns, *Pediatrics, 96,* 730.

88. Maisels, M.J. & Newman, T.B. (1998). Jaundice in full-term and near-term babies who leave the hospital within 36 hours. The pediatrician's nemesis. *Clin Perinatol, 25,* 295.

89. Maisels, M.J., et al. (1988). Jaundice in the healthy newborn infant: A new approach to an old problem. *Pediatrics, 81,* 505.

90. Martinez, J.C., et al. (1993). Hyperbilirubinemia in the breast-fed newborn: a controlled trial of four interventions. *Pediatrics, 91,* 470.

91. Martinez J.C., et al. (1999). Control of severe hyperbilirubinemia in full-term newborns with the inhibitor of bilirubin production Sn-mesoporphyrin. *Pediatrics, 103,* 1.

92. McDonagh, A.F. & Lightner, D.A. (1985). "Like a shriveled blood orange"—Bilirubin, jaundice and phototherapy. *Pediatrics, 75,* 443.

93. McDonagh, A.F. (1990). Is bilirubin good for you? *Clin Perinatol, 17,* 359.

94. McLean, M., et al. (2000). Expression of the heme oxygenase-carbon monoxide signaling system in human placenta. *J Clin Endocrinol Metab, 85,* 2345.

95. Melton, K. & Akinbi, H.T. (1999). Neonatal jaundice: Strategies to reduce bilirubin-induced complications. *Postgrad Med, 106,* 167.

96. Modi, N. (1989). Jaundice. In D. Harvey, R.W.I. Cooke, & G.A. Levitt (Eds.). *The baby under 1000 g.* Kent, England: Wright.

97. Moyer, V.A., Ahn, C. & Sneed, S. (2000). Accuracy of clinical judgement in neonatal jaundice. *Arch Pediatr Adolesc Med, 154,* 301.

98. National Institute of Child Health and Human Development. (1985). Randomized controlled trial of phototherapy for neonatal hyperbilirubinemia. *Pediatrics, 75,* 365.

99. Nava, S., et al. (1996). Aspects of fetal physiology from 8 to 37 weeks' gestation as assessed by blood sampling. *Obstet Gynecol, 87,* 975.

100. Nelson, C.A. & Horowitz, F.D. (1982). The short-term behavioral sequelae of neonatal jaundice treated with phototherapy. *Infant Behavior Dev, 5,* 289.

101. Newman, T.B. & Klebanoff, M.A. (1993). Neonatal hyperbilirubinemia and long-term outcome: Another look at the Collaborative Perinatal Project. *Pediatrics, 92,* 651.

102. Newman, T.B. & Maisels, M.J. (1990). Does hyperbilirubinemia damage the brain of healthy full-term infants. *Clin Perinatol, 17,* 331.

103. Newman, T.B. & Maisels, M.J. (1992). Evaluation and treatment of jaundice in the term newborn: A kinder, gentler, approach. *Pediatrics, 89,* 809.

104. Newman, T.B. & Maisels, M.J. (2000). Less aggressive treatment of neonatal jaundice and reports of kernicterus: Lessons about practice guidelines. *Pediatrics, 105,* 242.

105. Nicoll, A., Ginsburg, G. & Tripp, J.H. (1982). Supplementary feeding and jaundice in newborns. *Acta Paediatr Scand, 71,* 759.

106. Ostrea, M., et al. (1983). Influence of free fatty acids and glucose infusion on serum bilirubin and bilirubin binding to albumin. *J Pediatr, 102,* 426.

107. Paludetto, R. (1983). The behavior of jaundiced infants treated with phototherapy. *Early Human Dev, 8,* 259.

108. Poland, R. & Schultz, G. (1980). High milk lipase activity associated with breast milk jaundice. *Pediatr Res, 14,* 1328.

109. Ramsay, M.M., et al. (1996). *Normal values in pregnancy.* Philadelphia: W.B. Saunders.

110. Robertson, A., Carp, W., & Broderson, R. (1991) Bilirubin displacing effect of drugs used in neonatology, *Acta Paediatr Scand, 80,* 119.

111. Romagnoli, C., et al. (1988). Phototherapy for hyperbilirubinemia in preterm infants: Green versus blue or white light. *J Pediatr, 112,* 476.

112. Sarici S., et al. (1999). Comparison of the efficacy of conventional special blue light phototherapy and fiberoptic phototherapy in the management of neonatal hyperbilirubinemia. *Acta Paediatr, 88,* 1249.

113. Sarici S., et al. (2000). Double versus single phototherapy in term newborns with significant hyperbilirubinemia. *J Trop Pediatr, 46,* 1, 36.

114. Scheidt, P.C., et al. (1990). Phototherapy for neonatal hyperbilirubinemia: Six year follow-up of the NICHD clinical trial. *Pediatrics, 85,* 455.

115. Schneider, A.P. (1986). Breast milk jaundice in the newborn. *JAMA, 255,* 3270.

116. Schumacher, R.E. (1990). Noninvasive measurements of bilirubin in the newborn. *Clin Perinatol, 17,* 417.

117. Seidman, D.S., et al. (1999). Predicting the risk of jaundice in full-term healthy newborns: a prospective population-based study. *J Perinatol, 19,* 564.

118. Seidman, D.S., et al. (2000). A new blue light-emitting phototherapy device: A prospective randomized controlled study. *J Pediatr, 136,* 771.

119. Sisson, T.R.C. (1978). Bilirubin metabolism. In U. Stave (Ed.). *Perinatal physiology.* New York: Plenum.

120. Spear, M.L., et al. (1985). The effect of 15-hour fat infusions of varying dosage on bilirubin binding to albumin. *J Parenter Enteral Nutr, 9,* 144.

121. Steffensrud, S. (1998). Tin-metalloporphyrins: an answer to neonatal jaundice? *Neonatal Net, 17,* 5, 11.

122. Stocker, R., et al. (1987). Bilirubin is an antioxidant of possible physiologic importance. *Science, 235,* 1043.

123. Tan, K.L. (1989). Efficacy of fluorescent daylight, blue and green lamps in the management of nonhemolytic hyperbilirubinemia. *J Pediatr, 114,* 132.

124. Tan, K.L. (1997). Efficacy of bi-directional fiber-optic phototherapy for neonatal hyperbilirubinemia. *Pediatrics, 99,* 5.

125. Tan, K.L. (1998). Decreased response to phototherapy for neonatal jaundice in breast-fed infants. *Arch Pediatr Adolesc Med, 152,* 1187.

126. Tayaba, R., et al. (1998). Noninvasive estimation of serum bilirubin. *Pediatrics, 102,* E28.

127. Tudehope, D., et al. (1991). Breastfeeding practices and severe hyperbilirubinemia. *J Pediatr Child Health, 27,* 240.

128. Valaes, T., et al. (1994). Control of jaundice in preterm newborns by an inhibitor of bilirubin production: Studies with tin-mesoporphyrin. *Pediatrics, 93,* 1.

129. Valaes, T.N. & Harvey-Wilkes, K. (1990). Pharmacological approaches in the prevention and treatment of neonatal hyperbilirubinemia. *Clin Perinatol, 17,* 245.

130. Van Kaam, A. H. L. C., et al., (1998). Fibre optic versus conventional phototherapy for hyperbilirubinemia in preterm infants. *Eur J Pediatr, 157,* 132.

131. Vohr, B. (1990). New approaches to assessing the risks of hyperbilirubinemia. *Clin Perinatol, 17,* 293.

132. Vreman, H.J. & Stevenson, D.K. (1990). Metalloporphyrin-enhanced photodegradation of bilirubin in vitro. *Am J Dis Child, 144,* 590.

133. Waffarn, F., et al. (1982). Fetal exposure to maternal hyperbilirubinemia. *Am J Dis Child, 136,* 416.

134. Watchko, J.F. & Classen, D. (1994). Kernicterus in premature infants: Current prevalence and relationship to NICHD phototherapy study exchange criteria. *Pediatrics, 93,* 996.

135. Wiley, C.C., et al. (1998). Nursery practices and detection of jaundice after newborn discharge. *Arch Pediatr Adolesc Med, 152,* 972.

136. Wolf, J.L. (1996). Liver disease in pregnancy. *Med Clin North Am, 80,* 1167.

137. Wu, P.Y.K. (1981). Phototherapy update: Factors effecting efficiency of phototherapy. *Perinatol Neonatol, 5*(5), 45.

138. Wu, P.Y.K. (1982). Phototherapy: In vivo side effects. *Perinatol Neonatol, 6*(2), 21.

139. Wu, P.Y.K., et al. (1983). Metabolic aspects of phototherapy. *Pediatrics, 75*(suppl), 427.

140. Yamauchi, Y. & Yamanouchi, H. (1989). Transcutaneous bilirubinometry. *Acta Paediatr Scand, 78,* 844.

141. Yamauchi, Y. & Yamanouchi, H. (1990). Breast-feeding frequency during the first 24 hours after birth in full-term neonates. *Pediatrics, 86,* 171.

142. Yamauchi, Y. & Yamanouchi, I. (1990). Clinical application of transcutaneous bilirubin measurement. Early prediction of hyperbilirubinemia. *Acta Paediatr Scand, 79,* 385.

Pituitary, adrenal, and thyroid function and the hypothalamic-pituitary-adrenal (HPA) and hypothalamic-pituitary-thyroid (HPT) axes are critical for normal function and adaptation during pregnancy, growth, and development of the fetus, and adaptation of the newborn to the extrauterine environment. The HPA axis function of the mother and fetus are closely interrelated with placental function. The hormones of the HPA and HPT axes (see Figure 2-7) are necessary for many body functions, for development of the central nervous system (CNS) and other growth processes, and for reproductive function. Disorders of these axes are associated with infertility, alterations in normal changes at puberty, and complications of pregnancy. Concentrations of HPA and HPT axis hormones are altered in pregnant women and neonates. In the neonate marked changes in adrenal and thyroid function occur with birth. This chapter examines changes in the glands of the HPA and HPT axes and their hormones during pregnancy; development of neuroendocrine function in the fetus and neonate; and implications for the mother, fetus, and neonate.

MATERNAL PHYSIOLOGIC ADAPTATIONS

Pregnancy is associated with significant alterations in the morphology of the pituitary, adrenal, and thyroid glands. Concentrations of adrenocorticotropin (ACTH), corticotropin-releasing hormone (CRH), growth hormone (GH), cortisol, thyroid hormones (thyroxine [T_4] and triiodothyronine [T_3]), and thyroxine-binding globulin (TBG) are altered during pregnancy. Placental hormones, particularly estrogen, human chorionic gonadotropin (hCG), placental growth hormone, and placental CRH, and alterations in liver and kidney function influence these changes.

Antepartum Period
Hypothalamic-Pituitary-Adrenal Axis

Marked changes occur in the HPA axis during pregnancy. These changes are mediated primarily by placental hormones, including placental ACTH, GH, and CRH. (See Figure 2-1

for an illustration of the HPA axis). Maternal hypothalamic and pituitary function are discussed further in Chapter 2 along with the hypothalamic-pituitary-ovarian axis.

Anterior pituitary function. The anterior pituitary is composed of six cell types, each of which produces different hormones. These types of cells and their major hormones are lactotroph (prolactin), corticotroph (ACTH), somatotroph (GH), gonadotroph (follicle-stimulating hormone [FSH] and luteinizing hormone [LH]), thyroid-stimulating hormone (TSH) (thyrotropin), and "other." The anterior pituitary gland increases in size and weight (from 660 mg in the nonpregnant woman to 760 mg during pregnancy) due to an estrogen-induced increase in the lactotroph cells.[10,11,34,55,110] The changes in the shape of the anterior pituitary may cause it to bulge upward in some women, compressing the optic chiasma. For these pregnant women, this can result in a transient hemianopia.[10] Changes in pituitary function during pregnancy are summarized in Table 18-1.

In the nonpregnant women the prolactin-producing lactotroph cells make up approximately 20% of the anterior pituitary; this increases to around 60% during pregnancy.[11] Prolactin isoforms increase during pregnancy, with the nonglycosylated forms exceeding the N-linked glycosylated form that is most common in nonpregnant women.[10,11] The nonglycosylated form may be more bioactive and function to prepare the breast for lactation.[7] Prolactin increases during pregnancy to peak at delivery.[55] Most of the increase in prolactin is from the maternal anterior pituitary, although prolactin is also produced by the maternal decidua. Prolactin levels in the amniotic fluid peak in the second trimester.[11,55]

Corticotroph cells do not change in size during pregnancy.[11] However, ACTH secretion and plasma ACTH levels increase two- to fourfold (Figure 18-1), from approximately 10 pg/ml in nonpregnant women to 50 pg/ml at term.[11] ACTH secretion is stimulated by CRH and, in turn, stimulates release of cortisol by the adrenal gland. Changes in ACTH parallel the increase in free and total cortisol

TABLE **18-1**   Normal Pituitary Function Changes in Pregnancy

HORMONE	BASAL SERUM LEVEL CHANGES	DYNAMIC TESTING
Luteinizing hormone	Suppressed	Flat response to gonadotropin-releasing hormone
Follicle-stimulating hormone	Suppressed	Flat response to gonadotropin-releasing hormone
Prolactin	Elevated	
Growth hormone	Suppressed	Blunted response to hypoglycemia
Thyroid-stimulating hormone	Unchanged	Increased response to thyrotropin-releasing hormone
Adrenocorticotropin	Small rise	Blunted response to metyrapone
β-Melanocyte stimulating hormone	Elevated	
Arginine vasopressin	Unchanged	Normal response to water deprivation
Oxytocin	Vary considerably	Variable increase during labor

From Garner, P.R. (1991). Pituitary disorders in pregnancy. *Curr Obstet Med, 1,* 48.

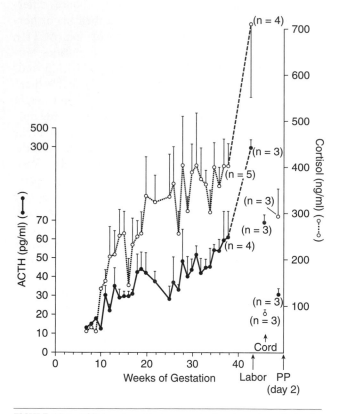

FIGURE **18-1** ACTH and cortisol concentration in maternal circulation throughout gestation. (From Carr, B.R., et al. (1981). Maternal plasma adrenocorticotropin [ACTH] and cortisol relationships throughout human pregnancy. *Am J Obstet Gynecol, 139,* 416.)

(Figure 18-1).[10,55,110] The increase in ACTH in the face of increased cortisol suggests a change in the set point for cortisol release that alters the ACTH-cortisol feedback (Figure 18-2).[10,65] ACTH maintains its circadian rhythm during pregnancy.[22,110] Placental ACTH increases in the second and third trimesters, but most of the increased maternal serum ACTH is thought to come from the maternal anterior pituitary.[55] The effects of ACTH on the adrenal gland and changes in cortisol during pregnancy are described further in the section Adrenal Function.

The increased ACTH secretion during pregnancy is due primarily to increased placental (and some decidual and fetal membrane) CRH, rather than maternal hypothalamic CRH (Figure 18-3).[20,55,110,159] Maternal serum CRH increases markedly beginning by 8 to 10 weeks and rises from nonpregnant values of 10 to 100 pg/ml to 300 to 1000 pg/ml by the third trimester.[11,27,110,159] CRH-binding protein (CRH-BP) decreases the bioactivity of the increased CRH throughout most of gestation. CRH-BP levels are similar to nonpregnant levels until the third trimester, then fall by two thirds in preparation for parturition (see Chapter 4).

Somatotroph and gonadotroph cells of the anterior pituitary decrease during pregnancy.[8] Hypothalamic gonadotropin-releasing hormone (GnRH) is suppressed in pregnancy, with a blunted response of the pituitary to GnRH and low LH and FSH levels by 6 to 7 weeks. By midpregnancy, LH and FSH levels are undetectable.[10,11,55,124] Gonadotropin function is described in Chapter 2.

Pituitary GH (GH-N) decreases in late pregnancy as placental GH (GH-V) increases (Figure 18-4).[55,103] GH-V is a GH variant that stimulates bone growth and regulates maternal insulin-like growth factor–I (IGF-I), which in turn alters maternal metabolism, stimulating

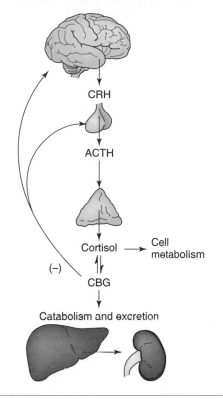

FIGURE **18-2** Regulation of cortisol. Neural stimuli trigger release of corticotropin-releasing hormone (CRH), which discharges adrenocorticotropin (ACTH) from the anterior pituitary, leading to adrenal cortisol secretion. The secreted cortisol has one of several fates: (1) it becomes bound to corticotropin-binding globulin (CBG), (2) it binds to cortisol receptors at target tissues, (3) it is catabolized by the liver or kidney, or (4) it induces feedback inhibition of the pituitary or central nervous system. (From Griffing G.T. & Melby, J.C. [1994]. The maternal adrenal cortex. In D. Tulchinsky & A.B. Little (Eds.). *Maternal-fetal endocrinology* [2nd ed.]. Philadelphia: W.B. Saunders.)

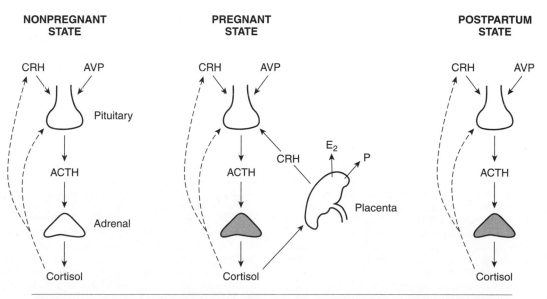

FIGURE **18-3** Schematic representation of the hypothalamic-pituitary-adrenal (HPA) axis in the non-pregnant, pregnant, and postpartum woman. *CRH,* corticotropin releasing hormone; *AVP,* arginine vaso-pressin; *ACTH,* adrenocorticotropin; E_2, estradiol; *P,* progesterone. Shaded areas represent relative hypertrophy of the adrenals. (From Mastorakos, G. & Ilias, I. [2000]. Maternal hypothalamic-adrenal axis in pregnancy and the postpartum period: Postpartum-related disorders. *Ann N Y Acad Sci, 900,* 100.)

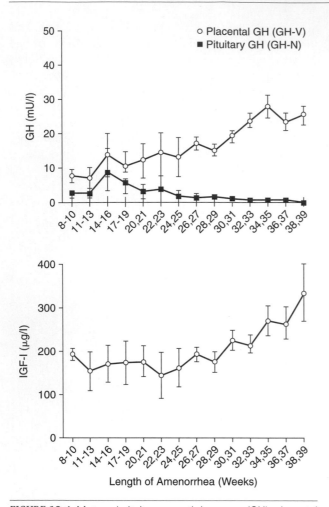

FIGURE **18-4** Maternal pituitary growth hormone (GH), placental growth hormone, and insulin-like growth factor-I (IGF-I) during pregnancy. (Adapted from Mirlesse, V., et al. [1993]. Placental growth hormone levels in normal and pathologic pregnancies. *Pediatr Res,34,* 439, by Evian-Brion, D. [1999]. Maternal endocrine adaptations to placental hormones in humans. *Acta Paediatr Suppl, 428,* 12.)

gluconeogenesis and lipolysis.[106] GH-V is secreted continuously, as opposed to the pulsatile secretion characteristic of GH-N.[1] GH-N is the main maternal GH until 15 to 20 weeks; then it decreases and becomes undetectable by term. GH-V increases from 15 to 20 weeks until term. GH-V stimulates IGF-I, with negative feedback suppression of maternal GH-N.[1,10,41,118]

Posterior pituitary function. The major posterior pituitary hormones are arginine vasopressin (AVP) and oxytocin. Posterior pituitary function changes are associated with osmoregulatory changes and parturition. AVP levels are within normal ranges during pregnancy; however, the threshold at which AVP is secreted is reset (see Chapter 10).[124] AVP also modulates ACTH release.[22] Oxytocin levels progressively increase during pregnancy, with further increase at term (see Chapter 4) and with lactation (see Chapter 5).[55,124]

Adrenal function. Pregnancy is characterized by a transient hypercortisolism (Figure 18-3).[110] Both total and free cortisol increase to peak at levels two to three times higher by term.[55,103] Urinary cortisol also increases threefold by term.[55] The diurnal secretion of cortisol—with higher levels in the morning versus evening—is blunted but maintained.[103,110,124] The increase in cortisol parallels the increase in ACTH (see Figure 18-1). Even though both ACTH and cortisol are elevated during pregnancy, normal cortisol responses to stress are maintained.[10,65,155]

The increase in total cortisol is primarily due to an estrogen-stimulated increase in cortisol-binding globulin (CBG) that increases to twice normal levels by the second trimester.[103v] Increased CBG reduces liver catabolism of cortisol, yielding a twofold increase in cortisol half-life.[110] The increase in free cortisol is also due in part to displacement of cortisol from CBG by progesterone.[55]

The adrenal gland becomes hypertrophic as the zona fasciculata widens, with no changes in the size of the zona glomerulosa or reticularis (see the box below).[54,55] Levels of

Adrenal Hormones

The adrenal gland is composed of the outer adrenal cortex and the inner adrenal medulla. The adrenal cortex is divided into three zones: zona fasciculata, zona glomerulosa, and zone reticularis. Although the adrenal cortex produces over 50 steroid hormones, the major hormones are cortisol and aldosterone.[139] The zona fasciculata is the site of glucocorticoid production that is regulated by corticotropin-releasing hormone (CRH) and adrenocorticotropin (ACTH) (see Figure 18-2). ACTH binds to membrane receptors on cells of the adrenal gland, activating adenylate cyclase. This increases movement of cholesterol, a precursor for pregnenolone, into the cells. Pregnenolone is metabolized in the smooth endoplasmic reticulum to cortisol, the main glucocorticoid.[86] Glucocorticoids regulate metabolism and blood glucose, increase with stress, and suppress immune functions. The zona glomerulosa produces mineralocorticoids, the major one being aldosterone. Mineralcorticoids regulate fluid and electrolyte balance (see Chapter 10). The zona reticularis produces androgens that are important for sexual differentiation, although the major source of androgens is the gonads (see Chapter 2). The adrenal medulla is the source of epinephrine and norepinephrine that are also involved in stress responses.

both cortisol (the primary glucocorticoid) and aldosterone (the primary mineralocorticoid) (see Chapter 10) are markedly increased in pregnancy. Synthesis of androgens and dehydroepiandrosterone sulfate (DHEA-S) by the zona reticularis also increase, but less so than the glucocorticoids and mineralocorticoids. Maternal serum DHEA-S levels remain low due to placental uptake and metabolism.[65]

Hypothalamic-Pituitary-Thyroid Axis

Marked changes are also seen in the HPT axis during pregnancy. Adaptations during pregnancy related to thyroid physiology mimic hyperthyroidism. The pregnant woman can be described as being in a state of euthyroid hyperthyroxinemia, however, since thyroid function per se does not change during pregnancy. This state is associated with periods of increased estrogen (pregnancy, oral contraceptives, or estrogen replacement therapy), liver dysfunction, and use of drugs (heroin and methadone).[112] Thyroid hormone changes are important in supporting the altered carbohydrate, protein, and lipid metabolism of pregnancy (see Chapter 15). The factors primarily responsible for changes in HPT axis function during pregnancy are the elevated hCG and TBG levels and increased urinary iodide excretion that lowers maternal plasma iodine.[22] The boxes below and Figure 18-5 review thyroid hormone production and regulation.

Thyroid hormones are transported in the blood bound to binding proteins, such as TBG, transthyretin, and thyroxine-binding prealbumin (TPBA). Under the influence of estrogen, hepatic synthesis and sialyation of TBG increases two- to threefold beginning within a few weeks after fertilization and plateauing by mid-gestation.[12,20,42,44,67,103,162]

Thyroid Function

The thyroid gland consists of multiple colloid-filled follicles that serve as a storage site for thyroid hormone (see Figure 18-5). The major component of the colloid is thyroglobulin. Thyroid cellular mechanisms for iodine transport and thyroxine (T_4) and triiodothyronine (T_3) formation and release into the blood. Iodide is actively transported into the thyroid cell, stored, and oxidized. Oxidized iodide is bound to tyrosine to form iodotyrosines. These substances are held within the thyroglobulin and used to form T_4 and T_3. T_4 and T_3 are stored in the thyroid, bound to thyroglobulin. Under the influence of thyroid-stimulating hormone (TSH), T_4 and a small amount of T_3 are cleaved from thyroglobulin and secreted. In peripheral tissue, T_4 is deiodinated to T_3 (70% to 80% of T_3 in tissues is derived from this process). Released iodine is reconcentrated by the thyroid or excreted by the kidneys. T_4 can also be metabolized to reverse T_3 (rT_3), which is an inactive compound. T_3 and rT_3 are in a reciprocal relationship. Nearly all of the thyroid hormones circulate in plasma bound to proteins, including thyroxine-binding globulin (TBG) (the major carrier), thyroxine-binding prealbumin (TBPA), or albumin. Changing levels of TBG, such as occurs during pregnancy, alter serum thyroxine levels without changing thyroid status. The small amounts of free T_3 and T_4 in the blood form the physiologically active fraction. Three types of the mondeiodinase (MDI) enzymes catabolize T_4: (1) type I MDI (found in the liver, kidney, thyroid, and pituitary); (2) type II MDI (found in the brain, pituitary, brown adipose tissue, keratinocytes, and placenta; and (3) type III MDI (found in the placenta, brain, and epidermis). Type I and II act on the outer (phenolic) ring of the iodothyronine molecule; type III acts primarily on the inner (tyroyl) ring. MDI action on the inner rings catabolizes T_4 to the inactive rT_4 or T_3 to the inactive T_2. MDI action on the outer ring converts T_4 to T_3.

From Guyton, A.C. (1991). *Textbook of medical physiology* (8th ed.). Philadelphia: W.B. Saunders.

Regulation of Thyroid Hormone Secretion

Thyroid-stimulating hormone (TSH) acts through receptors on the thyroid cell membrane to activate adenyl cyclase. This stimulates formation of cyclic adenosine monophosphate (cAMP), which activates cellular systems to alter thyroid processes. TSH secretion is stimulated by thyrotropin-releasing hormone (TRH) or factor. TRH is secreted primarily by paraventricular nuclei of the hypothalamus and is released into the hypothalamic-pituitary portal system. TRH binds to receptors on the plasma membrane of thyrotropic cells within the anterior pituitary to activate synthesis and secretion of TSH. Secretion of thyroid hormones decreases the responsiveness of the pituitary to TRH. Secretion of TSH is also influenced by circulating levels of free thyroid hormone and intrapituitary triiodothyronine (T_3) levels via negative feedback to the pituitary gland; that is, increased free thyroid hormone levels decrease secretion of TSH by the pituitary and vice versa. Circulating thyroxine (T_4) regulates TSH primarily through intrapituitary deiodination of T_4 to T_3. The pituitary-thyroid axis is controlled in turn by the hypothalamus and TRH. TSH is inhibited by excess circulating thyroid hormone.

From Guyton, A.C. (1991). *Textbook of medical physiology* (8th ed.). Philadelphia: W.B. Saunders.

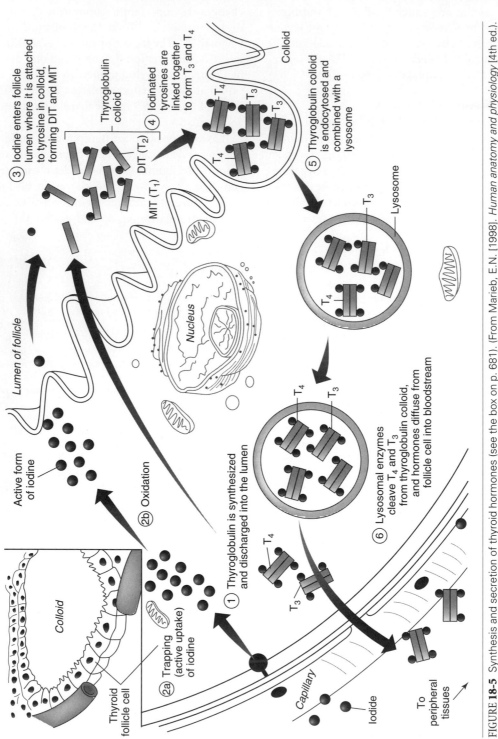
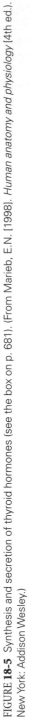

FIGURE **18-5** Synthesis and secretion of thyroid hormones (see the box on p. 681). (From Marieb, E.N. [1998]. *Human anatomy and physiology* [4th ed.]. New York: Addison Wesley.)

TABLE **18-2**   **Biochemical Parameters of Thyroid Function during Gestation**

PARAMETER (NONPREGNANT VALUE)	FIRST TRIMESTER	SECOND TRIMESTER	THIRD TRIMESTER
Total T_4 (3.9-11.6 µg/dl)	10.7 ± 0.2	11.5 ± 0.2*	11.5 ± 0.2†
Total T_3 (90.9-208 ng/dl)	205 ± 2.0	231 ± 3.0*	233 ± 2.0†
Molar T_3/T_4 (10-23 × 10³)	23.1 ± 0.3	24.3 ± 0.3†	24.8 ± 0.3†
Thyroxine-binding globulin (11-21 mg/l)	21.2 ± 0.3	28.5 ± 0.4*	31.5 ± 0.3*
Thyroxine-binding globulin saturation (28%-60%)	39.3 ± 0.6	30.9 ± 0.4*	27.9 ± 0.3*
Free T_4 (0.8-2.0 ng/dl)	1.4 ± 0.02	1.1 ± 0.01*	1.0 ± 0.01*
Free T_3 (190-710 pg/dl)	330 ± 0.06	270 ± 0.06*	250 ± 0.06*
Thyroid-stimulating hormone (0.2-4.0 mU/l)	0.75 ± 0.04	1.1 ± 0.04*	1.29 ± 0.04*
Human chorionic gonadotropin (IU/l × 10³)	38.5 ± 1.5	16.4 ± 0.9*	13.0 ± 1.5H

From Seely, B.L. & Burrow, G.N. (1999). Thyroid disease and pregnancy. In R.K. Creasy & R. Resnik (Eds). *Maternal-fetal medicine* (4th ed.). Philadelphia: W.B. Saunders.
*p <0.001.
†p = NS.
‡p <0.005.

Increased sialyation increases the half-life of TBG from 15 minutes to 3 days.[18,42,59] The ability of TBG to bind thyroxine doubles during this period; TBPA binding capacity, also influenced by estrogen, decreases.[22] These changes increase serum TBG levels, decrease the percent of T_4 bound to prealbumin, and increase total T_4 and T_3 (Table 18-2 and Figure 18-6). Although results are conflicting, most studies demonstrate a transient increase in free T_4 in the first trimester, related to the increase in hCG, and a 25% decrease in free T_3 and free T_4 in the second and third trimesters; however, levels remain within the low normal range.[42,67,97] Variations in findings are probably due to the iodine status of the populations studied and measurement techniques.[42,58,103] Thus concentrations of free T_3 and free T_4, although low, remain within normal physiologic limits.[90,112] The exact basis for these changes is unclear but thought to be related to the interaction of estrogen, TSH, and thyroid-binding proteins.

Resin T_3 uptake (RT$_3$U) decreases during pregnancy. RT$_3$U measures TBG-binding capacity, quantifies the number of unbound sites, and approximates the amount of free T_4. Although T_4-binding sites and binding capacity increase in pregnancy, the number of binding sites exceeds the available T_4. The increased number of unbound sites is reflected by decreased RT$_3$U.[90]

In contrast to the decrease in free T_3 and free T_4, total T_3 and T_4 increase, peaking at 10 to 15 weeks' gestation (Figure 18-6) and then plateauing at levels 30% to 100% higher than nonpregnant values.[42] This increase is primarily due to increases in TBG and hCG and possibly to an increase in type III monodeiodinase (MDI) production (see the box on p. 681) by the placenta. This enzyme converts T_4 to reverse T_3 (rT$_3$), an inactive compound, and T_3 to T_2, another inactive compound.[42] The increased T_3 and

T_4 are also related to increased TSH bioactivity stimulated by hCG, which peaks at about the same time. hCG has a mild TSH-like activity (the alpha subunits of hCG and TSH are similar) that increases secretion of T_4. Levels of T_3 are elevated because of the increased availability of T_4 for deiodination to T_3 in peripheral tissue rather than due to increased T_3 production per se. Elevated T_3 and T_4 suppress endogenous TSH secretion by the anterior pituitary.[44] TSH decreases slightly at 9 to 13 weeks' gestation at the time of the hCG peak (Figure 18-7), returning to nonpregnant levels by the second trimester.[11,20,21,42,59,83] Occasionally some otherwise healthy pregnant women will experience a transient hyperthyroxinemia associated with higher than usual hCG levels in the first trimester.[42,97] Because the increase in total T_3 and T_4 is less than the increase in TBG, resulting in an decreased T_4/TBG ratio, pregnancy has been described as a state of "relative hypothyroxinemia."[59]

The increased T_4 and T_3 stimulate increased serum protein-bound iodine (PBI).[112] Since circulating levels of free thyroid hormone are not significantly altered, increased PBI does not reflect maternal hyperthyroidism.[12] Thyroid iodine uptake increases because of a decrease in the total body iodine pool. This pool is altered because of increased renal iodide clearance secondary to the increased glomerular filtration rate (see Chapter 10) and placental transfer of iodine to the fetus.[20,22,42,162,166]

The thyroid compensates for the increased loss of iodine by hyperplasia and increased plasma iodine clearance. Iodine is stored as thyroglobulin (a prohormone) in the colloid of the thyroid gland follicles (see Figure 18-5). With TSH stimulation the thyroglobulin returns to the cell, where it is catabolized to form T_4 and T_3.[162] Serum thyroglobulin increases in the first trimester but is most marked in later pregnancy. This increase is associated with

Mother

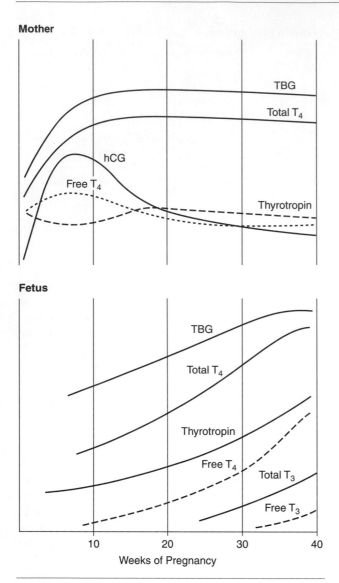

Fetus

FIGURE **18-6** Relative changes in maternal and fetal thyroid function during pregnancy. The effects of pregnancy on the mother include a marked and early increase in hepatic production of thyroxine-binding globulin (TBG) and placental production of human chorionic gonadotropin (hCG). The increase in serum TBG increases serum thyroxine (T$_4$) concentrations; hCG has a thyrotropin-like activity and stimulates maternal T$_4$ secretion. The transient hCG-induced increase in serum free T$_4$ inhibits maternal secretion of thyrotropin (thyroid-stimulating hormone [TSH]). (From Burrow, G.N., et al. [1994]. Maternal and fetal thyroid function. *N Engl J Med, 331,* 1072.)

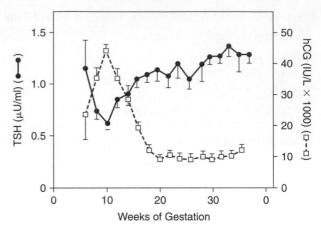

FIGURE **18-7** Serum thyroid-stimulating hormone (TSH) and human chorionic gonadotropin (hCG) as a function of gestational age from a cohort of 606 healthy pregnant women. (Adapted from Glinoer, D., et al. [1990]. Regulation of maternal thyroid during pregnancy. *J Clin Endocrinol Metab, 71,* 276, by Inzuvcchi, S.E. & Burrow, G.N. [1999]. The thyroid gland and reproduction. In S.S.C. Yen, R.B. Jaffe, & R.L. Barbieri (Eds.). *Reproductive endocrinology: Physiology, pathophysiology and clinical management* (4th ed.). Philadelphia: W.B. Saunders.

to marked thyroid enlargement in these women cannot be considered normal and requires further evaluation. The World Health Organization recommends an iodine intake of 200 μg/day during pregnacy.[59] Goiter is generally not a risk if iodine levels are greater than 0.08 μg/dl; in North America, levels average 0.3 μg/dl.[20] Goiter is a significant risk in areas with low iodine intake. In pregnant women with iodine deficiency, the thyroid gland may increase two to threefold.[60]

Intrapartum Period

The HPA and HPT axes undergo further alterations during the intrapartum period. CRH appears to be a trigger in the initiation of labor, and activation of the HPA axis may serve as a "biologic clock" timing the length of gestation.[113] Maternal plasma CRH, ACTH, and cortisol levels increase further during labor.[14,55,110] For example, ACTH increases from 50 pg/ml at term to 300 pg/ml in labor.[11] Further increases in ACTH and cortisol are seen in women with poor progress in labor.[50]

Levels of total and free T$_3$ increase during labor.[12] This change probably reflects the energy demands of labor on the maternal system. T$_3$ and T$_4$ have similar functions, but T$_3$ is 3 to 5 times more active. T$_3$ and T$_4$ increase intracellular enzymes (increased cellular metabolism), the number and activity of mitochondria (to provide energy for cellular enzyme systems), and Na-K adenosine triphosphatase

an increase in thyroid volume.[42,162] The degree of hyperplasia is related to the iodine intake. Mild thyroid hyperplasia (10% to 15% increase) and increased vascularity are seen in areas such as North America, where diets are generally iodine sufficient.[15,20,60,83,162] Therefore, moderate

(ATPase) (because of the increased energy use for myometrial contractions).[68,168]

Postpartum Period

The alterations in the HPA and HPT axes during pregnancy are reversed during the postpartum period. CRH levels drop rapidly with removal of the placenta and placental CRH.[11] Maternal ACTH and cortisol levels decrease by 4 days postpartum.[14,110] The HPA axis is depressed with a reduction in hypothalamic CRH for 3 to 6 weeks, returning to normal levels by 12 weeks.[107] This depression of the HPA axis may play a role in postpartum mood disorders or in exacerbation of autoimmune disorders in the postpartum period.[14,31,125] The lactotrophs of the anterior pituitary gland decrease in size by 1 month postpartum, but do not return to nonpregnant size.[124] Prolactin falls at delivery and returns to nonpregnant values by 3 months; in breastfeeding women, prolactin increases after delivery.[11,55] Postpartum changes in prolactin, FSH, and LH are described in Chapter 5.

After delivery and removal of the placenta and reduction in estrogen, hepatic synthesis of TBG decreases, as does the renal excretion of iodine. As a result, the metabolic alterations in thyroid processes gradually reverse, but they may persist for up to 6 to 12 weeks.[22] TRH is a (minor) stimulus of prolactin release and has been used to induce relactation.[96] Transient disorders in thyroid function are seen in some postpartum women (see the next section).

Thyroid hormones are secreted in breast milk. Levels are low initially; they then rise to mean levels of 4.3 μg/dl, equivalent to approximately 40 to 50 μg of T_4 per day.[170] Breast milk T_4 and T_3 have been reported to delay the development of hypothyroidism in some infants with this disorder.[51,153] These hormones may also mask clinical symptoms and impede the diagnosis of congenital hypothyroidism.[170]

CLINICAL IMPLICATIONS FOR THE PREGNANT WOMAN AND HER FETUS

Changes in the HPA and HPT axes are critical for maintenance of pregnancy. In addition, the maternal and fetal HPA axes and the interrelationship between maternal and fetal-placental function are essential for initiation of labor (see Chapter 4). Alterations in the HPA axis with infection or stress may lead to preterm labor. These risks are discussed further in Chapter 4. Thyroid disorders are more common in women and are not uncommon in pregnant women, being the second most common endocrine disorders (after diabetes mellitus) seen during pregnancy, whereas disorders of the adrenal and pituitary gland are uncommon.[103] Diagnosis of thyroid dysfunction during pregnancy may be more difficult since symptoms of thyroid disorders often

TABLE 18-3 Thyroid Function Tests during Pregnancy

PHYSIOLOGIC CHANGE	RESULTING CHANGE IN THYROID ACTIVITY
↑Serum estrogens ↑Serum TBG	↑Serum TBG ↑Demand for T_4 and T_3 ↑In total T_4 and T_3
↑hCG	↑TSH (in reference range unless hCG is >50,000 IU/L) ↓Free T_4 (in reference range unless hCG is >50,000 IU/L)
↑Iodine (I) clearance	↑In dietary requirement for I⁻ ↑In hormone production in I⁻ deficient areas ↓Goiter in I⁻ deficient areas
↑Type III deiodinase	↑T_4 and T_3 degradation ↑Demand for T_4 and T_3
↑Demand for T_4 and T_3	↑Serum thyroglobulin ↑Thyroid volume ↑Goiter in I⁻ deficient areas

Modified from Brent, G.A. (1997). Maternal thyroid function: Interpretation of thyroid function test in pregnancy. *Clin Obstet Gynecol, 40,* 3, by Fantz, C.R., et al. (1999). Thyroid function during pregnancy. *Clin Chem, 45,* 2250.
hCG, human chorionic gonadotropin; *T_3,* triiodothyronine; *T_4,* thyroxine; *TBG,* thyroxine-binding globulin; *TSH,* thyroid-stimulating hormone.

mimic some of the usual physiologic changes of pregnancy, and radioactive iodine tests cannot be used because of fetal risks. Implications of alterations in thyroid function and changes in laboratory tests during pregnancy are discussed in this section, along with disorders of thyroid function unique to the postpartum period.

Thyroid Function Tests during Pregnancy

Changes in TBG and thyroid hormones during pregnancy alter parameters for many tests used to assess thyroid status (see Table 18-2). These alterations, which vary with trimester, must be considered when evaluating thyroid function in pregnant and postpartum women. Free T_3 and T_4 assays are generally preferred because of the increased TBG.[21,82,103] Table 18-3 summarizes the changes in thyroid function during pregnancy that lead to alterations in these tests.

Thyroid Function and Nausea and Vomiting in Pregnancy

Nausea and vomiting in pregnancy (NVP) has been linked to alterations in T_4, TSH, and hCG (which has TSH-like activity). hCG stimulates receptors for both TSH (increases

T_4) and hCG (increases estriol and possibly NVP).[63] NVP severity has been correlated with increased free T_4 and decreased TSH, with values returning to normal pregnant ranges as the nausea and vomiting resolve.[121] These findings may lead to or be a consequence of emesis during early pregnancy. NVP is discussed further in Chapter 11.

Hyperemesis gravidarum in women without any history or evidence of thyroid dysfunction has also been associated with increased free T_4 and decreased TSH. These findings, seen in about 60% of women with hyperemesis, are similar to those of the euthyroid sick syndrome seen with severe illness.[42] T_4 levels in women with hyperemesis return to usual values in 1 to 4 weeks with or without treatment with antithyroid drugs.[12,20,22,39,42,97]

The Pregnant Woman with Hyperthyroidism

A transient hyperthyroidism is seen in about 15% of otherwise healthy pregnant women during the first trimester; this may be associated with increased hCG levels, multiple gestation, or NVP.[42,97,116] This subclinical hyperthyroidism is characterized by normal free T_4 and decreased TSH. A transient clinical hyperthyroidism (increased free T_4 and decreased TSH) is seen less frequently and may be associated with multiple gestation, hyperemesis gravidarum, and gestational trophoblast disorders with markedly increased hCG production.[42,97,116] Trophoblast disorders such as a molar pregnancy occasionally cause biochemical and sometimes (5% to 64%) clinical findings of hyperthyroidism because of the high levels of hCG secreted by the trophoblastic mass.[42,59] Biochemical hyperthyroidism (elevated free T_3, free T_4, and decreased TSH) has been reported to occur with hCG levels over 100,000 mIU/ml, with clinical findings of hyperthyroidism seen with hCG levels over 300,000 mIU/ml.[112]

Chronic hyperthyroidism occurs in up to 0.2% of pregnant women.[42,97,116] The diagnosis of hyperthyroidism during pregnancy may be difficult since many of the signs and symptoms associated with this disorder are often seen normally during pregnancy. Findings common to hyperthyroidism and certain stages of pregnancy include fatigue, heat intolerance, warm skin, emotional lability, insomnia, increased appetite, sweating, breathlessness, ankle edema, palpitations, and increased pulse pressure.[20,22,90,112,116,162] Failure to gain weight with a good appetite and persistent tachycardia (>100) are most suggestive of hyperthyroidism in pregnancy.[22,116] Increased free T_3 and total T_4 (over 15 µg/dl) and increased or high-normal RT_3U are seen with hyperthyroidism. Alterations in thyroid function tests during pregnancy (see Table 18-3) must be considered when interpreting test results. For example, since RT_3U is

decreased in pregnancy, values in the nonpregnant range suggest hyperthyroidism. TSH levels less than 0.05 µU/L and increased free T_4 levels greater than 11.6 µg/dl are diagnostic.[20,42,162]

Hyperthyroidism in pregnant women in North America is usually due to either an autoimmune disorder or an unknown cause; it is rarely due to goiter. The risk of goiter during pregnancy is attributed to increased avidity of the thyroid for iodine in response to increased renal loss and placental transport. In most women these losses are compensated for by a higher dietary iodine intake.

Hyperthyroidism in pregnant women is almost always (85% to 90%) due to Graves disease.[20,42,97,112] Graves disease is an autoimmune disorder in which a group of thyroid-stimulating immunoglobulins (TSIs) attach to and activate TSH receptors on the thyroid follicular cells. This leads to increased production of thyroid hormones and the clinical finding of hyperthyroidism.

Women with mild hyperthyroidism generally do well during pregnancy since increased serum TBG offsets the increased secretion of thyroid hormones. In women with Graves disease, their disorder may be aggravated in the first trimester (due to the increased hCG) and then improve, with remission and occasionally complete resolution in some women, during the third trimester.[20,34,42,112,116] This improvement is related to suppression of the maternal immune system (see Chapter 12) by fetal cytokines with lower TSI levels and decreased thyroid hormone production. Relapse or exacerbation generally occurs postpartum, usually within several weeks of delivery, as immune system alterations and production of TBG return to prepregnancy levels.[20,112]

Hyperthyroidism is treated with antithyroid drugs (thioamides), surgical removal, or thyroid ablation with [131]I. The most common thioamides are propylthiouracil (PTU) and methimazole (Tapazole or carbimazole that is metabolized to methimazole). Thioamides cross the placenta and can block synthesis of thyroid hormones by the fetus. The incidence of hypothyroidism in exposed infants is 1 in 100. The lower hormone levels stimulate increased TSH production, which can lead to goiter and tracheal obstruction. Infants of mothers treated with thioamides may have decreased T_4 and increased TSH levels after birth. These values are generally within normal neonatal limits by 4 to 5 days of age and later development is usually normal.[27,168] Methimazole has the advantage of less frequent dosing and fewer tablets per dose but is associated with a risk (less than 1%) of fetal scalp defects (cutis aplasia).[116] Pharmacologic effects must be monitored carefully, particularly during the third trimester in women with Graves disease, when remission can lead to decreased thyroid hormone production and a transient decrease in required drug dosage by 32 to 36 weeks.[4,116,120,162] In approximately 30% of women, these drugs can be transiently discontinued in late pregnancy.[116]

Pregnant women with hyperthyroidism will usually require a caloric intake that is higher than that generally recommended during pregnancy to compensate for their increased metabolic rate. These women are also at risk for fluid loss and dehydration as a result of the diarrhea and tachycardia that often accompany hyperthyroidism.[163] Pregnancy complicated by hyperthyroidism, particularly if this disorder is poorly controlled, is associated with intrauterine growth restriction and preterm labor.[20,97,116] Transplacental passage of TSIs can lead to a transient neonatal hyperthyroidism (see Chapter 12). TSIs are present even in women with Graves disease who are currently euthyroid due to thyroid ablation.

Pregnant women may also develop a transient subacute thyroiditis that often occurs in association with viral infections. The inflammation and destruction of thyroid tissue leads to release of stored thyroid hormone into serum and a transient hyperthyroxinemia. As the disorder resolves, the woman may develop hypothyroidism since the released thyroid hormones are used up before the thyroid gland can produce an adequate new supply. If treatment is initiated, beta-blockers such as propranolol are required rather than antithyroid drugs that block thyroid hormone production, since with subacute thyroiditis the thyroid is not making hormones.[22,90,97] Propranolol is generally not indicated for long-term treatment of pregnant women with hyperthyroidism. This drug crosses the placenta and has been associated with fetal growth restriction and impaired response to anoxia and neonatal hypoglycemia and bradycardia.

The Pregnant Woman with Hypothyroidism

Hypothyroidism in pregnant women is usually secondary to autoimmune disorders (after surgical removal or ablation of the thyroid with ^{131}I for Graves disease and idiopathic myxedema) or Hashimoto thyroiditis.[90] Women with untreated hypothyroidism have a high incidence of infertility and spontaneous abortion.[22,42,163] The diagnosis of hypothyroidism during pregnancy may be missed since some of the signs and symptoms associated with this disorder—such as fatigue, weight gain, constipation, and amenorrhea—are also seen normally during pregnancy.[22,112,162,163] The increase in TBG in pregnancy may mask the decrease in thyroid hormones; however, levels are usually still low for pregnant norms. In addition, free T_4 is low and TSH is elevated.[103]

In the absence of severe iodine deficiency or exposure to teratogenic drugs, fetal thyroid development often proceeds normally because the fetal thyroid is not dependent on maternal hormones for development.[23] However, several recent studies suggest that maternal thyroid hormones may be important for fetal neurologic development in the first trimester; untreated maternal hypothyroidism in early gestation has been associated with significant decreases in the intelligence quotient (IQ) of offspring in some studies.[70,97,99,131] Pregnancy in women with hypothyroidism may be complicated by an increased risk of fetal loss or prolonged pregnancy, however, possibly due to compromised placental blood flow or the inability of the thyroid gland to meet the metabolic demands of pregnancy.[163] Weight gain patterns must be carefully monitored in the woman with hypothyroidism.[163] These women may also have difficulty with fatigue and constipation during pregnancy. Thyroid hormone replacement doses usually need to be increased as a result of the increased TBG.[42,97]

Postpartum Thyroid Disorders

The postpartum period is associated with transient thyroid disorders. Physiologic alterations and experiences of pregnancy can mask clinical findings of hypo- or hyperthyroidism. As a result, these disorders may first become apparent in the postpartum period.[23] For example, up to 60% of childbearing women who develop Graves disease do so in the postpartum period, especially in the first 3 to 9 months postpartum.[80]

Postpartum thyroid disorder (PPTD) is a transient disorder seen in 5% to 9% of postpartum women.[19,97] PPTD generally appears in the first 6 months (usually by 6 to 8 weeks after delivery). PPTD (Figure 18-8) is characterized by weeks or months (average, 2 to 4 months) of mild hyperthyroidism, followed by weeks or months of hypothyroidism, and finally a return to normal thyroid function in most women— usually by 12 months postpartum.[22,23,42,90,97,112]

The exact cause of PPTD is unclear but has been described as a "model of aggravation of an autoimmune state."[5] The initial hyperthyroid phase is characterized by thyroid cell destruction with excessive release of thyroid hormone. PPTD may reflect postpartum exacerbation of a subclinical autoimmune disorder that, with release of pregnancy-induced immunosuppression, leads to rebound of immune components with excessive production of thyroid autoantibodies.[5,19,22,34] The subsequent hypothyroid phase is due to decreased thyroid hormones from excessive loss of thyroid cells during the first phase. As the thyroid cells regrow, normal function returns.[34]

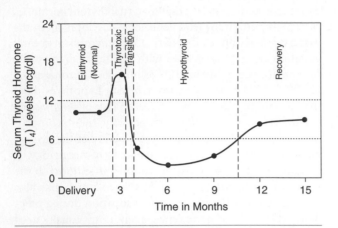

FIGURE 18-8 Thyroid function during postpartum thyroiditis. T_4, thyroxine. (From Smallridge, R.C., et al. (1988). Postpartum thyroiditis. *The Bridge, 3*, 3. Newsletter of the Thyroid Foundation of America, Inc.)

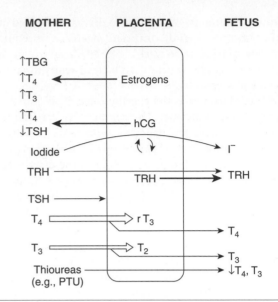

FIGURE 18-9 Placental role in maternal and fetal thyroid function. Heavy arrows indicate placental production of estrogens and human chorionic gonadotropin (hCG), predominately into maternal blood, and thyroid-releasing hormone (TRH), primarily into fetal blood. Iodide is actively transported from mother to fetus. The placenta is impermeable to thyroid-stimulating hormone (TSH) in either direction. Transfer of thyroxine (T_4) and triiodothyronine (T_3) is limited by inherent placental barriers and the type III iodothyronine deiodinase, which convert T_4 to rT_3 and T_3 to T_2 (rT_3 and T_2 are inactive compounds). Small amounts of active hormone are transported. The relatively free transport of antithyroid drugs (propylthiouracil [PTU] and methimazole) can inhibit fetal thyroid hormone production. (From Fisher, D.A. & Polk, D.H. [1994]. The ontogenesis of thyroid function and actions. In D. Tulchinsky & A.B. Little (Eds.). *Maternal-fetal endocrinology* (2nd ed.). Philadelphia: W.B. Saunders.)

Up to 25% of women with PPTD remain hypothyroid.[22,97] Biochemical abnormalities include elevated free T_4, suppression of TSH, presence of microsomal antibodies, and a low ^{131}I uptake.[97,112] PPTD may be misdiagnosed as postpartum depression and often recurs with subsequent deliveries.[23,97,180] Transient hypothyroidism is also seen occasionally during the postpartum period. Findings include fatigue, weight gain, low free T_4 and elevated TSH levels, and elevated antimicrosomal and antithyroglobulin antibody titers.[23]

Breastfeeding in Women with Thyroid Disorders

Breastfeeding is generally not contraindicated in women with hypothyroidism, because thyroid hormones cross in only small amounts and the infant should receive a dose no higher than that from a euthyroid woman.[96] Breastfeeding in women with hyperthyroidism is controversial, primarily because of passage of antithyroid medications in breast milk.[16,78,88] PTU is excreted in breast milk in relatively small amounts (0.025% to 0.077% of the maternal dose).[96] Most sources suggest that breastfeeding is not routinely contraindicated in women on PTU who are carefully monitored, but that each women needs to weigh the risks and benefits and the infant must be carefully monitored. PTU is usually preferred over methimazole (Tapazole), which crosses in much higher amounts.[12] Propranolol and

thiouracil cross in significant amounts and are generally contraindicated in breastfeeding women.[96]

The mammary glands actively take up, concentrate, and secrete iodine in breast milk. Thus breastfeeding is interrupted if the woman requires thyroid uptake studies or scans involving use of ^{123}I or [131]I. McDougall recommends that breastfeeding not be resumed unless the dose of radioactivity in the milk is below 1 rad of exposure to the infant's thyroid.[112] If radioactive iodine is needed, ^{123}I is preferred over ^{131}I, since breastfeeding generally needs to be stopped for only about 48 hours with ^{123}I but for a prolonged period of time with [131]I.[19,22]

Use of Radioiodine and Iodides

Iodine is actively transported across the placenta and taken up by the fetal thyroid (Figure 18-9). Avidity of the fetal thyroid for iodine is 20 to 50 times greater than that of the mother.[22] Administration of any form of iodine to pregnant women results in significantly higher concentrations per weight in fetal tissues and can lead to development of a goiter, especially after 12 weeks' gestation, when the fetal thyroid begins to concentrate iodine.[64,116] Fetal risks of radioactive substances include thyroid damage, microcephaly, intrauterine growth restriction, mental retardation, later malignancy, and death. As a result, radioiodine has been contraindicated during pregnancy. Radioiodine also alters spermatogenesis, so a 120-day period is recommended in males between therapy and fertilization.[64]

All women should have a pregnancy test before radioactive iodine studies. If these studies are done in a woman who is later found to be pregnant, however, the risks are minimal since the dose of ^{123}I used is generally low. The use of ^{131}I for definitive diagnosis and therapy of Graves disease is associated with increased pregnancy loss and destruction of the fetal thyroid; thus this agent is not used during pregnancy.

The use of nonradioactive iodides has also been reported to increase the risk of fetal goiter, tracheal obstruction, and hypothyroidism. Iodides are found in Betadine-containing vaginal suppositories and douches, saturated solution of potassium iodide (SSKI), iodinized medications for asthmatics, and some contrast materials.[22,64,116] The incidence of drug-induced fetal goiter is 1 in 10,000 and is seen primarily with daily iodide doses over 12 μg.

Maternal-Fetal Endocrine Relationships

Maternal, fetal, and placental HPA functions are closely interrelated. The placenta produces significant amounts of some hypothalamic and pituitary hormones such as CRH and GH. The fetus and placenta—via CRH production—influence the timing of parturition (see Chapter 4). Large quantities of steroids are produced by interaction of the mother, placenta, and fetus. Some of these substances are dependent upon the viability and well-being of the fetus and placenta, whereas others, such as progesterone, do not require the fetus to be viable for production to continue. Steroid-producing cells appear early in placental development. They can be seen first in the trophoblast tissue of the placenta; however, the syncytiotrophoblast lacks several of the key enzymes necessary for steroid metabolism. Therefore the placenta is an incomplete steroidogenic tissue and must receive precursors from exogenous sources (i.e., the fetus or maternal system) (see Chapter 3).

As a result of the limits on placental permeability to maternal TSH, T_4, and T_3, the fetal HPT axis develops and functions relatively independent of maternal influences.[47,66,84,142] However, the fetus is dependent on the

mother for iodides—either via direct transfer or breakdown of maternal T_4 by the placenta (see Figure 18-9).[47] Maternal TRH does cross the placenta but does not seem to have a major influence on fetal pituitary or thyroid function, probably because maternal TRH levels are low and much of the maternal TRH is degraded in the placenta.[48] Administration of thyroid hormone to the mother does not significantly increase fetal hormone levels.[47] Lack of significant transfer of T_3 and T_4 may be due to the presence in the placenta of α-iodothyronine, which increases levels of the inactive reverse T_3, or to deiodinase enzymes, which deiodinate (degrade) T_3 and T_4 into inactive products.[48,83,142,148]

Some maternal T_4 does reach the fetus both early and late in pregnancy. Maternal T_4 appears to have a role in fetal development, but the exact role is still unclear.[20,22,37,48] Early in gestation, from 6 to 12 weeks, before the fetal thyroid is functional, maternal thyroid hormone may diffuse into amniotic fluid. This source of thyroid hormone may be important for neural development.[20,47,162] Increased T_4 transfer has been reported in late gestation with fetuses with severe congenital hypothyroidism. Athyroid fetuses have T_4 levels that are 20% to 50% of normal.[30,47,177] The placenta is permeable to commonly used antithyroid drugs (PTU and methimazole), beta-blockers (propranolol) and iodine.[112] Placental permeability to TSIs can lead to development of transient neonatal hyperthyroidism in infants of women with Graves disease (see Chapter 12).

SUMMARY

Changes in the HPA axis during pregnancy enhance maternal adaptations and availability of nutrients to the fetus. Maternal HPA function is interrelated with placental function, because the placenta produces hypothalamic and pituitary hormones such as CRH and GH. Placental CRH plays a major role in initiation of parturition (Chapter 4). Changes in HPA and HPT function can alter reproductive processes. The pregnant woman is in a state of euthyroid hyperthyroxinemia and transient hypercortisolism, although control set points are reset so the women responds to stress in a manner that is similar to that of nonpregnant individuals. As a result, values for some endocrine function tests are altered. These changes must be considered when evaluating neuroendocrine function during pregnancy. Thyroid disorders are not uncommon in pregnant women. Knowledge of the effects of these disorders and their treatment is important to optimize fetal and neonatal outcome. Clinical recommendations related to thyroid function during pregnancy are summarized in Table 18-4.

TABLE **18-4**   Recommendations for Clinical Practice Related to Changes in Thyroid Function in Pregnant Women

Recognize the usual changes in pituitary and adrenal function during pregnancy (pp. 677-681, 684-685). Recognize the usual changes in thyroid function during pregnancy (pp. 681-685). Assess and monitor maternal nutrition in terms of iodine intake (pp. 683-684). Monitor fetal growth in women with normal and abnormal thyroid function (p. 689). Know the usual parameters for pituitary function during pregnancy (pp. 677-680 and Table 18-1). Know the usual parameters for thyroid function tests during pregnancy (p. 685 and Table 18-2). Recognize the signs and symptoms of thyroid dysfunction and similarities with certain pregnancy-related findings (pp. 686-687).	Counsel women with hyperthyroidism and hypothyroidism regarding the effects of their disorder on pregnancy and the fetus and of pregnancy on the thyroid disorder (pp. 686-687). Monitor medication levels and requirements in the pregnant woman with hyperthyroidism (pp. 686-687). Know the fetal and neonatal risks of maternal iodide and radioactive iodine administration (pp. 688-689). Avoid the use of iodides and radioactive iodine in pregnant women (pp. 688-689). Know the fetal and neonatal risks associated with the use of thyroid and antithyroid agents (pp. 686-688). Recognize and monitor for transient postpartum thyroid disorders (pp. 687-688 and Figure 18-8). Counsel women with hypothyroidism and hyperthyroidism regarding breastfeeding considerations (pp. 686-688).

DEVELOPMENT OF HYPOTHALAMIC, PITUITARY, ADRENAL, AND THYROID FUNCTION IN THE FETUS

Anatomic Development

Hypothalamus and Pituitary Gland

The hypothalamus and anterior pituitary glands develop simultaneously but independently of each other. As a result, growth of the various cells types within the anterior pituitary is not dependent on the presence of the hypothalamus. For example, anencephalic infants do not have a hypothalamus but have TSH cells with their rudimentary anterior pituitary gland.[142]

The hypothalamus develops from 6 to 12 weeks from the ventral portion of the diencephalon. Hypothalamic nuclei and supraoptic track fibers develop by 12 to 14 weeks, with maturation of the hypothalamic neurons by 30 to 35 weeks.[47,103,142] The anterior pituitary arises from the anterior wall of the Rathke pouch, an upward offshoot of the primitive oral cavity.[10,66] The posterior pituitary and stalk develop from the infundibulum, a thickening on the floor of the diencephalon.[154] The anterior pituitary can be seen by 4 weeks and is independent of the oral cavity by 12 weeks. During the fifth week the primitive anterior pituitary becomes connected with the infundibulum. Cellular differentiation within the anterior pituitary gland begins at 7 to 8 weeks, under the influence of Pit-1 (a transcription regulator) that activates expression of genes encoding GH and prolactin and differentiation of the different anterior pituitary cell types.[66] Thyrotrophic cells appear at 12 to 13 weeks. A marked increase in TSH-secreting cell volume occurs by 23 weeks.[142]

Adrenal Glands

The adrenal cortex arises in the fifth week from the mesoderm in the notch between the primitive urogenital ridge and the dorsal mesentary.[115] These cells proliferate and form cords migrating medially and laterally to the cranial end of the mesonephros (primitive interim kidneys).[78,123] Neural crest cells form a medial mass on the primitive cortex. These cells are surrounded by the cortex cells and differentiate into the adrenal medulla. Later, another wave of cells surround the initial cortical cells to form the definitive cortex.[115,154] By 8 weeks the cortex is organized into the fetal zone, with the definitive zone appearing a week later.[78,115,123] The fetal zone increases in size from 10 to 15 weeks and dominates from 16 to 20 weeks. By 28 to 30 weeks, a transitional zone appear between the fetal and definitive zones. The transitional zone is initially similar to the fetal zone. During the second and third trimesters, the adrenal glands enlarge, with hypertrophy of the fetal zone and hyperplasia of the definitive zone.[78]

By mid-gestation the fetal zone occupies 80% to 90% of the adrenal volume and is highly vascularized.[78,123] The adrenals double in size between 20 to 30 weeks and double again between 30 and 40 weeks as steroidogenic activity increases.[115] At term the adrenal glands weigh 3 to 4 g and, relative to adult proportions, are 20 to 30 times larger.[78,115,123] After birth the adrenal undergoes extensive remodeling, with a decrease in size and disappearance of the fetal zone.

Thyroid Gland

The thyroid gland develops during the first 12 weeks of gestation. The thyroid begins as an epithelial thickening at the base of the tongue. As the primordial gland migrates down the trachea, it becomes bilobular with a small median isthmus. The thyroid initially descends in front of the pharyngeal gut. Later the thyroid descends in front of the hyoid bone and larynx to reach its final position in front of the trachea by 7 weeks.[154]

Functional Development

Maturation of thyroid and adrenal function is interrelated with that of the hypothalamic and pituitary glands and the HPA and HPT axes. This process can be divided into three overlapping phases: embryogenesis (phase I), hypothalamic maturation (phase II), and maturation of thyroid and adrenal system function (phase III).[49,57,142] During the first phase (10 to 12 weeks), the adrenal and thyroid gland develop morphologically. Hypothalamic function matures during phase II (from 4 to 5 until about 35 weeks). TRH, gonadotropin-releasing hormone (GnRH), and somatostatin are detected in the hypothalamus by 10 to 12 weeks (by radioimmunoassay) and in fetal blood in the third trimester.[61,142] Phase III lasts from mid-gestation until term or 1 month after birth if transitional changes are considered. This stage involves increasing maturation and integration of endocrine system function.

Hypothalamic and Pituitary Function

The HPA axis is essential for regulating intrauterine homeostasis and maturation of the lungs, liver, and central nervous system; in conjunction with the placenta, it is essential in the timing of parturition.[102,117,128] The hypothalamus and pituitary gland also play major roles in regulating the principal fetal steroid-secreting glands (adrenal gland and gonads) via a negative feedback mechanism. Figure 18-10 summarizes the HPA axis in the fetus and its interaction with placental function.

In general, most of the hormones of the HPA axis are active by 10 to 16 weeks' gestation (Table 18-5).[78] Plasma concentrations of these hormones rise for the first half of gestation. At this time the negative feedback loop comes into operation and the production and release of pituitary hormones become more finely regulated.[70] CRH from the fetus and placenta stimulate ACTH, which controls growth, differentiation, and function of the adrenal cortex in conjunction with growth factors (GFs) and other mediators.[128]

GnRH appears by 18 weeks and increases to 30 weeks.[78] LH and FSH appear in the fetal pituitary gland during the tenth week and reach their peaks at about 20 to 22 weeks' gestation. The concentration of LH is higher than that of FSH, and females have higher levels than males.[77] FSH promotes development of follicles in females; it stimulates growth of seminiferous tubules and initiates spermatogenesis in males. LH increases the synthesis and secretion of testosterone in the male embryo and stimulates steroid synthesis in ovarian cells.

Fetal GH levels are higher than after birth due to immature inhibitory control and lack of GH receptors on fetal tissues.[61] Increases in cortisol before delivery are thought to induce GH receptors and changes in IGF-I.

Adrenal Function

The fetal adrenal gland initially consists of two zones: the fetal zone and the definitive zone. The fetal zone contains large lipid-containing steroidogenic cells. The fetal zone is the major source of dehydroepiandrosterone (DHEA) and its sulfate (DHEA-S), which serve as precursors of estrone and estradiol-17β in the placenta. DHEA-S is also the precursor for 16-hydroxydehydroepiandrosterone, which is needed for estriol production by the placenta (see Chapter 3).

The placenta does not produce these precursors, so it is dependent on the fetal adrenal (primary source) or mother. In fetuses with decreased adrenal function, such as anencephalic fetuses, estriol production by the placenta remains low. Enzymes to synthesize DHEA-S are present by 6 to 8 weeks.[78,117] High levels of 17α-hydroxylase (17-OH) and probably 21-hydroxylase (21-OH) are seen early in gestation (Figure 18-11). 17-OH and 21-OH are cytochrome P-450 enzymes not expressed by the placenta.[181] Deficiency of 21-OH is the most common cause of congenital adrenal hyperplasia; a lack of 21-OH can result in virilization of the female external genitalia. Since the genital tract differentiates at 7 to 10 weeks (see Chapter 1), it is assumed that this enzyme must be present early in gestation.[115] Levels of 3β-hydroxysteroid dehydrogenase (involved in cortisol production) are low in the fetus.[115] The large size of the adrenal glands allows the fetus to secrete up to 200 mg of adrenal androgens daily, predominantly DHEA-S, as compared with the adult, who secretes only 20 to 30 mg of DHEA-S.[165] The fetus supplies 90% of the DHEA-S to the placenta after 16-hydroxylation by the fetal liver (see Figure 18-10).[165]

De novo synthesis of glucocorticoids, such as cortisol, from cholesterol begins by 30 weeks in the transitional zone.[78,115] Cortisol is produced as early as 8 to 12 weeks but in small amounts and primarily from progesteones.[78,115] Cortisol is essential for fetal maturation of the lungs, gut, liver, and central nervous system.[101,128] Cortisol is also found in amniotic fluid. Most fetal tissues as well as the placenta contain enzymes to deactivate cortisol; this probably serves as a protective mechanism. Although maternal cortisol crosses the placenta, about 85% is deactivated.[123] Fetal cortisol levels are low from 15 to 30 weeks, gradually

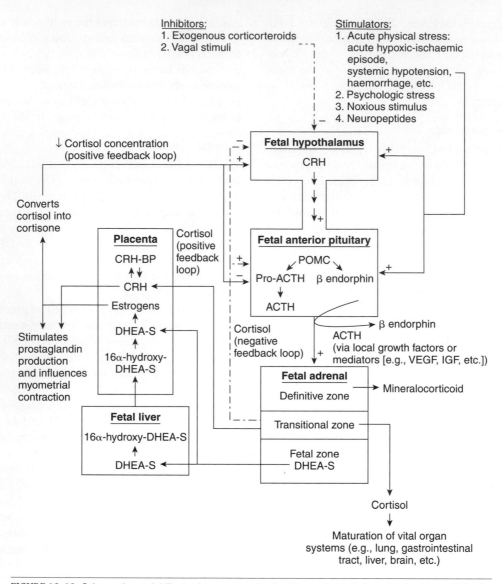

FIGURE **18-10** Schematic model illustrating neuroendocrine interaction between the fetal hypothalamic-pituitary-adrenal axis and the placenta. The *solid arrows* represent positive stimulatory pathways and the *broken arrows* represent negative inhibitory pathways. *ACTH*, adrenocorticotropin; *CRH*, corticotropin-releasing hormone; *CRH-BP*, cortictropin-releasing hormone binding protein; *DHEA-S*, dehydroxy-epiandrosterone sulfate; *IGF*, insulin-like growth factor; *POMC*, pro-opiomelanocortin; *pro-ACTH*, pro-adenocorticotrophin; *VEGF*, vascular endothelial growth factor. (From Ng, P.C. [2000]. The fetal and neonatal hypothalamic-pituitary-adrenal axis. *Arch Dis Child Fetal Neonatal Ed, 82,* F250.)

TABLE **18-5**   Ontogeny of Human Fetal Hypothalamic and Pituitary Hormones

HORMONE	AGE DETECTED (WEEKS)
HYPOTHALAMIC	
Gonadotropin-releasing hormone	14.0
Thyrotropin-releasing hormone	10.0
Somatostatin	14.0
Dopamine	11.0
Growth hormone-releasing hormones	18.0
Corticotropin-releasing hormone	16.0
PITUITARY	
Prolactin	16.5
Growth hormone	10.5
Adrenocorticotropin	7.0
Thyroid-stimulating hormone	13.0
Luteinizing hormone	10.5
Follicle-stimulating hormone	10.5

From Jaffe, R.B. (1999). Neuroendocrine metabolic regulation of pregnancy. In S.S.C. Yen, R.B. Jaffe, & R.L. Barbieri (Eds). *Reproductive endocrinology: Physiology, pathophysiology and clinical management* (4th ed.). Philadelphia: W.B. Saunders.

increasing to term; during labor, the fetal cortisol level doubles (Figure 18-12).[123] Intrauterine stress may activate adrenal cortisol secretion, but this often occurs at the cost of decreased DHEA-S production and thus lowered estriol production. The fetus also responds to stress after 18 to 19 weeks by increasing β-endorphin (BE) levels.[137,144]

CRH from the fetal hypothalamus and, in particular, from the placenta stimulates pituitary ACTH production that in turn stimulates the fetal adrenal to produce cortisol, DHEA, and DHEA-S. The placenta converts cortisol to cortisone, keeping fetal cortisol levels low and limiting negative feedback that would normally reduce CRH levels. This maintains CRH levels and DHEA-S synthesis.[101,117,128]

Growth of the adrenal glands is probably not dependent on ACTH, since the anencephalic fetus with low ACTH levels develops adrenal glands, but ACTH is required for adrenal function.[115] ACTH may exert its effect via local GFs and other mediators such as basic fibroblast GF, epidermal GF, transforming growth factor–α (TGF-α), IGF-I, IGF-II, transforming growth factor–β (TGF-β), activin, and inhibin.[76,78,115]

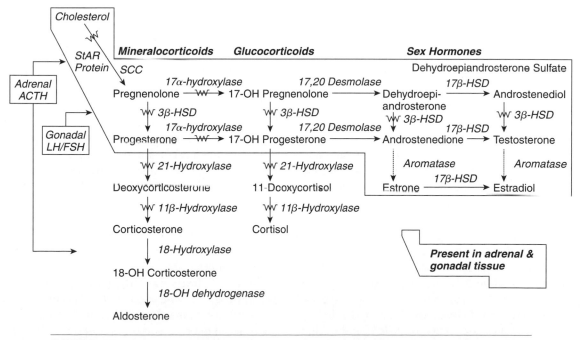

FIGURE **18-11**   Adrenal and gonadal steroidogenesis. *Solid line* represents a major pathway; *dotted line* represents a major pathway in ovaries and minor pathway in adrenals. ⌁, One of the potential areas of deficient enzymatic activity causing congenital adrenal hyperplasia. *StAR*, steroidogenic auto regulatory protein. *SCC*, cholesterol side chain cleavage enzyme. *3β-HSD*, 3β–hydroxysteroid dehydrogenase. *17β-HSD*, 17β-hydroxysteroid dehydrogenase. (From Pang, S. [1997]. Congenital adrenal hyperplasia. *Endocrinol Metab Clin North Am, 26,* 854.)

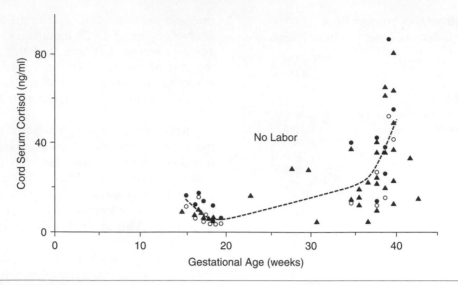

FIGURE **18-12** Cortisol concentrations in human umbilical arterial *(filled circles)*, venous *(open circles)* or mixed *(triangles)* cord serum obtained at cesarean section without labor. Results in ng/mg can be converted to nmol/l by multiplying by 2.8. (From Murphy, B.E.P. [1982]. Human fetal serum cortisol levels related to gestational age: Evidence of a mid-gestational fall and a steep late gestational rise, independent of sex or mode. *Am J Obstet Gynecol, 144,* 278.)

Thyroid Function

TRH synthesis begins in the hypothalamus by 6 to 8 weeks and is found in fetal serum by 10 to 12 weeks.[78,95] TRH is also synthesized by the placenta, fetal pancreas, and gut. Fetal serum TRH levels are high during the first and second trimesters due to these extrahypothalamic sources; hypothalamic TRH production probably matures nearer to term.[128] TSH can be detected in fetal serum by 13 weeks. Levels are low until 18 weeks, then increase to 28 weeks, then plateau and decrease to term.[22,78]

By 10 to 12 weeks, the thyroid gland accumulates and concentrates iodine, and begins to synthesize and secrete iodothyronines.[78] T_4 can be detected in fetal serum by 10 weeks after fertilization.[22] Thyroxine-binding proteins can be found from 12 weeks.[51] Fetal thyroid function remains at basal levels until mid-gestation, even though the capacity to secrete these hormones as well as TSH and TRH develops earlier.[22,44,47,78] After 18 to 20 weeks, TSH increases rapidly, followed at 20 to 22 weeks by increases in T_4 and reverse T_3 (rT_3).[22,48,61,78,168] T_4 and free T_4 increase progressively to term.[78] At term, T_4 levels are similar to or slightly higher than maternal values.[96] TBG parallels T_4 and reaches term values at mid-gestation.[51] Changes in fetal thyroid hormones are summarized in Figure 18-6.

TSH has been detected in amniotic fluid by 16 to 19 weeks, although the usefulness of this hormone for evaluating fetal thyroid function is unclear.[142,162,183]

Amniotic fluid T_4 levels peak at 25 to 30 weeks, then decrease; T_3 levels increase slowly throughout pregnancy.[88] Reverse T_3 also increases in amniotic fluid and peaks at 17 to 20 weeks. At term, levels are approximately three times higher than maternal serum concentrations.[22]

Serum T_3 levels remain low until 30 weeks, then increase slightly, but never approach maternal values.[47,142] At term, maternal free T_3 levels are two to three times higher than those of the fetus.[47] T_3 levels remain low because the fetus is unable to convert T_4 to T_3 peripherally, due to incomplete enzyme systems. The increase in T_3 after 30 weeks is associated with maturation of these enzymes.[47] Type II and III MDIs (see the box on p. 681) are present by mid-gestation; type I MDI (which converts T_4 to T_3) matures later. As a result, a greater proportion of T_4 is converted to rT_3 in the fetus than in the adult. Inactive metabolites are seven times higher in fetal serum than in maternal serum.[47]

Serum rT_3 levels rise early in the third trimester, then progressively decrease to term as MDI activity increases.[78] As noted earlier, the elevated serum rT_3 levels in the fetus are believed to be a result of increased type III MDI activity (see the box on p. 681).[32,44,47,84] Type III MDI is the predominant MDI in the fetus and placenta.[47,49] This increases conversion of T_4 to the biologically inactive rT_3 (rather than to biologically active T_3) and T_3 to the inactive T_2; this may be a way the fetus counteracts high T_4

TABLE **18-6** Characteristics of Fetal Thyroid Function

Limited placental transport of iodothyronines
Extrahypothalamic production of thyrotropin-releasing hormone by the placenta and selected fetal tissue
Progressive maturation of T_4 production and T_4 negative feedback control of thyroid-stimulating hormone (thyrotropin) secretion
Predominant metabolism of T_4 to inactive reverse T_3 and sulfated analogues
Local monodeiodinase type II mediated T_3 production from T_4 in selected fetal tissues including brain
Developmentally programmed maturation of thyroid hormone nuclear receptors in individual fetal tissues
Developmentally programmed maturation of thyroid hormone gene transcription in individual fetal tissues

From Fisher, D.A. (1999). Hypothyroxinemia in premature infants: Is thyroxine treatment necessary? *Thyroid, 9,* 715.

T_3, Triiodothyronine; T_4, thyroxine.

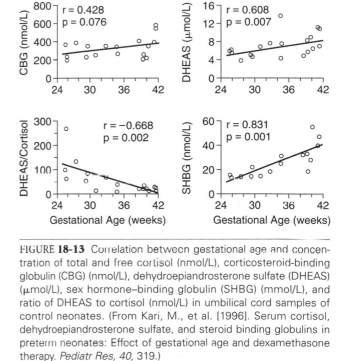

FIGURE **18-13** Correlation between gestational age and concentration of total and free cortisol (nmol/L), corticosteroid-binding globulin (CBG) (nmol/L), dehydroepiandrosterone sulfate (DHEAS) (μmol/L), sex hormone–binding globulin (SHBG) (mmol/L), and ratio of DHEAS to cortisol (nmol/L) in umbilical cord samples of control neonates. (From Kari, M., et al. [1996]. Serum cortisol, dehydroepiandrosterone sulfate, and steroid binding globulins in preterm neonates: Effect of gestational age and dexamethasone therapy. *Pediatr Res, 40,* 319.)

levels and maintains metabolic homeostasis.[47,48,49,168] Thyroid maturation in the late fetal and early neonatal period is related to progressive increases in hypothalamic TRH secretion, TRH responsiveness by the pituitary (by 26 to 28 weeks, the fetus responds to TRH in a manner similar to that of adults), sensitivity of the thyroid to TSH, and maturation of feedback mechanisms.[44,47,84,87] Fetal thyroid function is summarized in Table 18-6.

NEONATAL PHYSIOLOGY

Transitional Events

Catecholamines surge at birth to levels 20 times greater than those of adults.[136] The increase is greater with vaginal delivery than with cesarean delivery. Levels decrease after the first few hours. The catecholamine surge promotes extrauterine cardiorespiratory adaptation (see Chapters 8 and 9) and is accompanied by a surge in other hormones, including renin, angiotensin II, AVP (see Chapter 10), ACTH, BEs, and cortisol (see next section). BE is increased with fetal distress. Cord blood and maternal BE levels are not correlated.[137]

Hypothalamic-Pituitary-Adrenal Axis

Remodeling of the adrenal glands after birth occurs via apoptosis of the fetal zone, remodeling of the fetal zone cells, first and development of the other zones.[78,115,181] Apoptosis of the fetal zone is mediated by activin and TGF-β.[76] The size of the adrenals decrease 25% in the first 4 days after birth.[181]

At birth the infant's cortisol levels are about one third or less of maternal levels, possibly related to higher levels of CBG in the mother. Cortisol levels double during labor and increase further in the first 1 to 2 hours after birth, then gradually fall during the first week.[123] Changes in cortisol in relation to gestational age and postbirth age are illustrated in Figures 18-13 and 18-14. There is an inverse relationship between cortisol levels and gestational age.[161] Healthy term infants have relatively low basal cortisol levels that rapidly increase with stress.[71] ACTH and cortisol levels are higher in infants delivered vaginally than in those delivered by cesarean birth.[149] ACTH and BE levels are elevated in cord blood and decrease significantly by 24 hours and reach adult levels by 4 to 5 days in healthy infants.[57,100,106,137]

BEs are endogenous opioid-like substances that are derived, along with ACTH and other substances, from a large precursor molecule (proopiomelanocortin). BEs increase markedly with birth in both term and preterm infants. The

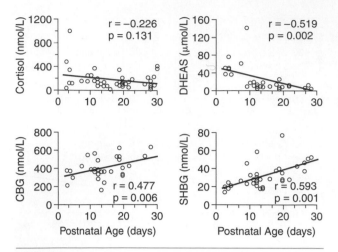

FIGURE **18-14** Correlation between postnatal age and concentration of cortisol (nmol/L), corticosteroid-binding globulin (CBG) (nmol/L), dehydroepiandrosterone sulfate (DHEAS) (μmol/L), and sex hormone–binding globulin (SHBG) (mmol/L) in neonates of preterm control and placebo group. (From Kari, M., et al. [1996]. Serum cortisol, dehydroepiandrosterone sulfate, and steroid binding globulins in preterm neonates: Effect of gestational age and dexamethasone therapy. *Pediatr Res, 40,* 319.)

TABLE **18-7**	Changes in Thyroid Function Associated with Fetal Transition to Extrauterine Life at Term

Neonatal TSH surge
Increased T_4 and T_3 production
Stimulation of brown adipose tissue thermogenesis
Increased T_4 to T_3 conversion
Permanently increased serum T_3 level
Decreased production of inactive thyroid hormone analogues (rT_3, T_4S, rT_3S, T_2S)
Decreased extrahypothalamic thyrotropin-releasing hormone production
Decreased TSH concentration
Resetting of hypothalamic-pituitary free T_4 setpoint for control of TSH secretion

From Fisher, D.A. (1999). Hypothyroxinemia in premature infants: Is thyroxine treatment necessary? *Thyroid, 9,* 715.
T_3, Triiodothyronine; T_4, thyroxine; *TSH*, thyroid-stimulating hormone (thyrotropin).

BE increase at birth is greater with perinatal asphyxia or other stress such as forceps delivery; it is reported to be inversely related to PO_2.[21,137,144,169] Other endogenous opioids, such as the enkephalins, are also increased at birth and further increased with asphyxia.[21,100]

Both term and preterm infants in the neonatal intensive care unit (NICU) have higher BE levels than healthy term infants. Preterm infants (especially preterm males) have higher BE levels than both healthy term and ill term infants.[100] Elevated BE levels are seen in stressed preterm infants with apnea, but not in nonstressed infants.[21,106] Release of BE is a component of neonatal respiratory control and is triggered by hypoxia.[21,106] BE levels are also higher in infants with respiratory distress.[100] Lower BE levels with birth have been associated with altered neurologic and motor development.[144] This may be a reflection of altered pituitary function or altered neuromotor development due to lack of the usual BE trophic effect.[144]

A transient adrenal cortex insufficiency is seen in some extremely low–birth weight (ELBW) infants. These infants have poor or limited ability to respond to shock with hypotension unresponsive to fluid and pressor management.[158] In these infants the adrenal may be unable to produce enough cortisol to maintain their blood pressure.[128] ELBW infants were reported to have elevated ACTH and cortisol following CRH administration and increased cortisol after ACTH administration, which are expected responses. However, some of the ELBW infants in this study, especially those who were ill, had very low serum cortisol levels that remained low even under stimulation.[71]

The standard administration of antenatal corticosteroids (see Chapter 9) leads to a transient suppression of the pituitary and adrenal glands, with recovery by 1 week. Even with this suppression, healthy, preterm infants respond to stress with increased cortisol.[128] The ill infant, however, is less able to respond to stress and more vulnerable to stress-related morbidity.

GH decreases rapidly after birth as free fatty acids, which block GH release, increase with nonshivering thermogenesis.[61] GH levels are higher in preterm infants than in term infants. Somatostatin levels in preterm infants are higher during the second week but decrease by the third to fourth weeks. Levels are even higher in infants with respiratory distress syndrome.[79]

Prolactin increases in the late fetal and early neonatal periods. Levels are higher in preterm infants than in term infants due to increased sensitivity to TSH and estrogens, pituitary insensitivity to dopaminergic inhibition, and reduced renal excretion by the immature kidney (with its lower glomerular filtration rate).[169] Prolactin may have a role in lung maturation and fluid homeostasis with transition. Dopamine levels are twice those of adults and function as a prolactin release–inhibiting factor.[78]

Hypothalamic-Pituitary-Thyroid Axis

The newborn is in a state of relative hyperthyroidism because of marked changes in thyroid function at birth (Table 18-7

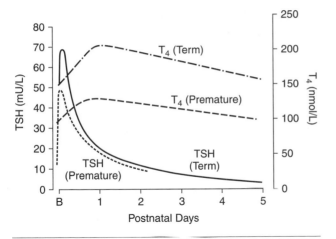

FIGURE **18-15** Changes in serum thyrotropin or thyroid-stimulating hormone (TSH) and thyroxine (T₄) in term and preterm infants during the first 5 days of life. Both TSH and T₄ increments are lower in preterm infants than in term infants. (Adapted from Fisher, D.A. & Klein, A.H. [1981]. Thyroid development and disorders of thyroid function in the newborn. *N Engl J Med, 304,* 702, by LaFranchi, S. [1999]. Thyroid function in the preterm infant. *Thyroid, 9,* 71.)

and Figure 18-15). TSH levels increase rapidly after birth. Exposure of the newborn to the cooler extrauterine environment is believed to stimulate skin thermal receptors, release of TRH by the hypothalamus, and TSH release by the pituitary gland. The TSH surge may also be related to cutting of the umbilical cord, since this surge has been reported to occur even if cooling is prevented.[152] TSH increases from 9 to 10 μU/ml at birth to peak values of 70 to 80 μU/ml by 15 to 60 (mean, 30) minutes after birth.[22,47,95] TSH rapidly decreases to 50% of peak values by 2 hours and to 20% by 24 hours, followed by a progressive decrease over the next 2 to 3 days to levels similar to cord blood values (see Figure 18-15).[122,47,48,78] During the first week, periodic oscillations in serum TSH have been reported, possibly reflecting establishment of a new equilibrium in the negative feedback exerted by thyroid hormone on the anterior pituitary.[142] In some infants, TSH may remain somewhat elevated for several months.[95]

The TSH surge leads to a rapid increase in T₄ and T₃ secretion (see Figure 18-15). T₄, T₃, and rT₃ levels are correlated with gestational age and birth weight. Cord blood levels of total and free T₄ in term infants are similar to adult values.[51] T₄ levels peak at 24 to 36 hours after birth (see Figure 18-15), then slowly decrease over the next few weeks.[95,168] Newborn T₄ levels are usually 10% to 20% less than maternal values.[51]

Cord blood T₃ values average 45 to 50 ng/dl (30% to 50% of maternal values). The newborn quickly changes from a state of T₃ deficiency to T₃ excess. T₃ levels increase

rapidly with birth and peak at 24 hours at 260 to 300 ng/ml (values exceeding those in adults) in most infants, then gradually fall.[47,84,95] T₃ increases more than T₄ because some T₄ is converted to T₃ by the liver and peripheral tissues. The increase in T₃ is due to the TSH surge and increased MDI I activity (see the top box on p. 681), with increased conversion of T₄ to T₃ and removal of the placenta (with its high levels of MDI III that convert T₃ to inactive forms).[49] The increase in T₃ may also be related to early cutting of the umbilical cord, which increases liver blood flow and conversion of T₃ to T₄.[168] T₃ and T₄ levels gradually fall to high-normal adult values by 4 to 6 weeks.[47,51,162]

Levels of rT₃ remain high for 3 to 5 days, then gradually decrease to adult values by 2 weeks.[51,168] TBG tends to be high because of transplacental passage of estrogens that stimulate its production. TBG-binding capacity in the infant is higher than in the pregnant woman and about 1.5 times that of the adult.[51] Radioactive iodine uptake by the thyroid is higher in the newborn because of increased avidity of the neonatal thyroid for iodine.

The TSH surge is seen in term, preterm, and SGA (small for gestational age) infants and seems unrelated to type of delivery.[151] Thyroid hormones in preterm infants follow patterns similar to those in term infants but may take longer to reach stable values.[22,51,95] Thyroid hormone levels are inversely related to gestational age.[49,95,162] Free T₄ and T₃ levels are lower and rT₃ levels higher in preterm and SGA infants than in term infants.[52] Lower cord blood T₄ levels are probably related to lower TBG levels, since free T₄ levels, though reduced, are not reduced as much as total T₄ in preterm infants.[95] TSH levels and response are generally similar to term infants.[162] Serum T₄ and T₃ levels may decrease to below birth levels in very-low–birth-weight (VLBW) preterm infants during the first week.[95] In addition, some ill and VLBW preterm infants develop a characteristic syndrome with elevated TSH and low T₄ levels without other evidence of hypothyroidism (see Transient Alterations in Thyroid Function in Preterm Infants).[48,49,84,95,162,173]

CLINICAL IMPLICATIONS FOR NEONATAL CARE

Endocrine adaptation at birth is influenced by gestational age, stresses of delivery, postnatal disease states, and degree of perinatal asphyxia.[169] Normal endocrine function is critical for normal growth and development both before and after birth. For example, biochemical maturation of the lungs and surfactant production is dependent on the HPA axis and its hormones, including CRH and cortisol, as well as thyroid hormones (see Chapter 9). Thyroid hormones are needed for lung development and surfactant production, bone growth, thermogenesis, and CNS maturation.

Within the CNS, these hormones are critical for dendritic arborization, synaptogenesis, and cerebellar cell migration and growth (see Chapter 14).[43,68] Effects on bone growth and CNS development continue into early childhood. An intact HPA axis is necessary for the infant to respond appropriately to stress and to prevent maladaptation.

Alterations in HPA and HPT function influence the transition to extrauterine life. For example, thyroid function is closely linked to thermoregulation and production of heat from brown adipose tissue. Alterations in health status from immaturity or acute illness can result in transient adrenal or thyroid dysfunction. Screening for hypothyroidism and congenital adrenal hyperplasia and recognition of hyper- and hypothyroidism has important ramifications for the infant's future growth and development. This section examines implications of these events.

Neonatal Stress

Although definitions and depictions of the stress response may vary, all or most posit an integrated biologic response pattern during or after stressor exposure. Activation of endocrine and neurotransmitter systems represent the major mechanisms upon which other aspects of this response is built. Responses to stressors are normally of short duration (acute stress) and are aimed at survival followed by a return to a state of dynamic homeostasis. Stress responses that go on for extended periods (chronic stress) can produce long-term changes in stress response systems, leading to decreases in adaptive capacity and increased risk for physical and psychologic disorders.[182]

The NICU has the potential for significant stress during a period of critical brain development. There are many sources of stress in the NICU from both internal (e.g., pain, distress, pathologic processes) and external (e.g., physical environment, caregiver interventions, medical or surgical procedures, multiple simultaneous modes of stimulation) demands. Stress and pain (see Chapter 14) interact. Preterm infants may be simultaneously exposed to pain stimuli and other noxious sensations (such as handling, light, sound, and temperature changes) that cause further activity in nociceptive pathways and systemic stress responses. An infant's stress tolerance may be reached or exceeded repeatedly, contributing to short- and long-term morbidity. Infants in the NICU experience both acute and chronic stress. Anand notes that most handling procedures in small and sick infants lead to stress, which if not controlled, may cause cumulative harm.[7]

Baseline responses to stress are set early in life and can influence later responses and adaptation. Stress activates the HPA axis with release of catecholamines, CRH, ACTH, BEs, and cortisol. Stress responses affect many systems: cardiovascular (increased blood pressure and heart rate), gastrointestinal (increased gut motility and splanchnic vasoconstriction), renal (sodium and water retention), and respiratory (increased oxygen consumption, decreased tidal volume, and functional residual capacity or ventilation-perfusion mismatch). Stress can alter coagulation, immune function, and cytokine production. Stress has profound metabolic consequences; metabolic stability may be more difficult to maintain in the neonate, especially in immature infants.[6] Stress can lead to hyper- or hypoglycemia in the neonate. Stress increases counterregulatory hormones (e.g., glucagon, ACTH, catecholamines, cortisol) that decrease insulin excretion. Glucagon, fat, and protein are converted to glucose, which—in the face of insulin resistance from the counterregulatory hormones—results in hyperglycemia. In immature infants, this response and the infant's nutrient stores may become exhausted, so over time the infant becomes hypoglycemic.[6]

Term infants, whether healthy or ill, have an intact HPA axis and can identify and respond to stress.[132] Healthy preterm infants older than 28 weeks' gestational age respond to stress with increased cortisol secretion, although at lower levels than in term infants.[132] However, in preterm infants who are ill or younger than 28 weeks' gestational age, the HPA is suppressed during the first few weeks after birth. These VLBW infants seem unable to "recognize" stress and to respond by increasing cortisol secretion.[71] Preterm infants—especially those who are ill or weigh less than 1000 g—have lower basal cortisol levels and are less able to increase cortisol production with stress. In these infants there is an increase in precursors but not in cortisol, suggesting immature activity of enzymes to convert these precursors to cortisol.[72,74,98]

Several reports suggest that early stress in the fetus and neonate may produce permanent changes in neural pathways, increasing the risk of later disorders such as adult psychopathology and hypertenesion.[3,8,29,155,165] Maternal stress in the third trimester is associated with increased ACTH and cortisol and increased placental CRH. Since CRH is a primary factor in labor onset, this may lead to preterm labor and decrease the sensitivity of the fetal-neonatal anterior pituitary to CRH, with permanent elevations in cortisol and BEs.[155]

Thyroid Function and Thermoregulation

Thyroid function and neonatal temperature regulation are interrelated (see Chapter 19). T_3 and T_4 increase basal metabolic rate and heat production, whereas T_4 and norepinephrine stimulate metabolism of brown adipose tissue (BAT). Occlusion of the umbilical cord activates BAT via

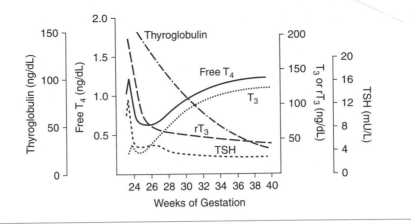

FIGURE **18-16** Maturation of thyroid function parameters in the very-low–birth-weight (23 to 35 weeks' gestation) premature infant. (Data from van Wassenaer, A.G., et al. [1997]. *Pediatr Res, 42,* 604; and Ares, S., et al. [1997]. *J Clin Endocrinol Metab, 82,* 1704. From Fisher, D.A. [1998]. Thyroid function in premature infants. The hypothyroxinemia of prematurity. *Clin Perinatol, 25,* 1008.)

a catecholamine surge and withdrawal of placental prostaglandins and adenosine.[47,49] T$_4$ enhances the effects of catecholamines to increase oxygen consumption (and metabolic rate) and increases BAT lipolysis. Within 6 hours of birth, the term neonate can respond to cold stress by increasing his or her metabolic rate 100%; by 6 to 9 days, this increase may be 170%. The preterm infant responds similarly to cold stress, although at a slower rate and lower percentage increase (~40%).[61]

Transient Alterations in Thyroid Function in Preterm Infants

In healthy preterm infants, cord blood T$_4$ levels range from 5.5 to 6 μg/dl, increasing to 7 to 9 μg/dl by 21 to 28 days and reaching values similar to those of term infants by 4 to 6 weeks.[89] As a result, preterm infants are more likely (1 in 6000) to have below normal values on thyroid screening tests compared with term infants.[51,53] Thyroid hormone values after birth are correlated with gestational age. For example, infants of 25 to 27 weeks' gestation have free T$_4$ levels that are two to three times lower than those of term infants.[49] Maturation of thyroid function in VLBW infants is illustrated in Figure 18-16.

Some preterm infants develop transient thyroid alterations in the early weeks after birth. T$_4$ and T$_3$ levels may fall in the first week to values lower than at birth. Possible causes include decreased liver TBG production, immaturity of the hypothalamic-pituitary-thyroid axis, inadequate nutrition, decreased MDI type I, decreased BAT, and immature tissue thyroid systems (Table 18-8).[48,49,95,173] This disorder is similar to the euthyroid sick syndrome seen in severely ill adults and children.[48]

TABLE **18-8**   Limitations of Thyroid Function in Very-Low–Birth-Weight Infants

Low thyroxine-binding globulin concentration
Obtunded neonatal thyroid-stimulating hormone surge and thyroxine increment
Limited brown adipose tissue thermogenesis
Minimal thyroxine to triiodothyronine conversion
Continued production of inactive thyroid hormone analogues
Immature thyroid hormone biogenesis
Limited thyroglobulin stores
Immature hypothalamic-pituitary-thyroid axis

From Fisher, D.A. (1999). Hypothyroxinemia in premature infants: Is thyroxine treatment necessary? *Thyroid, 9,* 715.

Thyroid function tends to return to normal as the infant matures or recovers from the underlying illness, with achievement of stable serum T$_4$ values by 6 to 7 weeks.[51] At 1 year, intellectual development has been reported as similar to that of infants without transient hypothyroidism in some studies; however, other studies suggest that low T$_4$ levels may impair neurologic development.[35,69,114,140,178] Three transient patterns of altered thyroid function have been described in preterm infants: physiologic hypothyroxinemia, transient primary hypothyroidism, and transient secondary/tertiary hypothyroidism.[48,49] These are more likely to occur in VLBW infants who weigh less than 1000 g and infants who are ill or stressed.

Physiologic hypothyroxinemia is seen in 70% or more of infants younger than 35 weeks' gestational age. These infants have low T_4 levels secondary to low to normal TBG and TSH levels.[48,95] This is a transient phenomenon that generally does not require treatment unless TSH levels are elevated.[49] Thus most preterm infants are hypothyroxinemic ("hypothyroxinemia of prematurity"). The frequency increases with decreasing gestational age. The mechanism and pattern of this disorder varies with gestational age.[48]

In infants older than 30 to 32 weeks' gestational age, T_4 and free T_4 increase transiently after birth in conjunction with the TSH surge (which is similar to the pattern seen with term infants), then decrease. This is followed by a gradual increase in TBG, T_4, free T_4, and T_3, reaching term values by 38 to 42 weeks.[9,38,48] These infants probably have immaturity of the thyroid's ability to respond to TSH and ability to convert T_4 to T_3.[48]

In VLBW infants younger than 30 weeks' gestational age, there is a limited TSH surge and an increase in T_4 and T_3, followed by a decrease in T_4 and free T_4 to a nadir at 1 to 2 weeks.[9,38,48,131,142] These infants usually achieve cord blood levels of serum T_4 by 3 to 4 weeks.[48] The cause of the hypothyroxinemia in these infants is primarily decreased TBG and probably an inability to increase iodine uptake and T_4 production with extrauterine adaption.[9,48] Because of immaturity, these infants also have inefficient production of thyroglobulin (see the top box on p. 681) and a decreased ability to convert T_4 to T_3 due to low levels of liver MDI I activity.[9,48]

Transient primary hypothyroidism is seen in 0.12% of LBW and 0.4% of VLBW infants.[48] These infants have low T_4 and free T_4, with increased TSH levels during the first 2 to 3 weeks after birth. Thyroglobulin and iodine stores are low, with increased T_4 utilization and demand. Fisher suggests that these infants need treatment if their TSH levels are greater than 20 mU.[48] The frequency of transient secondary/tertiary hypothyroidism is unknown but may occur in up to 10% of VLBW infants. These infants have low T_4 and free T_4 levels without changes in TSH during the first 1 to 2 weeks after birth.[48,49] There may be some benefit to treating these infants.[174]

The decision of whether to treat healthy or ill preterm infants with transient hypothyroidism is controversial.[51,52,174] Exogenous TRH significantly increases serum T_4 and TSH levels. Most studies of use of T_4 for thyroid hormone replacement do not demonstrate significant differences in the age at which serum T_4 values normalize or in infant growth parameters.[174] However, there is some evidence suggesting that this therapy may improve developmental outcome in the infant younger than 27 weeks' gestational age.[91,171,174] LaFranchi notes that if infants have low T_4 and increased TSH levels, they should be treated; infants with low T_4 but normal TSH and who are otherwise healthy may not need to be treated, depending on institutional protocol.[95]

Neonatal Hyperthyroidism

Neonatal hyperthyroidism is rare and is usually a transient disorder associated with transplacental passage of maternal TSIs in women with Graves disease (see Chapter 12). This may occur even in euthyroid women after thyroid removal or ^{131}I thyroid ablation, since TSIs are still present in the woman's system. TSI levels correlate positively with development of neonatal hyperthyroidism; thus maternal screening can identify the infant at risk. An increased fetal heart rate (greater than 160) after 22 weeks is of concern.[97] The mother may be treated with antithyroid drugs, if she is not already being treated, to maintain the fetal heart rate around 140.[75] The incidence of neonatal effects is 0.6% to 9.5%.[97,186] Although this disorder is usually transient, increased mortality has been reported, usually as a result of respiratory obstruction, difficult delivery due to the enlarged thyroid, or high-output cardiac failure secondary to tachycardia (heart rates greater than 200 beats/min).[97] T_4 and free T_4 levels are increased, but they are also increased in the normal newborn.

Clinical findings such as low birth weight, irritability, hunger, tachycardia, diarrhea, sweating, and arrhythmias may be present at birth. If the mother is on antithyroid medication, manifestations may be delayed for 2 to 10 days.[22,186] These infants have an advanced bone age and occasionally craniosynostosis. Clinical effects, although transient, last for 1 to 5 months (generally 2 to 3 months) or up to 10 months in some infants.[22]

Neonatal Hypothyroidism

The most common cause of congenital hypothyroidism in North America is thyroid dysgenesis, with an incidence of 1 in 4000 live births.[78,84,94,97] The cause is often unclear. In some infants the hypothyroidism is due to a single gene defect or familial autoimmune factors. In the majority (85%) of infants, the cause is a nonfamilial embryogenic defect.[94] In some infants this may be due to mutations in genes coding transcription factors that are needed for thyroid gland morphogenesis and differentiaiton.[94] Females are affected twice as often as males. Hypothyroidism and cretinism secondary to endemic goiter are rare in North America. Infants with intrauterine hypothyroidism may not experience significant impairment of somatic or brain growth before birth, because some maternal T_4 crosses the placenta and enough is catabolized to T_3 for normal fetal brain development.[47]

Most infants appear normal at birth, with clinical signs apparent in fewer than 5% to 30%. Common findings such as a large fontanel, hypotonia, macroglossia, and umbilical hernia may not develop for several weeks or months.[22,51,122,142] By the time these findings are apparent, significant neurologic damage has already occurred, since inadequate thyroid hormone during fetal life and early infancy alters CNS development. The exact mechanism of injury is not well understood, but the degree of neurologic abnormality correlates with the duration and severity of the hypothyroidism.[22,127]

Neonatal Screening for Hypothyroidism

Diagnosis and treatment of congenital hypothyroidism before 1 to 3 months of age are associated with an increased likelihood of normal mental development.[126] Therefore, routine screening of newborns for hypothyroidism has been implemented in the United States and many other countries. Screening involves evaluating T_4 or TSH levels. Infants with congenital hypothyroidism have decreased T_4 levels because of the thyroidal dysgenesis and elevated TSH levels. TSH levels are elevated because the low T_4 level does not provide the usual negative feedback inhibition of the anterior pituitary.[47,94] TSH screening is more useful to detect subclinical hypothyroidism; T_4 screening is most useful in detecting central hypothalamic-pituitary hypothyroidism and for infants with a delayed TSH rise.[97]

Screening for hypothyroidism is done at 2 to 5 days and again at 2 to 6 weeks of age. Approximately 10% of affected infants are detected only on the second screening.[94] Specimens taken immediately after birth are avoided because of the usual TSH surge. If T_4 values are below 10%, TSH values are measured. If these are elevated, the infant is recalled for further evaluation.[51,122] This test has a high selectivity and low (1% to 2%) recall rate.[351] Infants with a positive diagnosis are treated with thyroid hormone replacement therapy to normalize serum T_4 levels.[23]

Congenital Adrenal Hyperplasia

Congenital adrenal hyperplasia (CAH) comprises a group of autosomal recessive genetic disorders with a frequency of 1 in 15000 live births in North America.[129] These infants have a defect in cortisol synthesis. Without adequate cortisol negative feedback (Figure 18-2), ACTH levels are elevated, especially in the last half of gestation. The excess ACTH stimulates the adrenal glands to overproduce precursors for cortisol and leads to adrenal hyperplasia.[123,129] CAH is due to a complete or partial block in one of the enzymes involved in synthesis of adrenal cortex hormones (see Figure 18-11). Depending on the enzyme involved and the severity of the enzyme block, some female infants may have ambiguous genitalia due to virilization. Since some of the same enzymes are found in the gonads as the adrenals, both tissues are affected.[123] Prenatal therapy with maternal corticosteroids may prevent or minimize virilization of female genitalia if begun before 10 weeks.[127] In infants with partial enzyme defects, results may not be apparent until later in childhood or adolescent. Table 18-9 summarizes the effects of various enzyme blocks.

The most common block (90% to 95%) is in the cytochrome P-450 type enzyme 21-hydroxylase (21-OH), in

TABLE 18-9 Enzyme Deficiencies in Congenital Adrenal Hyperplasia

Deficient Enzyme	Effects on Hormones	Effect in the Newborn
21-Hydroxylase	Inability to synthesize glucocorticoids and aldosterone; increased androgen production in response to increased adrenocorticotropin	Ambiguous genitalia (females), hyponatremia, hyperkalemia, weight loss, acidosis, shock
11-Hydroxylase	Inability to synthesize glucocorticoids; suppression of renin activity	Ambiguous genitalia (females), hypertension, hypernatremia, hypokalemia, alkalosis
3β-Hydrosteroid dehydrogenase	Decreased androgen production; decreased glucocorticoid production	Incomplete genital development (males), mild virilization (females), hypotension, hypoglycemia, hyponatremia, hyperkalemia, acidosis, shock
17α-Hydroxylase	Impaired glucocorticoid and androgen production	Ambiguous genitalia (males), hypernatremia, hypokalemia, hypertension
Lipoid adrenal hyperplasia	Decreased glucocorticoid, mineralcorticoid, and androgen production	Ambiguous genitalia (males), hyponatremia, hyperkalemia, hypoglycemia, acidosis, shock

From Witt, C.L. (1999). Adrenal insufficiency in the term and preterm neonate. *Neonatal Network, 18*(5), 25.

which multiple types of mutations and clinical phenotypes are seen.[111,123,129] 21-OH mutations blocks conversion of progesterone to precursors needed for production of aldosterone and cortisol (Figure 18-11), with lower levels of these hormones. The excess precursors are instead converted to androgens that therefore increase. CAH is one of the disorders evaluated in newborn screening. CAH screening has traditionally been done by measuring levels of 17α-hydroxy-progesterone (see Figure 18-11). Newer DNA analysis techniques allow for identification of specific mutant gene forms; these are more effective in predicting disease severity.[111] Treatment involves glucocorticoid therapy to suppress ACTH. Aldosterone may be needed if the infant has a salt-wasting form of the disorder (see Table 18-9).

MATURATIONAL CHANGES DURING INFANCY AND CHILDHOOD

HPA maturation continues during infancy and childhood, followed by marked changes at puberty. Involution of the adrenal gland is most prominent in the first month after birth and is complete during the first year of life. By 1 month the adrenal is 50% of the size at birth.[181]

Adrenarche is maturation of the adrenal gland, with increased production of DHEA, DHEA-S, and other androgens and development of the zona reticularis. DHEA rises to a maximum around 25 years of age, then declines gradually thereafter.[17,147,175] Adrenarche begins in the prepubertal period around 8 years of age. Steroid hormones increase progressively and are associated with a transient increase in linear growth and bone maturation.[130] Adrenarche increases production of androgens and estrogens needed for puberty changes and occurs several years before the onset of puberty. The exact trigger for this change is unknown. It may be related to a decrease in levels of 3β-hydroxysteroid dehydrogenase (3β-HSD) in the zona reticularis.[56] Gonadal maturation and changes in the HPA axis with puberty are discussed in Chapter 2.

HPT function gradually changes during infancy and childhood. Thyroid hormones are critical for continued CNS maturation and bone growth. The critical period for thyroid hormone influences on the CNS continues to 6 to 8 months after birth. It has been estimated that infants with significant hypothyroidism lose 3 to 5 IQ points per month if untreated during this period.[47] The ability of the infant to convert T_4 to T_3 matures over the first month. Twenty-four-hour ^{131}I uptake by the thyroid at 1 month is similar to adult values.[51] During childhood, TSH levels tend to remain higher than adult levels. Maturation of negative feedback control of TSH secretion occurs by 2 months.[142] The T_4 turnover rate is higher in infants and children, accounting for the increased requirement of children for thyroid hormone per unit weight.[51] TBG levels gradually fall over the first few years. Thyroid hormones fall to high adult values by 4 to 6 weeks, but they do not reach mean adult values until puberty.[51]

SUMMARY

Maturation of the HPA and HPT axes and neuroendocrine function in the fetus and infant is essential for development of the CNS, lungs, bones, and other systems. These functions undergo significant changes during the transition to extrauterine life. In addition, thyroid function is interrelated with thermoregulation and changes dramatically at birth. Newborns normally have a relative hyperthyroidism, but immaturity or illness can lead to transient hypothyroidism. Screening for congenital hypothyroidism and congenital adrenal hyperplasia is a part of newborn metabolic screening. Use of this screening is essential for early identification and reduction of mortality and morbidity in these infants. All neonates should be monitored for stress, and protective interventions should be initiated. Preterm infants—especially those who are ill or younger than 28 weeks' gestational age—are particularly vulnerable to the adverse consequences of stress. Table 18-10 summarizes clinical recommendations related to neonatal thyroid function.

TABLE **18-10**   **Recommendations for Clinical Practice Related to Thyroid Function in Neonates**

Know the usual changes in pituitary and adrenal function in the fetus and during the neonatal period (pp. 691-697 and Figure 18-11).

Know usual changes in thyroid function during the neonatal period in term infants (pp. 696-697, Figure 18-15, and Table 18-7).

Know usual changes in thyroid function during the neonatal period in preterm infants (pp. 696-697, 699-700 and Figure 18-13, and Table 18-8).

Recognize the normal parameters related to thyroid function in term and preterm neonates (pp. 696-697, 699-700).

Recognize and monitor for transient alterations in thyroid function in the preterm infant (pp. 699-700 and Figure 18-13).

Recognize the signs of and monitor for transient hyperthyroidism in infants of mothers with Graves disease (pp. 686-687, 689, 700).

Recognize the clinical signs of hypothyroidism in infants (pp. 700-701).

Screen newborns for congenital hypothyroidism and congenital adrenal hyperplasia (pp. 700-702).

Monitor growth and neurologic status in infants with congenital hypothyroidism (pp. 700-701).

Monitor for signs of stress and pain in neonates (p. 698 and Chapter 14).

REFERENCES

1. Alsat, E., et al. (1997). Human placental growth hormone. *Am J Obstet Gynecol, 177,* 1526.
2. Alkalay, A., et al. (1996). Evaluation of hypothalamic-pituitary-adrenal axis in premature infants treated with dexamethasone. *Am J Perinatol, 13,* 473.
3. Alves, S.E., et al. (1997). Neonatal ACTH administration elicits long-term changes in forebrain monoamine innervation. *Ann N Y Acad Sci, 814,* 226.
4. Amino, N., et al. (1978). Changes of serum antithyroid antibodies during and after pregnancy in autoimmune thyroid diseases. *Clin Exp Immunol, 31,* 30.
5. Amino, N., Tada, H. & Hidaka, Y. (1999). Postpartum autoimmune thyroid syndrome: A model of aggravation of autoimmune disease. *Thyroid, 9,* 705.
6. Anand, K.J. (1990). Neonatal stress response to anesthesia and surgery. *Clin Perinatol, 17,* 207.
7. Anand, K.J. (2000). Effects of perinatal pain and stress. *Prog Brain Res, 122,* 117.
8. Anand, K.J. & Scalzo, F.M. (2000). Can adverse neonatal experiences alter brain development and subsequent behavior? *Biol Neonate, 77,* 69.
9. Ares, S., et al. (1997). Neonatal hyperthyroxinemia: Effects of iodine intake and premature birth. *J Clin Endocrinol Metab, 82,* 1704.
10. Barbieri, R.L. (1994). The maternal adenohypophysis. In D. Tuchinsky & A.B. Little (Eds.). *Maternal-fetal endocrinology* (2nd ed.). Philadelphia: W.B. Saunders.
11. Barbieri, R.L. (1999). Endocrine disorders in pregnancy. In S.S.C. Yen, R.B. Jaffe, & R.L. Barbieri (Eds.). *Reproductive endocrinology; physiology, pathophysiology and clinical management* (4th ed.). Philadelphia: W.B. Saunders.
12. Becker, R.A. (1987). Thyroid disease in pregnancy. In C.J. Pauerstein (Ed.). *Clinical obstetrics.* New York: John Wiley & Sons.
13. Benyo, Z. & Wahl, M. (1996). Opiate receptor-mediated mechanisms in the regulation of cerebral blood flow. *Cerebrovasc Brain Metab Rev, 8,* 326.
14. Bergant, A.M., et al. (1998). Childbirth as a biological model for stress? Associations with endocrine and obstetric factors. *Gynecol Obstet Invest, 45,* 181.
15. Berghout, H., et al. (1998). Thyroid size and thyroid function during pregnancy: An analysis. *Eur J Endocrinol, 138,* 536.
16. Berkowitz, G. S., et al. (1996). Corticotropin-releasing factor and its binding protein: Maternal serum levels in term and preterm deliveries. *Am J Obstet Gynecol, 174,* 1477.
17. Bonney, R.C., et al. (1984). The interrelationship between plasma 5-ene adrenal androgens in normal women. *J Steroid Biochem, 20,* 1353.
18. Brent, G.A. (1997). Maternal thyroid function: Interpretation of thyroid function test in pregnancy. *Clin Obstet Gynecol, 40,* 3.
19. Browne-Martin, K. & Emerson, C.H. (1997). Postpartum thyroid dysfunction. *Clin Obstet Gynecol, 40,* 90.
20. Burrow, G.N. (1993). Thyroid function and hyperfunction during gestation. *Endocr Rev, 14,* 194.
21. Burrow, G.N., et al. (1994). Maternal and fetal thyroid function. *N Engl J Med, 331,* 1072.
22. Burrow, G.N. (1999). Thyroid diseases. In G.N. Burrow & T.P. Duffy (Eds.). *Medical complications during pregnancy* (5th ed.). Philadelphia: W.B. Saunders.
23. Camargo, C. A. (1989). Hypothyroidism and goiter during pregnancy. In S.A. Brody & K. Ueland (Eds.). *Endocrine disorders in pregnancy.* Norwalk, CT: Appleton & Lange.
24. Cao, L., et al. (1993). Endogenous opioid-like substances in perinatal asphyxia and cerebral injury due to anoxia. *Chin Med J (Engl), 106,* 783.
25. Challis, J.R.G., et al. (1995). The placental corticotrophin-releasing hormone-adrenocorticotrophin axis. *Placenta, 16,* 481.
26. Chan, E., et al. (1993). Plasma corticotropin-releasing hormone, endorphin and cortisol inter-relationships during human pregnancy. *Acta Endocrinol, 126,* 339.
27. Cheron, R.G., et al. (1981). Neonatal thyroid function after propylthiouracil therapy for maternal Graves' disease. *N Engl J Med, 304,* 525.
28. Chrousos, G.P., et al. (1998). Interactions between the hypothalamic-pituitary-adrenal axis and the female reproductive system: clinical implications. *Ann Intern Med, 129,* 229.
29. Clark, P.A. (1998). Programming of the hypothalamic-pituitary-adrenal axis and the fetal origins of adult disease hypothesis. *Eur J Pediatr, 157,* S7.
30. Contempre, B., et al. (1993). Detection of thyroid hormones in human embryonic cavities during the first trimester of pregnancy. *J Clin Endocrinol Metab, 77,* 1719.
31. Copper, P.J., et al. (1998). Postnatal depression, *Br Med J, 316,* 1884.
32. Darras, V.M., Hume, R. & Visser, T.J. (1999). Regulation of thyroid hormone metabolism during fetal development. *Mol Cell Endocrinol, 25,* 37.
33. Davidson, S., et al. (1987). Cardiorespiratory depression and plasma beta-endorphin levels in low-birth-weight infants during the first day of life. *Am J Dis Child, 141,* 145.
34. Davies, T.F. (1999). The thyroid immunology of the postpartum period. *Thyroid, 9,* 675.
35. den Ouden, A.L., et al. (1996). The relationship between neonatal thyroxine levels and neurodevelopmental outcome at age 5 and 9 years in a national cohort of very preterm and/or very low birth weight infants. *Pediatr Res, 39,* 142.
36. Deshpande, S., Platt, M.P. & Aynsley-Green, A. (1993). Patterns of the metabolic and endocrine stress response to surgery and medical illness in infancy and childhood. *Crit Care Med, 21,* S359.
37. De Zegher, F., et al. (1995). The prenatal role of thyroid hormone evidenced by fetomaternal Pit-1 deficiency. *J Clin Endocrinol Metab, 80,* 3130.
38. Diamond, F.B. & Root, A.W. (1991). Thyroid function in the preterm infant. *Adv Exp Med Biol, 299,* 227.
39. Dozeman, R., et al. (1983). Hyperthyroidism appearing as hyperemesis gravidarum. *Arch Int Med, 143,* 2202.
40. Eriksson, L., et al. (1989). Growth hormone 24 hour profiles during pregnancy—lack of pulsatility for the placental variant. *Br J Obstet Gynecol, 96,* 949.
41. Evian-Brion, D. (1999). Maternal endocrine adaptations to placental hormones in humans. *Acta Paediatr Suppl, 428,* 12.
42. Fantz, C.R., et al. (1999). Thyroid function during pregnancy. *Clin Chem, 45,* 2250.
43. Ferreiro, B., et al. (1988). Estimation of nuclear thyroid hormone receptor saturation in human fetal brain and lung during early gestation. *J Clin Endocrinol Metab, 67,* 853.
44. Fisher, D.A. (1983). Maternal-fetal thyroid function in pregnancy. *Clin Perinatol, 10,* 615.
45. Fisher, D.A. (1986). The unique endocrine milieu of the fetus. *J Clin Invest, 78,* 603.
46. Fisher, D.A. & Polk, D.H. (1994). The ontogenesis of thyroid function and its relationship to neonatal thermogenesis. In D. Tulchinsky & A.B. Little (Eds.). *Maternal-fetal endocrinology* (2nd ed.). Philadelphia: W.B. Saunders.

47. Fisher, D.A. (1997). Fetal thyroid function: diagnosis and management of fetal thyroid disorders. *Clin Obstet Gynecol, 40,* 16.

48. Fisher, D.A. (1998). Thyroid function in premature infants. The hypothyroxinemia of prematurity. *Clin Perinatol, 25,* 999.

49. Fisher, D.A. (1999). Hypothyroxinemia in premature infants: is thyroxine treatment necessary. *Thyroid, 9,* 715.

50. Florido, J., et al. (1997). Plasma concentrations of β-endorphin and adrenocorticotropic hormone in women with and without childbirth preparation. *Eur J Obstet Gynecol Reprod Biol, 73,* 121.

51. Foley, T.P. & Morishima, A. (1997). Thyroid disorders. In A.A. Fanaroff & R.J. Martin (Eds.). *Neonatal-perinatal medicine: Diseases of the fetus and infant* (6th ed.). St. Louis: Mosby.

52. Forest, M.G. (1987). Endocrine disorders in the newborn. Problems related to thyroid and adrenal disorders in the neonatal period. In L. Stern & P. Vert (Eds.). *Neonatal medicine.* Chicago: YearBook Medical Publishers.

53. Frank, J.E. (1996). Thyroid function in very low birth weight infants: effects on neonatal hypothyroid screening. *J Pediatr, 28,* 548.

54. Garner, P.R. (1993). Disorders of the adrenal cortex in pregnancy. *Curr Obstet Med, 2,* 143.

55. Garner, P.R. (1999). Adrenal and pituitary disorders. In G.N. Burrow & T.P. Duffy (Eds.). *Medical complications during pregnancy* (5th ed.). Philadelphia: W.B. Saunders.

56. Gell, J.S., et al. (1998). Adrenarche results from development of a 3β-hydroxysteorid dehydrogenase-deficient adrenal reticularis. *J Clin Endocrinol Metab, 83,* 3695.

57. Gemelli, M., et al. (1988). Correlation between plasma levels and ACTH and beta-endorphin in the first seven days of postnatal life. *J Endocrinol Invest, 11,* 395.

58. Glinoer, D., et al. (1990). Regulation of maternal thyroid during pregnancy. *J Clin Endocrinol Metab, 71,* 276.

59. Glinoer, D. (1997). The regulation of thyroid function in pregnancy: pathways of endocrine adaptation from physiology to pathology. *Endocr Rev, 18,* 404.

60. Glinoer, D. (1997). Maternal and fetal impact of chronic iodine deficiency. *Clin Obstet Gynecol, 40,* 102.

61. Gluckman, P.D., et al. (1999). The transition from fetus to neonate—an endocrine perspective. *Acta Paediatr Suppl, 88,* 7.

62. Goland, R.S., et al. (1988). Biologically active corticotrophin-releasing hormone in maternal and fetal plasma during pregnancy. *Am J Obstet Gynecol, 159,* 884.

63. Goodwin, T.M., et al. (1992). The role of chorionic gonadotropin in transient hyperthyroidism of hyperemesis gravidarum. *J Clin Endocrinol Metab, 75,* 1333.

64. Gorman, C.A. (1999). Radioiodine and pregnancy. *Thyroid, 9,* 721.

65. Griffing G.T. & Melby, J.C. (1994). The maternal adrenal cortex. In D. Tuchinsky & A.B. Little (Eds.). *Maternal-fetal endocrinology* (2nd ed.). Philadelphia: W.B. Saunders.

66. Grumbach, M. & Gluckman, P.D. (1994). The human fetal hypothalamus and pituitary gland: The maturation of neuroendocrine mechanisms controlling the secretion of fetal pituitary growth hormone, prolactin, gonadotropins, adrenocorticotropin-related peptides, and thyrotropin. In D. Tuchinsky & A.B. Little (Eds.). *Maternal-fetal endocrinology* (2nd ed.). Philadelphia: W.B. Saunders.

67. Guillaume, J. (1985). Components of the total serum thyroid hormones concentrations during pregnancy: High free thyroxine and blunted thyrotropin (TSH) response to TSH-releasing hormone in the first trimester. *J Clin Endocrinol Metab, 60,* 678.

68. Guyton, A.C. & Hall, J.E. (1996). *Textbook of medical physiology* (9th ed.). Philadelphia: W.B. Saunders.

69. Hadeed, A.J., et al. (1981). Significance of transient postnatal hypothyroxinemia in premature infants with and without respiratory distress syndrome. *Pediatrics, 68,* 494.

70. Haddow, J.E., et al. (1999). Maternal thyroid deficiency during pregnancy and subsequent neuropsychological development of the child. *N Engl J Med, 341,* 549.

71. Hanna, C.E., et al. (1993). Hypothalamic-pituitary adrenal function in the extremely low birth weight infant. *J Clin Endocrinol Metab, 76,* 384.

72. Helbock, H.J., et al. (1993). Glucocorticoid-responsive hypotension in extremely low birth weight newborns. *Pediatrics, 92,* 715.

73. Heinrichs, W.L. & Gibbons, W.E. (1989). Endocrinology of pregnancy. In S.A. Brody & K. Ueland (Eds.). *Endocrine disorders in pregnancy.* New York: Appleton & Lange.

74. Hingre, R.V., et al. (1994). Adrenal steroidogenesis in very low birth weight preterm infants. *J Clin Endocrinol Metab, 78,* 266.

75. Hobel, C., et al. (1999). Maternal plasma corticotropin-releasing hormone associated with stress at 20 weeks' gestation in pregnancies ending in preterm delivery. *Am J Obstet Gynecol, 180*(suppl), 257S.

76. Jaffe, R.B., et al. (1998). The regulation and role of fetal adrenal development in human pregnancy. *Endocr Res, 24,* 191.

77. Jaffe, R.B. (1986). Endocrine physiology of the fetus and fetoplacental unit. In S.S.C. Yen & R.B. Jaffe (Eds.). *Reproductive endocrinology: Physiology, pathophysiology and clinical management.* Philadelphia: W.B. Saunders.

78. Jaffe, R.B. (1999). Neuroendocrine metabolic regulation of pregnancy. In S.S.C. Yen, R.B. Jaffe, & R.L. Barbieri (Eds.). *Reproductive endocrinology: physiology, pathophysiology and clinical management* (4th ed.). Philadelphia: W.B. Saunders

79. Jain, L., et al. (1995). Somatostatin in preterm infants: postnatal changes and response to stress. *Biol Neonate, 68,* 81.

80. Jansson, R., et al. (1987). The postpartum period constitutes an important risk for the development of clinical Graves' disease in young women. *Acta Endocrinol, 116,* 321.

81. Jones, M.O., et al. (1994). Postoperative changes in resting energy expenditure and interleukin-6 in infants. *Br J Surg, 81,* 536.

82. Kaplan, M.M. (1992). Assessment of thyroid function during pregnancy. *Thyroid, 2,* 57.

83. Kaplan, M.M. (1994). The maternal thyroid and parathyroid glands. In D. Tuchinsky & A.B. Little (Eds.). *Maternal-fetal endocrinology* (2nd ed.). Philadelphia: W.B. Saunders.

84. Kaplan, S.A. (1983). Ontogenesis of hormone action: Insulin, adrenal corticoids, thyroid hormones and growth hormone. In J.B. Warshaw (Ed.). *The biological basis of reproductive and developmental medicine.* New York: Elsevier Biomedical.

85. Kari, M., et al. (1996). Serum cortisol, dehydroepiandrosterone sulfate, and steroid binding globulins in preterm neonates: Effect of gestational age and dexamethasone therapy. *Pediatr Res, 40,* 319.

86. Karlsson, R., et al. (1999). Timing of peak serum cortisol values in preterm infants in low-dose and the standard ACTH test. *Pediatr Res, 45,* 367.

87. Klein, A.H., et al. (1982). Developmental changes in pituitary-thyroid function in the human fetus and newborn. *Early Hum Devel, 6,* 321.

88. Klein, A.H., et al. (1980). Amniotic fluid thyroid hormone concentrations during human gestation. *Am J Obstet Gynecol, 136,* 626.

89. Klein, A.H., et al. (1979). Thyroid hormone and thyrotropin responses to parturition in premature infants with and without the respiratory distress syndrome. *Pediatrics, 63,* 380.

90. Kohler, P.O. (1987). Thyroid function and reproduction. In D.H. Riddick (Ed.). *Reproductive physiology in clinical practice.* New York: Thieme Medical Publishers.

91. Kok, J.H., et al. (1995). Randomized placebo controlled trial of thyroxine administration to infants <30 weeks in relation to mortality and morbidity. *Pediatr Res, 37*(suppl), 218A.

92. Korebrits, C., et al. (1998). Maternal corticotropin releasing hormone is increased with impending preterm birth. *J Clin Endocrinol Metab, 83,* 1585.

93. LaFranchi, S. & Mandel, S.H. (1996). Graves' disease in the neonatal period and childhood. In L.E. Braverman & R.D. Untiger (Eds.). *Werner & Ingbar's the thyroid* (7th ed.). Philadelphia: Lippincott Raven.

94. LaFranchi, S. (1999). Congenital hypothyroidism: Etiologies, diagnosis, and management. *Thyroid, 9,* 735.

95. LaFranchi, S. (1999). Thyroid function in the preterm infant. *Thyroid, 9,* 71.

96. Lawrence, R.A. (1989). Breastfeeding and medical disease. *Med Clin North Am, 73,* 583.

97. Lazarus, J.H. & Kokandi, A. (2000). Thyroid disease in relation to pregnancy: a decade of change. *Clin Endocrinol, 46,* 381.

98. Lee, M.M., et al. (1989). Serum adrenal steroid concentrations in premature infants. *J Clin Endocrinol Metab, 69,* 1133.

99. Leung, A.S., et al. (1993). Perinatal outcome in hypothyroid pregnancies. *Obstet Gynecol, 81,* 349.

100. Leuschen, M.P., et al. (1991). Plasma beta-endorphin in neonates: effect of prematurity, gender, and respiratory status. *J Clin Endocrinol Metab, 73,* 1062.

101. Levine, S. (1994). The ontogeny of the hypothalamic-pituitary-adrenal axis. The influence of maternal factors. *Ann N Y Acad Sci, 30,* 275.

102. Linton, E.A., et al. (1993). Corticotropin-releasing hormone binding protein (CRH-BP): plasma levels decrease during the third trimester of normal human pregnancy. *J Clin Endocrinol Metab, 76,* 260.

103. Lockitch, G. (1997). Clinical biochemistry of pregnancy. *Crit Rev Clin Lab Sci, 34,* 67.

104. Lockwood, C.J. (1999). Stress-associated preterm delivery: The role of corticotropin-releasing hormone. *Am J Obstet Gynecol, 80,* S264-S266.

105. Lockwood, C.J., et al. (1996). Corticotropin releasing hormone and related pituitary-adrenal axis hormones in fetal and maternal blood during the second half of pregnancy. *J Perinat Med, 24,* 243.

106. MacDonald, M.G., et al. (1990). Cerebrospinal fluid and plasma beta-endorphin-like immunoreactivity in full-term neonates and in preterm neonates with and without apnea of prematurity. *Dev Pharmacol Ther, 15,* 8.

107. Magiakou, M.A., et al. (1996). Hypothalamic CRH suppression during the postpartum period: implications for the increase of psychiatric manifestations in this period. *J Clin Endocrinol Metab, 81,* 1912.

108. Magiakou, M. A., et al. (1996). The maternal hypothalamic-pituitary-adrenal axis in the third trimester of human pregnancy. *Clin Endocrinol, 44,* 419.

109. Majzoub, J. A., et al. (1999). A central theory of preterm and term labor: Putative role for corticotropin-releasing hormone. *Am J Obstet Gynecol, 180,* 232S.

110. Mastorakos, G. & Ilias, I. (2000). Maternal hypothalamic-adrenal axis in pregnancy and the postpartum period. Postpartum-related disorders. *Ann N Y Acad Sci, 900,* 95.

111. McCabe, E.R. & McCabe, L.L. (1999). State-of-the-art for DNA technology in newborn screening. *Acta Paediatr Suppl, 88,* 58.

112. McDougall, I.R. (1989). Hyperthyroidism and maternal-fetal thyroid hormone metabolism. In S.A. Brody & K. Ueland (Eds.). *Endocrine disorders in pregnancy.* Norwalk, CT: Appleton & Lange.

113. McLean, M., et al. (1995). A placental clock controlling the length of human pregnancy. *Nat Med, 1,* 460.

114. Meijer, W.J., et al. (1992). Transient hyperthyroxinemia associated with developmental delay in very preterm infants. *Arch Dis Child, 67,* 944.

115. Mesiano, S. & Jaffe, R.B. (1997). Developmental and functional biology of the primate fetal adrenal cortex. *Endocr Rev, 18,* 378.

116. Mestman, J.H. (1998). Hyperthyroidism in pregnancy. *Endocrinol Metab Clin North Am, 27,* 127.

117. Miller, W.L. (1998). Steroid hormone biosynthesis and actions in the materno-feto-placental unit. *Clin Perinatol, 25,* 799.

118. Mirlesse, V., et al. (1993). Placental growth hormone levels in normal and pathological pregnancies. *Pediatr Res, 34,* 439.

119. Mitchell, M.L., et al. (1982). Pitfalls in screening for neonatal hypothyroidism. *Pediatrics, 70,* 16.

120. Momolani, N., et al. (1994). Relationship between silent thyroiditis and recurrent Graves' disease in the postpartum period. *J Clin Endocrinol Metab, 79,* 285.

121. Mon, M., et al. (1988). Morning sickness and thyroid function in normal pregnancy. *Obstet Gynecol, 72,* 355-359.

122. Moshand, T. & Thronton, P.S. (1999). Endocrine disorders of the newborn. In G.B. Avery, M.A. Fletcher, & Macdonald, M.G. (Eds.). *Neonatology-pathophysiology and management of the newborn* (5th ed.). Philadelphia: J.B. Lippincott.

123. Murphy, B.E.P. & Branchaud, C.L. (1994). The fetal adrenal. In D. Tuchinsky & A.B. Little (Eds.). *Maternal-fetal endocrinology* (2nd ed.). Philadelphia: W.B. Saunders.

124. Nader, S. (1999). Other endocrine disorders of pregnancy. In R.K. Creasy & R. Resnik (Eds.). *Maternal–fetal medicine* (4th ed.). Philadelphia: W.B. Saunders.

125. Nanacs, R., et al. (1996). Postpartum mood disorders: diagnosis and treatment guidelines. *J Clin Psychiatry, 59*(suppl 2), 34.

126. New England Congenital Hypothyroidism Collaborative. (1981). Effects of neonatal screening for hypothyroidism: prevention of mental retardation by treatment before clinical manifestations. *Lancet, 2,* 1095.

127. New England Congenital Hypothyroidism Collaborative. (1985). Neonatal hypothyroidism screening: Status of patients at 6 years of age. *J Pediatr, 107,* 915.

128. Ng, P.C. (2000). The fetal and neonatal hypothalamic-pituitary-adrenal axis. *Arch Dis Child Fetal Neonatal Ed, 82,* F250.

129. Pang, S. (1997). Congenital adrenal hyperplasia. *Endocrinol Metab Clin North Am, 26,* 853.

130. Parker, L.N. (1991). Adrenarche. *Endocrin Metab Clin North Am, 20,* 71.

131. Pavelka, S., et al. (1997). Tissue metabolism and plasma levels of thyroid hormone in critically ill very premature infants. *Pediatr Res, 42,* 812.

132. Peters, K.L. (1998). Neonatal stress reactivity and cortisol. *J Perinat Neonat Nurs, 11,* 45-59.

133. Pierro, A. (1999). Metabolic response to neonatal surgery. *Curr Opin Pediatr, 11,* 230.

134. Pokela, M.L. (1993). Effects of opioid-induced analgesia on beta-endorphin, cortisol and glucose responses in neonates with cardiorespiratory problems. *Biol Neonate, 64,* 360.

135. Pop, V.J., et al. (1999). Low maternal free thyroxine concentrations during early pregnancy associated with impaired psychomotor development in infancy. *Clin Endocrinol, 50,* 149.

136. Quinn, M.W., et al. (1998). Stress response and mode of ventilation in preterm infants. *Arch Dis Child Fetal Neonatal Ed, 78,* F195.

137. Radunovic, N., et al. (1992). Beta-endorphin concentrations in fetal blood during the second half of pregnancy. *Am J Obstet Gynecol, 167,* 740.

138. Raffin-Sanson, M.L., et al. (1999). High precursor level in maternal blood results from alternate mode of proopiomelanocortin processing in human placenta. *Clin Endocrinol, 50,* 85.

139. Ramanathan, S., Puig, M.M. & Turndorf, H. (1989). Plasma beta-endorphin levels in the umbilical cord blood of preterm human neonates. *Biol Neonate, 56*, 117.

140. Reuss, M.L., et al. (1996). The relation of transient hypothyroxinemia in preterm infants to neurologic development at two years of age. *N Engl J Med, 334*, 821.

141. Romaguera J., et al. (1990). Responsiveness of the L-S ratio of the amniotic fluid to intra-amniotic administration of thyroxine. *Acta Obstet Gynecol Scand, 69*, 119.

142. Rooman, R.P., et al. (1996). Low thyroxinemia occurs in the majority of very low birth weight preterm newborns, *Eur J Pediatr, 155*, 211.

143. Rosendahl, W., et al. (1995). Surgical stress and neuroendocrine responses in infants and children. *J Pediatr Endocrinol Metab, 8*, 187.

144. Rothenberg, S.J., et al. (1996). Umbilical cord beta-endorphin and early childhood motor development. *Early Hum Dev, 20*, 83.

145. Roti, E., Gnudi, A., & Braverman, L.E. (1983). The placental transport, synthesis and metabolism of hormones and drugs that affect thyroid function. *Endocrinol Rev, 4*, 131.

146. Roti, E. (1988). Regulation of thyroid-stimulating hormone (TSH) secretion in the fetus and neonate. *J Endocrinol Invest, 11*, 145.

147. Rotter, J.I., et al. (1985). A genetic component to the variation of dehydroepiandrosterone. *Metab Clin Exp, 34*, 731.

148. Rovet, J.F. (1990). Does breast-feeding protect the hypothyroid infants whose condition is diagnosed by newborn screening? *Am J Dis Child, 144*, 319.

149. Ruth, V., et al. (1993).Corticotropin-releasing hormone and cortisol in cord plasma in relation to gestational age, labor and fetal distress. *Am J Perinatol, 10*, 115.

150. Ruth, V. (1991). Neonatal stress or distress. *J Perinat Med, 19*(suppl 1), 151.

151. Sack, J., Fisher, D.A., & Wang, C.C. (1976). Serum thyrotropin, prolactin and growth hormone levels during the early neonatal period in the human infant. *J Pediatr, 89*, 298.

152. Sack, J., et al. (1976). Umbilical cord cutting triggers hypertriiodothyroninemia and nonshivering thermogenesis in the newborn lamb. *Pediatr Res, 10*, 169.

153. Sack, J., et al. (1977). Thyroxine concentrations in human milk. *J Clin Endocrinol Metab, 45*, 171.

154. Sadler, T. (1990). *Langman's medical embryology* (6th ed.). Philadelphia: Williams & Wilkins.

155. Sandman, C.A., et al. (1997). Maternal stress, HPA activity, and fetal/infant outcome. *Ann N Y Acad Sci, 24*, 266.

156. Sankaran, K., Hindmarsh, K.W., & Tan, L. (1989). Diurnal rhythm of beta-endorphin in neonates. *Dev Pharmacol Ther, 12*, 1.

157. Santiago, L.B., et al. (1996). Longitudinal analysis of the development of salivary cortisol rhythm in infancy. *Clin Endocrinol (Oxf), 44*, 157.

158. Sasidharan, P. (1998). Role of corticosteroids in neonatal blood pressure homeostasis. *Clin Perinatol, 25*, 723.

159. Saski, A., et al. (1987). Immunoreactive corticotropin-releasing hormone in human plasma during pregnancy, labor, and delivery. *J Clin Endocrinol Metab, 64*, 224.

160. Scholle, S., et al. (1990). Plasma levels of beta-endorphin and substance P in the first year of life full-term and preterm infants. *Acta Paediatr Scand, 79*, 1237.

161. Scott, S.M. & Watterberg, K.L. (1995). Effect of gestational age, postnatal age, and illness on plasma cortisol concentrations in premature infants. *Pediatr Res, 37*, 112.

162. Seely, B.L. & Burrow, G.N. (1999). Thyroid disease and pregnancy. In R.K. Creasy & R. Resnik (Eds.). *Maternal–fetal medicine* (4th ed.). Philadelphia: W.B. Saunders.

163. Smith, J.E. (1990). Pregnancy complicated by thyroid disease. *J Nurs Midwifery, 35*, 143.

164. Smith, R.P., et al. (2000). Pain and stress in the human fetus. *Eur J Obstet Gynecol Reproduct Biol, 92*, 161.

165. Smyth, J.W., et al. (1996). Median eminence corticotropin-releasing hormone content following prenatal stress and neonatal handling. *Brain Res Bull, 40*, 195.

166. Smyth, P.P.A., et al. (1997). Maternal iodine status and thyroid. Volume during pregnancy: correlation with neonatal iodine intake, *J Clin Endocrinol Metab, 82*, 2840.

167. Sonir, R.R., et al. (2000). The emergence of salivary cortisol circadian rhythm and its relationship to sleep activity in preterm infants. *Clin Endocrinol, 52*, 423.

168. Speroff, L., Glass, R.H., & Kase, N.G. (1999). *Clinical gynecologic endocrinology and infertility* (6th ed.). Philadelphia: Lippincott, Williams & Wilkins.

169. Sulyok, E. (1989). Endocrine factors in the neonatal adaptation. *Acta Physiol Hung, 74*, 329.

170. Tulchinsky, D. (1994). Postpartum lactation and resumption of reproductive functions. In D. Tulchinsky & A.B. Little (Eds.). *Maternal-fetal endocrinology* (2nd ed.). Philadelphia: W.B. Saunders.

171. Vanhole, C. (1997). Thyroxine treatment of preterm newborns: clinical and endocrine effects. *Pediatr Res, 42*, 87.

172. Van Reempts, P.J., et al. (1996). Stress responses in preterm neonates after normal and at-risk pregnancies. *J Paediatr Child Health, 32*, 450.

173. van Wassenaer, A.G., et al. (1997). Thyroid function in very preterm infants: influences of gestational age. *Pediatr Res, 42*, 604.

174. van Wassenaer, A.G., et al. (1997). Effects of thyroxine supplementation on neurologic development in infants born at less than 30 weeks gestation. *N Engl J Med, 336*, 21.

175. Vermeulin, A. (1980). Adrenal androgens and aging. In A.R. Genazzani, J.H. Thijssen, & P.K. Siiteri (Eds.). *Adrenal androgens.* New York: Raven.

176. Vermiglio, F., et al. (1995). Maternal hypothyroxinemia during the first half of gestation in an iodine deficient area with endemic cretinism and related disorders. *Clin Endocrinol, 42*, 409.

177. Vulsma, T., et al. (1989). Maternal-fetal transfer of thyroxine in congenital hypothyroidism due to a total organification defect or thyroid agenesis. *N Engl J Med, 321*, 13.

178. Vulsma, Y & Kok, J.K. (1996). Prematurity-associated neurological and developmental abnormalities and neonatal thyroid function. *N Engl J Med, 334*, 857.

179. Vyas, J. & Kotecha, S. (1997). Effects of antenatal and postnatal corticosteroids on the preterm lung. *Arch Dis Child Fetal Neonatal Ed, 77*, F147.

180. Walfish, P.G. & Chan, J.Y.C. (1985). Postpartum hyperthyroidism. *J Clin Endocrinol Metab, 14*, 417.

181. Winter, J.S.D. (1998). Fetal and neonatal adrenocortical physiology. In R.A. Polin & W.W. Fox (Eds.). *Fetal and neonatal physiology* (2nd ed.). Philadelphia: W.B. Saunders.

182. Yehuda, R., et al. (1993). Long-lasting hormonal alterations to extreme stress in humans: normative or maladaptive? *Psychosomatic Med, 55*, 287.

183. Yoshida, K., et al. (1986). Measurement of TSH in human amniotic fluid diagnosis of fetal thyroid abnormality in utero. *Clin Endocrinol, 25*, 313.

184. Zagon, I.S., Tobias, S.W., & McLaughlin, P.J. (1997). Endogenous opioids and prenatal determinants of neuroplasticity. *Adv Exp Med Biol, 429*, 289.

185. Zanardo, V., et al. (2001). Labor pain effects on colostral milk beta-endorphin concentrations of lactating mothers. *Biol Neonate, 79*, 87.

186. Zimmerman, D. (1999). Fetal and neonatal hyperthyroidism. *Thyroid, 9*, 727.

Thermoregulation

Thermoregulation is the balance between heat production and heat loss involved in maintaining thermal equilibrium. Heat is produced by the body as a by-product of metabolic processes and muscular activity; thus a major function of the thermoregulatory system is dissipation of this heat.[20] The thermoregulatory system must also respond appropriately to alterations in environmental temperature to preserve thermal equilibrium. Maintenance of thermal stability is particularly critical in the newborn since exposure to cold environments and lowered body temperatures are closely correlated with survival, especially in very-low–birth-weight (VLBW) infants. Maternal temperature changes are also important in relation to fetal well-being and the potential adverse consequences of maternal hyperthermia. Regulation of body temperature is summarized in Figure 19-1 and the box on p. 708.

MATERNAL PHYSIOLOGIC ADAPTATIONS

Hormonal and metabolic alterations during pregnancy result in changes in maternal temperature. These changes are transient and may cause discomfort but are generally not associated with significant physiologic alterations.

Antepartum Period

The amount of heat generated increases 30% to 35% during pregnancy because of the thermogenic effects of progesterone, alterations in maternal metabolism and basal metabolic rate (BMR) (see Chapter 15), and maternal dissipation of heat generated by the fetus.[26,103] As a result, many pregnant women develop an increased tolerance for cooler weather and decreased tolerance for heat. The additional heat is dissipated by peripheral vasodilation with a four- to sevenfold increase in cutaneous blood flow and increased activity of the sweat glands (see Chapter 13). Cutaneous vasodilation leads to skin warmth.

The maternal temperature usually increases by 0.5° C (0.3° F). Both core and skin temperature increase during pregnancy. The core temperature peaks by midpregnancy and may decrease by late pregnancy.[87] This decrease may

be related to the decrease in progesterone and physical activity (which generates heat) in later pregnancy. The rise in skin temperature is particularly evident in the hands and feet, probably due to arteriovenous shunting in these areas.[137] A slight decrease in skin temperature may be noted by late pregnancy.[87] In general, heat accumulation may be slower and heat dissipation faster in later pregnancy than before pregnancy or in early pregnancy. The increased plasma volume of pregnancy provides a greater area for heat storage and may enhance heat transfer from the fetus to the mother.[87]

The pregnant woman has decreased vasoconstriction in response to cold during pregnancy. This may alter her ability to conserve heat during cold stress.[32,87]

Body temperature increases with exercise from heat by the increased metabolic energy. Some of this heat is dissipated by increased skin blood flow; the remainder is stored transiently, increasing the core temperature. Changes in temperature with exercise during pregnancy are moderate, as compared with changes in nonpregnant women, suggesting that the enhanced thermoregulatory capacity of the pregnant woman may protect her against hyperthermia.[87] The increased plasma volume in pregnancy may assist in maintaining uterine and placental blood flow during exercise and in maximizing heat transfer from the fetus and heat dissipation in the mother. Aerobic exercise in water is associated with minimal changes in either core or skin temperature.[87,137]

Intrapartum Period

An increase in body temperature may also occur during labor as a result of physical activity with uterine contractions and the release of fetal-placental products that may stimulate the maternal hypothalamic thermoregulatory center.[78,96] In some women the increase in temperature during labor is high enough to generate concern that the mother is infected. Although this may sometimes be the case, the most common cause for maternal fever during labor is use of epidural analgesia, not infection. In general, women with

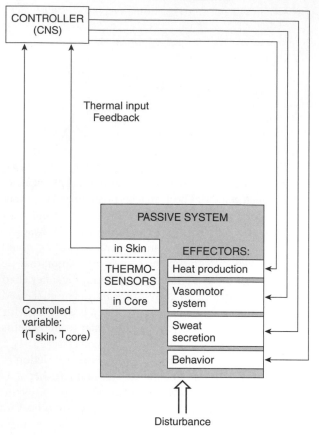

FIGURE **19-1** Regulation of body temperature. The diagram represents the biocybernetic concept of temperature regulation in humans. Temperature is sensed at various sites of the body, and the temperature signals are fed into the central controller (multiple input system). (From Bruck, K. [1998]. Neonatal thermal regulation. In R.A. Polin & W.W. Fox [Eds.]. *Fetal and neonatal physiology* [2nd ed.]. Philadelphia: W.B. Saunders.)

epidural analgesia are more likely to develop a fever during labor than women without this form of analgesia (16.6% versus 0.6%).[74] Epidural analgesia inhibits peripheral vasoconstriction and sweating in the lower body. The impairment of sweating and behavioral responses may decrease heat loss, although the exact mechanism for fever with epidural analgesia is unknown.[77,96]

The laboring woman is also at risk for hypothermia during the intrapartum period due to vasodilation of pregnancy (limiting usual vasoconstrictive responses to cold); administration of anesthetics, narcotics, and other pharmacologic agents; and rapid fluid replacement, especially if cool fluids are used. Prolonged exposure to a cool environment can aggravate heat loss. Hypothermia can result in shivering, hypotension, and hemodynamic and cardiorespiratory instability.[32,96]

Postpartum Period

Maternal temperature is monitored closely during the postpartum period since elevations may indicate infection or dehydration. A transient postpartum chill or shivering is often experienced about 15 minutes after birth of the infant or delivery of the placenta. The cause of this chill is unknown and various causes have been proposed. This phenomenon may represent muscular exhaustion or result from disequilibrium between the internal and external thermal gradients secondary to muscular exertion during labor and delivery, sudden changes in intraabdominal pressure with emptying of the uterus, or small amniotic fluid emboli. Most women who experience early postpartum shivering are normothermic, suggesting that this phenomenon is nonthermoregulatory in origin.[96] Shivering is seen in about 20% of women who did not receive neuraxial analgesia and more frequently in women after epidural analgesia.[96]

Body Temperature Regulation

Regulation of temperature depends on the ability to: (1) sense temperature changes in the external environment by skin receptors; (2) regulate heat production by increasing or decreasing metabolic rate; (3) conserve or dissipate heat (by sweating or altering skin blood flow); and (4) coordinate sensory input about environmental changes with appropriate body-temperature regulating responses.[66] Thermoregulation involves a "multiple-input system" controlled by the anterior and posterior portions of the hypothalamus. The anterior hypothalamus is temperature-sensitive and controls heat loss mechanisms. The preoptic nucleus of the anterior hypothalamus is the site of the set-point or threshold temperature. The set-point is a mechanism through which heat production and loss are regulated to maintain the core temperature within a narrow range. The posterior hypothalamus—the central controller of responses (heat production or dissipation) to cold or heat stimuli—receives input from central and peripheral receptors (skin, abdomen, spinal cord, hypothalamic preoptic nuclei, internal organs). With cold stress the thermoregulatory center acts to conserve heat (through cutaneous vasoconstriction and abolition of sweating) or increase heat production (through voluntary skeletal muscle activity, shivering, or nonshivering thermogenesis). This center dissipates heat by activation of sweat glands to increase evaporative loss, peripheral vasodilation, and respiration.

Transient maternal temperature elevations up to 38° C (100.4° F) occur in up to 6.5% of vaginally delivering women during the first 24 hours after delivery. In most women this resolves spontaneously and is secondary to noninfectious causes such as dehydration or a transient bacterial endometritis.[35,49] Maternal fever in the postpartum period may be a sign of puerperal infection, mastitis, endometritis, or urinary tract infection, although these infections are usually the cause of fever after 24 hours. Any temperature elevation merits close monitoring, especially with increasingly early discharge.[4,26,103]

CLINICAL IMPLICATIONS FOR THE PREGNANT WOMAN AND HER FETUS

Fetal Thermoregulation

The fetal ambient environmental temperature is the maternal temperature. Since fetal temperature is linked to maternal temperature and the maternal-fetal thermal gradient, the fetus cannot control its temperature independently Under normal resting conditions, the temperature of the fetus is approximately 0.5° C (0.9° F) higher (range, 0.3° to 1° C) than that of the mother, or about 37.6° to 37.8° C (99.7° to 100.0 °F).[74,109,116] Fetal core and skin temperature and the temperature of amniotic fluid are all similar. The fetal temperature must be higher than the maternal temperature to maintain a gradient to offload heat from the fetus to mother. Fetal heat dissipation is influenced by fetal and placental metabolic activity, thermal diffusion capacity of heat exchange sites within the placenta, and rates of blood flow in the umbilical cord, placental, and intervillous spaces.[74,87]

Heat generated by fetal metabolism is dissipated by the amniotic fluid to the uterine wall (conductive pathway) or via umbilical cord and placenta to maternal blood in the intervillous spaces (convective pathway). The majority (85%) of heat is transferred via the convective pathway through the placenta via the umbilical circulation. The large placental surface area, thin membrane barrier, and high blood flow rate enhance thermal exchange. Transfer of heat is facilitated by the maternal-fetal temperature gradient. If the mother has an elevated temperature (from exercise, illness, or exposure to hot environments such as a sauna), this gradient may be reduced or reversed, leading to an increase in the fetal temperature. Changes in fetal temperature lag behind maternal changes since the amniotic fluid provides some insulation.[57,60]

Fetal heat production and loss mechanisms are suppressed in utero. Fetal temperature is "heat clamped" to the maternal system, preventing the fetus from independent thermoregulation prior to birth.[48,102,116] Fetal responses to cooling are minimal and primarily involve shivering-like muscle contractions and endocrine response. Cooling of the fetus does not activate nonshivering thermogenesis (NST).[95,115] The inability to initiate NST is thought to be linked to placental inhibitors of thermogenin, a protein essential for brown adipose tissue (BAT) metabolism (see Brown Adipose Tissue Metabolism). These placental inhibitors, primarily prostaglandin E_2 and adenosine, decrease rapidly with clamping of the umbilical cord at birth.[43,112,116,134]

The fetal-maternal temperature gradient is sustained during labor, although it may widen with prolonged labor or decrease with compression of the umbilical cord (decreasing blood flow from the fetus and thus the ability of the fetus to dissipate heat).[102,109] If the maternal temperature rises in labor, as often occurs with epidural analgesia, the fetal temperature will also increase.[77,109] In the second and third trimester, increased fetal temperature leads to increased fetal heart rate but not to other thermoregulatory responses. Maternal fever in labor, in noninfected women, has been associated with transient neonatal side effects such as lower Apgar scores and increased need for resuscitation and oxygen at birth.[74,97]

Maternal Hyperthermia and Fever

There has been concern in recent years about the effects of elevated maternal temperature on the fetus. Maternal fever has three potential effects on the fetus: hypoxia secondary to maternal and fetal tachycardia and altered hemodynamics; teratogenesis; and preterm labor either from the fever per se, underlying infection, or associated hemodynamic alterations.[26] Maternal hyperthermia increases maternal oxygen consumption and shifts the oxygen-hemoglobin dissociation curve to the right. Although this latter change increases the oxygen supply to the placenta, fetal oxygen uptake becomes more difficult because of the altered thermal gradient.[57]

Research regarding adverse fetal effects has focused on three causes of maternal temperature elevations: fever secondary to illness, exercise, and the use of saunas or hot tubs. Although animal studies show specific effects of maternal hyperthermia, many of the human studies have been retrospective and suggestive but inconclusive.[22,33,87,66]

Maternal exercise is associated with increased heat production and temperature that may alter the maternal-fetal thermal gradient and fetal heat dissipation. In addition, uterine blood flow decreases during exercise, further altering the ability of the mother to dissipate fetal heat.[57,60,125] The ability of the mother to dissipate the heat generated by exercise may improve as pregnancy progresses.[24,87] The risks from temperature changes during exercise in late pregnancy are related to decreased uterine

TABLE **19-1**   Clinical Recommendations Related to Clinical Practice in Pregnant Women

Counsel pregnant women regarding basis for heat intolerance during pregnancy and intervention strategies (p. 707).

Counsel pregnant women to avoid activities that may lead to hyperthermia (pp. 709-710).

Encourage adequate fluid intake prior to and during exercise (pp. 709-710).

Discourage prolonged exercise especially in a hot, humid environment (pp. 709-710).

Maintain adequate ambient temperature in the delivery area (pp. 707-708).

Protect from cold drafts during delivery (pp. 707-708).

Avoid infusing cold solutions (pp. 707-708).

Avoid contact of maternal skin with wet drapes and towels (pp. 707-708).

Monitor maternal temperature and assess thermoregulatory status during the intrapartum and postpartum periods (pp. 707-709).

Evaluate women with elevated temperatures for signs of infection (p. 709).

blood flow, which can be potentiated by dehydration. Prolonged exercise or exercise in heat (increased ambient heat reduces the thermal gradient between the skin and environment) or high humidity (decreases evaporative heat loss) may result in a higher maternal temperature than exercise in a cool, dry environment or water environment (e.g., aerobic exercise in water).[87,137] Physical conditioning prior to pregnancy can improve thermoregulatory capacity and may decrease the effect of heat stress.[87]

Elevated maternal temperature secondary to illness-induced fever during early pregnancy, especially around the time of neural tube closure (22 to 28 days), has been associated with increased risk of anencephaly, microcephaly, and other central nervous system disorders; alterations in growth; cleft lip; and facial dysmorphogenesis in humans.[22,44,88,144] Whether these disorders are primarily due to the elevated temperature, the underlying infection, or a combination of these events is unclear. In a prospective study, Chambers et al reported a tenfold increase in neural tube defects in women who had a fever of 38.9° C (102° F) or greater lasting for more than 24 hours in the first month of pregnancy.[22] Several studies have reported similar patterns of defects in infants born to women whose extended heat exposure was secondary to sauna or hot tub use, suggesting that an elevated temperature may be the critical factor.[24,22,122] Milunsky et al found that the hot tub exposure posed a greater risk than sauna use, with no risk from electric blanket use.[89] Prospective studies from Finland of sauna use in pregnancy have not shown an increase risk. However, in these studies, maximal temperature was 38.1° C (100.6° F), below the value of 38.9° C (102° F) thought to be critical.[87]

SUMMARY

Alterations in thermal status during pregnancy increase the risk of alterations in fetal health and development. Ongoing assessment and monitoring of thermal status in the pregnant woman and neonate and initiation of appropriate interventions to maintain thermal stability can prevent or minimize these risks. Clinical recommendations related to maternal thermoregulation are summarized in Table 19-1.

NEONATAL PHYSIOLOGY

Thermoregulation is a critical physiologic function in the neonate that is closely linked to the infant's survival and health status.[63,123] An understanding of transitional events and neonatal physiologic adaptations is essential for provision of an appropriate environment to maintain thermal stability. Heat losses are greater and more rapid and can easily exceed heat production in both term and preterm neonates if they are left unclothed in an environment comfortable for an adult. This is because of the infant's larger surface area–to–body mass ratio, decreased insulating subcutaneous fat, increased skin permeability to water, and small radius of curvature of exchange surfaces.[28] Newborns (even most preterm infants) have a relatively well-developed thermoregulatory capacity. Their major thermoregulatory limitation is a narrow control range that makes them more vulnerable to alterations in the thermal environment.[63]

Transitional Events

With birth the fetus moves from the warm intrauterine environment to the colder extrauterine environment. Fetal thermoregulation is linked to the mother, and thermoregulatory processes are suppressed. These processes, especially initiation of NST, must be activated rapidly after birth if the infant is to survive the transition to extrauterine life. Stimulation of cutaneous cold receptors, which activate the sympathetic nervous system with norepinephrine release, and occlusion of the umbilical cord, which removes placental factors that suppress NST, activate BAT metabolism (see Brown Adipose Tissue Metabolism) and heat production.[6,47,48,108,112,134]

Newborns lose heat rapidly after birth, especially through evaporative losses from their moist body surface, as well as via convection (cool air in delivery area) and radiation to cooler room walls. A newborn's temperature may fall 0.2° to 1° C/min.[63] Rutter estimated that in a cool room, the body temperature of a 1000-g preterm infant falls 1° C every 5 minutes.[109] Interventions in the delivery room to reduce evaporative and other losses support transition, reduce cold stress, and have been associated with a higher PO₂ at 1 hour of age, lower mortality, and decreased morbidity.[63,99] An effective way to conserve heat after birth in the healthy term infant is to wrap the infant in a warm, dry towel and either give him or her to the mother for skin-to-skin contact or place him or her under a radiant warmer or in a prewarmed incubator.[40,138] Other interventions are listed in Table 19-2.

The infant's temperature may fall 2° to 3° C after birth, triggering cold-induced metabolic responses and heat production.[20] Term newborns can increase their metabolic rate by 100% by 15 to 30 minutes after birth and 170% at 1 week. This response is delayed in larger preterm infants, who do not approximate term values until 2 to 3 weeks of age; further delay is seen in VLBW infants.[2,70] Thermal transition at birth is interrelated with thyroid function (see Chapter 18).

Heat Transfer

The usual rectal temperature for a newborn is 36.5 to 37.5° C (97.5° to 99.5° F); skin temperature is 36° to 36.5° C (96.8° to 97.5° F) in term infants and 36.2° to 37.2° C (97.2° to 98.7° F) in preterm infants; axillary temperature is 36.5° to 37.3° C (97.5° to 99.1° F).[4,12,83,108,109] Heat transfer involves two interrelated processes: the internal and external gradients. The internal gradient involves transfer of heat from within the body to the surface and relies primarily on blood flow within an extensive capillary and venous plexus. Tissue insulation (subcutaneous fat) and convective movement of heat through blood influence efficiency of heat conduction. Heat conduction can be altered by vasomotor control processes mediated by the sympathetic nervous system that change skin blood flow with peripheral vasoconstriction to conserve heat and vasodilation to eliminate heat.

Heat transfer through the internal gradient is increased in neonates because of their thinner layer of subcutaneous fat (i.e., less insulation) and a larger surface-to-body mass ratio, especially in preterm infants. The subcutaneous layer of insulating fat accounts for only 16% of body fat in infants compared with 30% to 35% in adults.[29] The body mass of the neonate is about 5% of adult mass, whereas the surface area is 15%. In term infants the surface area–to–body mass ratio may be three times, and in preterm infants five times, greater than that of adults.[126] This ratio is even higher in extremely low–birth weight (ELBW) infants. For example, the surface area–to–body mass ratio of a

500-g infant may be six times greater than that of an adult and twice as great as that of a 1500-g infant.[56]

The external gradient involves transfer of heat from the body surface to the environment. The rate of heat loss is directly proportional to the magnitude of the difference between skin temperature and the environmental temperature and can be expressed as: heat loss = h (skin temperature − environmental temperature) × (surface area).[20,98] In this equation, h is the thermal transfer coefficient (the rate at which heat leaves the body surface) and is influenced by body size, tissue conductance, skin blood flow, and vasoactivity.[98] Heat loss per unit of body mass is inversely proportional to body size.[20] The mechanisms by which heat is transferred from the body surface are conduction, convection, radiation, and evaporation.

Heat transfer by the external gradient is also increased in the neonate because of increased surface area and an increased thermal transfer coefficient.[98] In terms of heat loss, the amount of exposed surface area is most critical; thus an infant who is not in an incubator or radiant warmer will lose less heat if he or she is diapered or swaddled. Factors that increase the thermal transfer coefficient (and thus heat loss), such as decreased skin thickness and altered conductance, are present in the neonate. The threshold for heat production in the newborn is more closely linked to skin temperature than in the adult. As a result, cold responses, especially in preterm infants, are related primarily to skin rather than core temperature changes.[20]

Heat Production and Conservation

Heat production is a result of metabolic processes that generate energy by oxidative metabolism of glucose, fats, and proteins. The amount of metabolic heat produced varies with activity, feeding (calorigenic or specific dynamic action), state (greater heat is produced in awake than sleep and in active versus deep sleep), health status, and environmental temperature.[20,113] Organs that generate the greatest amount of metabolic energy are the brain, heart, and liver. To maintain a constant body temperature, heat production must equal heat loss from the body surface over a given time. Basal heat production to maintain this stability is generated by body metabolic processes. In the event of cold stress, heat above basal needs can be generated by physical or chemical mechanisms. Because of their surface area to body mass ratio (which is an important determinant of heat loss), heat production in infants is low relative to heat loss.[109] In the term infant, heat production at rest (estimated by oxygen consumption) in a thermoneutral environment is similar to that of adults per unit of weight, but approximately half that of the adult per

TABLE **19-2**   Prevention of Heat Loss and Overheating in the Neonate

Mechanisms	Sources of Heat Loss/Overheating	Interventions
Conduction	Cool mattress, blanket, scale, table, x-ray plate, or clothing	Place warm blankets on scales, x-ray plates, and other surfaces in contact with the infant.
		Warm blankets and clothing before use.
		Preheat incubators, radiant warmers, and heat shields.
	Heating pads, hot water bottles, chemical bags	Avoid placing infant on any surface or object that is warmer than the infant.
Convection	Cool room, corridors, or outside air	Maintain the room temperature at levels adequate to provide a safe thermal environment for the infant (72° to 76° F).
		Transport the infant in an enclosed, warmed incubator through internal hallways and between external environments (e.g., ambulance to nursery).
		Open incubator portholes only when necessary and for brief periods.
		Use plastic sleeves on portholes.
		Swaddle with warm blankets (unless under radiant warmer) or stretch transparent plastic across the infant between the radiant warmer side guards; use caps with adequate insulation quality or hooded blankets.
	Convective air flow incubator	Monitor the incubator temperature to avoid temperatures warmer than the infant's body temperature.
	Drafts from air vents, windows, doors, heaters, fans, and air conditioners	Place infants away from air vents, drafts, and other sources of moving air particles.
		Use side guards on radiant warmers to decrease cross-current air flow across infant; stretch transparent plastic across the infant between the radiant warmer side guards.
	Cold oxygen flow (especially near facial thermal receptors)	Warm oxygen and monitor the temperature inside the oxygen hood
Evaporation	Wet body surface and hair in the delivery room or from bathing	Dry the infant, especially the head, immediately after birth with a warm blanket or towel.
		Use caps with adequate insulation quality or hooded blankets.
		Replace wet blankets with dry, warm ones and place in a warm environment.
		Delay the initial bath until the infant's temperature has stabilized, then give a sponge bath.
		Bathe the infant in a warm, draft-free environment, place on warmed towels and dry immediately; bathe under a radiant warmer.
	Application of lotions, solutions, wet packs, or soaks to the infant	Prewarm solutions and soaks; maintain warmth during use.
		Avoid overheating solutions and soaks.
	Water loss from lungs	Warm and humidify oxygen.
	Increased insensible water loss in very-low–birth-weight (VLBW) or ill infants	Remember that increased incubator humidity levels may be necessary, especially in dry climates or with VLBW infants.
Radiation	Placement near cold or hot external windows or walls; placement in direct sunlight	Place incubators, cribs, and radiant warmers away from external walls and windows and direct sunlight.
		Use thermal shades on external windows.
		Line the incubator with aluminum foil.
	Cold incubator walls	Use double-walled incubators or heat shields, or cover with plastic film.
		Prewarm incubators, radiant warmers, and heat shields,
	Heat lamps	Avoid use whenever possible; if used, monitor temperature every 10 to 15 minutes to avoid burns.

unit of surface area. This is further decreased in preterm infants, who have an even greater surface area to body mass ratio.[109]

Physical mechanisms include involuntary (shivering) and voluntary muscular activity. Shivering is the most important mechanism for the generation of additional heat in adults. The neonate uses physical methods (shivering and increased muscular activity) to some extent to generate additional heat. Shivering, which is controlled via the somatomotor system, is not as important in the neonate as in the adult, and the shivering threshold is probably at a lower body temperature.[21] Shivering in neonates is primarily seen as a late event associated with decreased spinal cord temperature after prolonged cold exposure. The cervical spinal region is protected from cold stress and preferentially receives heat generated by NST through metabolism of BAT in the intrascapular area. If NST is blocked or the infant is unable to generate adequate heat to compensate for severe or prolonged cold stress, the temperature of the spinal cord eventually decreases.[20]

Infants produce some heat by increasing muscular activity with restlessness, hyperactivity, or crying. Infants may try to conserve heat by postural changes such as flexion that reduce the surface area and heat loss through the internal gradient. The ability to produce heat by physical methods can be markedly reduced or obliterated with the use of anesthetics, muscle relaxants, sedatives, or tight restraints and in infants with brain injury.[3,12,20,25,29]

Heat can be generated by chemical or NST through increased metabolic rate and, in neonates, BAT metabolism. Both infants and adults can generate heat by increasing their metabolic rate above basal levels. An adult can increase heat production by 10% to 15% by NST; the neonate can have an increase of 100% or more.[49] NST is mediated by epinephrine in the adult and by norepinephrine in the neonate.[124] This results in activation of an adipose tissue lipase and splitting of triglycerides into glycerol and nonesterified fatty acids (NEFA), which are oxidized to produce heat, esterified to form triglycerides, or released into the circulation.[120,124,136] NST is triggered when the mean skin temperature falls to 35° to 36° C (95° to 96.8° F).[120]

NST is the major mechanism through which the infant produces heat above basal needs. Increasing the metabolic rate may lead to further problems in immature or compromised neonates, since any increase in metabolic rate increases oxygen consumption. Stressed infants may be unable to provide enough oxygen; oxygen debt with lactic acidosis from anaerobic metabolism and finally exhaustion can result.

Thermal receptors in the skin are important mediators of the hypothalamic thermal center's response to temperature changes or cold stress. Stimulation of these receptors initially leads to heat-conserving responses with peripheral vasoconstriction. This may lead to acrocyanosis in the neonate. In the infant, thermal receptors are most prominent and sensitive over the trigeminal area of the face. For example, cooling the face of an infant who is normothermic causes a responsive rise in metabolic rate. Conversely, warming the facial skin (i.e., use of warmed oxygen in an oxygen hood) when an infant is cold may suppress the usual increase in metabolic rate and other heat-generating mechanisms and can be dangerous.[98]

Brown Adipose Tissue Metabolism

The neonate relies primarily on BAT metabolism for NST. Large amounts of BAT are found in human and animal newborns, hibernators, and in adult animals after cold acclimatization.[29,91,136] Small amounts of BAT remain in the human adult and can be found around the kidneys and possibly the great vessels. However, with increasing age, most BAT deposits are replaced by white adipose tissue.[104] In the adult, BAT produces minimal energy. In the term newborn, BAT accounts for 2% to 7% of the infant's weight.[20] The major function of BAT is heat production. BAT is found in the midscapular region; nape of the neck; around the neck muscles extending under the clavicles into the axillae; in the mediastinum; and around the trachea, esophagus, heart, lungs, liver, intercostal and mammary arteries; abdominal aorta; kidneys; and adrenal glands. The largest deposits of BAT are around the kidneys and adrenals, with smaller amounts around the great vessels, extending to the neck and from the thoracic cavity to the axillae and clavicles.[29,36] The total amount of heat produced by BAT metabolism in the neonate is unknown, but it may account for nearly 100% of the infant's needs.

BAT cells begin to differentiate by 26 to 30 weeks' gestation and continue developing until 3 to 5 weeks after birth. BAT stores increase up to 150% during this time and account for one tenth of the adipose tissue in term infants.[124] BAT stores are lower in preterm and minimal in VLBW infants.

In appearance and composition, BAT is markedly different from white adipose tissue (Table 19-3).[20,29,91,104,124,136] These characteristics promote rapid metabolism, heat production, and heat transfer to the peripheral circulation. The lipolysis rate in BAT is three times higher than in white adipose tissue.[136] The unique structure of BAT gives it the ability to generate more energy than any other tissue in the body.[36]

TABLE **19-3**   Characteristics of Brown Adipose Tissue and their Significance

CHARACTERISTIC	SIGNIFICANCE
Many small fat vacuoles	Large fat-to-cytoplasm ratio, enhancing the rapidity of fat use
Many mitochondria	Production of energy (i.e., adenosine triphosphate [ATP]) for rapid metabolic turnover and heat production
Glycogen stores	Source of glucose for production of ATP and energy
Abundant blood supply	Brings nutrients to cell and transports heat produced to other areas of the body
Abundant sympathetic nerve supply	Metabolism of brown adipose tissue mediated by norepinephrine

Compiled from references 20, 29, 91, 104, 124, and 136.

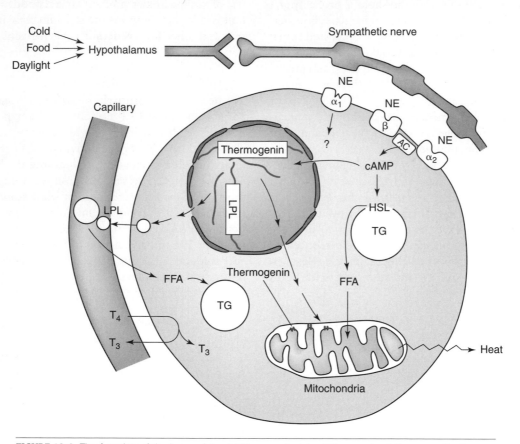

FIGURE **19-2** The function of the brown fat cell. When postnatal cold is perceived, the sympathetic nervous system is activated, and released norepinephrine (NE) interacts with adrenergic receptors, leading to the release of fatty acids that are combusted in the mitochondria. This combustion is possible as a result of the presence of the uncoupling protein thermogenin. Further substrate is provided by action of lipoprotein lipase. Brown adipose tissue may also produce triiodothyronine (T_3) from thyroxine (T_4), leading to local and systemic effects. *AC,* Adenylyl cyclase; *cAMP,* cyclic adenosine monophosphate; *FFA,* free fatty acids; *HSL,* hormone-sensitive lipase; *LPL,* lipoprotein lipase; *TG,* triglycerides. (From Nedergaard, J. & Cannon, B. (1998). Brown adipose tissue: Development and function. In R.A. Polin & W.W. Fox [Eds.]. *Fetal and neonatal physiology* [2nd ed.]. Philadelphia: W.B. Saunders.)

Heat production within the BAT cell is regulated by an uncoupling protein (UCP) called *thermogenin* (Figure 19-2) located along the inner membrane of brown adipocyte mitochondria. UCP permits protons to pass across the mitochondrial membrane without the need to conserve energy. UCP uncouples oxidative phosphorylation; thus more energy is used for heat and less is conserved for adenosine triphosphate (ATP) regeneration.[21,76,91,116,120]

Activation of UCP is controlled by the hypothalamus. The sympathetic nervous system and hormonal mediators control BAT metabolism. Changes in temperature are transmitted from peripheral cutaneous receptors to the posterior hypothalamus (see Figure 19-1). The sympathetic nervous system is stimulated to release norepinephrine within BAT stores and to stimulate catecholamine release from the adrenal medulla.

Norepinephrine released at the surface of the brown adipocytes interacts with α_1-, β_1-, and β_3-adrenergic receptors to increase cyclic adenosine monophosphate (AMP). The cAMP activates lipolysis of triglycerides and phospholipids within the brown adipocytes. The free fatty acids released activate UCP.[76,104] This process is enhanced by triiodothyronine (T_3) and thyroxine (T_4), which increase thermogenin levels. The thyroid gland is also stimulated by the pituitary release of thyroid-stimulating hormone to produce T_4. T_4 enhances the effect of norepinephrine on the BAT cells and may also act directly on BAT.[20,29,36] Prior to birth, placental PGE_2 and adenosine block this catecholamine-induced increase in cAMP that is needed to initiate NST.[76,112,134] Occlusion of the umbilical cord with cord clamping removes this inhibition.

Production of heat from BAT metabolism involves breakdown of triglycerides into glycerol and NEFAs. Approximately 30% of the NEFAs are oxidized, with formation of energy and metabolic heat. Since oxidation of NEFA is dependent on the availability of oxygen, glucose, and ATP, the ability of the neonate to generate heat can be altered by pathologic events such as hypoxia, acidosis, and hypoglycemia.

Heat Dissipation and Loss

The neonate can dissipate heat by peripheral vasodilation or by sweating. As the infant's core temperature rises above 37.3° C (99.1° F), cutaneous blood flow and skin thermal conductance increase along with heat loss through the external gradient.[129,130]

Sweating increases evaporative loss. Each milliliter of water evaporated results in 0.58 cal of heat loss.[98] Term infants can increase evaporative losses up to 100% but are less effective at sweating than adults.[81] Although the density of sweat glands is six times greater in the neonate, the capacity of these glands is only about one third of adult values.[39] Sweat appears first on the infant's forehead, generally beginning after 35 to 40 minutes of exposure to an ambient temperature above 37° C (98.6° F) and rectal temperature greater than 37.2° C (98.7° F). By 70 to 75 minutes, evaporative water losses increase four times. In the term small-for-gestational-age (SGA) infant, the onset of sweating is slower (55 to 60 minutes), but evaporative losses increase more rapidly to five times basal levels.[129]

Sweating is also altered in infants with central nervous system dysfunction and in preterm infants. In preterm newborns over 30 weeks' gestation, the onset of sweating is delayed. SGA infants demonstrate thermoregulatory potential similar to that in infants of comparable gestations but are limited by their body size. Infants of mothers on opiates such as heroin and methadone may have early maturation of sweating.[109] In preterm infants the maximal rate of sweating is less than that of either term or SGA infants.[129] Sweating is minimal or nonexistent in infants of less than 30 weeks' gestation because of inadequate development of sweat glands.[39] Even without large numbers of functional sweat glands, these infants have significant transepidermal water and heat losses (see Chapter 13).[51,120] These losses are significantly increased in infants cared for in a radiant warmer or receiving phototherapy. Neonates also lose heat by radiation, conduction, and convection (discussed in the next section).

CLINICAL IMPLICATIONS FOR NEONATAL CARE

Prevention of cold stress and hypothermia is critical for the intact survival of the neonate. Lowered body temperatures are inversely correlated with survival, especially in VLBW infants.[12,63,98,103] Exposure to cool environments and subsequent cold stress often result in physiologic changes that significantly alter the infant's health status. Major components of neonatal care include maintenance of infant thermoregulatory processes, provision of an appropriate thermal environment, and prevention of heat loss, hypothermia, and cold stress.

Neutral Thermal Environment

Body temperature and oxygen consumption are closely related. As the body temperature falls, the amount of oxygen needed for survival increases rapidly. Oxygen consumption is minimal in two thermal regions: the neutral thermal environment and with severe hypothermia (Figure 19-3). The neutral thermal environment (thermoneutrality) is an idealized setting defined as a range of ambient temperatures within which the body temperature is normal, metabolic rate is minimal, and thermoregulation is achieved by basal nonevaporative physical processes alone.[20,28,110,117] Within this range the person is in thermal equilibrium with the environment (Figure 19-4). Since all newborns lose fluid through their skin continuously, evaporative loss is always present. Darnell proposes the following clinical definition of thermoneutrality for infants: "that environment (usually a range of air temperatures in an incubator or abdominal skin temperature under a radiant warmer) in which the infant, when quiet or asleep, is not required to increase heat production above 'resting' levels to maintain body temperature."[28] Figure 19-3 illustrates the relationships between thermoneutrality, body temperature, and metabolism.

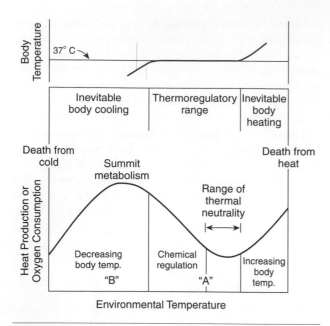

FIGURE 19-3 Effects of environmental temperature on oxygen consumption and body temperature. (From Klaus, M.H., Fanaroff, A.A., & Martin, R.J. [2001]. The physical environment. In M.H. Klaus & A.A. Fanaroff [Eds.]. *Care of the high-risk neonate*. [5th ed.]. Philadelphia: W.B. Saunders.)

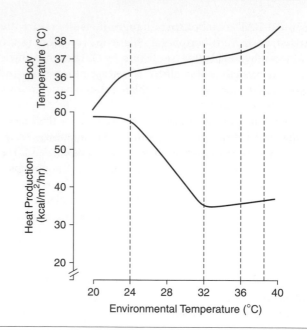

FIGURE 19-4 The effect of environmental temperature on heat production and body temperature of a 1.9 kg infant of 34 weeks' gestation, nursed naked in surroundings of uniform temperature and moderate humidity. Between 32° and 36° C heat production is minimal, there is no sweating, and body temperature is normal (neutral thermal range). When the environmental temperature exceeds 36° C, the infant sweats, and above 38° C, body temperature rises rapidly. Below 32° C, heat production increases by non-shivering thermogenesis, but below 24° C, heat production has reached its maximum and body temperature rapidly falls. (From Rutter, N. [1999]. Temperature control and its disorders. In J.M. Rennie & N.R.C. Robertson [Eds.]. *Textbook of neonatology* [3rd ed.]. London: Churchill Livingstone.)

In the thermoneutral state an infant is neither gaining nor losing heat, oxygen consumption is minimal, and the core-to-skin temperature gradient is small. A normal skin or core temperature does not necessarily mean that the infant is in a thermal neutral zone, since an infant may be maintaining that temperature by increasing metabolic rate and BAT metabolism. Thus body temperature is not a very sensitive indicator of neutral thermal environment stability.[109]

Thermoneutrality is generally achieved at environmental temperatures of 25° to 30° C (77° to 86° F) in the adult, at 32° to 33.5° C (89.6° to 92.3° F) in the term infant, at 34° to 35° C (93.2° to 95° F) in preterm infants at 30 weeks (1500 g), and at higher temperatures in more immature infants.[20,109,124] Environmental conditions that do not tax an adult may require increased metabolic work by the neonate. The thermoneutral range is narrowest for infants of lowest birth weight.[87] Guidelines for determining neutral thermal zones for infants of varying ages and weights are available.[52,63,85,98,117] These guidelines were developed for healthy infants at set environmental conditions and must be used in conjunction with evaluation of the temperature of the incubator walls and external environment; humidity; air velocity; posture; clothing; infant weight; health status and activity level; and, especially in the first week, gesta-

tional age.[98,109,110] These guidelines are not appropriate for ELBW infants because these infants require higher neutral temperatures because of increased evaporative losses.[50,82,106] The most immature infant may require an environmental temperature equal to or higher than skin and core temperature.[98] Hey and Katz provide a formula for increasing ambient temperature if incubator wall and air temperatures are unequal: Operative temperature for T (neutral) = 0.4 T (air) + 0.6 T (wall).[52]

Preterm infants cared for in environments outside the thermoneutral zone do not grow as well as infants with similar caloric intakes cared for in a thermoneutral environment.[42] VLBW infants may respond to temperatures outside the thermoneutral zone by a change in body temperature unaccompanied by an increase in oxygen consumption. Data indicate that there may not be a thermoneutral range for extremely preterm infants. The very high transepidermal water losses in these infants seem to be the major factor in determining their appropriate thermal environment.[82] Sauer and associates propose a redefinition of the neutral thermal environment for VLBW infants as "the ambient temperature at which the core temperature of the infant at rest is between 36.7° and 37.3° C (98.1° to 99.1° F) and the core and mean skin temperatures are changing less than 0.2° and 0.3° C an hour respectively."[110] Perlstein has estimated that an infant is in a minimal metabolic state if the incubator environment is less than 2.5° C cooler than the infant's skin temperature. Since it is difficult to determine environmental temperature, he suggests that for a rough estimate in a single wall incubator, one can assume that the incubator temperature is approximately 1° C cooler than the incubator air for each 7° C gradient between the incubator and nursery ambient temperature.[98]

Use of a neutral thermal environment in the early weeks after birth is associated with smaller feeding and caloric requirements.[63,120] However, Klaus et al suggest that as infants get ready for discharge, they may need opportunities for a less optimal temperatures as preparation for developing cold resistance needed for the home environment.[63]

Prevention of Heat Loss and Excessive Heat Gain

The four mechanisms by which heat is transferred to and from the body surface are conduction, convection, radiation, and evaporation. Examples of each mechanism in the neonate and appropriate interventions are listed in Table 19-2.

Conduction

Conduction involves transfer of heat from the body core to the surface through body tissue and from the body surface to objects in contact with the body (mattress, clothing, and scales). The rate at which heat is transferred is directly proportional to the size of the temperature gradient.[9] Conductive loss can be minimized through insulation such as blankets or clothing or through skin-to-skin contact and is increased by placing the infant on conductive surfaces such as metal.[40] The 1-inch foam rubber mattress used in most incubators and radiant warmers has a low conductivity. Room temperature blankets and mattresses can be associated with significant heat loss, especially in the preterm infant, and must be warmed before use.[67,69]

Heat can also be transferred from an object to the infant through conduction. Thus, if an infant is placed on a heated pad or hot water bottle that is warmer than the infant, hyperthermia or burns can develop.[80] Heat is also conducted to the surrounding stable air (boundary layer) in direct contact with the infant's body. This form of heat loss is minimal unless the air around the infant is moving such that the warmed air is constantly being replaced with cooler air, leading to convective losses.[49]

Convection

With convective losses, heat is dissipated from the interior of the body to the skin surface through the blood, conducted from the body surface to surrounding air (boundary layer), and carried away by diffusion to moving air particles (drafts, colder room or outside air) at the skin surface. Natural or passive convection involves movement of heat molecules into the boundary layer and then gradually away from the infant. Forced convection occurs when a mass of air is physically moving over the infant, conveying heat away from the body.[9,70] Transfer is dependent on ambient temperature, air flow velocity, and relative humidity (which determines the air's thermal density). In low birth weight (LBW) infants, convective losses are increased by the shorter radius of curvature of the body surface.[130] Heat can be lost by convective means through transfer of warmed inspired air to colder exterior air (or unheated oxygen) through exhalation. During resuscitation, use of cool oxygen (which removes warm carbon dioxide from the lungs) can decrease body temperature.[63] Measurements of air temperature should be made close to the infant's skin surface, since air temperature within an incubator or between incubator and hood temperatures may vary.

Convective losses are increased at higher air-flow velocities.[70] This is known as the wind-chill factor and may also be induced by incubator air circulation or gas flow into an oxygen hood. Environments with higher air temperatures and minimal air circulation can reduce convective loss by up to two thirds.[124] Heat can also be gained by convection if ambient temperature is higher than the infant's skin temperature. Incubators use this principle to warm infants by circulating warm air around the infant.

Convective heat losses can be minimized by swaddling or using caps on infants in cribs, warming oxygen, and placing infants away from drafts or air vents (see Table 19-2). Warming of oxygen used in oxygen hoods is essential because of the sensitivity of the thermal receptors in the trigeminal area. If the infant's environment is well heated below the neck but cool around the face, the infant will react as if cold stressed. This can lead to metabolic alterations and hyperthermia.[98] If the infant's face is warmer than the body, apnea may result.

Evaporation

Evaporative heat loss occurs as moisture on the body surface or respiratory tract mucosa vaporizes. These losses depend on air speed and relative humidity.[50,93,133] Evaporative loss is the major source of heat loss immediately after delivery or during bathing, accounting for up to 25% of the total heat loss.[126] A wet newborn in the delivery room loses heat and lowers his or her skin temperature at a rate of 0.3 °C/min (0.5 °F/min) and rectal temperature by 0.1° C/min (0.2° F/min). This change is equivalent to a temperature loss of 3° C (5° F) over 10 minutes.[120]

Evaporative losses are correlated with gestational age. Transepidermal water loss (TEWL) is up to six times higher per unit of surface area in VLBW infants than in term infants.[106] In immature infants, higher evaporative loss due to poor skin resistance to water passage from a lack of skin keratinization within the stratum corneum (see Chapter 13) constitutes a significant portion of overall heat loss (Figure 19-5).[12] The stratum corneum normally provides the greatest resistance to diffusion of water from the skin. In the term newborn the keratin in the stratum corneum creates resistance to water diffusion that is 1000 times greater than the resistance of the dermis.[84] In VLBW infants, evaporative losses in the first days exceed all other sources of heat loss and often exceed heat production.[10,70] VLBW infants may lose up to 120 ml/kg/day through skin water loss. This represents a loss of up to 72 kcal/kg/day, a significant portion of the infant's total caloric intake.[34] However, the degree of TEWL depends on the humidity, so infants in environments with greater humidity will lose less water and calories. For example, TEWL at 85% to 95% humidity is approximately 10% that at 50% humidity.[84] Evaporative insensible water loss (IWL) increases with activity and tachypnea, under radiant warmers, or with phototherapy (see Chapter 17).[56] Rapid maturation of the skin occurs in the first few weeks after birth in infants of all gestational ages, reducing the degree of TEWL (see Chapter 13). However, even at 4 weeks of age, TEWL is still twice as high in preterm versus term infants.[50] The term and older preterm infant can increase evaporative losses via the skin by sweating in response to a warm environment.[109]

Evaporative losses may be minimized by drying infants immediately after delivery or bathing, the use of sponge baths, warming soaks and solutions, use of polyethylene wraps, and warming and humidifying oxygen (see Table 19-2). In term and preterm infants the evaporative heat loss is inversely proportional to the partial pressure of water vapor.[70,111] The neutral thermal environment temperature has been calculated to be reduced approximately 0.5° C for each 1 mm increase in water vapor pressure.[120] Increasing relative humidity reduces evaporative losses; at a relative humidity of 100%, evaporative loss is nonexistent.[128,130] Incubator humidity levels may need to be increased to reduce evaporative losses in VLBW infants. These infants may have subnormal temperatures in spite of incubator temperatures above their body temperatures. The elevated air temperature reduces convective and radiant losses but does little to reduce the extremely high transepidermal evaporative loss in these infants.[82] Vapor pressure increases with higher temperatures, so as long as the infant's skin is warmer than the environment, evaporative losses can occur even with 100% humidity.[98]

Evaporative losses also increase with turbulent air currents, as can occur with hoods or higher air velocities. Thus using incubators with lower air speeds or heat shields closed at one end can also reduce evaporative loss. Evaporative water losses in infants under radiant warmers can be reduced by stretching a layer of plastic wrap or bubble wrap around the infant or across the infant between the side guards of the radiant warmer, which can reduce IWL up to 75%.[9,10,11,27,109] Hey and Scopes estimate that increasing the humidity of the VLBW infant by 50% is similar to increasing the ambient temperature 1.5° C.[12] Rutter recommends use of humidity in the first week after birth for infants less than 30 weeks' gestation and less than 1000 g.[108]

Evaporative losses can also be reduced by use of epidermal barriers and emollients. Semiocclusive polyurethane dressings (e.g., Tegaderm, Op-Site) and topical petroleum-based, preservative-free emollients (Aquaphor) have been used to decrease both IWL and evaporative heat loss in VLBW infants.[12,64,92,101,139] Concerns with use of these barriers include skin irritation, infection, and absorption by the permeable skin of the VLBW infant.

Radiation

The major form of heat loss in infants in incubators is radiation. Radiation involves the transfer of radiant energy

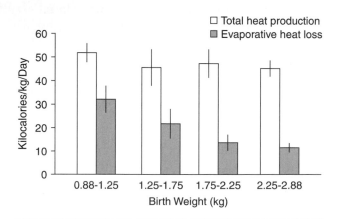

FIGURE **19-5** The relative role of evaporative heat loss at different birth weights. (From Klaus, M.H., Fanaroff, A.A., & Martin, R.J. [1993]. The physical environment. In M.H. Klaus & A.A. Fanaroff [Eds.]. *Care of the high-risk neonate* [3rd ed.]. Philadelphia: W.B. Saunders.)

from the body surface (through absorbance and emission of infrared rays) to surrounding cooler or warmer surfaces (walls, windows, heat lamps, light bulbs) not in contact with the infant. The rate of transfer depends on the temperature gradient, surface absorption, and geometry (the amount and angle of the infant's surface area facing the object).[9,70] Radiant heat losses are independent of ambient temperature, air speed and other heat loss mechanisms.[124] The infant can also gain heat by radiation, which is the principle of radiant warmers in which the (cooler) infant is placed under the warm radiant heat source.

Regulating incubator temperature only does not prevent heat loss by radiation. Thus infants can get cold in a room containing air warmer than the infant if the walls and windows are cold. Infants in warm incubators can be cold stressed if they radiate body heat to cooler incubator walls or cooler windows and walls or to the cool outside air during transport. The amount of radiant loss is related to the temperatures of the window and walls rather than the temperature of the air in the incubator. Conversely, a baby in a cool incubator can get overheated if the incubator walls or room windows or walls are too hot.[12,63,94]

Incubators tend to act as greenhouses by trapping heat. The acrylic walls of the incubator are opaque to infrared rays. The walls allow short light waves to enter the incubator and subsequently the infant's body. The infant converts the short waves to heat and re-emits them as longer infrared rays. Since these rays cannot escape from the incubator, they heat the incubator and then the infant ("greenhouse effect"). Infants in incubators can become hyperthermic even if they are not subjected to obvious heating and without a change in incubator temperature.[124] Radiant heat losses can be reduced by placing vulnerable infants away from the cooler exterior walls and windows, and by the use of thermal shades and heat shields or double-walled incubators. Overheating of infants by radiation can be prevented by placing infants away from windows and walls that are warmer than the infant and by avoiding or carefully monitoring the use of heat lamps.[12,63,94]

Monitoring Temperature

Neonatal temperature is usually monitored by rectal, skin, or axillary measurements, and by manual or servocontrol methods. Other methods occasionally used include tympanic and inguinal temperatures. Electronic and infrared thermometers have both predictive (algorithm predicts temperature after 60 seconds) and manual (probe is held in place until the temperature stabilizes) modes.[33,73] The mean length of time for manual modes is 3 minutes, although many infants require longer times. All sites are in-

fluenced by environmental temperature.[27,31,73] Studies of use of infrared tympanic temperature in neonates have demonstrated moderate correlations with skin and rectal measurements but wide variability in measurements, poor sensitivity for fever detection, and higher temperatures in infants cared for in radiant warmers.[55,73] Tympanic measurements are influenced by local metabolism, blood temperature, air movement, and temperature of the external auditory canal.[73,132]

Rectal temperature provides an approximation of core temperature. The reading varies depending on the depth of insertion, with greatest variation found in the first 3 cm. The reading is higher as the depth of insertion increases. For example, increasing the depth of insertion from 1 to 5 cm may result in a variation in temperature of up to 1.5° C.[98] Shallow insertion may give falsely low reading because blood from the legs circulates in venous plexuses around the anus. If used, the thermometer should be inserted downward and backward at a 30-degree angle to a depth of 3 cm in a term infant and 2 cm in a preterm infant.[61,109] Because of the risks of rectal temperatures, including trauma, perforation, and cross-contamination with repeated insertions, routine use is rare and other methods are preferred.

Axillary temperatures are noninvasive and approximate core temperature. Although axillary and rectal temperatures are correlated in neonates, reported mean differences have ranged from −0.05° C (axillary higher) to +0.55° C (rectal higher).[13,19,85,115] The optimal length of time to obtain an accurate assessment of temperature with axillary measurement using a mercury glass thermometer carefully placed in the axilla is 3 to 5 minutes in most studies, but the length of time can range up to 11 minutes.[73,85,118,127,135]

In a cold environment, core temperature may not indicate thermal stability. In a cold-stressed infant, the core temperature may be within normal limits because the infant has successfully compensated by increasing chemical thermogenesis. By the time the rectal temperature falls, the infant may be significantly compromised and difficult to rewarm.[98] Skin temperature measurement is frequently used with preterm and other neonates at risk for thermoregulatory problems. Skin temperature changes provide an early indication of cold or heat stress (Figure 19-6) since an early mechanism to preserve body heat is peripheral vasoconstriction detected by measuring skin temperature.[63]

Thermocouplers or thermistors must be carefully placed since skin temperature can vary widely. The best area for probe placement is not known, although sites usually recommended in textbooks are the skin surface over the liver, between the umbilicus and pubis, or the back in a prone infant. Another method that has been

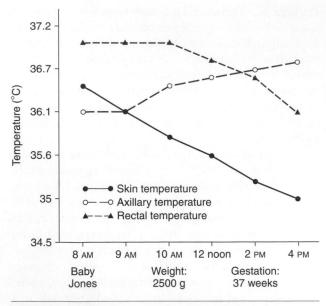

FIGURE **19-6** Temperature measurement at various sites during cold stress. In an environment that is less than thermal neutral, cold stress begins as skin temperature decreases (9 AM) because of vasoconstriction of the skin. Axillary temperature increases (10 AM) as the infant burns brown adipose tissue to keep warm. Rectal temperature is unchanged because the core temperature is maintained. At noon the infant is still cold stressed (decreased skin temperature), and axillary temperature is up as the infant continues to compensate (burns brown adipose tissue). Rectal temperature is still in the normal range. From 2 PM to 4 PM, the skin temperature reflects severe cold stress; the axilla is warm but the baby is cold, and rectal temperature (core temperature) falls as the body decompensates (severe cold stress). (From Merenstein, G.B. & Gardner, S.L. [1989]. *Handbook of neonatal intensive care* [2nd ed.]. St. Louis: Mosby.)

used involves placing the probe between the mattress and the infant's skin. Commonly suggested sites to avoid are areas of BAT, poorly vasoreactive areas, and excoriated or bruised areas or near transcutaneous gas monitoring transducers.[16,100] However, there have been few probe placement site studies to determine either the best areas or which areas to avoid. Differences have been reported between various sites used for probe placement, with lower temperatures in sites not exposed to radiant heat.[73,100] Lying on the probe may raise temperature by increasing skin insulation and lead to variable skin temperatures with repositioning.[100]

Disadvantages of skin temperature include accidental displacement of the probe, risk of skin irritation, misleading values with rapid temperature changes, and artifacts altering accuracy of measurement.[4,12,100] Artifacts that can alter readings include inadvertent insulation of the probe and the underlying skin; partial loss of skin contact with the probe; radiant or convective heating or cooling of the probe; increased probe temperature if covered with clothing or blankets or if the infant is lying on the probe (producing falsely high readings); and alteration in evaporative loss in skin covered with probes, especially with use of probe covers so that the temperature of the skin under the probe may be different than the skin temperature at other sites.[4,16,18,69,98,109,114,132] Insulated probes provide different information from exposed probes.[98,132] Insulated probes may result in probe temperatures greater than skin temperatures in either a radiant warmer or incubator and have been reported to alter incubator servocontrol with lower incubator temperatures and a higher skin-to-environment temperature gradient.[98,109,132] Therefore it is important to follow the manufacturer's directions regarding the type of probe and probe covers.

Servocontrol. Servocontrol methods have been used with increasing frequency to maintain an infant's temperature within specified ranges. Types of servocontrol include air servocontrol and infant servocontrol using proportional control units.[17] Air and skin servocontrol produce different thermal environments and may have different effects on emerging infant biorhythms.[18,132] Air servocontrol tends to provide a more stable thermal environment with greater infant temperature variability, whereas skin servocontrol leads to greater variability in air temperature but is more effective in maintaining an NTE.[79,121,132] With infant servocontrol, the temperature from either a skin or rectal probe (not currently recommended) is electronically monitored and used to control heater output decisions in either a convectively heated incubator or radiant warmer. Considerations related to use of skin probes and probe artifacts are discussed in the preceding section. Risks of servocontrol include hyperthermia if the probe becomes detached or is left in the manual mode, and failure to detect early signs of sepsis since alterations in body temperature are masked.

Servocontrol is less effective in immature infants because of their higher evaporative water losses. The servocontrol system is based on the assumption that the temperature of the skin under the probe represents that of the surrounding skin; however, attaching the probe to the skin reduces evaporative losses at the site where temperature is being monitored. Thus the servocontrol system may record skin temperatures that are higher than that of the rest of the infant's body and fail to keep the infant warm.[12,98] Increasing humidity may reduce these differences. Opening of the portholes may get an overdampening of the servocontrol system, with under- or overshooting of the air temperature for up to 1 hour later.[12]

TABLE **19-4**   Mechanisms of Supporting Thermoregulation in the Very-Low–Birth-Weight Infant

METHOD OF CONTROL	ADVANTAGES	DISADVANTAGES
RADIATION		
Radiant warmer	Infant is easily accessible	Large insensible water loss
	Efficient and powerful	Room drafts may cool infant
	Accommodates change rapidly	Dislodged temperature probe may cause overheating or cooling
Heat shield	Keeps infant visible	Decreases access
Double-walled incubator	Maintains access and visibility	Less efficient than other methods
CONVECTION		
Air-controlled incubator	Maintains steady environmental temperature	Water reservoir may promote bacterial growth
	Easy, safe	Does not regulate to infant's needs
	Provides humidity	Air temperature fluctuated when care delivered
	Maintains thermoneutral state at lower ambient temperature	
Skin-controlled incubator	Maintains set skin temperature	Displaced probe can cause temperature fluctuations
	Provides humidity	Air temperature fluctuates when care delivered
	Easy, safe	Water reservoir may promote bacteria growth
Warm room temperature	Easily maintained	May be uncomfortable for staff and parents who wear gowns
CONDUCTION		
Heating pad	Rapid	May cause burns
	Use in transport when other methods less efficient	Can be used only in combination with other methods
		Warming equipment may be cumbersome
Prewarmed linens	Easy	Time-consuming
EVAPORATION		
Head and body wraps	Inexpensive	Interferes with direct observation of all body surfaces
	Can maintain care by unwrapping only what is needed	Does not aid and may prevent rewarming of infant
Skin protection (e.g., barriers, creams, ointments)	No interference with observation or care	Can cause skin irritation
		Maybe source of infection

From Brueggemeyer, A. (1995) Thermoregulation. In L.P. Gunderson & C. Kenner (Eds.). *Care of the 24-25 week gestational age infant: Small baby protocol* (2nd ed.). Petaluma, CA: NICU Ink.

Methods of Promoting Thermal Stability

A major consideration in monitoring thermal status and promoting thermal stability in the neonate involves issues related to the various types of equipment that are currently available. High-risk neonates are generally cared for in either convectively heated incubators or open, radiantly heated beds. Each of these pieces of equipment and methods has inherent advantages and disadvantages, as do adjuncts to these beds such as humidity and heat shields, thermal blankets, occlusive dressings, and warmed mattresses. Unfortunately there are few good controlled studies that provide data to address most of these issues. Preterm and other high-risk infants are usually cared for in closed, convectively warmed incubators or open, radiant warmers. There is no consistent evidence supporting either as more effective in reducing morbidity or mortality and each has advantages and disadvantages, especially for VLBW infants (Table 19-4).[38,75]

Infant incubators. Standard single-walled or double-walled convective incubators operate by circulation of warmed air. Air entering the incubator is filtered, providing a barrier against airborne pathogenic organisms from the environment. Air leaving the incubator is not filtered, so personnel or infants in open warmers and cribs are not protected from airborne organisms in the incubator air. In newer double-walled incubators, walls are warmed by a

layer of warm water or by computer-controlled, electrically conductive plastic panels.[63,75]

Up to 60% to 70% of total heat loss in infants cared for in convectively heated incubators is radiation.[52,53,130,140] Since Plexiglas is relatively opaque to radiant waves, infants radiate their body heat primarily to the inner side of the incubator wall. In a single-walled incubator, the temperature of this wall is midway between the incubator and room air temperatures. In most nurseries, room air is considerably cooler than incubator air, which can lead to significant radiant heat loss, particularly in immature infants.

Radiant losses can be reduced by the use of double-walled incubators or heat shields.[82,143] These devices place a second layer of Plexiglas between the infant and the outer incubator wall. The infant radiates heat to the inner wall or shield, which is surrounded on both sides by warmed incubator air. Heat shields should have closed ends to prevent a wind-tunnel effect, which further increases convective losses. Increasing the ambient temperature of the room and placing the infant away from windows or exterior walls can also reduce radiant losses in infants in incubators. Further alterations in radiant losses occur when infants are clothed or incubators are covered with blankets or quilts to reduce light and noise levels.[3] As a result of extremely high transepidermal evaporative losses, VLBW infants may have subnormal temperatures in spite of incubator temperatures above their body temperatures and the use of heat shields and double-walled incubators. Semiocclusive dressings and emollients have also been used to decrease evaporative heat loss; warmed mattresses have been used to promote conductive heat gain.[12,64,92,101,139]

A major disadvantage of convective incubators is temperature fluctuations that occur with opening and closing of the portholes or hood. When the portholes are open, the temperature of the air in the incubator falls rapidly and recovers slowly. Temperature changes with opening of the portholes can be reduced by the use of plastic sleeves. Laminar flow incubators also minimize these fluctuations. Double-walled incubators provide a better balance between convective and radiant losses. The drop in air temperature when opening the incubator is less in double-walled than single-walled incubators, providing a more stable thermal environment during caregiving. The inner wall in a double-walled incubator acts as a heat reservoir, while in some models warm air is redirected across the front of the incubator when it is opened.[18] The air thermometer or thermistor in an incubator should be near to the infant's body and protected from being covered with bedding, clothing, or cool air flow from a resuscitation bag left in the incubator.[69,71]

Convective losses can also occur in incubators due to either natural convection or forced air convection. Natural convection is the thermal gradient between the skin surface and the surrounding air. Warm air rises from the infant's skin, carrying heat and moisture. This air then cools and falls back to the infant's surface, especially over the curvature of the body. Infants positioned in flexion have less exposed surface area and less heat loss than infants in an extended posture.[12] Forced convection usually occurs at air velocities equal to or greater than 0.27 m/sec. Lower air velocities can minimize these losses. In most incubators currently in use, the primary route of convective loss is through natural convection, since the air velocities near the infant's body are minimal.[12] Methods to enhance thermal stability in infants cared for in incubators are summarized in Table 19-5.

Air in the incubator can be humidified by active or passive methods. Passive methods involve an integral humid-

TABLE **19-5**   **Measures to Promote Thermoregulation in Incubators and Radiant Warmers**

BED	BASIS	MEASURES
Incubator	Decrease evaporative water and heat loss	Increase humidity Plastic heat shield Thermal blanket Semiocclusive dressings or emollients
	Reduce radiant and convective losses	Double-walled incubator Heat shield Thermal blanket
	Promote conductive heat gain	Heated mattress
Radiant warmer	Decrease evaporative water and heat loss	Heat shield Plastic wrap Thermal blanket
	Reduce radiant or convective losses	Heat shield Plastic wrap Thermal blanket

Compiled from Sinclair, J. (1992). Management of the thermal environment. In J.C. Sinclair & M.B. Brocker (Eds.). *Effective care of the newborn infant.* Oxford: Oxford University Press.

ifier, usually with heat passing over a water reservoir. Active methods use a modular integral or external humidifier, so water vapor is continuously added to the circulating air via vaporization. This method generally uses servocontrol, and the amount of humidity can be individualized. Advantages of active humidification include reduction in infection risk, easier cleaning, and reduced recovery time after incubator doors are opened.[84]

Radiant warmers. Radiant warmers maintain the infant's temperature using a proportional servocontrol system that maintains skin temperature at a constant level. The optimal skin temperature is not known and may vary from infant to infant.[18] For example, differences have been reported in individual infants in the temperature at which oxygen consumption is minimal.[18] Radiant heat is produced in the infrared spectrum and penetrates below the skin surface, where epidermal cells with a high water content absorb the radiant energy and convert it to heat. This heat is transferred to deeper tissues by conduction and circulating blood. The heat source is usually about 90 cm from the infant's surface.[109]

Radiant warmers are convenient to use, allow direct access to the infant, decrease radiant losses, and eliminate temperature fluctuations with opening of the portholes. Evaporative and convective losses are increased, however, with a risk of dehydration.[8,38,62,79,90,140] Evaporative losses are primarily increased due to the lower humidity and can be reduced by use of plastic wrap or blankets. IWL in infants in radiant warmers is increased 50% to 200%.[49,59,142] These losses may counteract the reduction in radiant losses in VLBW infants. Further IWL occurs if infants are simultaneously being treated with phototherapy (see Chapter 17). Although it may be possible to compensate for variations in evaporative and convective heat losses, the increased evaporative water losses are more difficult to manage.[12] Radiant warmers have been associated with an increase in oxygen consumption and metabolic rate, although the increase has not been statistically significant in most trials.[81,109,120] Other issues in use of radiant warmers include those associated with servocontrol and probe use, discussed earlier.

Convective losses can be reduced by using the sides on the warming bed or by stretching a layer of plastic wrap across the infant between the radiant warmer's side guards or on a special frame.[9,10,11,37] Plastic wrap does not block radiant heat waves as does Plexiglas; thus heat shields made from this material are not recommended for use with radiant warmers.[120] Plastic wrap also reduces IWL; plastic shields do not have a similar effect.[10,11,17] Methods to enhance thermal stability in infants cared for in radiant warmers are summarized in Table 19-5.

Skin-to-skin care. At birth, term infants who are dried and covered with a warm blanket and placed skin to skin against their mother maintain their temperature as well as infants cared for in standard heating units.[27,40,141] Studies of skin-to-skin (kangaroo) care with stable preterm infants demonstrate that most infants maintain adequate thermal control during this type of holding, especially if the infant is wearing a hat and covered with a blanket, and both skin and rectal temperature may increase.[1,7,18,23,72,120,141] The parent's clothing around the sides and back of the infant forms a "pouch" that provides insulation and reduces nonevaporative losses (and possibly evaporative losses).[120]

Use of head coverings, clothing, and blankets. Clothing and head coverings can provide thermal insulation, reducing radiant and convective losses, and can, depending on the fabric, also reduce evaporative loss.[18] In the neonate the head accounts for one fifth of the total body surface area. Brain heat production is estimated to account for 55% of total metabolic heat production in the newborn.[105] Thus the neonate's head is poorly insulated and accounts for a significant proportion of total heat loss. Head coverings are often used to reduce heat loss from this area. Head coverings or caps made of stockinette, which is a poor insulator, are relatively ineffective in reducing heat losses.[45,105] More effective materials include caps made of insulated fabrics, wool, or polyolefin; lined with Gamgee; or insulated with a plastic liner. Head coverings have been found to significantly decrease heat loss after delivery and in neonates cared for in cribs and incubators.[45,83,105,107,131] These coverings are most effective in a cool environment and are less effective in a thermoneutral environment or with use of infant servocontrol.[18,107] Head coverings and clothing interfere with radiant heat loss and gain and are not appropriate for infants under radiant warmers.

Clothing and blankets alter the thermal environment by both widening and lowering the neutral thermal range.[109] Insulation from swaddling with blankets decreases evaporative loss by reducing the amount of exposed surface area and by changing airflow patterns and skin emissivity. In addition, swaddling and nesting maintain flexion, which reduces exposed surface area and thus convective and radiant losses.[9,11,83] For example, swaddled infants in servocontrolled double-walled incubators have been reported to have higher abdominal skin temperatures and require lower incubator temperatures.[119] Swaddling appears to have a greater effect on skin than core temperature.[46] Others have found that nested infants have closer approximation of skin and rectal temperatures.[73]

TABLE 19-6   Infants at Risk for Problems in Thermoregulation

Infant Category	Basis for Risk
Preterm infants	Decreased subcutaneous fat for insulation
	Decreased BAT and ability to mobilize norepinephrine and fat
	Large surface area to weight ratio
	Inadequate caloric intake
	Inability to effectively increase oxygen consumption
	Increased open resting posture with less flexion
	Immature thermal regulatory mechanisms
	Increased evaporative water losses and higher body water content
Infants with neurologic problems	Alterations in hypothalamic control of body temperature
Infants with endocrine problems	Impairment of BAT metabolism because of inadequate catecholamines, thyroxine, or other hormones
Hypoglycemic infants	Decreased substrate for energy and ATP production in BAT
	Decreased metabolic response to cold stress
Infants with cardio-respiratory problems	Inability to increase oxygen consumption or minute ventilation further
	Inability to increase metabolic rate and reduce metabolic response to cold
	Impairment of BAT metabolism by hypoxia (impaired with PO_2 of 45 to 55 torr; essentially ceases at values below 30 torr)[99]
	Inadequate caloric intake to meet metabolic demands
	Increased risk of metabolic acidosis
	Increased temperature losses through evaporation of water from lungs
Infants with nutritional problems	Inadequate caloric intake to meet increased metabolic demands
Infants with electrolyte imbalances	Alterations in sodium and potassium may lead to sodium pump failure interfering with BAT metabolism
Infants with congenital anomalies (e.g., meningomyelocele, omphalocele, gastroschisis)	Increased surface area for heat loss
	Increased evaporative losses
Small-for-gestational-age infants	Decreased subcutaneous fat for insulation
	Increased surface area for weight
	Higher basal metabolic rate and energy demands
Sedated infants or maternal intrapartal analgesia	Limited physical activity to generate heat
	Maternal diazepam (over 30 mg within 15 minutes of delivery) or meperidine (200 to 400 mg within 3 to 5 hours of delivery) administration associated with decreased newborn temperature for up to 20 hours [25]

Compiled from references 12, 20, 25, 29, 63, 98, 124, and 126.
ATP, Adenosine triphosphate; *BAT,* brown adipose tissue.

Neonatal Hypothermia and Cold Stress

Alterations in health status or maturity can compromise the ability of the newborn to efficiently and effectively regulate heat production and respond to cold stress. Infants at risk and the basis for this risk are summarized in Table 19-6.

Signs of hypothermia are often absent or nonspecific in neonates. Clinical findings may include lethargy, restlessness, pallor, cool skin, tachypnea, grunting, poor feeding, or decreased weight gain.[98,124] With severe cold stress the infant may develop peripheral edema and sclerema. Cold stress can also interfere with interpretation of pH, since pH

is temperature dependent.[109] The initial temperature decrease is peripheral with stimulation of cutaneous receptors and initiation of NST. If the heat generated by this method is insufficient, the core (rectal) temperature will drop.

The hypothermic or cold-stressed neonate tries to compensate by conserving heat and increasing heat production. These compensatory mechanisms can lead to physiologic alterations that may set off a series of adverse metabolic events (Figure 19-7). If uninterrupted, this chain of events can result in hypoxemia, metabolic acidosis, glycogen depletion, hypoglycemia,

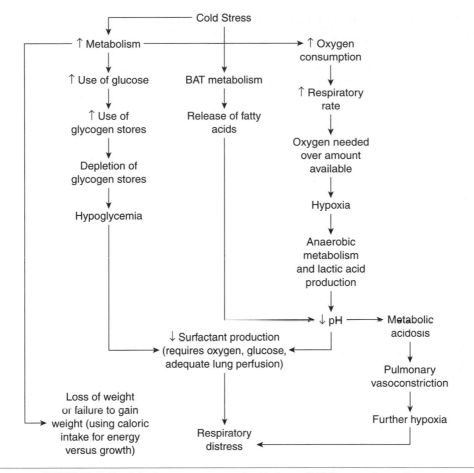

FIGURE 19-7 Physiologic consequences of cold stress. *BAT,* Brown adipose tissue.

and altered surfactant production. Physiologic effects of hypothermia and their consequences are summarized in Table 19-7.

Prevention of hypothermia and cold stress is a major component of neonatal health care. Strategies include careful monitoring of all infants, especially those at increased risk for hypothermia; decreasing heat losses by preventing evaporative, convective, conductive, and radiant losses; reducing the frequency and duration of cold exposure; and monitoring both infant and environmental temperatures.

Rewarming the Hypothermic Infant

The goal of rewarming a hypothermic infant in an incubator is to provide an environment in which the infant's temperature can increase through heat generated by the infant's internal mechanism while reducing sources of heat loss.[98] A radiant warmer may be more effective than an incubator for some infants, since it heats the baby, whereas an incubator reduces heat loss. Specific approaches to re-

warming are controversial, since both slow and rapid rewarming have inherent limitations. Slow rewarming prolongs the hypothermia and pathologic consequences of cold stress. Very rapid rewarming has been associated with heat-induced apnea and decreased blood pressure and shock due to rapid vasodilation with shunting and pooling of blood.[98,99,127]

Rutter, as cited by Sinclair, suggests rewarming at a rate of 1° to 2° C/hour, since somewhat faster rewarming has been associated with lower mortality.[120] Perlstein recommends a pragmatic approach to rewarming based on the principle of producing heat gain from the environment while eliminating further heat loss from the infant, with a goal of rewarming the infant using heat generated by the infant: (1) warm incubator air over the infant, and simultaneously increase the humidity to reduce evaporative losses while decreasing radiant losses by protecting the incubator walls or using a heat shield; (2) monitor incubator air temperature near infant's body while monitoring infant tempera-

TABLE **19-7**   Consequences of Neonatal Hypothermia

PHYSIOLOGIC EFFECT	PHYSIOLOGIC CONSEQUENCE
Peripheral vasoconstriction	Increased internal (core to skin) gradient and tissue insulation
	Persistent vasoconstriction can lead to reduced tissue perfusion and metabolism with accumulation of ketone bodies and development of metabolic acidosis
Increased metabolic rate	Increased oxygen consumption by increasing minute ventilation and respiratory rate
	Risk of hypoxia and respiratory failure in infants unable to increase oxygen intake (e.g., infant with respiratory distress syndrome or other respiratory problems, very low birth weight)
Increased requirements for oxygen, glucose, and calories	Exhaustion of supplies with subsequent development of hypoglycemia, hypoxia, aggravation of respiratory distress syndrome, or weight loss
Increased production of ketone bodies and accumulation of lactic acid from anaerobic metabolism	Metabolic acidosis with subsequent pulmonary vasoconstriction with further reduction in pulmonary perfusion
	Risk of hypoxia and altered surfactant synthesis
Norepinephrine release	Increased pulmonary vascular resistance with altered ventilation perfusion relationships and increased right-to-left shunting through the patent ductus arteriosus
	Risk of hypoxia and altered surfactant synthesis
Elevation in plasma non-esterified fatty acids	Alteration in glucose/fatty acid relationship with fall in blood glucose
	Risk of hypoglycemia and altered surfactant synthesis
	Competition with bilirubin for albumin binding sites with risk of bilirubin encephalopathy
Dissociation of albumin and bilirubin because of acidosis	Increased indirect (unbound) bilirubin
	Risk of bilirubin encephalopathy

Compiled from references 12, 20, 29, 63, 98, and 124.

ture with simultaneous skin and rectal temperatures (skin temperature should not be more than 1° C warmer than rectal temperature); (3) if the temperature ceases to decrease or begins to slowly rise, maintain the infant and continue to monitor, keeping infant skin temperature no more than 1° C warmer than rectal temperature; (4) if the infant's temperature continues to fall, raise the incubator temperature to 37° C (98.6° F), evaluate for missed sources of heat loss, and ensure that the humidity is greater than 70%; (5) if the infant's temperature is still falling 15 minutes later, raise the incubator temperature to 38° C (100.4° F) and reevaluate for missed source of heat loss; (6) if this fails, add a radiant warmer over the incubator to increase the external wall temperature; and (7) if the infant becomes apneic or shocky due to vasodilation with pooling of blood, slow the rate of rewarming.[98]

Hyperthermia in the Neonate

Although discussions regarding alterations in neonatal thermoregulation often focus primarily on hypothermia, the neonate is also at risk for hyperthermia. Hyperthermia increases metabolic demands, so even a slight increase in temperature can result in a significant increase in oxygen con-

sumption, especially in preterm infants. Other consequences of hyperthermia include increased heart, respiratory, and metabolic rates; increased IWL; dehydration; peripheral vasodilation with a risk of decreased blood pressure; alteration in weight gain; and the risk of hypoxia and metabolic acidosis.[63,98,126] Neonatal hyperthermia (i.e., temperature above 37.5° C [99.5° F]) is primarily due to overheating and less often to hypermetabolism. Hyperthermia also results from dehydration, drugs, or alterations in hypothalamic control mechanisms secondary to birth trauma.

Overheating because of increased environmental temperatures or radiant gains from exposure to sunlight or heat lamps is associated with peripheral vasodilation, a "flushed" appearance especially prominent in extremities, warm extremities, increased activity, irritability, increased IWL, extended posture, and sweating in older preterm or term infants. Skin temperatures are higher than core temperatures. Foot temperature is no more than 2° to 3° C cooler than abdominal skin temperature.[98,109] Infants, particularly VLBW infants, are at risk for thermal injury from environmental sources (see Table 19-6)

The neonate is more vulnerable to overheating than are older individuals because the infant has a lower capacity

TABLE **19-8**   **Recommendations for Clinical Practice Related to Thermoregulation in Neonates**

Know the mechanisms of heat production and dissipation in the neonate (pp. 711-715).	Use infant incubators and radiant warmers appropriately to maintain neonatal thermal status and reduce heat loss (pp. 720-723 and Table 19-5).
Initiate interventions to conserve body heat and reduce neonatal heat loss during transition (pp. 710-711 and Table 19-2).	Monitor insensible water loss in infants cared for in radiant warmers (p. 723).
Recognize the usual values for neonatal temperature (p. 711).	Use head coverings made of appropriate materials to reduce heat loss in infants in incubators and cribs (p. 723).
Avoid overheating or cooling the trigeminal area of the neonate's face (pp. 713, 717).	Recognize infants at risk for hypothermia and cold stress (pp. 723-725 and Table 19-6).
Recognize and monitor for events that increase heat loss by conduction, convection, evaporation, and radiation (pp. 717-719 and Table 19-2).	Monitor neonates for signs of hypothermia and cold stress (pp. 723-726).
Institute interventions to reduce heat loss in term and preterm infants by conduction, convection, evaporation, and radiation (pp. 717-719 and Table 19-4).	Monitor hypothermic or cold-stressed infants for adverse physiologic effects (pp. 723-726, Table 19-7, and Figure 19-6).
Provide term and preterm neonates with an appropriate thermal environment (pp. 715-717).	Monitor infants during rewarming (pp. 725-726).
Know the methods for monitoring thermal status and their advantages and limitations (pp. 719-720).	Recognize infants at risk for hyperthermia and thermal injury (pp. 726-727).
Understand the differences between and implications of core versus skin temperature (pp. 719-720).	Monitor neonates for signs of hyperthermia (pp. 726-727).
Know the advantages and limitations of different types of infant incubators and radiant warmers (pp. 720-723).	Monitor hyperthermic infants for adverse physiologic effects (pp. 726-727).
	Implement interventions to prevent thermal injury (pp. 717-719).

for normothermic heat storage, a larger surface-to-volume ratio, and narrower control range than an adult does.[63] At environmental temperatures above the neutral thermal zone, thermal equilibrium is reestablished by increasing evaporative losses.[20] The adult responds by increasing skin water losses and sweating. The neonate's initial response is to increase respiratory water loss (tachypnea). Infants over 30 weeks' gestation can sweat if the environmental temperature exceeds their threshold.[39,51]

Hyperthermia secondary to hypermetabolism can result from sepsis, cardiac problems, drug withdrawal, or other metabolic alterations. Clinical signs include peripheral vasoconstriction; pale, cool extremities; and a core body temperature that is higher than skin temperature.[98] Foot temperature is more than 3° C cooler than abdominal skin temperature.[98,109] Fever is less commonly seen with infections in neonates due to an immature, weak, or absent response to fever-producing substances such as bacterial endotoxins. Regardless of the cause, hyperthermia can lead to heat stroke, dehydration, and brain damage in the neonate.

MATURATIONAL CHANGES DURING INFANCY AND CHILDHOOD

NST is thought to be the major mechanism for thermoregulation in the first 3 to 6 months.[136] With increasing age, NST becomes less prominent and the infant begins to rely more on physical methods of heat generation such as activity and shivering.[20] BAT gradually disappears within the first year of life as it is replaced by white adipose tissue. This change is correlated with the switch in the major thermoregulatory mechanism from NST to shivering.[124] Sweating becomes more efficient as a method of heat dissipation. The threshold body temperature for sweating decreases and maximal sweat production increases.[130] Infants continue to have a decreased hypothalamic response to pyrogens for the first 2 to 3 months.[86]

Higher rectal temperatures predominate in infants. Average temperatures at 18 months of age are 37.7° C (99.8° F), with marked daily variations seen in some children.[13] Body temperatures gradually decrease from 2 years to puberty, stabilizing at 13 to 14 years of age in girls and 16 to 17 years in boys.[58,65]

SUMMARY

Thermal stability is one of the most critical processes during the transition to extrauterine life. Thermoregulation is essential for survival and has priority over most other metabolic demands. The infant who does not achieve thermal stability after birth or who is cold stressed in the neonatal period is more likely to experience health problems, poor growth, and increased morbidity and mortality. Ongoing assessment and monitoring of thermal status in the neonate and initiation of appropriate interventions to maintain thermal stability can prevent or minimize these risks. Clinical recommendations related to neonatal thermoregulation are summarized in Table 19-8.

REFERENCES

1. Acolet, D., Stern, K., & Whitelaw, A. (1989). Oxygenation, heart rate and temperature in very low birthweight infants during skin-to-skin contact with their mothers. *Acta Paediatr Scand, 78,* 189.

2. Adamsons, K. (1966). The role of thermal factors in fetal and neonatal life. *Pediatr Clin North Am, 13,* 599.

3. Adamsons, K., Gandy, G.M. & James, L.S. (1965). The influence of thermal factors upon oxygen consumption of the newborn human infant. *J Pediatr, 66,* 495.

4. American Academy of Pediatrics and American College of Obstetricians and Gynecologists (1988). *Guidelines for perinatal care* (2nd ed.). Elk Grove, IL: American Academy of Pediatrics; and Washington, DC: American College of Obstetricians and Gynecologists.

5. Anderson, G.C. (1991). Current knowledge of skin-to-skin (kangaroo) care for preterm infants. *J Perinatol, 11,* 216.

6. Ball, K.T., et al. (1995). A potential role for adenosine in the induction of nonshivering thermogenesis in the fetal sheep. *Pediatr Res, 37,* 303.

7. Bauer, K et al. (1997). Body temperatures and oxygen consumption during skin-to-skin (kangaroo) care in stable preterm infants weighing less than 1500 grams. *J Pediatr, 130,* 240.

8. Baumgart, S. (1985). Partitioning of heat losses and heat gains in premature newborn infants under radiant warmers. *Pediatrics, 75,* 89.

9. Baumgart, S. (1987). Current concepts and clinical strategies for managing low-birth-weight infants under radiant warmers. *Med Instrum, 21,* 23.

10. Baumgart, S., Fox, W.W. & Polin, R.A. (1982). Physiologic implications of two different heat shields for infants under radiant warmers. *J Pediatr, 100,* 787.

11. Baumgart, S., et al. (1981). Effect of heat shielding on convection and evaporation, and radiant heat transfer in the premature infant. *J Pediatr, 97,* 948.

12. Baumgardt, S., Nirrsch, S.C., & Touch, S.M. (1999). Thermal Regulation. In G.B. Avery, M.A. Fletcher, & M.G. Macdonald (Eds.). *Neonatology-pathophysiology and management of the newborn* (5th ed.). Philadelphia: J.B. Lippincott.

13. Bayley, N. & Stolz, H.R. (1937). Maturational changes in rectal temperatures of 61 infants from 1 to 36 months. *Child Dev, 8,* 195.

14. Belgaumkar, T.K. & Scott, K.E. (1975). Effects of low humidity on small premature infants in servo control incubators. II: Increased severity of apnea. *Biol Neonate, 26,* 348.

15. Bell, E.F. (1983). Infant incubators and radiant warmers. *Early Hum Develop, 8,* 351.

16. Bell, E.F. & Rios, G.R. (1983). Air versus skin temperature servo control of infant incubators. *J Pediatr, 103,* 954.

17. Bell, E.F., Weinstein, M.R., & Oh, W. (1980). Heat balance in premature infants: Comparative effects of convectively heated incubator and radiant warmer with and without plastic shields. *J Pediatr, 96,* 460.

18. Bell, E.F. & Glatzl-Hawlik, M-A. (1998). Environmental temperature control. In R.A. Polin & W.W. Fox (Eds.). *Fetal and neonatal physiology* (2nd ed.). Philadelphia: W.B. Saunders.

19. Bliss-Holtz, J. (1989). Comparison of rectal, axillary and inguinal temperatures in full-term newborns, *Nurs Res, 36,* 85.

20. Bruck, K. (1978). Heat production and temperature regulation. In U. Stave (Ed.). *Perinatal physiology.* New York: Plenum.

21. Bruck, K. (1998). Neonatal thermal regulation. In R.A. Polin & W.W. Fox (Eds.). *Fetal and neonatal physiology* (2nd ed.). Philadelphia: W.B. Saunders.

22. Chambers, C.D., et al. (1998). Maternal fever and birth outcome: A prospective study. *Teratol, 58,* 251.

23. Charpak, N., et al. (1997). Kangaroo mother versus traditional care for newborn infants A randomized, controlled trial. *Pediatrics, 100,* 682.

24. Clapp, J., Wesley, M. & Sleamaker, R. (1987). Thermoregulatory and metabolic responses to jogging prior to and during pregnancy. *Med Sci Sports Exerc, 19,* 124.

25. Cree, J.E., Meyer, J. & Hailey, D.M. (1973). Diazepam in labour: Its metabolism and effect on the clinical condition and thermogenesis of the newborn. *Br Med J, 4,* 251.

26. Cunningham, F.G & Whitridge, W.J. (1997). *Williams obstetrics* (20th ed.). Stamford, CT: Appleton & Lange.

27. Cusson, R., Madonia, J.A., & Tackman, J.B. (1997). The effect of environment on body site temperatures in full-term neonates. *Nurs Res, 46,* 202.

28. Darnell, R.A. (1987). The thermophysiology of the newborn infant. *Med Instrum, 21,* 16.

29. Davis, V. (1980). The structure and function of brown adipose tissue in the neonate. *J Obstet Gynecol Neonatal Nurs, 9,* 368.

30. Dollberg, S. (1994). Effect of insulated skin probes to increase skin-to-environment temperature gradients of preterm infants cared for in convective incubators. *J Pediatr, 124,* 799.

31. Dollberg, S., Atherton, H.D., & Hoath, S.B. (1995). Effects of different phototherapy lights on incubator characteristics and dynamics under three modes of servocontrol. *Am J Perinatol, 12,* 55.

32. Dunn, P.A., York, R., Cheek, T.G. & Yeboah, K. (1994). Maternal hypothermia: Implications for obstetrical nurses. *J Obstet Gynecol Neonatal Nurs, 23,* 238.

33. Fallis, W.M. & Christiani, P. (1999). Neonatal axillary temperature measurements: A comparison of electronic thermometer predictive and monitor modes. *J Obstet Gynecol Neonatal Nurs, 28,* 389.

34. Fanaroff, A.A., et al. (1972). Insensible water loss in low birth weight infants. *Pediatrics, 50,* 236.

35. Filker, R. & Monif, G.R.G. (1979). The significance of temperature during the first 24 hours postpartum. *Obstet Gynecol, 53,* 358.

36. Fisher, D.A. & Polk, D.H. (1994). The ontogenesis of thyroid function and activity. In D. Tulchinsky & A.B. Little (Eds.). *Maternal-fetal endocrinology* (2nd ed.). Philadelphia: W.B. Saunders.

37. Fitch, C.W. & Korones, S.B. (1984). Heat shield reduces water loss. *Arch Dis Child, 59,* 886.

38. Flenady, V.J. & Woodgate, P.G. (2000). Radiant warmers versus incubators in newborn infants. *Cochrane Database Syst Rev, 2,* CD000435.

39. Foster, K.G., Hey, E.N., & Katz, G. (1969). The response of the sweat glands of the newborn baby to thermal stimuli and to intradermal acetylcholine. *J Physiol, 203,* 13.

40. Gardner, S. (1979). The mother as an incubator after delivery. *J Obstet Gynecol Neonatal Nurs, 8,* 174.

41. Gibbs, R.S. (1987). Fever and infections. In C. J. Pauerstein (Ed.). *Clinical obstetrics.* New York: John Wiley & Sons.

42. Glass, L., Silverman, W.A., & Sinclair, J.C. (1968). Effect of the thermal environment on cold resistance and growth of small infants after the first week of life. *Pediatrics, 41,* 1033.

43. Gluckman, P.D., Sizonenko, S.V., & Bassett, N.S. (1999). The transition from fetus to neonate—An endocrine perspective. *Acta Paediatr Suppl, 88*(428), 7.

44. Graham, JM, Edwards, M.J., & Edwards, M.J. (1998). Teratogen update: gestational effects of maternal hyperthermia due to febrile illness and resultant patterns of defects in humans. *Teratol, 58,* 209.

45. Greer, P.S. (1988). Head coverings for newborns under radiant warmers. *J Obstet Gynecol Neonatal Nurs, 17,* 265.

46. Grover, M G., et al. (1994). The effects of bundling on infant temperature. *Pediatrics, 94*, 600.

47. Gunn, T.R., Ball, K.T., & Gluckman, P.D. (1993). Withdrawal of placental prostaglandins permits thermogenic response in fetal sheep brown adipose tissue. *J Appl Physiol, 74*, 998.

48. Gunn, T.R. & Gluckman, P.D. (1995). Perinatal thermogenesis. *Early Hum Dev, 42*, 169.

49. Guyton, A.C. & Hall, J.E. (1996). *Textbook of medical physiology* (9th ed.). Philadelphia: W.B. Saunders.

50. Hammarlund, K., et al. (1980). Transepidermal water loss in newborn infants versus evaporation from the skin and heat exchange during the first hours of life. *Acta Paediatr Scand, 69*, 385.

51. Hey, E.N. & Katz, G. (1969). Evaporative water loss in the new-born baby. *J Physiol, 200*, 605.

52. Hey, E.N. & Katz, G. (1970). The optimal thermal environment for naked babies. *Arch Dis Child, 45*, 328.

53. Hey, E.N. & Mount, L.E. (1967). Heat losses from babies in incubators. *Arch Dis Child, 42*, 75.

54. Hey, E.N. & O'Connell, B. (1970). Oxygen consumption and heat balance in the cot-nursed baby. *Arch Dis Child, 45*, 335.

55. Hicks, M.A. (1996). A comparison of tympanic and axillary temperatures of the preterm and term infant. *J Perinatol, 16*, 261.

56. Horns, K. (1994). Physiological and methodological issues: Neonatal insensible water loss. *Neonatal Net, 13*(5), 83.

57. Huch, R. & Erkkola, R. (1990). Pregnancy and exercise—exercise and pregnancy. A short review. *Br J Obstet Gynaecol, 97*, 208.

58. Iliff, A. & Lee, V.A. (1952). Pulse rate, respiratory rate and body temperature of children between two months and 18 years of age. *Child Dev, 23*, 238.

59. Jones, R.W., Rocheforst, M.J. & Baum, J.D. (1976). Increased insensible water loss in newborn infants nursed under radiant heaters. *Br Med J, 2*, 1347.

60. Jones, R., et al. (1985). Thermoregulation during aerobic exercise in pregnancy. *Obstet Gynecol, 65*, 340.

61. Karlberg, P. (1949). The significance of the depth of insertion of the thermometer for recording rectal temperatures. *Acta Paediatr Scand, 38*, 359.

62. Kjartansson, S., et al. (1995). Water loss from the skin of term and preterm infants nursed under a radiant warmer. *Pediatr Res, 37*, 233.

63. Klaus, M.H., Fanaroff, A.A., & Martin, R.J. (1993). The physical environment. In M.H. Klaus & A.A. Fanaroff (Eds.). *Care of the high risk infant*. Philadelphia: W.B. Saunders.

64. Knauth, A., et al. (1989) A semipermeable polyurethane dressing as an artificial skin in premature neonates. *Pediatrics, 83*, 943.

65. Kornienko, I.A. & Gokhblit, I.I. (1980). Age differences of temperature regulation in children age 5-12 years. *Human Physiol, 6*, 443.

66. Kruse, J. (1988). Fever in children. *Am Fam Physician, 37*, 127.

67. LeBlanc, M.H. (1984). Evaluation of two devices for improving thermal control of premature infants in transport. *Crit Care Med, 12*, 3.

68. LeBlanc, M.H. (1987). The physics of thermal exchange between infants and their environment. *Med Instrum, 21*, 11.

69. LeBlanc, M.H. & Edwards, N.K. (1985). Artifacts in the measurement of skin temperature under infant radiant warmers. *Ann Biomed Eng, 13*, 443.

70. LeBlanc, M.H. (1987). The physics of thermal exchange between infants and their environment. *Med Instrum, 21*, 11.

71. LeBlanc, M.H. (1991). Thermoregulation: Incubators, radiant warmers, artificial skins, and body hoods. *Clin Perinatol, 18*, 403.

72. Legault, M. & Goulet, C. (1995). Comparison of kangaroo and traditional methods of removing preterm infants from incubators. *J Obstet Gynecol Neonatal Nurs, 24*, 501.

73. Leick-Rude, M.K. & Bloom, L.F. (1998). A comparison of temperature taking methods in neonates. *Neonatal Net, 17*(5), 21.

74. Lieberman, E., et al. (2000), Intrapartum maternal fever and neonatal outcome. *Pediatrics, 105*, 8.

75. Libert, J.P., Bach, V., & Farges, G. (1997). Neutral temperature range in incubators: performance of equipment in current use. *Crit Rev Biomed Eng, 25*, 287.

76. Lowe, N.K. & Reiss, R. (1996). Parturition and fetal adaptation. *J Obstet Gynecol Neonatal Nurs, 25*, 339.

77. Macauley, J.H., Bond, K. & Steer, P.J (1992). Epidural analgesia in labor and fetal hyperthermia. *Obstet Gynecol, 80*, 665.

78. Macauley, J.H., Randall, N.R., Bond, K., & Steer, P.J (1992). Continuous monitoring of fetal temperature by non-invasive probe and its relationship to maternal temperature, fetal temperature, and cord arterial oxygen and pH. *Obstet Gynecol, 79*, 469.

79. Main, S.W. & Baumgart, S. (1987). Optimal thermal management for low birth weight infants nursed under high-powered radiant warmers. *Pediatrics, 79*, 47.

80. Malloy, M.B. (1989). High risk skin and high tech care: Skin care of the very low birthweight neonate. *NAACOG Update Series* (vol. 6, lesson 8). Princeton, NJ: Continuing Professional Education Center.

81. Marks, K.H., et al. (1986). Energy metabolism and substrate utilization in low birth weight neonates under radiant warmers. *Pediatrics, 78*, 465.

82. Marks, K.H. (1987). Incubators. *Med Instrum, 21*, 29.

83. Marks, K.M., et al. (1985). Thermal head wrap for infants. *J Pediatr, 107*, 956.

84. Marshall, A. (1997). Humidifying the environment for the premature neonate: Maintenance of a thermoneutral environment. *J Neonatal Nurs, 3*(1), 32.

85. Mayfield, S.R., et al. (1984). Temperature measurement in term and preterm neonates. *J Pediatr, 104*, 271.

86. McCarthy, P.L. (1998). Fever. *Pediatrics in Review, 19*, 401.

87. McMurray, R.G., Katz, V.L., Meyer-Goodwin, W.E., & Cefalo, R.C. (1993). Thermoregulation of pregnant women during aerobic exercise on land and in the water. *Am J Perinatol, 10*, 178.

88. Miller, P., Smith, D.W., & Shepherd, T.H. (1978). Maternal hyperthermia as a possible cause of anencephaly. *Lancet, 1*, 519.

89. Milunsky, A., et al. (1992). Maternal heat exposure and neural tube defects. *JAMA, 268*, 882.

90. Motil, K.J., Blackburn, M.G., & Pleasure, J.R. (1974). The effects of four different radiant warmer temperature set points used for rewarming neonates. *J Pediatr, 85*, 546.

91. Nedergaard, J. & Cannon, B. (1998). Brown adipose tissue: Development and function. In R.A. Polin & W.W. Fox (Eds.). *Fetal and neonatal physiology* (2nd ed.). Philadelphia: W.B. Saunders.

92. Nopper A.J., et al., (1996), Topical ointment therapy benefits premature infants. *J Pediatr, 128*, 660.

93. Okken, A., et al. (1982). Effects of forced convection of heated air on insensible water loss and heat loss in preterm infants in incubators. *J Pediatr, 101*, 108.

94. Okken, A. & Koch, J. (1995). *Thermoregulation of sick and low birth weight neonates*. Berlin: Springer-Verlag.

95. Oya A., et al. (1997). Thermographic demonstration of nonshivering thermogenesis in human newborns after birth: its relation to umbilical blood gases. *J Perinat Med, 25*, 447.

96. Panzer, O., et al. (1999). Shivering and shivering-like tremor during labor with and without epidural anesthesia. *Anesthesiology, 90*, 1609

97. Perlman. J.M. (1999). Maternal fever and neonatal depression: Preliminary observations. *Clin Pediatr, 38*, 287.

98. Perlstein, P.H. (1997). Physical environment. In A.A. Fanaroff & R.J. Martin (Eds.). *Neonatal-perinatal medicine: Diseases of the fetus and infant* (6th ed.). St. Louis: Mosby.

99. Perlstein, P.H., Edwards, N.K. & Sutherland, J.M. (1970). Apnea in premature infants and incubator-air-temperature changes. *N Engl J Med, 282,* 461.

100. Pacific Northwest Association of Neonatal Nurses (PNANN). Research Committee. Neonatal nursing thermal care. III: The effect of position and temperature probe placement. *Neonatal Net, 20*(3), 25.

101. Porat, R. & Brodsky, N. (1993). Effect of Tegederm use on outcome of extremely low birth weight (ELBW) infants. *Pediar Res, 33,* 231A.

102. Power, G.G. (1998). Perinatal thermal physiology. In R.A. Polin & W.W. Fox (Eds.). *Fetal and neonatal physiology* (2nd ed.). Philadelphia: W.B. Saunders.

103. Prichard, J.A., MacDonald, P.C., & Gant, N.F. (1985*). Williams obstetrics* (17th ed.). Norwalk, CT: Appleton-Century-Crofts.

104. Riquier, D. (1998). Neonatal brown adipose tissue, UCP1 and the novel uncoupling protein, *Biochem Soc Trans, 26,* 120.

105. Rowe, M.E., Weinberg, G., & Andrew, W. (1983). Reduction of neonatal heat loss by an insulated head cover. *J Pediatr Surg, 18,* 909.

106. Rutter, N. & Hull, D. (1979). Water loss from the skin of term and preterm babies. *Arch Dis Child, 58,* 858.

107. Rutter, N., Brown, S.M. & Hull, D. (1977). Variations in resting oxygen consumption of small babies. *Arch Dis Child, 53,* 850.

108. Rutter, N. (1999) Thermal adaptation to extrauterine life. In C.H. Rodeck & M.J. Whittle (Eds.). *Fetal medicine: Basic science and clinical practice.* London: Churchill Livingstone.

109. Rutter, N. (1999). Temperature control and its disorders. In J.M. Rennie & N.R.C. Robertson (Eds.). *Textbook of neonatology* (3rd ed.). London: Churchill Livingstone.

110. Sauer, P.J.J., Dane, H.J. & Visser, H.K.A. (1984). New standards for neutral thermal environment of healthy very low birthweight infants in week one of life. *Arch Dis Child, 59,* 18.

111. Sauer, P.J.J., Dane, H.J. & Visser, H.K.A. (1984). Influences of variations in ambient humidity on insensible water loss and thermoneutral environment of low birth weight infants. *Acta Paediatr Scand, 73,* 615.

112. Sawa, R., Asakura, H., & Power, G.G. (1991). Changes in plasma adenosine during stimulated birth of fetal sheep. *J Appl Phys, 70,* 1524.

113. Scher, M.S., et al. (1994). Rectal temperature changes during sleep state transitions in term and preterm neonates at postconceptional term ages. *Pediatr Neurol, 10,* 191.

114. Seguin, J. (1992). Effects of transcutaneous monitor electrode heat on skin servo-controlled environments. *J Perinatol, 12,* 276.

115. Schiffman, R.F. (1982). Temperature monitoring in the neonate: A comparison of axillary and rectal temperatures. *Nurs Res, 31,* 274.

116. Schroder, H.J. & Power, G.G. (1977). Engine and radiator: fetal and placental interactions for heat dissipation. *Exp Physiol, 82,* 403.

117. Scopes, J.W. & Ahmed, J. (1966). Range of critical temperatures in sick and premature newborn infants. *Arch Dis Child, 41,* 417.

118. Sheenan, M.S. (1996). Obtaining an accurate axillary temperature measurement. *J Neonatal Nurs, 2*(4), 6.

119. Short, M. (1998). A comparison of temperature in VLBW infants swaddled versus unswaddled in a double-walled incubator in skin control mode. *Neonatal Net, 17*(3), 25.

120. Sinclair, J. (1992). Management of the thermal environment. In J.C. Sinclair & M.B. Brocker (Eds.). *Effective care of the newborn infant.* Oxford: Oxford University Press.

121. Sinclair, J. (2000). Servo-control for maintaining abdominal skin temperature at 36C in low birth weight infants. *Cochrane Database Sys Rev, 2,* CD001074.

122. Smith, D.W., Clarren, S.K., & Harvey, M.A. (1978). Hyperthermia as a possible teratogenic agent. *J Pediatr, 92,* 878.

123. Stern, L. (1977). Thermoregulation in the newborn. Physiologic and clinical consequences. *Acta Paediatr Belg, 30,* 3.

124. Stern, L. (1979). Clinical aspects of thermoregulation in the newborn. *Contemp Obstet Gynecol, 13,* 109.

125. Sternfeld, B. (1997). Physical activity and pregnancy outcome: review and recommendations. *Sports Med, 23,* 33.

126. Streeter, N.S. (1986). *High-risk neonatal care.* Rockville, MD: Aspen.

127. Stephen, S.B. & Sexton, P.R. (1987). Neonatal axillary temperatures: Increases in readings over time. *Neonatal Net, 5*(6), 25.

128. Sulyok, E., Jequier, E. & Ryser, G. (1982). Effect of relative humidity on the thermal balance of the newborn infant. *Biol Neonate, 21,* 210.

129. Sulyok, E., Jequier, E., & Prod'hom, L.S. (1973). Thermal balance of the newborn infant in a heat gaining environment. *Pediatr Res, 7,* 888.

130. Swyer, P.R. (1987). Thermoregulation in the newborn. In L. Stern & P. Vert (Eds.). *Neonatal medicine.* New York: Masson.

131. Templeman, M.C. & Bell, E.F. (1986). Head insulation for premature infants in servocontrolled incubators and radiant warmers. *Am J Dis Child, 140,* 940.

132. Thomas, K.A. & Burr, R. (1999). Preterm infant thermal care: Differing thermal environments produced by air versus skin servo-control incubators. *J Perinatol, 19,* 264.

133. Thompson, M.H., Strothers, J.K. & McLellan, N.J. (1984). Weight and water loss in the neonate in natural and forced convection. *Arch Dis Child, 59,* 951.

134. Thornburn, G.D. (1992). The placenta, PGE2, and parturition. *Early Hum Dev, 29,* 63.

135. Torrance, J.T. (1968). Temperature readings of premature infants. *Nurs Res, 17,* 312.

136. Trayhurn P. & Nicholls, G.D. (1986). *Brown adipose tissue.* London: Edward Arnold.

137. Vaha-Eskeli, K., Erkkola, R. & Seppanen, A. (1991). Is the heat dissipating ability enhanced during pregnancy? *Eur J Obstet Gynecol Reprod Biol, 39,* 169.

138. Vaughans, B. (1990). Early maternal-infant contact and neonatal thermoregulation. *Neonatal Net, 8*(5), 19.

139. Vernon, H.J., et al. (1990). Semipermeable dressing and transepidermal water loss in premature infants. *Pediatrics, 86,* 357.

140. Wheldon, A.E. & Rutter, N. (1982). The heat balance of small babies nursed in incubators and under radiant warmers. *Early Hum Develop, 6,* 131.

141. Whitelaw A., et al. (1981). Skin-to-skin contact for very low birthweight infants and their mothers. *Arch Dis Child, 63,* 1377.

142. Wu, P.Y.K. & Hodgman, J.E. (1974). Insensible water losses in preterm infants: Changes with postnatal development and non-ionizing radiant energy. *Pediatrics, 54,* 704.

143. Yeh, T.F., et al. (1980). Oxygen consumption and insensible water loss in premature infants in single- versus double-walled incubators. *J Pediatr, 97,* 967.

Index

b, Box; *f*, figure; *t*, table.

Acknowledgments

Twin Studies is a novel, a work of fiction. I cannot emphasize too strongly that the university which appears in this novel, the one where Erica teaches, is entirely fictitious and should not be confused with *my* university, the real one where I have taught for many years. The mangaka Kaneshiro Mitsuko and her work *Two from One Fire* are fictitious; the other mangaka and their works are real. Some familiar public figures mentioned in passing are also real. All of the other characters and events in the book are fictitious, and any resemblance they might have to real characters or events is purely coincidental.

While researching this novel, I read a large number of articles and books. It would be pretentious to list all of them, but I do have to mention Nancy L. Segal's beautifully written *Entwined Lives: Twins and What They Tell Us about Human Behavior*, a popular and essential introduction to twin studies.

Writing is a social act, and I could not have written this novel without assistance. I want to thank at least some of the people who helped me. If I have got anything wrong, it's certainly not their fault, and the listing of their names should not be taken as endorsement. First of all, I should mention the twins who graciously talked to me. I regard my conversations with them as confidential, but they know who they are. Thank you.

Dr. Lynne Quarmby helped me to get the science right and to imagine careers for Erica and Stacey. Dr. Jay Hosking explained to me about working in a Psychology department. Drs. Margaret Nowaczyk, Karen McAssey, and Karen Shklanka answered my questions about genetics, endocrinology, and emergency medicine. My colleague in Asian Studies, Dr. Sharalyn Orbaugh, patiently responded to all of my off-the-wall email queries about Japanese culture.

Annabel Lyon helped me to imagine Karen's adolescence in the '80s. Lindy Vega gave me samples of colloquial Mexican Spanish. Jane Henderson explained Canadian family law to me. Dr. Michael Thompson answered, in exhaustive and valuable detail, my many questions about Tasmania. If Bryan Lynas sounds like a real contemporary Australian, it's because of the help I received from Rhett Davis. Chloe Chan introduced me to the wonderful world of manga. Since then, I have read over two hundred tankōbon, mostly shōjo, and what I have absorbed from them informs this book.

Alicia, known as "Brickme" on Tumblr, has an encyclopedic knowledge of old-school shōjo; she helped me enormously in creating my mangaka, Kaneshiro Mitsuko. Tetsuro Shigematsu suggested "*Two from One Fire*" as the title of my fictitious manga. Dr. Ray Hsu, Nancy Lee, and Anna Ling Kaye helped me to imagine my characters Stacey Chou and Jacqueline Ma. Holly Millar explained girls' soccer in West Vancouver, went over my soccer scene in meticulous detail, and suggested the play that ends that scene.

A special thanks goes to Aaron Biro and his family. They hosted me in Medicine Hat and went out of their way to help me to saturate myself in the ambience of the city. Aaron and I sat in his car for well over an hour and worked out the details of the accident that kills Annalise. Aaron also introduced me to Jennifer Davies who talked to me for an entire afternoon about growing up in the Hat. Her career in softball inspired Erica's.

Maureen Evans and Rachel Rose read the entire manuscript of *Twin Studies* in earlier and longer versions. Their comments were utterly invaluable. Ed Carson went over my manuscript just as thoroughly as he would have done back in the day when he was my editor, and his input improved the book enormously. My literary agent, John Pearce, has worked tirelessly on my behalf and has been a constant source of sage advice.

My wife Mary is my constant companion and best critic. She grew up in West Vancouver, and if she hadn't, I doubt that I would have even thought about writing this book. Every word of it passed before her eyes, and I couldn't have written it without her. My daughters, Jane and Elizabeth, contributed many tales of their own experiences of West Van. Liz helped me to get the dialogue of the younger characters right.

A most heartfelt thanks goes out to Kelsey Attard who responded to *Twin Studies* with such empathy and enthusiasm, and to the entire team at Freehand who have done such a fine job in bringing the book into the world, and finally, to my editor, Lee Shedden. Lee has the uncanny ability to sink right down into the text as deeply as the author. He's helped me out of many a tight corner, suggested many a new and refreshing take on things, and without him, my novel would be far inferior to the one that appears here.